Innovations in CBT for Childhood Anxiety, OCD, and PTSD

Childhood anxiety, OCD, and PTSD represent some of the most common mental health disorders affecting young people, often leading to major life impairments. This book brings together the world's leaders in treatment science to provide evidence-based psychosocial interventions for these disorders. It supplies practitioners and researchers with innovations in clinical science, highlighting advances in technology and neuroscientific discovery that have informed the development of these novel treatment advances. The authors tackle the two main challenges facing the field of childhood psychopathology: improving access to evidence-based CBT through innovations in treatment delivery, and increasing the positive outcomes for youth through unique therapies. Any reader who wants to be informed on the latest approaches to cognitive and behavioral interventions and how to apply them will benefit from this book.

LARA J. FARRELL is a clinical psychologist and Associate Professor in the School of Applied Psychology at Griffith University, Australia, where she contributes to the clinical training of students, conducts clinical research, and provides patient consultations.

THOMAS H. OLLENDICK is University Distinguished Professor in Clinical Psychology and Director of the Child Study Center at Virginia Polytechnic Institute and State University, United States.

PETER MURIS is Full Professor at Maastricht University, The Netherlands, where he combines research and educational activities with clinical work at the Academic Department of Child and Youth Care in Lucertis Maastricht.

Innovations in CBT for Childhood Anxiety, OCD, and PTSD

Improving Access and Outcomes

Edited by

Lara J. Farrell
Griffith University, Queensland

Thomas H. Ollendick
Virginia Tech

Peter Muris
Maastricht University

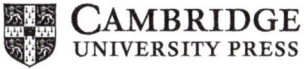

CAMBRIDGE
UNIVERSITY PRESS

University Printing House, Cambridge CB2 8BS, United Kingdom

One Liberty Plaza, 20th Floor, New York, NY 10006, USA

477 Williamstown Road, Port Melbourne, VIC 3207, Australia

314–321, 3rd Floor, Plot 3, Splendor Forum, Jasola District Centre,
New Delhi – 110025, India

79 Anson Road, #06–04/06, Singapore 079906

Cambridge University Press is part of the University of Cambridge.

It furthers the University's mission by disseminating knowledge in the pursuit of education, learning, and research at the highest international levels of excellence.

www.cambridge.org
Information on this title: www.cambridge.org/9781108416023
DOI: 10.1017/9781108235655

© Cambridge University Press 2019

This publication is in copyright. Subject to statutory exception and to the provisions of relevant collective licensing agreements, no reproduction of any part may take place without the written permission of Cambridge University Press.

First published 2019

Printed and bound in Great Britain by Clays Ltd, Elcograf S.p.A.

A catalogue record for this publication is available from the British Library.

Library of Congress Cataloging-in-Publication Data
Names: Farrell, Lara J., 1976– editor. | Ollendick, Thomas H., editor. | Muris, Peter, editor.
Title: Innovations in CBT for childhood anxiety, OCD and PTSD : improving access and outcomes / edited by Lara J. Farrell, Thomas H. Ollendick, Peter Muris.
Description: Cambridge, United Kingdom ; New York, NY : University Printing House, 2019. | Includes bibliographical references.
Identifiers: LCCN 2018027179| ISBN 9781108416023 (hardback) | ISBN 9781108401326 (paperback)
Subjects: | MESH: Anxiety Disorders – therapy | Stress Disorders, Post-Traumatic – therapy | Cognitive Therapy – methods | Child | Adolescent
Classification: LCC RJ506.A58 | NLM WM 172 | DDC 618.92/8522–dc23
LC record available at https://lccn.loc.gov/2018027179

ISBN 978-1-108-41602-3 Hardback
ISBN 978-1-108-40132-6 Paperback

Cambridge University Press has no responsibility for the persistence or accuracy of URLs for external or third-party internet websites referred to in this publication and does not guarantee that any content on such websites is, or will remain, accurate or appropriate.

Contents

List of Figures	*page* ix
List of Tables	x
List of Contributors	xi
Preface	xv
Acknowledgments	xviii

Part I Anxiety Disorders

1 Phenomenology and Standard Evidence-Based Care of Anxiety Disorders in Children and Adolescents 3
JENNIFER L. HUDSON, JODIE ANAGNOS, AND VICTORIA INGRAM

2 Evidence-Based Assessment 28
ANDRES DE LOS REYES AND BRIDGET A. MAKOL

3 Self-Help Treatment of Childhood Anxiety Disorders 52
LAUREN F. MCLELLAN, SALLY FITZPATRICK, CAROLYN ANNE SCHNIERING, AND RONALD M. RAPEE

4 New Technologies to Deliver CBT: Computer and Web-Based Programs, Mobile Applications, and Virtual Reality 73
SUSAN H. SPENCE, SONJA MARCH, AND CAROLINE L. DONOVAN

5 Cognitive Bias Modification Strategies for Anxious Children: Attention and Interpretation Bias Retraining 106
JENNIE M. KUCKERTZ AND NADER AMIR

6 Brief Intensive Treatments 130
DONNA B. PINCUS AND CHRISTINA HARDWAY

7 Pharmacologic-Enhanced Approaches for the Anxiety Disorders 160
JANKI MODI AVARI, MIA GINTOFT COHEN, DESPINA HATZIERGATI, AND JOHN T. WALKUP

8 Enhanced Family Approaches for the Anxiety Disorders 182
MICHAEL W. LIPPERT, VERENA PFLUG, KRISTEN LAVALLEE, AND SILVIA SCHNEIDER

9 Treatment of Comorbid Sleep Problems in Anxious Children 206
CANDICE A. ALFANO, ROGELIO GONZALEZ, AND JESSICA MEERS

10 Transdiagnostic Approaches to the Treatment of Anxiety Disorders in Children and Adolescents 226
JILL M. NEWBY AND ANNA C. MCKINNON

11 Dissemination and Implementation of Evidence-Based Programs for the Prevention and Treatment of Childhood Anxiety 248
SATOKO SASAGAWA AND CECILIA A. ESSAU

12 Innovations in the Treatment of Childhood Anxiety Disorders: Mindfulness and Self-Compassion Approaches 265
MARIJA MARIC, CHRISTOPHER WILLARD, MAJA WRZESIEN, AND SUSAN M. BÖGELS

Part II Obsessive-Compulsive Disorder

13 Phenomenology and Standard Care of OCD in Children and Adolescents 289
ERICA L. GREENBERG AND DANIEL A. GELLER

14 Evidence-Based Assessment of Child Obsessive-Compulsive Disorder (OCD): Recommendations for Clinical Practice and Treatment Research 313
ADAM B. LEWIN

15 Self-Help Treatments for Childhood Obsessive-Compulsive Disorder Including Bibliotherapy 332
GEORGINA KREBS AND CYNTHIA TURNER

16 New Technologies to Deliver CBT for Young Children with Obsessive-Compulsive Disorder 348
KRISTINA ASPVALL, FABIAN LENHARD, EVA SERLACHIUS, AND DAVID MATAIX-COLS

17 Interpretation and Attentional Bias Training 365
ELSKE SALEMINK, LIDEWIJ WOLTERS, AND ELSE DE HAAN

18 Innovations in Treating OCD: Brief, Intensive Treatments 392
KATELYN M. DYASON, LARA J. FARRELL, AND ALLISON M. WATERS

19 Pharmacologic-Augmented Treatments 407
SOPHIE C. SCHNEIDER AND ERIC A. STORCH

20	Enhanced Family Approaches in Childhood OCD	428
	JEFFREY J. SAPYTA AND COLLEEN M. COWPERTHWAIT	
21	Treatments for Obsessive-Compulsive Disorder and Comorbid Disorders	444
	TORD IVARSSON AND BERNHARD WEIDLE	
22	Transdiagnostic Approaches	467
	YOLANDA E. MURPHY, ANNA LUKE, AND CHRISTOPHER A. FLESSNER	
23	Pediatric OCD: Dissemination and Implementation	489
	MARTIN E. FRANKLIN, JORDAN A. KATZ, BRADLEY C. RIEMANN, AND SIMONE BUDZYN	
24	New Wave Therapies for Pediatric OCD	506
	R. LINDSEY BERGMAN AND MICHELLE ROZENMAN	

Part III Post-Traumatic Stress Disorder

25	Trauma-Focused Cognitive Behavioral Therapy: An Evidence-Based Approach for Helping Children Overcome the Impact of Child Abuse and Trauma	525
	MELISSA K. RUNYON, ELIZABETH RISCH, AND ESTHER DEBLINGER	
26	Advances in the Assessment of PTSD in Children and Young People	550
	DAVID TRICKEY AND RICHARD MEISER-STEDMAN	
27	New Technologies to Deliver CBT (Including Web-Based CBT, Mobile Apps, and Virtual Reality)	570
	DANIELLE WEISS AND MEGHAN L. MARSAC	
28	Eye Movement Desensitization and Reprocessing (EMDR)	590
	KERSTIN BERGH JOHANNESSON, MARGARETA FRIBERG WESCHKE, AND ABDULBAGHI AHMAD	
29	Innovation in Early Trauma Treatment: The Child and Family Traumatic Stress Intervention (CFTSI)	610
	STEVEN MARANS, CARRIE EPSTEIN, HILARY HAHN, AND MEGAN GOSLIN	
30	Pediatric Post-Traumatic Stress Disorder: Pharmacological Augmented Treatments	629
	ANTRA BAMI, JUDITH FERNANDO, AND CRAIG L. DONNELLY	
31	Enhanced Family-Based Interventions for Children Who Have Been Traumatized by Physical Abuse and Neglect	650
	CYNTHIA CUPIT SWENSON	

32	Treatment of PTSD and Comorbid Disorders VANESSA E. COBHAM AND RACHEL HILLER	671
33	Transdiagnostic Treatment for Youth with Traumatic Stress HILIT KLETTER, VICTOR G. CARRION, AND CARL F. WEEMS	697
34	Dissemination and Implementation of Evidence-Based Treatments for Childhood PTSD ALISON SALLOUM	715
35	New Wave Therapies for Post-Traumatic Stress Disorder in Youth MICHELLE R. WOIDNECK, ELLEN J. BLUETT, AND SARAH A. POTTS	731

Index   748

Figures

I Anxiety Disorders

3.1	Amelia's Symptoms of Anxiety and Depression	*page* 63
4.1	BRAVE-ONLINE Illustrations	96
4.2	BRAVE-ONLINE Illustrations	97
7.1	Treatment Algorithm for Anxiety Disorders in Children and Adolescents	163
8.1	3-Level Taxonomy of Parental Involvement in Treatment of Child Anxiety	186

II Obsessive-Compulsive Disorder

16.1	Screenshots from OCD? Not me!	352
16.2	Screenshots from BiP OCD	355
17.1	Completion of the top of an OCD Questionnaire and one Question by a 9-year-old Boy with OCD	368
17.2	VAS Scores of Case 1 Saf During the 12-Session CBM-I Training (pre-CBT)	381
17.3	VAS scores of Case 2 Joan During the 12-Session CBM-I Training (pre-CBT)	383

III Post-Traumatic Stress Disorder

26.1	Session by Session Symptom Tracking Using the CRIES-8	559
27.1	Sample Content from Coping Coach Intervention Levels and Adventure Log	573
27.2	Sample Content from Kids and Accidents Intervention	575
27.3	Sample Content from Bounce Back Now	576
27.4	Potential Steps to PTSD Prevention/Early Intervention/Treatment using Web-/Mobile-Based Technology	583
30.1	Pharmacologic Treatment Algorithm for Pediatric PTSD	633

Tables

I Anxiety Disorders

2.1	Rating Scales for Assessing Youth Anxiety	*page* 35
3.1	Overview of *Chilled Plus Online* modules	64
4.1	Summary of Randomized Controlled Trials Evaluating the Treatment of Clinically Anxious Children and/or Adolescents	77
7.1	List of the Agents Most Commonly Used in the Treatment of Anxiety Disorders in Children and Adolescents and Patient Properties	173
10.1	Examples of Currently Available Transdiagnostic Treatment Protocols for Anxiety Disorders in Children and Youth and Overview of Key Components	229
12.1	Mindfulness Exercises Commonly Used in Youth with Anxiety	272

II Obsessive-Compulsive Disorder

14.1	Recommended Empirical Measures	325
16.1	Treatment Chapters and Content of BiP OCD	353

III Post-Traumatic Stress Disorder

26.1	Measures for use with Traumatized Children and Young People	551
27.1	Summary of Evaluations of Web-Based PTSD Interventions for Children	578
30.1	Current Psychopharmacological Treatments for PTSD in Children and Adolescents: Levels of Evidence for Medication use and their Specific Target Symptoms and Response	640
34.1	Case example (Thomas): Assessment data as Obtained During the Stepping Together Treatment	724
34.2	Scary Ladder and Next step Activities for case Example	725

Contributors

ABDULBAGHI AHMAD, Uppsala University
CANDICE A. ALFANO, University of Houston
NADER AMIR, San Diego State University; University of California, San Diego
JODIE ANAGNOS, Macquarie University
KRISTINA ASPVALL, Karolinska Institute
JANKI MODI AVARI, Weill Cornell Medicine, New York-Presbyterian Hospital Westchester Division
ANTRA BAMI, Dartmouth-Hitchcock Medical Center
R. LINDSEY BERGMAN, UCLA Semel Institute for Neuroscience and Human Behavior
ELLEN J. BLUETT, VA Salt Lake City Health Care System
SUSAN M. BÖGELS, University of Amsterdam
SIMONE BUDZYN, University of Pennsylvania School of Medicine
VICTOR G. CARRION, Stanford University School of Medicine
VANESSA E. COBHAM, University of Queensland
MIA GINTOFT COHEN, Weill Cornell Medicine, New York-Presbyterian Hospital Westchester Division
COLLEEN M. COWPERTHWAIT, Duke University Medical Center
ELSE DE HAAN, University of Amsterdam
ANDRE DE LOS REYES, University of Maryland, College Park
ESTHER DEBLINGER, Rowan University School of Osteopathic Medicine
CRAIG L. DONNELLY, Dartmouth-Hitchcock Medical Center
CAROLINE DONOVAN, Griffith University
KATELYN M. DYASON, Griffith University
CARRIE EPSTEIN, Yale School of Medicine
CECILIA A. ESSAU, University of Roehampton
LARA J. FARRELL, Griffith University
JUDITH FERNANDO, Dartmouth-Hitchcock Medical Center
SALLY FITZPATRICK, Macquarie University
CHRISTOPHER A. FLESSNER, Kent State University
MARTIN E. FRANKLIN, University of Pennsylvania School of Medicine; Rogers Memorial Hospital, Philadelphia
DANIEL A. GELLER, Massachusetts General Hospital; Harvard Medical School
ROGELIO GONZALEZ, University of Houston

MEGAN GOSLIN, Yale School of Medicine
ERICA L. GREENBERG, Massachusetts General Hospital; Harvard Medical School
HILARY HAHN, Yale School of Medicine
CHRISTINA HARDAWAY, Merrimack College
DESPINA HATZIERGATI, Weill Cornell Medicine, New York-Presbyterian Hospital Westchester Division
RACHEL HILLER, University of Bath
JENNIFER L. HUDSON, Macquarie University
VICTORIA INGRAM, Macquarie University
TORD IVARSSON, Center for Child and Adolescent Mental Health, Eastern and Southern Norway
KERSTIN BERGH JOHANNESSON, Uppsala University
JORDAN A. KATZ, Rogers Memorial Hospital, Philadelphia
HILIT KLETTER, Stanford University School of Medicine
GEORGINA KREBS, King's College London
JENNIE M. KUCKERTZ, San Diego State University; University of California, San Diego
KRISTEN LAVALLEE, Ruhr University Bochum
FABIAN LENHARD, Karolinska Institute
ADAM B. LEWIN, University of South Florida
MICHAEL W. LIPPERT, Ruhr University Bochum
ANNA LUKE, Kent State University
BRIDGET A. MAKOL, University of Maryland, College Park
STEVEN MARANS, Yale School of Medicine
SONJA MARCH, University of Southern Queensland
MARIJA MARIC, University of Amsterdam
MEGHAN L. MARSAC, College of Medicine, University of Kentucky; Kentucky Children's Hospital
DAVID MATAIX-COLS, Karolinska Institute
ANNA C. MCKINNON, Macquarie University
LAUREN F. MCLELLAN, Macquarie University
JESSICA MEERS, University of Houston
RICHARD MEISER-STEDMAN, University of East Anglia
YOLANDA E. MURPHY, Kent State University
JILL M. NEWBY, University of New South Wales
VERENA PFLUG, Ruhr University Bochum
DONNA B. PINCUS, Boston University
SARAH A. POTTS, Utah State University; Boys Town Center for Behavioral Health
RONALD M. RAPEE, Macquarie University
BRADLEY C. RIEMANN, Rogers Memorial Hospital, Oconomowoc, WI
ELIZABETH RISCH, University of Oklahoma Health Sciences Center
MICHELLE ROZENMAN, UCLA Semel Institute for Neuroscience and Human Behavior
MELISSA K. RUNYON, Private Practice Prospect, KY
ELSKE SALEMINK, University of Amsterdam

ALISON SALLOUM, University of South Florida
JEFFREY J. SAPYTA, Duke University Medical Center
SATOKO SASAGAWA, Mejiro University
SILVIA SCHNEIDER, Ruhr University Bochum
SOPHIE C. SCHNEIDER, University of South Florida
CAROLYN ANNE SCHNIERING, Macquarie University
EVA SERLACHIUS, Karolinska Institute
SUSAN H. SPENCE, Griffith University
ERIC A. STORCH, University of South Florida
CYNTHIA CUPIT SWENSON, Medical University of South Carolina
DAVID TRICKEY, Anna Freud National Centre for Children and Families
CYNTHIA TURNER, Australian Catholic University
JOHN T. WALKUP, Ann and Robert H. Lurie Children's Hospital of Chicago
ALLISON M. WATERS, Griffith University
CARL F. WEEMS, Iowa State University
BERNHARD WEIDLE, Norwegian University of Science and Technology
DANIELLE WEISS, University of Maryland, Baltimore County
MARGARETA FRIBERG WESCHKE, Private Practice Prospect, Sweden
CHRISTOPHER WILLARD, Harvard Medical School
MICHELLE R. WOIDNECK, Boys Town Center for Behavioral Health
LIDEWIJ WOLTERS, Norwegian University of Science and Technology
MAJA WRZESIEN, University of Amsterdam

Preface

Anxiety and related disorders, including obsessive-compulsive disorder (OCD) and post-traumatic stress disorders (PTSD), are among the most common mental health disorders affecting children and adolescents (e.g., Merikangas et al., 2010). In 2013, with the publication of the current version of the *Diagnostic and Statistical Manual for Mental Disorders*, 5th Edition (APA, 2013), a major recategorization of these disorders (previously grouped together under the category anxiety disorders) led to the definition of these disorders under three different diagnostic categories – (1) anxiety disorders, (2) obsessive-compulsive and related disorders, and (3) trauma- and stressor-related disorders. Still, anxiety disorders, OCD, and PTSD in childhood and adolescence remain frequently comorbid with one another; anxiety continues to play an important role in all presentations to varying degrees across individuals; and critical to this volume, each responds similarly to the same broad therapeutic approach, namely cognitive behavioral therapy (CBT).

The experience of these emotional disorders during childhood and adolescence can be highly debilitating to the individual and their family, and frequently results in significant disruptions to healthy development, including problems scholastically, vocationally, and interpersonally. Furthermore, they tend to be chronic and are predictive of a host of other mental health problems later in life. Indeed, these disorders are costly to individuals, families, and society in more ways than one. For these reasons, basic and applied research into these emotional disorders in children and youth has proliferated over the past few decades, leading to notable advances in science and practice, in particular, treatment and implementation science. While the prevalence and burden of these disorders remains high, prognosis is generally good when a child has access to an evidence-based treatment such as CBT.

CBT is the single most effective treatment for childhood anxiety disorders, OCD, and PTSD. Over the past 25 years, empirical research has provided accumulative support for the efficacy of CBT in various forms (e.g., parent-focused, child-focused, family-focused) and modalities of delivery (e.g., individual, group) as an effective and durable therapy for children and their families with all forms of anxiety, and its related disorders (i.e., OCD and PTSD). However, there are two major challenges that our field has been faced with. The first is that children and youth largely do not have access to this evidence-based treatment despite the established evidence in support of its efficacy. And secondly, it is clear from the cumulative randomized controlled trials (RCTs) across child anxiety, OCD, and PTSD, that CBT, while generally effective, is simply not good enough for a substantive proportion of youth who do receive this intervention. These two major limitations to the field of child anxiety research have led to a shift in treatment research, leading to significant advancements in innovative approaches of improving access to care and enhancing patient outcomes.

Access to care for children and youth remains problematic for numerous reasons, from all points of access, including barriers from the point-of-service provision, therapist contact, and family-related constraints. Evidence-based treatments are costly, frequently limited to major metropolitan centers, and attract only limited funding and rebates from insurance providers. Furthermore, despite an increase in dissemination efforts of evidence-based practice guidelines, there remains poor uptake of such approaches by therapists in the community. For example, Nair and colleagues (2015) examined whether there was an increase in the uptake of evidence-based treatments for pediatric OCD (including selective serotonin reuptake inhibitor [SSRI] medication and CBT) in national mental health OCD services in London, following the publication of the National Institute of Health and Care Excellence (NICE) guidelines for the management of pediatric OCD in the United Kingdom in 2005. Strikingly, results found no increase in CBT, a significant decrease in the use of selective serotonin reuptake inhibitors (SSRIs), and an increase in non-CBT psychological therapies following the publication of these evidence-based guidelines. These results highlight the ongoing, real-world challenges for the dissemination of CBT, and the distinct void in the translation from science to service for evidence-based practice. Much work needs to be done at the roots of psychology training, and the provision of supervision for the psychological workforce.

Beyond the barriers to accessing treatment at the service level, and the challenges encountered with therapist skill level and preferences, there remain further challenges for families in regard to access. Families are busy entities and scheduling of weekly, clinic-based appointments can be problematic, especially for those parents who work, and for children who are involved in numerous extracurricular activities. And moreover, parents and children present to services with their own preferences, fears, and biases regarding different treatment approaches, which may prevent children receiving an evidence-based intervention. For these reasons (and more), innovations in the delivery of CBT have thrived over the past two decades and led to the development of technological advances and self-help modalities of CBT, as well as brief interventions of high-intensity CBT. Each of these innovations provides exciting opportunities to increase the reach of evidence-based interventions, which may indeed provide benefit over traditional CBT for some patients. The field is flourishing with possibilities in improving access to CBT, and with constant advances in technology, this domain of research will surely continue to be at the forefront of innovation.

Improving youth outcomes to CBT has, however, proven to be a more challenging endeavor. Partly, the challenge in finding a treatment with superior outcomes to standard CBT lies in the fact that effect sizes and response rates to CBT, while not perfect, are actually already quite good. Achieving superior outcomes over and above what CBT already delivers is therefore difficult, and requires both a robust, novel stand-alone or augmented intervention, and a very large sample size to achieve power to detect clinically meaningful and statistically significant incremental benefits in RCTs. To date there have been two major approaches to improve treatment outcomes via novel therapies. One is the development of treatment approaches that target *different mechanisms* from those proposed as central in cognitive behavioral therapies associated with either the pathogenesis of the disorder (i.e., biological processes in the case of pharmacological treatments) or based on a different theoretical formulation of the disorder etiology and maintenance of symptoms (e.g., third wave therapies). The second approach to treatment innovation has been the development of novel strategies that target known underlying mechanisms proposed as central in CBT models (e.g., cognitive biases, family processes), or central to the mechanisms associated with CBT therapy outcomes (e.g., pharmacological agents that enhance extinction learning), both of which aim to leverage the established therapeutic benefits of CBT. Each of these innovations has to date provided promise as an emerging alternative to CBT, or has the potential to augment CBT for those youth who may not respond to standard CBT. While the preliminary evidence to date is favorable, there remains substantive empirical work to be done in order to determine *how* these novel approaches may be optimally delivered (i.e., as stand-alone treatments, or augmented with CBT, and in what order), and for *whom* they exert the most powerful therapeutic benefits. Large RCTs of novel interventions with long-term follow-up of patient outcomes and careful examination of predictors, moderators, and mediators of outcome are the next frontier. Furthermore, basic and applied research aimed at elucidating and measuring the underlying mechanisms by which CBT, and more specifically exposure therapy, exerts its therapeutic effects is also critically needed in order to refine approaches or inform novel therapies. In these pursuits, the future for research in our field calls for large international, multisite collaborations, in order to deal with these complex, yet clinically critical, treatment questions.

The aim of the current scholarly volume was to compile international expert commentaries by the leaders in these innovations, highlighting progress to date in empirical evidence, the application of these approaches through clinical case descriptions, and directions for future science and practice. This volume therefore synthesizes the accumulative evidence toward improved, empirically supported novel interventions and modes of delivery of CBT for children and youth with anxiety and related disorders (including OCD and PTSD) aimed at improving access to care and patient outcomes. Each chapter includes real-world applications of these novel approaches to delivery of treatments and enhanced care, and highlights key practice points for practitioners. Finally, each chapter provides a summary and directions for future research, serving to pave the way forward for further refinements to these innovations, as well as inspire next-generation innovations in science and practice. It is our hope that this volume serves to inform current practice, and provide therapists with novel approaches to helping children and youth overcome the emotional distress and burden associated with anxiety, OCD, and PTSD.

Acknowledgments

I wish to dedicate this book to the men in my life who have supported and inspired me. In loving memory of my dad, who was proud beyond words. To my beautiful family, Andrew, Ollie, and Eli, for filling my life with love and laughter. Thank you for bringing me joy every single day and inspiring me to be a better human being.

I also wish to thank my good friend and mentor, Tom Ollendick, for influencing me, guiding me, and supporting me. You have led our field in science and practice, but also in the spirit of friendship and generosity. Thank you also Peter, for joining us on this project, and for your wisdom and good-heartedness throughout the entire process.

Lara Farrell

I wish to give thanks to my good friends and colleagues, Lara Farrell and Peter Muris, who eagerly joined me as coeditors in this important, exciting, and timely venture. This has been a rewarding project and one that would not have been possible without their vision, energy, and dedication. I also wish to thank my wife, Mary, our daughters, Laurie and Katie, and our sons-in-law, David and Billy, as well as our six grandchildren, Braden, Ethan, Calvin, Addison, Victoria, and William. They have taught me much about childhood and adolescence over the years. Without them, my life would be so much less interesting, enjoyable, and rewarding. I thank them for being who they are and for their love and support over the years.

Tom Ollendick

To my beautiful young ladies, Jip and Kiki

Peter Muris

From all of us – our most sincere gratitude to the contributors of each of the chapters herein. You are the superstars of our field – the leaders and the trailblazers. It is our hope that your innovations in science and practice translate to a better future for the children and families we care for.

Thank you finally to the wonderful team at Cambridge University Press, in particular Stephen Accera, Matthew Bennett, Emily Watton, and Bethany Johnson, for providing us the opportunity to create this exciting and important book, and for bringing it to life.

Lara, Tom, and Peter

PART I

Anxiety Disorders

1 Phenomenology and Standard Evidence-Based Care of Anxiety Disorders in Children and Adolescents

Jennifer L. Hudson, Jodie Anagnos, and Victoria Ingram

Introduction

Collectively, anxiety disorders are the most common mental disorders in children and adolescents (Merikangas et al., 2010). This finding is largely replicated in epidemiological studies throughout the world (Lawrence et al., 2015; Polanczyk et al., 2015). However, specific prevalence rates can vary, sometimes dramatically, due to differences in assessment methods, recall periods, and populations. Nevertheless, in childhood and adolescence, prevalence rates of anxiety disorders range from 2.5 to 8.3 percent (Lawrence et al., 2015; Merikangas et al., 2010; Rapee, Schniering, & Hudson, 2009). Over a lifetime, more than one in four individuals will experience an anxiety disorder, with the majority of individuals having experienced clinically significant symptoms before they reach adulthood (Kim-Cohen et al., 2003). In fact, anxiety disorders have the earliest onset of the mental disorders, and reported prevalence rates are typically higher during adolescence than childhood (e.g., Merikangas et al., 2010). Although some prevalence studies fail to find gender differences in prevalence of anxiety, on the whole, anxiety disorders tend to be more prevalent in girls than boys (Rapee, Schniering, & Hudson, 2009).

Anxiety disorders are responsible for significant disease burden not just in childhood but across the lifespan (Baxter et al., 2014; Erskine et al., 2015). Despite their prevalence and impact, historically these disorders have been overlooked and most children with anxiety disorders go unrecognized and untreated. This has been in part due to the lack of knowledge about these disorders and the mistaken belief that they are transient in nature. Although this may be true about normal childhood fears and separation anxiety, this is not the case for anxiety disorders. Without access to evidence-based treatment, these disorders tend to persist, often leading to a range of other mental disorders such as major depression and substance abuse (Birrell et al., 2015; Seligman & Ollendick, 1998). Overall, the evidence suggests that anxiety disorders in children and young people are relatively stable, chronic, and disabling conditions that warrant attention (Craske et al., 2017; Rapee, Schniering, & Hudson, 2009).

The last 25 years have seen an increased interest in these disorders in children and as a result we have a significantly greater understanding of these high-prevalence disorders. Much of the research focus in young people has been on this disorder group as a whole, with less attention paid to individual anxiety disorders. This is in contrast to the research in the adult field, which has largely focused on separate anxiety disorders (Barlow et al., 1985; Clark et al., 2006; Wells, 2005). Rather than focusing on specific disorders, child research has tended to consider these disorders collectively, as broad-based anxiety disorders.

This differing approach across the lifespan is in part due to the high rate of comorbidity between the anxiety disorders in children. In clinical samples, children presenting for treatment for anxiety rarely present with one anxiety disorder. During assessment, the clinician may identify one group of anxiety symptoms that is more severe and more interfering than other symptoms but typically these primary symptoms do not occur in isolation and will present with other types of anxiety. For example, at the Centre for Emotional Health at Macquarie University (Sydney, Australia), very few children seeking treatment for anxiety present with one disorder (8.9 percent; Hudson, Rapee et al., 2015). In fact, the majority of children are diagnosed with more than one anxiety disorder (87.3 percent). This type of comorbidity is not uncommon in other university clinics around the world. For example, in the largest randomized clinical trial of treatment of anxiety disorders in young people involving six clinics in the United States, 78.7 percent of children had more than one primary anxiety disorder (Walkup et al., 2008). Comorbidity among the anxiety disorders in community clinics is also very common. For example, Southam-Gerow and colleagues (2010) demonstrated that children presenting for treatment for anxiety at community child mental health clinics in the United States were diagnosed on average with more than three disorders. In addition to the primary anxiety disorder, at least 72.9 percent of children also met criteria for co-occurring specific phobia and 52.1 percent for separation anxiety disorder.

Despite the high comorbidity, separate anxiety disorders can be adequately differentiated in childhood and adolescence and can be reliably diagnosed. There are a number of added benefits for making distinct diagnoses such as assisting in the tailoring of treatment plans and identifying the most interfering problems to determine which symptoms warrant prioritizing. The anxiety disorders most commonly diagnosed in children and young people include separation anxiety disorder, social anxiety disorder, generalized anxiety disorder, and specific phobia. Less common disorders include selective mutism, agoraphobia, and panic disorder.

At the core of all of these disorders is anxiety. A child with an anxiety disorder experiences persistent fear or worry in certain environments that is excessive compared to typically developing children of a similar age. Importantly, the child avoids certain environments that elicit fear and may engage in specific behaviors to increase safety (such as reassurance seeking, avoiding eye contact). Anxiety itself is a very normal emotion. As fears are common in young children it can often be difficult to differentiate between normal and pathological anxiety. As it can be challenging for parents and teachers to determine whether the child's anxiety is part of normal development, anxiety disorders are often overlooked. The key to differentiating normal and abnormal anxiety is the extent to which the fears and worries have been enduring (e.g., typically at least six months) and the extent to which they interfere with the child's and/or the family's functioning. If the child experiences fear but this does not impact on day-to-day functioning, such as attending school, making friendships, keeping friendships, or attending certain activities, then we would not call the anxiety a "disorder." If the child's anxiety is enduring and impacting on the child and family, then treatment is warranted. We will now review the phenomenology of different types of anxiety disorders that present in children and young people.

Types of Anxiety Disorder in Children and Young People

Social Anxiety Disorder

Social anxiety disorder is characterized by an excessive fear of situations in which there is potential for negative evaluation. The child's fear can be specific to performance situations but more often occurs across a range of social situations. Children with social anxiety disorder tend to dislike being the center of attention and will avoid answering or asking questions in class, speaking to new people, public speaking, and attending social activities. Young people who are socially anxious frequently have difficulty making friends and, although they have close friends, often have a smaller network of friends. These children may be quiet and appear shy and hence these behaviors and the accompanying distress can go unnoticed.

Social anxiety disorder can occur in childhood, yet it is more common in adolescence, with the mean age of onset around early to middle adolescence (Cohen, Cohen, & Brook, 1993; Otto et al., 2001; Strauss & Last, 1993). Social anxiety disorder is one of the more stable anxiety disorders and is associated with significant risk for later anxiety and depression (Pine et al., 1998; Stein et al., 2001; Yonkers, Dyck, & Keller, 2001). Specific prevalence rates for social anxiety disorder across childhood and adolescence range from 0.3 to 1.5 percent (Merikangas et al., 2010; Rapee, Schniering, & Hudson, 2009).

Selective Mutism

With the introduction of the fifth edition of DSM, selective mutism was for the first time conceptualized as a unique anxiety disorder (Muris & Ollendick, 2015). Selective mutism is characterized by a persistent failure to speak in social situations that is not explained by a communication disorder or other disorder such as an autism spectrum disorder. A child with selective mutism is comfortable talking at home with parents and siblings but is unable to talk at school or to friends outside the family or close network. Selective mutism is a rare disorder with a prevalence rate of less than 1 percent and it is twice as common in girls as in boys (Muris & Ollendick, 2015; Viana, Beidel, & Rabian, 2009). This disorder, compared to other anxiety disorders, tends to have a shorter course, but is typically associated with other anxiety disorders throughout childhood and adolescence. Many authors argue that selective mutism is another form of social anxiety disorder characterized by social avoidance in situations involving communication with unfamiliar people (Black, 1996).

The high comorbidity rates between selective mutism and social anxiety disorder support this notion.

Separation Anxiety Disorder

Children with separation anxiety disorder exhibit excessive, inappropriate, and lasting anxiety about separation from the child's main attachment figures (American Psychiatric Association, 2013). Separation anxiety disorder is characterized by an excessive fear that the child or the child's attachment figure will come into some form of harm or danger. Children with separation anxiety disorder experience significant arousal when separation from parents is discussed or experienced, as well as persistent worry that an unexpected event may lead to separation (Kossowsky et al., 2012). They may become clingy and refuse to leave their attachment figure, and often follow parents around the house, refusing to go anywhere without their parents. Children with separation anxiety disorder may also have significant difficulties around bedtime such as refusing to sleep alone, long drawn-out bedtime routines, and frequent nightmares about separation.

Like many anxiety disorders, separation anxiety disorder is underdiagnosed in school-aged children, which prevents appropriate treatment for children with the disorder. Children with separation anxiety disorder may also exhibit a number of physical symptoms, such as nausea and vomiting, that can be particularly pronounced just before separation (Brand et al., 2011). Separation anxiety disorder may also be associated with a refusal to attend school, with one study finding approximately one-third of school refusal cases meeting criteria for this disorder (Heyne, King, & Tonge, 2004). As such, separation anxiety disorder may prevent children from developing normal social relationships with peers, as well as result in low academic performance due to poor school attendance. Separation anxiety disorder has been consistently found to have the earliest age of onset of common anxiety disorders, peaking at the age of 7 years old (Beesdo, Knappe, & Pine, 2009). Prevalence rates range from 0.2 to 1.5 percent, with typically lower prevalence rates in adolescence (Merikangas et al., 2010; Rapee, Schniering, & Hudson, 2009).

Generalized Anxiety Disorder

Generalized anxiety disorder is characterized by pervasive and uncontrollable worry about a variety of issues or events (American Psychiatric Association, 2013). This excessive worry occurs most days and is accompanied by at least one somatic symptom in children such as nausea, headaches, heart palpitations, muscle tension, and restlessness (Payne, Bolton, & Perrin, 2011; Ramsawh, Chavira, & Stein, 2010). In children and young people, generalized anxiety disorder may manifest as undue worry about their competence and performance at school or sporting events. Children with generalized anxiety disorder may constantly seek reassurance, ask a multitude of "what if" questions, and have unrealistic concerns about day-to-day activities. Such children may also demonstrate perfectionistic traits, fear criticism or making mistakes, and have frequent unfavorable assessments of their own abilities.

Unlike developmentally appropriate fears and worries, a child with generalized anxiety disorder is unable to "switch off" worries.

The typical age of onset for generalized anxiety disorder is during adolescence but can occur earlier as well (Beesdo et al., 2010). Prevalence rates for generalized anxiety disorder range from 0.3 to 0.9 percent, with girls being twice as likely as boys to experience the disorder (Merikangas et al., 2010; Rapee, Schniering, & Hudson, 2009). Generalized anxiety disorder is also among the most highly occurring comorbid anxiety disorders, with young people commonly seeking treatment for generalized anxiety disorder comorbid with separation anxiety disorder, social anxiety disorder, specific phobia, panic disorder, and obsessive-compulsive disorder (Kendall et al., 2010). Generalized anxiety disorder during childhood also significantly increases the risk of developing depression and other anxiety disorders during adolescence (Payne, Bolton, & Perrin, 2011). Furthermore, when generalized anxiety disorder is comorbid with depression, this often leads to worse outcomes for young people's school attendance, employment capabilities, and mental health service utilization (Hirschfeld, 2001).

Specific Phobia

Specific phobias in children involve an irrational and intense fear of certain objects or situations, with the fear often manifesting as crying, clinging behavior, freezing up, or tantrums (American Psychiatric Association, 2013). A diagnosis of specific phobia is given if children experience strong, persistent fear for more than six months, and if it is accompanied by intense physiological symptoms, avoidance, or distress. Some common examples of specific phobias for children include spiders, water, strangers, or heights (Muris et al., 2002). Children with specific phobias will become extremely distressed when confronted with the feared situation or object, and often fail to recognize that the fear is irrational. Importantly, specific phobias differ from common childhood fears in that the former involves increased fear toward the specific object or situation as children mature, whereas common childhood fears tend to dissipate with age (Gullone, 2000).

Unlike common childhood fears, specific phobias also do not decrease with appropriate reassurance. For example, an escalator phobia will persist despite reassurance from a parent that it is safe to walk on. The age of onset for many specific phobias begins in middle childhood, with the disorder typically affecting more girls than boys, and prevalence ranging from 0.6 to 1.9 percent (Merikangas et al., 2010; Rapee, Schniering, & Hudson, 2009).

Panic Disorder

Children and adolescents with panic disorder experience unexpected and reoccurring periods of discomfort and intense fear, known as panic attacks, which are not triggered by an identifiable stimulus (American Psychiatric Association, 2013). Physical symptoms of panic attacks may include feelings of a rapidly accelerated heart rate, dizziness, sweating, shaking, trembling, and a feeling of being smothered or an inability to breathe (Queen, Ehrenreich-May, & Hershorin, 2012; Ramsawh, Chavira, & Stein, 2010). Concurrently, the physical symptoms of panic attacks are often accompanied by terrifying thoughts of losing control and fear of fainting or dying. Panic disorder is diagnosed if young people experience at least one panic attack, followed by a month of persistent worry or concern over the negative consequences of experiencing another panic attack. Cued panic attacks can occur as a feature of many different anxiety disorders (e.g., in social or separation situations), but panic attacks in panic disorder appear to "come out of the blue." Children with panic disorder often make maladaptive behavioral changes as a result of their panic attacks, such as avoiding unfamiliar situations that may induce a panic attack.

The prevalence of panic disorder in younger children is fairly low, with age of onset often occurring in mid to late adolescence (Ollendick, Mattis, & King, 1994). Prevalence studies of panic disorder in adolescents range from 0.3 percent (Costello et al., 2003) to 1.2 percent (Wittchen, Nelson, & Lachner, 1998). Similar to other anxiety disorders, panic disorders are more common in adolescent females than males (Costello, Copeland, & Angold, 2011).

Agoraphobia

Agoraphobia in young people is characterized by a persistent fear of being trapped without a possibility to escape from certain situations or places (American Psychiatric Association, 2013). Typical situations that young people with agoraphobia find challenging include: using public transport, standing in a class line, or sitting in the middle of a crowded classroom. Children with agoraphobia may experience a panic attack in such a situation, or simply feel a sense of discomfort and unease. For agoraphobia to be diagnosed, the young person must exhibit, for six months, significant fear and anxiety in more than one situation or place from which he or she may not be able to easily escape, and avoid such locations accordingly.

Unlike previous editions, the DSM-5 has reclassified agoraphobia so that it is no longer linked to the presence of panic disorder and thus is a stand-alone diagnosis. Similarly, the DSM-5 has also tightened the definition of agoraphobia, so that children must experience fear/anxiety in at least two distinct situational domains such as: public transportation, being in enclosed places, being in open spaces, standing in line, being outside of the home, or being in a crowd (Cornacchio et al., 2015). Agoraphobia is found in 2.4 percent of adolescents and similar to other anxiety disorders, is more prevalent in young females than males (Merikangas et al., 2010).

Treatment of Anxiety Disorders Using a Standard Evidence-Based Approach

Given the comorbidity of anxiety disorders, treatments have tended to be transdiagnostic in their approach; that is, rather than targeting a specific anxiety disorder, treatment programs have largely been designed to treat a range of anxiety disorders. This makes sense clinically: if a child presents with both separation anxiety and social anxiety disorder, it does not seem adequate to deliver a treatment that focuses solely on one disorder and excludes the other. Thus, a transdiagnostic approach has been widely adopted in the management of anxiety disorders in children and adolescents. It is generally agreed that the underlying construct of anxiety, which is present in all anxiety disorders, can be treated with the same treatment protocol (Barlow, 2002). As mentioned earlier, the core features of anxiety disorders include an inaccurate perception of threat in a situation and excessive avoidance. The continued avoidance of potentially threatening situations serves to maintain the child's anxiety because the child is prevented from learning accurate information about the likelihood that something bad or dangerous will happen and about his or her ability to cope with the situation. Thus, CBT specifically addresses these underlying core cognitive processes and behaviors that serve to maintain anxiety. Using a cognitive-behavioral approach, anxious cognitions can be targeted via cognitive restructuring, and avoidance of feared stimuli can be addressed through gradual exposure. These are the core features of standard evidence-based care for all anxiety and related disorders (e.g., post-traumatic stress disorder, obsessive-compulsive disorder). There are a number of other techniques that are often used to support exposure and cognitive restructuring such as psychoeducation, problem solving, parent management, and relaxation. Manual-based treatments for anxiety disorders, usually between 10 and 16 sessions, are utilized to teach these techniques. The skills in the program are typically taught through verbal instruction, activities, role-plays, and/or modeling. Children are encouraged and rewarded for practice outside the session. This homework, or weekly between-session practice, is considered a key component of treatment success (Hudson, Kendall, & Davis, in press). Each of the key techniques utilized in standard evidence-based care will be discussed as follows.

Psychoeducation

As part of the standard treatment protocol, children and parents are provided with information about the fundamental components of their anxiety disorder; this includes the thoughts, behaviors, and physiological symptoms associated with the disorder, and in particular the way in which these factors interact to develop and maintain the disorder. Initial sessions are spent identifying the physiological experience of anxiety, so that the child can recognize the emotion when it occurs and know when to employ the new strategies he or she will learn throughout the program. These initial sessions also focus on working through practice examples linking thoughts with emotion and behavioral outcomes. By ensuring that parents and children understand the theoretical principles underlying treatment, they are better able to grasp the purpose behind the numerous tasks and experiments requested of them during treatment. This is particularly important if homework compliance is to be maintained. Similarly, collaboration and active participation is emphasized, to ensure that families recognize their own role in the therapy process. The goal of treatment is to provide the clients with skills they can utilize beyond the treatment, thereby reducing the burden of fear, anxiety, and worry and increasing function through reduced avoidance.

Parents and children are informed that fear, anxiety, and worry are normal experiences. This, in particular, highlights that the child is not alone in experiencing these anxiety-related phenomena. In this way, the therapist attempts to avoid or reduce the potentially stigmatizing effect of assessment or diagnosis. A functional level of anxiety is distinguished from anxiety that "gets in the way of doing things" that are appealing to the child. In this way, an attempt is made to engage the child's motivation and compliance in treatment, so that together the therapist, child, and parent can help reduce the impact the anxiety is having on the child's life.

Cognitive Restructuring

Cognitive restructuring is a technique that addresses maladaptive thoughts that are considered to maintain the expression of anxiety (Beck, 1976). The practice involves initially identifying the negative thoughts associated with the feared stimulus and considering their utility and accuracy. By reinterpreting the fear-provoking stimulus, and addressing negative thoughts and core beliefs that are unhelpful, new more accurate thoughts or evaluations of the feared stimulus can be acquired. As a result, the irrational thought is defused and a reduction in negative emotion is experienced when the feared item is subsequently encountered (Arch et al., 2012).

Developing more helpful thoughts can be challenging and relies upon the child's comprehension of the relationship between thoughts and outcomes, which is addressed in early sessions to impart an understanding of anxiety. This occurs through the use of therapist-led examples, in which the child practices identifying thoughts that lead to particular outcomes or feelings. For example, a child whose thoughts focus on "being laughed at" during a speech is likely to experience distress and avoid going to school on the day of the speech. The therapist may also help the child to identify thoughts that would lead to the reverse emotion or behavior, in the same scenario.

In the *Cool Kids* program, developed at Macquarie University in Sydney, Australia, children are encouraged to consider themselves a scientist or detective, and to collect evidence for their thoughts (Rapee et al., 2006). This evidence is utilized to determine the degree of fact or accuracy associated with the thought, and whether an alternate thought might be more accurate or useful. The process involves a number of steps, including: 1) identifying the feared event; 2) determining the worried thought; 3) considering the evidence or validity of the thought; 4) predicting the likelihood of the outcome; and 5) establishing a new more useful thought.

To aid this procedure, the therapist in conjunction with parents might pose provocative questions that aid the child's investigation of the thought. These are typically inspired by Socratic style questioning and can be supplemented with procedural worksheets available in many treatment manuals or workbooks. Some children find that particular questions or considerations are especially useful in their analysis of cognitions (e.g., "What happened last time?", "How likely is it to happen?") and might choose to print these on small cards that they can carry with them as reminders during anxiety-inducing situations.

Gradual Exposure

Exposure is a core feature of CBT and is often considered to be a primary mechanism by which CBT leads to reduced fear and anxiety (Meuret et al., 2012). Exposure is based on learning theory, and relies upon the premise that when a feared stimulus is experienced in the absence of an aversive event, the previous association between the stimulus and threat is reduced and the stimulus can now be experienced in the absence of fear (Wolpe, 1973). As explained earlier, the phenomenology of anxiety is maintained by avoidance of potential threat. As a result, the child attempts to avoid or limit any experience with the feared stimulus, and subsequently lacks sufficient opportunity to disprove fears that are disproportionate with actual events. Parents and children are taught that exposure serves to reduce avoidance and actively exposes the child to the feared item or situation, allowing the child to experience an accurate or "realistic" consequence, and providing the child with an opportunity to learn and apply coping skills.

Typically, exposure strategies are used in conjunction with a fear hierarchy. This is a list of fears devised by parent and child and rated from least to most fear-inducing or interfering. Each fear is broken down into a series of smaller steps of increasing difficulty. Due to the subjective nature of fear, each step is rated by the child on a subjective unit of distress scale (SUDS), and these are then addressed in hierarchical fashion, commencing with the step associated with the lowest level of distress or fear. Each step is completed until the fear experienced, or SUDS rating, is substantially reduced. At this point, each subsequent step is completed until the goal of experiencing the primary fear stimulus is achieved. This is often referred to as a stepladder, and its application aids compliance and motivation in children. An example of a stepladder may involve a child who completes schoolwork with an excessive degree of perfectionism and employs safety behaviors, such as checking homework repeatedly before school, because of a fear of making mistakes and getting in trouble. Through collaboration with parent and child, a series of goals may be formulated that graduate in difficulty toward the ultimate goal of submitting homework with deliberate mistakes, which seeks to address the child's fear belief of "making mistakes" and "getting in trouble." The stepladder may include a series of smaller steps, such as halving the time committed to completing homework, reducing the number of occasions that homework is checked by the child in the morning prior to school, or reducing the frequency with which parents check homework for errors. A reward is distributed by the parent for successful completion of each step, based on a previously agreed-upon list of rewards (see Child Management section). Difficulty completing a step may necessitate the use of other strategies discussed previously, such as relaxation techniques and cognitive restructuring. Some creativity or planning is often required on the part of the parent and/or therapist to provide the child with an opportunity to complete each step. On some occasions, exposure is imaginal, due to the difficulty or safety of replicating the feared stimulus in real life. On these occasions, the parents or therapist may assist the replication of a fear by role-playing a situation, either in place of a real-life exposure, or as practice, prior to engaging with the stimulus in vivo.

Historically, the active component of change associated with exposure was understood to be habituation (Foa & Kozak, 1986), necessitating that an individual experience fear activation, maintain prolonged exposure to the feared stimulus until a reduction in distress was experienced, and repeat these exposures between treatment sessions. As a result, the child learns the stimulus is not associated with threat or an aversive outcome, and also that anxiety will resolve over time. According to this theory, exposures provide experience of reduced fear and physiological arousal in the presence of the fear stimulus, thereby breaking the association between the stimulus and feared response (Groves & Thompson, 1970). More recent studies suggest that successful exposure occurs due to inhibitory learning (Bouton, 1993), which is not contingent on fear reduction during exposure trials. This premise ascribes reduction in fear as occurring when the feared stimulus acquires a new secondary meaning; that is, when safety information is newly associated with the feared stimulus. As a result, the feared stimulus has two competing meanings, the original fear and threat association, and a newly acquired meaning that associates safety with the stimulus (inhibitory learning). The intention of exposure therapy is then to obtain a stronger activation of the safety (inhibitory) response to the feared stimulus and reduce the activation of the threat response. Research conducted over the previous two decades has focused on the range of circumstances that lead to renewal of the threat association in response to the feared stimulus, despite successful learning during exposure. These include context change, spontaneous recovery due to time, or reinstatement due to related or unrelated adverse events following exposure. For this reason, application of inhibitory learning during exposure tasks is aimed at enhancing retrieval of the inhibitory or safe association in an effort to prevent the return to a threat association (Craske et al., 2014).

These tasks emphasize that successful exposure maximally violates the expectancy or intensity of the aversive outcome when the feared stimulus is encountered (Davey, 1992). Therefore, duration of exposure is determined sufficient at the point in which this violation has been achieved, as opposed to when fear has reduced, as would be the case in a habituation model. In addition, fear hierarchies are not typically employed, because maximal salience or opportunity to violate feared expectancies with actual events is desired. If the feared expectancy is only minimally likely, or minimally fear activating, as the case may be in the lower tier of a fear hierarchy, the opportunity to emphasize the discrepancy between expectancy and outcome is reduced. For this reason, some aspects of cognitive restructuring or relaxation techniques are not used in this style of exposure, because they could reduce the expectancy of a negative outcome and therefore reduce the opportunity for maximal violation between expectancy and outcome during the event. Learning is deemed successful when the expected outcome has not occurred, and if so, whether it was as aversive as initially believed (Craske et al., 2014).

Relaxation

Relaxation techniques encompass a range of strategies to reduce intense affect, which can inhibit the thoughtful application of CBT techniques. Numerous applications of CBT for children and adolescents include controlled breathing, and progressive muscular desensitization, or broader forms of muscular relaxation. The physiological description of anxiety explained to children and parents during psychoeducation is utilized to explain the effect of anxiety on increased heart rate and breathing. Training diaphragmatic breathing commences with distinguishing between shallow breathing and deep breathing that allows the lungs to be fully inflated with air. This can sometimes be illustrated by instructing children to place a hand on their stomach to observe its rise and fall when diaphragmatic breathing is engaged. Using relaxation can be useful in situations that are very anxiety-inducing and as a method to obtain affective relief. However, it is important that relaxation doesn't become another distraction technique that the child uses to avoid difficult situations. Importantly, the child and the parent need to know that anxiety itself, while uncomfortable, is normal and is not harmful and can be tolerated. Children however, often find these techniques useful in situations that are unavoidably stressful like exams or important speeches.

Protocols for breathing techniques are numerous, but typically involve inhalation and exhalation of breath at a prescribed rate, and sometimes counting is advised, to ensure consistent intake and out breath. Children are encouraged to practice for a set number of breaths and to do so either on a regular basis, such as at a prescribed time each day, e.g., before breakfast, or during and before events known to be challenging. For example, before a speech, or at bedtime (Taylor, 2001). Relaxation strategies, such as diaphragmatic breathing, are skills that require repeated practice for them to be useful.

Muscular desensitization is a similar technique in which clients are systematically taught to release muscular tension, most commonly by tensing and relaxing a sequence of muscles. Like breathing techniques, this strategy is often included in treatment to assist clients to reduce anxiety sensations sufficiently to engage in an anxiety inducing activity or exposure task. The task requires children to assume a position they find relaxing and if desired, close their eyes. The child is directed to select a series of muscle groups (e.g., arm muscles), focus on tensing these muscles for a number of seconds, and subsequently releasing those same muscles for a number of seconds. The child is advised to complete this activity with the remaining muscle groups in their body. It is sometimes easier to commence at the top of the body and progressively move downward toward the feet. Typically, children and their parents are instructed to practice this technique on a regular basis, or sometimes prior to or during an especially anxiety-inducing event (Öst, 1987; Ollendick & Cerny, 1981).

Similar to other skills acquired during treatment, the therapist emphasizes the need for practice and skill acquisition so the client is sufficiently practiced, and is better able to apply the selected form of relaxation in a critical moment of high anxiety. As mentioned, some debate exists over the use of relaxation as a component during exposure, with some researchers considering it a form of safety behavior, preventing a complete experience of the fear necessary for extinction to occur. However, regardless of its application during exposure, the techniques may be helpful to sufficiently prepare and motivate the child to participate in challenging situations that are often involved in exposure, especially so when anxiety is at a high level.

Problem Solving

Problem solving is taught to children as a method of identifying a more functional and less avoidant response to provocative situations. Anxious children have a tendency to overestimate the difficulty or threat associated with a situation and subsequently arrive at fewer potential solutions and have greater difficulty participating in fact-finding sessions. During problem solving, parents and therapist encourage the child view the problem as a scientific experiment, in which a number of potential explanations or solutions are applied and evaluated, before determining the best fit. The initial task is to identify as many solutions as possible through brainstorming sessions without excluding even the most outlandish suggestions. Thereafter, each suggestion is considered more carefully, with attention to the benefits and limitations or appropriateness of each before settling on a desired response that approximates the most useful and reasonable outcome. In some cases, for the purposes of training, a non-anxiety-inducing problem may be selected to engage and familiarize the child with the procedure. Parents and therapist must avoid providing solutions to the child, and instead allow the child to generate their own potential solutions.

Some children may find the formulation of the solution relatively straightforward, but find it challenging when application of the solution is required. For this reason, problem solving often involves developing a series of specific sub-goals that can be completed in sequence. By completing the smaller steps, the child is able to experience success, and by reflecting on successful completion of the earlier steps, they are able to challenge cognitive distortions associated with the task. On some occasions, problem solving is combined with social skills training and/or role play. Where problem-solving steps cannot be completed without a relevant skill, the focus of therapy is briefly centered around communication skills until the client obtains sufficient skills to attempt the next stage of their problem-solving tasks. The use of problem solving supplements other CBT strategies, by further removing the maladaptive avoidant response.

Child Management

Parents with anxious children often exhibit a number of unique behaviors. An important part of treatment is providing skills to parents that allow them to combat a tendency to modify family routines that accommodate the anxious child, for example co-sleeping with a child due to separation anxiety or taking responsibility for their communication with members of the community to reduce symptoms of social anxiety. Parents are trained in proactive anxiety management strategies they can use with their children during periods of acute anxiety. This primarily involves contingency management in which the child's behavior is shaped by preparing the parent to attend to behavior that is consistent with brave or courageous styles of acting, thereby reversing embedded patterns of attending to children when they exhibit anxiety and associated distress. A key focus of parental behavior is to reduce expressions of reassurance toward the anxious child, particularly in response to repeated requests for reassurance from the child, which is associated with maintenance of anxiety and reduced application of coping skills. One technique is the collaborative development of a reward system that promotes and recognizes goals and efforts toward confronting fears and reducing avoidance. This can be an essential tool to harness motivation and mastery. To further demonstrate the utility of newly learned skills, parents are encouraged to model brave behavior to their children, by completing tasks they themselves find worrying, or negotiating challenging situations using skills such as cognitive restructuring or problem solving. Similarly, it is useful to encourage parents to promote independence in their children, by providing children with opportunity to apply coping skills and negotiate challenges using problem-solving strategies. This can often be simply allowing the child to experience the natural consequences of their behavior, in place of the parent acting on their behalf (e.g., being responsible for phoning a friend to decline a party invitation or completing a purchase in a store). The child's increased opportunity to independently determine behavior or address problems, and reduced reliance on parents for direction and reassurance, can assist children to integrate and practice the skills learned during treatment.

Efficacy of Standard Care

Clinical trials evaluating the efficacy of CBT for anxious youth typically recruit heterogeneous groups of anxious children diagnosed primarily with GAD, SAD, and SoAD (Barrett, Dadds, & Rapee, 1996; Hudson et al., 2009; Kendall et al., 2008). Consequently, these trials provide information about the efficacy of CBT for anxiety disorders in general rather than for specific disorders. Considering anxiety disorders collectively, there is rigorous support for CBT as an efficacious method of reducing the presence of anxiety disorders and symptoms in children and adolescents (Bennett et al., 2016). There are a number of therapeutic guidelines that recommend CBT as the first line of treatment for anxious youth (Connolly & Bernstein, 2007; Hudson, Creswell, & McLellan, 2014; National Institute for Health and Care Excellence, 2013). Systematic reviews have demonstrated recovery rates of approximately 60 percent following treatment (Cartwright-Hatton et al., 2004; James et al., 2015). Further, there is some evidence to suggest that cognitive behavioral treatments produce better outcomes not only compared to wait-list conditions but also to psychological placebo interventions in which key CBT ingredients have been removed (Hudson et al., 2009). However, further research comparing CBT with active treatment conditions is needed (Bennett et al., 2016). There are few controlled studies evaluating the long-term efficacy of CBT, yet the uncontrolled long-term studies have shown the maintenance of positive treatment outcomes and reduction of mental health problems such as suicidal ideation and substance abuse later in life (Barrett et al., 2001; Kendall et al., 2004; Wolk, Kendall, & Beidas, 2015). These results suggest that when treatment is effective in childhood and adolescence, the skills learned in the program can better equip the child throughout their life to cope with anxiety-provoking and stressful situations.

Parental Involvement. Most treatment programs for child anxiety involve parents to some degree. As noted previously, the rationale for involving parents is that parents play an important role in the development and/or maintenance in the child's anxiety. We know that anxiety runs in families, thus, it is often likely that parents of the child in treatment also experience clinically significant anxiety. In such circumstances, the parent's anxiety and associated avoidance can serve to maintain the child's anxiety. The parent may communicate inaccurate information about threat and coping to the child and may be reluctant to engage in treatment if it involves situations the parent finds anxiety-provoking. In addition, parents can enhance the child's anxiety by rushing in too quickly to reduce the child's distress or providing too much assistance or reassurance to their child. Over time, this parent behavior serves to unintentionally increase anxiety because the child is prevented from learning accurate information about the situation and their ability to cope with it. For these reasons, it makes sense to involve the parents in therapy to ensure that these issues are addressed and monitored to avoid impacting on the child's treatment success.

Yet the extent to which parents are involved in manualized treatment programs varies extensively, with some programs including parents minimally in one or two sessions to other programs in which parents are a central part of the program. Ultimately, the research has tended to show that outcomes are not related to the amount of parental involvement. That is, children show similar outcomes regardless of whether parents are involved in minimal ways. More recently, there has been some evidence to suggest that the type of parental involvement is important. An individual patient data meta-analysis involving over 1300 children has shown improved child outcomes when parents are taught contingency management strategies (such as the use of attention and rewards to shape non-anxious behavior) or treatments that use a transfer of control model (whereby initially the therapist teaches the parent and the child and as treatment progresses the parent increases their involvement in the delivery of the treatment strategies; Manassis et al., 2014). These results suggest that better outcomes are produced when parents are included in treatment in this active way compared to minimal parental involvement. This finding did however fail to replicate in another analysis of a multisite database (Hudson et al., 2015) and thus further research is required to determine whether including parents in treatment adds any value to child outcomes.

Group or Individual Treatment. Although there is evidence from adult anxiety treatment research that individual treatment delivers superior outcomes compared to group delivery of CBT (Stangier et al., 2003), there is limited evidence in the child literature that suggests delivery method has an impact on outcome. A recent systematic review of randomized clinical trials comparing delivery methods failed to show that individual treatment leads to enhanced outcomes compared to group delivery (James et al., 2015). In contrast, one review utilizing child-reported outcomes showed significantly larger effect sizes for individual compared to group therapy (Reynolds et al., 2012). One of the significant limitations of research examining differential outcomes for children receiving CBT for anxiety disorders are the relatively small sample sizes that prevent the examination of possible moderators of treatment outcome. In a recent attempt to address this issue, a number of research clinics from around the world have contributed clinical research trial data to examine both genetic and clinical predictors of treatment outcome for anxious children (Hudson, Keers et al., 2015). In a recent study emerging from this collaboration, Keers and colleagues (2016) have provided preliminary evidence that polygenic risk scores of environmental sensitivity moderate children's response to different treatment types. Environmental sensitivity is defined as genetic risk associated with being less robust to either negative or positive environments. A child with high polygenic risk for environmental sensitivity is theorized to struggle in negative environments, yet flourish in positive environments. A child with low environmental sensitivity is predicted to be more immune to changes in environment. Consistent with this, Keers and colleagues found that children with high environmental sensitivity (that is, less robust to the environment) actually had better outcomes in individual therapy compared to group therapy or parent-led low intensity therapy. This finding suggests that children with higher environmental sensitivity may require more intensive therapy whereas the intensity of treatment may matter less for children with low environmental sensitivity. Further research is needed to explore whether outcomes following different delivery methods of standard CBT may vary based on individual characteristics of the child.

Predictors of Outcome in Standard Evidence-Based Care. Recently, evidence has emerged from large multisite studies identifying a number of factors that can predict which children are likely to respond more favorably to standard evidence-based care (Bennett et al., 2013; Compton et al., 2014; Hudson, Keers et al., 2015; Hudson et al., 2013). For example, one of these studies has shown that age does not appear to impact on treatment outcomes and thus, standard CBT can work well for both children and adolescents (Bennett et al., 2013). A number of studies have also identified that children who present with a diagnosis of social anxiety disorder have poorer outcomes and slower change than children with other anxiety disorders (Compton et al., 2014; Hudson, Keers et al., 2015; Hudson, Rapee et al., 2015). Importantly, children with social anxiety disorder do respond favorably to CBT, yet evidence suggests that this change may not be as great as children with other anxiety disorders. Thus, a standard approach may prove less effective for children with social anxiety.

Currently, it is unclear why children with social anxiety respond less favorably. It is possible that these children have poorer alliance with their therapists and this then may impact on engagement and treatment efficacy. Evidence from our research group suggests that this is in fact the case. Children with a social anxiety disorder diagnosis were observed during treatment to have a poorer therapeutic alliance than anxious children with other anxiety diagnoses (Ross & Hudson, 2016). Children with social anxiety disorder also differ from most other anxious children, in that the feared stimulus may be, in fact the therapist. This brings with it unique challenges for the therapist and the child. Our current transdiagnostic treatments may not address these issues sufficiently and may be providing a therapeutic environment that prevents greater change from occurring. It is also possible that our current treatments do not allow sufficient time or opportunity for challenging exposures (i.e., steps that allow the child to be exposed to possible costs of negative evaluation to learn that even if negative evaluation occurs it can be tolerated). As previously mentioned, the degree to which the therapist conducted challenging exposures during therapy, the better the child's outcome following CBT (Peris et al., 2017).

In adult treatments of social anxiety disorder, cognitive therapies that target specific social cognitions have produced superior outcomes compared to standard exposure-based therapy (Clark et al., 2006; Rapee, Gaston, & Abbott, 2009). Theoretically, disorder-specific techniques may result in greater change for these children. A handful of studies have started to examine this research question in children with anxiety disorders. For example, using a meta-analytic technique, Reynolds et al. (2012) showed superior outcomes based on child-reported measures for disorder-specific treatments for anxiety in general compared to transdiagnostic approaches. A preliminary clinical trial of social anxiety disorder in adolescents also showed superior outcomes for a disorder-specific cognitive therapy compared to transdiagnostic exposure-based treatment (Ingul, Aune, & Nordahl, 2013). In contrast to these preliminary findings, Spence and colleagues (2017) compared a disorder-specific treatment to a generic treatment for children with social anxiety and failed to find a significant difference between the two conditions, suggesting that a disorder-specific approach does not necessarily lead to better outcomes. Future research is required to develop and test innovative treatment solutions for children with social anxiety disorder.

There are a number of other factors that also may reduce the efficacy of a standard evidence-based treatment for children with anxiety disorders. For example, children with comorbid disorders such as depression have been shown to demonstrate poorer endpoints than children without co-occurring mood problems, suggesting that additional treatment that targets both anxiety and depression may be beneficial for these children (Hudson et al., 2015; Rapee et al., 2013). Evidence has also emerged to suggest pretreatment severity impacts on treatment outcome, that is, the more severe the child's anxiety prior to treatment the more likely they will have more severe anxiety after the completion of the treatment program (Hudson et al., 2015). Finally, there is evidence, albeit inconsistent, to suggest that parental psychopathology can impact the treatment outcomes for children following CBT for anxiety. A number of studies have demonstrated that anxious children whose parents are anxious are likely to have poorer outcomes following CBT compared to anxious children whose parents are not highly anxious (Cobham, Dadds, & Spence, 1998; Hudson, Newall et al., 2014). Yet, a number of studies have failed to show parental psychopathology is related to child outcome following CBT (Cobham et al., 2010; Kendall et al.,

2008). Again, perhaps the inconsistency across studies occurs because of different follow-up periods in studies, and sample sizes in clinical trials are rarely adequately powered to detect predictors. In our recent analysis of 1,519 children, there was no significant difference in symptom change immediately following treatment between children whose parents had high or low anxiety or depression symptoms, yet 12 months after treatment, some differences did emerge (Hudson, Keers et al., 2015). Controlling for initial severity, children whose parents were anxious or depressed at pretreatment were more likely to have high symptoms in the follow-up period compared to children whose parents were not anxious or depressed.

Future research needs to focus on developing treatment innovations for those children who are less likely to respond to standard evidence-based care. In this volume, there are numerous innovations that are described in detail that may help to improve outcomes for children with anxiety disorders as well as to improve access to evidence-based care for children with anxiety disorders.

Conclusions

In summary, anxiety disorders in children and young people are common and debilitating disorders that often go unnoticed and untreated. Recognizing and successfully treating anxiety problems in young people is important for lifelong mental health and well-being. Following numerous randomized clinical trials, there is now strong support for the use of cognitive behavioral therapy for the treatment of a range of anxiety disorders in young people. There is also evidence to suggest that the successful treatment of anxiety disorders in young people prevents further mental health disorders. To improve the mental health and well-being of children and adolescents, anxiety disorders in children need to be taken seriously. Providing clinicians with adequate training to deliver evidence-based practice is key to reducing the prevalence of anxiety disorders. Further, we need to invest in the development of treatment innovations that will work toward improving outcomes for those children who may respond less favorably to standard evidence-based care.

Key Practice Points

- Putting the child at ease: The first sessions can be challenging for the child and family. Spend time early on in therapy engaging in a brief nonthreatening fun activity. Give the child a clear understanding of what to expect from the session and the therapy.
- Understanding the fear: Clinicians should spend time conducting a comprehensive assessment of the anxiety to understand the child's core cognitions so that the exposure steps can be generated to sufficiently target the fear.
- Key treatment ingredient: Ensure that adequate therapy time is devoted to collaborative development of stepladders. Many therapists can become sidetracked by

other skills or issues that are perhaps easier to manage than facing fears. Facing fears is extremely difficult for everyone involved (child, parents, and therapists). For therapy to work, the child needs to be able to face the most difficult fears. Without this, therapy will be less successful.

- Practice: Practice between sessions is a key ingredient to long-term change. Clinicians should allow sufficient time at the beginning and end of every session to devote to reviewing and planning the weekly practice. Homework design should be done collaboratively with the child and parents to maximize the chance of successful completion. The expectations for homework completion need to be clear.
- Work collaboratively with parents: Clinicians should work collaboratively with the parents, initially modeling the ideal way to respond to the child's anxiety. Throughout therapy, the clinician can gradually decrease this as the parent becomes more confident with responding to the child's anxiety in a way that encourages approach rather than avoidance. The key messages to convey to parents include: understanding that rewards are important to motivate the child to face their fears, understanding the role the parents may be playing in maintaining the child's anxiety, and encouraging parents to change their reactions to anxiety to scaffold brave behavior and encourage independence.
- Group format: When running the program in groups, consider matching (where possible) similar ages as well as an even gender ratio. This will ensure children can maximize the normalizing process of the group and avoid a specific child feeling isolated.

References

American Psychiatric Association. (2013). *Diagnostic and statistical manual of mental disorders (DSM-5)* (5th ed.). Arlington, VA: American Psychiatric Association.

Arch, J. J., Wolitzky-Taylor, K. B., Eifert, G. H., & Craske, M. G. (2012). Longitudinal treatment mediation of traditional cognitive behavioral therapy and acceptance and commitment therapy for anxiety disorders. *Behaviour Research and Therapy*, 50 (7–8), 469–478. doi:10.1016/j.brat.2012.04.007

Barlow, D. H. (ed.) (2002). *Anxiety and its disorders: The nature and treatment of anxiety and panic* (2nd ed.). New York: Guilford Press.

Barlow, D. H., Vermilyea, J., Blanchard, E. B., Vermilyea, B. B., Di Nardo, P. A., & Cerny, J. A. (1985). The phenomenon of panic. *Journal of Abnormal Psychology*, 94(3), 320–328.

Barrett, P. M., Dadds, M. R., & Rapee, R. M. (1996). Family treatment of childhood anxiety: A controlled trial. *Journal of Consulting and Clinical Psychology*, 64(2), 333–342.

Barrett, P. M., Duffy, A. L., Dadds, M. R., & Rapee, R. M. (2001). Cognitive-behavioral treatment of anxiety disorders in children: Long-term (6-year) follow-up. *Journal of Consulting and Clinical Psychology*, 69(1), 135–141.

Baxter, A. J., Vos, T., Scott, K. M., Ferrari, A.J., & Whiteford, H.A. (2014). The global burden of anxiety disorders in 2010. *Psychological Medicine*, 44(11), 2363–2374. doi:10.1017/s0033291713003243

Beck, A.T. (1976). *Cognitive therapy and the emotional disorders*. New York: International Universities Press.

Beesdo, K., Knappe, S., & Pine, D.S. (2009). Anxiety and anxiety disorders in children and adolescents: Developmental issues and implications for DSM-V. *The Psychiatric Clinics of North America, 32*(3), 483–524. doi:10.1016/j.psc.2009.06.002

Beesdo, K., Pine, D.S., Lieb, R., & Wittchen, H. (2010). Incidence and risk patterns of anxiety and depressive disorders and categorization of generalized anxiety disorder. *Archives of General Psychiatry, 67*(1), 47–57. doi:10.1001/archgenpsychiatry.2009.177

Bennett, K., Manassis, K., Duda, S., Bagnell, A., Bernstein, G.A., Garland, E.J., ... Wilansky, P. (2016). Treating child and adolescent anxiety effectively: Overview of systematic reviews. *Clinical Psychology Review, 50*, 80–94.

Bennett, K., Manassis, K., Walter, S.D., Cheung, A., Wilansky-Traynor, P., Diaz-Granados, N., ... Wood, J.J. (2013). Cognitive behavioral therapy age effects in child and adolescent anxiety: An individual patient data metaanalysis. *Depression and Anxiety, 30*(9), 829-841. doi:10.1002/da.22099

Birrell, L., Newton, N.C., Teesson, M., Tonks, Z., & Slade, T. (2015). Anxiety disorders and first alcohol use in the general population: Findings from a nationally representative sample. *Journal of Anxiety Disorders, 31*(Supplement C), 108–113. doi:https://doi.org/10.1016/j.janxdis.2015.02.008

Black, B. (1996). Social anxiety and selective mutism. In L.J. Dickstein, M.B. Riba, & J.M. Oldham (eds.), *Review of psychiatry* (Vol. 15, pp. 469–495). Washington, DC: American Psychiatric Press Inc.

Bouton, M.E. (1993). Context, time, and memory retrieval in the interference paradigms of Pavlovian learning. *Psychological Bulletin, 114*(1), 80–99. doi:10.1037/0033-2909.114.1.80

Brand, S., Wilhelm, F.H., Kossowsky, J., Holsboer-Trachsler, E., & Schneider, S. (2011). Children suffering from separation anxiety disorder (SAD) show increased HPA axis activity compared to healthy controls. *Journal of Psychiatric Research, 45*(4), 452–459. doi:10.1016/j.jpsychires.2010.08.014

Cartwright-Hatton, S., Roberts, C., Chitsabesan, P., Fothergill, C., & Harrington, R. (2004). Systematic review of the efficacy of cognitive behaviour therapies for childhood and adolescent anxiety disorders. *British Journal of Clinical Psychology, 43*(4), 421–436.

Clark, D.M., Ehlers, A., Hackmann, A., McManus, F., Fennell, M., Grey, N., Waddington, L., & Wild, J. (2006). Cognitive therapy versus exposure and applied relaxation in social phobia: A randomized controlled trial. *Journal of Consulting and Clinical Psychology, 74*(3), 568–578.

Cobham, V.E., Dadds, M.R., & Spence, S.H. (1998). The role of parental anxiety in the treatment of childhood anxiety. *Journal of Consulting and Clinical Psychology, 66*(6), 893–905.

Cobham, V.E., Dadds, M.R., Spence, S.H., & McDermott, B. (2010). Parental anxiety in the treatment of childhood anxiety: A different story three years later. *Journal of Clinical Child and Adolescent Psychology, 39*(3), 410–420. doi:10.1080/15374411003691719

Cohen, P., Cohen, J., & Brook, J. (1993). An epidemiological study of disorders in late childhood and adolescence: II. Persistence of disorders. *Journal of Child Psychology and Psychiatry, 34*(6), 869–877.

Compton, S.N., Peris, T.S., Almirall, D., Birmaher, B., Sherrill, J., Kendall, P.C., ... Albano, A.M. (2014). Predictors and moderators of treatment response in childhood anxiety disorders: Results from the CAMS trial. *Journal of Consulting and Clinical Psychology, 82*(2), 212–224. doi:10.1037/a0035458

Connolly, S.D., & Bernstein, G.A. (2007). Practice parameter for the assessment and treatment of children and adolescents with anxiety disorders. *Journal of the American Academy of Child and Adolescent Psychiatry, 46*(2), 267–283.

Cornacchio, D., Chou, T., Sacks, H., Pincus, D., & Comer, J. (2015). Clinical consequences of the revised DSM-5 definition of agoraphobia in treatment-seeking anxious youth. *Depression and Anxiety, 32*(7), 502–508.

Costello, E.J., Copeland, W., & Angold, A. (2011). Trends in psychopathology across the adolescent years: What changes when children become adolescents, and when adolescents become adults? *Journal of Child Psychology and Psychiatry, 52*(10), 1015–1025.

Costello, E., Mustillo, S., Erkanli, A., Keeler, G., & Angold, A. (2003). Prevalence and development of psychiatric disorders in childhood and adolescence. *Archives of General Psychiatry, 60*(8), 837–844.

Craske, M., Treanor, M., Conway, C.C., Zbozinek, T., & Vervliet, B. (2014). Maximizing exposure therapy: An inhibitory learning approach. *Behaviour Research and Therapy, 58*, 10–23. doi:10.1016/j.brat.2014.04.006

Craske, M.G., Stein, M.B., Eley, T.C., Milad, M.R., Holmes, A., Rapee, R.M., & Wittchen, H.-U. (2017). Anxiety disorders. *Nature Reviews Disease Primers, 3*, 17024. doi:10.1038/nrdp.2017.24

Davey, G.C.L. (1992). Classical conditioning and the acquisition of human fears and phobias: A review and synthesis of the literature. *Advances in Behaviour Research and Therapy, 14*(1), 29–66. doi:10.1016/0146-6402(92)90010-L

Erskine, H.E., Moffitt, T.E., Copeland, W.E., Costello, E.J., Ferrari, A.J., Patton, G., ... Scott, J.G. (2015). A heavy burden on young minds: The global burden of mental and substance use disorders in children and youth. *Psychological Medicine, 45*(07), 1551–1563. doi:doi:10.1017/S0033291714002888

Foa, E.B., & Kozak, M.J. (1986). Emotional processing of fear: Exposure to corrective information. *Psychological Bulletin, 99*(1), 20–35. doi:10.1037/0033-2909.99.1.20

Ford, T., Goodman, R., & Meltzer, H. (2003). The British Child and Adolescent Mental Health Survey 1999: The prevalence of DSM-IV disorders. *Journal of the American Academy of Child and Adolescent Psychiatry, 42*(10), 1203–1211.

Groves, P.M., & Thompson, R.F. (1970). Habituation: A dual-process theory. *Psychological Review, 77*(5), 419–450. doi:10.1037/h0029810

Gullone, E. (2000). The development of normal fear: A century of research. *Clinical Psychology Review, 20*(4), 429–451.

Heyne, D., King, N.J., & Tonge, B.J. (2004). School refusal. In T.H. Ollendick & J.S. March (eds.), *Phobic and anxiety disorders in children and adolescents: A clinician's guide to effective psychosocial and pharmacological interventions* (pp. 236–271). New York: Oxford University Press.

Hirschfeld, R.M.A. (2001). The comorbidity of major depression and anxiety disorders: Recognition and management in primary care. *Primary Care Companion to The Journal of Clinical Psychiatry, 3*(6), 244–254.

Højgaard, D.R.M.A., Mortensen, E.L., Ivarsson, T., Hybel, K., Skarphedinsson, G., Nissen, J.B., ... Thomsen, P.H. (2017). Structure and clinical correlates of obsessive–compulsive symptoms in a large sample of children and adolescents: A factor analytic study across five nations. *European Child and Adolescent Psychiatry, 26*(3), 281–291. doi:10.1007/s00787-016-0887-5

Hudson, J.L., Creswell, C., & McLellan, L. (2014). A clinician's quick guide of evidence-based approaches: Childhood anxiety disorders. *Clinical Psychologist, 18*(1), 52–53.

Hudson, J. L., Keers, R., Roberts, S., Coleman, J. R., Breen, G., Arendt, K., ... Eley, T. C. (2015). Clinical predictors of response to cognitive-behavioral therapy in pediatric anxiety disorders: The Genes for Treatment (GxT) study. *Journal of the American Academy of Child & Adolescent Psychiatry, 54*(6), 454–463.

Hudson, J.L., Kendall, P.C. & Davis, J.P. (in press). Homework in CBT with children. In N. Kazantzis, F. (Ed.). *Using Homework Assignments in Cognitive Behavior Therapy.* New York, NY: Routledge.

Hudson, J.L., Lester, K.J., Lewis, C.M., Tropeano, M., Creswell, C., Collier, C., ... Eley T.C. (2013). Predicting outcomes following cognitive behaviour therapy in child anxiety disorders: The influence of genetic, demographic and clinical information. *Journal of Child Psychology and Psychiatry, 54*(10), 1086–1094.

Hudson, J.L., Newall, C., Rapee, R.M., Lyneham, H.J., Schniering, C.C., Wuthrich, V.M., ... Gar, N.S. (2014). The impact of brief parental anxiety management on child anxiety treatment outcomes: A controlled trial. *Journal of Clinical Child and Adolescent Psychology, 43*(3), 370–380.

Hudson, J.L., Rapee, R.M., Deveney, C., Schniering, C.A., Lyneham, H.J., & Bovopoulos, N. (2009). Cognitive-behavioral treatment versus an active control for children and adolescents with anxiety disorders: A randomized trial. *Journal of the American Academy of Child and Adolescent Psychiatry, 48*(5), 533–544. doi:http://dx.doi.org/10.1097/CHI.0b013e31819c2401

Hudson, J.L., Rapee, R.M., Lyneham, H.J., McLellan, L.F., Wuthrich, V.M., & Schniering, C.A. (2015). Comparing outcomes for children with different anxiety disorders following cognitive behavioural therapy. *Behaviour Research and Therapy, 72*, 30–37.

Ingul, J.M., Aune, T., & Nordahl, H.M. (2013). A randomized controlled trial of individual cognitive therapy, group cognitive behaviour therapy and attentional placebo for adolescent social phobia. *Psychotherapy and Psychosomatics, 83*(1), 54–61.

James, A.C., James, G., Cowdrey, F.A., Soler, A., & Choke, A. (2015). Cognitive behavioural therapy for anxiety disorders in children and adolescents. Cochrane Database of Systematic Reviews 2015, Issue 2. Art. No.: CD004690. DOI: 10.1002/14651858.CD004690.pub4.

Keers, R., Coleman, J.R., Lester, K.J., Roberts, S., Breen, G., Thastum, M., ... Eley, T.C. (2016). A genome-wide test of the differential susceptibility hypothesis reveals a genetic predictor of differential response to psychological treatments for child anxiety disorders. *Psychotherapy and Psychosomatics*, *85*(3), 146–158.

Kendall, P.C., Compton, S.N., Walkup, J.T., Birmaher, B., Albano, A.M., Sherrill, J., ... Piacentini, J. (2010). Clinical characteristics of anxiety disordered youth. *Journal of Anxiety Disorders*, *24*(3), 360–365.

Kendall, P.C., Hudson, J.L., Gosch, E., Flannery-Schroeder, E., & Suveg, C. (2008). Cognitive-behavioral therapy for anxiety disordered youth: A randomized clinical trial evaluating child and family modalities. *Journal of Consulting and Clinical Psychology*, *76*(2), 282–297.

Kendall, P.C., Safford, S., Flannery-Schroeder, E., & Webb, A. (2004). Child anxiety treatment: Outcomes in adolescence and impact on substance use and depression at 7.4-year follow-up. *Journal of Consulting and Clinical Psychology*, *72*(2), 276–287.

Kim-Cohen, J., Caspi, A., Moffitt, T.E., Harrington, H., Milne, B.J., & Poulton, R. (2003). Prior juvenile diagnoses in adults with mental disorder: Developmental follow-back of a prospective-longitudinal cohort. *Archives of General Psychiatry*, *60*(7), 709–717. doi:10.1001/archpsyc.60.7.709

Kossowsky, J., Wilhelm, F.H., Roth, W.T., & Schneider, S. (2012). Separation anxiety disorder in children: Disorder-specific responses to experimental separation from the mother. *Journal of Child Psychology and Psychiatry*, *53*(2), 178–187. doi:10.1111/j.1469-7610.2011.02465.x

Lawrence, D., Johnson, S., Hafekost, J., Boterhoven de Haan, K., Sawyer, M., Ainley, J., & Zubrick, S.R. (2015). The mental health of children and adolescents: Report on the second Australian Child and Adolescent Survey of Mental Health and Wellbeing.

Lewinsohn, P.M., Hops, H., Roberts, R.E., Seeley, J.R., & Andrews, J.A. (1993). Adolescent psychopathology: I. Prevalence and incidence of depression and other DSM-III-R disorders in high school students. *Journal of Abnormal Psychology*, *102*(1), 133–144.

Manassis, K., Lee, T.C., Bennett, K., Zhao X.Y., Mendlowitz., S., Duda, S., ... Wood, J. J. (2014). Types of parental involvement in CBT with anxious youth: A preliminary meta-analysis. *Journal of Consulting and Clinical Psychology*, *82*(6), 1163–1172.

Merikangas, K.R., He, J.-p., Burstein, M., Swanson, S.A., Avenevoli, S., Cui, L., ... Swendsen, J. (2010). Lifetime prevalence of mental disorders in U.S. adolescents: Results from the National Comorbidity Survey Replication-Adolescent Supplement (NCS-A). *Journal of the American Academy of Child & Adolescent Psychiatry*, *49*(10), 980–989. doi:http://dx.doi.org/10.1016/j.jaac.2010.05.017

Meuret, A.E., Wolitzky-Taylor, K.B., Twohig, M.P., & Craske, M. (2012). Coping skills and exposure therapy in panic disorder and agoraphobia: Latest advances and future directions. *Behavior Therapy*, *43*(2), 271–284. doi:10.1016/j.beth.2011.08.002

Muris, P., Merckelbach, H., de Jong, P.J., & Ollendick, T.H. (2002). The etiology of specific fears and phobias in children: A critique of the non-associative account. *Behaviour Research and Therapy*, *40*(2), 185–195.

Muris, P., & Ollendick, T.H. (2015). Children who are anxious in silence: A review on selective mutism, the new anxiety disorder in DSM-5. *Clinical Child* and *Family Psychology Review, 18*(2), 151–169. doi:10.1007/s10567-015-0181-y

National Institute for Health and Care Excellence. (2013). Social anxiety disorder: recognition, assessment and treatment. *Clinical Guideline [CG159]*.

Ollendick, T. H., & Cerny, J. A. (1981). *Clinical behavior therapy with children*. New York: Plenum Press.

Ollendick, T.H., Mattis, S.G., & King, N.J. (1994). Panic in children and adolescents: A review. *Journal of Child Psychology & Psychiatry & Allied Disciplines, 35*(1), 113–134.

Öst, L.-G. (1987). Applied relaxation: Description of a coping technique and review of controlled studies. *Behaviour Research and Therapy, 25*(5), 397–409.

Otto, M.W., Pollack, M.H., Maki, K.M., Gould, R.A., Worthington, J.J., Smoller, J.W., & Rosenbaum, J.F. (2001). Childhood history of anxiety disorders among adults with social phobia: Rates, correlates, and comparisons with patients with panic disorder. *Depression and Anxiety, 14*, 209–213.

Payne, S., Bolton, D., & Perrin, S. (2011). A pilot investigation of cognitive therapy for generalized anxiety disorder in children aged 7–17 years. *Cognitive Therapy and Research, 35*(2), 171–178. doi:10.1007/s10608-010-9341-z

Peris, T.S., Piacentini, J., Bergman, R.L., Caporino, N.E., O'Rourke, S., Kendall, P.C., … Compton, S. (2017). Therapist-reported features of exposure tasks that predict differential treatment outcome for youth with anxiety. *Journal of the American Academy of Child and Adolescent Psychiatry, 56*(12), 1043-1052.

Piacentini, J., Bergman, R.L., Keller, M., & McCracken, J. (2003). Functional impairment in children and adolescents with obsessive-compulsive disorder. *Journal of Child and Adolescent Psychopharmacology, 13*(2, Supplement 1), 61–69.

Pine, D.S., Cohen, P., Gurley, D., Brook, J., & Ma, Y. (1998). The risk for early-adulthood anxiety and depressive disorders in adolescents with anxiety and depressive disorders. *Archives of General Psychiatry, 55*, 56–64.

Polanczyk, G.V., Salum, G.A., Sugaya, L.S., Caye, A., & Rohde, L.A. (2015). Annual Research Review: A meta-analysis of the worldwide prevalence of mental disorders in children and adolescents. *Journal of Child Psychology and Psychiatry, 56*(3), 345–365.

Queen, A.H., Ehrenreich-May, J., & Hershorin, E.R. (2012). Preliminary validation of a screening tool for adolescent panic disorder in pediatric primary care clinics. *Child Psychiatry and Human Development, 43*, 171–183.

Ramsawh, H.J., Chavira, D.A., & Stein, M.B. (2010). Burden of anxiety disorders in pediatric medical settings: Prevalence, phenomenology, and a research agenda. *Archives of Pediatrics and Adolescent Medicine, 164*(10), 965–972.

Rapee, R.M., Gaston, J.E., & Abbott, M.J. (2009). Testing the efficacy of theoretically derived improvements in the treatment of social phobia. *Journal of Consulting and Clinical Psychology, 77*(2), 317–327. //doi:http://dx.doi.org/10.1037/a0014800

Rapee, R.M., Lyneham, H.J., Hudson, J.L., Kangas, M., Wuthrich, V.M., & Schniering, C.A. (2013). Effect of comorbidity on treatment of anxious children and adolescents:

Results from a large, combined sample. *Journal of the American Academy of Child and Adolescent Psychiatry, 52*(1), 47–56.

Rapee, R.M., Lyneham, H.J., Schniering, C.A., Wuthrich, V.M., Abbott, M.J., Hudson, J.L., & Wignall, A. (2006). *The Cool Kids Anxiety Treatment Program*. Sydney, Australia: Centre for Emotional Health, Macquarie University.

Rapee, R.M., Schniering, C.A., & Hudson, J.L. (2009). Anxiety disorders during childhood and adolescence: Origins and treatment. *Annual Review of Clinical Psychology, 5*, 335–365.

Reynolds, S., Wilson, C., Austin, J., & Hooper, L. (2012). Effects of psychotherapy for anxiety in children and adolescents: A meta-analytic review. *Clinical Psychology Review, 32*(4), 251–262. doi:https://doi.org/10.1016/j.cpr.2012.01.005

Ross, C., & Hudson, J.L. (2016). *Alliance, child involvement and therapist flexibility in the treatment of childhood anxiety disorders: The impact of primary anxiety diagnosis and comorbidity*. Sydney, Australia: Macquarie University.

Seligman, L.D., & Ollendick, T.H. (1998). Comorbidity of anxiety and depression in children and adolescents: An integrative review. *Clinical Child and Family Psychology Review, 1*(2), 125–144.

Southam-Gerow, M.A., Weisz, J.R., Chu, B.C., McLeod, B.D., Gordis, E.B., & Connor-Smith, J.K. (2010). Does CBT for youth anxiety outperform usual care in community clinics? An initial effectiveness test. *Journal of the American Academy of Child and Adolescent Psychiatry, 49*(10), 1043–1052. doi:10.1016/j.jaac.2010.06.009

Spence, S.H., Donovan, C.L., March, S., Kenardy, J.A., & Hearn, C.S. (2017). Generic versus disorder specific cognitive behavior therapy for social anxiety disorder in youth: A randomized controlled trial using internet delivery. *Behaviour Research and Therapy, 90*, 41–57.

Stangier, U., Heidenreich, T., Peitz, M., Lauterbach, W., & Clark, D.M. (2003). Cognitive therapy for social phobia: Individual versus group treatment. *Behaviour Research and Therapy, 41*(9), 991–1007. doi:https://doi.org/10.1016/S0005-7967(02)00176-6

Stein, M.B., Fuetsch, M., Müller, N., Höfler, M., Lieb, R., & Wittchen, H. (2001). Social anxiety disorder and the risk of depression: A prospective community study of adolescents and young adults. *Archives of General Psychiatry, 58*(3), 251–256. doi:10.1001/archpsyc.58.3.251

Strauss, C.C., & Last, C.G. (1993). Social and simple phobias in children. *Journal of Anxiety Disorders, 7*, 141–152.

Taylor, S. (2001). Breathing retraining in the treatment of panic disorder: Efficacy, caveats and indications. *Scandinavian Journal of Behaviour Therapy, 30*(2), 49–56. doi:10.1080/02845710118895

Viana, A.G., Beidel, D.C., & Rabian, B. (2009). Selective mutism: A review and integration of the last 15 years. *Clinical Psychology Review, 29*(1), 57–67.

Walkup, J.T., Albano, A.M., Piacentini, J., Birmaher, B., Compton, S.N., Sherrill, J.T., ... Kendall, P.C. (2008). Cognitive behavioral therapy, sertraline, or a combination in childhood anxiety. *New England Journal of Medicine, 359*(26), 2753–2766.

Wells, A. (2005). The metacognitive model of GAD: Assessment of meta-worry and relationship with DSM-IV generalized anxiety disorder. *Cognitive Therapy and Research, 29*(1), 107–121.

Wittchen, H.-U., Nelson, C.B., & Lachner, G. (1998). Prevalence of mental disorders and psychosocial impairments in adolescents and young adults. *Psychological Medicine, 28*(1), 109–126.

Wolk, C.B., Kendall, P.C., & Beidas, R.S. (2015). Cognitive-behavioral therapy for child anxiety confers long-term protection from suicidality. *Journal of the American Academy of Child and Adolescent Psychiatry, 54*(3), 175–179. doi:http://dx.doi.org/10.1016/j.jaac.2014.12.004

Wolpe, J. (1973). *The practice of behavior therapy* (2nd edn.). New York: Pergamon Press.

Yonkers, K.A., Dyck, I.R., & Keller, M.B. (2001). An eight-year longitudinal comparison of clinical course and characteristics of social phobia among men and women. *Psychiatric Services, 52*(5), 637–643.

2 Evidence-Based Assessment

Andres De Los Reyes and Bridget A. Makol

Evidence-Based Assessment

In order to deliver sound services to the children and adolescents in their care and monitor the progress of these services, mental health professionals require sound tools for quantifying and classifying the thoughts, emotions, and behaviors of children and adolescents (hereafter collectively referred to as "youth" unless otherwise specified). As others have noted (Silverman & Ollendick, 2005), assessment is the bedrock of service delivery. As with the research initiatives developed to identify evidence-based treatments (e.g., Chambless & Ollendick, 2001), it is incumbent on mental health professionals to leverage the considerable force and rigor of empiricism to guide identification, selection, and use of evidence-based assessments (Hunsley & Mash, 2007). These principles can be illustrated clearly in the research on evidence-based assessments for youth anxiety. This chapter begins with a discussion of conceptual models of anxiety that guide evidence-based assessment. Next, we delineate key considerations when selecting instruments. We use these considerations as the foundation for highlighting a select set of instruments for use in clinical work and research. We conclude by highlighting important directions for future research. Throughout this chapter, we highlight approaches to assessing signs and symptoms of anxiety conditions that commonly manifest among youth; these include such conditions as generalized anxiety disorder (GAD), separation anxiety disorder (SepAD), social anxiety disorder (SocAD), and specific phobia (SP) (e.g., American Psychiatric Association [APA], 2013).

How Conceptual Models Inform Assessment

A key component of the evidence-based approach to assessing anxiety is the deep conceptual foundation upon which this approach rests. A thorough discussion of these anxiety concepts is beyond the scope of this chapter, and good descriptions of these concepts exist elsewhere (see Barlow, 2002; Silverman & Ollendick, 2005; Lang, 1968). Thus, we focus specifically on elements of anxiety conceptualizations that inform key factors we considered with regard to the evidence-based assessments we describe as follows. Four elements are particularly relevant to this chapter.

First, Barlow (2002) highlights several key elements germane to defining anxiety, and one that warrants discussion here is the idea that, as a "future-oriented emotion," the anxious response includes a heavy dose of maladaptive subjective perceptions about one's environment. In particular, among environments deemed as potentially aversive or distressful, increased anxiety goes hand-in-hand with perceiving the environment as unpredictable and uncontrollable, as well as with an increased focus or hypervigilance toward either potentially threatening events (e.g., objects, physical environments, animals, social situations), or bodily responses to these events. Thus, an evidence-based approach to assessing anxiety ought to include sound estimates of subjective experiences with anxiety.

Second, because anxiety is a future-oriented emotion, a key element of definitions of anxiety involves understanding the consequences or outcomes of these emotions. When anxiety becomes a maladaptive response to one's environment and/or internal states, individuals may take measures to cope with the aversive nature of this anxiety in an effort to minimize distress (Barlow, 2002; Silverman & Ollendick, 2005). These coping mechanisms most often take the form of avoidance behaviors (e.g., missing out on a party or social event, averting eye contact in one-on-one conversations) and persistent thought patterns or cognitions revolving around worry about anxiety. Consequently, the evidence-based approach to assessing anxiety also includes efforts to measure behavioral and cognitive manifestations of the anxious response.

Third, as mentioned previously, a key element of the anxiety response involves perceptions stemming from real or apparent threat in the environment. Indeed, even when the anxiety response stems from internal experiences, one also experiences emotional responses that arise from internal bodily mechanisms that allow for detections of imminent theat. Maladaptive versions of these "fears," which Barlow (2002) termed as "panic," involve the tipping off of the body's fight or flight response: physiological efforts to prepare for defense against environmental threats, or otherwise flee from such threats. An important note is that behavioral, cognitive, and physiological anxiety response systems "feed" off of each other; they do not exist in isolation of each other and the presence of activity in one response system may contribute to the development and maintenance of activity in another system. The result of the omnidirectional nature of this "triple response system" is that points of activity from each of these systems should factor prominently in evidence-based approaches to assessing anxiety (e.g., Barlow, 2002; Lang, 1968; Silverman & Ollendick, 2005).

Fourth, activity from the anxiety response systems should not be interpreted uniformly across development. That is, among youth some anxiety responses stem from normative changes in the environment within and across developmental periods (e.g., for young children, lengthy separations from caregivers while at school; for adolescents, efforts to develop romantic relationships). Through assessment we strive to detect maladaptive anxiety responses, identify youth in need of care, and/or determine whether the care delivered to them improves their mental health. Consequently, "best practices" in evidence-based approaches to assessing anxiety necessitate measurement of a youth's anxiety responses, with an eye toward interpreting these responses relative to what would be expected from someone within that youth's developmental level who displays normative or healthy behavior. In line with these best practices and wherever possible, we highlight components of anxiety measures that allow for developmental considerations. These components include use of developmental modifications for instruments originally developed for adults (e.g., Anxiety Disorders Interview Schedule for Children and Adolescents [ADIS]; Silverman, 1991), and use of standardized scores norm-referenced to an assessed youth's gender and school grade level (e.g., Revised Child Anxiety and Depression Scales [RCADS]; Chorpita, Moffitt, & Gray, 2000).

Considerations When Selecting Evidence-Based Assessments

Overall, conceptualizations of anxiety inform evidence-based assessments insofar as anxiety is seen as future-oriented and multifaceted. Further, for a few anxiety conditions (e.g., SocAD, SepAD), concerns stemming from these conditions may illustrate context-dependency, such as the "performance-only" specifier of the condition delineated in the latest version of the *Diagnostic and Statistical Manual of Mental Disorders* (*DSM-5*; APA, 2013) for SocAD. As such, we stipulate three considerations that drove our review of instruments for assessing anxiety among youth.

Modalities

A key component of evidence-based approaches to assessing anxiety is a logical extension of the anxiety conceptualizations described previously. Specifically, if anxiety consists of multiple constituent response systems, then by definition no single index of anxiety can meaningfully capture activity in all of these systems simultaneously (Hunsley & Mash, 2007). This necessitates an assessment approach that incorporates anxiety measurements from multiple modalities (e.g., surveys and checklists, clinical interviews, behavioral observations, measures of physiological functioning) that collectively tap into the three response systems described previously (Silverman & Ollendick, 2005). Granted, multimodal approaches introduce uncertainty in clinical decision-making and interpreting findings from research, as mental health professionals often observe low between-modality correspondence in estimates of anxiety and anxiety-related responses (e.g., Achenbach, 2017; De Los Reyes & Aldao, 2015). This low correspondence often translates into inconsistent findings in clinical assessments and in the outcomes of research studies (e.g., De Los Reyes et al., 2013; De Los Reyes & Kazdin, 2006). Nevertheless, researchers are beginning to build an evidence base for how to integrate data across modalities (for reviews, see De Los Reyes & Aldao, 2015; De Los Reyes et al., 2015b; De Los Reyes &

Ohannessian, 2016). Along these lines, we will be highlighting measures across multiple modalities relevant to assessing anxiety responses among youth.

Type of Clinical Decision

A core principle of evidence-based assessment is that psychometric support for scores taken from a measure is not fixed (Hunsley & Mash, 2007; Nunnally & Bernstein, 1994). One can infer that scores taken from a measure reliably and validly reflect a youth's level of anxiety when screening for clinically relevant anxiety concerns. Yet, that same inference may not be correctly applied to scores taken from the measure when it is used to monitor treatment response. Similarly, scores taken from a measure may evidence psychometric support via reports from one information source to a greater degree than the reports from other information sources (cf. criterion-related validity for adolescent vs. parent vs. teacher report; Achenbach & Rescorla, 2001; Deros et al., 2018; Rausch et al., 2017). In light of this variation in psychometric properties of scores taken from clinical measures, when applicable we highlight evidence-based assessments for anxiety based on the clinical decision(s) for which the assessments have been tested.

Availability

Researchers have long contended that there exists a large gap between the evidence base gathered for efficacious mental health interventions and the evidence base available for mental health assessments in routine clinical practices (Hunsley & Mash, 2007). An additional challenge is that like evidence-based treatments, there exists a large gap between the availability of evidence-based assessments and the use of these assessments in clinical practice settings (Jensen-Doss & Hawley, 2010). In fact, mental health professionals from different training backgrounds (e.g., psychiatrists, psychologists, social work) and care settings (e.g., private practice, school, inpatient, outpatient) may vary in the value they place on making specific clinical decisions (e.g., diagnoses), and they prefer some modalities over others to obtain clinical information (e.g., structured vs. unstructured interviews; Jensen-Doss & Hawley, 2011). Although many factors likely account for the research-practice gap in use of evidence-based assessments, researchers recently highlighted one set of pertinent factors that deal with the availability of evidence-based measures. By "availability" we refer to those measures highlighted by Beidas and colleagues (2015) as "free, easily accessible, and brief," where "brief" – using their criterion – means that the measure contains less than 50 items. In our review of measures that follows, we highlight those measures that meet the availability criteria used by Beidas and colleagues (2015). Of course, basing reviews of evidence-based measures solely on availability might limit lists of the measures we discuss. Thus, we also review recent psychometric work of well-established measures as identified by others in prior work (Silverman & Ollendick, 2005, 2008; Hunsley & Mash, 2011).

Modalities

Traditional Clinical Tools

Semi-Structured Interviews. Best practices for determining whether youth meet diagnostic criteria for anxiety disorders entail use of structured and semi-structured diagnostic interviews. Obtaining accurate diagnoses is important for treatment planning as it facilitates the appropriate selection of evidence-based treatments (Silverman & Ollendick, 2005) and is associated with better youth treatment engagement and outcomes (Jensen-Doss & Weisz, 2008). For anxiety disorders in particular, it is important to assess the specific disorders for which youth meet diagnostic criteria, in order to appropriately plan treatment targets and exposures. Further, given the high rates of co-occurring mental health problems among youth, diagnostic interviews comprise a key component of evidence-based assessment in that they can be used to screen for other disorders that commonly co-occur with anxiety and anxiety-related conditions, leading to a more complete and accurate assessment (Silverman & Ollendick, 2005).

There are several advantages to using structured and semi-structured diagnostic interviews. First, unlike unstructured clinical interviews, structured and semi-structured interviews include structured question prompts that increase the reliability and validity of mental health professionals' diagnoses (Jensen-Doss & Weisz, 2008). Second, in addition to obtaining categorical information about the presence or absence of diagnoses, structured and semi-structured interviews gather clinical information about severity, course, and functional impairment. Third, structured interviews, and to a lesser extent semi-structured interviews, can be administered with minimal interviewer training. However, these interviews are not without limitations. First, the interviews can be time-consuming to administer and score, making them less feasible for use in low-resourced mental health settings (Beidas et al., 2015). Second, for difficult-to-observe conditions (e.g., anxiety and mood disorders), others have noted that semi-structured interviews may yield relatively higher quality data than highly structured interviews. This is because, relative to structured interviews, responses to semi-structured interviews place greater weight on the clinical judgments of interviewers, who will likely have a greater sense of the conditions being assessed and their constituent symptoms than the interview respondent (e.g., parent or youth) (Klein, Dougherty, & Olino, 2005). Consistent with this notion, in this section we focus on the semi-structured diagnostic interviews available to assess and diagnose youth anxiety and anxiety-related conditions. We know of no published psychometric research on the *DSM-5* versions of the interviews reviewed as follows, and thus we review available evidence based on their *DSM-IV* versions.

Anxiety Disorders Interview Schedule for DSM-IV: Child and Parent Versions (ADIS-IV-C/P; Silverman & Albano, 1996). The ADIS-IV-C/P is the most widely used diagnostic interview for youth anxiety disorders and includes parallel parent and youth forms. The interview includes modules for *DSM-IV* anxiety and mood disorders, externalizing disorders including attention deficit/hyperactivity disorder (ADHD), and a screener for a wide range of other disorders (e.g., eating disorders). A diagnosis is obtained if the interviewer finds that data collected from at least one informant (i.e., parent or youth) indicates the presence of the disorder. For each diagnosis, the interviewer completes a clinician severity rating (CSR), which is used to identify the principal (i.e., most severe) diagnosis. The ADIS-IV-C/P (Silverman & Albano, 1996) demonstrates moderate to high test-retest reliability over 1–2 weeks for youth ($\kappa = .63–.80$), parent ($\kappa = .65–.88$), and combined ($\kappa = .81–.92$) anxiety diagnoses (Silverman, Saavedra, & Pina, 2001), and high inter-rater agreement for principal ($\kappa = .92$) and specific anxiety disorder diagnoses ($\kappa = .80–1.0$) (Lyneham, Abbott, & Rapee, 2007). In addition, the ADIS-4-C/P anxiety disorder modules exhibit concurrent validity with parent and youth reports on an established measure of anxiety (Wood et al., 2002). Reliability and validity estimates of a DSM-5 version of the ADIS have yet to be established.

Schedule for Affective Disorders and Schizophrenia for School-Age Children (K-SADS; Kaufman et al., 1997). The K-SADS is a diagnostic interview administered to parents and youth to assess 33 current and past *DSM-IV* (APA, 1994) disorders and impairments. Parents and youth are interviewed separately, and a diagnosis is obtained by integrating both informants' reports. There are three versions of the K-SADS, including the Present State (K-SADS-P IVR), Epidemiologic (K-SADS-E), and Present and Lifetime (K-SADS-PL) versions, all of which can be used to assess current disorders. In addition, the K-SADS-P IVR assesses for worst past year episodes and the K-SADS-E and K-SADS-PL assess for lifetime diagnoses. The K-SADS-P IVR is particularly useful for monitoring treatment response, as it is the only K-SADS version that assesses for both categorical diagnoses and dimensional measures of symptom severity. The K-SADS demonstrates moderate to high inter-rater (98 percent agreement) and test-retest ($\kappa = .60–.90$) reliability for current and lifetime anxiety disorder diagnoses (Ambrosi, 2000; Kaufman et al., 1997; Birmaher et al., 2009). The convergent and divergent validity of the K-SADS anxiety disorder modules are supported by the strength of association between anxiety disorder diagnoses and established measures of internalizing and externalizing problems, and diagnoses converge with those found using established structured and semi-structured diagnostic interviews (Birmaher et al., 2009). Further, compared to youth without a K-SADS anxiety disorder diagnosis, youth with a diagnosis obtain higher scores on an independent measure of anxiety symptom severity.

Mini International Neuropsychiatric Interview for Children and Adolescents (MINI-KID/MINI-KID-P; Sheehan et al., 1997). The MINI-KID is a relatively efficient diagnostic interview. The most current version assesses 24 *DSM-5* disorders, although as mentioned previously, psychometric evidence is only available for the *DSM-IV* version. The interview is designed to be administered to the parent and youth together, although it can be administered to adolescents individually. A version designed for administration to parents only (MINI-KID-P) is also available. For each MINI-KID module, all symptom and impairment questions are only administered if screener questions are endorsed. For anxiety disorders diagnoses, the interviewer only assesses for current diagnoses. The MINI-KID demonstrates high inter-rater ($\kappa = .88-1.00$) and test-retest ($\kappa = .69-.98$) reliability for any anxiety disorder diagnosis (Sheehan et al., 2010). In addition, the MINI-KID and MINI-KID-P demonstrate high levels of agreement for these diagnoses ($AUC = .73-.88$). Further, despite taking approximately a third of the time as the K-SADS, the MINI-KID shows moderate to high agreement with the K-SADS-PL for these same diagnoses ($AUC = .69-.94$), with the MINI-KID overall obtaining higher rates of diagnoses (Sheehan et al., 2010).

Rating Scales. A wide variety of rating scales are available for assessing youth anxiety. Rating scales can be used to assess anxiety dimensionally and provide valuable information about subthreshold symptoms that do not meet diagnostic criteria but are key pieces of information to gather within an evidence-based assessment. Thus, rating scales can serve a host of purposes including screening, treatment monitoring and/or treatment evaluation, or as supplements to corroborate data retrieved from other modalities including semi-structured interviews (Hunsley & Mash, 2007). Depending on the measure, a single score or multiple scores (e.g., subscales from a multidimensional measure) can be obtained from rating scales that indicates the level or magnitude of the component of anxiety being assessed. Rating scales can be administered to a variety of individuals who have opportunities to observe youths' thoughts and behaviors, including youths themselves, parents, teachers, and mental health professionals, and thus are an efficient method for obtaining multi-informant reports (Achenbach, 2017). It is important to note that because most rating scales do not assess for impairment caused by the symptoms they assess, they cannot be used solely to arrive at diagnoses. Relatedly, prior work indicates that within treatment studies of youth anxiety, researchers test for the efficacy of treatments using subjective measures of anxiety symptoms to a far greater extent than measures of other components of the anxiety response (e.g., behavior, cognition, physiology; Davis et al., 2011). Consistent with prior work, the rating scales that follow largely assess anxiety symptoms and fears.

Consistent with recent recommendations for promoting dissemination and implementation in clinical practice (Beidas et al., 2015), we place particular emphasis on freely available measures, as described previously. In addition, we provide updated research on rating scales deemed exemplary, based on previous reviews (Silverman & Ollendick, 2005, 2008). A summary of our review of rating scales can be found in Table 2.1.

Multidimensional Anxiety Scale for Children (MASC; March et al., 1997; March, Sullivan, & Parker, 1999; March, 2012). The MASC is a widely used self-report measure of anxiety symptoms that has several scales (and subscales) including: Physical Symptoms (Tense/Restless, Somatic/Autonomic), Harm Avoidance (Perfectionism, Anxious Coping), Social Anxiety (Humiliation/ Performing in Public), and Separation Anxiety. Among youth in clinical and nonclinical samples, moderate to high internal consistency is found for the MASC total ($\alpha = .89-.93$) and scale ($\alpha = .74-.91$) scores (Anderson et al., 2009; Baldwin & Dadds, 2007; Grills-Taquechel, Ollendick, & Fisak, 2008; March et

Table 2.1 *Rating Scales for Assessing Youth Anxiety*

Rating Scale	Items	Ages	Informant	Brief (<50 Items) and Freely Available	Symptoms Assessed
FSSC-R-SF	25	4–17	S/P	✓	Fears of failure and criticism, the unknown, animals, danger and death, medical affairs
MASC	39	8–19	S		Physical symptoms, harm avoidance, SocAD, SepAD,
PARS	50	6–17	MHP		SocAD, SepAD, GAD
PSWQ-C	16	7–17	S	✓	Worry
RCADS	47	6–18	S/P	✓	GAD, SepAD, SocAD, PD, OCD, MDD
RCMAS	37	6–19	S		Physiological arousal, worry/oversensitivity, concentration
SCARED/ SCARED-R	41	6–18	S/P	✓	GAD, PD, SepAD, SocAD, school phobia
SPAI-C	26	8–17	S/P		SocAD
SCAS	44	7–19	S/P	✓	GAD, PD/agoraphobia, SocAD, SepAD, OCD, physical injury fear
YAM-5	50	8–18	S/P		SepAD, SocAD, selective mutism, PD, GAD, specific phobias (animals, natural environment, blood-injection-injury, situational/agoraphobia, and other types)

Note. FSSC-R-SF = Short Form of the Fear Survey Schedule for Children–Revised (Muris et al., 2014); MASC = Multidimensional Anxiety Scale for Children (March et al., 1997; March, Sullivan, & Parker, 1999; March, 2012); PARS = Pediatric Anxiety Rating Scale (Research Units on Pediatric Psychopharmacology Anxiety Study Group); PSWQ-C = Penn State Worry Questionnaire for Children (Chorpita et al., 1997); RCADS = Revised Child Anxiety and Depression Scales (Chorpita et al., 2000); RCMAS = Revised Children's Manifest Anxiety Scale (Reynolds & Richmond, 1985); SCARED = Screen for Child Anxiety Related Emotional Disorders (Birmaher et al., 1997, 1999); SPAI-C = Social Phobia and Anxiety Inventory for Children (Beidel et al., 1995); SCAS = Spence Children's Anxiety Scale (Spence, 1998); YAM-5 = Youth Anxiety Measure for DSM-5 (Muris et al., 2017); S = Self; P = Parent; MHP = Mental Health Professional.

al., 1997). Further, moderate to high test-retest reliability is found for the MASC total ($ICC = .88$) and scale ($ICC = .76–.92$) scores over 3 weeks (March, Sullivan, & Parker, 1999). Supporting the MASC's convergent and divergent validity, the measure shows strong associations with established measures of anxiety and weaker associations with established measures of depression and ADHD (March et al., 1997; Wood et al., 2002; Anderson et al., 2009; Baldwin & Dadds, 2007). The MASC can discriminate between youth with and without an anxiety disorder diagnosis (March, Sullivan, & Parker, 1999; Grills-Taquechel, Ollendick, & Fisak, 2008), and Receiver Operating Characteristic (ROC) analyses have been conducted to determine the sensitivity and specificity of the

MASC total and scale scores (see Anderson et al., 2009; van Gastel & Ferdinand, 2008). However, mixed support has been found for the validity of the MASC as a screening tool (van Gastel & Ferdinand, 2008; Grills-Taquechel, Ollendick, & Fisak, 2008), and mental health professionals should avoid using the MASC alone to determine whether to further assess for anxiety disorders. However, the MASC is a useful tool for monitoring treatment response (Wood et al., 2006; Kendall et al., 2008). Further, although the MASC was originally developed as a self-report instrument, psychometric evidence supports use of a parent-report version of the measure (Baldwin & Dadds, 2007).

Revised Child Anxiety and Depression Scales Youth and Parent Versions (RCADS/RCADS-P; Chorpita et al., 2000). The RCADS/RCADS-P is a measure of anxiety and depressive symptoms that can be used for screening and diagnosing anxiety and anxiety-related conditions including GAD, SepAD, SocAD, panic disorder (PD), and major depressive disorder (MDD). Parent-report and youth self-report versions are available. In both clinical and school-based samples, the RCADS/RCADS-P demonstrates moderate to high internal consistency ($\alpha = .61–.84$) and test-retest reliability over 1 to 3 weeks ($r = .65–.93$) (Chorpita et al., 2000; Chorpita, Moffitt, & Gray, 2005; Ebesutani et al., 2010, 2011; Ebesutani, Tottenham, & Chorpita, 2015). The convergent and divergent validity of the RCADS/RCADS-P is supported by the strength of correlations between the RCADS/RCADS-P and established measures of anxiety, depression, and oppositional behaviors (Chorpita et al., 2000; Chorpita, Moffitt, & Gray, 2005; Ebesutani et al., 2010; 2011; Ebesutani, Tottenham, & Chorpita, 2015). Further, the measure can discriminate between youth with and without the disorders assessed in each subscale (Chorpita et al., 2000; Ebesutani et al., 2010). To obtain maximum sensitivity and specificity when using the RCADS/RCADS-P, ROC analyses have been conducted for each subscale (see Chorpita, Moffitt, & Gray, 2005; Ebesutani et al., 2010). The RCADS/RCADS-P is also sensitive to treatment response (Muris, Meesters, & van Melick, 2002b; Queen, Barlow, & Ehrenreich-May, 2014).

Revised Children's Manifest Anxiety Scale (RCMAS; Reynolds & Richmond, 1985). The RCMAS is a youth self-report measure of anxiety symptoms and includes subscales assessing physiological arousal, worry/oversensitivity, and social concerns/concentration. The measure includes a lie scale designed to identify the presence of social desirability biases. The RCMAS demonstrates moderate to high internal consistency for the total ($\alpha = .78–.89$) and subscale scores ($\alpha = .60–.79$), although most reliability evidence was found using community samples of youth (Reynolds & Richmond, 1985; Reynolds & Paget, 1983; Muris et al., 2002c; Varela & Biggs, 2006). In addition, RCMAS total and subscale scores show moderate to high test-retest reliability ($r = .64–.76$) (Reynolds & Richmond, 1985). Supporting the convergent and divergent validity of the RCMAS, the total and subscale scores exhibit strong associations with established measures of anxiety symptoms and moderate associations with an established measure of depressive symptoms (Lee et al., 1988; Muris et al., 2002c). Meta-analytic findings suggest that the RCMAS discriminates between clinically anxious and control youth when using the total score ($d = 1.30$) as well as physiological arousal ($d = 1.27$), worry/oversensitivity ($d = 1.10$), and social concerns/concentration ($d = 0.71$) subscales (Seligman et al., 2004). Further supporting the RCMAS's sensitivity to the effects of treatment, a large effect ($d = 0.80$) has been found for the RCMAS total score from pre- to posttreatment.

Screen for Child Anxiety Related Emotional Disorders/Screen for Child Anxiety Related Emotional Disorders-Revised (SCARED/SCARED-R; Birmaher et al., 1997, 1999; Muris et al., 1999). The SCARED is a youth- and parent-report measure of anxiety symptoms with subscales for GAD, PD, SepAD, SocAD, and school phobia, and the SCARED-R also includes subscales for specific phobias, obsessive-compulsive disorder (OCD), and post-traumatic stress disorder (PTSD). The measure is useful for screening for specific anxiety disorders and evaluating and monitoring treatment outcomes. Across informants and sample types, the SCARED/SCARED-R total and subscale scores demonstrate moderate to high internal consistency ($\alpha = .64–.94$) and test-retest reliability over 5 weeks ($\alpha = .70–.90$) (Birmaher et al., 1997; Muris et al., 1999; Muris, Schmidt, & Merckelbach, 2000; Muris et al., 2002c). The convergent and divergent validity of the SCARED/SCARED-R is supported by the strength of correlations between SCARED subscales and established measures of anxiety, depression, and externalizing problems (Birmaher et al., 1999; Muris et al., 2000, 2004). Further, evidence supports the measurement invariance of both parent and youth versions of the instrument (Dirks et al., 2014). Demonstrating discriminant validity, the SCARED/SCARED-R subscales distinguish between clinically anxious and depressed youth, as well as between specific anxiety disorders (Birmaher et al., 1997, 1999; Muris et al., 2000). The SCARED is sensitive to the effects of treatment (Cohen, Mannarino, & Iyengar, 2011).

Spence Children's Anxiety Scale for Children and Parents (SCAS/SCAS-P; Spence, 1998). The SCAS/SCAS-P is a youth- and parent-report measure of six domains of anxiety, including GAD, panic/agoraphobia, SocAD, SepAD, OCD, and physical injury fears. The measure includes six positive filler items designed to minimize response biases. When administered to youth and parents, the SCAS/SCAS-P total ($\alpha = .89–.92$) and subscale ($\alpha = .60–.80$) scores demonstrate moderate to high internal consistency (Spence, 1998; Spence, Barrett, & Turner, 2003; Nauta et al., 2004). However, SCAS/SCAS-P subscales demonstrate only low to moderate test-retest reliability over 4 to 6 months ($r = .45–.75$). Convergent and divergent validity is evidenced by the strength of correlations between the SCAS/SCAS-P and established measures of anxiety, depression, and externalizing problems (Spence, 1998; Spence et al., 2003; Nauta et al., 2004; Muris et al., 2000). The SCAS/SCAS-P total score can discriminate between clinically anxious youth and those without any mental health disorder, and the SepAD, SocAD, and OCD subscales can discriminate between youth with and without these primary diagnoses (Spence, 1998; Nauta et al., 2004). Finally, the SCAS/SCAS-P is sensitive to symptom change over the course of treatment (Hudson et al., 2009; Keehn, Lincoln, Brown, & Chavira, 2013).

Fear Survey Schedule for Children–Revised/Short Form of the Fear Survey Schedule for Children–Revised (FSSC-R /FSSC-R-SF; Ollendick, 1983; Muris, Ollendick, Roelofs, & Austin, 2014). The FSSC-R/FSSC-R-SF is a widely used youth- and parent-report measure of youth fears. The FSSC-R includes subscales for fears of the unknown, injury and small animals, danger and death, failure and criticism, and medical affairs, and the short-form version includes subscales for fears of failure and criticism, the unknown, animals, danger and death, and medical affairs. When administered to parents and youth, the FSSC-R/FSSC-R-SF demonstrates moderate to high internal consistency for the total ($\alpha = .87–.95$) and subscale ($\alpha = .63–.92$) scores (Ollendick, 1983; Muris et al., 2014; Weems et al., 1999). Further, the FSSC-R demonstrates high test-retest reliability over 1 week ($r = .82$) (Ollendick, 1983). Convergent and divergent validity is evidenced by the strength of correlations between the FSSC-R/FSSC-R-SF and established measures of anxiety and depression (Muris et al., 2002c; Muris et al., 2014). The measure can discriminate between youth with and without school phobia as well as the specific phobias assessed by the subscales (Ollendick, 1983; Weems et al., 1999; Last, Francis, & Strauss, 1989; Muris et al., 2014). The FSSC-R/ FSSC-R-SF is sensitive to treatment response (Kendall et al. 1997; Muris et al., 2014).

Penn State Worry Questionnaire for Children (PSWQ-C; Chorpita et al., 1997). The PSWQ-C is a freely available self-report measure of the frequency and controllability of worry that is useful for screening for anxiety disorders characterized by excessive worry, particularly GAD. In clinical and community samples of youth, the PSWQ-C demonstrates high internal consistency ($\alpha = .89$) and test-retest reliability over 1 week ($r = .92$) (Chorpita et al., 1997; Pestle, Chorpita, & Schiffman, 2008). Convergent and divergent validity is evidenced by the strength of correlations between the PSWQ-C and established measures of anxiety, depression, and social desirability (Chorpita et al., 1997; Muris, Meesters, & Gobel, 2001; Pestle et al., 2008). In addition, the PSWQ-C can discriminate between youth diagnosed with GAD or any anxiety disorder with youth not meeting diagnostic criteria for any mental health disorder, as well as youth with an anxiety or mood disorder (Chorpita et al., 1997; Pestle et al., 2008). The PSWQ-C is sensitive to treatment response (Muris, Meesters, & Gobel, 2002a).

Social Phobia and Anxiety Inventory for Children (SPAI-C/SPAI-C-P; Beidel, Turner, & Morris, 1995). The SPAI-C/SPAI-C-P is a measure of somatic, cognitive, and behavioral symptoms of SocAD and can be administered to parents or youth. The measure exhibits high internal consistency ($\alpha = .93–.95$), and test-retest reliability over 2 weeks ($r = .86$) (Beidel, Turner, & Morris, 1995; Higa et al., 2006). Supporting the SPAI-C/SPAI-C-P's convergent and divergent validity, the measure is strongly associated with established measures of social anxiety and social competence and moderately associated with measures of externalizing problems (Beidel, Turner, & Morris, 1995; Higa et al., 2006; Morris & Masia, 1998). The SPAI-C can discriminate between youth with SocAD, an externalizing disorder, and no disorder (Beidel, Turner, & Morris, 1995; Beidel, Turner, & Fink, 1996; Beidel et al., 2000).

Finally, the SPAI-C/SPAI-C-P is sensitive to treatment response (Masia-Warner et al., 2007; Spence et al., 2017).

Recently Developed Rating Scales with Emerging Psychometric Data. Beyond the rating scales described previously, we found it useful to highlight recently developed rating scales that have yet to acquire sufficient psychometric data but nonetheless may hold promise for assessing youth anxiety concerns.

Pediatric Anxiety Rating Scale (PARS; Research Units on Pediatric Psychopharmacology Anxiety Study Group, 2002). The PARS is a clinician-rated measure of the severity of common anxiety disorder symptoms (i.e., SocAD, SepAD, GAD) and is administered to both youth and parent(s). The PARS can be used to assess seven dimensions of symptom severity including number of symptoms, physical symptoms, symptom frequency, severity of distress, avoidance, interference at home, and interference outside of the home. The measure's developers recommend summing all subscales except the number of symptoms and physical symptoms subscales to obtain a total severity score. The PARS exhibits moderate internal consistency for subscale scores ($\alpha = .64 - .91$) and moderate to high inter-rater reliability for the total severity and subscale scores ($ICC = .78 - .97$) (Research Units on Pediatric Psychopharmacology Anxiety Study Group, 2002; Ginsburg et al., 2011). However, the PARS exhibits low to moderate test-retest reliability over 3 weeks for the total severity ($ICC = .55$) and subscale scores ($ICC = .35 - .59$). (Research Units on Pediatric Psychopharmacology Anxiety Study Group, 2002). Supporting the PARS's convergent and divergent validity, the measure shows strong associations with established measures of anxiety symptoms and severity, and weaker associations with established measures of depression and externalizing problems (Research Units on Pediatric Psychopharmacology Anxiety Study Group, 2002; Ginsburg et al., 2011). The PARS can be used to discriminate between clinically anxious and non-anxious youth, and ROC analyses suggest that 11.5 is an optimal 5-item total severity score for differentiating between these two groups (Ginsburg et al., 2011). Signal detection analyses using a 6-item version of the PARS revealed that a reduction of 35 to 50 percent in PARS scores is associated with symptom remission (see Caporino et al., 2013). The PARS is sensitive to treatment response (Walkup et al., 2008; Lebowitz et al., 2014).

Youth Anxiety Measure for DSM-5 (YAM-5; Muris et al., 2017). The YAM-5 is a youth- and parent-report measure of anxiety disorder symptoms with two major scales (and subscales): anxiety disorders (i.e., SepAD, SocAD, selective mutism, PD, GAD) and specific phobias (i.e., animals, natural environment, blood-injection-injury, situational/agoraphobia, and other types). In clinical and community samples of youth and their parents, the YAM-5 exhibits moderate to high internal consistency for the scale and most subscale scores for anxiety disorders ($\alpha = .76 - .92$) and phobias ($\alpha = .53 - .89$), with the exception of subscale scores for selective mutism ($\alpha = .41 - .64$), animal phobia ($\alpha = .47 - .67$), situational type/agoraphobia ($\alpha = .35 - .72$), and other phobias ($\alpha = .41 - .72$), which demonstrate a range from low to moderate internal consistency depending on the sample employed (Muris et al., 2017; Muris, Mannens, Peters, & Meesters, in press). The measure exhibits moderate to high test-retest reliability over 1 month for the scale and subscale scores for anxiety disorders ($r = .78–.86$) and specific phobias ($r = .73–.89$), with the exception of the selective mutism subscale ($r = .54$) (Simon et al., 2017). The convergent and divergent validity of the YAM-5 is supported by the strength of correlations between the YAM-5 anxiety disorders and specific phobias scores and measures of trait anxiety, specific phobias, depression, and internalizing and externalizing problems (Muris et al., 2017; Muris et al., in press; Simon et al., 2017). The YAM-5 anxiety disorders scale can discriminate between youth with and without an anxiety disorder, although the specific phobia subscales cannot (Muris et al., 2017).

Behavioral Observations. Measures that fall under this modality include ratings of observed behaviors across various situations, and these contexts can range from highly unstructured to structured. Behavioral observations can provide useful clinical information about the presence and frequency of maladaptive anxiety-related behaviors, as well as the precipitating events and consequences of these behaviors. After gathering information about these patterns of youth behaviors and their contextual determinants, mental health professionals can generate hypotheses about how to change youth behaviors, particularly those that maintain anxiety (e.g., avoidance of feared situations). Mental health professionals often gather this information during the clinical interview process by asking questions about the presence of avoidance behaviors (e.g., school absenteeism), precipitants to behaviors (e.g., nausea), and resulting functional impairments (e.g., academic difficulties). Given that naturalistic observations (e.g., school observations) of youth can prove challenging to obtain, laboratory-based tasks and tasks involving role-play scenarios (e.g., giving a speech, interacting with a stranger) are most common. Behavioral observations address some limitations of structured interviews and ratings scales, such as social desirability biases that might impact the extent to which youth self-report their anxiety symptoms (for a review, see De Los Reyes et al., 2015b).

There are a number of behavioral observation tasks available to assess youth anxiety and anxiety-related conditions, and an even greater number of coding schemes. Providing an exhaustive list of tasks and coding schemes is beyond the scope of this chapter. For that reason, we will discuss a few examples of behavioral observation paradigms that can be used in evidence-based assessment of youth anxiety. Beyond the following review, we recommend reading Vasey and Lonigan's (2000) review for further information about behavioral observation tasks and their applications.

Behavioral Assessment Tests (BATs). In BATs, youth are exposed to anxiety-provoking situations. The extent to which a youth approaches, avoids, or engages in other anxiety-relevant behaviors (e.g., use of coping self-statements) is rated by youth themselves, or a trained observer such as a mental health professional (e.g., clinical interviewer) or another independent observer (e.g., research personnel). In many cases, these tasks are audiotaped or videotaped and later coded. Many BATs are completed in a set amount of time during which youth participate in a highly structured and contrived situation (i.e., so as to facilitate comparisons between youths or a single youth across multiple time points) and are instructed to behave as they normally would in such situations. These tasks reliably produce behaviors in youth that can be easily and consistently coded by independent raters (Vasey & Lonigan, 2000). In addition, BATs can be adapted for a wide range of anxieties and fears (e.g., dogs, school), and thus can be used to assess most anxiety disorders. However, it is important to note that BATs can be difficult to implement in clinical practice given that they require time, an appropriate confederate (e.g., appearing close in age to the youth being assessed), training, and a coding scheme.

When assessing SocAD, BATs are often used to gain information about youths' social anxiety symptoms and social skills. For example, Mesa, Beidel, and Bunnell (2014) administered two BATs to adolescents with SocAD and nonclinical controls. In their impromptu speech task, adolescents spoke for a minimum of 3 minutes and a maximum of 10 minutes about various topics in front of four audience members. The impromptu speech task assessed anxiety and behavioral avoidance while public speaking, and independent coders reliably rated the adolescents' speaking latency, duration of speaking, escape behaviors, and number of topics discussed (ICCs greater than or equal to .98). In their 10-minute social interaction task (SIT), adolescents interacted with a confederate using standardized question prompts while playing a video game. This task assessed social skills, and independent coders reliably rated the adolescents' speaking latency, time to spontaneous verbalization, and number of comments and questions (ICCs greater than or equal to .94). Supporting the discriminant validity of these BATs, adolescents with SocAD exhibited greater speech latency and less speech during the impromptu speech task and required more speech prompts to initiate interactions during the SIT than non-socially anxious adolescents. Further, adolescents with SocAD reported greater subjective distress and exhibited greater physiological arousal (i.e., skin conductance) during these tasks. Changes in behaviors during observation tasks such as these can also be used to evaluate changes in social anxiety symptoms and social skills from pre- to posttreatment for youth with SocAD (Beidel, Turner, Young, & Paulson, 2005; Herbert et al., 2009).

Emerging Technologies

Measures of Cardiovascular Physiology. An exciting area of research focuses on developing paradigms for incorporating cardiovascular physiology into assessments of youth anxiety (De Los Reyes & Aldao, 2015; Youngstrom & De Los Reyes, 2015). A key component of clinical anxiety is heightened physiological arousal (e.g., racing heart, perspiration, difficulty breathing) that is difficult for youth to regulate when anticipating or being exposed to anxiety-provoking situations (e.g., public speaking). The most commonly assessed metrics of cardiovascular physiology that are relevant to youth anxiety include heart rate (HR), heart rate variability (HRV), vagal tone, and blood pressure (for review, see Thomas, Aldao, & De Los Reyes, 2012). The metric selected depends on the purpose of the assessment, as each measure of cardiovascular physiology can provide unique, although correlated, information about anxiety relevant physiological functioning. Physiological symptoms of anxiety are most commonly assessed using subjective measures (e.g., youth self-reports), whereas more objective measures (e.g., HR monitors) are rarely used (Thomas et al., 2012). However, it is important to note that subjective and objective measures of physiological arousal do not go hand-in-hand. For example, socially anxious adolescents show a tendency to report stable and high levels of physiological arousal throughout a social stressor task despite objective physiological measures indicating task habituation (Anderson & Hope, 2009). Thus, subjective and objective measures of physiology are both important components in evidence-based assessment of youth anxiety, with neither alone providing a comprehensive picture of physiological functioning.

A key barrier to the increased use of measures of cardiovascular physiology in the assessment of youth anxiety is the lack of physiological expertise (i.e., scoring and interpreting physiological data) among mental health professionals in routine clinical settings. Increased use of cardiovascular physiology in youth anxiety assessment thus depends on the development of easy-to-implement and interpretable tools that validly and reliably inform evidence-based assessment. Recent work demonstrates that low-cost and feasible methods can be used for collecting in-vivo cardiovascular physiology. In several recent studies, novice raters were able to use graphical depictions of HR data to obtain accurate and reliable interpretations of adolescent cardiovascular physiology (De Los Reyes et al., 2015a; 2017 et al; Dunn, Aldao, & De Los Reyes, 2015). For example, these graphical representations were used to accurately and reliably make judgments about whether adolescent HR was above clinical norms and identify contextual variation in HR across social stressors (i.e., baseline, speech preparation, speech delivery). These clinically feasible paradigms have important implications for clinical practice. In fact, we encourage future research on whether these paradigms provide mental health professionals with objective indicators of physiological symptoms of anxiety, as well as allow them to determine whether treatments meaningfully change these symptoms.

Measures of Neural Physiology. A second emerging technology has important implications for distinguishing anxiety disorders from often comorbid conditions, namely mood disorders. Indeed, in addition to distinguishing different anxiety conditions from each other (e.g., SocAD vs. GAD), mental health professionals and researchers often encounter difficulty with not only determining the presence of co-occurring mood disorders but also determining primary diagnoses for the purposes of treatment (e.g., should anxiety be targeted for treatment first relative to mood or vice versa?; American Psychiatric Association, 2013; Silverman & Ollendick, 2005). In work that leverages assessments of neural activity via event related potentials measured using the electroencephalogram (EEG/ERP), researchers find that increased anxiety tends to relate to increased activity in a brain component that responds to error commission (i.e., error-related negativity [ERN]; for a review, see Olvet & Hajcak, 2008). Conversely, increased depression tends to relate to decreased activity in a brain component that responds to exposure to rewarding stimuli (i.e., feedback negativity [FN]; Foti & Hajcak, 2009).

In recent work with youth, increased ERN activity uniquely related to increased anxiety when controlling for FN activity and depressive symptoms, whereas decreased FN activity uniquely related to increased depressive symptoms when controlling for ERN activity and anxiety symptoms (Bress, Meyer, & Hajcak, 2015). Granted, the road toward clinical use of EEG/ERP assessments still requires a great deal of additional study including establishing clinical norms for these assessments and demonstrating that they provide incrementally valuable information in clinical decision-making, over-and-above less costly and time-intensive tools (e.g., behavioral checklists and diagnostic interviews; Youngstrom & De Los Reyes, 2015). That being said, an interesting direction for future research may be to test whether use of ERN/FN data improves mental health professionals' accuracy rates in clinical decisions regarding differential diagnosis for anxiety and mood disorders (e.g., in predicting the decisions made by a diagnostic consensus team), or whether therapists' use of ERN/FN data facilitates treatment planning, and thus improves clinical outcomes. The clinical implications of ERN/FN data merit further study.

Concluding Comments

In this chapter, we provided an overview of evidence-based approaches to assessing youth anxiety. We briefly reviewed the conceptual models that inform evidence-based approaches to assessing these mental health problems. We also outlined important considerations for measure selection, and in doing so highlighted evidence-based tools across a host of modalities and clinical uses, with an eye toward the availability of these tools. In addition to reviewing evidence-based measures that leverage traditional modalities (e.g., semi-structured interviews, surveys, behavioral observations), we briefly reviewed emerging technologies that in the future may bring clinical practice and research closer toward integrating measures of the physiological components of anxiety, which historically have been underrepresented in both clinical practice and research (i.e., relative to rating scales of anxiety symptoms and direct measures of anxiety-related behaviors; Davis, May, & Whiting, 2011; De Los Reyes & Aldao, 2015). In so doing, we outlined important directions for future research. In particular, we encourage future research that seeks to improve the clinical feasibility of emerging technologies for assessing physiological processes relevant to anxiety.

References

Achenbach, T. M. (2017). Future directions for clinical research, services, and training: Evidence-based assessment across informants, cultures, and dimensional hierarchies. *Journal of Clinical Child and Adolescent Psychology, 46*, 159–169. doi: 10.1080/15374416.2016.1220315

Achenbach, T. M., & Rescorla, L. (2001). *Manual for the ASEBA school-age forms and profiles*. Burlington: University of Vermont Research Center for Children, Youth, and Families.

Ambrosini, P. J. (2000). Historical development and present status of the Schedule for Affective Disorders and Schizophrenia for School-Age Children (K-SADS). *Journal of the American Academy of Child & Adolescent Psychiatry, 39*, 49–58. doi:10.1097/00004583-200001000-00016

American Psychiatric Association. (1994). *Diagnostic and statistical manual of mental disorders (DSM-IV)* (4th ed.). Washington, DC: Author.

American Psychiatric Association. (2013). *Diagnostic and statistical manual of mental disorders (DSM-5)* (5th ed.). Washington, DC: American Psychiatric Association.

Anderson, E. R., Jordan, J. A., Smith, A. J., & Inderbitzen-Nolan, H. M. (2009). An examination of the MASC social anxiety scale in a non-referred sample of adolescents. *Journal of Anxiety Disorders, 23*, 1098–1105.

Baldwin, J. S., & Dadds, M. R. (2007). Reliability and validity of parent and child versions of the Multidimensional Anxiety Scale for Children in community samples. *Journal of the American Academy of Child & Adolescent Psychiatry, 46*, 252–260.

Barlow, D. H. (2002). *Anxiety and its disorders: The nature and treatment of anxiety and panic* (2nd ed.). New York: Guilford.

Beidas, R. S., Stewart, R. E., Walsh, L., Lucas, S., Downey, M. M., Jackson, K., ... & Mandell, D. S. (2015). Free, brief, and validated: Standardized instruments for low-resource mental health settings. *Cognitive and Behavioral Practice, 22*, 5–19. doi:10.1016/j.cbpra.2014.02.002

Beidel, D. C. (1996). Assessment of childhood social phobia: Construct, convergent, and discriminative validity of the Social Phobia and Anxiety inventory for Children (SPAI–C). *Psychological Assessment, 8*, 235.

Beidel, D. C., Turner, S. M., Hamlin, K., & Morris, T. L. (2000). The Social Phobia and Anxiety Inventory for Children (SPAI–C): External and discriminative validity. *Behavior Therapy, 31*, 75–87. doi:10.1016/S0005-7894(00)80005-2

Beidel, D. C., Turner, S. M., & Morris, T. L. (1995). A new inventory to assess childhood social anxiety and phobia: The Social Phobia and Anxiety Inventory for Children. *Psychological Assessment, 7*, 73–79. doi:10.1037/1040-3590.7.1.73

Birmaher, B., Brent, D. A., Chiappetta, L., Bridge, J., Monga, S., & Baugher, M. (1999). Psychometric properties of the Screen for Child Anxiety Related Emotional Disorders (SCARED): A replication study. *Journal of the American Academy of Child & Adolescent Psychiatry, 38*, 1230–1236. doi:10.1097/00004583-199910000-00011

Birmaher, B., Ehmann, M., Axelson, D. A., Goldstein, B. I., Monk, K., Kalas, C., ... & Brent, D. A. (2009). Schedule for Affective Disorders and Schizophrenia for school-age children (K-SADS-PL) for the assessment of preschool children—A preliminary psychometric study. *Journal of Psychiatric Research, 43*, 680–686. doi:10.1016/j.jpsychires.2008.10.003

Birmaher, B., Khetarpal, S., Brent, D., Cully, M., Balach, L., Kaufman, J., & Neer, S. M. (1997). The Screen for Child Anxiety Related Emotional Disorders (SCARED): Scale construction and psychometric characteristics. *Journal of the American Academy of Child & Adolescent Psychiatry, 36*, 545–553. doi:10.1097/00004583-199704000-00018

Bress, J. N., Meyer, A., & Hajcak, G. (2015) Differentiating anxiety and depression in children and adolescents: Evidence from event-related brain potentials. *Journal of Clinical Child and Adolescent Psychology, 44*, 238–249. doi: 10.1080/15374416.2013.814544

Caporino, N. E., Brodman, D. M., Kendall, P. C., Albano, A. M., Sherrill, J., Piacentini, J., . . . & Rynn, M. (2013). Defining treatment response and remission in child anxiety: Signal detection analysis using the pediatric anxiety rating scale. *Journal of the American Academy of Child & Adolescent Psychiatry, 52*, 57–67. doi: 10.1016/j.jaac.2012.10.006

Chambless, D. L., & Ollendick, T. H. (2001). Empirically supported psychological interventions: Controversies and evidence. *Annual Review of Psychology, 52*, 685–716. doi: 10.1146/annurev.psych.52.1.685

Chorpita, B. F., Moffitt, C. E., Gray, J. A. (2005). Psychometric properties of the Revised Child Anxiety and Depression Scale in a clinical sample. *Behaviour Research and Therapy, 43*, 309–322. doi: 10.1016/j.brat.2004.02.004

Chorpita, B. F., Tracey, S. A., Brown, T. A., Collica, T. J., & Barlow, D. H. (1997). Assessment of worry in children and adolescents: An adaptation of the Penn State Worry Questionnaire. *Behaviour Research and Therapy, 35*, 569–581. doi:10.1016/S0005-7967(96)00116-7

Chorpita, B. F., Yim, L., Moffitt, C., Umemoto, L. A., & Francis, S. E. (2000). Assessment of symptoms of DSM-IV anxiety and depression in children: A Revised Child Anxiety and Depression Scale. *Behaviour Research and Therapy, 38*, 835–855.

Davis, T. E., May, A., & Whiting, S. E. (2011). Evidence-based treatment of anxiety and phobia in children and adolescents: Current status and effects on the emotional response. *Clinical Psychology Review, 31*, 592–602. doi: 10.1016/j.cpr.2011.01.001

De Los Reyes, A., & Aldao, A. (2015). Introduction to the special issue: Toward implementing physiological measures in clinical child and adolescent assessments. *Journal of Clinical Child and Adolescent Psychology, 44*, 221–237. doi: 10.1080/15374416.2014.891227

De Los Reyes, A., Aldao, A., Qasmieh, N., Dunn, E. J., Lipton, M. F., Hartman, C., Dougherty, L. R., Youngstrom, E. A., & Lerner, M. D. (2017). Graphical representations of adolescents' psychophysiological reactivity to social stressor tasks: Reliability and validity of the Chernoff Face approach and person-centered profiles for clinical use. *Psychological Assessment, 29*, 422–434. doi: 10.1037/pas0000354

De Los Reyes, A., Augenstein, T. M., & Aldao, A. (2017). Assessment issues in child and adolescent psychotherapy. In J. R. Weisz and A. E. Kazdin (eds.), *Evidence-based psychotherapies for children and adolescents* (3rd ed.) (pp. 537–554). New York: Guilford.

De Los Reyes, A., Augenstein, T. M., Aldao, A., Thomas, S. A., Daruwala, S. E., Kline, K., & Regan, T. (2015a). Implementing psychophysiology in clinical assessments of adolescent social anxiety: Use of rater judgments based on graphical representations of psychophysiology. *Journal of Clinical Child and Adolescent Psychology, 44*, 264–279. doi: 10.1080/15374416.2013.859080

De Los Reyes, A., Augenstein, T. M., Wang, M., Thomas, S. A., Drabick, D. A. G., Burgers, D., & Rabinowitz, J. (2015b). The validity of the multi-informant approach to assessing child and adolescent mental health. *Psychological Bulletin, 141*, 858–900. doi: 10.1037/a0038498

De Los Reyes, A., & Kazdin, A. E. (2006). Conceptualizing changes in behavior in intervention research: The range of possible changes model. *Psychological Review, 113*, 554–583. doi: 10.1037/0033-295X.113.3.554

De Los Reyes, A., & Ohannessian, C. M. (2016). Introduction to the special issue: Discrepancies in adolescent-parent perceptions of the family and adolescent adjustment. *Journal of Youth and Adolescence, 45*, 1957–1972. doi: 10.1007/s10964-016-0533-z

De Los Reyes, A., Thomas, S. A., Goodman, K. L., & Kundey, S. M. A. (2013). Principles underlying the use of multiple informants' reports. *Annual Review of Clinical Psychology, 9*, 123–149. doi:10.1146/annurev-clinpsy-050212-185617

Deros, D. E., Racz, S. J., Lipton, M. F., Augenstein, T. M., Karp, J. N., Keeley, L. M., ... De Los Reyes, A. (2018). Multi-informant assessments of adolescent social anxiety: Adding clarity by leveraging reports from unfamiliar peer confederates. *Behavior Therapy, 49*(1), 84–98. doi: 10.1016/j.beth.2017.05.001

Dirks, M. A., Weersing, V. R., Warnick, E., Gonzalez, A., Alton, M., Dauser, C., ... Woolston, J. (2014). Parent and youth report of youth anxiety: Evidence for measurement invariance. *Journal of Child Psychology and Psychiatry, 55*, 284–291. doi: 10.1111/jcpp.12159

Dunn, E. J., Aldao, A., & De Los Reyes, A. (2015). Implementing physiology in clinical assessments of adult social anxiety: A method for graphically representing physiological arousal to facilitate clinical decision-making. *Journal of Psychopathology and Behavioral Assessment, 37*, 587–596. doi: 10.1007/s10862-015-9481-2

Ebesutani, C., Bernstein, A., Nakamura, B. J., Chorpita, B. F., & Weisz, J. R. (2010). A psychometric analysis of the Revised Child Anxiety and Depression Scale – Parent Version in a clinical sample. *Journal of Abnormal Child Psychology, 38*, 249–260. doi:10.1007/s10802-009-9363-8

Ebesutani, C., Chorpita, B. F., Higa-McMillan, C. K., Nakamura, B. J., Regan, J., & Lynch, R. E. (2011). A psychometric analysis of the Revised Child Anxiety and Depression Scales – Parent Version in a school sample. *Journal of Abnormal Child Psychology, 39*, 173–185.

Ebesutani, C., Tottenham, N., & Chorpita, B. (2015). The Revised Child Anxiety and Depression Scale – Parent Version: Extended applicability and validity for use with younger youth and children with histories of early-life caregiver neglect. *Journal of Psychopathology and Behavioral Assessment, 37*, 705–718. doi:10.1007/s10862-015-9494-x

Foti, D., & Hajcak, G. (2009). Depression and reduced sensitivity to non-rewards versus rewards: Evidence from event-related potentials. *Biological Psychology, 81*, 1–8. doi:10.1016/j.biopsycho.2008.12.004

Ginsburg, G. S., Keeton, C. P., Drazdowski, T. K., & Riddle, M. A. (2011). The utility of clinicians ratings of anxiety using the Pediatric Anxiety Rating Scale (PARS). *Child & Youth Care Forum, 40*, 93–105. doi:10.1007/s10566-010-9125-3

Grills-Taquechel, A. E., Ollendick, T. H., & Fisak, B. (2008). Reexamination of the MASC factor structure and discriminant ability in a mixed clinical outpatient sample. *Depression and Anxiety, 25*(11), 942–950.

Herbert, J. D., Gaudiano, B. A., Rheingold, A. A., Moitra, E., Myers, V. H., Dalrymple, K. L., & Brandsma, L. L. (2009). Cognitive behavior therapy for generalized social anxiety disorder in adolescents: A randomized controlled trial. *Journal of Anxiety Disorders, 23*, 167–177. doi:10.1016/j.janxdis.2008.06.004

Higa, C. K., Fernandez, S. N., Nakamura, B. J., Chorpita, B. F., & Daleiden, E. L. (2006). Parental assessment of childhood social phobia: Psychometric properties of the Social Phobia and Anxiety Inventory for Children-Parent Report. *Journal of Clinical Child and Adolescent Psychology, 35*, 590–597. doi:10.1207/s15374424jccp3504_11

Hudson, J. L., Rapee, R. M., Deveney, C., Schniering, C. A., Lyneham, H. J., & Bovopoulos, N. (2009). Cognitive-behavioral treatment versus an active control for children and adolescents with anxiety disorders: A randomized trial. *Journal of the American Academy of Child & Adolescent Psychiatry, 48*, 533–544. doi:10.1097/CHI.0b013e31819c2401

Hunsley, J., & Mash, E. J. (2007). Evidence-based assessment. *Annual Review of Clinical Psychology, 3*, 29–51.

Hunsley, J., & Mash, E. J. (2011). Evidence-based assessment. In D. H. Barlow (ed.), *The Oxford handbook of clinical psychology* (pp. 76–97). New York: Oxford University Press.

Jensen-Doss, A., & Hawley, K.M. (2010). Understanding barriers to evidence-based assessment: Clinician attitudes toward standardized assessment tools. *Journal of Clinical Child and Adolescent Psychology, 39*, 885–896. doi:10.1080/15374416.2010.517169

Jensen-Doss, A., & Hawley, K.M. (2011). Understanding clinicians' diagnostic practices: Attitudes toward the utility of diagnosis and standardized diagnostic tools. *Administration and Policy in Mental Health and Mental Health Services Research, 38*, 476–485. doi: 10.1007/s10488-011-0334-3

Jensen-Doss, A., & Weisz, J. R. (2008). Diagnostic agreement predicts treatment process and outcomes in youth mental health clinics. *Journal of Consulting and Clinical Psychology, 76*, 711–722. doi:10.1037/0022-006X.76.5.711

Kaufman, J., Birmaher, B., Brent, D., & Rao, U. (1997). Schedule for Affective Disorders and Schizophrenia for School-Age Children-Present and Lifetime version (K-SADS-PL): Initial reliability and validity data. *Journal of the American Academy of Child & Adolescent Psychiatry, 36*, 980–988. doi:10.1097/00004583–199707000-00021

Kendall, P. C., Flannery-Schroeder, E., Panichelli-Mindel, S. M., Southam-Gerow, M., Henin, A., & Warman, M. (1997). Therapy for youths with anxiety disorders: A second randomized clinical trial. *Journal of Consulting and Clinical Psychology, 65*, 366–380. doi:10.1037/0022-006X.65.3.366

Kendall, P. C., Hudson, J. L., Gosch, E., Flannery-Schroeder, E., & Suveg, C. (2008). Cognitive-behavioral therapy for anxiety disordered youth: A randomized clinical trial evaluating child and family modalities. *Journal of Consulting and Clinical Psychology, 76*, 282–297.

Klein, D.N., Dougherty, L.R., & Olino, T.M. (2005). Toward guidelines for evidence-based assessment of depression in children and adolescents. *Journal of Clinical Child and Adolescent Psychology, 34*, 412–432. doi: 10.1207/s15374424jccp3403_3

Lang, P. J. (1968). Fear reduction and fear behavior. In J. Schlein (ed.), *Research in psychotherapy* (pp. 85–103). Washington, DC: American Psychological Association.

Last, C. G., Francis, G., & Strauss, C. C. (1989). Assessing fears in anxiety-disordered children with the Revised Fear Survey Schedule for Children (FSSC-R). *Journal of Clinical Child Psychology, 18*, 137–141. doi:10.1207/s15374424jccp1802_4

Lebowitz, E. R., Omer, H., Hermes, H., & Scahill, L. (2014). Parent training for childhood anxiety disorders: The SPACE program. *Cognitive and Behavioral Practice, 21*, 456–469. doi: 10.1016/j.cbpra.2013.10.004

Lee, S. W., Piersel, W. C., Friedlander, R., & Collamer, W. (1988). Concurrent validity of the Revised Children's Manifest Anxiety Scale (RCMAS) for adolescents. *Educational and Psychological Measurement, 48*, 429–433. doi:10.1177/0013164488482015

Lyneham, H. J., Abbott, M. J., & Rapee, R. M. (2007). Interrater reliability of the anxiety disorders interview schedule for DSM-IV: Child and parent version. *Journal of the American Academy of Child & Adolescent Psychiatry, 46*, 731–736. doi:

March, J. S. (2012). *Multidimensional Anxiety Scale for Children* (2nd ed.) Toronto, Canada: MultiHealth Systems.

March, J. S., Parker, J. D., Sullivan, K., Stallings, P., & Conners, C. K. (1997). The Multidimensional Anxiety Scale for Children (MASC): Factor structure, reliability, and validity. *Journal of the American Academy of Child & Adolescent Psychiatry, 36*, 554–565.

March, J. S., Sullivan, K., & Parker, J. (1999). Test-retest reliability of the Multidimensional Anxiety Scale for Children. *Journal of Anxiety Disorders, 13*, 349–358.

Masia-Warner, C., Fisher, P. H., Shrout, P. E., Rathor, S., & Klein, R. G. (2007). Treating adolescents with social anxiety disorder in school: An attention control trial. *Journal of Child Psychology and Psychiatry, 48*, 676–686. doi:10.1111/j.1469-7610.2007.01737.x

McNally Keehn, R. H., Lincoln, A. J., Brown, M. Z., & Chavira, D. A. (2013). The Coping Cat program for children with anxiety and autism spectrum disorder: A pilot randomized controlled trial. *Journal of Autism and Developmental Disorders, 43*, 57–67. doi:10.1007/s10803-012-1541-9

Mesa, F., Beidel, D. C., & Bunnell, B. E. (2014). An examination of psychopathology and daily impairment in adolescents with social anxiety disorder. *PloS One, 9*, e93668. doi:10.1371/journal.pone.0093668

Muris, P., Dreessen, L., Bögels, S., Weckx, M., & van Melick, M. (2004). A questionnaire for screening a broad range of DSM-defined anxiety disorder symptoms in clinically referred children and adolescents. *Journal of Child Psychology and Psychiatry, 45*, 813–820. doi:10.1111/j.1469-7610.2004.00274.x

Muris, P., Mannens, J., Peters, L., & Meesters, C. (2017). The Youth Anxiety Measure for DSM-5 (YAM-5): Correlations with anxiety, fear, and depression scales in non-clinical children. *Journal of Anxiety Disorders*. doi: 10.1016/j.janxdis.2017.06.001

Muris, P., Meesters, C., & Gobel, M. (2001). Reliability, validity, and normative data of the Penn State Worry Questionnaire in 8–12-yr-old children. *Journal of Behavior Therapy and Experimental Psychiatry, 32*, 63–72. doi:10.1016/S0005-7916(01)00022-2

Muris, P., Meesters, C., & Gobel, M. (2002a). Cognitive coping vs Emotional disclosure in the treatment of anxious children: A pilot-study. *Cognitive Behaviour Therapy, 31*, 59–67. doi: 10.1080/16506070252959490

Muris, P., Meesters, C., & van Melick, M. (2002b). Treatment of childhood anxiety disorders: A preliminary comparison between cognitive-behavioral group therapy and a psychological placebo intervention. *Journal of Behavior Therapy and Experimental Psychiatry, 33*, 143–158. doi:10.1016/S0005-7916(02)00025-3

Muris, P., Merckelbach, H., Ollendick, T., King, N., & Bogie, N. (2002c). Three traditional and three new childhood anxiety questionnaires: Their reliability and validity in a normal adolescent sample. *Behaviour Research and Therapy, 40*, 753–772. doi:10.1016/S0005-7967(01)00056-0

Muris, P., Merckelbach, H., Schmidt, H., & Mayer, B. (1999). The revised version of the Screen for Child Anxiety Related Emotional Disorders (SCARED-R): Factor structure in normal children. *Personality and Individual Differences, 26*, 99–112. doi:10.1016/S0191-8869(98)00130-5

Muris, P., Schmidt, H., & Merckelbach, H. (2000). Correlations among two self-report questionnaires for measuring DSM-defined anxiety disorder symptoms in children: The Screen for Child Anxiety Related Emotional Disorders and the Spence Children's Anxiety Scale. *Personality and Individual Differences, 28*, 333–346. doi:10.1016/S0191-8869(99)00102-6

Muris, P., Simon, E., Lijphart, H., Bos, A., Hale, W., & Schmeitz, K. (2017). The Youth Anxiety Measure for DSM-5 (YAM-5): Development and first psychometric evidence of a new scale for assessing anxiety disorders symptoms of children and adolescents. *Child Psychiatry & Human Development, 48*, 1–17. doi: 10.1007/s10578-016-0648-1

Nauta, M. H., Scholing, A., Rapee, R. M., Abbott, M., Spence, S. H., & Waters, A. (2004). A parent-report measure of children's anxiety: Psychometric properties and comparison with child-report in a clinic and normal sample. *Behaviour Research and Therapy, 42*, 813–839. doi:10.1016/S0005-7967(03)00200-6

Nunnally, J. C., & Bernstein, I. H. (1994). *Psychometric theory* (3rd ed.) New York: McGraw-Hill.

Ollendick, T. H. (1983). Reliability and validity of the Revised Fear Survey Schedule for Children (FSSC-R). *Behaviour Research and Therapy, 21*, 685–692. doi:10.1016/0005-7967(83)90087-6

Olvet, D. M., & Hajcak, G. (2008). The error-related negativity (ERN) and psychopathology: Toward an endophenotype. *Clinical Psychology Review, 28*, 1343–1354. doi:10.1016/j.cpr.2008.07.003

Pestle, S. L., Chorpita, B. F., & Schiffman, J. (2008). Psychometric properties of the Penn State Worry Questionnaire for Children in a large clinical sample. *Journal of Clinical Child and Adolescent Psychology, 37*, 465–471. doi:10.1080/15374410801955896

Queen, A. H., Barlow, D. H., & Ehrenreich-May, J. (2014). The trajectories of adolescent anxiety and depressive symptoms over the course of a transdiagnostic treatment. *Journal of Anxiety Disorders, 28*, 511–521. doi:10.1016/j.janxdis.2014.05.007

Rausch, E., Racz, S.J., Augenstein, T.M., Keeley, L., Lipton, M.F., Szollos, S., Riffle, J., Moriarity, D., Kromash, R., & De Los Reyes, A. (2017). A multi-informant approach to measuring depressive symptoms in clinical assessments of adolescent social anxiety using the Beck Depression Inventory-II: Convergent, incremental, and criterion-related validity. *Child and Youth Care Forum, 46*(5), 661–683. doi: 10.1007/s10566-017-9403-4

Research Units on Pediatric Psychopharmacology Anxiety Study Group. (2002). The Pediatric Anxiety Rating Scale (PARS): Development and psychometric properties. *Journal of the American Academy of Child & Adolescent Psychiatry, 41*, 1061–1069. doi:10.1097/00004583-200209000-00006

Reynolds, C. R., & Paget, K. D. (1983). National normative and reliability data for the revised Children's Manifest Anxiety Scale. *School Psychology Review, 12*, 324–336.

Reynolds, C. R., & Richmond, B. O. (1985). *Revised Children's Manifest Anxiety Scale: Manual.* Los Angeles: Western Psychological Services.

Seligman, L. D., Ollendick, T. H., Langley, A. K., & Baldacci, H. B. (2004). The utility of measures of child and adolescent anxiety: A meta-analytic review of the Revised Children's Anxiety Scale, the State-Trait Anxiety Inventory for Children, and the Child Behavior Checklist. *Journal of Clinical Child and Adolescent Psychology, 33*, 557–565. doi:10.1207/s15374424jccp3303_13

Sheehan, D., Lecrubier, Y., Sheehan, K. H., Janavs, J., Weiller, E., Keskiner, A., & . . . Dunbar, G. C. (1997). The validity of the Mini International Neuropsychiatric Interview (MINI) according to the SCID-P and its reliability. *European Psychiatry, 12*, 232–241. doi:10.1016/S0924-9338(97)83297-X

Sheehan, D. V., Sheehan, K. H., Shytle, R. D., Janavs, J., Bannon, Y., Rogers, J. E., . . . & Wilkinson, B. (2010). Reliability and validity of the Mini International Neuropsychiatric Interview for Children and Adolescents (MINI-KID). *The Journal of Clinical Psychiatry, 71*, 313–326. doi: 10.4088/JCP.09m05305whi

Silverman, W.K. (1991). *Anxiety disorders interview schedule for children.* Albany: Graywind.

Silverman, W.K., & Albano, A. (1996). *The Anxiety Disorders Interview Schedule for Children–IV (Child and Parent Versions).* San Antonio: Psychological Corporation/Graywind.

Silverman, W.K., & Ollendick, T.H. (2005). Evidence-based assessment of anxiety and its disorders in children and adolescents. *Journal of Clinical Child and Adolescent Psychology, 34*, 380–411. doi: 10.1207/s15374424jccp3403_2

Silverman, W. K., & Ollendick, T. H. (2008). Child and adolescent anxiety disorders. In J. Hunsley & E. J. Mash (eds.), *A guide to assessments that work* (pp. 181–206). New York: Oxford University Press.

Simon, E., Bos, A. E., Verboon, P., Smeekens, S., & Muris, P. (2017). Psychometric properties of the Youth Anxiety Measure for DSM-5 (YAM-5) in a community sample. *Personality and Individual Differences, 116*, 258–264. doi: 10.1016/j.paid.2017.04.058

Spence, S. H. (1998). A measure of anxiety symptoms among children. *Behaviour Research and Therapy, 36*, 545–566. doi:10.1016/S0005-7967(98)00034-5

Spence, S. H., Barrett, P. M., & Turner, C. M. (2003). Psychometric properties of the Spence Children's Anxiety Scale with young adolescents. *Journal of Anxiety Disorders, 17*, 605–625. doi:10.1016/S0887-6185(02)00236-0

Spence, S. H., Donovan, C. L., March, S., Kenardy, J. A., & Hearn, C. S. (2017). Generic versus disorder specific cognitive behavior therapy for social anxiety disorder in youth: A randomized controlled trial using internet delivery. *Behaviour Research and Therapy, 90*, 41–57.

Thomas, S. A., Aldao, A., & De Los Reyes, A. (2012). Implementing clinically feasible psychophysiological measures in evidence-based assessments of adolescent social anxiety. *Professional Psychology: Research and Practice, 43*, 510–519. doi:10.1037/a0029183

van Gastel, W., & Ferdinand, R. F. (2008). Screening capacity of the Multidimensional Anxiety Scale for Children (MASC) for DSM-IV anxiety disorders. *Depression and Anxiety, 25*, 1046–1052.

Varela, R. E., & Biggs, B. K. (2006). Reliability and validity of the Revised Children's Manifest Anxiety Scale (RCMAS) across samples of Mexican, Mexican American, and European American children: A preliminary investigation. *Anxiety,*

Stress & Coping: An International Journal, 19, 67–80. doi:10.1080/10615800500499727

Vasey, M. W., & Lonigan, C. J. (2000). Considering the clinical utility of performance-based measures of childhood anxiety. *Journal of Clinical Child Psychology, 29,* 493–508. doi: 10.1207/S15374424JCCP2904_4

Walkup, J. T., Albano, A. M., Piacentini, J., Birmaher, B., Compton, S. N., Sherrill, J. T., … & Iyengar, S. (2008). Cognitive behavioral therapy, sertraline, or a combination in childhood anxiety. *New England Journal of Medicine, 359,* 2753–2766. doi: 10.1056/NEJMoa0804633

Weems, C. F., Silverman, W. K., Saavedra, L. M., Pina, A. A., & Lumpkin, P. W. (1999). The discrimination of children's phobias using the Revised Fear Survey Schedule for Children. *Journal of Child Psychology and Psychiatry, 40,* 941–952. doi:10.1111/1469-7610.00511

Wood, J. J., Piacentini, J. C., Bergman, R. L., McCracken, J., & Barrios, V. (2002). Concurrent validity of the anxiety disorders section of the Anxiety Disorders Interview Schedule for DSM-IV: Child and parent versions. *Journal of Clinical Child and Adolescent Psychology, 31,* 335–342.

Wood, J. J., Piacentini, J. C., Southam-Gerow, M., Chu, B. C., & Sigman, M. (2006). Family cognitive behavioral therapy for child anxiety disorders. *Journal of the American Academy of Child & Adolescent Psychiatry, 45,* 314–321.

Youngstrom, E.A., & De Los Reyes, A. (2015). Commentary: Moving towards cost-effectiveness in using psychophysiological measures in clinical assessment: Validity, decision-making, and adding value. *Journal of Clinical Child and Adolescent Psychology, 44,* 352–361. doi: 10.1080/15374416.2014.913252

3 Self-Help Treatment of Childhood Anxiety Disorders

Lauren F. McLellan, Sally Fitzpatrick,
Carolyn Anne Schniering, and Ronald M. Rapee

Overview of the Issue – The Need for Innovation

Despite advances in the development of evidence-based interventions for child anxiety, dissemination and uptake of these interventions within the community remain suboptimal. The objective of this chapter is to examine innovative approaches in the use of self-help interventions for anxiety in children and adolescents. In particular, the evidence base for both bibliotherapy and computer-based interventions will be reviewed, with a focus on implications for clinicians in their own practice.

Cognitive behavioral therapy (CBT) is the recommended treatment for pediatric anxiety disorders (Bennett et al., 2016). However, up to 80 percent of children and adolescents do not receive any evidence-based treatment for their anxiety (Ebert et al., 2015; Pennant et al., 2015). Both person-centered and systemic factors have been identified as contributing to the poor uptake of treatment. Person-centered barriers that reduce participation in face-to-face treatment include a lack of symptom awareness or a lack of knowledge in identifying anxiety as a problem (March, Spence, & Donovan, 2009); reticence to seek help because of the perceived stigma associated with mental illness or discomfort discussing mental health problems (Gulliver, Griffiths, & Christensen, 2010); preference for self-help rather than seeking face-to-face treatment, particularly by adolescent populations (Gulliver, Griffiths, & Christensen, 2010); concerns about confidentiality (Spence et al., 2016); and a lack of time and loss of hours to participating in core therapeutic activities (Gulliver, Griffiths, & Christensen, 2010; Stallard et al., 2007). These challenges can be exacerbated by a range of systemic factors that contribute to the low engagement in traditional forms of therapy, such as high costs associated with face-to-face intervention (Ebert et al., 2015); lack of treatment availability or long wait-lists (Gulliver, Griffiths, & Christensen, 2010; Stallard et al., 2007); and the limited number and availability of trained CBT therapists (Gunter & Whittal, 2010; Stallard et al., 2007).

Self-help treatments such as bibliotherapy and the computerization of psychological interventions may address obstacles associated with attending traditional forms of therapy, as well as having the added benefit of relieving the burden on health care services (Jorm & Griffiths, 2006). Positive outcomes arising from self-help treatments for young people and their families include (Calear & Christensen, 2010; Ebert et al., 2015; Spence at el., 2016):

- ability to reach a larger and more diverse clientele across a wider geographic area;
- potentially reduced or negligible waiting lists (depending on the level of therapist involvement required);
- accessibility at any time and place provides greater convenience;
- anonymity / increased privacy for clients;
- reduced stigma associated with meeting a mental health professional in person;
- flexibility in self-direction and self-pacing results in greater user autonomy;
- the appeal of interactivity and visual attractiveness of internet-based programs for young people.

These benefits are further strengthened by the eagerness of young people to interact with their world via online modalities (Spence et al., 2016). Self-help interventions that use internet or mobile applications appear to be an acceptable method of intervention to young people and an effective way of engaging them in mental health treatments, and therefore have the potential to treat more children and young people than face-to-face forms of therapy (Spence et al., 2016). Current research is focused on understanding the extent to which these forms of therapies are efficacious and produce long-term improvements in the reduction of anxiety in children and adolescents. Overall, the research evidence suggests that bibliotherapy and computerized therapy programs are a useful adjunct to the range of services available for anxious young people.

Description of the Approach to Innovation

Traditionally, CBT has been delivered in person to individuals or groups by trained therapists. However, the highly structured nature of CBT, ease of manualization, and time-limited approach fostered the development of CBT self-help programs for children and adolescents. Self-help programs vary as to the type of self-help modality used (bibliotherapy compared to online), the level of guidance provided to children by their parents, and the extent to which therapist support is provided in implementing the program.

Historically, attempts to disseminate programs to a wider audience resulted in the development of self-help programs in which individuals address issues of concern with the assistance of video materials, audiotapes, or computerized programs (Rapee, Abbott, & Lyneham, 2006). The most widely developed form of self-help delivery has been through bibliotherapy, which provides written material to participants and instructions on how to practice skill development. More recently, the self-help content delivered in bibliotherapy programs has been adapted to an online environment. Initially, this involved the delivery of information on CD-ROM and videos. These programs did not require internet connection and therapist support was provided via telephone. Technological advances in recent years have seen CD-ROM programs give way to the development of internet-based therapy programs. Internet-delivered CBT involves the integration of information technology and psychological treatment (Vigerland et al., 2016). Online programs are delivered through treatment modules that may provide written texts, audio and video files, and interactive online features that enable participants to receive feedback and answers to questions.

Online therapy programs for adults have been shown to be as effective as face-to-face CBT programs for anxiety disorders (Spence et al., 2016). Vigerland and colleagues (2016) argue that while the evidence base for online therapy programs for children is increasing, the generalizability of findings from adult studies to pediatric populations is influenced by important developmental and practical differences. Content delivered through either bibliotherapy or online contexts must be appropriate to the developmental level of the child and take into account their cognitive ability as well as their reading and comprehension levels. In addition, outcomes may be influenced by the extent to which parents and children differ in their willingness to participate and their motivation for change.

Outcomes in bibliotherapy and online programs may also vary in the extent to which youth receive support in implementing the program. For younger children, most bibliotherapy and online self-help programs typically involve parents leading their children through the CBT program and guiding implementation of the CBT skills in day-to-day life. Benefits of guided parent-delivered CBT include less therapist contact, fewer resources than standard forms of CBT, and the capacity to be used in stepped-care models of intervention (Thirlwall, Cooper, & Creswell, 2017). In comparison, research suggests that adolescents require less guidance by parents or therapists in completing self-help programs and practicing skills on a daily basis (Spence et al., 2016).

Evidence Base for Self-Help Interventions for Anxiety

This chapter will focus on evaluating the evidence for self-help cognitive behavioral treatments for youth anxiety that are primarily, although not exclusively, delivered by written (e.g., book) or technological (e.g., CD-ROM or internet) mediums rather than by a therapist. An intervention is included in our summary if most of the program could be completed without direct presentation by, or discussion with, a therapist. Of course, this does not mean that therapists have no involvement, and most of the interventions described here include some degree of therapist input. In some cases, this is quite extensive. The interventions have been grouped into two broad categories: those where clinical delivery takes place via written material (bibliotherapy) and those where clinical delivery takes place using technology (e.g., CD-ROM, computer-assisted program, or internet). Programs with *some* therapist contact, whether in-person or using technology (e.g., feedback on electronic worksheets, email, telephone, or videoconferencing), were considered self-help in this chapter because the therapist contact was not the primary source for delivering the intervention. Furthermore, we focus on cognitive behavioral interventions because of their existing evidence base for treating youth anxiety, and review treatment research where participants initially met criteria for an anxiety disorder rather than subclinical symptoms or where interventions were aimed at prevention of anxiety.

Bibliotherapy

Research evaluating the efficacy of reading material for the treatment of childhood anxiety has somewhat understandably focused on material delivered to parents when treating children. Yet, interestingly, no research has evaluated the outcomes of printed material delivered directly to adolescents. Interventions with minimal therapist contact for teenagers have utilized technology, and these will be reviewed later in the chapter.

The first evaluation of parent-delivered self-help for child anxiety was published by Rapee and colleagues in 2006 (Rapee, Abbott, & Lyneham, 2006). This randomized controlled trial of 267 6- to 12-year-olds (60 percent male) with a DSM-IV anxiety disorder (generalized anxiety disorder (GAD), social anxiety disorder (SoAD), separation anxiety disorder (SAD), specific phobia (SPEC), obsessive-compulsive disorder (OCD), and panic disorder (PD)) found that providing parents with the self-help book *Helping Your Anxious Child* (HYAC; Rapee et al., 2000) led to almost 20 percent higher diagnostic remission (26 percent) than wait-list (7 percent), but less than completing a face-to-face family CBT group program (61 percent). Results were not always consistent for self-report, parent-report, or therapist symptom measures. Indeed, bibliotherapy at times demonstrated similar effects to both group CBT and wait-list, depending on the symptoms measured and/or whether the analysis involved intent-to-treatment or completer analyses only.

The self-help book HYAC provides information about and practical implementation strategies for CBT skills that children and parents can use to manage youth anxiety. In the trial, HYAC was accompanied by a child workbook with activities for parents and children to complete together. Interestingly, there was no therapist contact in this initial investigation of bibliotherapy for childhood anxiety and it remains the only study of pure self-help for youth anxiety.

In an effort to investigate methods to enhance outcomes of parent-led bibliotherapy for childhood anxiety, various types of therapist contact were provided along with the HYAC book in a second randomized trial (Lyneham & Rapee, 2006). Parents of 100 6- to 12-year-old children (51 percent male) with a primary DSM-IV anxiety disorder (i.e., GAD, SoAD, SAD, SPEC, OCD, and PD) from rural and remote communities in Australia were randomized to wait-list or one of three treatment conditions. The treatment material (bibliotherapy, HYAC) was identical in all three treatment conditions. Across the conditions, however, parents were allocated to receive either nine brief phone calls from a therapist, nine emails from a therapist, or they could contact a therapist as many times as they liked via phone or email during the 12-week treatment period (client-initiated contact). Results indicated that remission of primary anxiety disorder (and all anxiety disorders) was significantly greater when parents received consistent therapist phone support in addition to the parent self-help book (90 percent remission of primary anxiety disorder), compared with either of the other two conditions (respectively, 42 percent and 39 percent in the email and the client-initiated contact conditions). In this study all active treatments performed better than wait-list (1 percent remission), and similar results were found for child- and parent-reported symptom measures, as well as clinician severity rating scales.

These positive outcomes suggested that bibliotherapy, especially when supported by some therapist involvement, is a promising method to improve access to treatment. Some additional research has indicated that print-based interventions with therapist support can provide effects that are similar to those shown by face-to-face therapist-delivered interventions for DSM-IV anxiety disorders, although sample sizes in these studies were relatively small (Cobham, 2012; Leong et al., 2009). In the main outcome trial, Cobham (2012) randomly allocated 55 anxious children aged 7–14 years to three conditions: wait-list, face-to-face therapy, and bibliotherapy. Somewhat surprisingly, 95 percent of children in the bibliotherapy condition were free of all anxiety diagnoses immediately following treatment, and this figure was not significantly different to that in traditional treatment (78 percent), while both did better than a wait-list control condition (0 percent). A demonstration of the application of bibliotherapy to primary care settings was shown in a study comparing face-to-face therapy and therapist-supported, parent-led CBT for child anxiety (specifically, GAD, SoAD, SAD, SPEC, and OCD; Chavira et al., 2014). Although there was some suggestion that face-to-face therapy was superior (83 percent remission) to therapist-supported bibliotherapy (71 percent remission), the difference did not reach statistical significance with the relatively small sample ($N = 48$). Finally, in the largest study to date, data from a trial of stepped care for child anxiety were reanalyzed to allow comparison between self-help (mostly parent-led bibliotherapy, $N = 139$, primary diagnoses of DSM-5 anxiety disorders: SAD, SoAD, GAD, SPEC, other) and traditional, face-to-face treatment with a therapist ($N = 142$; Rapee et al., 2017). Immediately following treatment, 49 percent of children in the self-help condition were free of all anxiety disorders, which was significantly lower than the percentage of full remission in the traditional therapy group (66 percent). The key value of self-help though lay in its ease of delivery. Although it led to slightly less remission, delivery of self-help took 20 percent of the time that therapists required to deliver the traditional treatment.

Recent research has begun to evaluate the optimal amount of therapist guidance required for child-anxiety bibliotherapy. In a large sample ($N = 194$) of children with GAD, SoAD, SAD, SPEC, or PD/agoraphobia, Thirlwall and colleagues (2013) compared the same 8-session parent-guided self-help resource (*Overcoming Your Child's Fears and Worries: A Self-Help Guide Using Cognitive Behavioural Techniques* by Creswell and Willetts, 2007) with either weekly or fortnightly guidance. Weekly guidance involved four face-to-face sessions and four 20-minute phone sessions, whereas fortnightly guidance involved two face-to-face and two 20-minute phone sessions. Primary diagnostic remission and symptom improvement were superior to wait-list (25 percent) for the weekly guidance group (50 percent) but not for the fortnightly guidance group (39 percent). However, at 6-month follow-up both conditions showed continued and similar remission (76 percent vs. 71 percent).

Interestingly, guidance in this study involved some face-to-face sessions, limiting some of the advantages of self-help treatments, such as the utility of the intervention among populations unable to easily attend in-person sessions with therapists. Furthermore, this study excluded children whose parents had their own anxiety diagnosis or other serious mental health conditions. It is possible that therapist-led programs or heavily therapist-supported self-help may be required when parents meet criteria for their own psychopathology. However, further research is necessary in order to empirically evaluate this contention.

While most research on bibliotherapy for youth anxiety has targeted a range of common anxiety disorders within transdiagnostic intervention, a small amount of research has investigated disorder-specific programs. Results from case studies, for example, Lewis et al. (2015), indicate that disorder-specific bibliotherapy can also lead to reductions in the relevant disorder. Whether a focused, disorder-specific intervention will lead to larger effects than more generic, "transdiagnostic" interventions remains to be seen.

Overall, a small number of randomized controlled trials have evaluated bibliotherapy for children and none have investigated this treatment delivery method for adolescents. Among the small body of literature in children, bibliotherapy appears to be a promising treatment delivery method. That being said, the varying methodologies between studies make it difficult to draw firm conclusions about the amount and type of therapist guidance that would optimize treatment response. Future large-scale studies will be required to address this issue. Similarly, the impact of parent psychopathology needs to be more comprehensively evaluated in future bibliotherapy studies, particularly when minimal therapist guidance is provided.

Technology-Based Approaches

The initial attempts to evaluate the use of computer-based technology to deliver CBT for childhood anxiety relied on high levels of therapist involvement. For example, Spence et al. (2006) evaluated computer-augmented therapy against traditional face-to-face treatment and wait-list among 7- to 14-year-old anxious youth ($N = 72$, primary disorders of GAD, SoAD, SAD, and SPEC). Internet treatment involved five online sessions for the child and three for the parents, with an additional five child and three parent group sessions conducted face-to-face in the clinic. Face-to-face treatment involved 10 group sessions with children and six group sessions with parents (plus two booster sessions at 1 month and 3 months posttreatment). Not surprisingly, posttreatment remission was similar in the internet (52 percent) and traditional (59 percent) conditions and both were better than wait-list (13 percent).

A similar study by Khanna and Kendall (2010) compared computer-assisted therapy with traditional face-to-face treatment and a computer-assisted education support (i.e., placebo control) condition with 49 7- to 13-year-old children. Computer-assisted treatment included six child sessions and two parent sessions assisted by a therapist in addition to six child sessions spent independently on the computer. Traditional face-to-face treatment included 12 50-minute individual sessions of manualized CBT, while computer-assisted education support involved 12

50-minute sessions with 30 minutes of therapist contact and 20 minutes of time playing games on the computer. The computer-assisted intervention resulted in posttreatment remission of the primary disorder among 70 percent of children, which was not significantly different from those receiving traditional face-to-face intervention (81 percent), and both were better than the placebo control (19 percent).

Interestingly, both these studies indicated that computer-assisted therapy could produce outcomes of similar magnitude to traditional face-to-face therapy. However, both studies suffered two important limitations to address this question. First, both computer-assisted therapies included considerable contact with a therapist. The computer-assisted condition in Spence et al. (2006), in particular, involved a considerable component of traditional face-to-face therapy for which children had to attend the clinic. Second, both studies involved relatively small samples, leading to very low power by which to compare two active treatments. The sample size of the study by Khanna and Kendall (2010) was especially small with only around 15 participants per condition.

In an effort to reduce the resources required to deliver effective therapy, some research has begun to explore treatment provided by means of computer-based technology with minimal assistance from a therapist. Case studies in children and adolescents (Cunningham et al., 2008; Spence et al., 2008) provided early evidence for the potential benefits of CD-ROM (Cunningham et al., 2008; Cool Teens) and web-based (Spence et al., 2008; BRAVE for Teens) interventions with only minimal therapist support. Cunningham and colleagues provided five adolescents (14–16 years, four with GAD and one with SAD) with a 12-week (8-module) CBT-based CD-ROM, which they accompanied with brief biweekly calls from a therapist. After 3 months, 40 percent of the adolescents no longer met criteria for their primary disorder. Spence and colleagues (2008) reported outcomes from one child with primary SAD (10 years) and one adolescent with primary SoAD (17 years) who completed an online CBT program comprising 10 sessions with five additional sessions for parents, supported by weekly emails from therapists and two phone calls to the parents and child/adolescent. The online program also sent automated emails prior to and after each online session. Results suggested reliable change for the adolescent on most symptom measures and remission of all anxiety disorders (as well as dysthymia) at posttreatment. For the child, remission of anxiety disorders occurred by 6-month follow-up but not immediately following treatment and reliable change was observed on parent- but not child-reported symptoms of anxiety and internalizing.

A growing number of randomized controlled trials have now been conducted evaluating computer-based CBT programs for children and adolescents with various anxiety disorders. Using a sample of 43 14- to 17-year-old adolescents (GAD, SoAD, SAD, SPEC, OCD, PD), Wuthrich and colleagues (2012) compared an 8-module CD-ROM (Cool Teens) supported by brief (on average 16 minutes) weekly therapist calls to the teens and three to the parents against a wait-list. Following treatment there was significantly greater remission of the DSM-IV primary anxiety disorder (41 percent) among treated adolescents than among those on wait-list (0 percent). Similar differences were reported on all other measures reported by both the teenagers and their parents. Spence and colleagues (2011) evaluated the BRAVE for Teens web-based program comprising modules for both the adolescents and their parents, which was supported by weekly therapist emails and a single therapist support call. This internet program with minimal therapist support was compared to a traditional 10-session clinic program and a wait-list in a population of 115 anxious adolescents. Teens who demonstrated "moderate" or "severe" levels of depression were excluded. Treatment (regardless of delivery) resulted in greater remission of the primary disorder (GAD, SoAD, SAD, or SPEC; online = 34 percent; traditional = 30 percent) compared to wait-list (4 percent). Continuous measures showed slightly mixed outcomes, although most revealed larger effects for the two treatment conditions relative to wait-list. Overall, research evaluating technology-based self-help (with minimal therapist assistance) for adolescents is promising. The optimal extent of therapist assistance and the need to include parents still require further research in large randomized controlled trials.

Research on technology-based self-help CBT programs for children has found less consistent results. March, Spence, and Donovan (2009) tested the efficacy of their BRAVE online program by randomizing 73 7- to 12-year-old anxious children (with primary GAD, SoAD, SAD, or SPEC) to either immediate treatment or wait-list. Similar to the teen version, the program involved 10 1-hour online lessons for children and six 1-hour lessons for parents, accompanied by weekly emails from a therapist to review homework, two therapist support calls with parents and children, and automated emails prior to and after the availability of each lesson. The online treatment group (self-help with minimal therapist guidance) failed to show significantly greater remission of their primary disorder (30 percent) than wait-list (10 percent). However, greater improvement of active treatment over wait-list was demonstrated on clinician-rated measures of severity as well as parent- but not child-rated symptoms of anxiety.

Similar results were found by Vigerland and colleagues (2016) among 93 8- to 12-year-old anxious children (with primary GAD, SoAD, SAD, SPEC, or PD) who were randomized to receive immediate treatment or wait-list. Participants were excluded if they showed high depression (defined as a score of 20 or more on the Child Depression Inventory (CDI; Kovacs, 1985), or when the primary caretakers themselves reported "serious psychiatric disorders" or reported issues related to child risk or parent substance abuse. Treatment involved an 11-module web-based CBT program for Swedish children with anxiety (BarnInternetprojektet, BiP). Seven modules were delivered to parents and four to children. Modules were accompanied by three telephone calls from a therapist (at the beginning, middle, and end of treatment) and written feedback by therapists on worksheets and participant questions lodged onto the web-based platform. Although calls were infrequent, no information was provided about the length of calls or the time therapists spent providing feedback on platform worksheets or queries. Following treatment there was no significant difference in primary diagnostic remission between treatment (20 percent) and wait-list (7 percent) conditions. However, internet treatment did show stronger efficacy than wait-list according to clinician-rated disorder severity and overall functioning and parent-rated (but not child-rated) symptoms of anxiety. As with the adolescent technology-based self-help literature, more research is needed to understand the impact of depression comorbidity and parental psychopathology on outcomes, especially when interventions involve minimal therapist guidance.

One self-help program for preschool-aged children with anxiety disorders (GAD, SoAD, SAD, or SPEC) has also recently been evaluated. Donovan and March (2014) utilized online parent modules taken from the BRAVE online program for older children accompanied by a booklet containing age appropriate examples and explanations for preschool-aged children. This modified program was compared against wait-list among 52 children aged 3 to 6 years who had clinical anxiety disorders. There was no significant difference in remission between the active intervention (39 percent primary diagnosis and 35 percent all diagnoses) and wait-list (26 percent primary diagnosis and 26 percent all diagnoses), but children in the immediate treatment group showed greater reductions than those on wait-list in symptoms of anxiety and clinician-rated disorder severity. One other study holds some relevance to the current review. Morgan and colleagues (2017) developed an online version of the Cool Little Kids early intervention program (Rapee, Lau, & Kennedy, 2010) that involved 8 modules aimed directly at parents. Therapist involvement was minimal, comprising only automated emails and the availability of telephone support if requested. Preschool-aged children were included on the basis of anxiety risk due to high temperamental inhibition and hence this study is not directly relevant to the current review since the presence of anxiety disorders was not formally assessed prior to the intervention. However, the children had high levels of pretreatment anxiety symptoms and the majority probably met criteria for a disorder. Following intervention, significantly fewer children in the active intervention met criteria for an anxiety disorder (40 percent) than those on wait-list (54 percent). Parents in active treatment also reported that their children had fewer symptoms of anxiety and less life interference than those on wait-list.

While most research on technology-based self-help programs for anxiety has delivered broad-based anxiety programs (i.e., programs targeting a range of common anxiety disorders in the same intervention), a small amount of research has investigated disorder-specific programs. A CBT intervention for children with specific phobia (8–12 years) was evaluated in a small ($N = 30$) open trial using the previously described Swedish BiP web-based self-help program with minimal therapist guidance (Vigerland et al., 2013). Results at posttreatment indicated reductions in clinician-rated severity, remission of specific phobia (35 percent), and improvements in symptoms on parent and child reports. Furthermore, improvements were maintained at 3-month follow-up. However, the lack of a control group and randomization make it difficult to reach firm conclusions from this study. Finally, only one study to date has compared disorder-specific intervention against transdiagnostic treatment for young people aged 8–17 years with social anxiety disorder (Spence et al., 2017). The SAD-specific online intervention produced similar outcomes (13 percent remission) to a broad-based anxiety program, BRAVE Online (described previously) (15 percent remission), immediately following treatment, but both were significantly better than wait-list (3 percent remission). At 6-month follow-up, both conditions continued to show improvements (although limited) and did not differ significantly (specific – 30 percent; generic – 35 percent). Further research using larger randomized trials is required to determine whether disorder-specific self-help interventions might lead to larger effects than transdiagnostic or generic self-help programs.

The empirical evidence for technology-based self-help programs for children and adolescents with anxiety is not extensive. Among this small body of literature, variation in the type and extent of therapist involvement and crucial differences in participant inclusion limit the ability to draw firm conclusions. Most studies also include relatively small samples and there has been almost no comparison against placebo. Overall outcomes can at best be described as "promising." There is some hint that programs aimed at adolescents may provide more consistent benefits than those aimed at children, although the number of studies is still too few to draw firm conclusions. It is possible that the technology-based interventions provide a more appealing delivery method for this often difficult to engage group of anxious youth. Research with anxious children has shown treatment benefits on clinician-reported outcomes, but effects on symptom measures have been less consistent, especially when looking at children's reports. Surprisingly, few significant benefits have been demonstrated on the critical measure of diagnostic remission. Larger studies with longer-term follow-ups will allow empirical evaluation of the impact of child severity and parent psychopathology as potential moderators or predictors of self-help treatments for child anxiety. Studies evaluating technology-delivered interventions without therapist support are required. This is a yet-unanswered empirical question that has the potential to further improve access to, and cost-effectiveness of, self-help interventions for anxiety in young people.

Predictors of Change

Predictors of response to treatment have hardly been examined within trials of self-help for anxious youth since studies in this area to date have been focused on simply establishing the efficacy of these interventions. One of the logical potential predictors is age. Given the increased requirements for motivation and maturity within self-help, it may be expected that adolescents will manage self-help better than children (Spence et al., 2008). However, in reality, so-called "self-help" for children often follows a "parent as therapist" model (e. g., Rapee et al., 2006), whereas adolescents are expected to contribute more directly to their own progress (e.g., Wuthrich et al., 2012). Hence, it is more likely that children will respond more extensively to self-help than adolescents, because this form of intervention with children benefits from an external motivational agent (the parent). Empirically, such comparisons have not been made. The only empirical examination of the impact of age on outcomes in bibliotherapy evaluated results from a trial restricted to children aged 7–12 years (Thirlwall, Cooper, & Creswell, 2017). Within this restricted range there was no significant impact of age overall on outcome. However, younger children were more likely to be free of their primary diagnosis at posttreatment whereas older children showed a more favorable outcome at 6-month follow-up. The lack of significant impact of age on overall outcome in this study agrees with the results of a meta-analysis evaluating outcomes from internet programs for youth anxiety in which age was not identified as a significant predictor of differential efficacy between studies (Vigerland et al., 2016).

The reanalysis by Thirlwall, Cooper, & Creswell (2017) also examined the impact of other predictors. The only other significant predictor of outcome was primary diagnosis – there was no prediction from primary diagnosis to overall outcome, however, children with a primary diagnosis of GAD had better outcomes at post-treatment, but worse outcomes at 6-month follow-up. No other variables, including child gender or comorbidity, significantly predicted outcomes.

Finally, a recent analysis of online delivery of early intervention for inhibited preschool children showed that treatment outcome was uniquely predicted by participants' (parents') access to a printer (Morgan, Rapee, Salim, & Bayer, 2018). In turn, printer access predicted frequency of practice of skills taught in the program (a potential mediator). Aside from this one indication, at present we have little understanding of factors that might mediate self-help interventions and especially those that specifically mediate self-help relative to more generic treatment processes.

We have reached the stage where the basic efficacy of self-help interventions, both via printed materials and online, has now been established. Therefore, the field should now be ready to start to evaluate both the predictors of outcome and its potential underlying mechanisms. What will be particularly interesting will be to try and distinguish predictors and mechanisms of response to treatment that are general to all treatments for anxious youth from those factors that are specifically relevant to self-help delivery.

Clinical Case Illustration

Amelia is a 14-year-old girl who presented to the Centre for Emotional Health, Macquarie University, Sydney. She had a history of anxiety during childhood and, when she entered high school, she was overwhelmed by the new range of socially challenging situations. She felt like an "outcast," had few friends, and ate her meals alone. She was too scared to ask teachers for help and was worried about doing or saying the wrong thing and embarrassing herself. Amelia also "daydreamed" and found it hard to concentrate on her work. She began to fall behind in her grades and became increasingly isolated. Amelia experienced escalating distress, sometimes taking up to three hours to get ready for school due to perfectionism with her hair and make-up and she was having difficulty keeping up with daily tasks. Increasingly, her severe anxiety and a range of somatic problems such as stomachaches and headaches led to absences from school. As the year continued, Amelia experienced periods of depressed mood, poor self-esteem, and decreased interest in activities she previously enjoyed. Amelia's mother was unable to enforce regular school attendance. On days when Amelia did attend, she often would stay only an hour or two before calling her mother to collect her. Eventually, Amelia's distress and avoidance became so severe

```
                  Amelia's symptoms of anxiety and depression.
        40
        30
        20
        10
         0
              Pre treatment        Post treatment      6-month follow-up
                  ——  Spence Children's Anxiety Scale (Spence, 1998)
                  ——  Short Moods and Feelings Qre (Angold et al 1995)
```

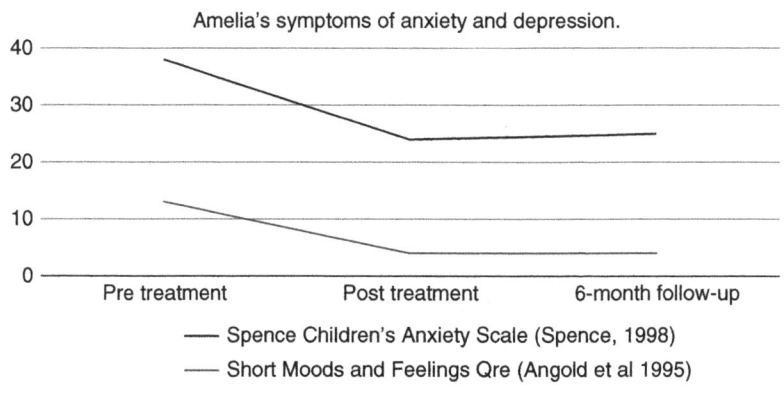

Figure 3.1 *Amelia's Symptoms of Anxiety and Depression*

that the school counselor recommended that she commence distance education. Her parents then contacted our clinic for an assessment.

A telephone-based diagnostic assessment, separately with Amelia and her mother, highlighted avoidance of a range of social and public situations including crowds, shopping centers, public transport, starting or joining conversations, and going to school. When she did attend school, she was quiet and failed to answer questions in class, didn't ask teachers for help, and spent the majority of time alone. These behaviors were underpinned by some extreme beliefs such as believing that others saw her as "stupid," having a "mental issue," or as being "different." The interview also picked up a wide range of worries including concerns about school performance, peer relationships, and family health. Amelia was quite perfectionistic, and her mother described how she often got "stuck" for long periods due to her fears of making a mistake. Aside from these fears, Amelia reported feeling sad most of the time, feeling worthless and guilty, and having "no energy." In sum, the information from her interview suggested that Amelia met criteria for social anxiety disorder (SoAD) as her principal diagnosis, in addition to generalized anxiety disorder (GAD) and persistent depressive disorder (PDD). Amelia had recently been prescribed an antidepressant by a psychiatrist; however, she had discontinued medication due to side effects. There was no evidence of suicide risk, and Amelia had a supportive family. Questionnaire data on symptoms were consistent with her interview responses (see Figure 3.1).

Amelia's family lived in a rural town with minimal access to mental health services. The family also could not afford to pay for lengthy psychological treatment. As a result, Amelia received treatment remotely via an online program for comorbid anxiety and depression in adolescents (i.e., *Chilled Plus Online*; Schniering et al., 2017). The program consists of eight modules, which are completed online over eight weeks, and each module is accompanied by a 30-minute therapist phone call. Parents receive a printed workbook and three 30-minute phone calls, as well as phone updates throughout. The content covered in each module is shown in

Table 3.1 *Overview of* Chilled Plus Online *modules*

Module	Content
1	Understanding Anxiety and Depression
2	Motivation, Goals and Increasing Enjoyment
3	Stepladders 1: Building Goal-Directed Action and Overcoming Avoidance
4	Stepladders 2 and Managing Emotions
5	Realistic Thinking and Stepladders
6	Positive Coping and Stepladders
7	Building Relationships and Stepladders
8	Review, Relapse and Maintenance

Table 3.1. More detail on the program components and the way in which we worked with Amelia follows.

Engagement and Motivation

A common problem for treatment is noncompletion of modules and lack of between-session practice. Strategies that have been employed with success in our program to address this problem include building strong rapport, persistence in phoning the client until contact is made, working with ambivalence as a mental state to be explored, and finding a small aspect of the problem to work on using graded steps. Throughout the program attention is paid to addressing the cycle of low motivation and avoidance drawing on motivational interviewing and behavioral activation principles. Adolescents develop goals that are related to their personal values, and they are taught to work with motivation as a fluctuating state of mind and to focus on boosting self-confidence with behavioral action. Weekly phone calls as well as text messages serve as cues for action and, where the youth agrees, parents are recruited to assist in providing increased structure for activities and rewards for change.

Initial sessions with Amelia focused on establishing rapport, developing appropriate expectations for the program and her role in it, and creating goals for change. During the first phone session, it became clear that Amelia had not completed module 1 online. As a result, sections of the module were completed with Amelia over the phone and she was asked to finish both modules 1 and 2 before the next phone session. At the second phone call, Amelia still had not completed either module. The therapist again completed some of module 2 with her and spent the remainder of the session discussing barriers to completion of modules and how she might overcome those. Avoidance was a key maintaining factor for Amelia and she was having difficulty breaking this pattern of avoidant coping in treatment. Amelia set goals for the program as follows: a) "I want to feel more relaxed and confident," and b) "I want to be able to engage in situations that I am avoiding, in particular social situations." Time was spent with her mother brainstorming strategies to facilitate the completion of modules, including rewards for effort and providing support. At this point it was decided to allow an extra week between the phone sessions for modules 2 and 3 to allow Amelia to complete the online content for the first three modules. At the phone call for module 3, Amelia had made good progress and had finished all online material and commenced practice around pleasant events. Motivational strategies as described previously were employed at every session thereafter in order to consolidate gains and to facilitate continued behavioral action.

Building Goal-Directed Action and Reducing Avoidance

Graded hierarchies are used throughout the program to build goal-directed action in situations that are avoided due to anxiety (e.g., not asking a question in class) as well as situations that are avoided due to low mood (e.g., withdrawal from friends). The development of goal-directed action progressed steadily over modules 3 to 8, and Amelia completed various hierarchies on social situations, including visiting public places such as restaurants and shopping centers, and using public transport. Stepladders also included more detailed social behaviors such as making telephone calls, speaking to her distance education teachers, engaging in online chat, and starting conversations with staff in stores. Hierarchies targeting situations related to low mood included developing increased social contact and friendships, and engaging in new interests and sport, such as drawing, music, and dance. At the completion of the main program, Amelia was far less avoidant in her schoolwork by speaking to teachers on the telephone, asking for help, attending face-to-face workshops with other students, and initiating online contact with students in her grade. All hierarchies were closely aligned with her personal program goals.

Managing Negative Emotion and Cognition

In the program, skills for managing negative emotion and cognition are covered transdiagnostically, such that they can be used to address components of both anxiety and depression. Emotion regulation skills in treatment include emotion awareness, the development of greater distress tolerance by having healthy beliefs around emotion, practicing staying with an emotion until it passes, and refocusing attention to the task at hand ("emotion surfing"). Amelia stated that the skill of emotion surfing (especially learning to accept moderate increases in negative emotions while maintaining her focus on whatever task she was doing) "changed her life" and that she used this daily as a means of coping with periods of low mood or stress. Realistic thinking skills are also taught in therapy to challenge both worried and negative thoughts, using a set of structured steps where adolescents look for "evidence" in order to challenge their thoughts and develop an alternative more realistic thought. Amelia was able to successfully challenge worries around schoolwork, and in particular, worked with her therapist to challenge several beliefs underlying her low self-esteem.

Building Relationships, Pleasant Events, and Positive Coping

Throughout treatment, depressive mood is targeted via activities that bring pleasure or mastery, by enhancing relationship skills and interpersonal connectedness, and via daily self-care (e.g., rest, diet, exercise). For Amelia, enjoyable activities were commenced in module 2, and continued throughout. Amelia used art as a method of self-expression and would often do pencil drawings as a means of riding her feelings out until they passed. Amelia needed help to improve her interpersonal skills in order to initiate new friendships. Following skill development, increased social contact assisted in boosting her mood, and at the conclusion of the program she had regular contact with two old friends with whom she had reconnected. Attention was also paid to sleep patterns as Amelia was going to bed at 1am and sleeping until nearly midday, and we worked with Amelia and her mother to establish more regular sleeping patterns using worry reduction and stimulus control principles.

Comorbidity and Treatment

As with other adolescents with comorbid presentations, one of the challenges we faced with Amelia was deciding how to treat her complex array of problems given the constraints of an 8-week program. One way in which we were able to address multiple problems concurrently was by targeting core common processes underpinning anxiety and depression, namely behavioral avoidance and difficulty managing negative thoughts and feelings. In addition, the focus on motivation and engagement throughout was essential to therapeutic outcomes. Given the 8-week time frame of therapy, we were able to address social anxiety and depressed mood; however, less therapy time was spent treating symptoms of generalized anxiety. While there was some generalization of treatment effects across disorders, Amelia would have likely benefited from additional therapy time targeting additional symptoms of generalized anxiety disorder.

Posttreatment Outcomes

Amelia rated all program modules and media components positively. She reported that she "loved working with us" and that "things were really getting better." Levels of avoidance had reduced markedly, and her mood had improved extensively. She reported having much greater energy and motivation to pursue positive activities. Measures of therapeutic alliance indicated a strong relationship with the therapist, and Amelia responded well to therapist guidance on exposure tasks. In the final phone call she stated, "I can't thank you enough" and "I never would have been able to come this far without you." Formal assessment information supported these impressions. At the end of treatment Amelia no longer met criteria for her pretreatment diagnoses of social anxiety disorder, generalized anxiety disorder, and persistent depressive disorder, although some symptoms of anxiety remained (see Figure 3.1).

In summary, this case illustrates the potential efficacy of a brief online intervention for comorbid anxiety and depression in youth. The program is currently in the final stages of evaluation and preliminary results indicate good efficacy (Schniering et al., 2016). This case has also demonstrated some of the benefits of an online format over traditional approaches in terms of increased accessibility and acceptability for a population that can be difficult to engage and retain in treatment. In line with the literature in the field, the case also illustrates the value of therapist involvement, even for this self-help intervention. Given the lack of engagement with the program early on, and the need for therapist intervention to boost initial uptake, it seems unlikely that Amelia would have achieved the outcomes seen here in the absence of therapist assistance.

Challenges and Future Development

The development and evaluation of self-help interventions for anxious youth, especially those involving newer technologies, have grown exponentially in a very short time. There is little doubt that this field will continue to move ahead at a great rate and that many of the existing questions will be addressed in the coming years. Compared to only a few years ago, we are already in a position where anxious young people in many parts of the world can easily access empirically validated treatments from the comfort of their own homes. As we have seen in the preceding review, the growing evidence base suggests that these self-help interventions can lead to marked reductions in anxiety, close to those seen in traditional face-to-face programs. At present, most of the available programs rely on some therapist involvement and in many cases, this is quite extensive. Evidence suggests that therapist supported self-help is associated with stronger outcomes than pure self-help. However, the optimal level of therapist involvement still requires extensive research. Pure self-help for anxiety has to date only been evaluated with printed materials (Rapee et al., 2006) and similarly, only studies using printed materials have compared different amounts of therapist support (Lyneham & Rapee, 2006; Thirlwall et al., 2013). Although mechanisms are unlikely to differ greatly between bibliotherapy and e-therapy, replication and extension to online programs would be valuable. Perhaps more importantly, research into the optimal type of therapist support is lacking. For example, through the advent of technology, a therapist can now be virtually present during an actual in vivo exposure session. Perhaps a single session of this type would be more efficacious than several sessions over the telephone, after the fact. Other aspects of therapist features also need to be evaluated. The optimal therapist training and qualifications, the types of materials that are best conducted virtually vs. face-to-face, and optimal means of building a relationship remotely are all issues that may impact on the efficacy of self-help treatments.

Along these lines, research into other moderators is critically important. Being able to identify who self-help will work best for and, more importantly, who it may not work for, will be critical to utilize resources most efficiently. This type of research requires large samples and may be best achieved through collaborative, cross-site studies. It is less likely that relevant variables will be the major ones (such as diagnosis, severity, duration) and more likely that critical moderators will reflect subtle variables such as the way the individual learns best, the relationship between parent and child, or simply patient preference. Similarly, research to identify underlying mechanisms of change will be critical to improve the efficacy and efficiency of self-help programs. Change following self-help is very likely to involve many of the same mechanisms that underpin many therapeutic programs. But there are also likely to be some unique mechanisms that specifically, or more extensively, mediate change within self-help delivery. Identification of these processes will be especially important.

Finally, a fitting way to close this chapter is by briefly examining the role of the therapist in a future (electronic) world. When e-therapies were first being developed, many therapists expressed fears and concerns about the future of their profession. This is less apparent these days but may still sit in the backs of some therapists' minds. As we have noted, so-called self-help therapies still work best when they are supported by therapists. Therefore, far from therapists losing their jobs, self-help treatments open up new methods of working with clients and new populations who may never have previously been able to reach a therapist. Hybrid therapies involving a mix of face-to-face and online sessions may also become a more common method of treatment. Of course, insurance providers will need to catch up to fund this mixed model. But there are several aspects of traditional therapy (such as psychoeducation) that are ideally delivered online and really don't require the cost of personal delivery by a highly qualified therapist. Similarly, virtual technology allows innovations in delivery that were previously unthought of. We earlier mentioned the possibility of virtual attendance of the therapist during exposure, but similarly the therapist could be "present" to assist with cognitive restructuring or relaxation at key times or may be able to provide faster feedback on monitoring forms. Some of the more experimental methods of treatment, such as virtual reality exposure or cognitive bias modification, can also be delivered online (Waters et al., 2016).

Another hybrid method of therapy that is beginning to be very widely discussed is stepped care. In brief, in a stepped care model, the idea is to begin treatment with the least costly and involved method and only increase to more resource-intensive therapy if the patient doesn't respond. To provide one example of how this might look, we recently completed a trial of stepped care for anxious young people (Rapee et al., 2017). After assessment, all youth went into step 1, which consisted of self-help (equivalent to that described earlier in Rapee et al., 2006 for children and Wuthrich et al., 2012 for adolescents). Following 12 weeks, they were reassessed and if they were doing well, that was all they needed. On the other hand, if they required further treatment, they then progressed to traditional treatment using our face-to-face, Cool Kids program. Twelve weeks later, following another assessment, any youth who required even more therapy were progressed to an individual, formulation-based, intervention with a highly experienced therapist. Using this model, we were able to produce the same outcomes as in standard, face-to-face treatment for everyone, but the stepped care model used significantly less therapist time.

This study was the first to evaluate stepped care for anxious young people and now paves the way for future research to explore the myriad of variations in the way a stepped care model could be constructed. These types of ideas potentially herald a new paradigm for service delivery that will include the optimal mix of self-help and face-to-face delivery.

Key Practice Points

- Due to recent developments in the field, we are now at a point where we have a number of evidence-based self-help interventions for anxiety disorders in youth.
- Increased comorbidity, in particular with depression and parental psychopathology, may predict poorer treatment response and relapse.
- Due to the limited number of studies available, the role of therapist involvement is somewhat unclear; however, a limited number of studies suggest that degree of involvement may influence treatment outcomes.
- Treatment planning in the use of self-help approaches may require joint consideration of client variables (e.g., comorbidity, parental psychopathology), therapist variables (e.g., therapist preferences, level of expertise), and program characteristics (e.g., degree of therapist/parent involvement, duration of treatment) to maximize treatment gains.

References

Achenbach, T. M. (1991). *Manual for the child behaviour checklist 4–18 and 1991 profile.* Burlington: Department of Psychiatry, University of Vermont.

Angold, A., Costello, E. J., Messer, S. C., Pickles, A., Winder, F., & Silver, D. (1995). The development of a short questionnaire for use in epidemiological studies of depression in children and adolescents. *International Journal of Methods in Psychiatric Research, 5,* 237–249.

Bennett, K., Manassis, K., Duda, S., Bagnell, A., Bernstein, G. A., Garland, E. J., ... Wilansky, P. (2016). Treating child and adolescent anxiety effectively: Overview of systematic reviews. *Clinical Psychology Review, 50,* 80–94. doi:http://doi.org/10.1016/j.cpr.2016.09.006

Calear, A. L., & Christensen, H. (2010). Review of internet-based prevention and treatment programs for anxiety and depression in children and adolescents. *The Medical Journal of Australia, 192,* S12–S14.

Cartwright-Hatton, S., McNicol, K., & Doubleday, E. (2006). Anxiety in a neglected population: Prevalence of anxiety disorders in pre-adolescent children. *Clinical Psychology Review, 26,* 817–833.

Chavira, D. A., Drahota, A., Garland, A., Roesch, S., Garcia, M., & Stein, M. B. (2014). Feasibility of two modes of treatment delivery for child anxiety in primary care. *Behaviour Research and Therapy, 60,* 60–66. Doi: 10.1016/j.brat.2014.06.010

Cobham, V. E. (2012). Do anxiety-disordered children need to come into the clinic for efficacious treatment? *Journal of Consulting and Clinical Psychology, 80,* 465–476. Doi: 10.1037/a0028205.

Costello, E.J., Angold, A., Burns, B.J., Stangl, D.K., Tweed, D.L., Erkanli, A., & Worthman, C.M. (1996). The Great Smoky Mountains Study of Youth: Goals, designs, methods and the prevalence of DSM-III-R disorders. *Archives of General Psychiatry, 53,* 1129–1136.

Creswell, C., & Willetts, L. (2007). *Overcoming your child's fears and worries: A self-help guide using cognitive behavioural techniques.* London: Constable & Robinson.

Cunningham M. J., Wuthrich, V. M., Rapee, R. M., Lyneham, H. J., Schniering, C. A., Hudson, J. L. (2008). The *Cool Teens* CD-ROM for anxiety disorders in adolescents: A pilot case series. *European Child and Adolescent Psychiatry, 18,* 125–129.

Donovan, C. L., & March, S. (2014). Online CBT for preschool anxiety disorders: A randomised control trial. *Behaviour Research and Therapy, 58,* 24–35. doi: 10.1016/j.brat.2014.05.001

Ebert, D. D., Zarski, A.-C., Christensen, H., Stikkelbroek, Y., Cuijpers, P., Berking, M., & Riper, H. (2015). Internet and computer-based cognitive behavioral therapy for anxiety and depression in youth: A meta-analysis of randomized controlled outcome trials. *PloS One, 10,* 1–15. doi:10.1371/journal.pone.0119895

Gulliver, A., Griffiths, K. M., & Christensen, H. (2010). Perceived barriers and facilitators to mental health help-seeking in young people: A systematic review. *BMC Psychiatry, 10,* 113. doi:10.1186/1471-244x-10–113

Jorm, A., & Griffiths, K. (2006). Population promotion of informal self-help strategies for early intervention against depression and anxiety. *Psychological Medicine, 36,* 3–6. doi:10.1017/S0033291705005659

Khanna, M. S., & Kendall, P. C. (2010). Computer-assisted cognitive behavioral therapy for child anxiety: Results of a randomised clinical trial. *Journal of Consulting and Clinical Psychology, 78,* 737–745. doi: 10.1037/a0019739

Kovacs, M. (1985). The Children's Depression, Inventory (CDI). *Psychopharmacology Bulletin, 21,* 995–998.

Leong, J., Cobham, V. E., deGroot, J., & McDermott, B. (2009). Comparing different modes of delivery: A pilot evaluation of a family-focused, cognitive-behavioral intervention for anxiety-disordered children. *European Child and Adolescent Psychiatry, 18,* 231–239. doi: 10.1007/s00787-008–0723-7

Lewis, K. M., Amatya, K., Coffman, M. F., & Ollendick, T. H. (2015). Treating nighttime fears in young children with bibliotherapy: Evaluating anxiety symptoms and monitoring behavior change. *Journal of Anxiety Disorders, 30,* 103–112.

Lyneham, H. J., & Rapee, R. M. (2006). Evaluation of therapist-supported parent-implemented CBT for anxiety disorders in rural children. *Behaviour Research and Therapy, 44,* 1287–1300. doi: 10.1016/j.brat.2005.09.009

March, S., Spence, S. H., & Donovan, C. L. (2009). The efficacy of an internet-based cognitive-behavioral therapy intervention for child anxiety disorders. *Journal of Pediatric Psychology, 34,* 474–487. doi: 10.1093/jpepsy/jsn099

Morgan, A. J., Rapee, R. M., Salim, A., & Bayer, J. K. (2018). Predicting response to an internet delivered parenting program for anxiety in early childhood. *Behavior Therapy, 49,* 237–248, doi: 10.1016/j.beth.2017.07.009

Morgan, A., Rapee, R. M., Salim, A., Goharpey, N., Tamir, E., McLellan, L. F., & Bayer, J. K. (2017). Internet-delivered parenting program for early intervention of anxiety problems in young children: Randomized controlled trial. *Journal of the American Academy of Child and Adolescent Psychiatry, 56,* 417–425. doi: 10.1016/j.jaac.2017.02.010

Muris, P., Merckelbach, H., Holdrinet, I., & Sijsenaar, M. (1998). Treating phobic children: Effects of EMDR versus exposure. *Journal of Consulting and Clinical Psychology, 66,* 193–198.

Pennant, M. E., Loucas, C. E., Whittington, C., Creswell, C., Fonagy, P., Fuggle, P., ... Kendall, T. (2015). Computerised therapies for anxiety and depression in children and young people: A systematic review and meta-analysis. *Behaviour Research and Therapy, 67,* 1–18. doi:http://doi.org/10.1016/j.brat.2015.01.009

Rapee, R. M., Abbott, M. J., & Lyneham, H. J. (2006). Bibliotherapy for children with anxiety disorders using written materials for parents: A randomized controlled trial. *Journal of Consulting and Clinical Psychology, 74,* 436–444. doi: 10.1037/0022-006X.74.3.436

Rapee, R. M., Lau, E. X., & Kennedy, S. J. (2010). *The Cool Little Kids Anxiety Prevention Program – Therapist Manual.* Sydney: Centre for Emotional Health, Macquarie University.

Rapee, R. M., Lyneham, H. J., Wuthrich, V., Chatterton, M. L., Hudson, J. L., Kangas, M., & Mihalopoulos, C. (2017). Comparison of stepped care delivery against a single, empirically validated cognitive-behavioral therapy program for youth with anxiety: a randomized clinical trial, *Journal of the American Academy of Child and Adolescent Psychiatry, 56,* 841–848. doi: 10.1016/j.jaac.2017.08.001

Rapee, R.M., Lyneham, H.J., Wuthrich, V., Chatterton, M.L., Hudson, J.L., Kangas, M., & Mihalopoulos, C. (2017). *Low intensity treatment for clinically anxious youth: A randomised controlled comparison against face-to-face intervention.* Manuscript in preparation.

Rapee, R. M., Spence, S. H., Cobham, V. E., & Wignall, A. (2000). *Helping your anxious child: A step-by-step guide for parents.* Oakland, CA: New Harbinger.

Schniering, C.A., Rapee, R.M., Einstein, D. & Kirkman, J. An internet-based treatment for adolescents with comorbid anxiety and depression: Results of a randomized controlled trial. Paper presented at the European Association of Behavioural and Cognitive Therapies annual congress. Stockholm, Sweden, Aug 31–Sept 3, 2016.

Schniering, C.A., Einstein, D.E., Rapee, R.M., & Kirkman, J. (2017). *Chilled Plus Online.* Sydney: Centre for Emotional Health, Macquarie University.

Shaffer, D., Gould, M. S., Brasic, J., Ambrosini, P., Fisher, P., Bird, H. R., & Aluwahlia, S. (1983). A Children's Global Assessment Scale (CGAS). *Archives of General Psychiatry, 40,* 787–792.

Silverman, W. K., & Albano, A. M. (1996). *Anxiety Disorders Interview Schedule for Children for DSM–IV: Child and Parent Versions.* San Antonio, TX: Psychological Corporation.

Spence, S.H. (1998). A measure of anxiety symptoms among children. *Behaviour Research and Therapy, 36*(5), 545–566.

Spence, S. H., Holmes, J. M., March, S., & Lipp, O. V. (2006). The feasibility and outcome of clinic plus internet delivery of cognitive–behavior therapy for childhood anxiety. *Journal of Consulting and Clinical Psychology, 74,* 614–621.

Spence, S. H., Donovan, C. L., March, S., Gamble, A., Anderson, R., Prosser, S., ... Kenardy, J. (2008). Online CBT in the treatment of child and adolescent anxiety disorders: Issues in the development of BRAVE–ONLINE and two case illustrations. *Behavioural and Cognitive Psychotherapy, 36,* 411–430. doi: 10.1017/S135246580800444X

Spence, S. H., Donovan, C. L., Gamble, A., Anderson, R. E., Prosser, S., & Kenardy, J. (2011). A randomized controlled trial of online versus clinic-based CBT for adolescent anxiety. *Journal of Consulting and Clinical Psychology, 79*, 629–642. doi: 10.1037/a0024512

Spence, S. H., Donovan, C. L., March, S., Kenardy, J., & Hearn, C. S. (2017). Generic versus disorder specific cognitive behavior therapy for social anxiety disorder in youth: A randomized controlled trial using internet delivery. *Behaviour Research and Therapy, 90*, 41–57. doi: 10.1016/j.brat.2016.12.003

Stallard, P., Udwin, O., Goddard, M., & Hibbert, S. (2007). The availability of cognitive behaviour therapy within specialist Child and Adolescent Mental Health Services (CAMHS): A National Survey. *Behavioural and Cognitive Psychotherapy, 35*, 501–505. doi:10.1017/S1352465807003724

Thirlwall, K., Cooper, P., & Creswell, C. (2017). Guided parent-delivered cognitive behavioral therapy for childhood anxiety: Predictors of treatment response. *Journal of Anxiety Disorders, 45*, 43–48. doi:https://doi.org/10.1016/j.janxdis.2016.11.003

Thirlwall, K., Cooper, P. J., Karalus, J., Voysey, M., Willetts, L., & Creswell, C. (2013). Treatment of child anxiety disorders via guided parent-delivered cognitive-behavioural therapy: Randomised controlled trial. *The British Journal of Psychiatry, 203*, 436–444. doi: 10.1192/bjp.bp.113.126698

Vigerland, S., Thulin, U., Ljotsson, B., Svirsky, L., Ost, L., Lindefors, N., et al. (2013). Internet-delivered CBT for children with specific phobia: A pilot study. *Cognitive Behaviour Therapy, 42*, 303–314. doi: 10.1080/16506073.2013.844201.

Vigerland, S., Ljotsson, B., Thulin, U., Ost, L., Andersson, G., & Serlachius, E. (2016). Internet-delivered cognitive behavioural therapy for children with anxiety disorders: A randomised controlled trial. *Behaviour Research and Therapy, 76*, 47–56. doi: 10.1016/j.brat.2015.11.006

Waters, A. M., Zimmer-Gembeck, M. J., Craske, M. G., Pine, D. S., Bradley, B. P., & Mogg, K. (2016). A preliminary evaluation of a home-based, computer-delivered attention training treatment for anxious children living in regional communities. *Journal of Experimental Psychopathology, 7*(3), 511–527.

Wuthrich, V. M., Rapee, R. M., Cunningham, M. J., Lyneham, H. J., Hudson, J. L., & Schniering, C. A. (2012). A randomised controlled trial of the *Cool Teens* CD-ROM computerized program for adolescent anxiety. *Journal of the American Academy of Child and Adolescent Psychiatry, 51*, 261–270.

4 New Technologies to Deliver CBT

Computer and Web-Based Programs, Mobile Applications, and Virtual Reality

Susan H. Spence, Sonja March, and Caroline L. Donovan

Introduction

The past decade has seen a surge of interest in the use of internet and computer-delivered programs and tools for the treatment of child and adolescent anxiety, and there are many position and review papers on the topic (Berry & Lai, 2014; Ebert et al., 2015; Pennant et al., 2015; Reyes-Portillo et al., 2014; Rooksby et al., 2015; Stasiak et al., 2016; Vigerland, Lenhard et al., 2016). Indeed, currently there are almost as many review papers as there are randomized controlled trials evaluating the impact of such interventions, with the research lagging substantially behind the enthusiasm. This chapter outlines the key developments in this exciting area, provides a pragmatic review of the empirical literature to date, and proposes some future directions for research and technological development, as well as guidelines for clinicians. The chapter will focus on CBT programs and tools delivered with the assistance of desktop computers, mobile devices, or other new technologies such as virtual reality. It will include internet-delivered CBT (ICBT), stand-alone computer-delivered CBT programs or tools (CCBT), and mobile device applications (APPS). To facilitate readability, ICBT, CCBT, and APPS will be referred to collectively as I/CCBT unless there is a need to differentiate. Some of the special issues relating to APPS are discussed in a separate section later in the chapter.

Rationale for Developing Effective I/CCBT Programs and Tools

Clinic-delivered CBT is a well-established, empirically supported treatment for anxiety in children and adolescents (Bennett et al., 2016; Reynolds et al., 2012). However, for a variety of reasons, only a minority of anxious youth receive treatment from mental health professionals (Chavira et al., 2004; Lawrence et al., 2015; Merikangas et al., 2010). There are many factors that act as barriers to the receipt of mental health services for young people. The relatively high prevalence of anxiety problems and cost of providing services is an obvious issue, as the number of anxious children and adolescents far exceeds the number of mental health practitioners with skills in evidence-based treatment of child anxiety, resulting in long wait lists

(Stallard et al., 2007). Other factors include a lack of parental awareness of their child's difficulties, lack of knowledge about available services, and lack of parental time or money to attend therapy (Salloum et al., 2016). Finally, some young people may be reluctant to participate in treatment for fear of embarrassment or stigma (Boyd et al., 2007).

Computer, mobile, and internet delivery methods have been proposed as potential ways of increasing young people's access to mental health treatment and preventive interventions (Reyes-Portillo et al., 2014). The majority of children in most Western societies now have access to the internet via a computer or a mobile device. For example, in Australia the 2014–2015 national census revealed that 97 percent of children under 15 years lived in a household with internet access, mostly through a desktop or laptop computer (Australian Bureau of Statistics, 2016). In the United States, estimates from the Pew Research Center in 2014–2015 suggested that 92 percent of 13–17-year-olds reported daily online activity, 73 percent had access to a smartphone, 87 percent to a desktop or laptop, and 58 percent to a tablet. Young people are highly skilled in the use of mobile and web technologies and, perhaps not surprisingly, they report the internet as being a key source through which they seek information about mental health issues (Livingstone & Bober, 2004; Mission Australia, 2017). Although the high level of youth internet connectivity seems impressive, it is important to note that cultural differences have been found in the way in which young people access online content. For example, young people from black or Hispanic backgrounds in the United States are less likely to have access to a computer and the internet at home, and are more likely to use a mobile phone for internet connection (Rideout & Katz, 2016), a finding that clearly has implications for the design and reach of these interventions.

Using technology to deliver CBT provides a relatively low-cost, flexible form of treatment delivery that can be completed in private, and is accessible 24/7 at times and places convenient for children and families (Ly et al., 2012). If effective, the use of technology has the potential to enable mental health professionals to assist a larger number of clients than is currently possible with traditional face-to-face therapy, as it generally requires less therapist time per patient. It can also provide better access to treatment for families who live in rural and remote areas where services are scarce and require long journeys to a clinic. Furthermore, the limited research to date suggests that children and parents are receptive to the concept of participating in I/CCBT for mental health issues, including child anxiety (Salloum et al., 2015; Stallard, Velleman, & Richardson, 2010). Clinicians tend to be a bit more skeptical, although the majority report favorable attitudes (Donovan et al., 2015; Stallard, Richardson, & Velleman, 2010; Vigerland et al., 2014).

Uses of I/CCBT Programs and Tools

Cognitive behavior therapy in particular is highly suited to translation for online and computerized delivery as it is highly structured and typically involves a series of clearly delineated therapy components that can be implemented in a sequential fashion or as elements within each session. For example, I/CCBT involves components designed to:

- provide psychoeducation about emotions and body signs of anxiety
- prompt completion of activities and home tasks
- monitor, record, and track (in real time or later data entry) events, child behavior, and activities such as:
  - the occurrence of feared situations
  - physiological signs of anxiety, behavior, thoughts, and feelings
  - the level of fear/anxiety/worry in specific situations
  - progress with homework assignments
- provide information on, and activities around, specific therapy components to teach skills such as:
  - relaxation and meditation skills
  - problem-solving skills
  - identifying the link between situations, thoughts, feelings, and behavior
  - cognitive restructuring
  - self-reinforcement
  - parenting skills
- give reinforcing messages for task completion and feedback about progress, and
- provide information about other treatment resources.

These elements can be combined either into full therapy programs involving multiple sessions, as adjuncts to therapy, or as stand-alone tools for a single component of I/CCBT. Interventions also vary in the degree of therapist involvement, ranging from fully self-help, to minimal therapist support, to full therapist involvement. There are many ways in which I/CCBT can be used in clinical practice such as (i) a fully self-help approach for early intervention and prevention, (ii) a stepped care approach whereby I/CCBT (either self-help or with clinician support) represents the first step, (iii) clinician supported I/CCBT as an alternative to face-to-face CBT, or (iv) an adjunct to clinic-delivered CBT.

The Effectiveness of I/CCBT: A Review of Randomized Controlled Trials of I/CCBT for Youth Anxiety Disorders

In reviewing the evidence regarding the effectiveness of I/CCBT with anxious children and adolescents, we will focus on those studies in which (i) participants were selected on the basis of at least one clinically diagnosed anxiety disorder, (ii) the focus of treatment was on anxiety reduction, (iii) the research design involved a randomized controlled trial, (iv) participants were children and/or adolescents, and (v) the results have been published in a refereed journal. The impact of I/CCBT in the prevention of anxiety disorders will be mentioned only briefly.

While there is a relatively large amount of research supporting the effectiveness of I/CCBT for anxiety in adults (Adelman et al., 2014), there have been considerably fewer studies conducted with children and adolescents. Table 4.1 provides a summary of the key randomized controlled trials to date evaluating the impact of ICBT with anxious youth. It is clear from this table that I/CCBT comes in many forms, with the extensive variation in content and the way that I/CCBT has been delivered making it very difficult to draw conclusions about what "works" and what does not. Studies vary according to factors such as:

- the amount and type of therapist support (e.g., fully self-help with no therapist support, brief therapist support through email or telephone, or face-to-face therapist support for all sessions),
- the level of parent involvement,
- the location in which the ICBT is completed (e.g., in the clinic, or at home),
- the medium through which the program is completed (e.g., fully interactive internet program, CD-ROM, or mobile APPs) and whether an internet connection is required,
- the types of CBT components included (e.g., relaxation, exposure, problem solving),
- the duration, number, and frequency of sessions, and use of booster sessions,
- the method of presentation of material and level of interactivity (e.g., use of video clips/text, quizzes, rewards, feedback regarding progress, chat rooms, discussion boards, avatars, computer gaming techniques),
- the severity and duration of symptoms of participants (prevention, early intervention, or treatment), types of presenting problem(s), and comorbidity,
- the personal characteristics of participants (e.g., age, gender, socioeconomic background, comorbid conditions), and
- the research methodology in terms of sample size, length of follow-up, type of control group, and outcome measures.

Given this variation in methodology and the small number of studies to date, we can make only tentative comments about the outcomes.

Impact upon Anxiety Diagnoses and Symptoms. The results of the studies outlined in Table 4.1 suggest that, at posttreatment, the percent of participants free of their primary diagnosis tended to be studies with greater levels of therapist contact. For example, where I/CCBT formed half of the intervention, with the remaining sessions involving clinic-based face-to-face therapy, the posttreatment effects for percent free of their primary anxiety diagnosis were between 56 and 80 percent (Khanna & Kendall, 2010; Spence, Holmes, March, et al., 2006; Storch et al., 2015). In these studies, effects for the combined I/CCBT plus clinic conditions were significantly greater than the wait-list control (WLC) (Spence, Holmes, March, et al., 2006), treatment as usual (Storch et al., 2015), and placebo (Khanna & Kendall, 2010) and equivalent to CBT delivered fully in the clinic (Khanna & Kendall, 2010; Spence, Holmes, March, et al., 2006).

Table 4.1 *Summary of Randomized Controlled Trials Evaluating the Treatment of Clinically Anxious Children and/or Adolescents*

Intervention Author(s) Year	Age and Anxiety Disorders	Aim of Intervention, Length of Intervention (sessions and duration), Therapist Support	Research Design	Completion, Compliance, Satisfaction	Intervention Outcomes upon Anxiety
The Brave Program Spence, Holmes, March, et al. (2006)	7–14 years GAD, SAD, SEP, SpPh	Half clinic and half internet delivery of CBT program 10 weekly sessions 5 clinic, 5 online (child) 3 clinic, 3 online (parents) 1-month booster (clinic) 3-month booster (internet) Internet sessions completed at home Recognizing body signs of anxiety, relaxation strategies, problem solving, self-reinforcement, cognitive challenging, exposure. Parenting skills Interactive tasks, games, quizzes, animations, cartoons, to illustrate concepts Exposure tasks – homework	RCT N=72 Brave Clinic CBT vs. half clinic/half ICBT sessions vs. WLC Assessed: pre, post, 6-month follow-up (for intervention groups) Measures: ADIS-C (parent), CSR, CGAS, SCAS-C/P, RCMAS, CBCL-Int	Retained 25/27 (93 percent) in combined clinic/internet condition at posttest. Children completed 91 percent and parents completed 91 percent of internet tasks. High parent and child satisfaction with half clinic/half ICBT, equivalent to full clinic condition.	56 percent clinic/internet group, 65 percent clinic, and 13 percent WLC primary diagnosis free at posttest. 89 percent clinic and 74 percent clinic/internet primary diagnosis free at 12-month follow-up. Clinic and clinic/internet conditions showed greater improvements on CSR, SCAS-P, CBCL-Int, and SCAS-C (not RCMAS) than WLC at posttreatment. No differences between clinic and clinic/internet except on SCAS-C (clinic/internet improvements > clinic alone). Treatment effects maintained or enhanced and no difference between treatments.

Table 4.1 (cont.)

Intervention Author(s) Year	Age and Anxiety Disorders	Aim of Intervention, Length of Intervention (sessions and duration), Therapist Support	Research Design	Completion, Compliance, Satisfaction	Intervention Outcomes upon Anxiety
BRAVE-ONLINE (Child and parent version) March et al. (2009)	7–12 years GAD, SAD, SEP, SpPh	Internet delivered CBT (ICBT): 10 child, 6 parent weekly sessions, 60 min duration. Plus 1- and 3-month boosters. Sessions completed online at home. Minimal therapist assistance – brief weekly emails, one midpoint phone call. Recognizing body signs of anxiety, relaxation strategies, problem solving, self-reinforcement, cognitive challenging, exposure. Parenting skills. Interactive tasks, games, quizzes, animations, cartoons, to illustrate concepts. Exposure tasks – homework	RCT $N=73$ ICBT vs. WLC Assessed: pre, post, 6-month follow-up (for intervention group) Measures: ADIS-C/P, CSR, CGAS, SCAS-C/P, CBCL-Int	Retained 30/34 (88 percent) in ICBT at post-assessment. At post-assessment 60 percent parents and 33.3 percent children had completed all 10 sessions (Mean 5.3/6 sessions for parents; 7.5/10 for children). By 6-month follow-up 72.3 percent parents and 62 percent children had completed all 10 sessions. Moderate parent and child satisfaction with ICBT.	30 percent ICBT and 10 percent WLC primary diagnosis free at posttest (NS). 75 percent ICBT primary diagnosis free at 6-month follow-up. ICBT showed greater improvements than WLC at post on CSR, CGAS, SCAS-P, and CBCL-Int, but not SCAS-C. Treatment effects maintained or enhanced at 6-month follow-up.

BRAVE-ONLINE (Teen and parent version) Spence et al. (2011)	12–18 years GAD, SAD, SEP, SpPh	ICBT: 10 teenage and 5 parent weekly, 60 min sessions. Plus 1- and 3-month boosters Minimal therapist assistance – brief weekly emails, one midpoint phone call. Content as for (March et al., 2009) adapted for teenagers. Clinic CBT (clinic) received equivalent content with face-to-face therapist.	RCT $N=115$ ICBT vs. Clinic CBT vs. WLC Assessed: pre, 12 weeks after start of treatment, 6-month and 12-month follow-ups (for intervention groups) Measures: ADIS-C/P, CSR, CGAS, SCAS-C/P, CBCL– Int, YSR- Int	Retained 41/44 (93 percent) in ICBT at 12-week assessment. At 12 weeks 66 percent of parents and 39 percent of teens had completed all 10 sessions (Mean 4.4/6 for parents; 7.5/10 for teens). Slower rate of session completion vs. clinic. By 12-month follow-up 79 percent parents and 79 percent teens had completed all 10 sessions. Moderate to high parent and teen satisfaction with ICBT. No difference vs. clinic CBT. No differences in therapeutic alliance between ICBT and clinic CBT (Anderson et al., 2012).	37 percent ICBT, 32.5 percent clinic, and 4.2 percent WLC primary diagnosis free at posttest. 62 percent ICBT and 58 percent clinic primary diagnosis free at 6-month follow-up. 78 percent ICBT and 81 percent clinic primary diagnosis free at 12-month follow-up. ICBT and clinic improvements > WLC at post on CSR, CGAS, and CBCL-Int but not SCAS-C; clinic > WLC for SCAS-P; ICBT> WLC for YSR-Int. Treatment effects maintained or enhanced at 6- and 12-month follow-ups. No significant differences in outcome between ICBT and clinic CBT.

Table 4.1 (cont.)

Intervention Author(s) Year	Age and Anxiety Disorders	Aim of Intervention, Length of Intervention (sessions and duration), Therapist Support	Research Design	Completion, Compliance, Satisfaction	Intervention Outcomes upon Anxiety
BRAVE-ONLINE (Child and parent version) Conaughton et al. (2017)	8–12 years High Functioning Autism Spectrum Disorder Plus Anxiety Disorder(s)	ICBT: 10 child and 6 parent weekly, 60 min sessions. Plus 1- and 3-month boosters Minimal therapist assistance – brief weekly emails, one midpoint phone call. Content as for (March et al., 2009).	RCT $N=42$ ICBT vs. WLC Assessed: pre, post, 3-month follow-up (for intervention group) Measures: ADIS-C/P, CSR, CGAS, SCAS-C/P, CBCL-Int	Retained 20/21 (95 percent) of ICBT group at posttreatment. Parents completed mean of 4.86/6 by posttreatment and 5.24/6 by 3 months. Children completed mean of 6.7/10 by posttreatment, 7.38/10 by 3 months. Moderate parent and child satisfaction ratings.	20 percent primary diagnosis free at post vs. 0 percent WLC. 39 percent primary diagnosis free at 3-month follow-up. ICBT showed significantly greater improvements pre- to posttreatment in number of diagnoses, CSR, SCAS-C, SCAS-P, and CBCL-Int and CGAS compared to WLC. Treatment effects maintained or enhanced at 3-month follow-up.
BRAVE-ONLINE for parents of preschoolers Donovan and March (2014)	3–6 years SEP, SAD, GAD, SpPh	BRAVE-ONLINE – Parent program plus 6 parent weekly internet sessions, 60 mins duration + preschool-specific booklet. 1- and 3-month boosters. Minimal therapist assistance – brief weekly emails, one midpoint phone call.	RCT $N=52$ ICBT vs. WLC Assessed: pre, post, 6-month follow-up (for intervention group) Measures: ADIS-C/P, CSR, CGAS, PAS, CBCL 1/5 – 5 Yrs-Int	Retained 23/23 (100 percent) in ICBT group at posttreatment. Parents completed mean of 4.14/6 by posttreatment and 4.65/6 by 6 months. Moderate to high parent satisfaction with program.	39 percent primary diagnosis free at post vs. 26 percent WLC (NS). 71 percent primary diagnosis free at 6-month follow-up. ICBT showed significantly greater pre- to posttreatment decrease in CSR, PAS, and CBCL-Int and increase in CGAS compared to WLC. Treatment effects maintained or enhanced at 6-month follow-up.

BarnInternetprojektet (BiP) (translated as the Stockholm Child Internet Project) Vigerland, Ljotsson, et al. (2016)	8–12 years GAD, panic, SEP, SAD, SpPh	Psychoeducation, parenting strategies to decrease anxious and increase "brave" behavior, relaxation and coping strategies, positive self-talk, exposure hierarchy, problem solving. ICBT 10 weeks, therapist support (written feedback on worksheets, 3 phone calls, with additional calls if required). 11 modules, Reading material, films, animations, illustrations, exercises, parent and child modules, psychoeducation, coping strategies, problem-solving skills, exposure.	RCT $N=93$ ICBT vs. WLC Assessed: pre, post, 3-month follow-up (for intervention group) Measures: ADIS-C/P, CSR, CGAS, SCAS-C/P, FSSC-R, PSWQ, SAI-C, and SPAI-C/P	Retained 46/46 (100 percent) ICBT group at posttreatment. Families completed mean of 9.7/11 modules. Children and parents were moderately satisfied with the treatment.	20 percent primary diagnosis free at post vs. 7 percent WLC (NS). 50 percent primary diagnosis free at 3 months. ICBT showed significantly greater pre- to posttreatment decrease in CSR and SCAS-P, and increase in CGAS compared to WLC (but no differences for SCAS-C, FSSC-R, PSWQ-C, PSWQ, SAI-C, and SPAI-C/P). Treatment effects maintained or enhanced at 3-month follow-up.
BarnInternetprojektet (BiP)	8–12 years GAD, panic, SEP, SAD, SpPh	As previously for Vigerland et al. (2016)	Long-term follow-up of Vigerland et al. (2016). Initial RCT: As previously for Vigerland et al. (2016)		55 percent primary diagnosis free at 3 months, and 73 percent at 12 months.

Table 4.1 (cont.)

Intervention Author(s) Year	Age and Anxiety Disorders	Aim of Intervention, Length of Intervention (sessions and duration), Therapist Support	Research Design	Completion, Compliance, Satisfaction	Intervention Outcomes upon Anxiety
Vigerland et al. (2017)		WLC children with continued anxiety disorder(s) admitted into treatment condition. 12-month follow-up of treated children.	ICBT vs. WLC, then WLC received treatment after post-assessment $N=84$ Assessed: pre, 3- and 12-month follow-up Measures: ADIS-C/P, CSR, CGAS, SCAS-P		Posttreatment improvements maintained or enhanced at 3 months and 12 months on CSR, CGAS, and SCAS-P. Lower long-term improvement predicted by ASD symptoms.
Tillfors et al. (2011)	15–21 years Social Anxiety Disorder	Internet-based CBT (ICBT) 9 weeks, 9 sessions Modules included information, exercises, 2 essay questions, interactive multiple-choice quiz, homework tasks. Therapist provided feedback on homework within 36 hours. Psychoeducation, cognitive restructuring, exposure, reducing self-focused attention, social skills, relapse prevention	RCT $N=19$ ICBT vs. WLC. (WLC started ICBT after post). Assessed: pre, post, 12-month follow-up (for ICBT) Measures: SPSQ-C, LSAS-SR, BAI	Retained 9/10 (90 percent) in ICBT at posttreatment. Low compliance. No students completed modules 7–9. Only 3/9 completed up to and including module 4. High satisfaction with program.	Greater pre- to posttreatment improvements for ICBT than WLC for SPSQ-C, LSAS-SR, and BAI. Effects maintained for ICBT at 12-month follow-up in original sample and treated WLCs.

Camp Cope-A-Lot Khanna and Kendall (2010)	7–13 years SEP, SAD, GAD, SpPh or Panic	Computer-assisted CBT (CACBT) 50 percent of sessions are therapist-guided in clinic. Sessions 1–6 completed independently by child (skill building); Sessions 7–12 completed with the therapist. Plus two parent sessions with therapist/coach. Psychoeducation, cognitive restructuring, relaxation training, exposure, homework, animations, audio, photographs, videos, text, cartoon characters, schematics, reward system.	RCT $N=49$ CACBT vs. clinic CBT (CBT) vs. attention placebo control. Assessed: pre, post, 3-month follow-up (for treatment groups) Measures: ADIS-C/P (joint), CSR, CGAS, MASC	Retained 16/16 (100 percent) in CACBT condition at posttreatment. 100 percent compliance for participants in CACBT. Higher parent and child satisfaction with both treatments compared to placebo, with no difference between treatments. No differences in therapeutic alliance between CACBT and CBT.	81 percent, 70 percent, and 19 percent (CACBT, CBT, and placebo, respectively) primary diagnosis free at posttreatment. CACBT and CBT showed greater pre- to posttreatment improvements than placebo on CSR and CGAS. No difference between treatments. No difference between either treatment and placebo on MASC. Benefits maintained at 3 months for CACBT and regular CBT. No differences between treatments. Higher therapist adherence but lower flexibility ratings for CACBT.
Camp Cope-A-Lot Storch et al. (2015)	7 – 13 years SEP, SAD, GAD, SpPh or Panic	Computer-assisted CBT (CACBT)	RCT $N=100$ CACBT vs. TAU	Retained 45/49 (92 percent) in CACBT at posttreatment.	55 percent CACBT vs. 17.6 percent TAU free of primary diagnosis (CSR <4) at posttreatment.

Table 4.1 (cont.)

Intervention Author(s) Year	Age and Anxiety Disorders	Aim of Intervention, Length of Intervention (sessions and duration), Therapist Support	Research Design	Completion, Compliance, Satisfaction	Intervention Outcomes upon Anxiety
		All 12 sessions delivered in clinic. Content described previously (Khanna & Kendall, 2010).	Assessed: pre, post, 1-month follow-up Measures: ADIS-C/P, PARS, CGI, CBCL-Int, MASC	No data provided about youth compliance with computer tasks. High parent and youth satisfaction with CACBT.	Greater pre- to posttreatment improvements for CACBT than TAU on CSR, PARS, CGI-severity, CBCL-Int. No difference on MASC. No long-term follow-up (only 1-month). Note: Only 55 percent of TAU received any treatment.
Cool-Teens Wuthrich et al. (2012)	14–17 years	Computerized CBT (CCBT) – CD-ROM, with 8 therapist telephone calls to youth (~ 15 mins each) and 3 calls to parents (~ 17 mins each). Total therapist phone contact < 3 hrs. 8 modules, 30 mins each, weekly. Cognitive restructuring, exposure, psychoeducation, goal setting. Audio and video material, text, cartoons, illustrations, parent handouts.	RCT $N=43$ CCBT vs. WLC Assessed: pre, post, 3-month follow-up Measures: ADIS-C/P, CSR, SCAS-C/P, SDQ-Emot	Retained 21/24 (87 percent) at posttreatment. Of those, 100 percent compliance with modules and 98.4 percent compliance with phone calls.	41 percent CCBT vs. 0 percent WLC free of primary diagnosis at posttreatment. 23.5 percent CCBT condition free of primary diagnosis at 3-month follow-up. Greater pre- to posttreatment improvement for CCBT than WLC on CSR, number of anxiety disorders, SCAS-C, SCAS-P.

Notes: Outcomes based on retained to posttreatment samples, unless otherwise stated.

Abbreviations:

TAU = Treatment as usual
WLC = Wait-list control
SEP = Separation Anxiety Disorder, SAD = Social Anxiety Disorder, SpPh = Specific Phobia, GAD = Generalized Anxiety Disorder
ADIS-C/P Anxiety Disorders Interview Schedule for Children/Parents (Silverman & Albano, 1996);
CBCL-Int Child Behavior Checklist – Internalizing Subscale (Achenbach & Rescorla, 2001);
YSR-Int Youth Self-Report – Internalizing Subscale (Achenbach & Rescorla, 2001);
CSR Clinical Severity Rating (Silverman & Albano, 1996);
CGAS Children's Global Assessment Scale (Shaffer et al., 1983);
SCAS-C/P Spence Children's Anxiety Scale (Spence, 1998);
PAS Preschool Anxiety Scale (Spence et al., 2001);
MASC Multidimensional Anxiety Scale for Children (March et al., 1997);
SDQ-Emot Strengths and Difficulties Questionnaire – Emotional Subscale (Goodman, 1997);
FSSC-R Fear Survey Schedule for Children – Revised (Ollendick, 1983);
PSWQ-C Penn State Worry Questionnaire (Chorpita et al., 1997);
SAI-C Separation Anxiety Inventory for Children (In-Albon, Meyer, & Schneider, 2013);
SPAI-C/P Social Phobia and Anxiety Inventory (Beidel, Turner, & Morris, 1995);
PARS Pediatric Anxiety Rating Scale (Riddle et al., 2002);
CGI Clinical Global Impressions (Guy, 1976);
SPSQ-C Social Phobia Screening Questionnaire – Child (Gren-Landell et al., 2009);
BAI Beck Anxiety Inventory (Beck et al., 1988);
LSAS-SR Liebowitz Social Anxiety Scale Self-Report (Liebowitz, 1987).

In contrast, for studies with only brief therapist support during the program, around 20 to 40 percent of youth were free of their primary diagnosis at posttreatment (e.g., March, Spence, & Donovan, 2009; Spence et al., 2011; Vigerland, Ljotsson, et al., 2016; Wuthrich et al., 2012). Although these effects were smaller than those typically found for clinic-based CBT at posttreatment (around 50 to 60 percent free of primary diagnosis) (Cartwright-Hatton et al., 2004; Ewing et al., 2015; James et al., 2015), they were significantly better than the WLC in the majority of studies. By 6- to 12-month follow-up, the level of therapist support did not appear to impact on the percent free of primary diagnosis, with around 70 to 80 percent remission of primary diagnosis in keeping with the literature for clinic-based CBT (Cartwright-Hatton et al., 2004). One study found no significant long-term differences in outcomes between fully online ICBT and full clinic delivery of CBT (Spence et al., 2011). Thus, it appears that I/CCBT, with at least brief therapist email contact, can produce strong reductions in anxiety, particularly at follow-up, with effects equivalent to those found with clinic-delivered CBT. However, it will be important to replicate this finding in future research.

A confounding factor was evident in comparing the results for I/CCBT and the WLC at posttreatment, in that youth and parents completing ICBT at home, with minimal therapist support, tended to be slower to complete their therapy sessions (Spence et al., 2011). Thus, when posttreatment assessments were completed at a set number of weeks equivalent to the wait-list period, a significant proportion of families in the ICBT condition had not actually finished treatment, and they continued to complete sessions over the next few weeks. This complicates comparability of the intervention with control conditions, as the WLC participants have generally commenced some form of treatment after the wait-list period and they are no longer included in the study at follow-up, making it impossible to adequately compare the longer-term outcomes.

Client Satisfaction and the Therapist-Client Relationship. The widespread uptake of I/CCBT programs will only occur if young people, their parents, and clinicians believe that the approach offers a credible, engaging, and effective form of treatment. The evidence summarized in Table 1 shows that children, adolescents, and parents were moderately to highly satisfied with I/CCBT in most studies. Indeed, for adolescents, treatment satisfaction ratings for ICBT delivered with only minimal therapist support (via email and one brief phone call) were equivalent to those for adolescents receiving face-to-face CBT in the clinic (Spence et al., 2011). Although parents indicated slightly higher satisfaction ratings for the clinic than the I/CCBT format, their perceptions of the internet format were still very positive.

Some clinicians express concern that the loss of face-to-face contact with a therapist in I/CCBT will have an adverse impact upon the therapist-client relationship, and that this in turn will result in reduced therapeutic outcomes, high drop-out rates, and low levels of compliance with therapy tasks (Stallard, Richardson, et al., 2010; Vigerland et al., 2014). As Table 1 suggests, however, it would seem that these feared consequences do not eventuate for I/CCBT when accompanied by brief therapist support by email and phone. Anderson et al. (2012) found that youth who received I/CCBT using BRAVE-ONLINE with minimal therapist support reported positive working alliance scores, with levels equivalent to those reported by their peers who received face-to-face CBT with a therapist. This finding is important as there was no face-to-face contact with the therapist for the BRAVE-ONLINE group, with only brief weekly email contact and a single phone call midway through the program. The parents who participated in BRAVE-ONLINE similarly reported positive working alliance scores, albeit slightly lower than those of parents who received the clinic format. Khanna and Kendall (2010) also found no adverse impact upon the quality of the therapist-client relationship when half the CBT sessions were delivered in the clinic and half using CCBT, compared to full clinic CBT delivery. Thus, a high level of face-to-face contact does not seem to be necessary for a young person to experience a positive relationship with their therapist.

Therapy Dropout and Compliance. Despite concerns expressed by therapists about high rates of therapy dropout and lack of treatment compliance, the data summarized in Table 1 suggest that, for those programs with at least minimal therapist support, these adverse consequences are not realized, with a high percentage (>80 percent) remaining in I/CCBT at the posttreatment assessment point and completing the majority of sessions. Exact compliance with treatment is difficult to determine as it has been measured in different ways in different studies. In general, the majority of children and parents had completed the majority of sessions by the post-assessment point, even in those studies with only minimal therapist support. However, Table 1 indicates that session completion rates tended to be higher in those studies with greater levels of therapist contact.

The Effectiveness of I/CCBT: Meta-Analyses

Four meta-analyses have examined the impact of I/CCBT for anxious youth versus a control condition over the same time period (typically a WLC) and include the studies described in Table 1 that had been published at the time when the meta-analyses were conducted. Although only a small number of studies were available for inclusion, in all instances the results indicated that the effect size (standardized mean difference) was statistically significant and favored I/CCBT. Ebert et al. (2015) reported an effect size = 0.68 from seven studies; Pennant et al. (2015) reported an effect size = 0.77 from six trials (although some of those were very small trials and included young adults); Rooksby et al. (2015) found an effect size of 0.69 from five trials (although two of the studies were targeting emotional disorders rather than anxiety disorders per se); and Ye et al. (2014) found an effect size of 0.52 from six studies (although three of the studies evaluated programs that were not specifically designed for anxiety and included the treatment of depression). Despite methodological differences in the meta-analyses and different criteria for study inclusion, the findings are similar and indicate a moderate effect size for I/CCBT compared to a wait-list or nontreatment control. To date, there are insufficient

The Effectiveness of I/CCBT: Open Trials and Non-RCT Designs

We have given emphasis in this chapter to those studies that involved RCT designs. However, there are additional studies that have involved open trials and other designs, from which valuable information can be gleaned. For example, Vigerland and colleagues (Vigerland et al., 2013) conducted an open trial of six sessions of ICBT with 30 children diagnosed with specific phobias. Statistically significant decreases were found in the severity of parent- and child-rated anxiety and fear from pre- to posttreatment, with improvements being maintained at 3-month follow-up. Silfvernagel et al. (2015) reported a very small open trial of an ICBT intervention that involved 6–9 online, individualized text modules, plus optional online therapist guidance, telephone support, and face-to-face sessions if required. The trial involved 11 participants aged 15–19 years. Although three participants dropped out, strong reductions in anxiety were found for those completing the intervention. The program was interesting as a total of 17 potential modules were designed and the number and type of modules completed by the young person were matched to their individual presenting problems.

March et al. (2018) reported on an open trial of 1095 young people with elevated symptoms of anxiety who enrolled in, and completed at least 3 sessions of, a 10-session, *entirely self-help version* (as opposed to the therapist-assisted versions trialed in the RCTs discussed previously) of BRAVE-ONLINE. Although on average, these young people completed 5–6 of the 10 sessions, only around 15 percent completed all 10 sessions. Thus, without some form of professional support, it would seem that anxious young people are at risk of not completing and dropping out of self-help I/CCBT. Nevertheless, those who completed at least three sessions showed significant reductions in anxiety symptoms, with the degree of decrease in anxiety increasing as the number of sessions completed increased as measured by a brief, 8-item Children's Anxiety Scale (CAS-8, Spence et al., 2014). Irrespective of the number of sessions completed, by their final recorded assessment, 35.4 percent showed reliable improvement in anxiety, and 42.2 percent showed a reduction from the elevated anxiety range into the "nonelevated" range from baseline to their final CAS-8 score. Reliable change and clinically significant improvement levels tended to be greater for children than adolescents and were greater for those who completed more sessions.

I/CCBT with Subgroups of Young People or Subtypes of Anxiety

To date, there have been only a few studies that have examined whether I/CCBT is effective with specific subgroups of the population or subtypes of anxiety. For example, Donovan and March (2014) adapted the BRAVE-ONLINE program for parents of anxious preschoolers. Fifty-two children aged 3 to 6 years were randomly allocated to ICBT or a wait-list control group. Results at posttreatment showed a significantly greater reduction in clinical severity, anxiety symptoms, and internalizing behavior, as well as a greater increase in overall functioning for children in the ICBT group compared to the WLC condition (see Table 1). Although ICBT did not differ from the WLC in terms of the percentage of children who lost their primary anxiety diagnosis from pre- to posttreatment, by 6-month follow-up reductions in anxiety in the ICBT group were maintained or enhanced, with 70.6 percent now being free of their primary diagnosis.

The BRAVE-ONLINE program was also evaluated in an RCT with young people who were diagnosed with comorbid anxiety and high-functioning autism spectrum disorder (Conaughton, Donovan, & March, 2017). As outlined in Table 1, ICBT showed significantly greater reductions in anxiety compared to the WLC at posttreatment, with effects being maintained or enhanced at follow-up. However, we note that the percent free of the primary diagnosis did not differ significantly from the WLC at posttreatment and continued to be lower at follow-up than in most other studies in Table 1. Thus, additional intervention components are suggested for this population.

A recent study examined the impact of I/CCBT with children and adolescents with social anxiety disorder (SAD) as their primary presenting problem (Spence et al., 2017). The researchers noted that there was convincing evidence that treatment outcomes for youth with SAD who received generic CBT in clinic contexts (that is, traditional CBT in which the same intervention is received irrespective of the type of anxiety disorder) tended to be weaker than outcomes for youth with other types of anxiety disorder (Hudson, Keers, et al., 2015; Hudson, Rapee, et al., 2015). The RCT included 125 clinically anxious youth aged 8–17 years, who were randomly assigned to (i) WLC, (ii) the generic ICBT program BRAVE-ONLINE, or (iii) an adapted version of BRAVE-ONLINE that was specifically tailored to SAD. The SAD-specific program included components for social skills training, reduction in self-focused attention, and cognitive-restructuring examples that illustrated specifically the social dimensions of anxiety and cognition, in addition to psychoeducation, relaxation skills, problem-solving skills, and self-reinforcement. Both treatment groups showed significantly greater reductions in clinician severity ratings (CSR) and parent and youth ratings of anxiety and social anxiety than the WLC from pre- to posttreatment, and there was no difference between the generic and disorder-specific treatments. However, the treatments did not differ from the WLC at posttreatment in terms of percent free of their primary diagnosis. By 6-month follow-up, reductions in anxiety were maintained or enhanced, and the percent free of their primary diagnosis had improved in both treatments, with 53 percent of the social phobia specific and 47 percent of the generic I/CCBT group reaching this indicator of remission. These figures are very similar to the percent free of SAD reported from clinic-based studies of generic CBT (Hudson, Keers, et al., 2015; Hudson, Rapee, et al., 2015). Thus, the addition of the social anxiety specific content did not appear to enhance the efficacy of generic ICBT as proposed.

Although these studies indicate emerging developments in research into the use of I/CCBT with different populations, there is a clear need for further investigations with other subgroups, such as youth from specific cultural or demographic backgrounds, to ensure that the findings are generalized. Adaptations to the programs can then be made on the basis of feedback from youth, parents, and clinicians.

Mediators and Moderators of Change

Given the relatively few evaluations of I/CCBT to date, it is not surprising that there is limited information about mediators and moderators of change. Furthermore, the sample sizes in most of the studies have been insufficient to enable valid examination of mediators and moderators of change. The limited evidence to date tends to raise more questions than it provides answers for. For example, Anderson et al. (2012) examined the impact of the therapist-client working alliance and treatment compliance in the prediction of outcome following ICBT with 132 anxious children and adolescents. The study found that, while overall levels of working alliance and treatment compliance did not predict response to ICBT, these effects were moderated by age. That is, higher working alliance and program compliance predicted better treatment outcome for teenagers, but not for children. Both were found to have direct effects upon reductions in anxiety symptoms, and compliance was not found to mediate the relationship between the working alliance and outcome. Gender, age of child, family income, and parental education were not found to moderate outcome. Vigerland, Ljotsson, et al. (2016) also did not find treatment compliance (in terms of session content completed) to predict outcome in their evaluation of ICBT with children. The other studies in Table 1 did not examine moderators and mediators of change, and this is clearly an area for future research. It would be valuable to determine whether factors such as anxiety severity, type of diagnosis, number of anxiety disorders and other comorbidity, motivation, client perceptions of credibility, expectancy, and satisfaction, or involvement of parents influence outcome.

Mobile Applications: Some Specific Issues

The studies reviewed above used CBT interventions delivered in real time over the internet (using a computer or mobile device) or using a stand-alone computer, rather than through mobile applications (APPs) on a mobile device. APPs have the advantage that they can be downloaded onto a mobile device such as a smartphone or tablet and used off-line without an internet connection for many activities. The APP can then reconnect with the internet at a future point when information can be synchronized, thereby providing greater flexibility for the user. In 2013, it was noted that more mobile APPs had been downloaded than there were people on the earth, and more than 13.4 billion downloads of APPs occurred in the first quarter of 2013 (Hides, 2014). No doubt this number has expanded since. A visit to mobile application stores reveals a phenomenal number of APPs providing information and treatment programs and tools for every conceivable mental health problem (Bakker et al., 2016; Sucala et al., 2017), including many relevant to child and adolescent anxiety.

A major issue in the selection of mobile APPs is that the vast majority have not been evaluated in terms of effectiveness (Anthes, 2016). To date, research into the use of APPs for the treatment of anxiety in children and adolescents has been limited to evaluations of client/therapist judgments of acceptability, utility, feasibility, and satisfaction, rather than the impact upon anxiety. For example, Pramana et al. (2014) reported the development of an APP to support clinician administered CBT for youth anxiety, with a view to potentially shortening the number of face-to-face sessions required. The APP included information and tasks designed to provide daily review of skills and information presented in sessions, prompt completion of home-based tasks, exposures, and use of CBT skills in real-life settings, and increase opportunities for communication between the youth, parents, and therapist via a secure portal. It included gamification techniques to increase youth engagement with the content and provided personalized, data-driven feedback about progress. In a small pilot study, anxious youth and therapists reported the APP to be useful and acceptable. Another example is the REACH for success APP. Stoll et al. (2016) reported the development of this APP, which aims to increase out-of-session activities to support clinic-based CBT. Some of the interesting design features included fillable forms that used an avatar, speech capture, gaming (progressive reward incentives), on-device recording of user responses, situations, and subjective units of distress, and a data export feature. The APP was highly rated by youth and clinicians in terms of usability, acceptability, and satisfaction. However, the impact upon youth anxiety is yet to be evaluated. Finally, Whiteside (2016) described the development of the Mayo Clinic Anxiety Coach, with modules covering self-evaluation, psychoeducation, and exposure. The APP can be used by adolescents and children with parental support, although it is also designed for use by adults. It includes 24 predetermined exposure hierarchies for Social Anxiety Disorder, Separation Anxiety Disorder, and Specific Phobias, with guidance for implementation. The available data are so far limited to usage statistics.

Given the proliferation of mobile APPs, it is extremely important that high-quality research is conducted to determine their effectiveness as either stand-alone interventions or adjuncts to clinic-based treatment. Unfortunately, young people tend to purchase and download them based on popularity rather than evidence (Hides, 2014). It is also important that research examines the impact of different strategies to increase client engagement and persistence with APP usage. Hides (2014) reported that initial enthusiasm for the use of APPs tends to wane quickly, and mental health APPs are rarely used for more than 10 occasions. Thus, we need an evidence base to assist young people and mental health practitioners to select those that are most likely to be of value.

Virtual Reality

Virtual reality (VR) allows the user to navigate and interact with a preprogrammed, 3D computer-generated environment that is experienced via either head-mounted displays or immersive rooms. The participant experiences a sense of presence and immersion, providing live opportunities for interactivity and skill rehearsal that are not possible in static I/CCBT programs. He or she may be able to move around, interact with characters and objects and, in more sophisticated programs, the environment can respond to the participant's actions. Thus, it provides an excellent opportunity to recreate contexts and experiences that can be controlled by the clinician, unlike real-world experiences.

Virtual Reality Exposure Therapy (VRET) provides opportunity to efficiently confront fears in less threatening virtual settings ("in virtuo"), providing safe and controlled opportunities for repeated exposure. Research examining the use of VRET in childhood anxiety is scarce, but emerging. With respect to spider phobia, a single case study (Bouchard et al., 2007) followed by a larger pilot study (St-Jacques, Bouchard, & Bélanger, 2010) demonstrated the initial feasibility of VR in the delivery of exposure therapy and reduction of fear in spider phobic children. In a small trial, Gutiérrez-Maldonado et al. (2009) demonstrated that children with school phobia receiving VRET showed significant reductions in school fears following treatment. The feasibility of VRET has also been demonstrated for social phobia in children. A small case series showed that four out of five adolescents completing VRET for social phobia (e.g., giving speeches to virtual classrooms) reported reductions in weekly anxiety over the course of treatment (Doré & Bouchard, 2006). Finally, in a recent study, Wong Sarver, Beidel, and Spitalnick (2014) examined the utility of an interactive virtual school environment for the exposure and skills rehearsal component of a CBT intervention for social anxiety disorder in children. The VR component was judged to be a highly credible and acceptable component of therapy.

The studies to date have involved only small sample sizes, and lack control conditions and therefore its use in the treatment of childhood anxiety cannot yet be endorsed with confidence. However, VR offers a promising technological approach to the delivery of exposure therapy in childhood anxiety, with promising pilot data suggesting the acceptability, utility, and potential efficacy of this approach for exposure therapy and skills rehearsal.

Future Directions for Research

Research into the effectiveness of I/CCBT for youth anxiety summarized previously tentatively suggests that outcomes are generally positive and that this approach does have a role to play in clinical service delivery. Nevertheless, there are considerable weaknesses in the research to date that need to be addressed in future studies before firm conclusions can be drawn. Most of the RCTs have been limited to comparisons with WLCs and therefore it is unclear whether the improvements demonstrated are simply nonspecific intervention effects. More RCTs are required that compare I/CCBT for youth anxiety with attention placebo, treatment as usual, and clinic-delivered CBT conditions. Sample sizes need to be larger so that studies have sufficient power to detect small effect size differences between conditions, and so that examinations of moderators and mediators of treatment outcome can be conducted. It is important that evidence is produced regarding the characteristics of those who respond well to I/CCBT versus those for whom this approach is not to be recommended. Ultimately, we need sufficient RCTs to enable the conduct of valid meta-analyses that enable examination of the impact of different dimensions of delivery, such as level and type of therapist support, parent participation, extent of program interactivity, use of audio and video clips, and the impact of different strategies to increase client engagement and compliance. Finally, economic analyses, in terms of costs and benefits of such interventions, are needed for both preventive and clinical I/CCBT interventions.

Clinical Issues

The Use of I/CCBT for Anxious Young People in Clinical Practice and Barriers to Uptake. Although children, parents, and clinicians generally hold positive views about the potential value of I/CCBT, mental health professionals have been slow to make use of new technologies in their clinical practice (Vigerland et al., 2014). There are various barriers to the adoption of I/CCBT including the exclusion of I/CCBT sessions from some health fund rebate schemes, reluctance of some health services to purchase access to I/CCBT programs or APPs for their clients, and therapist concerns about the suitability of I/CCBT. Clinicians tend to have particular worries about the use of I/CCBT with clients with more severe and complex issues where they perceive that a face-to-face therapist can better monitor progress, address comorbid or urgent issues, and adapt treatment in a more flexible way in response to challenging or urgent situations (Vigerland et al., 2014). To some extent, the concerns of therapists reflect their tendency to think of I/CCBT as a self-help approach that replaces clinic-based treatment and that is only suitable for mild cases, rather than an approach that can be used with clinician support to enhance clinic-based therapy (Stallard, Richardson, et al., 2010). The evidence reviewed in this chapter suggests that I/CCBT, when combined with at least a minimal level of clinician support, does not lead to high levels of dropout and low compliance, and that fears of an adverse impact upon the therapist-client relationship are unfounded.

Another factor that is likely to contribute to low levels of uptake of I/CCBT by clinicians relates to their belief that they lack the training, knowledge, and expertise to use I/CCBT, and are not aware about what is available, what is effective, and how to use such approaches (MacLeod, Martinez, & Williams, 2009). Indeed, there is relatively little evidence to inform practitioners about what programs are effective, and training in e-mental health interventions is not typically part of the curriculum of degree programs in mental health disciplines. Not surprisingly, knowledge relating to I/CCBT is found to predict clinician attitudes about the use of this approach, and more positive attitudes are acquired following the viewing of a brief information video (Donovan et al., 2015). Thus, in the future, it is important that clinical training and professional development programs include content relating to the various ways in which I/CCBT can be used, with supervised practice in actually implementing such interventions. Similarly, the clinical use of I/CCBT needs to be included in ongoing professional development programs. Some useful online resources and courses have already been developed for practitioners intending to use I/CCBT (e.g., https://schools.au.reachout.com/using-e-mental-health-services). Resources of this type provide information about what I/CCBT programs and tools are available for specific disorders and the associated evidence of effectiveness, along with information addressing common concerns of clinicians and guidelines about how to use I/CCBT in clinical practice. Material also covers ethical and professional issues regarding confidentiality of data, secure storage of client responses, monitoring treatment compliance and progress, mechanisms for dealing with crises, and ways of providing additional support if required.

Increasing Participant Engagement, Therapy Compliance, and Program Completion. Although participant engagement and compliance are relatively good for therapist-guided I/CCBT for youth anxiety, these are clearly areas of concern for I/CCBT when it is delivered in a fully self-help format. Drop out from therapy is not always a bad thing if the client has made rapid improvements in the early sessions and they feel that they no longer need assistance. However, for those who drop out despite continuing to experience high levels of anxiety, it is important that we identify ways to increase client engagement with the interventions and their motivation to complete sessions, particularly where there is no therapist to provide support and encouragement. In general, treatment compliance and therapy outcomes are found to be stronger for interventions that are supported by a therapist rather than those delivered on a purely self-help basis (Richards & Richardson, 2012). In the youth anxiety area, there are insufficient trials to allow firm conclusions to be drawn on this issue, as most outcome studies have included at least some monitoring by and/or feedback from a clinician (see Table 1). Furthermore, in many instances, I/CCBT for child and adolescent anxiety has included at least some parent involvement. Interestingly, there is emerging research from the adult literature suggesting that support provided by nonprofessionals (e.g., technicians) or professionals not trained in CBT can be as beneficial as support provided by specialist CBT clinicians (Titov, Andrews, Davies, et al., 2010). In the majority of I/CCBT programs, the core CBT components are built into the program and supported through multimedia mechanisms and interactive activities. Thus, specialized skills in CBT are not required from the support person and it may be possible to use nonclinicians, such as teachers, nurses, or youth workers, as support persons in treatment delivery without loss of efficacy. This is an area for future research.

A Program Illustration: Developing BRAVE-ONLINE

We will illustrate some of the practical aspects involved in the development and implementation of a particular program, namely BRAVE-ONLINE. This intervention was designed for the treatment of a range of anxiety disorders in 7–18-year-olds (Spence, Holmes, & Donovan, 2006; Spence, March, & Holmes, 2005). There are versions for children (7–12 years) and adolescents (13–18 years), with associated parent programs, all of which can be completed online using a desktop or laptop computer, tablet, or mobile device. More recently, an adapted version of the parent program has been trialled for preschoolers (Donovan & March, 2014), a self-help version has been implemented in an open trial (March et al., 2018), and a version that includes strategies specific to social anxiety disorder has been trialled with children and adolescents (Spence et al., 2017). Results from these trials were described in Table 4.1. The version presented as follows is "therapist assisted," in that a therapist is able to monitor the responses of youth and parents and has (minimal) email contact.

Program Content. The program includes 10 sessions for children and adolescents, and six sessions for parents (or five extended sessions for parents of adolescents). Sessions are completed once per week, providing time between sessions for practice of skills and completion of exposure tasks. The content of the BRAVE program includes evidence-based CBT components, namely psychoeducation, the detection of physiological signs of anxiety (B represents Body Signs), relaxation techniques (R represents Relax), cognitive strategies such as thought detection, cognitive restructuring, and coping statements (A represents Activate Helpful Thoughts), graded exposure and problem-solving skills (V represents Victory Over Your Fears), and self- and parent reinforcement (E represents Enjoy! Reward Yourself). The parent program provides an overview of material being learned by the child, and also includes parent strategies for parenting an anxious child (e.g., ignoring fearful behavior; prompting and rewarding "brave" responses).

Design Features. One of the key challenges in designing I/CCBT programs for youth is to present material in a way that facilitates learning, and that enhances client engagement and motivation to complete the sessions in the absence of face-to-face therapist contact. In both the child and adolescent BRAVE programs, participants are supported to complete the program with brief, weekly email feedback from a clinician, sent within 1–3 days of the youth or parent completing a session. The clinician is able to monitor participant activities and responses and uses a template system for their email communications. Participants also receive a 15–30-minute phone call from the clinician midway through the program to assist in developing the exposure hierarchy. In order to enhance the therapist-client relationship, we introduced the concept of a "Brave-Trainer" (rather than a therapist) in the adolescent program to whom participants are introduced in virtual terms through a web page (see Figure 4.1). Personalized, automated messages are also sent to the child throughout the program and signed from their "Brave-Trainer."

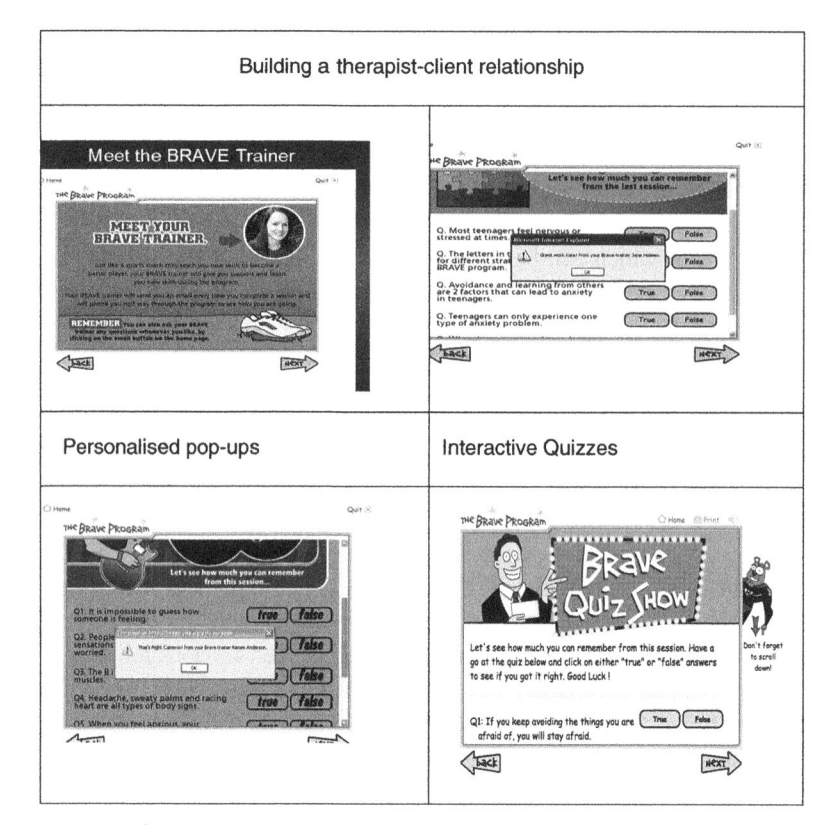

Figure 4.1 *BRAVE-ONLINE Illustrations.* © Copyright of The University of Queensland

In order to keep children engaged, the BRAVE-ONLINE sessions are not static web pages. The program presents the material in a stimulating and interactive way, with bright colors, sounds, animated cartoons, quizzes, and games. The sessions also include corrective/reinforcement messages, personalized messages/pop-ups, and automated feedback and reinforcement. The personalized pop-up messages aim to create a sense of contact with the therapist, even though they are computer generated.

Knowledge and skills are taught through vignettes, illustrated examples and stories, downloadable material, worksheets, quizzes, and home practice tasks. It was necessary to ensure that the material was age-appropriate, requiring different illustrations and examples for the child versus teen programs. The program makes use of a cartoon character (Brave Buddy) in the child program and hypothetical adolescents in the adolescent program to act as models in the demonstration of coping strategies and presentation of information (see Figure 4.2).

Developing a program of this type is not without its challenges. First, the cost of software development and graphic design is expensive, given that the number of web pages required for 10 child, 10 teen, six parent (children), and five parent (teens) sessions, plus two associated booster sessions, is extensive. In addition, technologies change over time requiring regular upgrades, some of which require extensive reprogramming. Also, children become more sophisticated in their use of internet

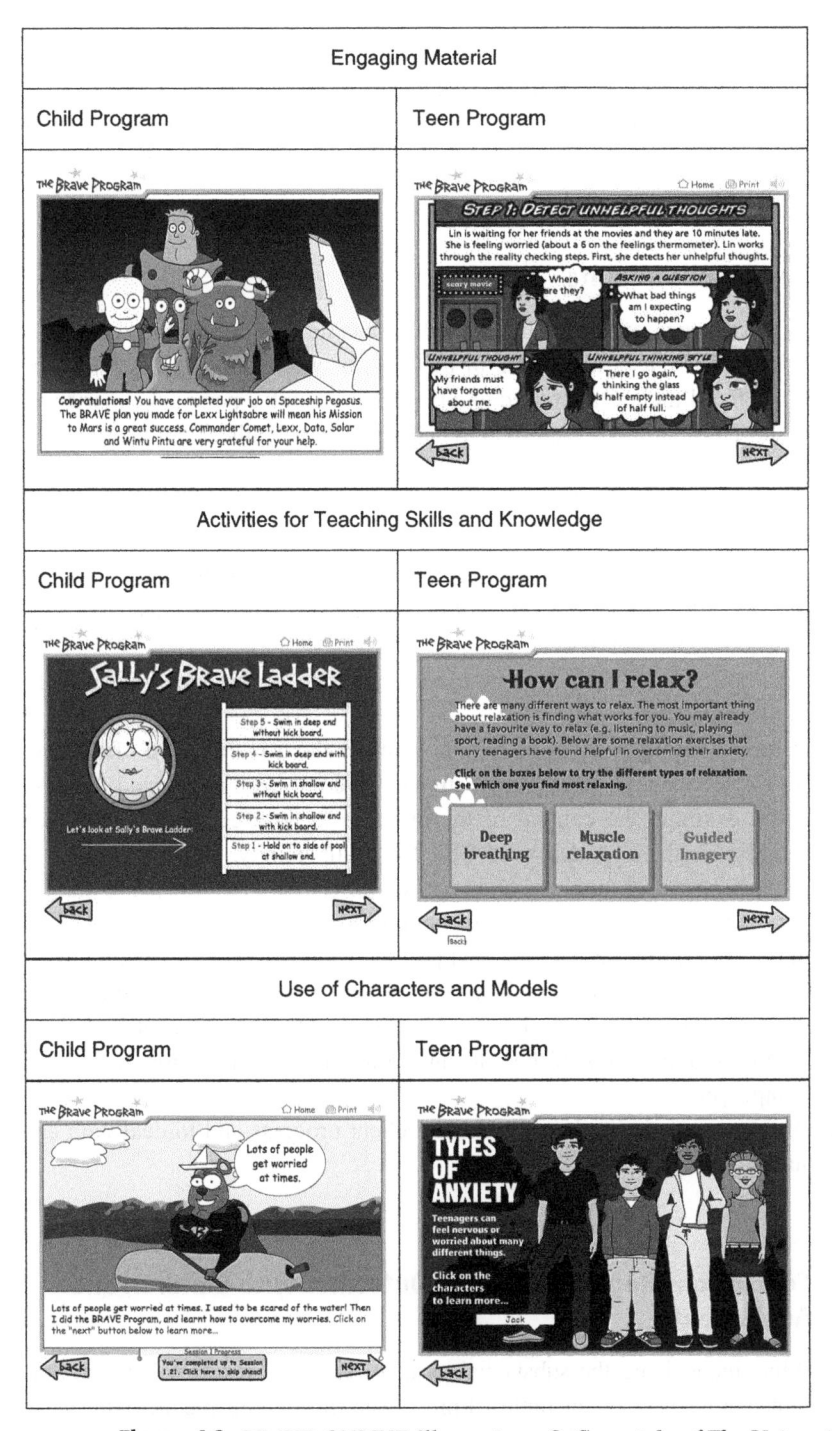

Figure 4.2 *BRAVE-ONLINE Illustrations.* © *Copyright of The University of Queensland*

programs and APPs, and their expectations change regarding the quality of graphics and the way in which material is presented. Furthermore, advances in knowledge about effective CBT strategies mean that these components should be integrated into I/CCBT interventions. Thus, we have the ongoing challenge and cost of upgrading the program to maintain high client satisfaction and to optimize treatment effectiveness.

Key Practice Points

In the absence of sufficient research to enable us to draw firm evidence-based conclusions about best-practice in I/CCBT for youth anxiety, the following guiding points for clinicians are based to a large degree on the personal experiences of the authors. They should therefore be regarded as "tips" rather than facts.

We suggest that, before implementing an I/CCBT program or tool in clinical practice, clinicians should:

- Complete an online training program for the use of I/CCBT with young people to increase your skills and knowledge in the area: https://schools.au.reachout.com/using-e-mental-health-services
- Clarify exactly how I/CCBT is to be used in practice as this will influence the selection of program or tools.
- Conduct some investigation to determine whether there is evidence of the program/tool's effectiveness. If empirical studies have not been conducted the clinician should examine the content of the program to ensure that it is based on evidence in line with clinic-delivered CBT for youth anxiety.
- Enroll in the program or purchase and use the tool yourself first to ensure that the content is appropriate for the age group and problem concerned.
- Select, if possible, programs or tools that provide feedback and information to the clinician so that one can monitor client progress and response to program tasks.
- Ensure that data provided by clients are securely stored and meet the client confidentiality requirements of the relevant professional organization, health service, or employer.
- Ensure that a system is in place to monitor client progress and to deal with any crises that may emerge.

Conclusions Regarding I/CCBT Outcomes with Children and Adolescents

While recognizing the substantial weaknesses in the research literature, the studies outlined previously and in Table 4.1 provide an encouraging picture of the value of I/CCBT in the prevention and treatment of anxiety in children and adolescents. We note that the surge of interest in I/CCBT and the proliferation of mobile applications relating to the treatment of youth anxiety have proceeded well ahead of the empirical support for their use. This is a particular issue for the use of APPs, as most of the research to date has made use of real-time internet programs or stand-alone computer programs rather than APPs on mobile devices. Also, we are a long way from knowing exactly which type of I/CCBT is likely to be effective for individual children with specific clinical and personal characteristics. The chapter also noted that, despite generally positive attitudes toward I/CCBT, clinicians have been relatively slow to make use of such programs and tools in their clinical practice. This was proposed to reflect their reservations and concerns about I/CCBT and lack of skills and knowledge about what is available, the evidence base, and how such programs and tools can be used in different contexts. There is a clear need to include I/CCBT approaches in training and continuing professional development programs for mental health professionals.

Despite the lag in empirical research, the promise held by the use of technology in therapy is enormous, with a myriad of exciting potential new ways that it could be incorporated into the delivery of CBT for anxious youth. Motivational interviewing (Titov, Andrews, Schwencke, et al., 2010), virtual "reward" systems, electronic prompts (e.g., SMS), avatars and computer gaming methods (Bobier et al., 2013), chat rooms, blogs, video meetings (e.g., Skype), and linked social media sites (e.g., Facebook, Twitter, Tumblr, or Instagram) could all be used to increase youth engagement and compliance with ICBT. Real-time personal tracking tools for recording locations, situations, activities, thoughts, and feelings, and providing instantaneous feedback are also becoming increasingly sophisticated and could be incorporated into ICBT programs. Undoubtedly yet more technological tools will be developed over the next decade that could also be used to enhance I/CCBT. The opportunities are endless, and we face exciting times ahead.

References

Achenbach, T. M., & Rescorla, L. A. (2001). *Manual for the ASEBA school-age forms and profiles*. Burlington: University of Vermont, Research Center for Children, Youth and Families.

Adelman, C. B., Panza, K. E., Bartley, C. A., Bontempo, A., & Bloch, M. H. (2014). A meta-analysis of computerized cognitive-behavioral therapy for the treatment of DSM-5 anxiety disorders. *The Journal of Clinical Psychiatry, 75*(7), e695-e704.

Anderson, R. E., Spence, S. H., Donovan, C. L., March, S., Prosser, S., & Kenardy, J. (2012). Working alliance in online cognitive behavior therapy for anxiety disorders in youth: Comparison with clinic delivery and its role in predicting outcome. *Journal of Medical Internet Research, 14*(3), 86–101.

Anthes, E. (2016). Pocket psychiatry: Mobile mental-health apps have exploded onto the market, but few have been thoroughly tested. *Nature, 532*(7597), 20–23.

Australian Bureau of Statistics. (2016). *Household Use of Information Technology, Australia, 2014–15 (8146.0)*. Canberra: Australian Bureau of Statistics.

Bakker, D., Kazantzis, N., Rickwood, D., & Rickard, N. (2016). Mental health smartphone apps: Review and evidence-based recommendations for future developments. *JMIR Mental Health, 3*(1), e7.

Beck, A. T., Epstein, N., Brown, G., & Steer, R. A. (1988). An inventory for measuring clinical anxiety: Psychometric properties. *Journal of Consulting and Clinical Psychology, 56*(6), 893–897.

Beidel, D. C., Turner, S. M., & Morris, T. L. (1995). A new inventory to assess childhood social anxiety and phobia: The Social Phobia and Anxiety Inventory for Children. *Psychological Assessment, 7*(1), 73–79.

Bennett, K., Manassis, K., Duda, S., Bagnell, A., Bernstein, G. A., Garland, E., . . . Wilansky, P. (2016). Treating child and adolescent anxiety effectively: Overview of systematic reviews. *Clinical Psychology Review, 50*, 80–94.

Berry, R. R., & Lai, B. (2014). The emerging role of technology in cognitive–behavioral therapy for anxious youth: A review. *Journal of Rational-Emotive and Cognitive-Behavior Therapy, 32*(1), 57–66.

Bobier, C., Stasiak, K., Mountford, H., Merry, S., & Moor, S. (2013). When 'e' therapy enters the hospital: Examination of the feasibility and acceptability of SPARX (a cCBT programme) in an adolescent inpatient unit. *Advances in Mental Health, 11*(3), 286–292.

Bouchard, S., St-Jacques, J., Robillard, G., & Renaud, P. (2007). Effectiveness of an exposure-based treatment for arachnophobia in children using virtual reality: A pilot study. *Journal de Thérapie Comportementale et Cognitive, 17*(3), 101–108.

Boyd, C., Francis, K., Aisbett, D., Newnham, K., Sewell, J., Dawes, G., & Nurse, S. (2007). Australian rural adolescents' experiences of accessing psychological help for a mental health problem. *Australian Journal of Rural Health, 15*(3), 196–200.

Cartwright-Hatton, S., Roberts, C., Chitsabesan, P., Fothergill, C., & Harrington, R. (2004). Systematic review of the efficacy of cognitive behaviour therapies for childhood and adolescent anxiety disorders. *British Journal of Clinical Psychology, 43*(4), 421–436.

Chavira, D. A., Stein, M. B., Bailey, K., & Stein, M. T. (2004). Child anxiety in primary care: Prevalent but untreated. *Depression and Anxiety, 20*(4), 155–164.

Chorpita, B. F., Tracey, S. A., Brown, T. A., Collica, T. J., & Barlow, D. H. (1997). Assessment of worry in children and adolescents: An adaptation of the Penn State Worry Questionnaire. *Behaviour Research and Therapy, 35*(6), 569–581.

Conaughton, R. J., Donovan, C. L., & March, S. (2017). Efficacy of an internet-based CBT program for children with comorbid High Functioning Autism Spectrum Disorder and anxiety: A randomised controlled trial. *Journal of Affective Disorders, 218*, 260–268.

Donovan, C. L., & March, S. (2014). Online CBT for preschool anxiety disorders: A randomised control trial. *Behaviour Research and Therapy, 58*(1), 24–35.

Donovan, C. L., Poole, C., Boyes, N., Redgate, J., & March, S. (2015). Australian mental health worker attitudes towards cCBT: What is the role of knowledge? Are there differences? Can we change them? *Internet Interventions, 2*(4), 372–381.

Doré, F., & Bouchard, S. (2006). *Using virtual reality to treat social anxiety disorders in adolescents*. Paper presented at The 11th Annual CyberTherapy Conference, Gatineau, Canada.

Ebert, D. D., Zarski, A.-C., Christensen, H., Stikkelbroek, Y., Cuijpers, P., Berking, M., & Riper, H. (2015). Internet and computer-based cognitive behavioral therapy for anxiety and depression in youth: A meta-analysis of randomized controlled outcome trials. *PloS One Vol 10 (3), 2015, ArtID e0119895, 10*(3).

Ewing, D. L., Monsen, J. J., Thompson, E. J., Cartwright-Hatton, S., & Field, A. (2015). A meta-analysis of transdiagnostic cognitive behavioural therapy in the treatment of child and young person anxiety disorders. *Behavioural and Cognitive Psychotherapy, 43*(5), 562–577.

Goodman, R. (1997). The Strengths and Difficulties Questionnaire: A research note. *Journal of Child Psychology and Psychiatry and Allied Disciplines, 38*(5), 581–586.

Gren-Landell, M., Björklind, A., Tillfors, M., Furmark, T., Svedin, C. G., & Andersson, G. (2009). Evaluation of the psychometric properties of a modified version of the Social Phobia Screening Questionnaire for use in adolescents. *Child and Adolescent Psychiatry and Mental Health, 3*(1), 36.

Gutiérrez-Maldonado, J., Magallón-Neri, E., Rus-Calafell, M., & Peñaloza-Salazar, C. (2009). Virtual reality exposure therapy for school phobia. *Anuario de Psicología, 40*(2), 223–236.

Guy, W. (ed.) (1976). *ECDEU Assessment Manual for Psychopharmacology.* Rockville, MD: US Department of Health, Education, and Welfare. Public Health Service. Alcohol, Drug Abuse, and Mental Health Administration.

Hides, L. (2014). Are SMART apps the future of youth mental health? *InPsych, June.*

Hudson, J. L., Keers, R., Roberts, S., Coleman, J. R. I., Breen, G., Arendt, K., ... Eley, T. C. (2015). Clinical predictors of response to cognitive-behavioral therapy in pediatric anxiety disorders: The genes for treatment (GxE) study. *Journal of the American Academy of Child and Adolescent Psychiatry, 54*(6), 454–463.

Hudson, J. L., Rapee, R. M., Lyneham, H. J., McLellan, L. F., Wuthrich, V. M., & Schniering, C. A. (2015). Comparing outcomes for children with different anxiety disorders following cognitive behavioural therapy. *Behaviour Research and Therapy, 72,* 30–37.

In-Albon, T., Meyer, A. H., & Schneider, S. (2013). Separation anxiety avoidance inventory-child and parent version: Psychometric properties and clinical utility in a clinical and school sample. *Child Psychiatry and Human Development, 44*(6), 689–697.

James, A. C., James, G., Cowdrey, F. A., Soler, A., & Choke, A. (2015). *Cognitive behavioural therapy for anxiety disorders in children and adolescents.* Cochrane Database Systematic Review.

Khanna, M. S., & Kendall, P. C. (2010). Computer-assisted cognitive behavioral therapy for child anxiety: Results of a randomized clinical trial. *Journal of Consulting and Clinical Psychology, 78*(5), 737–745.

Lawrence, D., Johnson, S., Hafekost, J., Boterhoven De Haan, K., Sawyer, M., Ainley, J., & Zubrick, S. R. (2015). *The Mental Health of Children and Adolescents. Report on the Second Australian Child and Adolescent Survey of Mental Health and Wellbeing.* Canberra: Department of Health.

Liebowitz, M. R. (1987). Social phobia. *Modern Problems of Pharmacopsychiatry, 22,* 141–173.

Livingstone, S., & Bober, M. (2004). Taking up opportunities? Children's uses of the internet for education, communication and participation. *E-learning, 1*(3), 395–419.

Ly, K. H., Dahl, J., Carlbring, P., & Andersson, G. (2012). Development and initial evaluation of a smartphone application based on acceptance and commitment therapy. *SpringerPlus, 1*(1), 1–11.

MacLeod, M., Martinez, R., & Williams, C. (2009). Cognitive behaviour therapy self-help: Who does it help and what are its drawbacks? *Behavioural and Cognitive Psychotherapy, 37*(1), 61–72.

March, J. S., Parker, J. D., Sullivan, K., Stallings, P., & Conners, C. (1997). The Multidimensional Anxiety Scale for Children (MASC): Factor structure, reliability, and validity. *Journal of the American Academy of Child and Adolescent Psychiatry, 36*(4), 554–565.

March, S., Spence, S. H., & Donovan, C. L. (2009). The efficacy of an Internet-based cognitive-behavioral therapy intervention for child anxiety disorders. *Journal of Pediatric Psychology, 34*(5), 474–487.

March, S., Spence, S. H., Donovan, C. L., & Kenardy, J. (2018). Large-scale dissemination of internet-based cognitive behavioral therapy for youth anxiety: Feasibility and acceptability study. *Journal of Medical Internet Research, 20*(7): e234.

Merikangas, K. R., He, J.-P., Brody, D., Fisher, P. W., Bourdon, K., & Koretz, D. S. (2010). Prevalence and treatment of mental disorders among US children in the 2001–2004 NHANES. *Pediatrics, 125*(1), 75.

Mission Australia. (2017). *Youth Mental Health Report: Youth Survey 2012–2016*. Sydney: Mission Australia.

Ollendick, T. H. (1983). Reliability and validity of the Revised Fear Survey Schedule for Children (FSSC-R). *Behaviour Research and Therapy, 21*(6), 685–692.

Pennant, M. E., Loucas, C. E., Whittington, C., Creswell, C., Fonagy, P., Fuggle, P., … Kendall, T. (2015). Computerised therapies for anxiety and depression in children and young people: A systematic review and meta-analysis. *Behaviour Research and Therapy, 67*, 1–18.

Pramana, G., Parmanto, B., Kendall, P. C., & Silk, J. S. (2014). The SmartCAT: An m-Health platform for ecological momentary intervention in child anxiety treatment. *Telemedicine and e-Health, 20*(5), 419–427.

Reyes-Portillo, J. A., Mufson, L., Greenhill, L. L., Gould, M. S., Fisher, P. W., Tarlow, N., & Rynn, M. A. (2014). Web-based interventions for youth internalizing problems: A systematic review. *Journal of the American Academy of Child and Adolescent Psychiatry, 53*(12), 1254–1270.e1255.

Reynolds, S., Wilson, C., Austin, J., & Hooper, L. (2012). Effects of psychotherapy for anxiety in children and adolescents: A meta-analytic review. *Clinical Psychology Review, 32*(4), 251–262.

Richards, D., & Richardson, T. (2012). Computer-based psychological treatments for depression: A systematic review and meta-analysis. *Clinical Psychology Review, 32*(4), 329–342.

Riddle, M. A., Ginsburg, G. S., Walkup, J. T., Labelarte, M. J., Pine, D. S., Davies, M., … Pediat Psychopharmacology, A. (2002). The Pediatric Anxiety Rating Scale (PARS): Development and psychometric properties. *Journal of the American Academy of Child and Adolescent Psychiatry, 41*(9), 1061–1069.

Rideout, V. J., & Katz, V. S. (2016). Opportunity for all? Technology and learning in lower-income families. A report of the Families and Media Project. New York: The Joan Ganz Cooney Center at Sesame Workshop.

Rooksby, M., Elouafkaoui, P., Humphris, G., Clarkson, J., & Freeman, R. (2015). Internet-assisted delivery of cognitive behavioural therapy (CBT) for childhood anxiety: Systematic review and meta-analysis. *Journal of Anxiety Disorders, 29*(1), 83–92.

Salloum, A., Crawford, E. A., Lewin, A. B., & Storch, E. A. (2015). Consumers' and providers' perceptions of utilizing a computer-assisted cognitive behavioral therapy for childhood anxiety. *Behavioural and Cognitive Psychotherapy, 43*(1), 31–41.

Salloum, A., Johnco, C., Lewin, A. B., McBride, N. M., & Storch, E. A. (2016). Barriers to access and participation in community mental health treatment for anxious children. *Journal of Affective Disorders, 196*, 54–61.

Shaffer, D., Gould, M. S., Brasic, J., Ambrosini, P., Fisher, P., Bird, H., & Aluwahlia, S. (1983). A Children's Global Assessment Scale (CGAS). *Archives of General Psychiatry, 40*(11), 1228–1231.

Silfvernagel, K., Gren-Landell, M., Emanuelsson, M., Carlbring, P., Andersson, G., Linköpings, u., ... Östergötlands Läns, L. (2015). Individually tailored internet-based cognitive behavior therapy for adolescents with anxiety disorders: A pilot effectiveness study. *Internet Interventions, 2*(3), 297–302.

Silverman, W. K., & Albano, A. M. (1996). *Anxiety disorders interview schedule for children for DSM-IV: Child and parent versions*. San Antonio, TX: The Psychological Corporation – Harcourt, Brace & Company.

Spence, S. H. (1998). A measure of anxiety symptoms among children. *Behaviour Research and Therapy, 36*(5), 545–566.

Spence, S. H., Donovan, C. L., March, S., Gamble, A., Anderson, R. E., Prosser, S., & Kenardy, J. (2011). A randomized controlled trial of online versus clinic-based CBT for adolescent anxiety. *Journal of Consulting and Clinical Psychology, 79*(5), 629–642.

Spence, S. H., Donovan, C. L., March, S., Kenardy, J. A., & Hearn, C. S. (2017). Generic versus disorder specific cognitive behavior therapy for social anxiety disorder in youth: A randomized controlled trial using internet delivery. *Behaviour Research and Therapy, 90*, 41–57.

Spence, S. H., Holmes, J. M., & Donovan, C. L. (2006). *BRAVE for Teenagers – ONLINE: An internet-based program for adolescents with anxiety*. Brisbane, Australia: School of Psychology, University of Queensland.

Spence, S. H., Holmes, J. M., March, S., & Lipp, O. V. (2006). The feasibility and outcome of clinic plus internet delivery of cognitive-behavior therapy for childhood anxiety. *Journal of Consulting and Clinical Psychology, 74*(3), 614–621.

Spence, S. H., March, S., & Holmes, J. M. (2005). *BRAVE for Children – ONLINE: An internet-based program for children with anxiety*. Brisbane, Australia: School of Psychology, University of Queensland.

Spence, S. H., Rapee, R., McDonald, C., & Ingram, M. (2001). The structure of anxiety symptoms among preschoolers. *Behaviour Research and Therapy, 39*(11), 1293–1316.

Spence, S. H., Sawyer, M. G., Sheffield, J., Patton, G., Bond, L., Graetz, B., & Kay, D. (2014). Does the absence of a supportive family environment influence the outcome of a universal intervention for the prevention of depression? *International Journal of Environmental Research and Public Health, 11*(5), 5113–5132.

St-Jacques, J., Bouchard, S., & Bélanger, C. (2010). Is virtual reality effective to motivate and raise interest in phobic children towards therapy? *Journal of Clinical Psychiatry, 71*(7), 924–931.

Stallard, P., Richardson, T., & Velleman, S. (2010). Clinicians' attitudes towards the use of computerized cognitive behaviour therapy (cCBT) with children and adolescents. *Behavioural and Cognitive Psychotherapy, 38*(05), 545–560.

Stallard, P., Udwin, O., Goddard, M., & Hibbert, S. (2007). The availability of cognitive behaviour therapy within specialist child and adolescent mental health services (CAMHS): A national survey. *Behavioural and Cognitive Psychotherapy, 35*(4), 501–505.

Stallard, P., Velleman, S., & Richardson, T. (2010). Computer use and attitudes towards computerized therapy amongst young people and parents attending child and adolescent mental health services. *Child and Adolescent Mental Health, 15*(2), 80–84.

Stasiak, K., Fleming, T., Lucassen, M. F., Shepherd, M. J., Whittaker, R., & Merry, S. N. (2016). Computer-based and online therapy for depression and anxiety in children and adolescents. *Journal of Child and Adolescent Psychopharmacology, 26*(3), 235–245.

Stoll, R. D., Pina, A. A., Gary, K., & Amresh, A. (2017). Usability of a smartphone application to support the prevention and early intervention of anxiety in youth. *Cognitive and Behavioral Practice, 24*(4), 393–404.

Storch, E. A., Salloum, A., King, M. A., Crawford, E. A., Andel, R., McBride, N. M., & Lewin, A. B. (2015). A randomized controlled trial in community mental health centers of computer-assisted cognitive behavioral therapy versus treatment as usual for children with anxiety. *Depression and Anxiety, 32*(11), 843–852.

Sucala, M., Cuijpers, P., Muench, F., Cardoş, R., Soflau, R., Dobrean, A., . . . David, D. (2017). Anxiety: There is an app for that. A systematic review of anxiety apps. *Depression and Anxiety, 34*(6), 518–525.

Tillfors, M., Andersson, G., Ekselius, L., Furmark, T., Lewenhaupt, S., Karlsson, A., & Carlbring, P. (2011). A randomized trial of internet-delivered treatment for social anxiety disorder in high school students. *Cognitive Behaviour Therapy, 40*(2), 147–157.

Titov, N., Andrews, G., Davies, M., McIntyre, K., Robinson, E., & Solley, K. (2010). Internet treatment for depression: A randomized controlled trial comparing clinician vs. technician assistance. *PloS One Vol 5 (6), Jun 2010, ArtID e10939, 5*(6).

Titov, N., Andrews, G., Schwencke, G., Robinson, E., Peters, L., & Spence, J. (2010). Randomized controlled trial of internet cognitive behavioural treatment for social phobia with and without motivational enhancement strategies. *Australian and New Zealand Journal of Psychiatry, 44*(10), 938–945.

Vigerland, S., Lenhard, F., Bonnert, M., Lalouni, M., Hedman, E., Ahlen, J., . . . Ljotsson, B. (2016). Internet-delivered cognitive behavior therapy for children and adolescents: A systematic review and meta-analysis. *Clinical Psychology Review, 50,* 1–10.

Vigerland, S., Ljótsson, B., Bergdahl Gustafsson, F., Hagert, S., Thulin, U., Andersson, G., & Serlachius, E. (2014). Attitudes towards the use of computerized cognitive behavior therapy (cCBT) with children and adolescents: A survey among Swedish mental health professionals. *Internet Interventions, 1*(3), 111–117.

Vigerland, S., Ljotsson, B., Thulin, U., Ost, L.-G., Andersson, G., & Serlachius, E. (2016). Internet-delivered cognitive behavioural therapy for children with anxiety disorders: A randomised controlled trial. *Behaviour Research and Therapy, 76,* 47–56.

Vigerland, S., Serlachius, E., Thulin, U., Andersson, G., Larsson, J.-O., & Ljotsson, B. (2017). Long-term outcomes and predictors of internet-delivered cognitive behavioral therapy for childhood anxiety disorders. *Behaviour Research and Therapy, 90,* 67–75.

Vigerland, S., Thulin, U., Ljotsson, B., Svirsky, L., Ost, L.-G., Lindefors, N., . . . Serlachius, E. (2013). Internet-delivered CBT for children with specific phobia: A pilot study. *Cognitive Behaviour Therapy, 42*(4), 303–314.

Whiteside, S. P. H. (2016). Mobile device-based applications for childhood anxiety disorders. *Journal of Child and Adolescent Psychopharmacology, 26*(3), 246–251.

Wong Sarver, N., Beidel, D., & Spitalnick, J. (2014). The feasibility and acceptability of virtual environments in the treatment of childhood social anxiety disorder. *Journal of Clinical Child and Adolescent Psychology, 43*(1), 63–73.

Wuthrich, V. M., Rapee, R. M., Cunningham, M. J., Lyneham, H. J., Hudson, J. L., & Schniering, C. A. (2012). A randomized controlled trial of the Cool Teens CD-ROM computerized program for adolescent anxiety. *Journal of the American Academy of Child and Adolescent Psychiatry, 51*(3), 261–270.

Ye, X., Bapuji, S. B., Winters, S. E., Struthers, A., Raynard, M., Metge, C., ... Sutherland, K. (2014). Effectiveness of internet-based interventions for children, youth, and young adults with anxiety and/or depression: A systematic review and meta-analysis. *BMC Health Services Research, 14*(1), 313.

5 Cognitive Bias Modification Strategies for Anxious Children
Attention and Interpretation Bias Retraining

Jennie M. Kuckertz and Nader Amir

Over the last decade, research on computerized interventions for anxiety disorders has advanced rapidly. Such research is the culmination of influences, including the increasing prominence of technology, an emerging understanding of the role of cognition in the etiology and maintenance of anxiety disorders, and a growing emphasis on mechanism-driven approaches to clinical interventions. Such interventions, borne out of the intersection of the cognitive, experimental, and clinical psychology literatures, emphasize modification of cognitive biases that are implicated in the etiology and maintenance of anxiety disorders. This class of interventions, referred to as cognitive bias modification (CBM), are defined as any program that includes "direct manipulation of a target cognitive bias, by extended exposure to task contingencies that favor predetermined patterns of processing selectivity" (MacLeod & Mathews, 2012, p. 191).

CBM comprises two subclasses of interventions: 1) those targeting attentional processes (attention bias modification, ABM), and 2) those targeting interpretation processes (interpretation bias modification, IBM). Although initial research on CBM programs focused predominantly on anxious adult populations, in recent years there has been an increased research focus on implementation of these programs for anxious children and adolescents. Several reviews have examined the preliminary efficacy of CBM interventions for youth (Cristea, Mogoase et al., 2015; Lowther & Newman, 2014), hence the goal of the current chapter is to briefly describe extant findings specifically from the child anxiety literature while commenting on directions for future research and clinical practice. As the CBM literature in clinically anxious child populations is not as extensive as the literature in adults, we also describe findings from the adult anxiety CBM literature in areas in which the child anxiety CBM literature is less developed. We also note that CBM may also include strategies designed to modify memory bias (Vrijsen, Hertel, & Becker, 2016) or automatic action tendencies (Huijding et al., 2009); however, these interventions have a much smaller evidence base and thus it is not currently possible to review their efficacy for anxious youth.

Overview of the Issue

Child anxiety disorders cause significant impairment across multiple domains of functioning, including school, social, and home/family life (Langley et al., 2014; Langley et al., 2004). In addition to the significant impairment associated with anxiety disorders, presence of an anxiety disorder in childhood confers risk for later psychopathology, including other anxiety disorders and depression (Bittner et al., 2007; Foley et al., 2004; Goldstein et al., 2006). Anxiety disorders are common, with approximately 17 percent of youths in primary care settings meeting criteria for an anxiety disorder in the last year (Chavira et al., 2004). Considering the impairment, chronicity, and prevalence of anxiety disorders in children, treatment represents a pressing public health need.

Evidence-based efficacious treatments for child anxiety disorders include cognitive behavioral therapy (CBT) and medication, most notably selective serotonin reuptake inhibitors (SSRIs) (Connolly, Bernstein, & The Work Group on Quality Issues, 2007; Manassis, Russell, & Newton, 2010; Walkup et al., 2008). Despite the existence of efficacious treatments, approximately 72 percent of children with an anxiety disorder do not receive any form of treatment (Chavira et al., 2004). Engagement in treatment is limited by a variety of factors, including lack of access to trained providers, skeptical provider attitudes toward evidence-based practices, high costs associated with CBT and/or SSRIs, wanting to handle treatment on one's own, parent concerns related to medication, and stigma associated with seeking treatment (Christiana et al., 2000; Collins et al., 2004; Gunter & Whittal, 2010). Attempts to address these barriers have been met with mixed success, leading some to express frustration that "for the past 50 years, calls for placing more behavioral and developmental health care providers in rural areas have failed" (Kelleher & Gardner, 2010, pp. 1301–1302).

An alternate approach may be to develop delivery methods and/or interventions that bypass these barriers. In recent years, the increasing presence of and familiarity with technology has led to considerable research aimed at delivering care for youth anxiety disorders via such platforms (Rooksby et al., 2015). Data from a nationally representative sample suggest that 69 percent of adolescents in the United States spend at least one hour per day on mobile phones, tablets, computers, or video games (Kenney & Gortmaker, 2017). In addition to their ability to be delivered at home via computer or mobile devices, CBM interventions do not require interaction with a therapist, are often reframed as "brain training," and have the potential to be delivered at low or no cost. Thus, CBM interventions offer the possibility of simultaneously addressing many barriers to access of care. In addition to lack of access, even with gold standard care for child anxiety (e.g., CBT with SSRI), approximately 2 in 5 children do not respond to treatment. Thus, CBM may represent a potentially useful adjunct to standard treatment (Beard, 2011; Hakamata et al., 2010).

Finally, CBM represents an interface between basic and applied science research. Neurocognitive models of attentional bias suggest that anxious youth demonstrate an early, amygdala-driven vigilance for threat related information, followed by later, more heterogeneous responding including either difficulty disengaging attention from threat mediated by deficient dorsolateral prefrontal cortex responding, attentional avoidance of threat mediated by the parietal cortex/striatum, or no consistent bias toward or away from threat (Roy, Dennis, & Warner, 2015). Research examining interpretation biases in the context of social anxiety has found that high and low anxious individuals differ in their neural activity in response to resolution of ambiguity in a positive or negative manner, specifically in terms of P600 – an event-related potential thought to be involved in violations of expectancy (Moser et al., 2008). Increasingly, research efforts have been directed toward the study of mechanism-driven clinical interventions across multiple levels of analysis that integrate brain and behavior findings (Insel, 2014; Insel & Gogtay, 2014). Given the theoretical specificity of CBM interventions, they are well-suited for this type of research.

Description of the Approach to Innovation

Attention Bias Modification (ABM)

Research suggests that clinically anxious children (Roy et al., 2008; Shechner et al., 2013) and adults (Bantin et al., 2016; Bar-Haim et al., 2007; Van Bockstaele et al., 2014) demonstrate an early and automatic attention bias for threat-relevant information.

Although a number of tasks have been used to assess attentional bias (spatial cueing task: Posner, 1980; visual search task: e.g., Gilboa-Schechtman, Foa, & Amir, 1999; Rinck et al., 2003), the most commonly used assessment paradigm in clinically anxious youth is the probe detection task (MacLeod, Mathews, & Tata, 1986). In a representative version of this task, Roy and colleagues (2008) presented clinically anxious children ages 7–18 with threat and neutral stimuli (i.e., angry and neutral faces) on opposite sides of a computer screen for a brief interval (i.e., 500 ms) and then the stimuli disappeared and a probe appeared either in the location of the threat or neutral face. Children were then instructed to respond to the probe by indicating its screen location (i.e., right or left) with a key press. Attentional bias for threat was defined as slower average reaction times for responding to trials in which the probe replaced the neutral face compared to trials in which the probe replaced the threat face, with anxious children demonstrating greater attentional bias scores relative to non-anxious youth. While the precise attentional mechanisms underlying this difference in reaction times remain unclear (Koster et al., 2004; Roy et al., 2015), it is commonly assumed that this difference reflects difficulty disengaging attention from the location where the threat stimulus had appeared in order to redirect attention to the location of the neutral stimulus.

Tasks used to assess attentional bias can also be adapted as training tasks to facilitate changes in attentional processing of threat (Mathews & MacLeod, 2002). For example, Eldar and colleagues (2012) presented clinically anxious youth ages 8–14 with a modified probe detection task for training attention. The probe detection training task was identical to the assessment version with one critical difference: these researchers built in contingency between the location of the threat face and the location of the probe, such that the probe always appeared in the same location as the neutral face. The rationale for this manipulation was that children would become more adept at directing their attention away from threat faces, thereby reducing symptoms of anxiety over time. Thus, ABM was predicated on two assumptions: (1) anxious individuals possess a bias toward threat stimuli, and (2) this bias can be reduced through training (Kuckertz & Amir, 2015; MacLeod & Clarke, 2015). Although the overall finding from a large set of studies supports these assumptions, the picture is less than clear upon close inspection.

For example, despite this clear set of assumptions, an increasing body of research suggests that many anxious youth present with a bias away from threat stimuli or inconsistent pattern of bias (for a review, see Roy et al., 2015). Such findings have led some to conclude that rather than the traditional ABM approach of training attention solely away from threat, training toward positive stimuli may be clinically useful (Waters et al., 2013, 2014, 2015, 2016). In addition, researchers have attempted to improve the ecological validity of ABM tasks by using visual search tasks. For example, Waters and colleagues (2013) presented participants with repeated trials consisting of a 3 × 3 matrix of happy and threat faces. Participants are trained to attend toward positive by clicking on the happy face in the matrix as quickly as possible. Of note, anxious children in attending toward positive conditions are still being trained not to attend to threat faces, as paradigms to date use the probe detection task with threat and positive stimuli (Waters et al., 2014) or the visual search task with threat and positive stimuli (Waters et al., 2013, 2015). While such designs may be clinically useful for a greater percentage of youth due to training away from threat as well as toward positive, it is difficult to assess the mechanism of action in such designs because bias toward threat and bias toward positive stimuli are inversely related.

Interpretation Bias Modification (IBM)

Consistent with cognitive models that posit an etiological and maintenance role of maladaptive interpretations in youth anxiety disorders (Daleiden & Vasey, 1997; Muris & Field, 2008), research suggests that anxious youths are more likely to endorse ambiguous information as threatening and/or less likely to endorse ambiguous information as benign relative to non-anxious peers (e.g., Bögels & Zigterman, 2000; Gifford et al., 2008).

A wide variety of assessment measures have been used to study interpretation biases in clinically anxious youth. The most common paradigm uses variations of ambiguous scenarios tasks, in which participants are presented with ambiguous sentences or short stories and asked to resolve the ambiguity by either (1) rating the likelihood of various threat or benign interpretations (Bögels & Zigterman, 2000; Waters, Craske et al., 2008; Waters, Wharton et al., 2008), (2) selecting the most likely outcome from a list of threat and benign interpretations (Blossom et al., 2013; Creswell, Schniering, & Rapee, 2005), and/or (3) generating an interpretation that is later coded as threatening or benign (Barrett et al., 2008; Bögels & Zigterman, 2000; Hughes & Kendall, 2008).

Other studies have assessed interpretation biases in anxious youth using homographs (i.e., words with the same spelling but different possible meanings) that have either a threat or neutral meaning (e.g., growth, chicken). Taghavi et al. (2000) found that clinically anxious youth were more likely to construct sentences out of homographs consistent with the threat interpretation of the homograph, relative to non-anxious youth. In another variant of this task, Gifford et al. (2008) presented recordings of ambiguous homographs or homophones and asked participants to select one of two pictures corresponding to either the threat or neutral interpretation. Anxious children were more likely to select pictures corresponding to threat interpretations, relative to non-anxious children.

Finally, several studies have utilized other performance-based tasks to assess interpretation bias in anxious youth (In-Albon et al., 2009; Rozenman, Amir, & Weersing, 2014). For example, Rozenman, Amir, & Weersing (2014) used a word-sentence association paradigm in which participants were presented with a threat or neutral word followed by an ambiguous sentence and asked to decide whether the word and sentence were related. This task assesses endorsement rate of threat vs. neutral interpretations, but also assesses interpretation bias at a more automatic level via speed of responding to threat vs. neutral interpretations.

Despite the relative variety of tasks that have been used to assess interpretation bias, the only training paradigm that has been used in clinically anxious youth populations is the ambiguous scenarios task. In the most common training variation of the ambiguous scenarios task, participants are presented with an ambiguous short vignette and asked to complete spelling of the last word in the sentence in a way that resolves the ambiguity in a neutral or positive manner (Fu et al., 2013; Klein et al., 2015; Reuland & Teachman, 2014; Salemink, Wolters, & De Haan, 2015). For example, Klein et al. (2015) presented clinically anxious youths with the following training scenario, "You help a friend to study for a class test. A little later you see him/her coming out of the test. Your friend is probably hap_y" (p. 81). In this scenario, the participant is expected to the type in the missing letter "p" in order to resolve the scenario in a positive way. After participant response was recorded, participants were asked a yes/no comprehension question that reinforced the positive or neutral interpretation of the scenario.

In the ambiguous scenarios training task described previously, the resolution of ambiguity as benign is obvious because children do not have a choice whether to resolve the ambiguity in a benign or threatening manner. Such training tasks may not closely represent the child's decision-making process in the resolution of ambiguity in everyday life. In another training variation of the ambiguous scenarios task, Orchard et al. (2017) presented socially anxious children with ambiguous scenarios and asked children to select what they thought happened from either a threatening or neutral (benign) choice. Children were either given feedback "This is correct" if they selected the benign interpretation or "This is incorrect" if they selected the threat interpretation. Children were then prompted to think about why the benign interpretation resolved the ambiguous situation. In contrast to word completion variants of the ambiguous scenarios task, participants in the Orchard et al. study may have been required to exercise greater cognitive resources and thus potentially better incorporate benign interpretations into their understanding of the situation.

Although variations of the homographs task and word-sentence association paradigm have been used successfully to assess interpretation biases in clinically anxious youth as well as to train clinically anxious adults (Amir & Taylor, 2012; Hayes et al., 2010), their utility as a training tool in youth populations remains unknown and represents an area for further research.

Evidence Base for Innovation

Attention Bias Modification (ABM)

Research on the clinical efficacy of ABM for anxious youth is limited. To date there are only a handful of randomized controlled trials (RCTs) conducted with clinically anxious youth, with studies split between those that examined ABM as a stand-alone (Eldar et al., 2012; Pergamin-Hight et al., 2016; Waters et al., 2013, 2015, 2016) versus adjunctive treatment (Britton et al., 2013; Riemann et al., 2013; Shechner et al., 2014; Waters et al., 2014; White et al., 2017). Of the stand-alone ABM trials, three studies compared ABM to a sham attention control condition in which there was no contingency between the probe location and threat stimulus (Eldar et al., 2012; Pergamin-Hight et al., 2016; Waters et al., 2013) and two studies compared ABM to a wait-list control condition (Waters et al., 2015, 2016). All of the adjunctive ABM trials compared ABM plus CBT to control condition plus CBT (Britton et al., 2013; Riemann et al., 2013; Shechner et al., 2014; Waters et al., 2014; White et al., 2017), with two of those studies including an additional CBT only comparison condition (Britton et al., 2013; Schechner et al., 2013).

In these studies, ABM yielded significant reductions in anxiety from pre- to posttreatment on at least one outcome measure across all RCTs. However, approximately half of these studies also found that the control condition resulted in similar reductions in anxiety (Britton et al., 2013; Pergamin-Hight et al., 2016; Shechner et al., 2014; Waters et al., 2014). Mixed findings on the superiority of ABM to the control condition exist for both stand-alone and adjunctive treatment studies. Although to date there are no meta-analyses examining the efficacy of ABM in clinically anxious youth populations, meta-analyses of CBM in youth populations broadly and/or ABM in adult populations have concluded relatively modest effects of ABM based on between-group effect sizes rather than within-group effect sizes (Cristea et al., 2015; Heeren et al., 2015; Mogoaşe, David, & Koster, 2014). Indeed, research consistently suggests that ABM results in significant anxiety reduction in anxious youth; however, extant control conditions have in some cases yielded comparable reductions.

Several possibilities may account for this pattern of results whereby ABM consistently results in symptom reduction for clinically anxious youth but does not consistently outperform the control condition. Cristea et al. (2015) suggested that reductions in symptoms following ABM may be explained by demand characteristics such as participant attunement to the researcher's expectation of symptom reduction. While demand characteristics represent a possible explanation that could entirely and/or partially account for symptom reductions in both ABM and control conditions, several factors warrant consideration. Given that both participants and assessors are typically blinded to treatment condition (e.g., Eldar et al., 2012; Pergamin-Hight et al., 2016; Riemann et al., 2013), there would be a 50 percent probability of the participant having been assigned to the control group. Moreover, research examining participant expectations has shown that the majority of participants believe that they are in the control group (Amir et al., 2009) and patient-reported credibility of ABM is generally low (Beard, Weisberg, & Primack, 2012). Moreover, Shechner et al. (2014) found that both ABM and control conditions yielded greater reductions in symptoms as an adjunctive to CBT rather than a CBT only condition. As all three groups would be expected to yield improvement in symptoms, it is somewhat unlikely that these findings would be driven solely by demand effects. Other explanations for these mixed findings include shared mechanisms of action between ABM and control conditions, including exposure to threatening stimuli, modification of attentional bias for threat, and/or improved general attentional control. We discuss these possible mechanisms further in the "Mediators and Moderators of Change" section that follows.

Interpretation Bias Modification (IBM)

Relative to the evidence base for ABM, even fewer studies have examined the efficacy of IBM in clinically anxious youth and hence merit being reviewed individually. All studies with anxious youth have used training variants of the ambiguous scenarios task with various study designs and control conditions.

Two studies compared a training IBM condition to a sham IBM condition. Fu et al. (2013) examined the effects of a single session IBM training of 60 trials in adolescents ages 12–17 diagnosed with social anxiety disorder (SAD) or generalized anxiety disorder (GAD). Relative to a sham condition in which participants resolved word fragments with a positive or negative meaning with equal frequency, the positive training condition did not affect mood ratings. Effect of training on interpretation bias was more mixed, with results suggesting that the training modified some but not all interpretation indices. In another RCT, Klein et al. (2015) examined the effects of IBM in children ages 7–12 with a primary anxiety disorder diagnosis. The intervention was self-administered in the participants' homes over a two-week period and comprised 15 IBM sessions of 10 trials each (total: 150 trials). Results suggested that relative to a control condition, the training condition was associated with reduced mother- and father-rated child social anxiety symptoms but had no effects on any other parent- or child-rated anxiety symptoms. While there was no overall group x time interaction effect on interpretation bias scores, the authors did report a significant training-related decrease in interpretation bias specifically for social scenarios when examining participants who demonstrated a threat bias at baseline.

A third study compared IBM to a wait-list condition among children ages 7–12 with a diagnosis of SAD (Orchard et al., 2017). The IBM condition consisted of three sessions of 15 scenarios each (total: 45 trials). Participants were not reassessed until a mean of 6.11 weeks after group allocation, suggesting that relatively few training trials were dispersed over a relatively long period of time. These authors did not find any group x time interaction effects for symptom measures. Effects on interpretation bias were mixed, with the authors reporting a marginally significant group x time interaction effect for benign but not threat ratings.

Two additional studies examining the effects of IBM in clinically anxious children are of note. Salemink, Wolters, and De Haan (2015) examined the efficacy of IBM versus a sham condition as an adjunct to CBT for adolescents diagnosed with obsessive compulsive disorder (OCD). Training comprised 8 sessions of 42 trials each (total: 336 trials) completed over 11 days. These authors reported greater reduction in obsessions in the training relative to sham condition, although this effect was only marginally significant. Condition-consistent effects were found for some, but not all, indices of interpretation bias. Finally, Reuland and Teachman (2014) examined the effect of training positive interpretation bias in children with SAD ages 10–15, their mothers, or both. Families (N=18) completed one of the three training conditions in a multiple baseline design. Training comprised 8 sessions of 50 trials each (total: 400 trials). Results from this pilot study generally suggested that all training conditions produced the expected effects in symptoms and interpretation bias and that conditions did not differ from one another on outcomes.

Together, results of IBM studies in clinically anxious youth present a mixed picture for the intervention's ability to effectively target both symptoms and purported mechanism(s) (i.e., increase in benign bias and/or reduction in threat bias). However, IBM studies with clinically anxious youth are limited in number and extant studies have methodological limitations including small sample sizes (range: 5–43 participants per condition) and relatively few training trials (range: 45–400). These limitations notwithstanding, these IBM studies provide preliminary evidence for possible efficacy of IBM in changing bias and symptoms.

A larger number of studies have examined the effects of IBM in healthy youth or youth with elevated anxiety. In a combined reanalysis of six IBM studies with 387 healthy youth, Lau and Pile (2015) demonstrated that over one session of training, IBM significantly reduced negative mood whereas control conditions did not. Similarly, adolescents completing IBM relative to control conditions reported fewer negative interpretations and greater positive interpretations at post-training. Another meta-analysis examined the effect of IBM in youth more broadly and collapsed across symptom measures and a wide range of populations (Cristea et al., 2015). Despite finding small and nonsignificant effects on symptoms, Cristea and colleagues reported that IBM had a moderate effect on interpretation bias. However, the authors also reported a moderate amount of heterogeneity among studies included in their analyses. This suggests that meta-analyses addressing more focused questions about the efficacy of IBM may be more informative than asking broadly whether IBM works under all conditions (e.g., diagnostic group, age group, delivery setting). The limited number of studies conducted to date precludes such analysis in clinically anxious youth populations.

Mediators and Moderators of Change

Attention Bias Modification (ABM)

Mediators. Few studies have examined the mediators of ABM efficacy in clinically anxious youth. Waters et al. (2013) examined attentional biases to threat and positive stimuli and found that changes in both types of biases were related to treatment outcome. In another study by Waters et al. (2014) examining augmentation effects of adding ABM to a one-session exposure treatment for specific phobia, positive bias at posttreatment was predictive of anxiety severity in the ABM group but not in the control condition at 3-month follow-up. Eldar et al. (2012) found that threat bias change did not mediate the effect of training condition on treatment outcome. However, these authors noted that their sample size was underpowered to detect a significant mediation effect.

In the broader ABM literature including adult studies, research supports a mechanistic role of bias change in predicting treatment outcome. While an early meta-analysis suggested a strong relationship between change in bias and anxiety symptoms (Hakamata et al., 2010), a later meta-analysis failed to find a significant relationship (Mogoaşe et al., 2014). In an attempt to reconcile these findings in the context of improved power, Price et al. (2016) conducted a pooled patient-level meta-analysis from 13 studies with 778 participants. In line with the notion of moderator-defined subgroups (Kraemer, 2010), Price et al. first identified subgroups in which ABM was clinically efficacious relative to the control condition. In those subgroups (e.g., younger patients, in-lab training, symptoms assessed by a clinician), there was evidence for mediation of threat bias on outcome. In another review of ABM, Clarke, Notebaert, and MacLeod (2014) examined 29 studies and reported that only three were inconsistent with the notion that when ABM successfully modifies bias, there is a corresponding impact on symptoms. Thus, existing research strongly suggests that when attentional bias is differentially reduced as a function of training condition, so too are symptoms.

However, as reviewed in the previous "Evidence Base for Innovation" section, at least some studies with both children and adults yield significant and comparable reductions in anxiety symptoms and attention bias for ABM and control groups (e.g., Britton et al., 2013; Shechner et al., 2014). Moreover, some studies suggest that ABM yields significant reductions in symptoms in the absence of bias change (Waters et al., 2015). Such findings suggest that additional mechanisms beyond modification of attention bias may produce symptom change. For example, McNally et al. (2013) suggested that both ABM and control conditions enhance one's ability to flexibly direct control of attention in general, rather than specifically away from threat and/or toward positive. Other research groups have proposed that dynamic changes in allocation to threat versus neutral stimuli within a given session may be more relevant to anxiety than static measurement that averages bias across many trials (Iacoviello et al., 2014; Zvielli, Bernstein, & Koster, 2015). In support of this notion, one study reported that changes in the plasticity of attentional bias within session, but not changes in traditional attention bias, mediated treatment effects (Kuckertz, Amir, et al., 2014). Thus, additional research is needed to determine the relative mechanistic contributions of threat attentional bias, positive attentional bias, attentional control, and dynamic attention bias. In addition, such mechanisms should be disentangled from potential demand effects.

Moderators. A number of studies have examined moderators of ABM efficacy in child or adult populations. Studies examining the role of baseline attention bias have been mixed. For example, Pergamin-Hight et al. (2016) reported that baseline threat bias did not moderate outcomes between ABM and the control groups, while Waters et al. (2014) reported that baseline threat bias moderated change in child-rated anxiety but not other clinical outcomes. Waters et al. also tested the moderating role of baseline positive bias, with nonsignificant findings. At the meta-analytic level, among predominantly adult samples there is support for the moderating role of baseline threat bias under some but not all conditions, including participants trained in a laboratory and whose symptoms were assessed by a clinician (Price et al., 2016).

In addition to examining baseline threat bias as a potential moderator, Pergamin-Hight et al. (2016) examined the potential moderating role of baseline attentional control. Results suggested a moderation effect whereby only children with low baseline attentional control benefited from ABM when compared to those assigned to the control condition. These findings are consistent with the possibility that ABM operates on attentional mechanisms other than threat bias alone.

Finally, studies have examined age as a moderator of symptoms. Pergamin-Hight et al. (2016) reported that among children ages 6–18, older but not younger children differentially benefited from ABM compared to the control condition. Meta-analyses based predominantly on adult samples have also suggested that younger adults benefit more from ABM relative to older adults (Mogoaşe et al., 2014; Price et al., 2016). These findings suggest that ABM may be most beneficial for adolescents and young adults, although replication is needed, particularly in youth samples. This pattern of enhanced efficacy is seemingly at odds with the finding that among clinically anxious children, threat bias is greater among younger compared to older children (Carmona et al., 2015). Such findings raise the possibility that among adolescents, mechanisms of symptom reduction other than change in threat bias may be in play.

Interpretation Bias Modification (IBM)

Mediators. To date one study has examined mediators of IBM outcome in clinically anxious youth. In that study, Orchard et al. (2017) reported that neither change in benign nor threat bias mediated reduction in social anxiety symptoms. However, given the brief intervention (45 trials) these findings should be interpreted with caution. More consistent with the purported mechanisms of IBM, in their reanalysis of six IBM studies with healthy youth, Lau and Pile (2015) reported small but significant relationships between changes for both positive and negative endorsement and changes in positive mood. This relationship was found in conditions in which participants were trained toward benign interpretations, but not in control conditions. However, neither changes in endorsement of positive nor threat interpretations were associated with changes in negative mood. Given that all studies in this reanalysis included healthy children trained over a single session, it is possible that floor effects on negative mood may have precluded an observed influence on symptoms.

Greater evidence supports a mechanistic link between changes in bias and symptoms in adult populations. In a recent meta-analysis, Menne-Lothmann et al. (2014) demonstrated a strong and significant correlation between changes in interpretation bias and negative mood/anxiety symptoms. Among adults diagnosed with SAD, Amir and Taylor (2012) found that after 12 IBM sessions of 220 trials each (total: 2,640 trials), changes in social threat interpretations mediated the relationship between group (IBM vs. control condition) and changes in social anxiety. Moreover, these data suggest that IBM only affects symptoms to the extent that it effects changes in interpretation bias.

Moderators. Few studies have examined moderators of IBM outcome. For example, Klein et al. (2015) reported that reductions in social threat bias were observed in the training group only for youths who presented with a bias at baseline. These results suggest that IBM may be ineffective in modifying the purported mechanism of action in children who do not have a preexistent bias.

Lau and Pile (2015) reviewed the possible influence of age and gender as moderators of IBM outcome among six studies of healthy youths ages 11–17. The authors divided their sample into early adolescence (11–14 years), mid-adolescence (15–16 years), and late adolescence (17–18 years). Training effectiveness differed by age as well as gender within each developmental period. Specifically, for females completing IBM, the most effective period for change in interpretations was early and late adolescence. For males the most effective age for changing interpretations was mid-adolescence. However, changes in mood state were not moderated by age or gender, likely due to overall weak effects of training on mood in healthy samples.

Clinical Case Illustration

Kristie is a 9-year-old female whose mother, Sarah, presented to our clinic in response to a study flyer advertising "computerized treatment for kids with anxiety." Kristie had never received previous psychiatric treatment. Sarah stated that Kristie's anxiety had gotten progressively worse in the past two years. Sarah reported that while Kristie had little difficulty interacting with children 1:1, she "shuts down" in larger groups such as birthday parties or family gatherings. Sarah also reported that Kristie had significant anxiety about speaking with adults including teachers or friends' parents. Additionally, Sarah reported that Kristie was very worried about "perfectionism" related to sports, homework, and tests. After completing a semi-structured interview, we diagnosed Kristie with SAD and GAD. We also administered the Pediatric Anxiety Rating Scale (PARS; Research Units on Pediatric Psychopharmacology Anxiety Study Group, 2002), a semi-structured interview measure of child anxiety severity. Kristie's six-item PARS score was at baseline at 15 (clinical cutpoint = 13; Walkup et al., 2008).

As part of the research study, children were randomized to complete either ABM or the control condition three times per week for four weeks (once/week in clinic, twice/week at home). During in-clinic visits, Kristie completed the training program in a private office with a research assistant present in the room to monitor program compliance. As instructed, Kristie completed the program twice/week on a USB drive at home between clinic sessions. Sarah was instructed to designate a quiet, distraction-free place in which Kristie could complete the training at home. Kristie, Sarah, and the assessing clinician were blind to child condition. Each session consisted of 160 dot-probe trials using paired disgust and neutral facial stimuli (Amir et al., 2009).

Post-Training Assessment. After four weeks, Kristie was assessed for clinical change. Sarah noted that she was better able to help Kristie "re-frame things" in anxiety-provoking situations and noted that Kristie had become "more flexible." Sarah reported clear behavioral examples of improvement in Kristie's anxiety. Sarah reported that Kristie was interacting more with her teachers and friends' parents and was no longer reporting muscle tension. Sarah stated that Kristie continued to be somewhat nervous in large groups or when interacting with unfamiliar adults, but that her nervousness typically lasted less than a minute. Sarah could not recall any recent instances in which Kristie expressed worry about perfectionism. Moreover, Kristie's PARS score at post-training was a 5. We determined that Kristie no longer met criteria for SAD or GAD.

Although Kristie reported that she found the task repetitive and boring, Sarah stated that she appreciated that she was able to seek treatment for her child without the use of medication. Following the assessment, the assessor was unblinded to condition and revealed to the family that Kristie had been randomized to the active ABM condition.

Follow-Up Assessment. The assessor completed a follow-up interview with the family approximately two months following the post-training assessment. At that time, Sarah noted that Kristie was continuing to function "much better," appeared more confident at soccer games, recently volunteered to help the class with math problems, and seemed more comfortable around adults. Kristie's PARS score at follow-up was a 3.

Challenges and Recommendations for Future Research

Current State of CBM Research

The first CBM study was conducted 15 years ago in an experimental context with nonclinical undergraduate students (Mathews & MacLeod, 2002). It was not until 2009 that CBM was first examined in a clinically anxious adult population (Amir et al., 2009; Schmidt et al., 2009) and 2011 when first examined in a clinically anxious youth population (Rozenman, Weersing, & Amir, 2011). In the short period of time since this class of interventions was introduced as a possible method of modifying symptoms (less than 10 years ago), an impressive amount of research in this area has been conducted. This research has examined several hypotheses about the circumstances that may lead to CBM effects in clinical outcomes and the methodology through which such effects are elicited. Researchers have examined the effects of CBM as a tool for prevention among children at risk for development of psychopathology (White et al., 2016), an intervention for treatment-seeking families (Rozenman et al., 2011), and a treatment for children who have been nonresponsive to gold-standard interventions (Bechor et al., 2014). CBM has been tested in labs (Eldar et al., 2012), schools (Fitzgerald, Rawdon, & Dooley, 2016), homes (Waters et al., 2016), and residential treatment settings (Riemann et al., 2013) across the developmental spectrum, and with populations ranging from healthy children (Lau & Pile, 2015) to a variety of clinical populations including disordered eating (Boutelle et al., 2014), anxiety disorders (Orchard et al., 2017), OCD (Salemink, Wolters, & De Haan, 2015), aggressive behavior (Vassilopoulos, Brouzos, & Andreou, 2015), and depression (Micco, Henin, & Hirshfeld-Becker, 2014).

Such enthusiasm for the potential clinical applications of CBM is not surprising given that gold-standard treatments (e.g., CBT, exposure-based treatment) for most psychological disorders are not accessed by the majority of patients nor do the majority of patients receiving these interventions evidence complete response. Nonetheless, the enthusiasm with which CBM research has been pursued has perhaps outpaced arguably less exciting yet critical research on the measurement and characterization of cognitive biases in various clinical populations.

Several research groups have conducted meta-analytic reviews (Cristea, Kok, & Cuijpers, 2015; Cristea et al., 2015; Hallion & Ruscio, 2011) about the efficacy of CBM as a broad class of interventions. While the overall place of CBM in our clinical arsenal of intervention strategies represents an interesting and relevant question, the relative infancy of CBM research has not consistently matched the level at which it has been reviewed. Questions such as whether CBM modifies symptoms among children regardless of clinical profile, outcome measure, type of bias targeted, methodology, or dose are unlikely to yield the types of specific implications and suggestions that are needed at this stage of research in a new field. When examining mechanisms of complex sets of mixed CBM findings, many of the premises on which CBM interventions are predicated have limited evidence supporting them. In order to meaningfully evaluate whether CBM succeeded in modifying symptoms relative to a control group, a number of prerequisites must be met. For example, it is important to establish that (1) the purported mechanism can be assessed reliably so as to examine questions of mechanism, (2) the purported mechanism of change is causally implicated in that disorder, (3) the purported mechanism of change can be modified, and (4) the methodology used is sufficient to modify that mechanism. We comment on these prerequisites as follows.

Reliability of Bias Measurement

Prior to examining whether interventions are successful in modifying the purported mechanisms, it is important to develop and establish reliable methods of measuring such mechanisms at the individual level. Currently, methods used to assess attentional and interpretation processes targeted in various CBM interventions have limited evidence of reliability. For example, ABM research has been predicated on 30 years of accumulated research using the probe detection paradigm (MacLeod et al., 1986). However, as reviewed by Price et al. (2015), test-retest reliability for the standard method of calculating attentional bias from the probe detection paradigm is poor (i.e., difference score between response latencies for responding to threat and neutral stimuli). However, reaction time measures are highly reliable. Therefore, it is important to develop new and reliable methods of assessing information processing biases at the individual level. Similar calls for establishing the reliability of physiological measures (Hajcak, Meyer, & Kotov, 2017) have begun to guide theoretical and empirical inquiries regarding measurement and modification of other types of biases. In a reanalysis of probe detection data from three studies, Price et al. (2015) found that specific analytic modifications increased the reliability of the probe detection task (e.g., only analyze trials in which the probe appears in the bottom half of the screen, combine multiple assessment points, Winsorize data instead of applying arbitrary outlier cutpoints).

Of course it has long been established that the reliability of the difference score (i.e., bias or change scores) is limited by the correlation between the constructs comprising the difference score (Furr & Bacharach, 2014). For example, assume a researcher is interested in examining rate of change in reading level across two consecutive years in school in predicting Scholastic Aptitude Test (SAT) scores at graduation. She hypothesized that children who show a faster rate of change will have higher SAT scores at graduation. To test this hypothesis, the researcher calculates a difference score (gain in reading score) to assess improvement in reading and uses this variable to predict SAT scores at graduation. Assuming that the reading scores in both years are reliable (e.g., alpha = .85) and valid and that the variance is equal across years, the question becomes what is the reliability of the difference score as this reliability will set a limit on the validity of the change scores, i.e., its correlation with any other measure—in this case SAT score. As Furr and Bacharach (2014, Chapter 6) demonstrate, the reliability of the difference score is determined by the reliability of the constituent scores but more importantly by the correlation between the two measures (two reading level scores). Assuming the correlation between the two reading level tests is .7, then the reliability of the difference score will be only .5 given the preceding assumptions,[1] thus having lower reliability than each score alone. If the correlation between the two reading scores increases to .9 (as is the case for reaction time measures), then the reliability of the difference score can approach 0 as the correlation between the measures approaches 1. The caution suggested by the counterintuitive fact that two reliable and valid measures can result in a difference score that has low reliability has not been heeded by CBM researchers interested in individual differences in information processing. As a result, reports on the unreliability of bias scores are treated as new findings when statisticians have long cautioned again their use.

A simple solution is not to use difference scores but to simply enter the two reading level scores into a regression equation in predicting SAT scores at graduation. Of course, these issues are not limited to cognitive measures and are present when one measures any psychological construct. Another solution is to predict what the reliability of the difference scores is likely to be in a particular experiment and then decide whether to use a difference score (Trafimow, 2015). Indeed, there are combinations of parameters that imply that difference scores are reasonably reliable, e.g., when the two tests have unequal variance.

Other research groups have proposed examination of dynamic rather than static forms of attentional bias measured in the context of the probe detection task (Iacoviello et al., 2014; Zvielli, Bernstein, & Koster, 2015), with initial evidence supporting improved reliability (Price et al., 2015; Zvielli et al., 2016). In addition, researchers should more clearly consider the statistical limitations associated with difference scores, including reduced reliability, correlated errors between difference components, and restricted variance (Lord, 1958; Peter, Churchill, & Brown, 1993). Thus, psychometric comparisons between difference scores, raw response latency averages, and other forms of bias calculation represent a critical area for future research.

Which Biases Do We Target?

Using reliable tools to assess cognitive biases, more specific characterization of these biases in specific clinical populations is needed. It is not sufficient to simply demonstrate the presence of an interpretation bias in anxious youth. Instead, questions of bias characterization warrant further research in order to target bias change more efficiently. For example, it is unclear whether interpretation biases are best described as a failure to favor benign interpretations, tendency to adopt threat interpretations, or a combination of both these biases (Amir et al., 2012; Huppert et al., 2003). That is, it may be the case that while healthy individuals typically interpret ambiguous situations as benign, anxious individuals fail to do so (lack of benign bias). Conversely, it may be the case that faced with ambiguous situations,

---

[1] Let X denote the reading level at first test and Y denote the reading level at second test, with R_{XX}: reliability of the first test; R_{YY}: reliability of the second test; s^2_{Xo}: variance of first test; s^2_{Yo}: variance of second test; $r_{Xo\ Yo}$: correlation between first and second test; and R_d: reliability of the difference score. Then $R_d = (s^2_{Xo} R_{XX} + s^2_{Xo} R_{yy} - 2\ r_{Xo\ Yo}\ s_{Xo}\ s_{Yo}) / (s^2_{Xo} + s^2_{Yo} - 2\ r_{Xo\ Yo}\ s_{Xo}\ s_{Yo})$ (Furr & Bacharach, 2014, formula 6.10).

anxious individuals consistently interpret those situations as threatening. Another theory-driven question underlying IBM concerns the relative advantages of training individuals to endorse positive rather than emotionally neutral interpretations of ambiguous situations (Holmes et al., 2006). Moreover with few exceptions (e.g., Rozenman et al., 2014), research on interpretation biases in anxious youths has not clearly delineated at which stage of processing these biases occur.

Context in Which Biases Are Most Malleable

Research suggests that some settings and developmental periods may be more robust in producing bias change. Perhaps the most examined contextual factor for CBM outcome relates to training setting. Several recent meta-analyses of ABM based on mostly adult data suggest that ABM yields poorer clinical outcomes when completed outside of the laboratory (Linetzky et al., 2015; Mogoaşe et al., 2014; Price et al., 2016). Such findings have yet to be established in clinically anxious youth populations or for other forms of CBM. Although there are many possible explanations for discrepant ABM outcomes across lab versus home settings, at least one study suggests that it may be possible to improve ABM outcomes in home settings by activating a fear structure prior to training completion (Kuckertz, Gildebrant, et al., 2014). In addition to training setting, developmentally sensitive periods for CBM training have yet to be fully delineated. Nonetheless, preliminary research suggests that even among youth, specific developmental periods may be associated with superior outcomes for both ABM (Pergamin-Hight et al., 2016) and IBM (Lau & Pile, 2015).

Key Practice Points

A number of questions remain regarding the characterization and modification of cognitive biases among clinically anxious youths; thus, we echo others in their emphasis on the need for caution in disseminating CBM for clinical practice (Cristea et al., 2015). However, we believe that such caution must be placed in balance with the urgent need for treatment and scarcity of providers for child anxiety disorders. As the majority of children with an anxiety disorder do not receive first-line treatment (Chavira et al., 2004), we see minimal harm and potentially significant benefit to making CBM interventions available to families of anxious children, with several caveats. Given the currently mixed state of the outcome literature, we strongly urge the need to not advertise CBM as a panacea that will work for all clinically anxious children under any conditions. Of course, CBT with or without SSRIs has been and should be the first line intervention for clinically anxious youth. Nonetheless, we suggest that it is reasonable to consider the role of CBM in some specific circumstances, such as when CBT or SSRIs are not available or acceptable to the family, or if families are placed on long wait lists to receive treatment.

Moreover, we encourage continued research examining moderators of the efficacy of ABM as a training tool for both anxious parents and anxious children. A large body of research has highlighted the bidirectional relationship between parent and child symptoms as well as suggested intervention upon parent anxiety (Barmish & Kendall, 2005; Breinholst et al., 2012), with mixed findings. In contrast to parent intervention strategies that may be perceived as relatively intrusive (i.e., including parent as a co-client in CBT), completion of ABM alongside their child may be a relatively less threatening intervention for parents.

Finally, we emphasize the critical need for further research on patient attitudes, and specifically child attitudes, toward CBM interventions. While dissemination of CBM is relatively innocuous in terms of potential side effects, exposing a child to treatment that is both ineffective and unpleasant may potentially discourage that child or family from pursuing further mental health treatment. Initial qualitative research in this area suggests that anxious adult patients expressed more positive attitudes toward IBM relative to ABM, and did not understand the purpose or relevance of the ABM task to their anxiety (Beard et al., 2012). Thus, we suggest that it may be most prudent to suggest a CBM trial for patients who indicate more positive attitudes toward and expectations of the program at pretreatment. In support of this notion, data from our research group suggest that a reliable, three-item measure of initial attitudes toward ABM predicts reduction in symptoms (Kuckertz et al., 2018). Moreover, important strides have been made over the last several years toward enhancing the enjoyableness of CBM programs (Dennis-Tiwary et al., 2016; Notebaert et al., 2015). Wolf (1978) emphasized the importance of patient attitudes toward behavioral techniques, arguing that "feedback from participants is not a trivial issue: that if the participants don't like the treatment then they may avoid it, or run away, or complain loudly. And thus, society will be less likely to use your technology, no matter how potentially effective and efficient it might be" (p. 206).

References

Amir, N., Beard, C., Taylor, C. T., Klumpp, H., Elias, J., Burns, M., & Chen, X. (2009). Attention training in individuals with generalized social phobia: A randomized controlled trial. *Journal of Consulting and Clinical Psychology, 77*(5), 961–973.

Amir, N., Prouvost, C., & Kuckertz, J. M. (2012). Lack of a benign interpretation bias in social anxiety disorder. *Cognitive Behaviour Therapy, 41*(2), 119–129.

Amir, N., & Taylor, C. T. (2012). Interpretation training in individuals with generalized social anxiety disorder: A randomized controlled trial. *Journal of Consulting and Clinical Psychology, 80*(3), 497–511.

Bantin, T., Stevens, S., Gerlach, A. L., & Hermann, C. (2016). Journal of Behavior Therapy and What does the facial dot-probe task tell us about attentional processes in social anxiety? A systematic review. *Journal of Behavior Therapy and Experimental Psychiatry, 50*, 40–51.

Bar-Haim, Y., Lamy, D., Pergamin, L., Bakermans-Kranenburg, M. J., & van IJzendoorn, M. H. (2007). Threat-related attentional bias in anxious and nonanxious individuals: A meta-analytic study. *Psychological Bulletin, 133*, 1–24.

Barmish, A. J., & Kendall, P. C. (2005). Should parents be co-clients in cognitive-behavioral therapy for anxious youth? *Journal of Clinical Child and Adolescent Psychology, 34*, 569–581.

Barrett, P. M., Farrell, L., Pina, A. A., Peris, T. S., & Piacentini, J. (2008). Evidence-based psychosocial treatments for child and adolescent obsessive-compulsive disorder. *Journal of Clinical Child and Adolescent Psychology, 37*, 131–155.

Beard, C. (2011). Cognitive bias modification for anxiety: Current evidence and future directions. *Expert Review of Neurotherapeutics, 11*, 299–311.

Beard, C., Weisberg, R. B., & Primack, J. (2012). Socially anxious primary care patients' attitudes toward cognitive bias modification (CBM): A qualitative study. *Behavioral and Cognitive Psychotherapy, 40*, 618–633.

Bechor, M., Pettit, J. W., Silverman, W. K., Bar-Haim, Y., Abend, R., Pine, D. S., ... Jaccard, J. (2014). Attention bias modification treatment for children with anxiety disorders who do not respond to cognitive behavioral therapy: A case series. *Journal of Anxiety Disorders, 28*, 154–159.

Bittner, A., Egger, H. L., Erkanli, A., Jane Costello, E., Foley, D. L., & Angold, A. (2007). What do childhood anxiety disorders predict? *Journal of Child Psychology and Psychiatry and Allied Disciplines, 48*, 1174–1183.

Blossom, J. B., Ginsburg, G. S., Birmaher, B., Walkup, J. T., Kendall, P. C., Keeton, C. P., ... Albano, A. M. (2013). Parental and family factors as predictors of threat bias in anxious youth. *Cognitive Therapy and Research, 37*, 812–819.

Bögels, S. M., & Zigterman, D. (2000). Dysfunctional cognitions in children with social phobia, separation anxiety disorder, and generalized anxiety disorder. *Journal of Abnormal Child Psychology, 28*, 205–211.

Boutelle, K. N., Kuckertz, J. M., Carlson, J., & Amir, N. (2014). A pilot study evaluating a one-session attention modification training to decrease overeating in obese children. *Appetite, 76*, 180–185.

Breinholst, S., Esbjorn, B. H., Reinholdt-Dunne, M. L., & Stallard, P. (2012). CBT for the treatment of child anxiety disorders: A review of why parental involvement has not enhanced outcomes. *Journal of Anxiety Disorders, 26*, 416–424.

Britton, J. C., Bar-Haim, Y., Clementi, M. A., Sankin, L. S., Chen, G., Shechner, T., ... Pine, D. S. (2013). Training-associated changes and stability of attention bias in youth: Implications for attention bias modification treatment for pediatric anxiety. *Developmental Cognitive Neuroscience, 4*, 52–64.

Carmona, A. R., Kuckertz, J. M., Suway, J., Amir, N., Piacentini, J., & Chang, S. W. (2015). Attentional bias in youth with clinical anxiety: The moderating effect of age. *Journal of Cognitive Psychotherapy, 29*, 185–196.

Chavira, D. A., Stein, M. B., Bailey, K., & Stein, M. T. (2004). Child anxiety in primary care: Prevalent but untreated. *Depression and Anxiety, 20*, 155–164.

Christiana, J. M., Gilman, S. E., Guardino, M., Mickelson, K., Morselli, P. L., Olfson, M., & Kessler, R. C. (2000). Duration between onset and time of obtaining initial treatment among people with anxiety and mood disorders: An international survey of members of mental health patient advocate groups. *Psychological Medicine, 30*, 693–703.

Clarke, P. J. F., Notebaert, L., & MacLeod, C. (2014). Absence of evidence or evidence of absence: Reflecting on therapeutic implementations of attentional bias modification. *BMC Psychiatry, 14*, 8.

Collins, K. A., Westra, H. A., Dozois, D. J. A., & Burns, D. D. (2004). Gaps in accessing treatment for anxiety and depression: Challenges for the delivery of care. *Clinical Psychology Review, 24*, 583–616.

Connolly, S. D., Bernstein, G. A., & The Work Group on Quality Issues. (2007). Practice parameter for the assessment and treatment of children and adolescents with anxiety disorders. *Journal of the American Academy of Child & Adolescent Psychiatry, 46*, 267–283.

Creswell, C., Schniering, C. A., & Rapee, R. M. (2005). Threat interpretation in anxious children and their mothers: Comparison with nonclinical children and the effects of treatment. *Behaviour Research and Therapy, 43*, 1375–1381.

Cristea, I. A., Kok, R. N., & Cuijpers, P. (2015). Efficacy of cognitive bias modification interventions in anxiety and depression: Meta-analysis. *The British Journal of Psychiatry: The Journal of Mental Science, 206*, 7–16.

Cristea, I., Mogoase, C., David, D., & Cuijpers, P. (2015). Practitioner review: Cognitive bias modification for mental health problems in children and adolescents: A meta-analysis. *Journal of Child Psychology and Psychiatry, 56*, 723–734.

Daleiden, E. L., & Vasey, M. W. (1997). An information processing perspective on childhood anxiety. *Clinical Psychology Review, 17*, 407–429.

Dennis-Tiwary, T. A., Egan, L. J., Babkirk, S., & Denefrio, S. (2016). For whom the bell tolls: Neurocognitive individual differences in the acute stress-reduction effects of an attention bias modification game for anxiety. *Behaviour Research and Therapy, 77*, 105–117.

Eldar, S., Apter, A., Lotan, D., Edgar, K. P., Naim, R., Fox, N. A., ... Bar-Haim, Y. (2012). Attention bias modification treatment for pediatric anxiety disorders: A randomized controlled trial. *The American Journal of Psychiatry, 169*, 213–220.

Fitzgerald, A., Rawdon, C., & Dooley, B. (2016). A randomized controlled trial of attention bias modification training for socially anxious adolescents. *Behaviour Research and Therapy, 84*, 1–8.

Foley, D. L., Pickles, A., Maes, H. M., Silberg, J. L., & Eaves, L. J. (2004). Course and short-term outcomes of separation anxiety disorder in a community sample of twins. *Journal of the American Academy of Child & Adolescent Psychiatry, 43*, 1107–1114.

Fu, X., Du, Y., Au, S., & Lau, J. Y. F. (2013). Reducing negative interpretations in adolescents with anxiety disorders: A preliminary study investigating the effects of a single session of cognitive bias modification training. *Developmental Cognitive Neuroscience, 4*, 29–37.

Furr, R. M., & Bacharach, V. R. (2014). *Psychometrics: An Introduction* (2nd edn.). SAGE.

Gifford, S., Reynolds, S., Bell, S., & Wilson, C. (2008). Threat interpretation bias in anxious children and their mothers. *Cognition & Emotion, 22*, 497–508.

Gilboa-Schechtman, E., Foa, E. B., & Amir, N. (1999). Attentional biases for facial expressions in social phobia: The face-in-the-crowd paradigm. *Cognition & Emotion, 13*, 305–318.

Goldstein, R. B., Olfson, M., Wickramaratne, P. J., & Wolk, S. I. (2006). Use of outpatient mental health services by depressed and anxious children as they grow up. *Psychiatric Services, 57*, 966–975.

Gunter, R. W., & Whittal, M. L. (2010). Dissemination of cognitive-behavioral treatments for anxiety disorders: Overcoming barriers and improving patient access. *Clinical Psychology Review, 30*, 194–202.

Hajcak, G., Meyer, A., & Kotov, R. (2017). Psychometrics and the neuroscience of individual differences: Internal consistency limits between-subjects effects. *Journal of Abnormal Psychology, 126*, 823–834.

Hakamata, Y., Lissek, S., Bar-Haim, Y., Britton, J. C., Fox, N. A., Leibenluft, E., ... Pine, D. S. (2010). Attention bias modification treatment: A meta-analysis toward the establishment of novel treatment for anxiety. *Biological Psychiatry, 68*, 982–990.

Hallion, L. S., & Ruscio, A. M. (2011). A meta-analysis of the effect of cognitive bias modification on anxiety and depression. *Psychological Bulletin, 137*, 940–958.

Hayes, S., Hirsch, C. R., Krebs, G., & Mathews, A. (2010). The effects of modifying interpretation bias on worry in generalized anxiety disorder. *Behaviour Research and Therapy, 48*, 171–178.

Heeren, A., Mogoase, C., Philippot, P., & McNally, R. J. (2015). Attention bias modification for social anxiety: A systematic review and meta-analysis. *Clinical Psychology Review, 40*, 76–90.

Holmes, E. A., Mathews, A., Dalgleish, T., & Mackintosh, B. (2006). Positive interpretation training: Effects of mental imagery versus verbal training on positive mood. *Behavior Therapy, 37*, 237–247.

Hughes, A., & Kendall, P. C. (2008). Effect of a positive emotional state on interpretation bias for threat in children with anxiety disorders. *Emotion, 8*, 414–418.

Huijding, J., Field, A. P., De Houwer, J., Vandenbosch, K., Rinck, M., & van Oeveren, M. (2009). A behavioral route to dysfunctional representations: The effects of training approach or avoidance tendencies towards novel animals in children. *Behaviour Research and Therapy, 47*, 471–477.

Huppert, J. D., Foa, E. B., Furr, J. M., Filip, J. C., & Mathews, A. (2003). Interpretation bias in social anxiety: A dimensional perspective. *Cognitive Therapy and Research, 27*, 569–577.

Iacoviello, B. M., Wu, G., Abend, R., Murrough, J. W., Feder, A., Fruchter, E., ... Charney, D. S. (2014). Attention bias variability and symptoms of posttraumatic stress disorder. *Journal of Traumatic Stress, 27*, 232–239.

In-Albon, T., Dubi, K., Rapee, R. M., & Schneider, S. (2009). Forced choice reaction time paradigm in children with separation anxiety disorder, social phobia, and nonanxious controls. *Behaviour Research and Therapy, 47*, 1058–1065.

Insel, T. R. (2014). The NIMH Research Domain Criteria (RDoC) Project: Precision medicine for psychiatry. *American Journal of Psychiatry, 171*, 395–397.

Insel, T. R., & Gogtay, N. (2014). National Institute of Mental Health clinical trials: New opportunities, new expectations. *JAMA Psychiatry, 71*, 745–746.

Kelleher, K. J., & Gardner, W. (2010). Out of sight, out of mind – Behavioral and developmental care for rural children. *New England Journal of Medicine, 376*(14), 1301–1303.

Kenney, E. L., & Gortmaker, S. L. (2017). United States adolescents' television, computer, videogame, smartphone, and tablet use: Associations with sugary drinks, sleep, physical activity, and obesity. *Journal of Pediatrics, 182*, 144–149.

Klein, A. M., Rapee, R. M., Hudson, J. L., Schniering, C. A., Wuthrich, V. M., Kangas, M., ... Rinck, M. (2015). Interpretation modification training reduces social anxiety in clinically anxious children. *Behaviour Research and Therapy, 75*, 78–84.

Koster, E. H. W., Crombez, G., Verschuere, B., & De Houwer, J. (2004). Selective attention to threat in the dot probe paradigm: Differentiating vigilance and difficulty to disengage. *Behaviour Research and Therapy, 42*, 1183–1192.

Kraemer, H. (2010). Moderators and mediators: The MacArthur updated view. In A. Steptoe (ed.), *Handbook of behavioral medicine: Methods and applications*. Springer.

Kuckertz, J. M., & Amir, N. (2015). Attention bias modification for anxiety and phobias: Current status and future directions. *Current Psychiatry Reports, 17*, 9.

Kuckertz, J. M., Amir, N., Boffa, J. W., Warren, C. K., Rindt, S. E. M., Norman, S., ... McLay, R. (2014). The effectiveness of an attention bias modification program as an adjunctive treatment for post-traumatic stress disorder. *Behaviour Research and Therapy, 63*, 25–35.

Kuckertz, J. M., Gildebrant, E., Liliequist, B., Karlström, P., Väppling, C., Bodlund, O., ... Carlbring, P. (2014). Moderation and mediation of the effect of attention training in social anxiety disorder. *Behaviour Research and Therapy, 53*, 30–40.

Kuckertz, J. M., Schofield, C. A., Clerkin, E. M., Primack, P., Boettcher, H., Weisberg, R. B., Amir, N., & Beard, C. (2018). Attentional bias modification for social anxiety disorder: What do patients think and why does it matter? *Behavioural and Cognitive Psychotherapy*. Advance online publication. doi:10.1017/S1352465818000231

Langley, A. K., Bergman, R. L., McCracken, J., & Piacentini, J. C. (2004). Impairment in childhood anxiety disorders: Preliminary examination of the Child Anxiety Impact Scale – parent version. *Journal of Child and Adolescent Psychopharmacology, 14*, 105–114.

Langley, A. K., Peris, T., Wiley, J. F., Kendall, P. C., Ginsburg, G., Birmaher, B., ... Piacentini, J. (2014). The Child Anxiety Impact Scale: Examining parent- and child-reported impairment in child anxiety disorders. *Journal of Clinical Child & Adolescent Psychology, 43*, 579–591.

Lau, J. Y. F., & Pile, V. (2015). Can cognitive bias modification of interpretations training alter mood states in children and adolescents? A reanalysis of data from six studies. *Clinical Psychological Science, 3*, 112–125.

Linetzky, M., Pergamin-Hight, L., Pine, D. S., & Bar-Haim, Y. (2015). Quantitative evaluation of the clinical efficacy of attention bias modification treatment for anxiety disorders. *Depression and Anxiety, 32*, 383–391.

Lord, F.-M. (1958). The utilization of unreliable difference scores. *Journal of Educational Psychology, 49*, 150–152.

Lowther, H., & Newman, E. (2014). Attention bias modification (ABM) as a treatment for child and adolescent anxiety: A systematic review. *Journal of Affective Disorders, 168*, 125–135.

MacLeod, C., & Clarke, P. J. F. (2015). The attentional bias modification approach to anxiety intervention. *Clinical Psychological Science, 3*, 58–78.

MacLeod, C., & Mathews, A. (2012). Cognitive bias modification approaches to anxiety. *Annual Review of Clinical Psychology, 8*, 189–217.

MacLeod, C., Mathews, A., & Tata, P. (1986). Attentional bias in emotional disorders. *Journal of Abnormal Psychology, 95*, 15–20.

Manassis, K., Russell, K., & Newton, A. S. (2010). The Cochrane Library and the treatment of childhood and adolescent anxiety disorders: An overview of reviews. *Evidence-Based Child Health, 5*, 541–554.

Mathews, A., & MacLeod, C. M. (2002). Induced processing biases have causal effects on anxiety. *Cognition and Emotion, 16*, 331–354.

McNally, R. J., Enock, P. M., Tsai, C., & Tousian, M. (2013). Attention bias modification for reducing speech anxiety. *Behaviour Research and Therapy, 51*, 882–888.

Menne-Lothmann, C., Viechtbauer, W., Höhn, P., Kasanova, Z., Haller, S. P., Drukker, M., ... Lau, J. Y. F. (2014). How to boost positive interpretations? A meta-analysis of the effectiveness of cognitive bias modification for interpretation. *PloS One, 9*(6), e100925.

Micco, J. A., Henin, A., & Hirshfeld-Becker, D. R. (2014). Efficacy of interpretation bias modification in depressed adolescents and young adults. *Cognitive Therapy and Research, 38*, 89–102.

Mogoaşe, C., David, D., & Koster, E. H. W. (2014). Clinical efficacy of attentional bias modification procedures: An updated meta-analysis. *Journal of Clinical Psychology, 70*, 1133–1157.

Moser, J. S., Hajcak, G., Huppert, J. D., Foa, E. B., & Simons, R. F. (2008). Interpretation bias in social anxiety as detected by event-related brain potentials. *Emotion, 8*, 693–700.

Muris, P., & Field, A. P. (2008). Distorted cognition and pathological anxiety in children and adolescents. *Cognition & Emotion, 22*, 395–421.

Notebaert, L., Clarke, P. J. F., Grafton, B., & MacLeod, C. (2015). Validation of a novel attentional bias modification task: The future may be in the cards. *Behaviour Research and Therapy, 65*, 93–100.

Orchard, F., Apetroaia, A., Clarke, K., & Creswell, C. (2017). Cognitive bias modification of interpretation in children with social anxiety disorder. *Journal of Anxiety Disorders, 45*, 1–8.

Pergamin-Hight, L., Pine, D. S., Fox, N. A., & Bar-Haim, Y. (2016). Attention bias modification for youth with social anxiety disorder. *Journal of Child Psychology and Psychiatry and Allied Disciplines, 57*, 1317–1325.

Peter, J. P., Churchill, Jr., G. a., & Brown, T. J. (1993). Caution in the use of difference scores in consumer research. *Journal of Consumer Research, 19*, 655. doi:10.1086/209329

Posner, M. I. (1980). Orienting of attention. *The Quarterly Journal of Experimental Psychology, 32*, 3–25.

Price, R. B., Kuckertz, J. M., Siegle, G. J., Ladouceur, C. D., Silk, J. S., Ryan, N. D., ... Amir, N. (2015). Empirical recommendations for improving the stability of the dot-probe task in clinical research. *Psychological Assessment, 27*, 365–376.

Price, R. B., Wallace, M., Kuckertz, J. M., Amir, N., Graur, S., Cummings, L., ... Bar-Haim, Y. (2016). Pooled patient-level meta-analysis of children and adults completing a computer-based anxiety intervention targeting attentional bias. *Clinical Psychology Review, 50*, 37–49.

Reuland, M. M., & Teachman, B. A. (2014). Interpretation bias modification for youth and their parents: A novel treatment for early adolescent social anxiety. *Journal of Anxiety Disorders, 28*, 851–864.

Riemann, B. C., Kuckertz, J. M., Rozenman, M., Weersing, V. R., & Amir, N. (2013). Augmentation of youth cognitive behavioral and pharmacological interventions with attention modification: A preliminary investigation. *Depression and Anxiety, 30*, 822–828.

Rinck, M., Becker, E. S., Kellermann, J., & Roth, W. T. (2003). Selective attention in anxiety: Distraction and enhancement in visual search. *Depression and Anxiety, 18*, 18–28.

Rooksby, M., Elouafkaoui, P., Humphris, G., Clarkson, J., & Freeman, R. (2015). Internet-assisted delivery of cognitive behavioural therapy (CBT) for childhood anxiety: Systematic review and meta-analysis. *Journal of Anxiety Disorders, 29*, 83–92.

Roy, A. K., Dennis, T. A., & Warner, C. M. (2015). A critical review of attentional threat bias and its role in the treatment of pediatric anxiety disorders. *Journal of Cognitive Psychotherapy, 29*, 171–184.

Roy, A. K., Vasa, R. A., Bruck, M., Mogg, K., Bradley, P., Sweeney, M., ... Team, C. (2008). Attention bias toward threat in pediatric anxiety disorders. *Journal of the American Academy of Child & Adolescent Psychiatry, 47*, 1189–1196.

Rozenman, M., Amir, N., & Weersing, V. R. (2014). Performance-based interpretation bias in clinically anxious youths: Relationships with attention, anxiety, and negative cognition. *Behavior Therapy, 45*, 594–605.

Rozenman, M., Weersing, V. R., & Amir, N. (2011). A case series of attention modification in clinically anxious youths. *Behaviour Research and Therapy, 49*, 324–330.

Salemink, E., Wolters, L., & De Haan, E. (2015). Augmentation of treatment as usual with online cognitive bias modification of interpretation training in adolescents with obsessive compulsive disorder: A pilot study. *Journal of Behavior Therapy and Experimental Psychiatry, 49*, 112–119.

Schmidt, N. B., Richey, J. A., Buckner, J. D., & Timpano, K. R. (2009). Attention training for generalized social anxiety disorder. *Journal of Abnormal Psychology, 118*, 5–14.

Shechner, T., Jarcho, J. M., Britton, J. C., Leibenluft, E., Pine, D. S., & Nelson, E. E. (2013). Attention bias of anxious youth during extended exposure of emotional face pairs: An eye-tracking study. *Depression and Anxiety, 30*(1), 14–21.

Shechner, T., Rimon-Chakir, A., Britton, J. C., Lotan, D., Apter, A., Bliese, P. D., ... Bar-Haim, Y. (2014). Attention bias modification treatment augmenting effects on cognitive behavioral therapy in children with anxiety: Randomized controlled trial. *Journal of the American Academy of Child and Adolescent Psychiatry, 53*, 61–71.

Taghavi, M. R., Moradi, A. R., Neshat-Doost, H. T., Yule, W., & Dalgleish, T. (2000). Interpretation of ambiguous emotional information in clinically anxious children and adolescents. *Cognition & Emotion, 14*, 809–822.

Taylor, C. T., & Amir, N. (2012). Modifying automatic approach action tendencies in individuals with elevated social anxiety symptoms. *Behaviour Research and Therapy, 50*, 529–536.

Trafimow, D. (2015). A defense against the alleged unreliability of difference scores. *Cogent Mathematics, 2*: 1064626.

Van Bockstaele, B., Verschuere, B., Tibboel, H., De Houwer, J., Crombez, G., & Koster, E. H. W. (2014). A review of current evidence for the causal impact of attentional bias on fear and anxiety. *Psychological Bulletin, 140*, 682–721.

Vassilopoulos, S. P., Brouzos, A., & Andreou, E. (2015). A multi-session attribution modification program for children with aggressive behaviour: Changes in attributions, emotional reaction estimates, and self-reported aggression. *Behavioural and Cognitive Psychotherapy, 43*, 538–548.

Vrijsen, J. N., Hertel, P. T., & Becker, E. S. (2016). Practicing emotionally biased retrieval affects mood and establishes biased recall a week later. *Cognitive Therapy and Research, 40*, 764–773.

Walkup, J. T., Albano, A. M., Ph, D., Piacentini, J., Birmaher, B., Compton, S. N., ... Kendall, P. C. (2008). Cognitive behavioral therapy or a combination in childhood anxiety. *The New England Journal of Medicine, 359*, 2753–2766.

Waters, A. M., Craske, M. G., Bergman, R. L., & Treanor, M. (2008). Threat interpretation bias as a vulnerability factor in childhood anxiety disorders. *Behaviour Research and Therapy, 46*, 39–47.

Waters, A. M., Farrell, L. J., Zimmer-Gembeck, M. J., Milliner, E., Tiralongo, E., Donovan, C. L., ... Ollendick, T. H. (2014). Augmenting one-session treatment of children's specific phobias with attention training to positive stimuli. *Behaviour Research and Therapy, 62*, 107–119.

Waters, A. M., Pittaway, M., Mogg, K., Bradley, B. P., & Pine, D. S. (2013). Attention training towards positive stimuli in clinically anxious children. *Developmental Cognitive Neuroscience, 4*, 77–84.

Waters, A. M., Wharton, T. A., Zimmer-Gembeck, M. J., & Craske, M. G. (2008). Threat-based cognitive biases in anxious children: Comparison with non-anxious children before and after cognitive behavioural treatment. *Behaviour Research and Therapy, 46*, 358–374.

Waters, A. M., Zimmer-Gembeck, M. J., Craske, M. G., Pine, D. S., Bradley, B. P., & Mogg, K. (2015). Look for good and never give up: A novel attention training treatment for childhood anxiety disorders. *Behaviour Research and Therapy, 73*, 111–123.

Waters, A. M., Zimmer-Gembeck, M. J., Craske, M. G., Pine, D. S., Bradley, B. P., & Mogg, K. (2016). A preliminary evaluation of a home-based, computer-delivered attention training treatment for anxious children living in regional communities. *Journal of Experimental Psychopathology, 7*, 511–527.

White, L. K., Sequeira, S., Britton, J. C., Brotman, M. A., Gold, A. L., Berman, E., ... Pine, D. S. (2017). Complementary features of attention bias modification therapy and cognitive-behavioral therapy in pediatric anxiety disorders. *American Journal of Psychiatry, 174*, 775–784.

White, L. K., Suway, J. G., Pine, D. S., Field, A. P., Lester, K. J., Muris, P., ... Fox, N. A. (2016). The cognitive and emotional effects of cognitive bias modification in interpretations in behaviorally inhibited youth. *Journal of Experimental Psychopathology, 7*, 499–510.

Wolf, M. M. (1978). Social validity: The case for subjective measurement or how applied behavior analysis is finding its heart. *Journal of Applied Behavior Analysis, 11*, 203–214.

Zvielli, A., Bernstein, A., & Koster, E. H. W. (2015). Temporal dynamics of attentional bias. *Clinical Psychological Science, 3*, 772–788.

Zvielli, A., Vrijsen, J. N., Koster, E. H. W., & Bernstein, A. (2016). Attentional bias temporal dynamics in remitted depression. *Journal of Abnormal Psychology, 125*, 768–776.

6 Brief Intensive Treatments

Donna B. Pincus and Christina Hardway

Introduction

Anxiety disorders are the most prevalent psychiatric disorders to affect children and adolescents (Beesdo, Knappe, & Pine, 2009; Comer & Olfson, 2010; Merikangas, Nakamura, & Kessler, 2009). Symptoms of child and adolescent anxiety frequently persist into adulthood and are associated with considerable burden, life impairment, dysfunction, and reduced quality of life (Comer et al., 2011; Copeland et al., 2014). An extensive search of cross-national studies examining the prevalence of anxiety disorders suggests that up to 10 percent of children and between 20 and 30 percent of adolescents in the general population suffer from an anxiety disorder at any given time (Essau & Gabbidon, 2013; Merikangas et al., 2010). Numerous aspects of child and adolescent functioning can be impaired by an untreated anxiety disorder. For example, youth may have difficulty attending school or staying in school, they may have problems attending school functions or staying in the classroom, they may avoid potentially enjoyable social situations or developmentally appropriate activities, and they may have negative interactions with parents. Some youth with anxiety report distressing physiological symptoms such as stomachaches, headaches, or pounding heart; some may be distracted by constant worry and may have disrupted sleep; and others may seem inattentive and show poor academic performance. It is not uncommon for children and adolescents to endorse a number of these impairing and distressing symptoms. Thus, it is not surprising that parents of children with anxiety disorders report high levels of stress and compromised quality of life for the entire family (Grills-Taquechel & Ollendick, 2012; Liberman et al., 2015). Given the distress and interference associated with anxiety disorders, and the fact that youth with untreated anxiety problems are at risk for other negative mental health problems, including major depression and substance use problems, it is imperative that youth with anxiety receive appropriate treatment as quickly and efficiently as possible.

Fortunately, there have been tremendous advances over the last few decades in the development of efficacious psychological treatments for youth anxiety (Higa-McMillan, et al., 2016; Silverman, Pina, & Viswesvaran, 2008; Walkup et al., 2008). These treatments have been shown to decrease lifelong symptoms, functional burden, cost, and the subsequent onset of comorbid problems such as depression and substance use (see Tolan & Dodge, 2005). Cognitive behavioral therapy (CBT) is considered the "gold standard" psychological treatment, with standard CBT protocols consisting of 11–18 sessions delivered weekly by trained therapists. Although there are minor variations across protocols, most of these treatments include a cognitive component where patients are taught to challenge catastrophic thinking, and a graduated exposure component that is either carried out in vivo, imaginally, or virtually. Roughly 60 to 75 percent of youth show a clinical response and global improvements in functioning after receiving CBT for an anxiety disorder (Higa-McMillan et al., 2016; Silverman, Pina, & Viswesvaran, 2008).

Overview of the Issue – The Need for Innovation

Unfortunately, the majority of children who suffer from anxiety disorders still do not receive any treatment, and the majority of those who do receive treatment do not receive evidence-based psychological treatments. In the United States, for example, fewer than 18 percent of adolescents with anxiety disorders are treated, though older adolescents and females are more likely to receive treatment, compared with younger children and males (Merikangas et al., 2011). One of the reasons children do not receive treatment is due to a shortage of available mental health treatment facilities. In the United States, for example, only 63 percent of counties have a mental health treatment facility that provides care on an outpatient basis to children and families (Cummings, Wen, & Druss, 2013). These shortcomings are even greater in rural areas, where treatment facilities for providing mental health treatment for youth are often nonexistent or difficult to access. Even when mental health facilities are accessible, many of these facilities do not provide youth and families with evidence-based treatment. This may be due to a shortage of therapists trained in evidence-based procedures for treating anxiety, or due to a tendency for medication to be prescribed as a monotherapy in outpatient child and adult mental health settings, despite patients' preferences for psychological treatments (Gallo, Comer, & Barlow, 2013; McHugh et al., 2013).

Parents report numerous other obstacles to their child receiving or completing treatment for their anxiety (Salloum et al., 2016). In addition to financial difficulties (Children's Defense Fund, 2009), logistical barriers impede children's ability to access or benefit from mental health care services (Bringewatt & Gershoff, 2010). Examining specific barriers to accessing and completing community-based mental health services for anxiety treatment, Salloum and colleagues (2016) identified several nonfinancial hindrances that are barriers to receiving appropriate mental health services. Work schedules, transportation, and lack of time to arrange appointments all present difficulties for parents. More than any other barrier to participation, parents cite "stress in their own lives" as an obstacle to getting their child to mental health treatment appointments. Even for youth who do receive treatment, barriers exist that prevent youth from attending sessions or completing homework associated with treatment. For example, over 20 percent of youth surveyed by Salloum and colleagues (2016) indicated they had trouble finding the time needed to complete treatment homework. The length of the treatment itself may also be problematic for some children and young adolescents, with over 20 percent of youth indicating that the 12-week program they were in to treat their anxiety "lasted too long," or that they just generally "lost interest in coming to sessions." Thus, while there is substantial and well-established evidence that supports the effectiveness of traditionally delivered CBT in treating anxiety disorders (e.g., Higa-McMillan et al., 2016), the number of weekly sessions included in this format is quite high. If treatments for anxiety could be delivered more efficiently, perhaps by delivering the same "dose" of treatment across shorter spans of time, it is possible that more youth could be treated, and youth might be better engaged in treatment and have fewer missed sessions. A more expedient format of treatment could help relieve stress on parents and families and help youth return more rapidly to healthier developmental trajectories.

It is also important to consider that despite all the advances that have been made in the development of evidence-based treatments for anxiety disorders, there is still considerable work to be done to optimize the treatments that already exist. This is especially important given that between 25 and 40 percent of youth who do in fact receive "standard" full-length CBT treatments do not show clinical response, or do not reach "diagnosis free" status (Ollendick & King, 2012; Reynolds et al., 2012). Many youth remain symptomatic following treatment, others are resistant to treatments, and a considerable number relapse at long-term follow-up (Ginsburg et al., 2014). Other families report not seeking treatment at all due to the stigma of being involved in lengthy psychological treatment. Thus, numerous questions remain regarding how to adapt treatments so that they are capable of treating complex clinical presentations, and how to modify treatment formats so that they can be delivered more efficiently to youth and families.

Examining the relative benefits of intensive and time-limited therapies is, therefore, an important and innovative step because it could broaden the number of children who access, complete, and benefit from cognitive behavioral therapies (Donovan, 2014). Furthermore, it is possible that delivering CBT across a relatively brief period of time could be helpful for youth with complex clinical presentations, as it may reduce the number of missed sessions and could more efficiently build clinical momentum for the patient. It could also provide opportunities for patients to experience more efficient and varied massed exposures to facilitate the process of inhibitory learning of the feared response and the acquisition of new learning (Bouton, 1993; Craske et al., 2012). In fact, Craske et al. (2012) suggest that anxiety exposures are optimized when sessions are close in proximity and situations are varied for new learning associations to form and replace the fear response.

Against this backdrop, there has been a movement in the last few decades to develop briefer, more intensive, and time-efficient therapies for youth with anxiety disorders, both to expand the "reach" of CBT treatments and to optimize outcomes. The purpose of this chapter is to describe the innovative approaches that researchers have utilized to develop brief, intensive, and concentrated cognitive behavioral treatments for youth. We will first describe the general approach that researchers have taken to develop new treatment formats that contain the same core treatment ingredients as standard full-length CBT treatments. We then summarize the evidence base for this innovative approach to treating child and adolescent anxiety by describing advances in intensive treatments that currently exist for DSM-5 anxiety disorders. Given the importance of expanding our understanding of *why* these treatments work, and *for whom* they work, we proceed to summarize research describing potential mediators and moderators of change in the intensive treatment approach. Using a case illustration (composite of several different patients), we will demonstrate how a brief, intensive treatment can be effective in reducing clinically severe levels of anxiety in an adolescent with panic disorder. Finally, the chapter closes with recommendations for future research in this area, as well as key practice points for those considering utilizing a brief, intensive, and concentrated approach to treat a child or adolescent with an anxiety disorder.

Description of the Approach to Innovation

Innovations in the delivery of CBT in the modern era have largely come from refinements to well-established treatment practices, which have led to more efficiency, allowing therapy to be delivered in fewer sessions, and sometimes even in a single treatment session. The elements of these briefer and more concentrated treatments still address the underlying physiological, behavioral, or cognitive components involved in traditionally delivered CBT (Davis, Ollendick, & Öst, 2009). The first of these abbreviated CBTs for anxiety was originated by Öst and colleagues in the late 1980s (Öst, 1989). These briefer and/or more intensive adaptations have reduced the time over which the therapy is delivered or the number of sessions included in the therapies, but have generally retained what are considered the two "key ingredients" of CBT: cognitive restructuring (helping participants address catastrophic thinking) and behavioral exposures (Öst & Ollendick, 2017).

In their review, Öst and Ollendick (2017) have distinguished between "brief, low intensity" treatments and "brief, intensive and concentrated" treatments. Brief low intensity interventions may be guided or unguided internet-based interventions or self-help books, whereas brief, intensive, and concentrated interventions involve a markedly reduced number of sessions compared to standard CBT and are carried out with a therapist providing the patient with an extended treatment session or more than one session within a short period of time. In the context of a stepped care approach, it is possible that some individuals might benefit from a brief, low intensity treatment such as a self-directed internet-based intervention, whereas others might require either a brief, intensive, and concentrated approach or a standard full-length CBT intervention.

There are many reasons why briefer treatment formats might help transcend some of the barriers to youth receiving evidence-based psychological treatment for anxiety disorders, and why they may be seen as acceptable and even preferable to youth and families. A number of researchers have highlighted patient preference for briefer treatments. For example, Pincus et al. (2010) and Angelosante et al. (2009) reported that one of the most common reasons that patients declined to participate in an 11-

week treatment for panic disorder was the long length of treatment; families reported wanting a treatment that could more quickly help their adolescent return more rapidly to healthy developmental functioning. For youth who are not attending school, the need for an efficient and expedient treatment approach is underscored. If youth could come in for therapy during one day, or one weekend, or one week, for example, and gain the same types of skills as in longer therapies, they would be able to return to developmentally appropriate activities more quickly and functional impairment could be reduced. Furthermore, for patients who have not responded to standard CBT, an intensive approach might provide just the "jumpstart" that they need to start the process of facing their fears. The more intensive approaches to child anxiety treatment also may be more cost-effective and may reduce the risk of attrition. Finally, if learning can be maximized through massed practice, it may make treatment more effective. Given all of these potential benefits, it is not surprising that researchers around the world have reexamined the standard delivery of 50-minute weekly sessions of CBT over a 3–6-month period and have developed briefer and more concentrated treatments. We now turn to reviewing the evidence base for the brief intensive treatments that have been developed for various types of anxiety problems faced by youth.

Evidence Base for Innovation

Intensive Treatment for Specific Phobias

Over the past 20 years that intensive treatments for anxiety have been available, more than 20 studies have investigated their relative benefits (Öst & Ollendick, 2017). Though abbreviated treatments have been developed for several disorders, including panic disorder with agoraphobia, separation anxiety disorder, and social anxiety disorder, considerably more evidence has been accumulated to support the efficacy of the intensive treatment for specific phobias (Öst & Ollendick, 2017). Specific phobias are characterized by an intense and out of proportion fear of a specific object or situation that causes an individual to avoid that stimulus (APA, 2013; Ollendick & Muris, 2015). Whereas the treatment of specific phobias had traditionally been delivered in multiple 50-minute sessions across months of treatment, a groundbreaking series of studies by Öst, Ollendick, and colleagues shows striking evidence that the treatment of phobias can actually be delivered in a single session. In One Session Treatment (OST) of specific phobias, the therapist provides the child and adolescent with psychoeducation and a set of simple skills and then leads the patient to engage in massed exposures during one three-hour session (Ollendick & Davis, 2013; Öst et al., 2001). After an initial assessment with the child in which the clinician assesses the child's associated catastrophic cognitions, discusses the details of the child's phobia, describes the plan for treatment to the child, and answers the child's questions, the one-session intervention is scheduled for about one week later. During that single intervention, a series of exposure exercises is completed to help the child gradually confront the feared stimulus. Using the principles of participant modeling, in vivo exposure, and social reinforcement, the child gains skills that are typically generalized to other situations and stimuli (Ollendick, King, & Chorpita, 2006). In the case of specific phobias, OST is considered a "well-established" treatment, with a great deal of research conducted across several countries supporting its efficacy (Ollendick & Davis, 2013; Ollendick & Muris, 2015; Ollendick et al., 2015; Ryan et al., 2017). While there is some evidence that suggests that OST may be more effective for treating animal phobias than other kinds of phobias, it is still considered to be an effective treatment for all phobias and one that may even help ameliorate other comorbid anxiety disorders (Ollendick & Davis, 2013). In fact, in their narrative meta-analysis, Ollendick and Davis (2013) determine that OST is the "treatment of choice" for young people exhibiting a specific phobia (Ollendick & Davis, 2013, p. 282). OST may be effective because it ameliorates negative cognitions and reduces both cognitive and behavioral avoidance (Davis, Ollendick, & Öst, 2009). Children receiving this treatment report that it is well-paced; it also seems to have a positive impact on children's self-efficacy (Ollendick & Davis, 2013). Overall, results of these studies are highly encouraging in that OST appears to produce similar treatment outcomes as longer, standard CBT packages, and helps youth return more quickly to developmentally appropriate activities.

Intensive Treatment for Separation Anxiety Disorder

As is the case with specific phobias, separation anxiety disorder (SAD) presents earlier than other anxiety disorders (Beesdo et al., 2009). It is marked by a developmentally inappropriate fear of being separated from attachment figures and manifests itself as an excessive distress associated with being alone and an avoidance of sleeping away from home or attachment figures (Mohr & Schneider, 2014). Different therapeutic approaches have been employed to treat children and adolescents with SAD, including various well-established cognitive behavioral treatment programs lasting several months in duration (e.g., "Cool Kids" Anxiety Treatment Program by Rapee and colleagues (Rapee, 2000; Rapee et al., 2006) or "Coping Cat" by Kendall and colleagues (Kendall, 1994; Kendall et al., 1997). However, a promising intensive treatment for separation anxiety disorder employed a one-week "summer camp" style of treatment. The Child Anxiety Multi-Day Program (CAMP) for separation anxiety disorder was specifically designed and tailored to treat school-aged girls aged 7 to 12 with SAD over the course of one week (Santucci et al., 2009; Santucci & Ehrenreich-May, 2013). This treatment program provided youth with the same "dose" of evidence-based treatment components that have been shown in longer treatments to reduce the frequency and intensity of separation anxiety but are delivered in a much shorter time span. The program also provided a camp-like, group structure for youth to engage in developmentally appropriate exposure practices requiring gradual separation from a caregiver, including field trips, movie nights, and social activities; the weeklong treatment culminated in a sleepover so the girls could practice being away from their parents for an entire evening. The program also incorporated peer support to reinforce youths' progress. Parents also received trainings on topics such as using differential reinforcement to shape approach behaviors and modeling nonavoidant behaviors in new situations. The program was quite successful; compared with a wait-list control group, the girls who received treatment showed significant improvements in clinical severity of separation anxiety. At the 6-week follow-up assessment, 50 percent of CAMP participants no longer met the criteria for a SAD diagnosis, compared with 0 percent of children in the wait-list group. Parents also reported that they were very satisfied with the treatment, indicating that it was a promising way of engaging children in numerous separation exposures across varying contexts (Santucci & Ehrenreich-May, 2013).

Intensive Treatment for Social Anxiety Disorder

There are also intensive or abbreviated treatments that have been developed to treat social anxiety disorder (also sometimes referred to as social phobia), a condition characterized by interfering levels of anxiety in social situations and avoidance of those situations (Donovan, 2014). Children with social anxiety disorder may avoid social situations or endure them with considerable distress; this anxiety inevitably impacts social relationships and can result in increased feelings of sadness and isolation. One of the first brief, intensive treatments to be developed for social anxiety disorder was a 3-week group CBT intervention treating children aged 8 to 11 (Donovan, 2014; Gallagher, Rabian, & McCloskey, 2004). This brief, intensive treatment included three, 3-hour sessions that focused on psychoeducation about the nature of anxiety, cognitive strategies, and exposures. It was found to be effective in alleviating the severity of children's social anxiety symptoms with identifiable and significant gains at the 3-week follow-up assessment. Children in the treatment group showed lower levels of social anxiety compared with the wait-list control group (Gallagher, Rabian, & McCloskey, 2004), although rates of remission of the diagnosis of social anxiety were lower than in standard weekly social anxiety treatments. Donovan (2014) posited that youth might have made even more substantial gains if the abbreviated group treatment protocol had incorporated social skills and parent training components. To examine this, Donovan et al. (2015) developed an intensive, group-based intervention for children ages 7 to 12 that was administered across the space of three weekends and included four, 3-hour sessions (for a total of 12 hours of treatment). This intensive treatment program included social skills training, exposures, cognitive restructuring, and problem solving along with a parent training element. Children who had received treatment showed a reduction in both anxiety and internalizing symptoms. At the conclusion of treatment, 52.4 percent of children in the treatment group no longer qualified for a diagnosis of social phobia, compared with 15.8 percent of children in the wait-list group. Moreover, several children in the treatment group continued to improve after the conclusion of treatment, with 76.9 percent of them achieving diagnosis-free status at the 6-month follow-up. Taken together, these results suggest that the positive effects of intensive treatments may emerge after the posttreatment assessment, but over time, their impact may increase and be similar to longer programs of treatment. Perhaps most impressive, 100 percent of the 21 participants in the pilot study completed the treatment, and both parents and children were satisfied with the program (Donovan et al., 2015). The authors suggest that more work in refining intensive treatments for this disorder be conducted, with future research examining whether the component social skills program should be spaced more across the treatment period, rather than grouped into one session. Additionally, research should examine whether emails or telephone calls from therapists after the completion of treatment would benefit patients. Moreover, researchers should investigate whether the treatment could be shortened further for social anxiety disorder, reducing the overall amount of time in therapy, rather than just amassed across a shorter duration of time (Donovan, 2014).

Intensive Treatment for Panic Disorder and/or Agoraphobia

Panic disorder (PD) is characterized by the presence of recurring, unexpected panic attacks, an intensive surge of intense fear and discomfort that reaches a peak within minutes, and causes both physical and cognitive symptoms (APA, 2013). Panic attacks may occur in school-aged children, but it is rare for youth of this age to meet criteria for panic disorder. Panic disorder prevalence rates begin to increase after the onset of puberty (Merikangas et al., 2010). Adolescents with panic often experience uncomfortable physical sensations, such as palpitations, pounding heart, trembling, dizziness, nausea, fears of dying, derealization, and shaking; they also frequently worry about the onset of a future attack and its potential negative and imagined consequences. Some adolescents with panic disorder also present with agoraphobia; these adolescents typically avoid places for fear of those places triggering uncomfortable physical sensations. Panic disorder and agoraphobia are considered to be highly debilitating disorders that have the potential to cause significant life impairment. Some adolescents with panic miss classes frequently due to the onset of panic attacks; in the most severe cases, adolescents do not attend school at all. Youth with panic also tend to avoid other developmentally appropriate activities such as going to the movies, going to the mall, or participating in social outings with friends. Thus, it is not surprising that youth with untreated panic disorder have an increased risk for depression as well as substance use disorders (Costello et al., 2003). Overall, PD is recognized as one of the most impairing anxiety disorders to affect adolescents and warrants treatment at its earliest stages (Ollendick & Pincus, 2008; Pincus et al., 2010).

Fortunately, over the past few decades, numerous iterations of panic treatment have been developed, tested, and specifically tailored for adolescents. In one of the first studies investigating the treatment of panic disorder in adolescents, Ollendick (1995) utilized a multiple baseline design to demonstrate that adult panic control treatment (PCT) could be developmentally tailored and successfully applied to adolescents in six to nine treatment sessions. All adolescents demonstrated a decrease in panic attacks at posttreatment in comparison to baseline. Given these promising and encouraging results, Hoffman and Mattis (2000) further developed panic control treatment for adolescents (PCT-A), an 11-week, cognitive behavioral treatment for adolescents aged 12–17 with panic disorder and their parents.

The treatment included several major components: (1) psychoeducation regarding the interplay of physiological, cognitive, and behavioral factors in the origin and maintenance of panic symptoms, (2) a cognitive component that covers cognitive distortions, cognitive restructuring, and hypothesis testing of feared cognitions, and (3) interoceptive and situational exposures to help youth reduce their avoidance. Youth also create a fear avoidance hierarchy with the therapist in-session but conducted in vivo exposures as homework on their own, without therapist assistance. Results of the first randomized controlled trial of this 11-session PCT-A treatment were quite positive; treatment improved panic severity, anxiety sensitivity, and depression relative to a wait-list control group. Treatment gains were maintained at 3 and 6 months posttreatment, and patients reported that the interference and distress associated with panic were significantly reduced (Pincus et al., 2010). Although this treatment provided symptom relief for many families, numerous families reported that they were concerned about the length of treatment, as the 11 sessions were delivered over 12 weeks, which was a long time to wait before youth could fully resume developmentally appropriate activities. These families requested a briefer treatment to more quickly alleviate their adolescents' panic and to help their family return to healthier functioning.

Subsequently, an intensive format of PCT-A was developed by Pincus and colleagues (Angelosante et al., 2009; Pincus et al., 2014; Pincus, Elkins, & Hardway, 2014) to provide families with quicker relief of panic symptoms; this treatment entailed longer sessions (each spanning 3 to 6 hours in length) delivered across a briefer period of time (8 days). The treatment included all of the components of treatment included in the regular, weekly PCT-A treatment, but also included massed therapist-assisted in vivo exposures to guide and encourage adolescents to enter previously avoided situations. The first three sessions each last 2–3 hours and cover psychoeducation (session 1), cognitive skills (session 2), and interoceptive exposure (session 3). Sessions 4 and 5 each last 6–8 hours and include therapist-assisted in vivo exposures, with gradual fading of the therapist involvement. Sessions 6 and 7 are devoted to adolescents completing independent in vivo exposures. Finally, session 8 is concerned with relapse prevention and future exposure practice planning. This intensive format of treatment is developed to overcome several barriers to care – for example, those living in locations with limited access to any mental healthcare and those who cannot receive care due to long wait-lists at overburdened clinics are able to receive specialty psychological treatment for panic disorder immediately and efficiently. Treatment also included a parent component so that parents can learn skills for supporting their adolescents' success. A recent randomized controlled trial (RCT) demonstrated the efficacy of intensive panic treatment for adolescents aged 11–17 compared to a wait-list control condition; this trial also investigated the relative efficacy of including parents in treatment. Results of the RCT showed that 63 percent of adolescents who received treatment no longer met diagnostic criteria for PD at posttreatment; this rate continued to improve at subsequent follow-up points (Pincus et al., 2014, 2017). This study also showed that parent involvement did not significantly impact the outcome of treatment, as all adolescents who received treatment showed improvement. However, a recent study showed that those adolescents who had mothers who were highly stressed did not improve as much, suggesting that future iterations of panic intensive treatment might include a module directly targeting parental stress (Fenley et al., 2017). The intensive format of treatment was also found to reduce the severity of comorbid anxiety disorder diagnoses, even though these diagnoses were not specifically targeted during treatment (Gallo et al., 2012). In a study examining the rate and shape of change in panic severity, fear, and avoidance across this 8-day intensive treatment, panic severity showed a linear decrease throughout treatment. In contrast, fear and avoidance ratings both showed cubic change, peaking slightly at the first session of treatment, decreasing slightly after the second session, and vastly declining through the end of the fourth day of treatment. These improvements were maintained through the end of the treatment (Gallo et al., 2013). Based on the extant literature, the 8-day intensive format of treatment showed comparable efficacy to the 3-month, weekly format of treatment (Chase, Whitton, & Pincus, 2012). Overall, the intensive treatment format was found to be a highly acceptable and promising format of treatment for teens and parents.

Intensive Treatment for Generalized Anxiety Disorder

Generalized anxiety disorder (GAD) is characterized by the presence of excessive, uncontrollable worry that occurs with (at least one) physiological symptom (APA, 2013). These persistent worries involve negative thoughts about potential dangers and their consequences, and they must also be distressing and interfere with day-to-day life. The prevalence of GAD rises as youth age, and this increase may partially be attributable to maturational increases in children's cognitive ability, which allows them to imagine a range of possible futures in more abstract ways as they grow older. GAD is highly related to other anxiety disorders, and it may also be related to the trait disposition of negative affect (Peters & Waters, 2014). While research on intensive treatments for children and adolescents has not directly targeted reducing the clinical severity of a GAD diagnosis, treatments designed to alleviate the severity of other anxiety disorders have been shown to also reduce the symptoms of GAD. For example, patients receiving the one session treatment (OST) for specific phobias showed improvements in the severity of their other anxiety disorders, including GAD (Ollendick et al., 2010). As many as 50 percent of participants receiving OST for their specific phobia who were also diagnosed with comorbid GAD were considered diagnosis-free at the posttreatment assessment, rising to 77.8 percent of participants being free of their GAD diagnosis at the 6-month follow-up assessment (Ryan et al., 2017). Intensive treatments aimed at reducing panic disorder and agoraphobia have also been shown to have a corollary benefit of reducing the clinical severity of other comorbid disorders, such as GAD (Peters & Waters, 2014). For example, Gallo et al. (2012) conducted an investigation of the changes in comorbid diagnoses following treatment of adolescent panic disorder and agoraphobia (PDA). Of the 55 adolescents included in the PDA intensive treatment, 33 percent (18/55) also met criteria for a diagnosis of GAD. Adolescents' clinical severity ratings on the Anxiety Disorders Interview Schedule (ADIS; Silverman & Albano, 1996) declined from a mean of 4.28 to 2.11 between the pretreatment and the posttreatment assessments, falling below clinically significant diagnostic levels of 4–8 on the scale.

While also not specifically targeting GAD, intensive treatments that are meant to impact a range of anxiety disorders have also been shown to improve the symptoms of GAD. In a pan-diagnostic protocol, Crawley and colleagues (Crawley et al., 2013; Peters & Waters, 2014) developed a brief version of CBT (8 sessions) and delivered it to children between the ages of 6 and 13 with diagnoses of separation anxiety disorder, generalized anxiety disorder, and/or social phobia. They found this treatment to be acceptable to the participants and, at the conclusion of the treatment, 42.3 percent of the treated youth did not meet criteria for their principal anxiety diagnosis. Given that treating comorbid disorders appears to also reduce levels of GAD, therapists treating youth with GAD might utilize existing brief treatment protocols but tailor exposures accordingly. This might be an approach that therapists could use while awaiting further research on intensive treatments for GAD. When other disorders are not present, Peters and Waters (2014) suggest that providing a range of exposure tasks for a range of worry domains (and consistent with the children's source of worry) may be an effective way to conduct GAD intensive therapy. Exposures for youth with GAD could be individually tailored to help the child or adolescent reduce avoidance and perseveration about their particular domains of worry (e.g., perfectionism, health, and personal appearance). Given the limited extant research devoted to investigating the merits of intensive treatment for GAD, this should be a focus of future research efforts.

Overall, there is considerable evidence that these intensive treatments hold promise. A meta-analysis of several brief, intensive, and concentrated CBTs suggests that these treatments are effective when compared with both a wait-list control group and a placebo control group such as education or nondirective therapy (Öst & Ollendick, 2017). Shorter treatment durations were even found to have a higher effect size than longer therapies. The effects of intensive and brief therapies also seem to endure across at least a year, and the rates of recovery and response compare well with regularly delivered CBT therapies (Öst & Ollendick, 2017). Furthermore, intensive treatment formats may reduce the risk of attrition, as research has shown that attrition increases with increasing length of therapy (Swift & Greenberg, 2012).

Mediators and Moderators of Change

Much is yet to be learned regarding both the mediating variables accounting for the benefits of brief and intensive CBT protocols as well as the moderators of this treatment, predicting which patient characteristics or contexts are associated with better or worse outcomes (Ollendick & Muris, 2015). A few demographic predictor variables have been identified; specifically, it is possible that girls may benefit more than boys from intensive therapies (Ollendick & Davis, 2013; Öst & Ollendick, 2017). Age may also be a moderator of treatment efficacy, with older children and adolescents benefiting more compared with younger children (Öst & Ollendick, 2017). Presence of comorbid anxiety disorders and presence of parental involvement in treatment have also been examined in numerous studies. Fortunately, there is some evidence to suggest that the presence of comorbid anxiety disorders does not impede patients' progress in short-term CBT. For example, a few studies indicate that the presence of other disorders does not interfere with the effectiveness of OST (Ollendick et al., 2010; Ryan et al., 2017). OST was even found to be effective for a child with water phobia who presented with other more severe problems, including developmental delays and behavioral problems (Davis et al., 2007; Ollendick & Davis, 2013). In general, however, the findings on non-anxiety comorbidity are more limited and less encouraging than studies on anxiety comorbidity. One study did investigate the effects of having a diagnosis of specific phobia and comorbid attention-deficit/hyperactivity disorder (ADHD) and found that children who have comorbid symptoms of ADHD may be less likely to respond to OST for a specific phobia, according to both the immediate posttreatment assessment and follow-up assessments years later (Halldorsdottir & Ollendick, 2016).

Several studies have also found that brief and intensive treatments may even ease the symptoms and severity of comorbid anxiety disorders when they are present. For example, Ollendick and colleagues (2010) found that OST for specific phobia reduces the severity of the other nontargeted phobias and anxiety disorders (Ollendick et al., 2010; Ryan et al., 2017). Ryan and colleagues (2017) further investigated these effects by examining the ways that OST ameliorated the severity of each of three comorbid diagnoses: GAD, SAD, or other nontargeted specific phobias. They found that, at the conclusion of treatment, all groups demonstrated improvement in their specific phobia, regardless of the co-occurring anxiety disorder. Although the SAD group showed initial poorer improvement than the other groups, this effect was not evident at 6-month follow-up. Thus, these comorbid anxiety disorders didn't interfere with specific phobia treatment and the comorbid anxiety disorders continued to improve as a corollary benefit. Severity of comorbid anxiety disorders (GAD, social phobia, and specific phobia) also improved after an intensive treatment for adolescents with PDA. After completing an intensive treatment for PDA, the percentage of patients qualifying for any clinical anxiety disorder diagnosis was reduced from 78.2 percent to 43.6 percent (Gallo et al., 2012).

Few studies have examined how pretreatment severity of fear and degree of avoidance impact treatment response to an intensive treatment. While it might be predicted that a child with high levels of baseline fear and avoidance might have less favorable outcome, one recent study showed that more moderate levels of baseline fear and avoidance, not more severe levels of fear and avoidance, predicted more favorable outcomes in a sample of youth who received an intensive treatment for panic disorder (Elkins et al., 2016). These findings suggest that this type of intensive treatment may be best suited for youth with more moderate initial anxiety. Future research should investigate the moderating role of pretreatment severity to help elucidate which subgroups of patients might respond best to this format of treatment.

Several researchers have discussed possible sources of mediation by which intensive CBT has a generalized impact on symptoms of other disorders. One such possible mechanism is patients' increased sense of self-efficacy. Patients' improved perception of their ability to cope with the unpleasant affect associated with anxiety may account for the effects of one treatment generalizing to other anxiety disorders (Gallo et al., 2012; Ollendick et al., 2010; Peters & Waters, 2014; Ryan et al., 2017). Other research has focused specifically on the potential mediation of inhibitory learning, in which unhealthy responses to an anxiety-provoking stimulus or context are still present but are inhibited and are replaced by healthier ones that are exhibited (Craske et al., 2012; Ollendick & Muris; 2015; Öst & Ollendick, 2017). Derived from the theoretical and empirical work of learning theorists, some have suggested the effectiveness of CBT in general may be attributable to the repeated exposures that are also incorporated into most abbreviated and intensive treatments (Ollendick & Muris; 2015; Öst & Ollendick, 2017). In this conceptualization, exposures that maximize the effects of inhibitory learning and regulation are predicted to produce superior outcomes (rather than those that focus more on habituation and fear reduction). These new pairings do not erase the originally feared stimulus, but the responses are inhibited by new pairings (Craske et al., 2012). From the perspective of this "learning-centered" theory of CBT, it is useful to deliver exposures by providing several triggers (Craske et al., 2012), a process well-aligned with the methods of intensive treatment (Öst & Ollendick, 2017; Ryan et al., 2017). Some have suggested that the best way to promote this kind of "extinction learning" is to provide exposures that are introduced repeatedly across a short span of time, and ideally, practiced across several contexts (Mohr & Schneider, 2014). Thus, brief and/or intensive CBT protocols provide an opportunity to administer several exposures across a short period of time, and as a result they may be especially effective for this kind of extinction learning. Briefer and more intensive CBT allows for these kinds of exposures to be administered in a more rapid succession, allowing the new associations to form over several situations that are spaced closely together (Öst & Ollendick, 2017).

From this theoretical view, higher levels of fear are sometimes important components of successful exposures, and therefore removing any potential safety behaviors or signals facilitates the development of new pairings. If the safety signal (sometimes the presence of another person) is present, the patient's levels of fear may be reduced, and thus, the opportunity to learn that the fear itself is not inherently threatening is lost (Craske et al., 2012). This may explain some of the mixed findings regarding the moderating variable of parent involvement in intensive CBT (Öst & Ollendick, 2017). Some evidence suggests that, when compared with the control wait-list condition, having a parent present does not produce significantly different outcomes (Ollendick & Davis, 2013; Ollendick & Muris, 2015; Ost et al., 2001; Pincus et al., 2014, 2017). Other research, however, suggests that parental presence may interfere with a child's progress in treatment. In their meta-analysis of intensive and abbreviated CBT, Öst and Ollendick (2017) found that lower parental involvement yielded greater effect sizes than higher levels of parental involvement across brief and intensive formats. It is possible that parents may be serving as a "safety" signal for their children, and possibly reduce the level of personal self-efficacy the patients are building during the course of treatment. It is also possible that parents who are more directly involved with therapy may develop unreasonable expectations for their children as a function of observing their progress while in treatment (Ollendick, et al., 2015; Ollendick & Muris, 2015). It has also been suggested that parents' inability to tolerate their own levels of stress and distress at seeing their child anxious may cause them to interfere in the exposure process (Fenley et al., 2017). Still other research concludes that parents can be incorporated successfully into treatment and trained to coach their children's exposures appropriately (Whiteside et al., 2015). In general, parental involvement in treatment for anxiety is a source of ongoing discussion in cognitive behavioral therapies, and the complicated array of findings may also arise, in part, because the parent involvement components differs across therapies and also diffuses the focus on exposures (Taboas et al., 2015).

Clinical Case Illustration

Background and Assessment

Kayla, age 16, stated during her initial assessment that she had been searching the internet for help for what she called the intense "tidal waves" of uncomfortable feelings that started when she was in middle school. She reported that despite the fact that she had a number of close friends, and good relationships with her teachers and her family, she had not told anyone about these "waves" of sheer panic that she experienced because she had always found ways to manage them herself. She reported that she started getting panic attacks at the age of 12, during her ballet classes. Specifically, Kayla described her first panic attack that occurred while doing regular barre work in ballet – her heart was racing already from dancing, and suddenly, "out of the blue" she felt dizzy, nauseous, and after a few minutes she felt very short of breath. She told her dance teacher that she didn't feel well and stopped dancing for the rest of the class. In subsequent dance classes, Kayla described that she would start to feel the uncomfortable feelings arise even before dance started. Sometimes Kayla worried that she was going crazy, her heart was malfunctioning, or that she was terribly out of shape. She stated that she combatted these feelings pretty successfully by taking frequent sips of her water bottle; she also reported that she cut out a tiny piece of her baby blanket that she kept tucked away and hidden in her ballet slipper. She described that whenever she had this blanket piece with her, nothing catastrophic seemed to happen, and her panic never got too "out of control" for her to manage. Kayla reported that she occasionally felt panicky in school but typically could ask for a pass to the bathroom when this happened. Kayla worried that something was very wrong with her body, or that she was at risk for a heart attack. But she did not want to worry her parents who already had a lot of stress in their lives, so she continued to manage these symptoms alone.

When Kayla turned 16, she started her first job waitressing at a local diner. She was excited to get a job in their town to make extra money; she also knew the family was often stretched thin in finances and that this job would help out. Kayla had two older sisters and one younger sister, and her parents worked hard and often long hours. Both of her older sisters had jobs waitressing too. Kayla's father was a salesman and her mother worked as a secretary at a middle school near their home. Kayla reported that she knew she needed help for her panicky feelings after she began waitressing. Kayla reported that she frequently felt her panic symptoms increase after she had taken a customer's order, and on several occasions, she felt she had to leave the restaurant and walk outside temporarily for the panic to subside. During her first few weeks of waitressing, she had many customers complain that she "took too long" to get their order. Kayla's anxiety continued to soar; her anxiety and worry about having a panic attack while waitressing caused her panic frequency to further increase. At the time that she searched for help, Kayla reported having approximately five "out of the blue" panic attacks per day. She also reported that her typical methods for feeling better (like drinking her water, texting a friend, or touching her piece of baby blanket) were no longer working. What alarmed Kayla most was that one Sunday morning, she experienced her worst panic attack while in her pajamas eating breakfast with her father. Typically, this was the most relaxed part of her day. Her worry about her panic increased at school. When she asked her teachers for passes to leave the classroom and use the restroom, they refused, noting that she had been "making a habit of leaving the class way too often." This caused Kayla to panic and she refused to return to school. She confided in her mother about how desperate she was for help. Kayla's mother began taking time off from work to accompany Kayla to school. She reported that Kayla's panic seemed to subside when she was nearby. On "bad days," Kayla's mother stated that she would just sit in the parking lot of the school in case Kayla needed her to take her home. Even on good days, Kayla's mother said she was constantly responding to texts from Kayla asking for reassurance that she was going to be ok. Kayla reported that she found the adolescent anxiety clinic after searching online and her mother agreed that things had gotten "out of hand" and that they needed help.

Kayla's mother accompanied Kayla to the assessment session and feedback session. During the feedback session, the therapist explained the symptoms of panic disorder and described several evidence-based treatment options. Kayla stated that she hoped that the treatment did not include medication, as she did not want to take anything else that might make her feel "not herself." The therapist described the types of skills that Kayla would learn in cognitive behavioral therapy for panic and described that the majority of teens respond well to learning CBT skills. The therapist also presented several options of formats for receiving CBT treatment. One option was an 11-week CBT treatment for panic disorder offered once per week (50 minutes per session). The other option was an 8-day intensive treatment option that would require Kayla to attend sessions every day for 8 consecutive days. Kayla, her mother, and the therapist discussed several pros and cons of each option. Kayla's mother feared that if they chose the 11-week option, they might miss sessions due to holidays, bad weather, or due to their busy schedules. Kayla worried that 11 weeks was a "long time" to wait to get better. She stated that if she could learn how to feel better quickly, perhaps she could get her old waitressing job back. Kayla's mom also expressed preference for a briefer treatment period, as she was watching her daughter's life "unravel" around her. Kayla and her mom decided that completing treatment across an 8-day period could work during the school vacation week. Kayla and her mother scheduled the one-week intensive treatment. At the end of the feedback session, Kayla stated that she was worried that she was going to be the "only person" that the treatment wouldn't work for.

Session 1

During the first day of treatment (Day 1, Monday), Kayla's therapist (who was the same therapist who conducted the assessment) welcomed her to treatment and engaged her in a discussion of her goals for therapy. Kayla reported wanting to "get rid" of her panic attacks so she could lead a normal life again. The therapist validated Kayla's desires to get better and acknowledged how difficult it must have been to make the call to get help. The therapist also acknowledged the fact that Kayla happened to find one of the best specialty clinics in the country to get help for anxiety, which Kayla said gave her a lot of comfort and helped her to not feel so alone. Kayla's therapist also utilized other motivational interviewing strategies such as asking Kayla how her life would be better if she could learn to manage her anxiety, and what the costs would be of things "staying the same." The therapist also described how getting better was going to require some hard work and dedication on Kayla's part; in addition to the daily sessions, Kayla would need to complete readings in her workbook each night and would be required to practice the skills she learned in session. Kayla articulated that she was willing to do hard work but feared that she would not be able to tolerate her panic. The therapist reassured Kayla that she would learn skills to help her and that she would never be forced to do anything she wasn't ready and willing to try. Prior to the first session, Kayla had already read portions of the adolescent panic workbook about the causes of panic and about the three-component model of panic, which was a depiction of the cognitive, physiological, and behavioral symptoms and their interactions. Kayla's mother also reported that she read Kayla's workbook, as she was desperate to learn better ways to help Kayla function better.

During the first session of the intensive treatment, which lasted approximately 3 hours, the therapist met with Kayla first and answered Kayla's questions about the three-component model. The therapist then presented psychoeducation about panic – why anxiety and panic are actually the fight or flight system, the body's way of protecting itself from danger. Kayla reported being surprised at how many symptoms of the fight or flight system (e.g., heart racing, shortness of breath, dizziness, sweatiness, nausea) were actually adaptive. What surprised Kayla most was the fact that her body was "hard wired" to sweat to ward off danger, and that by being sweaty, humans are "slippery" and protected from danger. Kayla also learned that panic does not actually come from "out of the blue," but that there were typically triggers for panic. Kayla learned that panic triggers could be a thought, physical feeling, or behavior. The therapist guided Kayla in identifying potential triggers to her panicky feelings. The therapist also emphasized that the frightening feelings that Kayla had been experiencing were actually harmless; they were simply evidence that the fight or flight system had been activated. At the end of the session, Kayla and the therapist constructed a Fear Avoidance Hierarchy (FAH) so that Kayla could begin thinking about the types of activities she currently avoided due to panic.

The therapist stated that they would track changes in her ratings of fear and avoidance of these activities and situations. The atmosphere in the session was quite collaborative; Kayla contributed situations to the FAH and also helped to put them in order from least to most anxiety-provoking. At the end of the session, the rationale and structure of the rest of the week of treatment was presented to Kayla, along with homework assignments. Kayla's mother was brought into the session during the last 30 minutes, and Kayla taught her mother some of the facts she had just learned about panic during the session. Kayla's mother was glad to be involved and included but recognized that getting better was going to mostly be up to Kayla. Kayla was assigned additional chapters of reading to do for homework to prepare her for the next day's session.

Session 2

The second session of treatment (Day 2, Tuesday) lasted two hours and was geared toward helping Kayla understand the cognitive distortions that could contribute to the three-component model of anxiety and panic. Kayla was particularly interested in learning to cope with probability overestimation and catastrophic thinking. Kayla was taught how to counter these distortions using cognitive restructuring and by learning to think more realistically. The therapist also covered topics such as overt avoidance and safety behaviors, and the reasons why both types of avoidant behaviors tend to maintain anxiety. Kayla recognized that her drinking water excessively was a safety behavior and not simply part of good hydration; she also quickly pointed out that her habit of carrying the little square of her baby blanket with her was also a safety behavior. She was eager to complete her homework assignment to identify and challenge her automatic thoughts.

Session 3

The third session of treatment (Day 3, Wednesday) lasted two hours. During this session, Kayla's therapist introduced the topic of interoceptive exposure by guiding Kayla through a series of symptom-induction exercises that purposely were meant to "bring on" panic. Kayla became tearful when running in place and breathing through a cocktail straw, as she stated that these exercises brought on her panic "full force." After several trials of each exercise, Kayla noticed that her anxiety about the symptoms was decreasing. She noticed that the symptoms seemed to dissipate within a few minutes and she stated that she was surprised at the fact that her body "knew" how to bring itself back to a "normal" state. The therapist described that the goal of the exercises was to help her learn that the feelings of anxiety are harmless, temporary, and can be overcome. Kayla's homework assignment for the evening was to continue practicing her interoceptive exposure exercises. Kayla's mom was invited into the session at the end of treatment and Kayla requested that her mom try out a few of the exercises that Kayla found to be the most difficult. Kayla's mother stated that she had "no idea" that the symptoms of panic were that intense, and that she was proud of her daughter for tolerating such intense physical feelings.

Session 4 and 5

Sessions 4 and 5 (Days 4 and 5, Wednesday and Thursday) of treatment each lasted 6–8 hours and were devoted to conducting in vivo exposures. Kayla stated that she realized she would have to practice her new skills while learning not to avoid. Kayla had decided that anyplace where she could not escape easily would be a good place to practice "bringing on panic," such as riding the subway, going to a movie and sitting in the middle of the auditorium, taking a several hour boat tour, going to dance classes, and sitting in crowded classrooms. The therapist started by taking away all safety objects (water bottle, square of baby blanket). The therapist then engaged Kayla in conducting exposures that elicited moderate anxiety to increase her confidence and then proceeded with more difficult and longer exposures. Kayla was occasionally resistant to conduct certain exposures (like visiting a college classroom and attending a lecture), but the therapist reminded Kayla of her overall goals for treatment and the costs she had outlined in session one of not getting better. Kayla was able to reiterate all the reasons why she wanted to get better, and why the short term "cost" of feeling uncomfortable was worth the long term "gains" of "getting her life back." She was successful at conducting exposures listed on her FAH and even repeated certain exposures in different contexts to facilitate her learning new behaviors. Kayla's mother was very proud to learn about all Kayla had accomplished in such a short time period.

Sessions 6, 7, and 8

During the weekend (Days 6 and 7), Kayla planned several exposures that her mom could take her to (e.g., more dance classes, and a sleepover at a friend's house). On the final session of treatment (Day 8), Kayla discussed her experience of conducting exposures on her own and with her mom. The final session of treatment lasted approximately 2 hours. Kayla stated that she felt much more confident in herself and her ability to understand her panic. She stated that although she was still having some panic attacks, she wasn't afraid of them. The therapist and Kayla talked about a plan for future exposure practices, and also talked about normal fluctuations in anxiety that she might expect over time. Kayla showed her mother her plan for future exposure practice, which Kayla's mother supported. At the end of treatment, Kayla's mother asked for a few moments alone with the therapist. She became tearful as she stated how grateful she was for the help for her daughter; she also described feeling sad that her daughter did not "need" her to help in the same way anymore. She reported wanting to be sure that their relationship continued to be strong despite the fact that Kayla's panic had subsided. Kayla and her mother discussed the importance of continuing to make time for each other, in addition to Kayla spending more time with friends. The therapist reminded Kayla's mother that she could still nurture a close relationship with her daughter while encouraging her independence to try new things. Kayla reported feeling much happier and was shocked at her "turn-around" in just a week's time. The therapist called Kayla once per week for four weeks after treatment; at each of these check-ins, Kayla reported that her panic frequency had decreased substantially, and that she was proud to say that she got a new waitressing job. She also was attending school. She proudly stated that the baby blanket had a special place in her room, but no longer was her "safety net." Overall, Kayla reported feeling happier, and that she was finally able to return to her favorite activities with her friends.

Challenges and Recommendations for Future Research in This Area

Research on Intensive Treatments for Other Anxiety Disorders and Ways to Augment or Optimize Intensive Treatments

Considerably more research has been devoted to brief and intensive treatments for specific phobias compared with the other anxiety disorders. In their meta-analysis of intensive treatments, Öst and Ollendick (2017) included 13 RCT studies targeting specific phobias and only one study focused on panic disorder with agoraphobia, one on separation anxiety, and one on social anxiety disorder, with another one focusing on mixed anxiety. More research investigating the effectiveness of these kinds of brief, intensive, and concentrated therapies for the other anxiety disorders in youth is necessary, especially for GAD, SAD, and PDA. In addition, no studies to date have reported the efficacy of intensive approaches for selective mutism, although studies are currently underway testing one-week treatment of selective mutism in preschool and school-aged children (e.g., Furr et al., 2017). Furthermore, transdiagnostic anxiety intensive treatment formats may hold promise as well; such treatments could be structured in a way that allows them to be tailored to treat a variety of anxiety disorders. Furthermore, given the success of initial research demonstrating ways to augment intensive treatment of specific phobias using attention training to positive stimuli, future research might further investigate ways to incorporate attention training to optimize children's responses (Waters et al., 2014). Ultimately, we need more trials to be conducted with youth with a variety of anxiety diagnoses in order to better understand why they work and for whom they work best.

Treatment Nonresponders

Despite the impressive results of brief, intensive, and concentrated treatments, a substantial portion of participants still do not respond to treatment. Promisingly, more participants show recovery when measured later at follow-up than on posttreatment assessment points; this improvement appears to be similar to standard CBT. While patients receiving intensive treatments tend to improve more than those who received wait-list and placebo comparison groups, additional treatment variations should be explored to help nonresponders (Öst & Ollendick, 2017). Even in the most well-established of these intensive treatments, OST for specific phobia, a substantial percentage of children do not respond at all or only partially respond (20 to 50 percent; Ollendick & Muris; 2015) to treatment. Research investigating ways to help this group of children and adolescents who do not show adequate response to standard or intensive treatments for anxiety is critically needed. Future research might focus on ways to optimize or augment treatment using techniques such as attention training or booster sessions delivered via phone or e-health methods. Other research could investigate ways to increase the salience and relevance of exposures.

While e-health methods have now been harnessed to expand the "reach" of many evidence-based treatments for youth, to date there have not been many known existing studies that have incorporated this technology into intensive treatments to further reduce barriers to patients' access to treatment. One such study is currently underway in which the psychoeducation portion of an intensive treatment for panic disorder in adolescents is delivered directly to youth in middle and high schools using an I-pad or tablet (Pincus, 2017). Adolescents aged 12–17 with panic disorder and agoraphobia access an online "course" in which they complete modules of treatment twice per week for four weeks. Each treatment module can be completed in 30 minutes. At the end of each module, the adolescent can access a therapist by utilizing WebEx teleconferencing software on the tablet. The therapist, who is specially trained in panic disorder treatment, conducts a 10-minute "check-in" to answer adolescents' questions about their newly acquired knowledge. Focus groups are being conducted with school personnel (principals, teachers, school psychologists, and nurses) to gain a better understanding of the barriers and facilitators of this type of treatment modality being sustainable in a school setting. Future research can continue to explore the utility of e-health methods to expand the reach of intensive treatments into children's and adolescents' natural settings (e.g., school, aftercare, pediatric primary care).

Long-Term Impact of Treatment

While a substantial portion of patients may not respond initially to intensive therapies for anxiety, it is important to note that several studies, across disorders, indicate that participants continued to improve at later follow-up assessments, sometimes months after the conclusion of an intensive therapy. Thus, more research should be conducted on the possible delayed impact of intensive treatment. For example, Santucci and Ehrenreich-May (2013) found that after an intensive treatment for SAD, 43 percent of participants no longer met criteria for the SAD diagnosis, but at 6-week follow-up, that number had risen to 61 percent. Likewise, Ryan et al. (2017) found continued improvement in the severity of comorbid anxiety disorders at 6 months following one session treatment (OST) for specific phobias. Moreover, Donovan (2014) reported that children with social anxiety disorder continued to improve more over time after intensive treatment, with up to 76.9 percent of youth achieving diagnosis-free status at the 6-month follow-up, suggesting that the effects may be slower to emerge than in a traditionally delivered format but over time, the impact is similar to longer programs of treatment (Donovan, 2014). Pincus et al. (2014) also reported that youth with panic disorder showed the largest response to treatment at 3 months following an intensive treatment for PDA. Although Ollendick and colleagues (2015) show lasting improvements in clinical severity of specific phobias up to 4 years posttreatment, most existing studies have not included follow-up assessments of functioning beyond one year. Future studies could investigate the durability of treatment effects after intensive treatments for PDA, social anxiety disorder, and separation anxiety disorder. Studies could also evaluate whether the use of booster sessions, either in person, by phone, or via e-health methods, can prevent future relapse.

Optimizing the Role of Parents in Intensive Treatments

Although research findings to date generally indicate that the degree of parental involvement in intensive treatment is inversely related to treatment outcomes, future studies with larger and more diverse samples might further investigate whether there are certain "optimal" levels of parental involvement based on several contextual variables, such as the child's anxiety at pretreatment, the age of the child, and parental variables such as levels of parental stress and psychopathology. Furthermore, it is possible that the content of the parent portion of treatment could be revisited or reconceptualized. For example, it may be helpful for parents to have separate meetings with a therapist in which they gain psychoeducation about anxiety being adaptive and unharmful, and learn to support children's and adolescents' nonavoidance of fear. It also may be helpful for parents to gain education about how to reduce stress and more effectively cope with stress and problems in their own lives. However, it may be necessary for parents not to be present during children's or adolescents' exposure practice so that they don't inadvertently serve as a safety signal. Overall, it would be helpful for future research to continue to investigate when to involve parents as well as the most appropriate ways to include parents (Taboas et al., 2015).

Research with Larger and More Diverse Samples

Across studies of intensive treatments there is a need for investigations that include larger and more diverse samples of patients in order to fully explore fine-grained analyses of mediators and moderators of change, and to better understand the ways that treatment might be tailored to better fit particular subgroups of patients. For example, it is possible that intensive treatments increase self-efficacy, and also decrease children's danger expectancies and behavioral approach tendencies; such investigations would be better powered with larger samples. Further, larger samples with more comorbidity would also afford us opportunities to explore the benefits of intensive treatments for youth for patients of different backgrounds and different pretreatment profiles. It would be helpful to understand which subgroups of patients might respond better to more traditional, longer CBT treatments and which might respond better to more intensive approaches. With more diverse samples, it will be possible to explore how the effectiveness of treatment might be impacted by the presence of impairing comorbid disorders such as behavioral disorders, learning disorders, or attentional problems. It is possible that the presence of these disorders may limit the teen's ability to focus and acquire necessary skills during long treatment sessions, for example. Future intensive treatments may explore how to adapt or tailor treatments so that they can accommodate youth with these types of disorders.

Appropriate Ways to Scale Intensive Interventions So They Can Be Delivered in Community-Based Settings

It is important to consider how these intensive treatments can be effectively scaled and disseminated to be delivered in more community-based settings, such as schools or primary care settings. Although some research on this topic is already underway, the field continues to need to develop ways that the very best treatments can be made available to greater numbers of youth. In addition, it is necessary for future research to investigate ways to increase the accessibility and affordability of such treatments (Albano, 2009). Despite the evidence base for brief and intensive treatments, there are challenges associated with making them more accessible to those in need, such as securing the support of third-party payers or finding ways to schedule 180 minutes, rather than the traditional 50-minute block more frequently used. Other challenges include generally gaining acceptability of these shorter-term treatments among the public (Albano, 2009; Davis, Ollendick, & Öst, 2009). Future research might engage community clinicians in research collaborations to discern whether intensive formats are transportable to these settings and whether further adaptation of these treatments is needed.

Key Practice Points

Building Rapport

There are a number of factors to consider when implementing an intensive treatment format. A number of researchers have pointed out that the intensive format of treatment, whether conducted over a few hours or a few weeks, does not allow therapists a lot of time to slowly develop a therapeutic alliance with a patient in the same way that could occur in a weekly therapy that spans several months. Some researchers, however, have raised the question of whether strong rapport between therapist and patient is even necessary for treatment to be effective (Whiteside & Storch, 2015). Nevertheless, therapists might consider a number of strategies for aligning with the patient and building trust quickly. One strategy involves using motivational enhancement techniques in the first session, as illustrated in the case of Kayla. Rapport can also be built with the child or adolescent and family if the therapist aligns with the child when talking about the goals for treatment (e.g., reducing fear, making life easier and happier). Therapists might also refer to themselves as a "coach" who is going to help teach the child skills for reducing their fears, rather than a "doctor" who is there to "fix" them. In this way, the therapeutic alliance is fostered while emphasizing the importance of the child's role in getting better. Some researchers have proposed that the therapeutic alliance may be built even more quickly in an intensive treatment due to the numerous sequential hours of in vivo exposure practice (Angelosante et al., 2009). As the child gradually completes new exposures and learns that his or her feared consequences do not happen, trust with the therapist is fostered.

Planning Time

The intensive treatment format does require more planning time "up front" for the therapist, who must plan exposures, teach skills, and manage patient care over a shorter period of time. Unlike weekly treatment that spans several months, therapists who conduct treatment in an intensive format will not have the benefit of having long spans of time between sessions to plan subsequent sessions. In many ways, this requires a good deal of energy on the part of the therapist, who may need to limit their caseload while conducting intensive treatment.

Advance planning is often required for intensive treatments to run smoothly and for patients to engage in several appropriate exposures in a limited time. For example, the process of conducting one session, intensive treatment of phobias involves more advanced planning so that therapists can provide the requisite elements to properly treat children's and adolescents' fears (Davis, Ollendick, & Öst, 2009). Therapists must be prepared to make certain that they themselves are comfortable with the stimulus, must plan where the exposures will take place, and must have a general familiarity with the stimulus including elevators or insects. Similar suggestions have been made for therapists conducting intensive treatment of panic disorder in adolescents (Angelosante et al., 2009). Thus, regardless of the anxiety diagnosis, it is good practice to make sure that the delivery of these short-term, intensive treatments is carefully planned. Therapists must know what is safe themselves (e.g., in the case of food allergies, or contact with particular types of animals). Additionally, the therapist must be prepared to deal with unexpected contingencies and, when they arise, use them skillfully as part of the treatment.

Special Developmental Considerations in Treating Children

When treating children, Ollendick and Davis (2013) suggest that therapists take into account the child's developmental level. For example, children may require more concrete examples and younger children may need more support in eliciting and recognizing their associated catastrophic cognitions. Very young children may not be able to access or articulate their feared cognitions; in these cases, the treatment might focus more on conducting in vivo exposures and providing the child with accurate information about the feared stimulus. Treatment formats that decrease the stigma of receiving mental health treatment (such as the CAMP for SAD described by Santucci and colleagues earlier in this chapter) may increase the chance that the treatment is seen as acceptable to youth and that youth are motivated to take part in it.

Another important practice point involves how much independence to give youth as they practice exposures. Children may need to have parents involved in at least some exposure planning; for example, in the case of conducting exposures for SAD, parents may need to drive youth to friends' houses or help plan sleepovers away from home. In the case of dog phobias, parents may need to take youth to dog walking parks or other places where they are likely to encounter dogs. However, parents may be coached on how and when to give youth "space" as the child plans and conducts exposures, so that parents do not inadvertently function as a safety person and reduce the exposure's efficacy. There are many exposures that children can engage in independently; taking charge of exposures could further reinforce the child's confidence and self-efficacy. In the case of an adolescent with panic who was avoiding movies, for example, the therapist had the parent drive the adolescent to the movie, but the parent did not sit with the adolescent during the movie. Therapists should help parents to navigate their role in the exposure process and teach parents methods for navigating their own distress as they watch their child experience the "temporary discomfort" of anxiety as the child faces his or her fears. Future research might explore whether parents with particular risk factors (i.e., high anxiety, overprotective parenting style) might benefit most from treatments that include parents.

It is not uncommon for any patient to express some resistance to change, and this may be especially evident in intensive treatments given that they require a good deal of motivation on the part of the patient. In the case of young children, this may be observable in the form of tantrums, and in the case of adolescents this may be observable in the form of refusal to engage in exposures. The therapist should be aware of using differential reinforcement (praising approach behaviors and ignoring tantrums), as well as helping youth break down exposures into manageable "steps" in case resistance is met. Moreover, therapists can encourage youth to revisit how life could be better without their particular fear or anxiety getting in the way.

Supporting Continued Success after Intensive Treatment

Given the delay in impact of intensive treatments, it is important to emphasize to patients the importance of continued exposure practice even after treatment has ended. For example, it has been suggested that therapists align with youth in planning a detailed list of self-directed exposure practices in the patient's home setting to help youth maintain and even increase treatment gains over the weeks and months following treatment. This can be accomplished by having the child (and parent) agree to plan out a specific schedule for practice exposures on a planning calendar. Patients could be encouraged to first brainstorm potential obstacles to exposure completion (e.g., lack of time due to busy schedule, inability to encounter a feared stimulus), and then for patients (and parents and the therapist) to brainstorm solutions together. Developing a detailed plan for when, how, and where the exposures could be conducted may increase the likelihood of compliance; furthermore, patients could be specifically educated about how continued practice keeps "reminding" one's brain on how to respond without fear. Brief telephone check-ins with a therapist could be scheduled and booster sessions could be implemented with a therapist as needed. Angelosante et al. (2009) recommend that parents continually reinforce a child's or adolescent's progress, even after treatment has terminated. As investigations of intensive treatments continue, it is likely that we will learn more about how to reduce barriers to care, how to engage parents most effectively in supporting treatment, and how to support youths' continued success so that their impairment is reduced and quality of life is improved.

References

Albano, A. M. (2009). Special Series: Intensive cognitive-behavioral treatments for child and adolescent anxiety disorders, *Cognitive and Behavioral Practice*, *16*, 358–362.

American Psychiatric Association. (2013). *Diagnostic and statistical manual of mental disorders* (5th edn.). Arlington, VA: American Psychiatric Publishing.

Angelosante, A. G., Pincus, D. B., Whitton, S. W., Cheron, D., & Pian, J. (2009). Implementation of an intensive treatment protocol for adolescents with panic disorder and agoraphobia. *Cognitive and Behavioral Practice*, *16*(3), 345–357. doi:10.1016/j.cbpra.2009.03.002

Beesdo, K., Knappe, S., & Pine, D. S. (2009). Anxiety and anxiety disorders in children and adolescents: Developmental issues and implications for DSM-V. *Psychiatric Clinics of North America*, *32*(3), 483–524. doi:10.1016/j.psc.2009.06.002

Bouton, M. E. (1993). Context, time and memory retrieval in the interference paradigms of Pavlovian learning. *Psychological Bulletin*, *114*, 80–99. http://dx.doi.org/10.1037/0033-2909.114.1.80

Bringewatt, E. H., & Gershoff, E. T. (2010). Falling through the cracks: Gaps and barriers in the mental health system for America's disadvantaged children. *Children and Youth Services Review*, *32*(10), 1291–1299. doi:10.1016/j.childyouth.2010.04.021

Chase, R. M., Whitton, S. W. & Pincus, D. B. (2012). Treatment of adolescent panic disorder: A nonrandomized comparison of intensive versus weekly CBT. *Child and Family Behavior Therapy*, *34*, 305–323.

Children's Defense Fund (2009). The barriers: Why is it so difficult for children to get mental health screens and assessments? Retrieved from http://www.childrensdefense.org/library/data/barriers-children-mental-health-screens-assesments.pdf

Comer, J. S. & Olfson, M. (2010). The epidemiology of anxiety disorders. In H. B. Simpson, F. Schneier, Y. Neria, & R. Lewis-Fernandez (eds.), *Anxiety disorders: Theory, research, and clinical perspectives* (pp. 6–19). New York: Cambridge University Press.

Comer, J. S., Blanco, C., Hasin, D. S., et al. (2011). Health-related quality of life across the anxiety disorders: Results from the National Epidemiologic Survey on Alcohol and Related Conditions (NESARC). *The Journal of Clinical Psychiatry*, *72*(1), 43–50.

Copeland, W. E., Angold, A., Shanahan, L., & Costello, E. J. (2014). Longitudinal patterns of anxiety from childhood to adulthood: The Great Smoky Mountains Study. *Journal of the American Academy of Child and Adolescent Psychiatry*, *53*(1), 21–33.

Costello, E. J., Mustillo, S., Erkanli, A., Keeler, G., & Angold, A. (2003). Prevalence and development of psychiatric disorders in childhood and adolescence. *Archives of General Psychiatry*, *60*(8), 837–844.

Craske, M. G., Liao, B., Brown, L., & Vervliet, B. (2012). Role of inhibition in exposure therapy. *Journal of Experimental Psychopathology*, *3*(3), 322–345. doi:10.5127/jep.026511

Crawley, S. A., Kendall, P. C., Benjamin, C. L., Brodman, D. M., Wei, C., Beidas, R. S., … Mauro, C. (2013). Brief cognitive-behavioral therapy for anxious youth: Feasibility and initial outcomes. *Cognitive and Behavioral Practice, 20*(2), 123–133. doi:10.1016/j.cbpra.2012.07.003

Cummings, J. R., Wen, H., & Druss, B. G. (2013). Improving access to mental health services for youth in the United States. *JAMA: Journal of the American Medical Association, 309*(6), 553–554. doi:10.1001/jama.2013.437

Davis, T. I., Kurtz, P. F., Gardner, A. W., & Carman, N. B. (2007). Cognitive-behavioral treatment for specific phobias with a child demonstrating severe problem behavior and developmental delays. *Research in Developmental Disabilities, 28*(6), 546–558. doi:10.1016/j.ridd.2006.07.003

Davis, T. I., Ollendick, T. H., & Öst, L. (2009). Intensive treatment of specific phobias in children and adolescents. *Cognitive and Behavioral Practice, 16*(3), 294–303. doi:10.1016/j.cbpra.2008.12.008

Donovan, C. L. (2014). Brief treatment of child social anxiety disorder. *Psychopathology Review 1*(1), 195–200. doi.org/10.5127/pr.033513

Donovan, C. L., Cobham, V., Waters, A. M., & Occhipinti, S. (2015). Intensive group-based CBT for child social phobia: A pilot study. *Behavior Therapy, 46*(3), 350–364. doi:10.1016/j.beth.2014.12.005

Ehrenreich, J. T., & Santucci, L. C. (2009). Special series: Intensive cognitive-behavioral treatments for child and adolescent anxiety disorders. *Cognitive and Behavioral Practice, 16*(3), 290–293. doi:10.1016/j.cbpra.2009.04.001

Elkins, R. M., Gallo, K.P., Pincus, D.B. & Comer, J.S. (2016). Moderators of intensive cognitive behavioral therapy for adolescent panic disorder: The roles of fear and avoidance, *Child and Adolescent Mental Health, 21*(1), 30–36.

Essau, C.A., & Gabbidon, J. (2013). Epidemiology, comorbidity, and mental health services utilization. In C.A. Essau, & T.H. Ollendick (eds.), *The Wiley-Blackwell handbook of the treatment of child and adolescent anxiety* (pp. 23–41). Chichester, UK: John Wiley & Sons, Ltd.

Fenley, A. R., Holly, L. E., Merson, R., Langer, D. A. & Pincus, D. B. (2017). An investigation of the association between parental stress and treatment outcomes in an intensive panic treatment for adolescents. Poster presented at the 51st Annual Convention of the Association for Behavioral and Cognitive Therapies, San Diego, CA.

Furr, J. M., delBusto, C. T., Kurtz, S., Merson, R., Avny, S. & O'Connor, E. E. (2017). Intensive group behavioral treatments for children and early adolescents with selective mutism. Panel presented at the 51st Annual Association for the Advancement of Cognitive and Behavioral Therapies, San Diego, CA.

Gallagher, H. M., Rabian, B. A., & McCloskey, M. S. (2004). A brief group cognitive-behavioral intervention for social phobia in childhood. *Journal of Anxiety Disorders, 18*(4), 459–479. doi:10.1016/S0887-6185(03)00027-6

Gallo, K. P., Comer, J. S. & Barlow, D. H. (2013). Direct-to-consumer marketing of psychological treatments for anxiety disorders. *Journal of Anxiety Disorders, 27*, 793–801.

Gallo, K. P., Chan, P. T., Buzzella, B. A., Whitton, S. W., & Pincus, D. B. (2012). The impact of an 8-day intensive treatment for adolescent panic disorder and agoraphobia on comorbid diagnoses. *Behavior Therapy, 43*(1), 153–159. doi:10.1016/j.beth.2011.05.002

Gallo, K. P., Cooper-Vince, C. E., Hardway, C. L., Pincus, D. B., & Comer, J. S. (2013). Trajectories of change across outcomes in intensive treatment for adolescent panic disorder and agoraphobia. *Journal of Clinical Child & Adolescent Psychology 0*(0), 1–9. DOI: 10.1080/15374416.2013.794701

Ginsburg, G. S., Becker, E. M., Keeton, C. P., Sakolsky, D., Piacentini, J., Albano, A. M. et al. (2014). Naturalistic follow-up of youths treated for pediatric anxiety disorders. *JAMA Psychiatry, 71*(3), 310–318.

Grills-Taquechel, A. E., & Ollendick, T. H. (2012). *Phobic and anxiety disorders in youth.* Cambridge, MA: Hogrefe & Huber Publishers.

Halldorsdottir, T., & Ollendick, T.H. (2016). Long-term outcomes of brief, intensive CBT for specific phobias: The negative impact of ADHD symptoms. *Journal of Consulting and Clinical Psychology, 84* (5), 465–471.

Higa-McMillan, C. K., Francis, S. E., Rith-Najarian, L., & Chorpita, B. F. (2016). Evidence base update: 50 years of research on treatment for child and adolescent anxiety. *Journal of Clinical Child & Adolescent Psychology, 45*(2), 91–113.

Hoffman, E. C., & Mattis, S. G. (2000). A developmental adaptation of panic control treatment for panic disorder in adolescence. *Cognitive and Behavioral Practice, 7*, 253–261.

Kendall, P. C. (1994). Treating anxiety disorders in children: Results of a randomized clinical trial. *Journal of Consulting and Clinical Psychology, 62*, 100–110.

Kendall, P. C., Flannery-Schroeder, E., Panichelli-Mindell, S. M., Southam-Gerow, M., Henin, A., & Warman, M. (1997). Therapy for youths with anxiety disorders: A second randomized clinical trial. *Journal of Consulting and Clinical Psychology, 65*, 366–380.

Liberman, L., Larsson, K., Altuzarra, M.P., Öst, L-G., & Ollendick, T. H. (2015). Self-reported life satisfaction and response style differences among children in Chile and Sweden. *Journal of Child and Family Studies, 24*, 66–75. http://dx.doi.org/10.1007/s100826-013–9814-2.

McHugh R. K., Whitton S.W., Peckham, A. D., Welge, J. A., Otto, M. W. (2013). Patient preference for psychological vs pharmacologic treatment of psychiatric disorders: A meta-analytic review. *Journal of Clinical Psychiatry, 74*, 595–602. doi: 10.4088/JCP.12r07757

Merikangas, K. R., He, J., Burstein, M. E., Swendsen, J., Avenevoli, S., Case, B., ... Olfson, M. (2011). Service utilization for lifetime mental disorders in U.S. adolescents: Results of the national comorbidity survey adolescent supplement (NCS-A). *Journal of the American Academy of Child and Adolescent Psychiatry, 50* (1), 32–45. doi.org/10.1016/j.jaac.2010.10.006

Merikangas, K. R., He, J., Burstein, M., Swanson, S. A., Avenevoli, S., Cui, L., ... Swendsen, J. (2010). Lifetime prevalence of mental disorders in US adolescents: Results from the National Comorbidity Study-Adolescent Supplement (NCS-A). *Journal of the American Academy of Child and Adolescent Psychiatry, 49*(10), 980–989. http://doi.org/10.1016/j.jaac.2010.05.017

Merikangas, K. R., Nakamura, E. F., & Kessler, R. C. (2009). Epidemiology of mental disorders in children and adolescents. *Dialogues in Clinical Neuroscience, 11*(1), 7–20.

Mohr, C., & Schneider, S. (2014). Intensive treatments for Separation Anxiety Disorder in children and adolescents. *Psychopathology Review, 1*(1), 201–208. doi:10.5127/pr.035013

Ollendick, T. H. (1995). Cognitive-behavioral treatment of panic disorder with agoraphobia in adolescents: A multiple baseline design analysis. *Behavior Therapy, 26*, 517–531.

Ollendick, T. H., King, N.J., & Chorpita, B. F. (2006). Empirically supported treatments for children and adolescents. In P.C. Kendall (ed.), *Child and adolescent therapy:*

Ollendick, T. H., & Pincus, D. (2008). Panic disorder in adolescents. In R. G. Steele, T. D. Elkin, & M. Roberts (eds.), *Handbook of evidence-based therapies for children and adolescents: Bridging science and practice* (pp. 83–102). New York: Springer.

Ollendick, T. H., & King, N.J. (2012). Evidence-based treatments for children and adolescents: Issues and controversies. In P.C. Kendall (ed.), *Child and adolescent therapy: Cognitive-behavioral procedures* (pp. 499–519). New Yok: Guilford Publications, Inc.

Ollendick, T. H., & Davis, T. I. (2013). One-session treatment for specific phobias: A review of Öst's single-session exposure with children and adolescents. *Cognitive Behaviour Therapy, 42*(4), 275–283. doi:10.1080/16506073.2013.773062

Ollendick, T. H., Halldorsdottir, T., Fraire, M. G., Austin, K. E., Noguchi, R. J., Lewis, K. M., & ... Whitmore, M. J. (2015). Specific phobias in youth: A randomized controlled trial comparing one-session treatment to a parent-augmented one-session treatment. *Behavior Therapy, 46*(2), 141–155. doi:10.1016/j.beth.2014.09.004

Ollendick, T. H., & Muris, P. (2015). The scientific legacy of Little Hans and Little Albert: Future directions for research on specific phobias in youth. *Journal of Clinical Child and Adolescent Psychology, 44*(4), 689–706. doi:10.1080/15374416.2015.1020543

Ollendick, T. H., Öst, L., Reuterskiöld, L., & Costa, N. (2010). Comorbidity in youth with specific phobias: Impact of comorbidity on treatment outcome and the impact of treatment on comorbid disorders. *Behaviour Research and Therapy, 48*(9), 827–831. doi:10.1016/j.brat.2010.05.024

Öst, L. (1989). One-session treatment for specific phobias. *Behaviour Research and Therapy, 27*(1), 1–7. doi:10.1016/0005-7967(89)90113-7

Öst, L., Svensson, L., Hellström, K., & Lindwall, R. (2001). One-session treatment of specific phobias in youths: A randomized clinical trial. *Journal of Consulting and Clinical Psychology, 69*(5), 814–824. doi:10.1037/0022-006X.69.5.814

Öst, L., & Ollendick, T.H. (2017). Brief, intensive, and concentrated cognitive behavioral treatments for anxiety disorders in children: A systematic review and meta-analysis. *Behavioral Research and Therapy, 97*, 134–145.

Peters, R. M., & Waters, A. (2014). Intensive treatments for generalized anxiety disorder in children and adolescents. *Psychopathology Review, 1*(1), 209–214. doi:http://dx.doi.org/10.5127/pr.033113

Pincus, D. B., Ehrenreich-May J.E., Whitton, S. W., Mattis, S. G., & Barlow, D. H. (2010). Cognitive-behavioral treatment of panic disorder in adolescence. *Journal of Clinical Child and Adolescent Psychology, 39*, 638–649.

Pincus, D. B., Leyfer, O., Hardway, C., Elkins, R., & Comer, J. (2014, November). *Recent advances in the development of psychological treatments for adolescents with panic disorder.* In A. Asnaani (Symposium Chair), "Novel and Innovative Applications of Evidence-Based Treatments for Emotional Disorders in Adolescent Patients." Paper presented at the 48th annual meeting of the Association for Behavioral and Cognitive Therapies. Philadelphia, PA.

Pincus, D. B., Elkins, R. M., & Hardway, C. (2014). Intensive treatments for adolescent panic disorder and agoraphobia: Helping youth move beyond avoidance. *Psychopathology Review, 1*(1), 189–194. doi:10.5127/pr.033313

Pincus, D. B. (2017). Treating youth with anxiety disorders in schools using e-learning and telehealth methods. Panel presentation (D. Pintello, moderator), Developing and deploying effective mobile and connected mental health intervention efforts for youth and families. 51st Annual Convention of the Association for Behavioral and Cognitive Therapies, San Diego, CA.

Pincus, D. B., Whitton, S. W., Gallo, K., Weiner, C. L., Chow, C., & Barlow, D. H., & Hardway, C. L. (2017). *Intensive treatment of adolescent panic disorder: Results of a randomized controlled trial*. Manuscript in preparation.

Rapee, R. M. (2000). Group treatment of children with anxiety disorders: Outcome and predictors of treatment response. *Australian Journal of Psychology, 52*, 125–129.

Rapee, R. M., Lyneham, H. J., Schniering, C. A., Wuthrich, V., Abbott, M. J., Hudson, J. L., & Wignall A. (2006). *The Cool Kids® Child and Adolescent Anxiety Program, Therapist Manual. Sydney*: Centre for Emotional Health, Macquarie University.

Reynolds, S., Wilson, C., Austin, J., & Hooper, L. (2012). Effects of psychotherapy for anxiety in children and adolescents: A meta-analytic review. *Clinical Psychology Review, 32*, 251–262. http://dx.doi.org/10.1016/j.cpr.2012.01.005

Ryan, S. M., Strege, M. V., Oar, E. L., & Ollendick, T. H. (2017). One session treatment for specific phobias in children: Comorbid anxiety disorders and treatment outcome. *Journal of Behavior Therapy and Experimental Psychiatry, 54*, 128–134. doi:10.1016/j.jbtep.2016.07.011

Salloum, A., Johnco, C., Lewin, A. B., McBride, N. M., & Storch, E. A. (2016). Barriers to access and participation in community mental health treatment for anxious children. *Journal of Affective Disorders, 196*, 54–61. doi:10.1016/j.jad.2016.02.026

Santucci, L. C., Ehrenreich, J. T., Trosper, S. E., Bennett, S. M., & Pincus, D. B. (2009). Development and preliminary evaluation of a one-week summer treatment program for separation anxiety disorder. *Cognitive and Behavioral Practice, 16*, 317–331.

Santucci, L. C., & Ehrenreich-May, J. (2013). A randomized controlled trial of the Child Anxiety Multi-Day Program (CAMP) for separation anxiety disorder. *Child Psychiatry and Human Development, 44*(3), 439–451. doi:10.1007/s10578-012-0338-6

Silverman, W. K., & Albano, A. M. (1996). *The Anxiety Disorders Interview Schedule for DSM-IV - Child and Parent versions*. San Antonio, TX: Psychological Corporation.

Silverman, W. K., Pina, A. A., & Viswesvaran, C. (2008). Evidence-based psychosocial treatments for phobic and anxiety disorders in children and adolescents. *Journal of Clinical Child and Adolescent Psychology, 37*(1), 105–130.

Storch, E. A., Geffken, G. R., Merlo, L. J., Mann, G., Duke, D., . . . Goodman, W. K. (2007). Family-based cognitive-behavioral therapy for pediatric obsessive compulsive disorder: Comparison of intensive and weekly approaches. *Journal of the American Academy of Child & Adolescent Psychiatry, 46*, 469–478. http://dx.doi.org/10.1097/chi.0b013e31803062e7.

Swift, J. K., & Greenberg, R. P. (2012). Premature discontinuation in adult psychotherapy: A meta-analysis. *Cognitive Behaviour Therapy, 43*, 33–45.

Taboas, W. R., McKay, D., Whiteside, S. H., & Storch, E. A. (2015). Parental involvement in youth anxiety treatment: Conceptual bases, controversies, and recommendations for intervention. *Journal of Anxiety Disorders, 30*, 3016–3018. doi:10.1016/j.janxdis.2014.12.005

Tolan, P. H., & Dodge, K. A. (2005). Children's mental health as a primary care and concern: A system for comprehensive support and service. *American Psychologist, 60*(6), 601–614. doi: 10.1037/0003-066X.60.6.601

Walkup, J. T., Albano, A. M., Piacentini, J., et al. (2008). Cognitive behavioral therapy, sertraline, or a combination in childhood anxiety. *The New England Journal of Medicine. 359*(26), 2753–2766.

Waters, A. M., Farrell, L. J., Zimmer-Gembeck, M. J., Milliner, E., Tiralongo, E., ... Ollendick, T. H. (2014). Augmenting one-session treatment of children's specific phobias with attention training to positive stimuli. *Behaviour Research and Therapy, 62,* 107–119. http://dx.doi.org/10.1016.j.brat.2014.07.020.

Whiteside, S. H., Ale, C. M., Young, B., Dammann, J. E., Tiede, M. S., & Biggs, B. K. (2015). The feasibility of improving CBT for childhood anxiety disorders through a dismantling study. *Behaviour Research and Therapy, 73,* 83–89. doi:10.1016/j.brat.2015.07.011

Whiteside, S. P., McKay, D., De Nadai, A. S., Tiede, M. S., Ale, C. M., Storch, E. A. (2014). A baseline controlled examination of a 5-day intensive treatment for pediatric obsessive-compulsive disorder. *Psychiatry Research, 220*(1–2), 441–446. http://www.ncbi.nlm.nih.gov/pubmed/25070176

7 Pharmacologic-Enhanced Approaches for the Anxiety Disorders

Janki Modi Avari, Mia Gintoft Cohen, Despina Hatziergati, and John T. Walkup

Introduction and Overview of the Issue

Anxiety disorders have an early onset and are among the most common psychiatric disorders in children and adolescents with a prevalence as high as 18 percent (Costello et al., 1996; Strawn et al., 2015). If left untreated, pediatric anxiety disorders result in ongoing suffering, accumulated impairment, difficulty transitioning into adulthood (Mohatt, Bennett, & Walkup, 2014), and the risk for substance use disorders, depression, and suicidal behavior (Pine et al., 1998; Rynn et al., 2015; Woodward & Fergusson, 2001).

The earliest study that included children with anxiety occurred in 1960 at Johns Hopkins, when Leon Eisenberg and Leon Cytryn examined the benefit of existing medications with tranquilizing properties – meprobamate and prochlorperazine – as compared to placebo in children ages 5 to 13 years (N=83) with a variety of psychiatric symptoms (Cytryn et al., 1960). The early work by Cyrtryn and colleagues laid the groundwork for later pharmacological treatment studies in general, and more specifically anxiety in children. A decade later, in 1971, a second pioneering trial of the antidepressant imipramine showed superiority over placebo in treating school phobic children with anxiety (Gittelman-Klein & Klein, 1971).

Very few studies of children with anxiety disorders occurred subsequently and, although somewhat effective, tricyclic antidepressants for treatment of pediatric anxiety disorders were essentially abandoned in the late 1980s with the marketing of the selective serotonin reuptake inhibitors (SSRIs). The SSRIs grew in popularity as they were considered to have a better side effect profile and were generally safer than tricyclics and other antidepressants. A number of SSRI trials have demonstrated their superiority over placebo in children with separation anxiety disorder (SAD), social phobia (social anxiety disorder) (SoP), and generalized anxiety disorder (GAD) with a milder side effect burden. These preliminary studies culminated in the Child/Adolescent Anxiety Multimodal Study (CAMS) (Walkup et al., 2008). CAMS was the first large, multicenter, comparative efficacy study of youth suffering from separation, social, and generalized anxiety disorders and evaluated the relative efficacy of cognitive behavioral therapy (CBT); the SSRI, sertraline; their combination; and pill placebo. More recently, the serotonin norepinephrine reuptake inhibitor

(SNRI) duloxetine was found to be effective in children and adolescents with generalized anxiety (Strawn et al., 2015). While the preponderance of evidence supports the use of SSRIs for pediatric anxiety disorders, the industry-sponsored Food and Drug Administration (FDA) registration trial of duloxetine (Strawn et al., 2015) led to an FDA indication for duloxetine in pediatric generalized anxiety disorder; the only medication with an FDA indication for the childhood anxiety disorders.

We have learned much about the pharmacological and psychosocial treatment of the pediatric anxiety disorders over the past 10 years; however, further research is needed. Specifically, identifying whether there are groups of children with anxiety disorders who have a differential responsiveness to CBT or medication is needed. If there was differential responsiveness, then treatment guidelines could more effectively inform patients' families and prescribers how best to initiate treatment. Moreover, the question – what is the best sequence of treatments for those who do not respond to initial treatment – has not yet been empirically explored. And perhaps most importantly, research is needed to address a very common parental question – how long should a child or adolescent remain on medication to optimize outcome and prevent recurrence when medication is discontinued (Pine, 2002). While the lack of long-term data regarding safety and efficacy of SSRIs and other medications is commonly cited as a future research need, we will likely never have the kind of data that we would like as it is difficult to design and implement controlled trials (i.e., drug vs. placebo) of long duration in affected individuals to definitively identify longer-term safety and efficacy.

Description of the Approach to Innovation

All treatment should begin with a thorough evaluation of the child and family that includes gathering a comprehensive history from the patient, the parents, and their collateral contacts (e.g., teachers, therapists). Underlying medical comorbidities, psychosocial stressors, and patients' developmental level should be reviewed, as this will guide initial treatment choices. Once a thorough history has been completed, clinicians should decide if treatment should start with either medication or psychotherapy alone or a combination of psychotherapy and medication. The availability of evidence-based psychotherapy in the community, illness severity, and current impairment will play a role in the decision whether to start with medication early in treatment or not. For patients with mild to moderate anxiety disorders, the clinician may decide to first start with cognitive behavioral therapy (CBT), which among the psychotherapies has the most empirical support. For those patients who have more severe anxiety disorders, or who have no access to CBT, or for those who have partially responded and failed to remit with an adequate trial of psychotherapy (e.g., 8–14 weeks), medication can be considered as a starting point.

Selective serotonin reuptake inhibitors (SSRIs) are the first line therapy for the treatment of anxiety disorders in children and adolescents, and have low side effect profiles. Medications such as serotonin norepinephrine reuptake inhibitors (SNRIs) are considered second line as there is relatively less data to support their use, even though one of the medications of this type (duloxetine) is FDA approved for generalized anxiety disorder in children and adolescents. SSRIs used for the treatment of childhood anxiety disorders include fluoxetine (Prozac, Sarafem, Symbyax), first introduced in 1988, followed by sertraline (Zoloft), paroxetine (Paxil, Paxil CR, Pexeva), fluvoxamine (Luvox, Luvox CR), citalopram (Celexa), and escitalopram (Lexapro)

As a class of medications, the antidepressants are all likely effective (with the exception of bupropion), but are less well studied. The use of an unstudied antidepressant can be useful, if the medication has an effect profile that matches what the child with anxiety treatment needs (e.g., an antidepressant with sedative properties for the child who struggles to fall asleep). These other antidepressant would include the tricyclic antidepressants and atypical antidepressants such as mirtazapine, and even the newer antidepressants vilazodone, levomilnacipran, and vortioxetine. Thus, for patients who do not respond, have partial response, or cannot tolerate SSRIs or SNRIs, other antidepressant medications can be considered to pursue response and remission.

Other medication classes are also used for anxiety and include the benzodiazepines, beta-blockers, alpha agonists, and antihistamines. While often used for anxiety, these medications lack data on efficacy, and these medications, even if effective in the short term, should not be routinely used as they have limited long-term utility and can have ongoing adverse effects. For example, the benzodiazepines cause sedation and have a risk for dependency and abuse.

Evidence Base for Innovation

Selective Serotonin Reuptake Inhibitors (SSRIs)

Uses in Children and Adolescents

SSRIs as a class are the first line medications used for the treatment of childhood anxiety disorders due to their established efficacy and mild adverse effects. Their benefits surpass the risk for adverse effects. The SNRI duloxetine is FDA approved for use in children with GAD but the evidence base is not as strong as that for the SSRIs. There is limited data for other medications that might be considered as having anxiolytic properties such as the benzodiazepines, beta-blockers, alpha-agonists, and antihistamines. Choosing an antidepressant is based on evidence of efficacy, side effect profile, the potential for drug-drug interactions, medication half-life (i.e., time it takes for the medication to be metabolized and excreted), and ease of administration, for example, pill or liquid or number of dose adjustments to get to a typical effective dose.

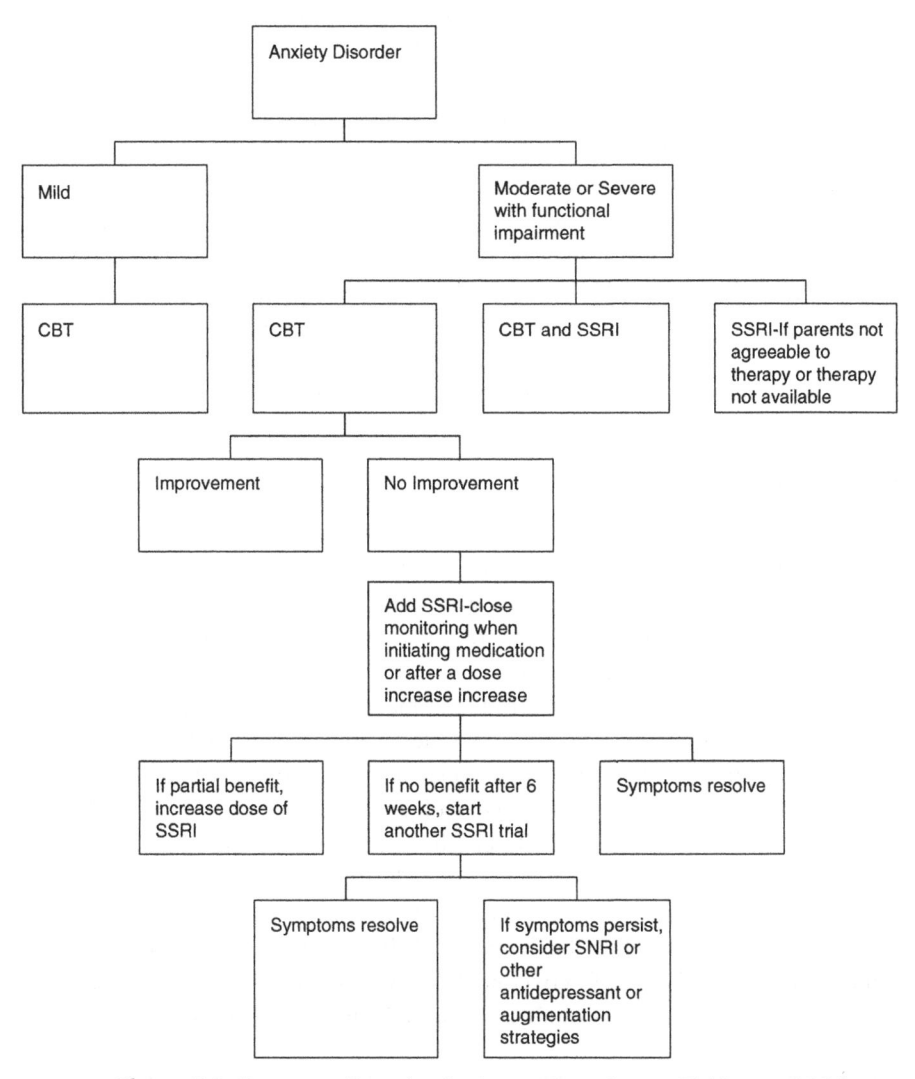

Figure 7.1 *Treatment Algorithm for Anxiety Disorders in Children and Adolescents*

Efficacy Studies

The first trial of an SSRI for the childhood anxiety disorders was conducted by the NIMH supported Research Units of Pediatric Psychopharmacology (RUPP) and demonstrated the efficacy of 8 weeks of fluvoxamine as compared to placebo in reducing the symptoms of anxiety in 128 children ages 6 to 17 years (Pine, Walkup et al., 2001). A similar trial of fluoxetine for 12 weeks in children 7 to 17 years proved to be a safe and efficacious medication for the treatment of anxiety disorders in children (Birmaher et al., 2003). These two studies set the stage for the Child/Adolescent Anxiety Multimodal Study (CAMS), a 6-year, multicenter, randomized, controlled study of 488 participants ages 7 to 17, with diagnoses of SAD, GAD, and

SoP. This trial demonstrated the efficacy of sertraline as compared to placebo in the treatment of anxiety disorders, and additionally established that combination treatment of psychotherapy and sertraline had the best results in improving anxiety symptoms (Walkup et al., 2008). Another comparative efficacy trial compared Social Effectiveness Therapy for Children (SET-C) for children and adolescents with social phobia to fluoxetine and to placebo in children 7 to 17 years old and demonstrated the efficacy of both fluoxetine and SET-C over placebo (Beidel et al., 2007). A number of industry sponsored clinical trials have also been published and support the efficacy of SSRIs and SNRIs for specific childhood onset anxiety disorders including sertraline (Rynn et al., 2001) and venlafaxine (Rynn et al., 2007) for generalized anxiety disorder, and paroxetine (Wagner et al., 2004) and venlafaxine (March et al., 2007) for social phobia (social anxiety disorder).

Pharmacokinetics

Even though each SSRI medication has a different chemical structure, they similarly inhibit the neuronal uptake pump for serotonin (5-HT). SSRIs increase the serotonin concentration at the synapse and because they have limited effects on alpha-1 adrenergic, histaminic, and muscarinic receptors they have a predictable and milder side effect profile compared to TCAs.

Even though the SSRIs are similar in their mechanism, efficacy, and side effects, they have different pharmacokinetic properties. SSRIs are metabolized in the liver by the Cytochrome P450 enzyme system and vary in the duration they remain in the bloodstream before being fully metabolized and excreted (i.e., half-life). A medication with a longer half-life can be beneficial in children or adolescents who are likely to miss occasional doses of medication, while a longer half-life can complicate things if initial side effects are troublesome or when switching to other medications. Fluoxetine has the longest half-life (1–4 days) and norfluoxetine, a potent, active metabolite of fluoxetine, has a half-life of 7–15 days. Fluvoxamine and sertraline have half-lives of about 1 day and citalopram has a half-life of about 36 hours.

The SSRIs while metabolized by Cytochrome P450 isoenzymes (CYP 450) can also inhibit that system and impact their own metabolism and that of other medications. For example, paroxetine has the shortest half-life after a single dose but with multiple doses the half-life becomes much longer as paroxetine, like fluoxetine, inhibits its own metabolism. Thus, its accumulation in the body is considered to be nonlinear. Nonlinear metabolism makes dosing much more unpredictable as a dose change from say paroxetine 10 to 20 mg might result in a 3–4-fold increase in blood level. Whether a medication inhibits CYP 450 also impacts the risk for drug-drug interactions. For example, fluoxetine inhibits the metabolism of aripiprazole, which can result in increases in aripiprazole blood levels by upward of 40 percent and result in unanticipated side effects of aripiprazole. Sertraline, citalopram, and escitalopram have short to medium duration half-lives and minimal risk for drug interactions. So, while fluoxetine has been on the market the longest and may have the greatest evidence of efficacy its pattern of nonlinear accumulation, extra-long half-life, and risk for drug-drug interactions might make it a good choice for a teen who might miss doses of medication consistently, but a poor choice for children with anxiety who may be sensitive to side effects or may require combination medication treatment. Sertraline on the other hand has a short half-life, linear pharmacokinetics, and low risk for drug interaction so would seem ideal for a child sensitive to side effects but not one who is likely to miss medication doses consistently. Thus, practicing evidence-based prescribing of the SSRIs for anxiety requires a review of not only efficacy but the critical pharmacokinetics of a given medication.

Dosing

Due to children's increased sensitivity to medications and in order to avoid side effects, most physicians prefer to start with low doses of medications and adjust upward as tolerated for children. Recommended starting doses are fluoxetine 10 mg/day, sertraline 25 mg/day, escitalopram 5 mg/day, citalopram 10 mg/day, and fluvoxamine 25 mg/day. Dose adjustments can be made every week, while monitoring for side effects. For children and adolescents, the final dose can be equal to that for adults if a higher dose is needed to enhance benefit and is well tolerated. SSRIs must be taken daily and it may take 4–6 weeks for benefit to be observed as long as the dose is in the targeted range. For example, in the pivotal CAMS trial optimal dosing of sertraline ~120 mg/daily was achieved by week 8 of the study (Walkup et al., 2008). Another factor in choosing an SSRI is how many dose changes are required before a stable effective dose of medication is achieved. Some medication such as sertraline would require 3–4 weeks of weekly increases to reach 100 mg/day whereas fluoxetine might take 1–2 weeks to go from 10 to 20 mg/day.

Assessing and Managing Partial Response or Treatment Failure

The most common causes of treatment failure with medication treatment include too low a dose, too short a duration of the treatment trial, premature discontinuation, or under dosing due to concerns about apparent side effects. There are different strategies to manage ongoing anxiety symptoms after treatment dose and duration have been fully optimized. It is important to recall that 80 percent of children in CAMS did well with combination treatment and perhaps the best strategy for a partial response is to make sure that the child is getting an appropriate dose of medication and a good trial of CBT by a qualified provider. If there is still no response, then there is the option of trying another SSRI or switching to an antidepressant medication from a different category, such as an SNRI like duloxetine, or some form of pharmacological augmentation strategy.

Changing from one medication to another can be done in one of two ways: either by discontinuing the first medication (i.e., a "washout") and subsequently starting a second medication, or by adding the second medication to the first one and allowing adequate time for the second medication to start working before making the decision to discontinue the first medication (i.e., cross tapering). Both methods have advantages and disadvantages. In the first case, the patient is left without any medication coverage for days to weeks as the new medication takes time to start working. Sometimes during the washout the patient may experience a return of symptoms even though there was the impression that the first medication was minimally effective. Cross tapering avoids the risk of returning symptoms by not discontinuing the first medication first but with a couple of caveats. For the cross taper to be effective the second medicine has to be on board long enough to establish its efficacy before removing or reducing the first medication. Premature reduction of the first medication may result in a return of symptoms while the patient is on both medications. It can be difficult to interpret the return of symptoms during a poorly executed cross taper as the patient will be on two medications and is having a worsening of symptoms. Is the worsening due to the premature lowering of the first medication, an adverse effect of the second medication, or a side effect of the two medications together? Usually it is related to premature discontinuation of the first medication but it can be a confusing time and often in the face of such confusion both medications are discontinued, leaving the patient without any medication support, and the patient family and prescriber are reluctant to try medications again. Understanding the potential complications of a cross taper is critical to implementing a cross taper successfully. Given the potential for drug-drug interaction and side effects when combining two antidepressants, two short half-life antidepressants with minimal risk for drug interactions is a better strategy than two longer acting meds that might interact with each other. For example, the combination of paroxetine and fluoxetine might be the most problematic combination of SSRIs as these two medications inhibit their own and each other's metabolism and would result in much higher blood levels of each than might be expected based on observed dose and greater risk for side effects. Clearly implementing a cross taper can be beneficial but it is critically important to understand how to interpret changes in clinical status and adverse events in the process.

Monitoring

SSRIs are relatively safe medications, with few side effects. They do not require blood levels, or prescreening with bloodwork or EKGs. However, they should be used in an evidence-based approach and require ongoing medical monitoring for potential side effects especially when initiating treatment and adjusting dose. Common side effects are behavioral activation (especially in younger children), sleep disturbance, headaches, gastrointestinal distress, and sexual side effects. Compared to adolescents being treated with SSRIs, children are more likely to experience side effects such as agitation, irritability, insomnia, impulsivity, and vomiting. For children, SSRIs were most often discontinued due to the previous side effects, which are usually observed shortly after starting or increasing the dose of medication (Rynn et al., 2015).

After FDA review of over 4000 children treated with SSRIs and placebo, ~4 percent experienced changes in suicidal thoughts (there were no completed suicides and there were very few suicide attempts) compared to ~2 percent of children on placebo (Hammad et al., 2006). Consequently, the FDA issued a "black box" label warning stating that children and adolescents who are being treated with SSRIs might experience an increase in suicidal thoughts or behavior. Therefore, children and adolescents being treated with SSRI medications should be carefully monitored for new onset or worsening suicidal thoughts and behavior. Thus, close monitoring is recommended the first few weeks after initiating SSRIs or when dose increases are being made. It is important that parents are educated about the preceding adverse reactions and are advised to seek medical advice when there are such concerns. Subsequent analyses with a larger number of studies have estimated the risk to be about 1 in 140 children treated to have changes in suicidal thoughts that could be attributed to medication (Bridge et al., 2007). Given the relatively high rates of suicidal thoughts among children and adolescents with anxiety and depression, sorting the cause of a child's or teen's suicidal thoughts and behavior is clinically challenging.

Discontinuation

Although SSRIs are not addictive medications, abrupt discontinuation is not recommended because it can result in withdrawal symptoms. As might be expected, shorter half-life SSRIs might be more associated with withdrawal symptoms than those with a longer half-life where there would be a much slower decline in blood level with abrupt discontinuation. Discontinuation side effects include flu-like symptoms, nausea, diarrhea, dizziness, tremor, lethargy, headache, insomnia, nightmares, and irritability (Hosenbocus & Chahal, 2011). Among SSRIs, paroxetine is most commonly reported to have the most frequent and problematic discontinuation symptoms due to its shorter half-life (see the previous text); sertraline and fluvoxamine are moderate (Hosenbocus & Chahal, 2011) and fluoxetine has the mildest discontinuation adverse effects due to its long half-life. For example, it might take upward of 4–6 weeks for fluoxetine to completely clear from the blood after discontinuation. Duloxetine has also been associated with withdrawal symptoms. Withdrawal symptoms are best prevented by slow tapering of short half-life medications or discontinuation and "self-tapering" of long half-life medications like fluoxetine. If withdrawal symptoms occur with abrupt discontinuation they can be treated with a resumption of medication at the prior dose and then slow tapering over an extended period of time.

One of the great challenges in interpreting withdrawal symptoms in patients with anxiety disorders is that withdrawal symptoms are similar to anxiety symptoms. In the evaluation of withdrawal symptoms, it is important to differentiate withdrawal symptoms from a return of anxiety symptoms when coming off of medication. Parents and patients should be informed about the potential effects of abrupt discontinuation and be educated as to how to proceed to avoid such reactions or to manage them effectively (i.e., resume medication at an appropriate dose).

How Long to Treat with Medication?

One of the most common questions parents ask prior to medicating their children is "how long will my child have to be on medication?" While there are no empirical studies determining how long to treat after a child with anxiety has remitted, it is recommended that treatment continue for at least one year before considering discontinuation. At that point, tapering of medications over several weeks is recommended, reducing by small amounts each week. It is also advisable to taper the medications during less stressful or demanding times of the year and when the child can be monitored for withdrawal symptoms or a return of anxiety symptoms. For example, it is best not to discontinue the medication when the child is away at summer camp or during exciting but stressful holiday seasons. In case the anxiety symptoms return during a therapeutic discontinuation, reinitiating or increasing the medication to recapture symptom control is the goal (Keeton, Kolos, & Walkup, 2009).

Serotonin Norepinephrine Reuptake Inhibitors (SNRIs)

SNRIs

In addition to the SSRIs, randomized controlled trials suggest benefit for the serotonin norepinephrine reuptake inhibitors (SNRIs), including venlafaxine (March et al., 2007) and duloxetine (Strawn et al., 2015). As noted, duloxetine has received FDA approval for the treatment of generalized anxiety disorder (GAD) in youth 7–17 years of age.

Uses in Children and Adolescents

As previously noted, SSRIs have typically been the first-line pharmacologic treatment for anxiety disorders because they have been the most studied class of medication and are generally well-tolerated. However, there are some situations that may lead the practitioner to choose an antidepressant medication with dual inhibiting actions on serotonin and norepinephrine (SNRI) over an SSRI. Since there are no comparative head-to-head RCTs of SSRIs or SNRIs, the choice of medication is typically guided by the patient's history, prior medication trials and response, side-effect profiles, interactions with other medications, and family history (Kodish et al., 2011).

Studies

Venlafaxine
The SNRI venlafaxine has been evaluated in two randomized placebo-controlled trials of 8-week duration in youth diagnosed with GAD, ages 6–17 years ($n = 323$) (Rynn et al., 2007). Venlafaxine ER 112.5–225 mg/day was found to be superior to

placebo in the pooled data from the two identically designed studies. Study participants who received venlafaxine were more likely than participants on placebo to experience side effects such as asthenia, pain, anorexia, somnolence, and weight loss.

The efficacy of venlafaxine ER as a treatment for social phobia has been evaluated in a randomized, double-blind, placebo-controlled trial of 293 outpatient children and adolescents (ages 8–17 years; mean, 13.6) (March et al., 2007). Venlafaxine ER 112.5–225 mg/d had a greater reduction in social anxiety symptoms compared with placebo, 56 vs. 37 percent, respectively. Common side effects were similar to Rynn and colleagues' report and included asthenia, pain, anorexia, somnolence, and weight loss. Of note, three patients treated with venlafaxine ER developed suicidal ideation, compared to no patients with suicidal ideation in the placebo group, which suggests that similar to SSRIs, patients started on SNRIs should be advised and closely monitored.

Duloxetine
The SNRI duloxetine was evaluated in a single, large ($N=272$), industry-sponsored randomized placebo-controlled trial in children and adolescents ages 7–17 years with generalized anxiety disorder. Duloxetine was significantly better than placebo on measures of anxiety severity, response rate (59 percent vs. 42 percent), and remission rates. Side effects differed from those typically observed in SSRIs with fewer activation side effects such as insomnia, restlessness, and agitation but more gastrointestinal symptoms (Strawn et al., 2015).

Dosing

As discussed previously, children with anxiety tend to be more sensitive to side effects in general. Similar to SSRIs, starting with lower doses of SNRIs may help reduce the rate of early side effects. Although it is common clinical practice to start low and go slow to reduce the possibility of side effects, it is important to not start too low or go too slow and put the patient at risk for nonresponse and treatment failure. Dosing in randomized-controlled trials is generally higher and faster than in clinical practice but offers a good guide for endpoint dosing. Thus, the clinician should individualize dosing to each patient in order to reach remission of anxiety symptoms and minimize side effects.

Monitoring

Benefits/Adverse Events
Meta-analyses have generally failed to detect treatment differences and side effect profiles between SSRIs and SNRIs (Ipser et al., 2009). The similarity in side effect profile is possible due to the heterogeneity in adverse event ascertainment across studies and relatively high rates of gastrointestinal symptoms, headaches, and other physical symptoms reported by children and adolescents with untreated anxiety

disorders (Crawley et al., 2014; Strawn et al., 2017). SNRI specific side effects include increases in heart rate and small increases in blood pressure in children and adolescents (Strawn et al., 2015). In addition, activation, which may include irritability, mild disinhibition, increased restlessness, and insomnia, occurs at higher rates in youth than adults and has been associated with both SSRIs and SNRIs (Strawn et al., 2015). With respect to changes in suicidality in youth with anxiety disorders, two meta-analyses failed to identify an increased risk of treatment-emergent suicidality (Bridge et al., 2007; Strawn et al., 2015). The reported number needed to harm (NNH) for treatment-emergent suicidality in youth with depressive disorders is 111, while the NNH for treatment-emergent suicidality in youth with anxiety disorders is 143 (Bridge et al., 2007). This means that 111 youth with depressive disorders and 143 youth with anxiety disorders would need to be treated with SSRIs or SNRIs for a single child to experience treatment-emergent suicidality.

Discontinuation

Due to Venlafaxine's relatively short half-life of about 3–13 hours (average 5 hours), more frequent and severe discontinuation reactions have been reported (Hosenbocus & Chahal, 2011). Fava and colleagues reported an incidence of 78 percent of discontinuation reactions within three days despite a taper of up to two weeks (Fava et al., 1997). Dizziness, lightheadedness, excessive sweating, irritability, dysphoria, and insomnia were among the reported discontinuation reactions. An 8-week, double-blind study comparing sertraline to venlafaxine revealed that venlafaxine was associated with an increased rate of discontinuation symptoms (Sir et al., 2005). Venlafaxine has also been reported to have more severe discontinuation reactions such as auditory and visual hallucinations, akathisia (Haddad, 2001), illusions (Louie et al., 1996), prolonged delusions (Koga et al., 2009), tinnitus (Farah & Lauer, 1996), palinopsia (persistent and recurrent visual images) (Spindler, 2008), and a transient narcolepsy-cataplexy syndrome (Nissen et al., 2005).

How Long to Treat with Medication?

The time to onset of symptom control and recommendations for treatment duration are similar for SNRIs and SSRIs (see the previous text). An extended period of time in treatment after remission has been achieved – up to one year – is recommended to ensure that the child has the best chance to come off medication without a return of symptoms (Hathaway et al., 2018).

Tricyclic Antidepressants (TCAs)

Amitryplyline (Elavil)
Axoxapine
Clomipramine (Anafranil)

Desipramine (Norpramin)
Doxepin (Sinequan)
Imipramine (Tofranil)
Nortriptyline (Pamelor)
Protriptyline (Vivactil)

In general, the use of TCAs for the treatment of anxiety disorders is limited. Only a few studies have showed their efficacy and it has been difficult to replicate these results. As a result, SSRIs have become the mainstay of treatment due to their clear efficacy and better side effect profile.

As noted earlier, the use of tricyclic antidepressants in the treatment of anxiety disorders started in the 1960s and 1970s, focusing on adult panic disorder. The earliest study in children was done by Gittleman-Klein in 1971 and compared imipramine 100–200mg vs. placebo with and without behavioral treatment in children ($N=35$) with school phobia over a 6-week period. Imipramine was found to be superior to placebo alone in helping the youth return to school (Gittleman-Klein & Klein, 1971). A replication study investigated the efficacy of imipramine in children and adolescents with separation anxiety disorder but failed to show benefit over placebo (Klein et al., 1992). Several factors may have contributed to negative findings including a smaller sample size, as well as a subset of patients with milder symptoms. Imipramine plus cognitive behavioral therapy (CBT) versus placebo with CBT were compared in the treatment of school phobia with anxiety and depression (Bernstein et al., 2000). School attendance and depression improved significantly for the children treated with the combination of imipramine plus CBT group compared to the placebo with CBT group (Bernstein, 2000). The patients in the Imipramine plus CBT arm also got better faster when compared to those in placebo plus CBT. A 12-week, double-blind, placebo-controlled trial of clomipramine for children and adolescents with school refusal and "neurotic" disorder ($N=46$) did not demonstrate superiority of clomipramine over placebo even though it did help treat co-occurring depression (Berney et al., 1981).

Other Medications Used for the Treatment of Childhood Anxiety Disorders

The data for the use of non-SSRI agents in the treatment of childhood anxiety disorders are limited. Medications such as buspirone, antihistamine medications such as diphendyramine and hydroxyzine, alpha agonists, and benzodiazepines have been occasionally used to treat anxiety disorders, but there is limited data on their efficacy and utility long-term. An unpublished industry-sponsored, randomized controlled trial of buspirone in children and adolescents with generalized anxiety disorder failed to differentiate drug from placebo due to high response rates in both intervention arms.

Antihistaminic medications such as diphenhydramine and hydroxyzine have been used extensively in psychiatry mostly for their sedative properties with some efficacy in the short term in treatment of acute anxiety (Effron, 1953). However, no follow-up or longer-term studies support antihistamines in chronic management of anxiety disorders. The sedation and anticholinergic effects also limit their use as a primary agent for management of anxiety.

The use of benzodiazepines is commonplace for acute anxiety symptoms, but such practices are not supported by large, high-quality clinical trials (Graae, 1994; Simeon, 1992). Furthermore, the side effect profile of benzodiazepines including sedation and risk for psychological and physical dependence do not make it a likely first choice or a long-term choice for the treatment of anxiety disorders in youth. Clinicians should be weary of benzodiazepines in general and particularly in patients with a history of substance abuse.

Informed Consent

The cornerstone of treating children, adolescents, and families is building a therapeutic alliance between the child, the parents, and the physician. Informed consent is integral to the therapeutic relationship when medicating children and adolescents with anxiety disorders. Informed consent involves educating parents about the risks and benefits of the specific agent being considered, including possible side effects and their management, expected time to and magnitude of treatment response, duration of treatment, management of partial response, and plan for ultimate discontinuation. Research suggests that educating families about these expectations and concerns regarding use of psychotropic medications often prevents them from abandoning medication trials prematurely (Kodish et al., 2011).

Clinical Case Illustration

Ashley is a 14-year-old 9th grader who is currently living with her parents and siblings. Ashley was brought into the local clinic regarding her recent decline in academic functioning and social difficulties. Ashley's parents have also been worried as they have noticed she has become much more anxious since transitioning to high school. Ashley has had difficulty making friends, keeping her grades up, and completing day to day tasks such as her homework, helping out babysitting the neighbor's child, and coping with a new volunteer job.

Ashley reports feeling worried about a variety of things during the day including school, friend relationships, and whether she will make her parents proud of her. She describes feeling very self-conscious at school and reports having a lot of difficulty concentrating and "freezing up" when required to do class work, which is upsetting and makes it difficult to sit still in class. She reports not wanting to speak to the other kids for fear that she will say the wrong thing and be embarrassed. She states that this worry has always been present but has only intensified as she has had to move to a much larger high school. She admits to sometimes leaving class when feeling overwhelmed and hanging out in the bathroom or even telling her parents she is not feeling well in order to stay home.

Table 7.1 *This Table is a List of the Agents Most Commonly Used in the Treatment of Anxiety Disorders in Children and Adolescents. The Tabs also Include Pertinent Properties of Each Medication Important for Clinicians to be Aware of.*

	FDA Approval	Mechanism of Action	Half-Life	Drug-Drug Interaction	Prominent Properties
Fluoxetine (Prozac) (Sarafem) (Selfemra)	*OCD (>7 years) Panic Dis.	Serotonin Reuptake Inh	14 days	-CYP 3A4 inh- increase aripiprazole levels -CYP 2D6 inh	-Multiple drug-drug interactions
Fluvoxamine (Luvox) (Faverin)	*OCD (>8 years)	Serotonin Reuptake Inh	9–28 hrs	-CYP 3A4 inh -CYP 2C9/19 inh -CYP 1A2 inh	
Sertraline (Zoloft) (Lustral)	*OCD (>6 years) Panic Dis. Social Anx Dis.	Serotonin Reuptake Inh	22–36 hrs	-CYP 3A4 inh -CYP 2D6 inh -interacts lethally with pimozide	
Citalopram (Celexa) (Cipramil)	GAD Social Anx Dis. Panic Dis. OCD	Serotonin Reuptake Inh	23–45 hrs	-CYP 2D6 inh	-Dose related QT prolongation
Escitalopram (Lexapro) (Cipralex)	GAD	Serotonin Reuptake Inh	27–32 hrs	No significant interactions	-Few drug-drug interactions
Paroxetine (Paxil) (Seroxat) (Brisdelle) (Pexeva)	OCD Panic Dis Social Anx Dis GAD	Serotonin Reuptake Inh	24 hrs	-CYP 2D6 inh	-Short half-life
Venlafaxine (Effexor)	Social Anx Dis Panic Dis GAD	Serotonin Norepinephrin Reuptake Inh	3–7 hrs- Parent drug 9–13 hrs- Active metabolite	-Few adverse drug interactions	-Short half-life
Duloxetine (Cymbalta) (Irenka)	*GAD (>7 years)	Serotonin Norepinephrin Reuptake Inh	12 hrs	-CYP 2D6 inh and also metabolized by CYP 2D6	

Table 7.1 (cont.)

	FDA Approval	Mechanism of Action	Half-Life	Drug-Drug Interaction	Prominent Properties
Clomipramine (Anafranil)	OCD	Serotonin and Norepinephrin Reuptake	17–28 hrs		
Imipramine (Tofranil)	Enuresis (>6 years)	Serotonin and Norepinephrin Reuptake	19 hrs		
Desipramine (Norpramine)	Anxiety Insomnia	Norepinephrine Reuptake Inh	24 hrs	-Metabolized by CYP 2D6-slow metabolizers need lower doses	-Active metabolite of Imipramine
Nortriptaline (Pamelor) (Aventyl)	Anxiety Insomnia	Norepinephrine Reuptake Inh	36 hrs		-Active metabolite of Amitrytaline
Buspirone (Buspar) (Vanspar)	Anxiety	Serotonin Receptor Partial Agonist	2–3 hrs		-No sexual side effects

She reports having trouble falling asleep at night but once asleep sleeps well and feels rested. She also describes frequent headaches or stomach aches when getting ready for school and when at school. Ashley often spends time in the nurse's office because of stomach pain or headache and has gone home because of these symptoms. She was seen by her pediatrician and the work up of the stomach pain and headache revealed tension headaches. There was no cause for the stomach pain found.

School reports indicate that Ashley is very quiet in the classroom setting. She tends to sit in the back and does not participate in class discussions. On the few occasions Ashley is called on, she looks down, speaks softly and sometimes is unable to answer. Ashley's guidance counselor has also noted that Ashley spends most of her time alone and has few friends. She does eat lunch with a couple of friends whom she has known since grade school and has not made any new friends since starting high school.

At home Ashley is more talkative and her mood appears full range with the capacity to enjoy herself with family activities. She spends time with her younger siblings and enjoys sports. Her parents have not noticed any change in her mood but have noted an increase in her anxiety about school. They report that she has always been a nervous child and even as a toddler and young school age child had trouble separating from them when having to go to day care. They report she had gone to a small elementary and middle school and knew all of the teachers and kids and had been able to manage her worries but now since she has moved to the much larger high school is no longer able to. They report that her grades have dropped. When she stays home, she completes her homework, which generally takes her more time than before. They report that she has always "taken hours" to do her homework because she wants it to be perfect and worries about getting "bad grades."

Ashley has stopped babysitting as she worries that something might happen to the neighbor's child for whom she is caring. Her parents were pleased when she volunteered at a soup kitchen to help the indigent but more recently she is unable to look the customers in the eye. When a patron asks her a question or makes a request, she becomes easily flustered and has difficulty speaking. Her volunteer supervisor has moved her to jobs in the soup kitchen that don't require her to interact with others.

Case Conceptualization

Upon reading the previous case, there are several symptoms that give the reader the pertinent facts to identify early separation anxiety as well as symptoms of generalized anxiety disorder and social anxiety disorder. Ashley is described as an anxious child starting from when she was about 3. She had difficulty separating from her parents and only had a few friends growing up. She was in a small elementary and middle school, which allowed her to manage her anxiety, but as she transitioned to a much larger high school, she was unable to adapt to this setting. Ashley has difficulty in social situations including making friends at school, babysitting, and volunteer activities. Her anxiety is pervasive and encompasses every aspect of her life. She reports worry about a variety of things ranging from friends and school to her parents' perception of her. She also reports frequent somatic symptoms that have no identified medical cause, a feature that is common among children with anxiety disorders. These symptoms have steadily worsened and are now impairing her ability to function in social settings. She has been unable to make new friends, does not participate in class, and cannot interact with patrons at the soup kitchen. She doesn't meet criteria for ADHD as the nature of her inattention and restlessness is related to worry and anxiety. She does not meet criteria for major depression as her low mood is situational and appears to be closely linked to the anxiety-related changes in her functioning.

The treatment of social anxiety disorder and generalized anxiety disorder is generally twofold. The results of CAMS showed that a combination of psychotherapy, specifically cognitive behavioral therapy, and SSRIs was shown to have the best outcome in treating patients with separation, social, and generalized anxiety disorders.

Having Ashley enrolled in cognitive behavioral therapy would help her begin to learn strategies to manage her anxiety. Cognitive behavioral therapy works on the premise that thoughts, feelings, and behaviors are linked. Exposure-based CBT would focus on improving her abilities to engage others socially in a variety of settings. With exposure-based treatment Ashely would learn that there is less reason to worry than she thinks and she would also develop better tolerance for her current distress. Given the prominent social anxiety, Ashley might also benefit from a group therapy experience. The pervasiveness of her anxiety symptoms and functional impairment also suggests that she might benefit from intensive outpatient CBT initially.

Ashley could also benefit from a trial of an SSRI. Medications such as sertraline and fluoxetine are first-line agents indicated to treat social anxiety, social phobia, and generalized anxiety. For example, if Ashley were to start sertraline, it would generally be started at 25mg daily with increases every week until a target dose of 100–150mg daily is reached. Common side effects Ashley's psychiatrist would look for include activation early in the course of treatment or shortly after dose changes. Activation presents as an experience of internal agitation and physical restlessness and could make it difficult for her to fall asleep. Activation is challenging to manage and may require discontinuation and a switch in medication strategy. Also, gastrointestinal side effects such as upset stomach, nausea, vomiting, or diarrhea and headaches would require close monitoring as Ashley already experiences these symptoms. These side effects are generally self-limited and occur when the medication is first started or when there is an increase in the dose so close monitoring and having patience during the start-up of medication is important as ultimately the medication should reduce the physical symptoms of anxiety and improve sleep quality. Ashley's parents should also be informed of the black box warning regarding the potential in a very small percentage of young people for an increase in suicidal ideation when starting SSRIs.

Six months later after CBT and starting medication Ashley is doing much better. She reports that she and her CBT therapist set goals for her and have worked at them successfully. She is babysitting again. Her neighbors have commented to Ashley's parents that she seems more confident and engaged with them and their daughter. She is serving food again at the soup kitchen. She has also made two friends at school. She reports school still makes her feel anxious but she isn't spending all of her time with the nurse. She has learned some relaxation techniques such as deep breathing to help her when she feels overwhelmed and is getting better grades while studying less hard. She also started taking sertraline, which was increased to 125mg daily. She reports that she did not feel activated initially when she started the medication but she did feel a little nauseous but this only lasted a few days. Overall, she feels more healthy as she has fewer headaches and stomach aches.

Challenges and Recommendations for Future Research in the Area

As previously discussed, children and their families greatly benefit from treatment of anxiety disorders. There are two fundamental questions that parents ask about treatment of their child with medications that are important targets for future research. The first is how long does one have to be on medication – "Do they have to be on medication for the rest of their life?" and the second is what are the risks of long-term treatment. We currently do not know how long a child with an anxiety disorder has to be on medication to reduce the risk of recurrence of symptoms after going into remission on medication. Addressing this through a large medication discontinuation trial is possible but would require a large sample size and could be expensive to implement. Currently, the duration of medication treatment is largely driven by whether the child goes into remission of their anxiety disorder. Children who have no or minimal anxiety disorder symptoms remaining may get treatment for an additional 6–12 months before undergoing therapeutic medication discontinuation. Children who don't go into remission may have more difficulty coming off medication. Thus, it is an important goal of treatment to assertively pursue optimal outcome and remission of anxiety disorder symptoms. The second question about long-term risk is very difficult to address via research as the best approach would require a very long-term placebo-controlled treatment trial in anxious youth. That is, youth would have to be randomized to medication or placebo over the duration of development (i.e., years) to identify differences in long-term outcomes of medication. Animal studies can also address longer-term effects of medication but there are limitations to the inferences that can be drawn from such studies. Similarly, large health care data sets can be analyzed but most available data sets were not developed to address the long-term risk of medications, making the interpretation of any study outcome challenging. We do have data about the long-term risk of not treating anxiety and those risks are real and quantifiable. Managing the known risks of not treating and the unknown risks of long-term treatment requires a very strong prescriber-patient-family relationship and good communications

Addressing these important but challenging questions will be difficult as funding for childhood psychiatric clinical research is not readily available. Federal research funding in psychiatry has generally decreased over the years, particularly for treatment research, and many of the medications we use clinically in child psychiatry are off-patent and pharmaceutical companies of those generic medications are not investing in research in this area. Streamlining or fast tracking the regulatory approval of new medications may encourage pharmaceutical companies to invest resources in this area.

Recruitment for clinical trials of childhood anxiety disorders may be more difficult than other populations because parents may be understandably reluctant to place their child on a pharmacological treatment in a research setting let alone a clinical setting. This is especially true for the anxiety disorders as the age of onset of anxiety disorders is prior to puberty and medication trials in this population require the prescriber to have good communication skills and sensitivity.

Given the early onset of the anxiety disorders and efficacy of both CBT and medication in the treatment of the anxiety, it is critical to reduce impairment and longer-term morbidity for professional organizations, such as the Anxiety and Depression Association of America, the American Academy of Child and Adolescent Psychiatry, and the Society of Clinical Child and Adolescent Psychology or their equivalents in other countries, to promote the benefit of current treatments and for the need of additional research.

Key Practice Points

- Prior to beginning treatment, a comprehensive evaluation that includes history and physical should be completed. Collateral from patient's family, school contacts, and prior treaters should be done if indicated.
- Clinician should decide whether the patient should begin with psychotherapy alone or whether a combination of psychotherapy and medication is indicated. Illness severity, prior treatment response, and ability to participate in psychotherapy should all be considered.
- Selective serotonin reuptake inhibitors have been shown to be the most effective medication for management of moderate to severe anxiety disorders in children and adolescents (Walkup et al., 2008).
- In cases where SSRIs or SNRIs cannot be used, clinicians should consider second- and third-line antidepressants, as antidepressants as a class of medication are likely to be effective despite the lack of definitive treatment trials. Benzodiazepines, buspirone, alpha agonists, and antihistaminic agents may be useful short term but lack data suggesting any longer-term efficacy.
- Risks and benefits should be carefully discussed with patients and their families as such informed consent is key to an effective therapeutic alliance.
- Treatment should focus initially on symptom reduction short term but focus on remission and maintenance of benefit longer term.

Medication discontinuation trials after an extended period of symptom remission are an important component of effective pharmacotherapy for children with anxiety.

References

Beidel D. C., Turner, S. M., Sallee, F. R., Ammerman, R. T., Crosby, L. A., Pathak, S. (2007). SET-C versus fluoxetine in the treatment of childhood social phobia. *J Am Acad Child Adolesc Psychiatry, 46*(12), 1622–1632. PubMed PMID: 18030084.

Berney, T., Kolvin, I., Bhate, S. R., Garside, R. F., Jeans, J., Kay, B., & Scarth, L. (1981). School phobia: A therapeutic trial with clomipramine and short-term outcome. *The British Journal of Psychiatry, 138*(2), 110–118.

Bernstein, G. A., Borchardt, C. M., Perwien, A. R., Crosby, R. D., Kushner, M. G., Thuras, P. D., & Last, C. G. (2000). Imipramine plus cognitive-behavioral therapy in the treatment of school refusal. *Journal of the American Academy of Child & Adolescent Psychiatry, 39*(3), 276–283.

Birmaher, B., Waterman, G. S., Ryan, N., Cully, M., Balach, L., Ingram, J., ... Schowalter, J. E. (1996). Fluoxetine for childhood anxiety disorders. *Year Book of Psychiatry & Applied Mental Health, 1996*(3), 46.

Birmaher, B., Khetarpal, S., Brent, D., Cully, M., Balach, L., Kaufman, J., & Neer, S. M. (1997). The screen for child anxiety related emotional disorders (SCARED): Scale construction and psychometric characteristics. *Journal of the American Academy of Child & Adolescent Psychiatry, 36*(4), 545–553.

Birmaher, B., Axelson, D. A., Monk, K., Kalas C., Clark, D. B., Ehmann, M., Bridge, J., Heo, J., Brent, D. A. (2003). Fluoxetine for the treatment of childhood anxiety disorders. *J Am Acad Child Adolesc Psychiatry, 42*(4), 415–423. PubMed PMID: 12649628.

Bridge, J. A., Iyengar, S., Salary, C. B., Barbe, R. P., Birmaher, B., Pincus, H. A., ... Brent, D. A. (2007). Clinical response and risk for reported suicidal ideation and suicide attempts in pediatric antidepressant treatment: A meta-analysis of randomized controlled trials. *Journal of the American Medical Association, 297*(15), 1683–1696.

Compton, S. N., Walkup, J. T., Albano, A. M., Piacentini, J. C., Birmaher, B., Sherrill, J. T., ... Iyengar, S. (2010). Child/adolescent anxiety multimodal study (CAMS): Rationale, design, and methods. *Child and Adolescent Psychiatry and Mental Health, 4*(1), 1.

Connolly, S. D., & Bernstein, G. A. (2007). Practice parameter for the assessment and treatment of children and adolescents with anxiety disorders. *Journal of the American Academy of Child & Adolescent Psychiatry, 46*(2), 267–283.

Costello, E. J., Angold, A., Burns, B. J., Stangl, D. K., Tweed, D. L., Erkanli, A., & Worthman, C. M. (1996). The Great Smoky Mountains Study of Youth: Goals, design, methods, and the prevalence of DSM-III-R disorders. *Archives of General Psychiatry, 53*(12), 1129–1136.

Crawley, S. A., Caporino, N. E., Birmaher, B., Ginsburg, G., Piacentini, J., Albano, A. M., ... McCracken, J. (2014). Somatic complaints in anxious youth. *Child Psychiatry & Human Development, 45*(4), 398–407.

Cytryn, L., Gilbert, A., & Eisenberg, L. (1960). The effectiveness of tranquilizing drugs plus supportive psychotherapy in treating behavior disorders of children: A double-blind study of eighty outpatients. *American Journal of Orthopsychiatry, 30*(1), 113.

Diaz-Guerrero, R., Feinstein, R., & Gottlieb, J. S. (1956). EEG findings following intravenous injection of diphenhydramine hydrochloride (benadryl R). *Electroencephalography and Clinical Neurophysiology, 8*(2), 299–306.

D'Souza, R. F., Uguz, S., George, T., Vahip, S., Hopwood, M., Martin, A. J., ... Burt, T. (2005). Randomized trial of sertraline versus venlafaxine XR in major depression: Efficacy and discontinuation symptoms. *Journal of Clinical Psychiatry*.

Effron, A. S., & Freedman, A. M. (1953). The treatment of behavior disorders in children with benadryl: A preliminary report. *The Journal of Pediatrics, 42*(2), 261–266.

Farah, A., & Lauer, T. E. (1996). Possible venlafaxine withdrawal syndrome. *The American Journal of Psychiatry*.

Fava, M., Mulroy, R., Alpert, J., Nierenberg, A. A., & Rosenbaum, J. F. (1997). Emergence of adverse events following discontinuation of treatment with extended-release venlafaxine. *American Journal of Psychiatry, 154*(12), 1760–1762.

Gittelman-Klein, R., & Klein, D. F. (1971). Controlled imipramine treatment of school phobia. *Archives of General Psychiatry, 25*(3), 204–207.

Graae, F., Milner, J., Rizzotto, L., & Klein, R. G. (1994). Clonazepam in childhood anxiety disorders. *Journal of the American Academy of Child & Adolescent Psychiatry, 33*(3), 372–376.

Haddad, P. M. (2001). Antidepressant discontinuation syndromes. *Drug Safety, 24*(3), 183–197.

Hammad, T.A., Laughren, T., Racoosin, J. (2006). Suicidality in pediatric patients treated with antidepressant drugs. *Arch Gen Psychiatry, 63*(3), 332–339.

Hathaway, E.E, Walkup, J.T, Strawn, J.R. (2018). Antidepressant treatment duration in pediatric depressive and anxiety disorders: How long is long enough? *Curr Probl Pediatr Adolesc Health Care, 48*(2), 31–39.

Hiemke, C., & Härtter, S. (2000). Pharmacokinetics of selective serotonin reuptake inhibitors. *Pharmacol Ther*, 85(1), 11–28.

Hosenbocus, S., & Chahal, R. (2011). SSRIs and SNRIs: A review of the discontinuation syndrome in children and adolescents. *Journal of the Canadian Academy of Child and Adolescent Psychiatry*, 20(1), 60.

Keeton, C. P., Kolos, A. C., & Walkup, J. T. (2009). Pediatric generalized anxiety disorder. *Pediatric Drugs*, 11(3), 171–183.

Klein, R. G., Koplewicz, H. S., & Kanner, A. (1992). Imipramine treatment of children with separation anxiety disorder. *Journal of the American Academy of Child & Adolescent Psychiatry*, 31(1), 21–28.

Kodish, I., Rockhill, C., & Varley, C., (2011). Pharmacotherapy for anxiety disorders in children and adolescents. *Dialogues in Clinical Neuroscience*, 13(4), 439–452.

Koga, M., Kodaka, F., Miyata, H., & Nakayama, K. (2009). Symptoms of delusion: the effects of discontinuation of low-dose venlafaxine. *Acta Psychiatrica Scandinavica*, 120(4), 329–331.

Louie, A. K., Lannon, R. A., Kirsch, M. A., & Lewis, T. B. (1996). Venlafaxine withdrawal reactions. *The American Journal of Psychiatry*, 153(12), 1652.

March, J. S., Entusah, A. R., Rynn, M., Albano, A. M., & Tourian, K. A. (2007). A randomized controlled trial of venlafaxine ER versus placebo in pediatric social anxiety disorder. *Biological Psychiatry*, 62(10), 1149–1154.

Mohatt, J., Bennett, S. M., & Walkup, J. T. (2014). Treatment of separation, generalized, and social anxiety disorders in youths. *American Journal of Psychiatry*, 171(7), 741–748.

Nissen, C., Feige, B., Nofzinger, E., Riemann, D., Berger, M., & Voderholzer, U. (2005). Transient narcolepsy-cataplexy syndrome after discontinuation of the antidepressant venlafaxine. *Journal of Sleep Research*, 14(2), 207–208.

Pine, D. S. (2002). Treating children and adolescents with selective serotonin reuptake inhibitors: How long is appropriate? *Journal of Child and Adolescent Psychopharmacology*, 12(3), 189–203.

Pine, D. S., Cohen, P., Gurley, D., Brook, J., & Ma, Y. (1998). The risk for early-adulthood anxiety and depressive disorders in adolescents with anxiety and depressive disorders. *Archives of General Psychiatry*, 55(1), 56–64.

Rahn, K. A., Cao, Y. J., Hendrix, C. W., & Kaplin, A. I. (2015). The role of 5-HT1A receptors in mediating acute negative effects of antidepressants: Implications in pediatric depression. *Translational Psychiatry*, 5(5), e563.

Reinblatt, S. P., and Walkup, J. T. (2005). Psychopharmacologic treatment of pediatric anxiety disorders. *Child and Adolescent Psychiatric Clinics of North America*. 877–908.

Rynn, M. A., Walkup, J. T., Compton, S. N., Sakolsky, D. J., Sherrill, J. T., Shen, S., ... Riddle, M. A. (2015). Child/Adolescent anxiety multimodal study: Evaluating safety. *Journal of the American Academy of Child & Adolescent Psychiatry*, 54(3), 180–190.0.

Rynn, M. A., Riddle, M. A., Yeung, P. P., & Kunz, N. R. (2007). Efficacy and safety of extended-release venlafaxine in the treatment of generalized anxiety disorder in children and adolescents: Two placebo-controlled trials. *American Journal of Psychiatry*, 164(2), 290–300.

Safer, D. J., & Zito, J. M. (2006). Treatment-emergent adverse events from selective serotonin reuptake inhibitors by age group: Children versus adolescents. *Journal of Child & Adolescent Psychopharmacology*, 16(1–2), 159–169.

Simeon, J. G., & Ferguson, H. B. (1987). Alprazolam effects in children with anxiety disorders. *The Canadian Journal of Psychiatry, 32*(7), 570–574.

Simeon, J. G., Knott, V. J., Dubois, C., Wiggins, D., Geraets, I., Thatte, S., & Miller, W. (1994). Buspirone therapy of mixed anxiety disorders in childhood and adolescence: A pilot study. *Journal of Child and Adolescent Psychopharmacology, 4*(3), 159–170.

Spindler, P. E. (2008). Palinopsia following discontinuation of venlafaxine. *Psychiatrische Praxis, 35*(5), 255–257.

Strawn, J. R., Dobson, E. T., & Giles, L. L. (2017). Primary pediatric care psychopharmacology: Focus on medications for ADHD, depression, and anxiety. *Current Problems in Pediatric and Adolescent Health Care, 47*(1), 3–14.

Strawn, J. R., Welge, J. A., Wehry, A. M., Keeshin, B., & Rynn, M. A. (2015). Efficacy and tolerability of antidepressants in pediatric anxiety disorders: A systematic review and meta-analysis. *Depression and Anxiety, 32*(3), 149–157.

Strawn, J. R., Prakash, A., Zhang, Q., Pangallo, B. A., Stroud, C. E., Cai, N., & Findling, R. L. (2015). A randomized, placebo-controlled study of duloxetine for the treatment of children and adolescents with generalized anxiety disorder. *Journal of the American Academy of Child & Adolescent Psychiatry, 54*(4), 283–293.

Wagner, K. D., Berard, R., Stein, M. B., Wetherhold, E., Carpenter, D. J., Perera, P., ... Machin, A. (2004). A multicenter, randomized, double-blind, placebo-controlled trial of paroxetine in children and adolescents with social anxiety disorder. *Archives of General Psychiatry, 61*(11), 1153–1162.

Walkup, J. T., Albano, A. M., Piacentini, J., Birmaher, B., Compton, S. N., Sherrill, J. T., ... Iyengar, S. (2008). Cognitive behavioral therapy, sertraline, or a combination in childhood anxiety. *New England Journal of Medicine, 359*(26), 2753–2766.

Walkup, J. T., Labellarte, M. J., Riddle, M. A., Pine, D. S., Greenhill, L., Klein, R., ... Klee, B. (2001). Fluvoxamine for the treatment of anxiety disorders in children and adolescents. *New England Journal of Medicine, 344*(17), 1279–1285.

Woodward, L. J., & Fergusson, D. M. (2001). Life course outcomes of young people with anxiety disorders in adolescence. *Journal of the American Academy of Child & Adolescent Psychiatry, 40*(9), 1086–1093.

8 Enhanced Family Approaches for the Anxiety Disorders

Michael W. Lippert, Verena Pflug, Kristen Lavallee, and Silvia Schneider

Introduction

Many child and adolescent psychotherapists are convinced that parental involvement is essential to ensuring and maintaining change in therapy for childhood anxiety disorders. This may be largely due to the common knowledge among therapists that anxiety disorders run in families. Having an immediate family member with an anxiety disorder (AD) is among the strongest and most well-documented risk factors for developing an AD (Seehagen, Margraf, & Schneider, 2014). Both top-down (investigations of the children of anxious parents) and bottom-up (investigations of the parents of anxious children) studies point to a strong link between parent and child anxiety disorders (Cooper et al., 2006; Micco et al., 2009). Familial transmission appears to flow both through genetic risk factors and early vulnerability risk factors, such as behavioral inhibition, and patterns of cognition developed within the family (Murray, Creswell & Cooper, 2009). Although the importance of the family in the development and maintenance of childhood anxiety is established (for a review, see Burt, 2009), and therapists commonly believe parental involvement is important in treatment, empirical support does not yet provide a definitive answer on how much or whether parental involvement can be considered an essential therapy component. In practice, parental involvement must be present at least to some extent in child therapy (i.e., scheduling and keeping appointments), but the relative impact of including, or even targeting, family members in cognitive behavioral therapy (CBT), the most effective treatment modality for childhood anxiety disorders (James et al., 2013), is in need of further exploration, and is therefore the topic of this chapter.

Overview of the Potential Need for Family-Based Innovation

Anxiety disorders are, as detailed in the previous chapters in this volume, highly prevalent in children (point-prevalence is 6.5 percent; lifetime prevalence is 8 to 19 percent), and indeed the most commonly diagnosed mental disorder category in children and youth (Grills-Taquechel & Ollendick, 2013; Polanczyk et al., 2015), causing children and their families distress and impairment in everyday living.

Unresolved childhood anxiety disorders may also lead to other mental disorders in later adolescence and adulthood, including depression, substance abuse, and, in particular, other anxiety disorders such as panic disorder (Kossowsky et al., 2013; Woodward & Fergusson, 2001). Several meta-analyses point to the effectiveness of CBT in treating anxiety disorders (Ewing et al., 2015; In-Albon & Schneider, 2007; James et al., 2013; Manassis et al., 2014; Reynolds et al., 2012), with recovery rates in intent-to-treat (ITT) analyses between 47.6 percent and 66.4 percent (Warwick et al., 2017; James et al., 2013). However, completer analyses show recovery rates of 64.1 to 76.9 percent (In-Albon & Schneider, 2007). Although these rates are considered good, and an indication of the successfulness of CBT, there are still many children who do not respond to therapy. Thus, there is room for improvement in the treatment of children with anxiety disorders. Determining the relative importance of therapeutic components and/or additions may be key in improving remission rates.

As improvements to therapy for anxiety disorders in children and adolescents are being sought, whether, when, and to what extent parents should be involved in, and/or targeted, in child therapy are important areas for exploration. Etiological research points to family factors in the development and maintenance of anxiety disorders. The family can both elicit and play a role in maintaining anxiety disorders (via modeling, reinforcing avoidance behavior, excessively controlling the child, etc.), especially when one or both parents suffer from an anxiety disorder themselves (Ginsburg et al., 2004). The presence of anxiety disorders is correlated among members of the same family (Micco et al., 2009). Several studies indicate that the odds of developing an anxiety disorder are increased if one or both parents have had an anxiety disorder themselves, with standardized incident ratios between 1.90 and 5.10 (Li, Sundquist, & Sundquist, 2008; Steinhausen et al., 2016). Twin studies are particularly well-suited to untangling the mechanisms underlying familial transmission. Interestingly, in one such twin study, Eley and colleagues (2015) found that the association between parental and child anxiety was better explained by environmental transmission than by direct genetic transmission.

The role of parenting in the development of childhood anxiety was first recognized decades ago (Marks, 1969; McLeod, Weisz, & Wood, 2007). Contemporary reviews (Bögels & Brechman-Toussaint, 2006; Ginsburg et al., 2004; Rapee, 2012) lend empirical support to the role of family environment influences, such as parenting style, parental control, family functioning, family quality, and social/vicarious learning in the development of childhood anxiety. Some research points to insecure attachment as a stronger predictor of childhood anxiety disorders than either child temperament or parental anxiety (Craword & Manassis, 2001; Warren et al., 1997). Parental cognitions and parental self-efficacy may influence parenting style and may be of particular interest for the development and maintenance of children's anxieties. Parental verbal behavior and conveyance of information about potentially threatening situations is associated with higher anxiety in children (Barrett et al., 1996), presumably through the mechanism of influencing child cognitions (Prins, 2001). Interpretation bias, attentional bias, and anxiety sensitivity have all been linked to childhood anxiety disorders, with findings supporting the existence of an overall biased information-processing style in anxious children (Barrett et al., 1996; Bögels & Zigterman, 2000; Chorpita, Albano, & Barlow, 1996). These cognitive styles may be learned at home, as parents' own dysfunctional cognitions are elevated (Schneider et al., 2002) and parenting self-efficacy and satisfaction diminished in parents of children with separation anxiety, for example, as compared with parents of healthy children (Herren, In-Albon, & Schneider, 2013). Importantly, these effects remain significant after controlling for parental anxiety and depression, suggesting direct transmission of cognition from parent to child.

Some of the strongest predictors of child anxiety are parental control and overprotection (overprotection versus promotion of autonomy) and parental rejection (as one end of a continuum, with acceptance and warmth on one pole, and rejection and criticism on the other). Indeed there is considerable evidence that parental overcontrol, and to lesser extent a rejecting family environment, is associated with elevated child anxiety levels (Bögels & Brechman-Toussaint, 2006; Rapee & Heimberg, 1997). Parental control covers a wide range of parent-child-interactions, such as overcontrol, lack of autonomy granting, encouragement of the child's dependence, and excessive and restrictive regulation of the child's behavior (Wei & Kendall, 2014), thereby actively or passively encouraging avoidance behavior (Moore, Whaley, & Sigman, 2004). Parents (primarily mothers have been studied) of children with, and at-risk for, anxiety disorders are more rejecting and controlling in interactions with their children than mothers of healthy control children are (e.g., Hudson & Rapee 2001; Schneider et al., 2009). Though not as well supported by empirical evidence, a systemic perspective focuses on another family factor as well. That is, families of children with separation anxiety disorder appear to have a low degree of cohesion (meaning family members are often disengaged from one another) and adaptability, presenting as highly rigid and inflexible (Bernstein et al., 1999), with this rigidity related to increased child pathology and somatization. However, this result could not be replicated in another study (Blatter-Meunier, Kreißl, & Schneider, 2016). Further research indicates that children with anxiety disorders may tend to have families that are less accepting and autonomy-granting (Siqueland, Kendall, & Steinberg, 1996), less sociable and supportive, and more conflictual and enmeshed (Stark et al., 1990) than families of children without anxiety disorders. Two meta-analyses report a moderate association between parental control and child anxiety (McLeod, Weisz, & Wood, 2007; van der Bruggen, Stams, & Bögels, 2008). Theoretical models of the development of ADs suggest that early experiences with parental overprotection and overcontrol might provide children with information that the world is a threatening place and prevent them from developing an adequate sense of control and mastery over their environments and thus increase their vulnerability for the development of an AD (Chorpita & Barlow, 1998; Ollendick & Grills, 2016; Rapee & Heimberg, 1997). Finally, parental psychopathology seems to affect their children's therapy outcomes. Wergeland et al. (2016), in studying predictors of therapy outcome, found that, in addition to several child factors, parental internalizing symptoms predicted poorer therapy outcomes.

In sum, the family environment plays a role in the development, maintenance, and treatment outcomes of childhood anxiety disorders. Attachment, parent transmission of cognitions and interpretation biases, parental overcontrol, parental rejection, and parents' own psychopathology all contribute to childhood anxiety. Most studies suggest a direction of effects that flows from parent to child, but there may be bidirectional effects as well, whereby child anxiety also increases parent anxiety, creating a feedback loop (Rapee, 2009; Seehagen et al., 2014). The involvement of parents in therapy thus seems intuitive. Yet, the empirical evidence for the utility of including parents in therapy, per se, is not as strong as one would predict (In-Albon & Schneider, 2007; Manassis et al., 2014; Reynolds et al., 2012; Thulin et al., 2014). While family involvement might not be absolutely essential for general therapeutic success, it may potentially be a candidate ingredient for improving therapeutic outcomes for those children who do not respond to treatment as usual. This may be especially true in cases of increased familial risk factors, such as parental anxiety, which potentially make standard child-focused treatment less effective (Wergeland et al., 2016). While the true utility for this approach in various contexts and with specific populations continues to be clarified through research, we give the topic of parental involvement, and how it has been operationalized so far, careful attention in the present chapter.

Description of Family-Based Therapy

There is no single formula for enhanced family treatment or parental involvement in therapy, though the modality has received much attention. There are nearly as many different approaches to parental involvement as there are studies that research the topic. Some approaches have much in common, but there are also marked theoretical divergences. The field would benefit greatly from a more unified understanding of the role family approaches can, or should, take in the treatment of childhood anxiety, and from a classification of family approaches built on a solid theoretical and empirical foundation. A recent meta-analysis offered such a classification of types of parental involvement used in 18 treatment studies so far (Manassis et al., 2014), which can be used to categorize differences between types of parental involvement. The classification differentiates active parental involvement focusing on transfer of control (TOC) and contingency management (CM) from active parental involvement without TOC and CM, and from a category of very limited/ no parental involvement, therefore comparing two types of parental involvement and one control group. The authors propose that TOC and CM, described in more detail later in this section, may be the most effective components of parental involvement. Although this classification system provides a rough organizational overview of the field of research in this area, it misses some approaches to how parents may be or have been involved in the child's psychotherapy.

Accordingly, the present chapter presents a new, more comprehensive taxonomy (Figure 8.1), based on a more thorough tally and coding of approaches used across multiple reviews and meta-analyses. The aim is to structure the current research

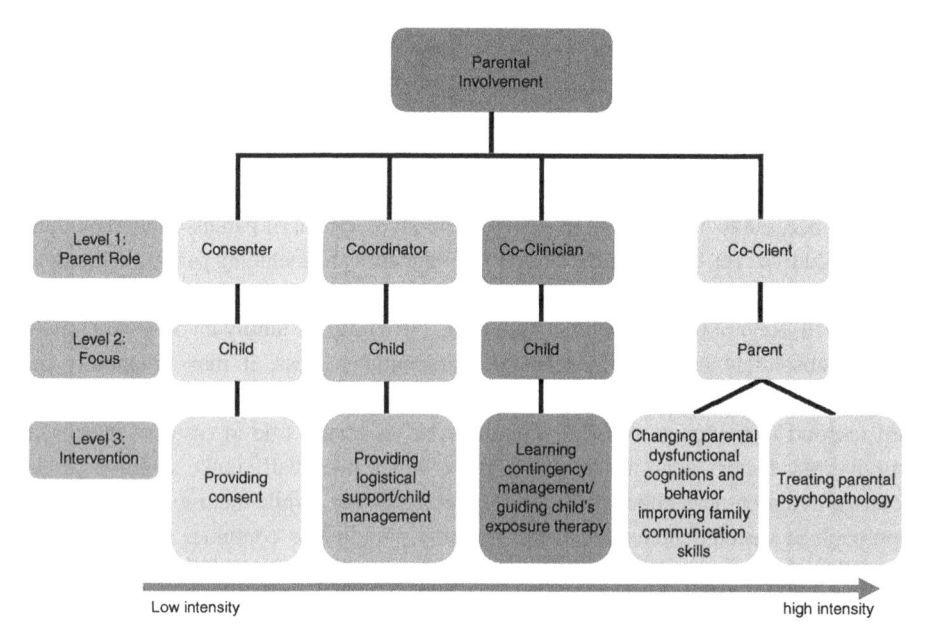

Figure 8.1 *3-Level Taxonomy of Parental Involvement in Treatment of Child Anxiety*

situation and thus lay the foundation for a systematic accumulation of knowledge. In contrast to the taxonomy proposed by Manassis et al., the current taxonomy is based on the widest possible net, including approaches to parental involvement found not only in the 18 clinical studies included in Manassis et al. (2014), but across 7 total reviews and meta-analyses (Breinholst et al., 2012; Manassis et al., 2014; Rapee, 2012; Reynolds et al., 2012; Taboas et al., 2015; Thulin et al., 2014; Wei & Kendall, 2014). While the Manassis classification exclusively focused on one aspect of parental involvement, that is the extent to which the parents support the treatment of the child as a co-clinician, the current taxonomy delineates three different levels and more possibilities for the involvement of parents in their child's therapy (see Figure 8.1). The levels are structured in the following way:

Level 1: Parent Role: The first level labels the role the parents have in relation to the therapy. The intensity in which parents are involved increases from left to right. The lowest and most fundamental necessary level of parent's involvement in the child's therapy is to provide consent. The next more intensive role is the role of a coordinator, helping their child to fulfill the basic conditions of therapy. When parents are more involved in the therapeutic context itself, they may take on the role of either co-clinician (supporting their child) or co-clients (working on their own behavior or cognitions). Within these roles, intensity can also vary from low to high.

Level 2: Focus of Parental Involvement: The second level in the taxonomy differentiates between two foci of parental involvement. This focus can either be on the child (in the form of consenter, coordinator, or co-clinician roles) or on the parent and the treatment of his or her own pathology (as in the case of the co-client role).

Level 3: Type of Intervention: The third level describes the specific interventions intended to enhance or facilitate therapy, falling under each role and focus.

In most studies, researchers use a combination of multiple approaches. Further, some categories are not completely distinct, as in the case of "Changing dysfunctional behavior" and "Changing dysfunctional cognitions," as there is some conceptual and practical overlap. Nevertheless, each subcategory in the classification system focuses on themes and strategies in the child's therapy that could be potentially enhanced by adding parental involvement. Each category will be described in detail in the following sections.

Consenter – Child-Focused – Providing Consent

While not an intervention component per se, parental consent is an essential and necessary form of parental involvement for child treatment. Although the exact legal parameters might vary slightly among countries, most of the time, therapy requires parental consent when the child is under a certain age. Therefore, consent as a form of parental involvement is not a choice, but a requirement.

Coordinator – Child-Focused – Providing Logistical Support and Child Management

The coordinator role refers to parental support of therapy that has no direct connection to the therapeutic content itself. Logistical support, in the form of transportation and supervision, is provided to most children, who are typically accompanied to the therapy center when under the age of 13 (or older in other countries where car transportation, rather than train or tram, is required). Without this logistical support, in most cases, therapy would not occur. Even in child-focused treatment, a basic level of structural parental involvement is necessary, especially for younger children.

Child management is another type of involvement in which the parents act as coordinators, and refers to structural support for the therapy, without direct involvement in the therapy. Parents can support therapy by giving reminders to complete therapeutic homework, motivating their child to go to therapy, reminding their child to bring therapy folders or workbooks to and from the session, and by providing opportunities to do exposure practice in the family's everyday life. As homework is an essential component of most CBT anxiety treatment programs (Hudson & Kendall, 2002), child management may be necessary for therapy completion and success, though research specifically into its effectiveness is rare. One study, analyzing in-session, as well as out-of-session involvement (including child management), showed that higher out-of-session parental involvement was associated with lower child anxiety symptoms (rated by the mother) (Pereira et al., 2016). While parents did not differ in in-session support, they did differ in out-of-session support, implying that out-of-session child-management support is an aspect of therapy that parents differ on, and that appears to have consequences for treatment success, and therefore should not be neglected when exploring the effects of parental involvement.

Co-Clinician – Child-Focused – Supporting Child's Therapy

While the previous roles mostly take place outside of the therapy room, the following interventions require active parental participation in the therapeutic context. The co-clinician role places parents in a position to learn, model, and practice therapeutic skills and to build knowledge in support of the child. This may be achieved via the process of transfer of control (TOC). TOC refers to the process of transferring therapeutic skills, methods, and knowledge from the clinician to the parents, thus enabling the parents to be in-situ therapists with the child at home (Ginsburg, Silverman, & Kurtines, 1995). One specific skill that parents may learn is the use of contingency management (CM) to encourage children to face (rather than flee) anxiety-eliciting situations (Silverman & Kurtines, 1999). CM is based on operant conditioning procedures and was originally used in a therapeutic context to reduce externalizing problems (Kazdin, 1997). Research supports the use of CM in encouraging and increasing courageous behavior in children with anxiety disorders (Ginsburg & Schlossberg, 2002). In therapy, the clinician encourages the child and the parents to develop a plan to reward all types of nonavoidant behavior during daily home life, specific exposure tasks, etc., increasing the child's motivation for entering high-anxiety situations. Coaching the parents to take control over exposure in daily life is a helpful way to encourage the transfer of skills and methods from therapy to the real world (Barmish & Kendall, 2005). In contrast to other modalities of parental involvement, TOC involve the parents by making them co-therapists, while not decreasing the percentage of time dedicated to exposure (Taboas et al., 2015). If exposure is the main component and the primary active ingredient of anxiety therapy (Craske et al., 2014; Tiwari et al., 2013), a combined TOC approach should theoretically be a good candidate for enhancing anxiety therapy with family involvement while not decreasing the child's exposure time.

Co-Client – Parent Focused

In contrast to child-focused parental involvement, parent-focused involvement targets parent risk-factors, with the parent as a co-client rather than a co-clinician (James et al., 2013).

Reframing of Parental Cognitions

The co-client role places the parents in the position of learning to change their own dysfunctional cognitions and behavior with regard to the child's pathology, receiving treatment for their own psychopathology, and/or improving deficits in parental skills. One approach to a parent-focused therapeutic component is to target the parents' dysfunctional cognitions and beliefs about the child's anxiety (Herren et al., 2013; Schneider et al., 2011). Dysfunctional cognitions in the parent about the child can serve to reinforce or encourage avoidance behavior in the child (Moore et al., 2004), and teaching the parent to reframe them is intended to produce change in the parents' interactions with the child around potentially anxiety-provoking situations. It is important to emphasize that the approach of reframing parent cognitions focuses on changing dysfunctional cognitions about the child's anxiety, and not necessarily changing dysfunctional cognitions regarding the parents' own psychopathology (this is addressed further on in this section).

Changing Parental Dysfunctional Behavior

In addition to changing dysfunctional cognitions, it is also possible to target dysfunctional parental behavior, once again with a focus on the child's anxiety. In anxiety-specific, parent behavior training programs or modules, which are often added to child-focused CBT (e.g., Bodden et al., 2008; Wood et al., 2006), anxiety-reducing parenting skills and behaviors are targeted and changed in complementary support of the child's own therapy. Parent training aims to reduce dysfunctional parental behavior, including overprotection and parental control, intrusiveness, and nonacceptance of the child's emotions. It also aims to increase the parent's trust in the child's skills, autonomy, and self-efficacy. Finally, it should encourage parents to serve as models for adaptive coping strategies when facing anxious situations themselves.

Improving Communication Skills

Improving communication skills may also be useful in enhancing the child's anxiety therapy, especially when the family climate is negative and parents often use negative communication skills (e.g., blaming, criticizing) (Ginsburg, Silverman, & Kurtines, 1995). The intervention aims to replace negative communication skills with positive communication such as active listening. Though not part of typical CBT treatments for anxiety, elements from existing parent training programs, such as the Positive Parenting Program (Sanders, 1999), can be used to improve family communication. One study, for example, showed that decreasing the level of negative expressed emotion (criticism, emotional overinvolvement) in parents of adolescents (13–18 years old) with social phobia in a family training program focusing on communication and contingency management leads to significantly better therapy outcomes in children (Garcia-Lopez et al., 2014).

Co-Client – Parent Focused – Treating Parental Psychopathology

Another parent-focused approach involves reducing the parents' own psychopathology, if present, with CBT for the parents themselves (e.g., Windheuser et al., 1977). In their own therapeutic sessions, parents may work on reducing their own psychopathology (i.e., anxiety, depression, obsessive compulsive disorder) through

> **Box 1 Does Treating Parental Psychopathology Influence the Child?**
>
> Although the association between parental and child anxiety is well documented, there are not many studies or therapy programs which explore the effects of parent treatment on child anxiety. In an exploratory study, with only 22 patients, Creswell and colleagues added eight individual CBT sessions for parents with anxiety disorders to the children's CBT (Creswell et al., 2008). Although the parental anxiety decreased, they found no significant effect on the child's anxiety in this small sample.
>
> Some other research does, however, point to beneficial effects of successful anxiety treatment on family members. In a pilot study by our group using a prospective naturalistic design, 37 parents with panic disorder received cognitive behavioral therapy for panic disorder (Schneider et al., 2013). Results indicated that even seven years after treatment, successful parental psychotherapy for panic disorder had a substantial positive influence on children's psychopathology, and was related to reduced anxiety sensitivity, agoraphobic cognitions and avoidance. In a similar vein, Weissman et al. (2006) found that effective psychopharmacological treatment of mothers with major depression led to a reduction of symptoms and diagnoses in their children after remission of maternal depression at one-year follow-up. While these studies showed top-down effects of parental treatment on child well-being, Kendall et al. (2008) looked at bottom-up effects of children's treatment on parental well-being. They found that psychotherapy of anxious children positively changed parental psychopathology in that 40 percent of treated children's mothers' AD diagnoses were no longer present at follow-up. Thus, treating ADs appears to have significant positive top-down and bottom-up influences on the psychopathology and well-being of first-degree family members. While more efficacy research is needed, treatment of parents' own pathology stands as one form of parental involvement used in therapy practice.

psychoeducation, cognitive restructuring, and exposure practice. Healthier parents can serve as models for coping, showing their children through their own actions that attending therapy sessions and doing exposure practice can lead to a reduction in the anxiety symptoms. Some evidence and further explanation of the treatment of parental psychopathology is found in Box 1.

Evidence Base for Family-Based Therapies

As noted previously, evidence for the involvement of parents in therapy for anxiety disorders is inconclusive. With regard to parental involvement as a potential moderating variable in the treatment of AD, meta-analyses generally indicate no significant differences in outcome between child- and family-based treatments for anxiety disorders in general, with both types of treatment equally effective across the broad spectrum of children with anxiety disorders (In-Albon & Schneider, 2007; James et al., 2013; Reynolds et al., 2012, Thulin et al. 2014). In-Albon and Schneider (2007) compared data from 17 child-based and 14 family-based treatments (defined as "four or more sessions including parents"), finding no significant differences regarding effect sizes or remission rates posttreatment between child- and family-based modalities. Reynolds et al. (2012) analyzed 55 trials including treatments with no parental involvement, minimal involvement, some involvement, and significant involvement. They also found no significant differences among the groups, indicating that treatment was generally successful regardless of the level of family involvement. In a subgroup-analysis, James et al. (2013) analyzed 31 studies (7 individual CBT, 13 group CBT, and 11 family CBT) and found no difference between these three CBT formats. The Thulin et al. (2014) meta-analysis was unique in that it analyzed 16 studies that directly compared child-only and parent-involved treatments within each study. This analysis again revealed no significant differences, with a slight, trend-level advantage in favor of child-only treatments. Though the overall trend favored child-focused treatment, there were some studies that favored family treatment. Some of the latter studies (Barrett et al., 1996; Wood et al., 2006) tended to include slightly younger children, but there was no statistical age difference in effectiveness of the modalities. In the same year, Manassis and colleagues (2014) compared 18 randomized control trial studies using CBT. Similar to Reynolds et al. (2012), Manassis et al. (2014) categorized the treatment studies by how the parents were involved. In this study, the categories included low parental involvement, active parental involvement focusing on transfer of control (TOC) and contingency management (CM), and active parental involvement without TOC and CM. Manassis et al. (2014) found no significant differences when analyzing therapy success posttherapy, consistent with prior meta-analyses. Interestingly, however, they did find that in the treatment group with active parental involvement (TOC and CM), anxiety diagnoses decreased further between posttreatment and 1-year follow-up, whereas the other groups merely maintained their posttreatment improvements. In line with the conclusions of Creswell and Cartwright-Hatton (2007), Manassis et al. (2014) conclude that family involvement does not necessarily lead to better outcomes at postintervention, but may help integrate therapy outcomes into daily life and encourage families to continue practicing their skills even after the therapy is finished, leading to continued improvements, and thus facilitating long-term gains after CBT is over.

It is possible that the level of family involvement in "child-only" therapy is already enough to transfer knowledge and cognition change to parents. It is typical, for example, for parents to receive information from therapists or the child him- or herself after each session. It is nearly impossible to parcel out all parental involvement, nor would it likely be desirable. Manassis et al. (2014) did attempt to differentiate among types of parental involvement (i.e., with and without TOC and CM); however, most of the meta-analyses offered a broad-based assessment of the effects of parental involvement without classifying or controlling for the specific ways in which parents were involved in their child's treatment. Identifying the specific components and types of family involvement should be an important next step in determining whether some types of family involvement may increase therapy effectiveness in certain circumstances. It is also possible that family-based therapy may benefit certain children who do not respond as well to child-only therapy.

In another recent study, Pereira et al. (2016) examined effects of parental involvement in session and out of session in a group therapy program for anxious youths. They administered the FRIENDS for Life program (Barrett, 2010) to anxious youth and assessed parental involvement via a therapist questionnaire (Pereira & Barros, 2013), assessing communication with the clinician, the parent's support of their child's homework activities, the parent's support of their child's exposure exercises, and attendance at the parent session. They reported that the overall parental involvement was only moderate. While most parents were rated as high on the items assessing communication and attendance of parents' sessions (in-session involvement) the out-of-session involvement (homework and exposure) was significantly lower. Nonetheless, when looking at the treatment outcome, results indicated significant decreases in mother-rated anxiety symptoms when the parents rated themselves higher in therapy involvement. No significant effects were found for the child's rating. Further, and interestingly, parents with more fearful reactions to physical anxiety symptoms and stronger negative beliefs regarding the child's anxiety were less involved in the therapy. While one study alone does not counterbalance the aggregate results of the meta-analyses, this study may serve to illustrate the possibility of multiple mediating and moderating effects of parental involvement in therapy. Finally, the TAFF (German: Trennungsangst fuer Familien; English: Separation Anxiety Program for Families) study (Schneider et al., 2013)[1] randomized 64 children with separation anxiety to either the child-focused Coping Cat program (Kendall, 1994) or the family-focused disorder-specific TAFF (Schneider et al., 2011) program, in which parents attended parent-only therapy sessions in addition to child-only sessions, joint sessions, and exposure sessions. Separation anxiety disorder directly involves the relationship between the child and the primary caregiver, and thus may be a prime candidate for family treatment, which also targets the parents' dysfunctional cognitions concerning the child's anxiety. The child-focused treatment and the enhanced family treatment were both successful in decreasing anxiety symptoms and diagnoses, with no significant differences in diagnoses or ratings of separation anxiety symptoms, and some trend level effects favoring the TAFF group. Tertiary analyses indicated that parental dysfunctional cognitions decreased in both groups, independent of the treatment condition, indicating that parents' cognitions improved, even when they were not the target of treatment. Parental cognitions are often the focus of cognitive treatments involving parents, yet do not appear to be a main mechanism for change through family involvement.

In sum, nearly all evidence points to the equivalence of child-focused therapies and those that involve parents. However, there may be some slight advantage of family-based therapy in continued improvements posttherapy (Manassis et al., 2014). Future research should examine potential moderating effects of family involvement. It may be that specific types of family involvement work better than others, and that family involvement may enhance outcomes for special subsets of anxious youth, such as those with highly anxious parents, or those resistant to therapy for some other reason. However, in the meantime, nearly all evidence for family

---

[1] For interested therapists, the TAFF manual is available in German from the last author and has been extensively described in English in Schneider and Lavallee (2013). Further, the principles and lessons from the TAFF program have recently been translated into a self-help guide in narrative workbook format for children and their parents, therapist, teacher, or caregivers to work through together, titled *What to Do When You Don't Want to Be Apart: A Kid's Guide to Overcoming Separation Anxiety* (Lavallee & Schneider, 2017). The guide is part of the American Psychological Association's What-to-do Guides for Kids. While this book doesn't include the parent in the co-client role used in TAFF, it does involve the parent or caregiver as co-clinician, and includes an educational introduction for parents and caregivers.

involvement points to it being equivalent to child-focused therapy in effectiveness. Thus, at this time, family involvement in child therapy for childhood anxiety disorders should generally be considered a choice related to the personal preferences of individual therapists and families, and not of substantial consequence for the anxious child, although child-only therapy might be more cost efficient.

Mediators and Moderators of Change

Following the lack of empirical evidence for an overall enhancing effect of parental involvement in CBT for anxious children, there are even fewer studies of moderators and mediators for parental involvement. Two of the meta-analyses on parental involvement in therapy (Manassis et al., 2014; Thulin et al., 2014) examined potential moderating factors such as age and comorbidity, with no significant effects found, overall. One study revealed moderating effects of age and gender in that female and younger children (7–10 years old) profited more from family-involved treatment than from child-only treatment (Barrett, Dadds, & Rapee, 1996), with effects significant through the 1-year follow-up, and then disappearing by the 6-year follow-up. Although it is intuitive that younger children might benefit more from family-enhanced treatments, more empirical data are needed to support this hypothesis. There are some data indicating that children with parents who suffer from anxiety disorders themselves may benefit more from a combined parent-child than child-based treatment (Cobham, Dadds, & Spence, 1998). The authors assigned children into two groups according to their parents' anxiety level (high versus low). They then underwent treatment either with or without additional parental anxiety management (PAM). Results indicated that children with low anxious parents benefited from CBT with and without parental anxiety management. However, those children with high anxious parents experienced significantly less improvement in the treatment without PAM than those with PAM. The effects were maintained at follow-up. Unfortunately, there are no meta-analytic data exploring a possible moderating role of parental psychopathology on family-enhanced treatment outcome. A single study attempted to treat parental psychopathology as an add-on to a child-focused treatment in a clinical trial (Creswell et al., 2008). The authors added eight individual CBT sessions for the parents. The treatment resulted in a decrease in parental psychopathology, but no significant effect on the child's treatment outcome. In sum, much more research with large samples, comparing different approaches to parental involvement, is needed to fully understand potential moderating factors in family-enhanced psychotherapy.

Clinical Case Illustration

Description of Symptoms

Ten-year-old "Sabrina" and her parents presented and were interviewed in our therapy center. The family recounted Sabrina's great difficulties spending time alone. During the day she was not able to play alone in her room if her mother was not with her. She would only go to her friends' homes if her mother accompanied her. Sleepovers were not possible. On some days, and especially on Mondays, Sabrina experienced a stomach ache and nausea before school. Her mother then called her in sick and spent the morning with her, intensively caretaking her (sitting together on the sofa, watching TV together, making her favorite food). On the other days, Sabrina was able to go to school, although she required an intensive farewell ritual with her mother. Up until the start of the therapy, Sabrina had never slept in her own bed. Sabrina told her therapists that she was afraid of losing her mother, either to an accident or to a burglar. When she was in school she often thought that terrible things were happening to her mother. At night, she only felt safe in her parents' bed.

Diagnostics

Sabrina and her parents underwent an extensive psychological diagnostic battery, including a structured interview as well as psychometric instruments. The results of the combined parent and child interview of the Kinder-DIPS (Schneider et al., 2017) indicated a single primary diagnosis, separation anxiety disorder, with a severity index of 7 on a scale ranging from 0 (no disorder) to 8 (very severe disorder). The questionnaire scores corroborated the outcome of the interview. Additional parent questionnaires indicated elevated overprotection and fearful parental cognitions concerning the fear of the child.

Psychoeducation Phase

Sabrina and her parents took part in a family-based cognitive behavioral therapy program (TAFF). The program consists of eight psychoeducational sessions, including four for the child and four for the parents separately, plus eight joint sessions for exposure with both parents and child. In the first sessions, Sabrina learned basic information about fear and anxiety and its adaptive origins and purpose. She was told that other children also suffer from anxiety to normalize her feelings. With the help of her therapist, she explored the three components of anxiety (thoughts, feelings, and behavior), and practiced reframing negative, catastrophic thoughts into more optimistic ones (cognitive restructuring). She then discovered how to overcome her fear by comparing successful experiences in which she had overcome nervousness or fear to separation situations. She learned that she has to face her fear and seek out anxiety-eliciting situations over and over again. An anxiety hierarchy of feared situations was developed ("being alone at home for 10 minutes, being alone at home for 30 minutes, being alone at a friend's place, sleeping in her own bed, sleepover at a friend's house") and these situations became the targets of the exposure sessions.

Parental Psychoeducation – Preparation of Transfer of Control, Identifying Dysfunctional Cognitions/Behavior

In contrast to other therapies that only deliver therapy to the child, the TAFF program also included four alternating parent-only psychoeducation sessions, in which Sabrina's parents entered the role of co-clients with their daughter. Sabrina's parents also learned about anxiety and the role they may play in either reinforcing or assuaging their child's anxiety. Via guided discovery, her parents learned that separation is a normal developmental task and that anxiety can have an adaptive purpose. They developed an understanding of the three-component model of the maintenance of anxiety (thoughts, feelings, and behavior) and the vicious circle of anxiety and avoidance. The therapist pointed out that in addition to child factors that led to anxiety, there are also parent factors that may contribute to Sabrina's anxiety, including their cognitions about her anxiety, any potential parent psychopathology (mother was anxious, but no disorder criteria were fulfilled), and their child-rearing style. Sabrina's parents identified their own dysfunctional conditions, such as "we will traumatize our child if we are not there to help her when she is afraid." Sabrina's mother was able to see that she herself was overprotective and had anxious thoughts about separating from her daughter (i.e., "someone will abduct her"), and thus reinforced her child's avoidance of separation situations. Sabrina's parents learned to restructure dysfunctional thoughts concerning separation into positive, fear-reducing thoughts (e.g., "If I trust her to make it through a separation, I can help my daughter overcome her fear"). Finally, the therapist explained the rationale for the exposure therapy sessions by illustrating various separation situations in which the child avoids separation, and then posing hypothetical alternative endings, in which the separation could not be avoided. The therapist helped the parents understand the principle of habituation and how fear can be overcome facing it (i.e., fear cannot rise indefinitely; but rather Sabrina would eventually habituate to the separation situation and experience a natural decrease in fear). The parents learned basic principles of contingency management (ignoring anxious behavior and praising courageous behavior) and other behavioral strategies to support their child. They identified everyday situations (e.g., buying some sweets at the bakery while the parents are waiting outside) in which Sabrina already showed courageous behavior and in which her parents were reinforcing her behavior with praise.

Exposure Phase – Transfer of Control, Reframing Parental Dysfunctional Cognitions, Changing Parental Dysfunctional Behavior

After the completion of the psychoeducation sessions, Sabrina and her parents were conjointly seen for the rest of the therapy sessions for exposure preparation, exposure itself, and relapse prevention. In these sessions, the parents moved from their role of co-clients to co-clinicians, following a transfer-of-control approach. In the first joint session, Sabrina and her parents outlined a final hierarchy of fear-eliciting situations. At the end of the session, the therapist discussed the dos and don'ts of exposure with the parents alone. Together with the child, they planned out the first exposure that was to take place during the next session. The next session took place at Sabrina's home because she chose "staying alone in her room" as her first exposure. The therapist guided Sabrina through the exposure session, while the parents were tasked with observing how the therapist introduced the task and reinforced Sabrina's behavior. The therapist took care to reinforce courageous behavior and reminded Sabrina to remember her positive thoughts ("Nothing will happen to my parents. I can do it!"). During the first session, Sabrina successfully stayed in her room for 10 minutes. Her parents and the therapist praised her for her efforts and success. She then wanted to do another exposure in which she stayed in the room for 15 minutes. Afterward, the exposures were reviewed with the help of anxiety graphs on which Sabrina rated her anxiety before, during, and after the practice, and observed that the anxiety decreased a little over time and over the two practice events. At the end of the session, Sabrina received the agreed-upon reward of playing a special board game with the therapist and her parents.

Starting in the next session, the parents took over the role of therapist and guided the child's exposure. Sabrina's mother worried that her own anxiety could be an obstacle in guiding the exposure, so the parents decided that Sabrina's father would initially coach Sabrina in the exposure practice. In the session, they once again practiced situations at home, starting with a situation in which Sabrina stayed in her own room for 15 minutes, repeating the already successful task from the previous session. Then, the parents and the therapist left the house while Sabrina stayed inside in the living room for 10 minutes. Sabrina managed to stay in the situation without running after her parents, although she reported high levels of fear. She was very proud after the practice sessions and was once again rewarded for facing the fear-eliciting situations. At the end of the session, the therapist planned further exposure practices to take place during the time between the therapist-guided sessions. Sabrina and her parents conducted these "homework" sessions on their own.

During the next sessions with the therapist, the family reported on their weekly exposure training and discussed problems and difficulties that had arisen. In addition, the therapist discussed the "meta-messages" the parents sent their daughter when they had fearful cognitions and worries about Sabrina having too much fear to handle certain situations. The therapist helped the parents to construct meta-messages that support autonomy (e.g., "We think you can walk to your friend's house alone. You can do it" instead of "I will bring Sabrina to her friend's. It's safer that way"). Sabrina and her parents continued working on the hierarchy of fearful situations at home. In the exposures, Sabrina made progress in staying at home alone and started to sleep in her own bed for some parts of the night. She no longer had difficulty going to school, and successfully helped herself cope with positive, optimistic thoughts. Her parents rewarded courageous behaviour. Sabrina told* the therapist that her ultimate goal was to have a sleepover at her best friend's house. The last two therapy sessions focused on relapse prevention and intervention.

Posttherapy and Follow-Up Assessment

The posttherapy assessment indicated that while some symptoms of the separation anxiety were still present, the diagnostic criteria were no longer fulfilled. The parents' and child's questionnaire responses revealed a considerable decrease in anxiety scores for separation situations. Sabrina and her parents returned to the therapy center for a 6-month follow-up. Sabrina reported that she was feeling proud because she had successfully joined a school trip for one week. She was regularly having sleepovers with her friends, and her parents were able to go to the supermarket or to visit neighbors during the day without her having a strong fear reaction. She was sleeping in her own bed, even though sometimes the worries and fearful thoughts about her parents returned. She then remembered and rehearsed her positive thoughts and managed to face her fears. The parents told the assessor that they had continued to practice coping with anxiety-eliciting situations. They were also able to taper off the reward system. Sabrina's mother emphasized that she had experienced personal change, and that she was able to support her daughter's autonomy, even though she still sometimes feared that something could happen to her. She told the assessor that she herself had overcome a lot of her own fears. The whole situation in the family was more relaxed and Sabrina continued to be diagnosis-free at follow-up.

Challenges and Recommendations for Future Research

The question of whether parents should be included in the psychotherapy of children and adolescents with anxiety disorders cannot be answered with a simple "yes" or "no." As parental involvement must be present at least to some extent in child therapy (giving their consent), especially with younger children, (i.e., logistical support, scheduling and keeping appointments), the more relevant question is rather *how* and how intensively parents should be involved. But the relative impact of including, or even targeting, family members in cognitive behavioral therapy is in need of further exploration. In general, it is unclear how and whether active parental involvement improves anxiety therapy for children in the aggregate. From a theoretical and etiological point of view, including parents in children's therapy appears intuitive and rational, especially given that anxiety runs in families and many family factors are associated with the child's anxiety. At the same time, the present therapeutic findings of equivalence may support the premise that the absence of parents in the therapy can help children to gain greater self-efficacy and autonomy, as parents' presence, when they are included, may serve to facilitate safety behavior (Ollendick et al., 2015) associated with increased anxiety. However, the research to date is somewhat mixed and has not identified a clear advantage of family-based therapy over child-focused therapy, with results usually pointing to equivalence.

As the treatment modalities and the amount of parental involvement vary widely, our current knowledge of the exact role and mechanisms of parental involvement is poor and needs far more theoretical and empirical refinement. A few studies (Barrett et al., 1996) indicate that there may be age effects on family-therapy effectiveness, in that younger children might benefit more from family-enhanced treatment. Nevertheless, the current body of research is lacking studies that explore this question in detail and with sufficient power to detect clear effects. Considerably more research is needed with sample sizes large enough to detect small effects, and examine subgroups, including age, gender, parental anxiety disorder, and subtypes of children's anxiety disorders. In an ongoing multi-center study by our group, using a randomized control study design, we will examine the disorder-specific efficacy of parental participation in a larger sample size of at least 300 children with anxiety disorders (age 8–14 years). The study compares two intensive exposure-based therapy programs: a child-focused therapy program with only one organizational session for the parents, and a family-based therapy program, in which the parents are present in each session. The latter is centered around transfer of control and contingency management therapy techniques. In contrast to preliminary studies, the study aims for a large sample size, in order to conduct subgroup analyses and identify factors that influence outcome. Conducting cost-effectiveness studies could be another way to analyze the impact of parental involvement. So far, child-based therapy seems to be more cost-efficient, because more intensive parental involvement usually requires additional sessions with the parents. From another point of view, parental involvement could be more cost-efficient, if it actually decreased the number of total sessions needed with the child, with the therapist making the parents co-clinicians, in effect outsourcing exposure sessions. Costs could further be reduced if parental involvement reduces relapse and stabilizes therapy success after the end of the therapy as proposed by Manassis et al. (2014).

We are still a long way from really understanding which family-related key factors may contribute to a change in therapy for childhood anxiety disorders. For example, the current body of research is lacking studies that explore the importance of fathers' role. Most of the studies including parental involvement treat and examine primarily mothers, not fathers. Thus, additional research is needed with a focus on fathers as they take on different, but also essential roles in the understanding of child's anxieties (Bögels & Phares, 2008). Further, although research has found associations between various family dynamics such as overprotection, parental anxiety or family quality, the full etiological picture of child anxiety is still being developed, with some mechanisms possibly missing from current models.

The field needs a cumulative research strategy that builds upon itself, instead of a juxtaposition of many individual studies that are not well connected to one another. To coordinate this, a theoretical framework is needed that structures the field and facilitates systematic examination of individual components of parental involvement. It is still unclear which family factors and which parental involvement strategies would be the agents of change in family-based enhancement of the child's psychotherapy. In a critical review concerning the failure of empirical research to find enhancing effects of parental involvement, Breinholst et al. (2012) conclude that the variability of family factors on which studies base their approaches, as well as the variability of the parental involvement approaches used in the studies, is rather high. Therefore, it is not possible to analyze them all together. A common, theoretical framework might be able to solve this problem. To further explore enhancement effects on treatment the first goal should be to dismantle the important active factors of parental involvement. Wei and Kendall (2014) even go further by proposing that parental involvement could be optimized by identifying the most important factors for each individual family. With such a profile of risk factors different family modules could be added to a standard CBT-exposure focused treatment. That would require reliable, theory-based psychological assessment and diagnosis and a scientifically tested catalogue of different family-focused therapy modules, from which the therapist can choose individual ingredients needed to enhance an individual child's therapy with regard to present risk factors. Unfortunately, the current database does not allow for any evidence-based customization but is based solely on clinical judgment.

In summary, the current empirical data do not support a unique role for parental involvement in the enhancement of child anxiety therapy. The data do show, however, that family-based cognitive behavioral therapy is at least as effective as child-focused treatment. In the future, more research is needed to further elucidate the major mechanisms in the ethology of childhood anxiety as well as in family treatment of anxiety disorders in children.

Key Practice Points

- The majority of the current empirical data indicate that family-based cognitive behavioral therapy is at least as effective as child-focused treatment. From a theoretical and etiological point of view, including parents in children's therapy appears to make sense, given that anxiety runs in families. From an economical point of view, however, child-based therapy might be more cost-efficient.
- A certain amount of minimal out-of-session parental involvement (logistical support, child management) must be present to some extent in child therapy.
- There are many different approaches to more active in-session parental involvement (i.e., transfer of control and contingency management, treating parental psychopathology, changing parental dysfunctional cognitions and/or behavior regarding the child's anxiety, and improving general communication skills).
- Empirical support does not yet provide a definitive answer on how much or whether parental involvement can be considered an essential therapy component. A framework and a research agenda are urgently needed to structure and coordinate more systematic research in this area.

References

Barmish, A. J., & Kendall, P. C. (2005). Should parents be co-clients in cognitive-behavioral therapy for anxious youth? *Journal of Clinical Child & Adolescent Psychology, 34* (3), 569–581. https://doi.org/10.1207/s15374424jccp3403_12

Barret, P. (2010). *FRIENDS for life for children. Participant workbook and leader's manual.* Brisbane: Barret Research Resources.

Barrett, P. M., Dadds, M. R., & Rapee, R. M. (1996). Family treatment of childhood anxiety: A controlled trial. *Journal of Consulting and Clinical Psychology, 64*(2), 333–342.

Barrett, P. M., Rapee, R. M., Dadds, M. M., & Ryan, S. M. (1996). Family enhancement of cognitive style in anxious and aggressive children. *Journal of Abnormal Child Psychology, 24*(2), 187–203. https://doi.org/10.1007/BF01441484

Bernstein, G. A., Warren, S. L., Massie, E. D., & Thuras, P. D. (1999). Family dimensions in anxious-depressed school refusers. *Journal of Anxiety Disorders, 13*(5), 513–528. Retrieved from http://www.ncbi.nlm.nih.gov/pubmed/10600052

Blatter-Meunier, J., Kreißl, M.W., & Schneider, S. (2016). Familienstrukturen in Familien von Kindern mit einer Störung mit Trennungsangst: Eine Untersuchung mit dem Familiensystemtest. *Zeitschrift für Klinische Psychologie und Psychotherapie.* 45, pp. 258–266. DOI: 10.1026/1616-3443/a000384.

Bodden, D. H. M., Bögels, S. M., Nauta, M. H., De Haan, E., Ringrose, J., Appelboom, C., ... Appelboom-Geerts, K. C. M. M. J. (2008). Child versus family cognitive-behavioral therapy in clinically anxious youth: An efficacy and partial effectiveness study. *Journal of the American Academy of Child & Adolescent Psychiatry, 47*(12), 1384–1394. https://doi.org/10.1097/CHI.0b013e318189148e

Bögels, S. M., & Zigterman, D. (2000). Dysfunctional cognitions in children with social phobia, separation anxiety disorder, and generalized anxiety disorder. *Journal of Abnormal Child Psychology, 28*(2), 205–211.

Bögels, S. M., & Brechman-Toussaint, M. L. (2006). Family issues in child anxiety: Attachment, family functioning, parental rearing and beliefs. *Clinical Psychology Review, 26*(7), 834–856. https://doi.org/10.1016/j.cpr.2005.08.001

Bögels, S., & Phares, V. (2008). Fathers' role in the etiology, prevention and treatment of child anxiety: A review and new model. *Clinical Psychology Review, 28*(4), 539–558. https://doi.org/10.1016/j.cpr.2007.07.011

Breinholst, S., Esbjørn, B. H., Reinholdt-Dunne, M. L., & Stallard, P. (2012, April). CBT for the treatment of child anxiety disorders: A review of why parental involvement has not enhanced outcomes. *Journal of Anxiety Disorders, 26*(3), 416–424.

Burt, S. A. (2009). Rethinking environmental contributions to child and adolescent psychopathology: A meta-analysis of shared environmental influences. *Psychological Bulletin, 135*(4), 608–637. https://doi.org/10.1037/a0015702

Chorpita, B. F., & Barlow, D. H. (1998). The development of anxiety: The role of control in the early environment. *Psychological Bulletin, 124*(1), 3–21.

Chorpita, B. F., Albano, A. M., & Barlow, D. H. (1996). Cognitive processing in children: Relation to anxiety and family influences. *Journal of Clinical Child Psychology, 25* (2), 170–176. https://doi.org/10.1207/s15374424jccp2502_5

Cobham, V. E., Dadds, M. R., & Spence, S. H. (1998). The role of parental anxiety in the treatment of childhood anxiety. *Journal of Consulting and Clinical Psychology, 66* (6), 893–905.

Cooper, P. J., Fearn, V., Willetts, L., Seabrook, H., & Parkinson, M. (2006). Affective disorder in the parents of a clinic sample of children with anxiety disorders. *Journal of Affective Disorders, 93*(1–3), 205–212. https://doi.org/10.1016/j.jad.2006.03.017

Craske, M. G., Treanor, M., Conway, C. C., Zbozinek, T., & Vervliet, B. (2014). Maximizing exposure therapy: An inhibitory learning approach. *Behaviour Research and Therapy, 58,* 10–23. https://doi.org/10.1016/j.brat.2014.04.006

Crawford, A. M., & Manassis, K. (2001). Familial predictors of treatment outcome in childhood anxiety disorders. *Journal of the American Academy of Child & Adolescent*

Creswell, C., & Cartwright-Hatton, S. (2007). Family treatment of child anxiety: Outcomes, limitations and future directions. *Clinical Child and Family Psychology Review, 10* (3), 232–252. https://doi.org/10.1007/s10567-007-0019-3

Creswell, C., Willetts, L., Murray, L., Singhal, M., & Cooper, P. (2008). Treatment of child anxiety: An exploratory study of the role of maternal anxiety and behaviours in treatment outcome. *Clinical Psychology & Psychotherapy, 15*(1), 38–44.

Eley, T. C., McAdams, T. A., Rijsdijk, F. V., Lichtenstein, P., Narusyte, J., Reiss, D., . . . Neiderhiser, J. M. (2015). The intergenerational transmission of anxiety: A children-of-twins study. *American Journal of Psychiatry, 172*(7), 630–637. https://doi.org/10.1176/appi.ajp.2015.14070818

Ewing, D. L., Monsen, J. J., Thompson, E. J., Cartwright-Hatton, S., & Field, A. (2015). A meta-analysis of transdiagnostic cognitive behavioural therapy in the treatment of child and young person anxiety disorders. *Behavioural and Cognitive Psychotherapy, 43*(5), 562–577. https://doi.org/10.1017/S1352465813001094

Garcia-Lopez, L. J., Díaz-Castela, M. del M., Muela-Martinez, J. A., & Espinosa-Fernandez, L. (2014). Can parent training for parents with high levels of expressed emotion have a positive effect on their child's social anxiety improvement? *Journal of Anxiety Disorders, 28*(8), 812–822. https://doi.org/10.1016/j.janxdis.2014.09.001

Ginsburg, G. S., & Schlossberg, M. C. (2002). Family-based treatment of childhood anxiety disorders. *International Review of Psychiatry, 14*(2), 143–154. https://doi.org/10.1080/09540260220132662

Ginsburg, G. S., Silverman, W. K., & Kurtines, W. K. (1995). Family involvement in treating children with phobic and anxiety disorders: A look ahead. *Clinical Psychology Review, 15*(5), 457–473. https://doi.org/10.1016/0272-7358(95)00026-L

Ginsburg, G. S., Siqueland, L., Masia-Warner, C., & Hedtke, K. A. (2004). Anxiety disorders in children: Family matters. *Cognitive and Behavioral Practice, 11*(1), 28–43. https://doi.org/10.1016/S1077-7229(04)80005-1

Grills-Taquechel, A. E., & Ollendick, T. H. (2013). *Phobic and anxiety disorders in children and adolescents*. Cambridge, MA: Hogrefe.

Herren, C., In-Albon, T., & Schneider, S. (2013). Beliefs regarding child anxiety and parenting competence in parents of children with separation anxiety disorder. *Journal of Behavior Therapy and Experimental Psychiatry, 44*, 53–60.

Hudson, J. L., & Rapee, R. M. (2001). Parent-child interactions and anxiety disorders: an observational study. *Behaviour Research and Therapy, 39*(12), 1411–1427.

Hudson, J. L., & Kendall, P. C. (2002). Showing you can do it: Homework in therapy for children and adolescents with anxiety disorders. *Journal of Clinical Psychology, 58* (5), 525–534. https://doi.org/10.1002/jclp.10030

In-Albon, T., & Schneider, S. (2007). Psychotherapy of childhood anxiety disorders: A meta-analysis. *Psychotherapy and Psychosomatics, 76*, 15–24. https://doi.org/10.1159/000096361

James, A. C., James, G., Cowdrey, F. A., Soler, A., & Choke, A. (2013). Cognitive behavioural therapy for anxiety disorders in children and adolescents. In A. C. James (ed.), *Cochrane Database of Systematic Reviews* (p. CD004690). Chichester, UK: John Wiley & Sons, Ltd. https://doi.org/10.1002/14651858.CD004690.pub3

Kazdin, A. E. (1997). Parent management training: evidence, outcomes, and issues. *Journal of the American Academy of Child and Adolescent Psychiatry, 36*(10), 1349–1356. https://doi.org/10.1097/00004583-199710000-00016

Kendall, P. C. (1994). Treating anxiety disorders in children: Results of a randomized clinical trial. *Journal of Consulting and Clinical Psychology, 62*(1), 100–110. Retrieved from http://www.ncbi.nlm.nih.gov/pubmed/8034812

Kendall, P. C., Hudson, J. L., Gosch, E., Flannery-Schroeder, E., & Suveg, C. (2008). Cognitive-behavioral therapy for anxiety disordered youth: A randomized clinical trial evaluating child and family modalities. *Journal of Consulting and Clinical Psychology, 76*(2), 282–297. https://doi.org/10.1037/0022-006X.76.2.282

Kossowsky, J., Pfaltz, M. C., Schneider, S., Taeymans, J., Locher, C., & Gaab, J. (2013). The separation anxiety hypothesis of panic disorder revisited: A meta-analysis. *American Journal of Psychiatry, 170*(7), 768–781. https://doi.org/10.1176/appi.ajp.2012.12070893

Lavallee, K. L., & Schneider, S. (2017). *What to do when you don't want to be apart: A kid's guide to overcoming separation anxiety.* Washington, DC: American Psychological Association.

Li, X., Sundquist, J., & Sundquist, K. (2008). Age-specific familial risks of anxiety. *European Archives of Psychiatry and Clinical Neuroscience, 258*(7), 441–445. https://doi.org/10.1007/s00406-008-0817-8

Manassis, K., Changgun Lee, T., Bennett, K., Yan Zhao, X., Mendlowitz, S., Duda, S., ... Wood, J. J. (2014). Types of parental involvement in CBT with anxious youth: A preliminary meta-analysis. *Journal of Consulting and Clinical Psychology, 82*(6), 1163–1172. doi: 10.1037/a0036969

Marks, I. M. (1969). *Fears and phobias.* New York: Academic Press.

McLeod, B. D., Weisz, J. R., & Wood, J. J. (2007). Examining the association between parenting and childhood depression: A meta-analysis. *Clinical Psychology Review, 27*(8), 986–1003. https://doi.org/10.1016/j.cpr.2007.03.001

Micco, J. A., Henin, A., Mick, E., Kim, S., Hopkins, C. A., Biederman, J., & Hirshfeld-Becker, D. R. (2009). Anxiety and depressive disorders in offspring at high risk for anxiety: A meta-analysis. *Journal of Anxiety Disorders, 23*(8), 1158–1164. https://doi.org/10.1016/j.janxdis.2009.07.021

Moore, P. S., Whaley, S. E., & Sigman, M. (2004). Interactions between mothers and children: Impacts of maternal and child anxiety. *Journal of Abnormal Psychology, 113*(3), 471–476. https://doi.org/10.1037/0021-843X.113.3.471

Murray, L., Creswell, C., & Cooper, P. J. (2009). The development of anxiety disorders in childhood: an integrative review. *Psychological Medicine, 39*(9), 1413. https://doi.org/10.1017/S0033291709005157

Ollendick, T. H., & Grills, A. E. (2016). Perceived control, family environment, and the etiology of child anxiety – Revisited. *Behavior Therapy, 47*, 633–642.

Ollendick, T. H., Halldorsdottir, T., Fraire, M. G., Austin, K. E., Noguchi, R. J. P., Lewis, K. M., ... Whitmore, M. J. (2015). Specific phobias in youth: A randomized controlled trail comparing one-session treatment to a parent-augmented one-session treatment. *Behavior Therapy, 46*, 141–155.

Pereira, A. I., & Barros, L. (2013). *Escala de envolvimento parental na terapia [Parental Involvement in Therapy Scale].* Lisbon: University of Lisbon.

Pereira, A. I., Muris, P., Mendonça, D., Barros, L., Goes, A. R., & Marques, T. (2016). Parental involvement in cognitive-behavioral intervention for anxious children:

Parents' in-session and out-session activities and their relationship with treatment outcome. *Child Psychiatry & Human Development, 47*(1), 113–123.

Polanczyk, G. V., Salum, G. A., Sugaya, L. S., Caye, A., & Rohde, L. A. (2015). Annual research review: A meta-analysis of the worldwide prevalence of mental disorders in children and adolescents. *Journal of Child Psychology and Psychiatry, 56*(3), 345–365. https://doi.org/10.1111/jcpp.12381

Prins, P. J. M. (2001). Affective and cognitive processes and the development and maintenance of anxiety and its disorders. In *Anxiety disorders in children and adolescents: Research, assessment and intervention* (pp. 23–44). New York: Cambridge University Press.

Rapee, R. M., & Heimberg, R. G. (1997). A cognitive-behavioral model of anxiety in social phobia. *Behaviour Research and Therapy, 35*(8), 741–56.

Rapee, R. M. (2009). Early adolescents' perceptions of their mother's anxious parenting as a predictor of anxiety symptoms 12 months later. *Journal of Abnormal Child Psychology, 37*(8), 1103–1112. https://doi.org/10.1007/s10802-009-9340-2

Rapee, R. M. (2012). Family factors in the development and management of anxiety disorders. *Clinical Child and Family Psychology Review, 15*(1), 69–80. https://doi.org/10.1007/s10567-011-0106-3

Reynolds, S., Wilson, C., Austin, J., & Hooper, L. (2012). Effects of psychotherapy for anxiety in children and adolescents: A meta-analytic review. *Clinical Psychology Review, 32*(4), 251–262. https://doi.org/10.1016/j.cpr.2012.01.005

Sanders, M. R. (1999). Triple P-Positive Parenting Program: Towards an empirically validated multilevel parenting and family support strategy for the prevention of behavior and emotional problems in children. *Clinical Child and Family Psychology Review, 2*(2), 71–90. https://doi.org/10.1023/A:1021843613840

Schneider, S. & Lavallee, K. L. (2013). Separation anxiety disorder. In C. A. Essau & T. Ollendick (eds.), *The Wiley-Blackwell handbook of the treatment of childhood and adolescent anxiety* (pp. 301–334). Chichester: Wiley-Blackwell.

Schneider, S., & Nündel, B. (2002). Familial transmission of panic disorder: The role of separation anxiety disorder and cognitive factors. *European Neuropsychopharmacology, 12*, 149–150. https://doi.org/10.1016/S0924-977X(02)80097-9

Schneider, S., Blatter-Meunier, J., Herren, C., Adornetto, C., In-Albon, T., & Lavallee, K. (2011). Disorder-specific cognitive-behavioral therapy for separation anxiety disorder in young children: A randomized waiting-list-controlled trial. *Psychotherapy and Psychosomatics, 80*(4), 206–215. https://doi.org/10.1159/000323444

Schneider, S., Blatter-Meunier, J., Herren, C., In-Albon, T., Adornetto, C., Meyer, A., & Lavallee, K. L. (2013). The efficacy of a family-based cognitive-behavioral treatment for separation anxiety disorder in children aged 8–13: A randomized comparison with a general anxiety program. *Journal of Consulting and Clinical Psychology, 81*(5), 932–940. https://doi.org/10.1037/a0032678

Schneider, S., Houweling, J. E. G., Gommlich-Schneider, S., Klein, C., Nündel, B., & Wolke, D. (2009). Effect of maternal panic disorder on mother-child interaction and relation to child anxiety and child self-efficacy. *Archives of Women's Mental Health, 12*(4), 251–259. https://doi.org/10.1007/s00737-009-0072-7

Schneider, S., In-Albon, T., Nuendel, B., & Margraf, J. (2013). Parental panic treatment reduces children's long-term psychopathology: A prospective longitudinal study. *Psychotherapy and Psychosomatics.* https://doi.org/10.1159/000350448

Schneider, S., Pflug, V., In-Albon, T. & Margraf, J. (2017). *Kinder-DIPS Open Access: Diagnostisches Interview bei psychischen Störungen im Kindes- und Jugendalter.* Bochum: Ruhr-Universität Bochum, Forschungs- und Behandlungszentrum für psychische Gesundheit.

Schneider, S., Unnewehr, S., Florin, I., & Margraf, J. (2002). Priming panic interpretations in children of patients with panic disorder. *Journal of Anxiety Disorders, 16*(6), 605–624.

Seehagen, S., Margraf, J., & Schneider, S. (2014). Developmental psychopathology. In P. Emmelkamp & T. Ehring (eds.), *The Wiley-Blackwell handbook of anxiety disorders* (pp. 148–171). Chichester: John Wiley & Sons.

Silverman, W. K., & Kurtines, W. M. (1999). *A pragmatic perspective toward treating children with phobia and anxiety problems* (pp. 505–521). Boston: Springer. https://doi.org/10.1007/978-1-4615-4755-6_26

Silverman, W. K., & Treffers, P. D. A. (2001). *Anxiety disorders in children and adolescents: Research, assessment, and intervention.* Cambridge: Cambridge University Press.

Siqueland, L., Kendall, P. C., & Steinberg, L. (1996). Anxiety in children: Perceived family environments and observed family interaction. *Journal of Clinical Child Psychology, 25*(2), 225–237. https://doi.org/10.1207/s15374424jccp2502_12

Stark, K. D., Humphrey, L. L., Crook, K., & Lewis, K. (1990). Perceived family environments of depressed and anxious children: Child's and maternal figure's perspectives. *Journal of Abnormal Child Psychology, 18*(5), 527–547. https://doi.org/10.1007/BF00911106

Steinhausen, H.-C., Jakobsen, H., Meyer, A., Jørgensen, P. M., & Lieb, R. (2016). Family aggregation and risk factors in phobic disorders over three-generations in a nation-wide study. *PloS One, 11*(1), e0146591. https://doi.org/10.1371/journal.pone.0146591

Taboas, W. R., McKay, D., Whiteside, S. P. H., & Storch, E. A. (2015). Parental involvement in youth anxiety treatment: Conceptual bases, controversies, and recommendations for intervention. *Journal of Anxiety Disorders, 30*, 16–18.

Thulin, U., Svirsky, L., Serlachius, E., Andersson, G., & Öst, L.-G. (2014). The effect of parent involvement in the treatment of anxiety disorders in children: A meta-analysis. *Cognitive Behaviour Therapy, 43*(3), 185–200.

Tiwari, S., Kendall, P. C., Hoff, A. L., Harrison, J. P., & Fizur, P. (2013). Characteristics of exposure sessions as predictors of treatment response in anxious youth. *Journal of Clinical Child & Adolescent Psychology, 42*(1), 34–43.

van der Bruggen, C. O., Stams, G. J. J. M., & Bögels, S. M. (2008). Research review: The relation between child and parent anxiety and parental control: A meta-analytic review. *Journal of Child Psychology and Psychiatry, 49*(12), 1257–1269.

Warren, S. L., Huston, L., Egeland, B., & Sroufe, L. A. (1997). Child and adolescent anxiety disorders and early attachment. *Journal of the American Academy of Child & Adolescent Psychiatry, 36*(5), 637–644.

Warwick, H., Reardon, T., Cooper, P., Murayama, K., Reynolds, S., Wilson, C., & Creswell, C. (2017). Complete recovery from anxiety disorders following Cognitive Behavior Therapy in children and adolescents: A meta-analysis. *Clinical Psychology Review, 52*, 77–91.

Wei, C., & Kendall, P. C. (2014). Parental involvement: Contribution to childhood anxiety and its treatment. *Clinical Child and Family Psychology Review, 17*(4), 319–339.

Weissman, M. M., Pilowsky, D. J., Wickramaratne, P. J., Talati, A., Wisniewski, S. R., Fava, M., ... Rush, A. J. (2006). Remissions in maternal depression and child psychopathology. *JAMA, 295*(12), 1389. https://doi.org/10.1001/jama.295.12.1389

Wergeland, G. J. H., Fjermestad, K. W., Marin, C. E., Bjelland, I., Haugland, B. S. M., Silverman, W. K., ... Heiervang, E. R. (2016). Predictors of treatment outcome in an effectiveness trial of cognitive behavioral therapy for children with anxiety disorders. *Behaviour Research and Therapy, 76*, 1–12.

Windheuser, H. J. (1977). Anxious mothers as models for coping with anxiety. *Behavioral Analysis and Modification, 2*, 39–58.

Wood, J., Piacentini, J. C., Southam-Gerow, M. A., Chu, B. C., & Sigman, M. (2006). Family cognitive behavioral therapy for child anxiety disorders. *Journal of the American Academy of Child & Adolescent Psychiatry, 45*(3), 314–321. https://doi.org/10.1097/01.chi.0000196425.88341.b0

Woodward, L. J., & Fergusson, D. M. (2001). Life course outcomes of young people with anxiety disorders in adolescence. *Journal of the American Academy of Child and Adolescent Psychiatry, 40*(9), 1086–1093. https://doi.org/10.1097/00004583-200109000-00018

9 Treatment of Comorbid Sleep Problems in Anxious Children

Candice A. Alfano, Rogelio Gonzalez, and Jessica Meers

Introduction

As evidenced by results from multiple randomized controlled trials, review papers, and meta-analyses, cognitive behavioral therapy (CBT) is the most effective psychosocial treatment available for childhood anxiety disorders irrespective of whether delivered in an individual, group, or family format (James et al., 2013; James, Soler, & Weatherall, 2005; Silverman, Pina, & Viswesvaran, 2008). A recent review of 26 treatment studies found an overall remission rate of 59 percent among anxious youth treated with CBT compared to 16 percent of wait-list controls (James et al., 2013). When compared to active control treatments or "treatment as usual" however, CBT remission rates do not differ meaningfully from outcomes associated with other interventions (James et al., 2013). Even fewer studies have examined the durability of CBT-based outcomes over time, but available findings are most disappointing. In the largest and longest follow-up study to date, rates of anxiety diagnoses, symptom severity, and global functioning among children who received CBT several years earlier did not differ from anxious youth receiving no treatment (Ginsburg et al., 2014). Clearly, there remains much room for improvement.

Against this backdrop, delineation of theoretically derived mechanisms of change during treatment is a requisite next step in the development and delivery of more potent interventions for early-onset anxiety. With this goal in mind, our chapter focuses on the role of sleep in childhood anxiety disorders – a topic that has seen tremendous growth in recent years – and specifically considers how sleep-wake processes might be leveraged to improve CBT outcomes. We begin with an overview of the interleaved nature of sleep and anxious arousal including description of their bidirectional associations. This is followed by a review of research examining the presence of sleep problems and sleep-wake patterns among clinically anxious samples of youth. We then summarize outcomes from the few studies that have explicitly examined changes in sleep following CBT for childhood anxiety and provide a case example of an integrated sleep-anxiety intervention for youth. In the second part of the chapter, we introduce findings from more recent, novel sleep research with clinically anxious children, as well as a few recent treatment studies among anxious adults with potential significance for the treatment of anxious youth. We conclude with specific suggestions for future clinical research and key points for clinical practice.

The Reciprocal Nature of Sleep Problems and Anxiety

Consideration of sleep among children with anxiety disorders would be incomplete without first acknowledging the complex relationships that exist between these two domains. The presence of sleep complaints among anxious youth is well-recognized, as is the fact that sleep problems constitute diagnostic symptoms for several specific disorders; however, youth with sleep disorders evidence high rates of anxiety disorders at alarming rates. For example, 75 percent of adolescents with sleep terrors and/or sleepwalking were found to have an anxiety disorder in one study (Gau & Soong, 1999). In another study, 65 percent of youth referred for insomnia had previously received an anxiety diagnosis (Ivanenko et al., 2004). While anxiety and sleep disorders share several overlapping features, findings from clinical and community samples of youth suggest that anxious cognition, particularly during the pre-sleep period, is one salient pathway through which sleep and anxiety may be connected (Alfano et al., 2009; Hiller et al., 2014).

Experimental manipulations of sleep also produce robust changes in anxious arousal (e.g., Dinges et al., 1997; Reddy et al., 2017; Talbot et al., 2010). For example, in healthy individuals dose-dependent increases in subjective anxiety are reported with cumulative hours of wakefulness (Dinges et al., 1997) and a worsening of panic and anxiety symptoms has been observed in adults with panic disorder (Roy-Byrne, Uhde, & Post, 1986). Sleep loss increases anxious arousal at the physiologic level (e.g., Franzen et al., 2009) as well as the cognitive level. For example, healthy adolescents and adults have been found to estimate the likelihood of potential catastrophes to be greater when sleep deprived and adolescents appraised their worries as more threatening overall when sleep deprived compared to when rested (Talbot et al., 2010).

Bidirectional relationships are also evident from longitudinal studies. Numerous investigations identify early sleep problems as a robust predictor of later anxiety (Gregory et al., 2004, 2005; Gregory & O'Connor, 2002; Leahy & Gradisar, 2012). Gregory et al. (2005) found nearly one half of school-aged children with persistent sleep-related problems between the ages of five and nine years met criteria for an anxiety disorder by age 21. In another study, difficulty in falling asleep and early morning awakenings in childhood were found to predict the onset of generalized anxiety disorder (GAD) in adolescence (Shanahan et al., 2014). In an adolescent sample, subjective short sleep duration predicted anxiety disorders one year later (Roberts & Duong, 2017).

Early anxiety similarly predicts later sleep problems and disorders (Goldman-Mellor et al., 2014; Johnson, Roth, & Breslau, 2006; Shanahan et al., 2014). A four-decade longitudinal study found adolescents with anxiety disorders were nearly twice as likely to experience insomnia in mid-adulthood (Goldman-Mellor et al., 2014). Overall however, more robust evidence exists to support childhood sleep problems as a precursor of anxiety than the opposite (McMakin & Alfano, 2015). For example, in one of the few longitudinal studies to objectively measure sleep, Kelly and El-Sheikh (2014) used three waves of childhood data to show shorter sleep duration and worse sleep quality predicted increased anxiety (and depressive) symptoms, whereas weaker pathways were detected for anxiety-sleep relationships.

The relative strength of temporal relationships from early sleep to subsequent problems with anxiety is surely rooted in sleep's central role in brain maturation (Dahl, 2007). By the time a child reaches the age of 2 years, more than one half of his/her life will have been spent sleeping, achieved through a polyphasic sleep-wake pattern (i.e., multiple sleep periods during a 24-hour day). Even upon school entry, children continue to require amounts of sleep comparable to wakefulness. This predominance of sleep during the infant and childhood years strategically coincides with critical developments in behavioral regulation, affect modulation, and emotional learning and memory (Dahl, 1996; Horne, 1993). As such, inadequate sleep, in duration and/or quality, during the formative years may have long-term implications for emotional health and well-being.

Sleep in Children with Anxiety Disorders

Children with anxiety disorders often complain of disturbed sleep and daytime tiredness (Alfano et al., 2006; Alfano, Ginsburg, & Kingery, 2007; Alfano et al., 2010; Hansen et al., 2011; Hudson et al., 2009), though these problems are more common in certain disorders. Children with GAD evidence the highest rates of subjective sleep complaints including greater insomnia, nightmares, bedtime resistance, and shorter sleep duration than controls (Alfano et al., 2006, 2007, 2010; Chase & Pincus, 2011; Hudson et al., 2009; Mullin et al., 2017). In one study, up to 90 percent of children with GAD reported a sleep problem, a significantly higher rate than found in children with separation anxiety disorder, social anxiety disorder (SOC), or obsessive-compulsive disorder (Alfano et al., 2010). In contrast, youth with SOC evidence the same rates of sleep problems found in the general population of children (Alfano et al., 2010; Mesa, Beidel, & Bunnell, 2014). Still, among children with other primary psychiatric disorders, the presence of comorbid anxiety is uniquely predictive of sleep problems (Hansen et al., 2011).

In light of evidence for pervasive sleep complaints among anxious youth, it is remarkable that most studies have assessed a relatively narrow range of potential problems falling under this broad category. In fact, "sleep-related problems" in children encompass problems that manifest at or around bedtime, such as resistance/avoidance of getting into bed, problems initiating sleep, and refusals to sleep independently, problems that manifest later in the night, such as parasomnias, nightmares, and prolonged nighttime awakenings, and problems awakening in the morning and maintaining wakefulness during the day. Thus, while available data suggest the transition to sleep from wake is highly problematic for anxious youth (McMakin

& Alfano, 2015), less is known about other types of sleep-related difficulties in this population.

An additional limitation of this body of research is the infrequent use of subjective and objective sleep measures in the *same* study. Available data nonetheless indicate poor correspondence between self-reported and objectively-measured sleep in anxious youth (Alfano, Patriquin & De Los Reyes, 2015). Alterations in sleep architecture and timing have been observed when anxious youth are studied in a novel setting such as a sleep laboratory (Alfano et al., 2013; Forbes et al., 2008), but naturalistic sleep assessments (i.e., conducted in the home environment) typically fail to show significant differences in the actual sleep-wake patterns of clinically anxious youth and healthy controls, including comparable estimates of total sleep duration, nighttime awakenings, bedtimes, and wake times (Alfano et al., 2015; Alfano et al., 2013; Forbes et al., 2006, 2008; Palmer & Alfano, 2017; Patriquin et al., 2014).

One exception is sleep onset latency. For the most part, objective findings corroborate subjective reports indicating anxious youth require significantly longer to fall asleep at night compared to controls. In fact, findings across several actigraphy-based studies reveal sleep onset latencies from 5 to 7 minutes longer on average among anxiety-disordered children (Alfano et al., 2015; Cousins et al., 2011; Mullin et al., 2017).

Reconciling Subjective-Objective Sleep Discrepancies

Why do anxious youth (and their parents) provide reports of problematic sleep in the absence of objective evidence? First, it must be acknowledged that actigraphy, unlike polysomnography (PSG), is not a direct measure of sleep. Actigraphy relies on accelerometer-measured movement to determine sleep-wake periods and cannot easily distinguish lack of movement from sleep. This may be particularly problematic in populations prone to worry, anxiety, and fear at night. Accordingly, actigraphy-derived estimates of sleep onset latency, and possibly other sleep variables, might underestimate sleep disruption.

Second, objective sleep measures do not provide information about the sleep environment, yet numerous factors including excessive noise or light, uncomfortable sleeping surfaces, and/or room temperatures that are too hot or cold can adversely affect sleep. Where children sleep, with whom they sleep, and social interactions that take place within the context of sleep also exert significant effects. Parent-child conflict and certain sleep practices including bed sharing/co-sleeping have generally been associated with child sleep problems (Alfano et al., 2013; Stein et al., 2001). In a recent study of school-age children aged 6 to 12 years, one-third of children with GAD co-slept with parents at least some of the time compared to only 5 percent of non-anxious controls (Palmer et al., 2018). Unfortunately, because most published studies of anxious youth have failed to account for sleep arrangements and nighttime interactions in the home, understanding of how these specific contexts impact the sleep of anxious children is lacking.

Third, child and parent-endorsed sleep problems tend to be retrospective. Well-established cognitive biases among anxious youth (Alfano, Beidel, & Turner, 2002; Barrett et al., 1996) might include biased recall of problematic rather than restful nights of sleep and/or exaggeration of these experiences. Example comes from a study directly comparing retrospective versus prospective reports of nightmares among children with GAD and healthy controls (Reynolds & Alfano, 2016). Children with GAD (and their parents) retrospectively endorsed significantly more frequent nightmares than controls, though prospective assessment across a one-week period revealed no group differences. It is possible that the daytime events, interactions, and symptoms experienced by anxious youth influence not only the valance and content of dream activity but its recall over time. Both anxious adults and children have been found to report more emotionally negative dream content than controls (McNamara et al., 2010; Nielsen et al., 2000). Dreams with a more negative emotional tone might also be recalled as more distressing when elevated levels of anxiety are present.

Lastly, anxious children might be highly sensitive to (i.e., less tolerant of) even mild disruptions in sleep. A body of research reveals robust inter-individual differences in the effects of sleep loss on sleepiness, impairment, and mood, irrespective of habitual sleep patterns (Van Dongen et al., 2004; Van Dongen & Belenky, 2009). Indeed, even when actual sleep duration is comparable, children with anxiety disorders report significantly greater levels of daytime sleepiness and sleeping too little than non-anxious youth (Alfano et al., 2015). Anxiety sensitivity, or the perception that physiological sensations associated with anxiety are uncontrollable and threatening, has been shown to predict sleep complaints in youth with anxiety disorders, whereby greater anxiety sensitivity is associated with longer (subjective) sleep onset latency (Weiner et al., 2015). Because sleep-wake processes are shaped by emotional and cognitive inputs (Saper, Cano, & Scammell, 2005; Walker, 2009), persistently elevated levels of anxiety throughout the day might increase homeostatic sleep pressure toward regulating the physiologic, biochemical, and emotional effects of arousal.

In summary, sleep complaints and reports of daytime tiredness are pervasive in children with anxiety disorders, particularly those with GAD. Available objective data often fail to corroborate parent and child sleep reports, but these inconsistencies should not diminish the significance of reported poor sleep. The basis of observed measurement discrepancies is assuredly complex and likely influenced by methodological, contextual, developmental, and/or phenomenological issues that have rarely been explored. In clinical populations such as anxious youth, understanding of sleep is further limited by assessment practices that center on deficiencies and disorders rather than on overall sleep health. A far more useful approach for clinicians and researchers is to consider sleep as a multidimensional concept that can be measured across multiple levels of analysis and aspects (Buysse, 2014).

Sleep-Based Outcomes Following CBT for Childhood Anxiety Disorders

In view of the bidirectional relationship between sleep and anxiety, it is possible that the sleep problems experienced by anxious individuals remit, at least to some extent, following CBT intervention for anxiety. Notably, CBT for childhood anxiety shares several intersecting components with behavioral interventions for insomnia and other child sleep problems, including strategies for reducing cognitive and somatic arousal and extinguishing sleep-related avoidance behaviors (e.g., co-sleeping). A meta-analysis of treatment studies including anxious adults revealed CBT had a moderate effect on coexisting sleep problems (Belleville et al., 2010). However, the authors caution that research in this area is nascent, evidenced by the fact that the review of more than 1200 potential studies for inclusion identified only 25 (2 percent) reporting sleep-related outcomes.

A few studies have examined sleep problems among anxious youth in relation to CBT outcomes (Clementi et al., 2016; Donovan, Spence, & March, 2017; Peterman et al., 2016; Wallace et al., 2017). Both Clementi and colleagues (2016) and Peterman and colleagues (2016) found significant improvements within the domains of bedtime resistance and sleep anxiety specifically following CBT; however, in both studies, most youth continued to exhibit sleep problem scores in the clinically significant range. Clementi et al. (2016) also found parent-reported daytime sleepiness to be most resistant to improvement during treatment, while Peterman et al. (2016) found improvements in parent- but not child-reported sleep problems. Based on sleep diary data, authors of the latter study concluded that CBT did not improve sleep via changes in sleep hygiene.

It is important to note that the studies described previously are limited by the inclusion of subjective sleep measures only, absence of comparison control groups, lack of follow-up assessment, and the wide age ranges of participants. Results from a recent study highlight the importance of the latter point in the context of sleep-based outcomes. Specifically, children but not adolescents demonstrated a significant decrease in sleep-related problems following an online CBT program for anxiety (Donovan, Spence, & March, 2017). This finding aligns with outcomes from sleep intervention trials suggesting sleep problems to be particularly resistant to change during adolescence (e.g., Cain, Gradisar, & Moseley, 2011; Schlarb, Liddle, & Hautzinger, 2011). Biologically mediated changes in sleep timing/preference, increased levels of independence, and heightened academic/social demands that occur during this developmental period likely underlie these developmental differences.

In sum, limited but emerging research suggests that anxiety-focused CBT reduces some of the sleep problems common among anxious children, including those that tend to occur at or around bedtime. However, evidence for more global improvements in sleep is lacking.

Targeting Sleep Directly in Anxiety-based Treatment

A small pilot study examined the utility of an integrated behavioral intervention for anxiety and sleep problems in four children with GAD, ages 7 to 11 years (Clementi & Alfano, 2014). Targeted Behavioral Therapy (TBT) included a 2-session prescriptive sleep intervention in addition to psychoeducation and exposures for anxiety. Following 14 weeks of treatment, improvements in both sleep and anxiety were observed. Specifically, two of four (50 percent) children lost their GAD diagnosis at posttreatment and none of the children had a diagnosis at the 3-month follow-up. In terms of sleep, three out of four children (75 percent) reported improvement at posttreatment, and two of three (67 percent) improved at follow-up. Based on parent reports, the number of children exceeding the clinical cut-off on a validated sleep problems measure decreased from three out of four children (75 percent) at baseline to one of the four children (25 percent) at posttreatment and one out of the three children (33 percent) at follow-up. Although the small sample size and lack of a comparison control group preclude specific conclusions, the authors proposed that the inclusion of only 2 sessions explicitly focused on sleep might have been inadequate for producing meaningful sleep-based changes.

Building on preliminary findings, a randomized controlled trial comparing TBT to a well-established, "gold standard" treatment for childhood anxiety disorders (Coping Cat; Kendall, 1994) was recently completed (Clementi & Alfano, 2017). A total of 20 children (ages 6–12) with primary GAD were assigned to 16 weeks of treatment with either TBT or Coping Cat and completed assessments at baseline, posttreatment, and 6-month follow-up. Each assessment included diagnostic interviews and one week of objective sleep monitoring using actigraphy. Preliminary results indicate that anxiety and global functioning significantly improved in both groups from baseline to posttreatment, and improvements were maintained at 6-month follow-up. Equivalent improvements in both child- and parent-reported sleep problems were also observed across the groups. In terms of objective sleep variables, only sleep onset latency improved, albeit marginally, after treatment, decreasing in both groups by approximately 6 minutes on average. Notably, the latter finding dovetails with previous work finding a 5–7 minute difference in sleep onset latency between untreated anxious children compared to healthy children (Alfano et al., 2015; Cousins et al., 2011). However, an overall lack of change in objective sleep parameters stands in contrast to outcomes based on CBT interventions for sleep that produce meaningful improvements in objectively measured sleep duration and sleep efficiency in addition to sleep onset latency (Blake et al., 2017).

Additionally, time series analyses revealed that nearly twice as many TBT participants compared to Coping Cat participants showed a significant linear decrease in nightly bedtime problems over the course of the 16-week treatment. Overall, findings from this study suggest that traditional CBT for childhood anxiety may produce improvements in sleep complaints even when they are not targeted directly. At the same time, findings highlight the potential role of differential mechanisms underlying sleep-based changes during an integrated sleep and anxiety intervention compared to anxiety-only treatment that warrants further study.

Case Example Using Targeted Behavioral Therapy (TBT)

Riley is a healthy 8-year-old girl with a history of nighttime fears and difficulty sleeping independently. On a nightly basis, Riley requests that one of her parents sit on her bed with her until she falls asleep. Riley tells her parents that she is afraid of something happening to her while everyone else is sleeping, such as a burglar breaking into the house and taking her away. She insists on sleeping with an overhead light on in her room. Even when a parent is present, Riley requires approximately 30 minutes to fall asleep. On the few occasions her parents have insisted she try to initiate sleep on her own, Riley stays in her bed for no more than 3 minutes before calling out to her parents and/or getting out of bed and leaving her room. As a result of these nighttime struggles, she is often tired during the day and falls asleep on car rides. Riley worries about her sleep (or lack thereof) and whether she will always have trouble sleeping. In fact, Riley worries about many things, including her school performance, getting injured, her parents getting hurt or dying, and contracting an illness. Other fears include being alone on one level of the house if family members are on another level and talking to strangers.

Riley's clinical evaluation included: 1) structured interviews with Riley and her parents regarding psychiatric symptoms, sleep behaviors and routines, current stressors, medical, developmental, social, and family history; 2) completion of several child- and parent-report questionnaires; and 3) completion of a daily sleep log during a one-week period prior to the clinical assessment. Based on the information collected, Riley was diagnosed with generalized anxiety disorder and primary insomnia.

Riley was treated with Targeted Behavioral Therapy (TBT) including 16 weekly 1-hour sessions. The first five sessions focused on psychoeducation and sleep. The concept of "Sleep Thieves" was introduced to describe specific behaviors that interfere or "steal" children's sleep (e.g., keeping inconsistent bed and wake times, exposure to bright light in the evening, worrisome thoughts in bed) and Riley was asked to track her own Sleep Thieves (with her parents' help) and continue keeping a sleep log. Over the next few weeks, identification of Riley's Sleep Thieves was used to design a prescriptive sleep intervention that included practicing good sleep hygiene, stimulus control (i.e., to strengthen the association between the bed and sleep), and graduated extinction. Specifically, Riley's parents were directed to sit in a chair next to her bed at bedtime without talking or interacting with Riley and to gradually move the chair away from the bed over successive nights, with the goal of removing the chair from the bedroom after one week. Over the next week, Riley's parents agreed to check in on her after bedtime at regular intervals (i.e., every 5 minutes) by standing in her bedroom doorway. Riley was told that provided she remain quiet and in her bed, her parents would continue to check on her regularly. Riley's therapist checked on the family's success in implementing the sleep plan each week, helping to identify ways to modify the plan as needed.

TBT sessions 6 through 16 included graduated exposures for anxiety. As part of her fear hierarchy, Riley completed several in vivo exposures that required her to stay in the therapy room alone for progressively longer periods of time and with a decreasing amount of light while the therapist waited outside. The same behavior was practiced during the day in her bedroom for homework. Throughout treatment, both sleep and anxiety were tracked using weekly worry and sleep logs as well as sticker charts (i.e., contingency management). Specifically, for every night Riley followed a healthy bedtime routine and slept in her own bed by herself she earned a sticker toward a bigger reward (i.e., a scooter). She earned a second sticker for completing weekly anxiety-based homework tasks. The number of stickers required to earn her reward was increased each week as she experienced greater success.

After 16 weeks of treatment, Riley was able to sleep in her own room by herself most nights without seeking or calling out to her parents. Worry and sleep logs indicated a significant reduction in worrisome thoughts, as well as an increase in total sleep and a reduced sleep onset latency.

Reconceptualizing the Sleep Problems of Anxious Youth

In contrast to previous data documenting the presence of sleep problems using one-time reports and/or broad objective sleep indices, more recent studies among anxious youth highlight a general shift in focus toward elucidating the ways in which more "micro" aspects of sleep relate to daytime symptoms and functioning. In a study including youth with anxiety disorders, depressive disorders, and no psychiatric disorders, one week of actigraphy data was collected in conjunction with daily affect monitoring to examine relationships between these domains (Cousins et al., 2011). Although anxious youth did not differ from controls in terms of total sleep time or time in bed, differential sleep-affective relationships were identified. For anxious youth only, increases in negative affect during the day predicted more time spent awake that night, and as positive affect *increased* during the day, total time in bed *decreased* that night. Potentially, the presence of greater positive daytime affect may result in anxious youth spending less time in bed worrying that night. In the opposite direction, more time awake spent at night was related to *greater negative* affect the following day among anxious youth (Cousins et al., 2011). These data reveal unique sleep-affective relationships among children with clinical levels of anxiety irrespective of quantitative sleep indices.

Our lab recently examined how affective and somatic symptoms across a one-week period relate to aspects of sleep architecture in $N=66$ youth with GAD and healthy controls (Palmer & Alfano, 2017). Although no group difference in total slow wave sleep (i.e., the deepest and most restorative sleep stage) was detected, a greater percentage of slow wave sleep was associated with significantly less negative affect in children with GAD. No such relation was observed among controls. This particular finding corresponds with findings from experimental sleep research suggesting slow wave sleep to attenuate the effects of negative emotional experiences that occur during the day (Talamini et al., 2013). Another study including children at-risk for depression showed a greater amount of slow wave sleep in childhood to be protective for the development of depression years later in adolescence (Silk et al., 2007). Our study also found a significant relationship between percentage of rapid eye moment (REM) sleep (i.e., the sleep stage most closely associated with emotion) and daytime somatic and depressive symptoms in children with GAD but not controls (Palmer & Alfano, 2017).

In light of the well-established role of sleep in learning and memory, particularly emotional memory (Walker & van der Helm, 2009), another study investigated memory reactivation during sleep and its potential role in long-term emotional memory consolidation in children with SOC (Groch et al., 2017). Both youth with SOC and healthy controls were taught associations between pictures of ambiguous social situations and positive or negative words. That night, some words were represented (i.e., cued) during sleep in the laboratory. Although "cueing" facilitated retention of positive and negative memories equally in both groups the next morning, SOC youth rated cued negative words less positively one week later. Consistent with the well-recognized social memory biases of SOC individuals (cf. Clark & Wells, 1995), this finding may reflect preferential abstraction of negative emotional information via sleep. Specifically, since the memory consolidation process includes incorporating newly acquired information into existing memory stores, which likely include more negative social experiences among SOC youth, Groch and team (2017) posit that previous social memories in this population could render newer social learning experiences to be recalled more negatively and resistant to alteration over time.

Using the same sample of socially anxious youth and healthy controls, Wilhelm and colleagues (2017) examined the presence of slow (9–12 Hz) and fast (13–16 Hz) sleep spindles. Sleep spindles, defined as bursts of oscillatory brain activity visible on EEG, have been shown to synchronize the flow of information from limbic structures to the cortex (Clemens et al., 2007; Siapas & Wilson, 1998), fostering consolidation of newly acquired information into durable memories (Schabus et al., 2004; 2006). The authors found a marked reduction in fast sleep spindles in the SOC group, as well as a significant negative relationship between fast spindle activity and social anxiety severity (Wilhelm et al., 2017). These results are bolstered by other findings linking sleep spindles with emotional functioning in childhood. For example, both at-risk and depressed youth show less spindle activity than healthy controls (Lopez, Hoffmann, & Armitage, 2010), and greater sleep spindles have been linked with better emotional health in preschool-aged children both concurrently and longitudinally (Mikoteit et al., 2013). Sleep spindles might therefore mark a child's ability to adequately process emotionally challenging information/events, in turn minimizing or increasing risk of emotional problems.

In summary, emerging research underscores a need for broader conceptualizations of sleep among clinically anxious children grounded in an understanding of sleep's fundamental role in emotional learning and memory. El-Sheikh and Buckhalt (2015) have specifically called for integrative models that cut across developmental psychology, affective neuroscience, and other domains in order to fully explicate the functions of sleep in the context of both healthy and maladaptive developmental trajectories. Youth with anxiety disorders possess preexisting vulnerabilities in emotional reactivity and regulation that may serve to magnify the (deleterious) daytime effects of even minor sleep-wake alterations.

Likewise, the transition from wake to sleep quite conceivably poses a challenge for children with high levels of trait anxiety based on an essential requirement of lowered vigilance and arousal. The extent to which these self-regulatory processes relate to alterations in micro aspects of sleep and their functions is only beginning to be explored.

Leveraging the Power of Sleep in Treatment

Emerging experimental research provides insight into some of the ways sleep might be harnessed to enhance CBT outcomes for children with anxiety disorders. For example, since exposure has been shown to be the "essential ingredient" of CBT (Walkup et al., 2008; Kendall et al.,1997) and sleep occupies an essential role in emotional learning and memory (Walker, 2009), several studies have explored sleep's potential to enhance extinction learning. Fear extinction – the goal of exposure – refers to the loss of a conditioned fear response following repeated, controlled presentation of a feared stimulus. Guided by the results of experimental studies showing that fear extinction trials flanked (i.e., followed) by sleep result in greater fear reduction (e.g., Graves et al., 2003; Hagewoud et al., 2010; Vecsey et al., 2009), two studies have investigated sleep-enhanced extinction in clinically anxious adults (Kleim et al., 2014; Pace-Schott et al., 2012). In one study, 20 spider phobic adults who napped after a single virtual-reality exposure session showed enhanced extinction compared to 20 phobic non-nappers during a behavioral assessment one week later (Kleim et al., 2014). In another study where spider phobics completed an exposure session either in the morning or in the evening (i.e., right before the overnight sleep period), evidence of greater extinction based on both subjective and physiological (e.g., skin conductance) decreases in fear/arousal was found the next morning among subjects who completed exposure in the evening (Pace-Schott et al., 2012). Overall, findings suggest sleep that closely follows extinction training (i.e., exposure) may facilitate learning stabilization and assist with memory consolidation (Stickgold & Walker, 2005).

Other studies suggest that cumulative waking hours might directly impact fear extinction. In a sample of healthy adults, Pace-Schott et al. (2013) found that exposure sessions conducted in the morning as compared to later in the day resulted in greater fear reduction. Similar findings were recently reported in a sample of adults with post-traumatic stress disorder (PTSD). Specifically, hours-since-waking was found to moderate the relationship between fear extinction and PTSD symptoms whereby participants with greater symptoms showed significantly poorer extinction learning with increasing hours spent awake (Zuj et al., 2016). Since homeostatic sleep pressure increases across the day, reducing efficiency of waking cognition, extinction potential may be heightened when sleep pressure is low (cf. Hobson & Pace-Schott, 2002). Overall, this growing body of research suggests that strategically timing exposure sessions could help optimize extinction learning and maximize treatment benefit.

Overall Summary

Disturbances of sleep are closely linked with anxious psychopathology and youth with anxiety disorders often complain of poor sleep. Common sleep-related problems reported by anxious children and their parents include difficulty initiating sleep, fear of/refusal to sleep alone, nightmares, and feeling overtired during the day, among others. Despite their pervasive presence, these nighttime problems have been more challenging to capture using objective sleep measures, as comparisons with healthy children (i.e., who do not complain of sleep problems) often reveal equivalent sleep-wake parameters. There are numerous, potentially mutually-inclusive reasons for such discrepancies, but none that diminishes the significance of perceived poor sleep and daytime tiredness in children with clinical levels of anxiety.

Based on the reciprocal nature of sleep and arousal, some sleep problems reported by anxious youth might improve following CBT for anxiety. Recent studies directly examining this question suggest that difficulties related to bedtime resistance and sleep anxiety specifically are reduced with treatment. However, agreement between children and parents regarding improvement is poor and overall sleep is not meaningfully improved. Fewer data are available at this time examining whether the addition of behavioral treatment components directly targeting sleep might produce greater improvement in sleep (and perhaps anxiety). However, clarity regarding distinct aspects of sleep health requiring clinical attention is similarly lacking.

Beyond a focus on self-reported sleep problems and broad quantitative sleep estimates, recent studies have begun to explore how certain aspects of sleep physiology interact with daytime symptoms and functioning in different populations of children. Novel findings from this growing body of research indeed highlight the presence of unique sleep-affective relationships among anxious youth, underscoring both the bidirectionality of these functions and how they might act to shape one another across development. Moreover, emerging experimental findings among adults provide insight into the ways sleep might help to augment the effects of CBT for anxiety and produce more durable treatment outcomes.

Recommendations for Clinical Research and Practice

Sleep occupies a central role in emotional development, influencing emotional appraisals, reactivity, and regulation, but much remains to be learned about the functions of sleep-wake processes in early-onset anxiety disorders. As a first step, it is essential for researchers and clinicians alike to view and conceptualize sleep through a broader, dimensional lens. Beyond specific, circumscribed types of sleep problems, Buysee (2014) recommends five specific aspects of sleep be assessed for understanding individual sleep health, including: *sleep duration* (total amount of sleep obtained in a 24-hour period), *sleep continuity/efficiency* (ease of falling asleep and returning to sleep), *sleep timing* (placement of sleep within the 24-hour day), *alertness/sleepiness* (ability to maintain attentive wakefulness), and *satisfaction/quality* (subjective assessment of "good" or "poor" sleep).

With regard to anxious children (all children, in fact) we would add one additional aspect of interest: the *sleep context*. Periodic co-sleeping, variable sleep-wake routines, and the overall "emotional tone" in which sleep occurs may be especially problematic for anxious youth who struggle with various regulatory processes (e.g., emotion and attentional regulation). Maintaining stable sleep-wake practices helps to strengthen sleep "cues" and contribute to healthy sleep patterns and practices over the long term. This broader conceptual approach to sleep also requires assessment strategies that favor multi-method approaches (over singular questionnaires) that offer potential information about aspects of restorative sleep and its associations with emotional health.

In light of the continuous changes in sleep that characterize the childhood years, greater attention to distinct developmental periods is also needed to guide research questions, experimental designs, and clinical assessment strategies. A large proportion of sleep-based research conducted among youth with anxiety disorders has included age ranges that span several developmental stages. When age-based differences are considered, dichotomous groups based on chronological age (e.g., 7–11 compared to 12–17 years) are typically examined. In addition to constant changes in overall sleep need, normative alterations in circadian preference and timing that occur with the onset of puberty exert influence in sleep-emotion relationships (e.g., Miller et al., 2015; Talbot et al., 2010) and might dictate differential intervention approaches. For example, educating both teens and parents about the biologically mediated sleep changes that typically occur during adolescence (i.e., a shift to later sleep and wake times) and the way these changes interact with emotion can set the stage for incorporating a sleep focus into CBT for anxiety. The extent to which developmentally typical changes in sleep might elevate risk for or amplify symptoms of anxiety during the teenage years is a question for future research.

Finally, a broader focus on "sleep health" including recognition of normative developmental changes in sleep is necessary for understanding the functions of sleep in the context of anxiety-based treatments for youth. Remarkably, sleep has rarely been explored as a potential mediator in randomized controlled trials among clinically anxious youth even though several dimensions of sleep might directly undermine CBT effectiveness. Sleep duration that is too short, for example, might result in less effort, motivation, and attention during treatment sessions and interfere with skill acquisition. Exposure sessions that are followed by delayed sleep onset at night might be less successful in reducing fear due to prolonged periods of waking between extinction learning and sleep-based memory consolidation. Clinicians should therefore attend to the ways different sleep parameters relate to progress (or lack thereof) in CBT and utilize sleep-based strategies that match the individual child.

References

Alfano, C. A., Beidel, D. C., & Turner, S. M. (2002). Cognition in childhood anxiety: Conceptual, methodological, and developmental issues. *Clinical Psychology Review, 22*(8), 1209–1238.

Alfano, C. A., Beidel, D. C., Turner, S. M., & Lewin, D. S. (2006). Preliminary evidence for sleep complaints among children referred for anxiety. *Sleep Medicine, 7*(6), 467–473. doi:10.1016/j.sleep.2006.05.002

Alfano, C. A., Ginsburg, G. S., & Kingery, J. N. (2007). Sleep-related problems among children and adolescents with anxiety disorders. *Journal of the American Academy of Child and Adolescent Psychiatry, 46*(2), 224–232. doi:10.1097/01.chi.0000242233.06011.8e

Alfano, C. A., Patriquin, M. A., & De Los Reyes, A. (2015). Subjective – objective sleep comparisons and discrepancies among clinically-anxious and healthy children. *Journal of Abnormal Child Psychology, 43*(7), 1343–1353. doi:10.1007/s10802-015-0018-7

Alfano, C. A., Pina, A. A., Zerr, A. A., & Villalta, I. K. (2010). Pre-sleep arousal and sleep problems of anxiety-disordered youth. *Child Psychiatry and Human Development, 41*(2), 156–167. doi:10.1007/s10578-009-0158-5

Alfano, C. A., Reynolds, K., Scott, N., Dahl, R. E., & Mellman, T. A. (2013). Polysomnographic sleep patterns of non-depressed, non-medicated children with generalized anxiety disorder. *Journal of Affective Disorders, 147*(1–3), 379–384. doi:10.1016/j.jad.2012.08.015

Alfano, C. A., Smith, V. C., Reynolds, K. C., Reddy, R., & Dougherty, L. R. (2013). The Parent-Child Sleep Interactions Scale (PSIS) for preschoolers: Factor structure and initial psychometric properties. *Journal of Clinical Sleep Medicine, 9*(11), 1153–1160. doi:10.5664/jcsm.3156

Alfano, C. A., Zakem, A. H., Costa, N. M., Taylor, L. K., & Weems, C. F. (2009). Sleep problems and their relation to cognitive factors, anxiety, and depressive symptoms in children and adolescents. *Depression and Anxiety, 26*(6), 503–512. doi:10.1002/da.20443

Barrett, P. M., Rapee, R. M., Dadds, M. M., & Ryan, S. M. (1996). Family enhancement of cognitive style in anxious and aggressive children. *Journal of Abnormal Child Psychology, 24*(2), 187–203.

Belleville, G., Cousineau, H., Levrier, K., St-Pierre-Delorme, M. E., & Marchand, A. (2010). The impact of cognitive-behavior therapy for anxiety disorders on concomitant sleep disturbances: A meta-analysis. *Journal of Anxiety Disorders, 24*(4), 379–386.

Blake, M. J., Sheeber, L.B., Youssef, G. J., Raniti, M B. & Allen, N B. (2017). Systematic review and meta-analysis of adolescent cognitive-behavioral sleep interventions. *Clinical Child and Family Psychology Review, 20*, 227–249.

Buysse, D. J. (2014). Sleep health: Can we define it? Does it matter? *Sleep, 37*(1), 9–17. doi:10.5665/sleep.3298

Cain, N., Gradisar, M., & Moseley, L. (2011). A motivational school-based intervention for adolescent sleep problems. *Sleep Medicine, 12*, 246–251. doi: 10.1016/j.sleep.2010.06.008.

Chase, R. M., & Pincus, D. B. (2011). Sleep-related problems in children and adolescents with anxiety disorders. *Behavioral Sleep Medicine, 9*(4), 224–236. doi:10.1080/15402002.2011.606768

Clark, D. M., & Wells, A. (1995). A cognitive model of social phobia. In R. G. Heimberg, M. R. Liebowitz, D. A. Hope, F. R. Schneier, R. G. Heimberg, M. R. Liebowitz, ... F. R. Schneier (eds.), *Social phobia: Diagnosis, assessment, and treatment* (pp. 69–93). New York: Guilford Press.

Clemens, Z., Mölle, M., Erőss, L., Barsi, P., Halász, P., & Born, J. (2007). Temporal coupling of parahippocampal ripples, sleep spindles and slow oscillations in humans. *Brain: A Journal of Neurology, 130*(11), 2868–2878. doi:10.1093/brain/awm146

Clementi, M., & Alfano, C. A. (2014). Targeted behavioral therapy for childhood generalized anxiety disorder: A time-series analysis of changes in anxiety and sleep. *Journal of Anxiety Disorders, 28*(2), 215–222. doi:10.1016/j.janxdis.2013.10.006

Clementi, M., & Alfano, C. A. (2017). Efficacy of an Integrated Sleep and Anxiety Intervention for Anxious Children. *Manuscript in Preparation*.

Clementi, M., Alfano, C., Holly, L., & Pina, A. (2016). Sleep-related outcomes following early intervention for childhood anxiety. *Journal of Child and Family Studies*, 1–8. doi:10.1007/s10826-016-0478-6

Cousins, J. C., Whalen, D. J., Dahl, R. E., Forbes, E. E., Olino, T. M., Ryan, N. D., & Silk, J. S. (2011). The bidirectional association between daytime affect and nighttime sleep in youth with anxiety and depression. *Journal of Pediatric Psychology, 36*(9), 969–979. doi:10.1093/jpepsy/jsr036

Dahl, R. E. (1996). The regulation of sleep and arousal: Development and psychopathology. *Development and Psychopathology, 8*(1), 3–27. doi:10.1017/S0954579400006945

Dahl, R. E. (2007). Sleep and the developing brain. *Sleep, 30*(9), 1079–1080.

Dinges, D. F., Pack, F., Williams, K., Gillen, K. A., Powell, J. W., Ott, G. E., . . . Pack, A. I. (1997). Cumulative sleepiness, mood disturbance, and psychomotor vigilance performance decrements during a week of sleep restricted to 4–5 hours per night. *Sleep, 20*(4), 267–277.

Donovan, C. L., Spence, S. H., & March, S. (2017). Does an online CBT program for anxiety impact upon sleep problems in anxious youth? *Journal of Clinical Child and Adolescent Psychology, 46*(2), 211–221. doi:10.1080/15374416.2016.1188700

El-Sheikh, M., & Buckhalt, J. A. (2015). Sleep and development: Advancing theory and research: II. Moving sleep and child development research forward: Priorities and recommendations from the SRCD-sponsored forum on sleep and child development. *Monographs of the Society for Research in Child Development, 80*(1), 15–32. doi:10.1111/mono.12142

Forbes, E. E., Bertocci, M. A., Gregory, A. M., Ryan, N. D., Axelson, D. A., Birmaher, B., & Dahl, R. E. (2008). Objective sleep in pediatric anxiety disorders and major depressive disorder. *Journal of the American Academy of Child and Adolescent Psychiatry, 47*(2), 148–155. doi:10.1097/chi.0b013e31815cd9bc

Forbes, E. E., Williamson, D. E., Ryan, N. D., Birmaher, B., Axelson, D. A., & Dahl, R. E. (2006). Peri-sleep-onset cortisol levels in children and adolescents with affective disorders. *Biological Psychiatry, 59*(1), 24–30. doi:10.1016/j.biopsych.2005.06.002

Franzen, P. L., Buysse, D. J., Dahl, R. E., Thompson, W., & Siegle, G. J. (2009). Sleep deprivation alters pupillary reactivity to emotional stimuli in healthy young adults. *Biological Psychology, 80*(3), 300–305. doi:10.1016/j.biopsycho.2008.10.010

Gau, S. F., & Soong, W. T. (1999). Psychiatric comorbidity of adolescents with sleep terrors or sleepwalking: A case-control study. *Australian and New Zealand Journal of Psychiatry, 33*(5), 734–739. doi:10.1080/j.1440-1614.1999.00610.x

Ginsburg, G. S., Becker, E. M., Keeton, C. P., Sakolsky, D., Piacentini, J., Albano, A. M., . . . Kendall, P. C. (2014). Naturalistic follow-up of youths treated for pediatric anxiety disorders. *JAMA Psychiatry, 71*(3), 310–318. doi:10.1001/jamapsychiatry.2013.4186

Goldman-Mellor, S., Gregory, A. M., Caspi, A., Harrington, H., Parsons, M., Poulton, R., & Moffitt, T. E. (2014). Mental health antecedents of early midlife insomnia: Evidence from a four-decade longitudinal study. *Sleep, 37*(11), 1767–1775. doi:10.5665/sleep.4168

Graves, L. A., Heller, E. A., Pack, A. I., & Abel, T. (2003). Sleep deprivation selectively impairs memory consolidation for contextual fear conditioning. *Learning and Memory, 10*(3), 168–176. doi:10.1101/lm.48803

Gregory, A. M., Caspi, A., Eley, T. C., Moffitt, T. E., O'Connor, T. G., & Poulton, R. (2005). Prospective longitudinal associations between persistent sleep problems in childhood and anxiety and depression disorders in adulthood. *Journal of Abnormal Child Psychology, 33*(2), 157–163.

Gregory, A. M., Eley, T. C., O'Connor, T. G., & Plomin, R. (2004). Etiologies of associations between childhood sleep and behavioral problems in a large twin sample. *Journal of the American Academy of Child & Adolescent Psychiatry, 43*(6), 744–751. doi:10.1097/01.chi/0000122798.47863.a5

Gregory, A. M., & O'Connor, T. G. (2002). Sleep problems in childhood: A longitudinal study of developmental change and association with behavioral problems. *Journal of the American Academy of Child and Adolescent Psychiatry, 41*(8), 964–971. doi:10.1097/00004583-200208000-00015

Groch, S., Preiss, A., McMakin, D. L., Rasch, B., Walitza, S., Huber, R., & Wilhelm, I. (2017). Targeted reactivation during sleep differentially affects negative memories in socially anxious and healthy children and adolescents. *The Journal of Neuroscience, 37*(9), 2425–2434. doi:10.1523/JNEUROSCI.1912-16.2017

Hagewoud, R., Whitcomb, S. N., Heeringa, A. N., Havekes, R., Koolhaas, J. M., & Meerlo, P. (2010). A time for learning and a time for sleep: The effect of sleep deprivation on contextual fear conditioning at different times of the day. *Sleep, 33*(10), 1315–1322. doi:10.1093/sleep/33.10.1315

Hansen, B. H., Skirbekk, B., Oerbeck, B., Richter, J., & Kristensen, H. (2011). Comparison of sleep problems in children with anxiety and attention deficit/hyperactivity disorders. *European Child and Adolescent Psychiatry, 20*(6), 321–330. doi:10.1007/s00787-011-0179-z

Henin, A., & Warman, M. (1997). Therapy for youths with anxiety disorders: A second randomized clinical trial. *Journal of Consulting and Clinical Psychology, 65*(3), 366–380. doi:10.1037/0022-006X.65.3.366

Hiller, R. M., Lovato, N., Gradisar, M., Oliver, M., & Slater, A. (2014). Trying to fall asleep while catastrophising: What sleep-disordered adolescents think and feel. *Sleep Medicine, 15*(1), 96–103. doi:10.1016/j.sleep.2013.09.014

Hobson, J. A., & Pace-Schott, E. F. (2002). The cognitive neuroscience of sleep: Neuronal systems, consciousness and learning. *Nature Reviews Neuroscience, 3*(9), 679–693.

Horne, J. A. (1993). Human sleep, sleep loss and behaviour. Implications for the prefrontal cortex and psychiatric disorder. *British Journal of Psychiatry, 162*, 413–419.

Hudson, J. L., Gradisar, M., Gamble, A., Schniering, C. A., & Rebelo, I. (2009). The sleep patterns and problems of clinically anxious children. *Behaviour Research and Therapy, 47*(4), 339–344. doi:10.1016/j.brat.2009.01.006

Ivanenko, A., Barnes, M. E., Crabtree, V. M., & Gozal, D. (2004). Psychiatric symptoms in children with insomnia referred to a pediatric sleep medicine center. *Sleep Medicine, 5*(3), 253–259. doi:10.1016/j.sleep.2004.02.001

James, A., James, G., Cowdrey, F. A., Soler, A., & Choke, A. (2013). Cognitive behavioural therapy for anxiety disorders in children and adolescents. *Cochrane Database of Systematic Reviews* (6), Cd004690. doi:10.1002/14651858.CD004690.pub3

James, A., Soler, A., & Weatherall, R. (2005). Cognitive behavioural therapy for anxiety disorders in children and adolescents. *Cochrane Database of Systematic Reviews* (4), Cd004690. doi:10.1002/14651858.CD004690.pub2

Johnson, E. O., Roth, T., & Breslau, N. (2006). The association of insomnia with anxiety disorders and depression: Exploration of the direction of risk. *Journal of Psychiatric Research, 40*(8), 700–708. doi:10.1016/j.jpsychires.2006.07.008

Kelly, R. J., & El-Sheikh, M. (2014). Reciprocal relations between children's sleep and their adjustment over time. *Developmental Psychology, 50*(4), 1137–1147. doi:10.1037/a0034501

Kendall, P.C. (1994). Treating anxiety disorders in children: Results of a randomized clinical trial. *Journal of Consulting and Clinical Psychology, 62*(1), 100–110. doi:10.1037/0022-006X.62.1.100

Kendall, P. C., Flannery-Schroeder, E., Panichelli-Mindel, S. M., Southam-Gerow, M., Henin, A., & Warman, M. (1997). Therapy for youths with anxiety disorders: A second randomized clinical trial. *Journal of Consulting and Clinical Psychology, 65*, 366–380.

Kleim, B., Wilhelm, F. H., Temp, L., Margraf, J., Wiederhold, B. K., & Rasch, B. (2014). Sleep enhances exposure therapy. *Psychological Medicine, 44*(7), 1511–1519. doi:10.1017/S0033291713001748

Leahy, E., & Gradisar, M. (2012). Dismantling the bidirectional relationship between paediatric sleep and anxiety. *Clinical Psychologist, 16*(1), 44–56. doi:10.1111/j.1742-9552.2012.00039.x

Lopez, J., Hoffmann, R., & Armitage, R. (2010). Reduced sleep spindle activity in early-onset and elevated risk for depression. *Journal of The American Academy of Child & Adolescent Psychiatry, 49*(9), 934–943. doi:10.1016/j.jaac.2010.05.014

McMakin, D. L., & Alfano, C. A. (2015). Sleep and anxiety in late childhood and early adolescence. *Current Opinion Psychiatry, 28*(6), 483–489. doi:10.1097/yco.0000000000000204

McNamara, P., Auerbach, S., Johnson, P., Harris, E., & Doros, G. (2010). Impact of REM sleep on distortions of self-concept, mood and memory in depressed/anxious participants. *Journal of Affective Disorders, 122*(3), 198–207. doi:10.1016/j.jad.2009.06.030

Mesa, F., Beidel, D. C., & Bunnell, B. E. (2014). An examination of psychopathology and daily impairment in adolescents with social anxiety disorder. *PLoS One, 9*(4), e93668. doi:10.1371/journal.pone.0093668

Mikoteit, T., Brand, S., Beck, J., Perren, S., von Wyl, A., von Klitzing, K., … Hatzinger, M. (2013). Visually detected NREM Stage 2 sleep spindles in kindergarten children are associated with current and future emotional and behavioural characteristics. *Journal of Sleep Research, 22*(2), 129–136. doi:10.1111/j.1365-2869.2012.01058.x

Miller, M. A., Rothenberger, S. D., Hasler, B. P., Donofry, S. D., Wong, P. M., Manuck, S. B., Kamarck, T. W., Roecklein, K. A. (2015). Chronotype predicts positive affect rhythms measured by ecological momentary assessment. *Chronobiology International, 32*(3), 376–384. doi:10.3109/07420528.2014.983602

Mullin, B. C., Pyle, L., Haraden, D., Riederer, J., Brim, N., Kaplan, D., & Novins, D. (2017). A preliminary multimethod comparison of sleep among adolescents with and without generalized anxiety disorder. *Journal of Clinical Child and Adolescent Psychology, 46*(2), 198–210. doi:10.1080/15374416.2016.1220312

Nielsen, T. A., Laberge, L., Paquet, J., Tremblay, R. E., Vitaro, F., & Montplaisir, J. (2000). Development of disturbing dreams during adolescence and their relation to anxiety symptoms. *Sleep, 23*(6), 727–736.

Pace-Schott, E. F., Spencer, R. C., Vijayakumar, S., Ahmed, N. K., Verga, P. W., Orr, S. P., ... Milad, M. R. (2013). Extinction of conditioned fear is better learned and recalled in the morning than in the evening. *Journal of Psychiatric Research, 47*(11), 1776–1784. doi:10.1016/j.jpsychires.2013.07.027

Pace-Schott, E. F., Verga, P. W., Bennett, T. S., & Spencer, R. C. (2012). Sleep promotes consolidation and generalization of extinction learning in simulated exposure therapy for spider fear. *Journal of Psychiatric Research, 46*(8), 1036–1044. doi:10.1016/j.jpsychires.2012.04.015

Palmer, C. A., & Alfano, C. A. (2017). Sleep architecture relates to daytime affect and somatic complaints in clinically anxious but not healthy children. *Journal of Clinical Child and Adolescent Psychology, 46*(2), 175–187. doi:10.1080/15374416.2016.1188704

Palmer, C. A., Clementi, M., Meers, J. M., Alfano, C.A. (2018). Co-sleeping among school-aged anxious and non-anxious children: Associations with sleep variability and timing. *Journal of Abnormal Child Psychology, 46*(6), 1321–1332. doi:10.1007/s10802-017-0387-1

Patriquin, M. A., Mellman, T. A., Glaze, D. G., & Alfano, C. A. (2014). Polysomnographic sleep characteristics of generally-anxious and healthy children assessed in the home environment. *Journal of Affective Disorders, 161*, 79–83. doi:10.1016/j.jad.2014.02.037

Peterman, J. S., Carper, M. M., Elkins, R. M., Comer, J. S., Pincus, D. B., & Kendall, P. C. (2016). The effects of cognitive-behavioral therapy for youth anxiety on sleep problems. *Journal of Anxiety Disorders, 37*, 78–88. doi:10.1016/j.janxdis.2015.11.006

Reddy, R., Palmer, C. A., Jackson, C., Farris, S. G., & Alfano, C. A. (2017). Impact of sleep restriction versus idealized sleep on emotional experience, reactivity and regulation in healthy adolescents. *Journal of Sleep Research, 26*(4), 516–525. doi:10.1111/jsr.12484

Reynolds, K. C., & Alfano, C. A. (2016). Things that go bump in the night: Frequency and predictors of nightmares in anxious and nonanxious children. *Behavioral Sleep Medicine, 14*(4), 442–456. doi:10.1080/15402002.2015.1017099

Roberts, R. E., & Duong, H. T. (2017). Is there an association between short sleep duration and adolescent anxiety disorders? *Sleep Medicine, 30*, 82–87. doi:10.1016/j.sleep.2016.02.007

Roy-Byrne, P. P., Uhde, T. W., & Post, R. M. (1986). Effects of one night's sleep deprivation on mood and behavior in panic disorder. Patients with panic disorder compared with depressed patients and normal controls. *Archives of General Psychiatry, 43*(9), 895–899.

Saper, C. B., Cano, G., & Scammell, T. E. (2005). Homeostatic, circadian, and emotional regulation of sleep. *Journal of Comparative Neurology, 493*(1), 92–98. doi:10.1002/cne.20770

Schabus, M., Gruber, G., Parapatics, S., Sauter, C., Klösch, G., Anderer, P., ... Zeitlhofer, J. (2004). Sleep spindles and their significance for declarative memory consolidation. *Sleep, 27*(8), 1479–1485.

Schabus, M., Hödlmoser, K., Gruber, G., Sauter, C., Anderer, P., Klösch, G., ... Zeitlhofer, J. (2006). Sleep spindle-related activity in the human EEG and its relation to general cognitive and learning abilities. *European Journal of Neuroscience*, *23*(7), 1738–1746.

Schlarb, A. A., Liddle, C. C., & Hautzinger, M. (2011). JuSt – A multimodal program for treatment of insomnia in adolescents: A pilot study. *Nature and Science of Sleep*, *3*, 13–20. doi:10.2147/nss.s14493

Shanahan, L., Copeland, W. E., Angold, A., Bondy, C. L., & Costello, E. J. (2014). Sleep problems predict and are predicted by generalized anxiety/depression and oppositional defiant disorder. *Journal of the American Academy Child and Adolescent Psychiatry*, *53*(5), 550–558. doi:10.1016/j.jaac.2013.12.029

Siapas, A. G., & Wilson, M. A. (1998). Coordinated interactions between hippocampal ripples and cortical spindles during slow-wave sleep. *Neuron*, *21*(5), 1123–1128.

Silk, J. S., Vanderbilt-Adriance, E., Shaw, D. S., Forbes, E. E., Whalen, D. J., Ryan, N. D., & Dahl, R. E. (2007). Resilience among children and adolescents at risk for depression: Mediation and moderation across social and neurobiological context. *Development and Psychopathology*, *19*(3), 841–865. doi:10.1017/S0954579407000417

Silverman, W. K., Pina, A. A., & Viswesvaran, C. (2008). Evidence-based psychosocial treatments for phobic and anxiety disorders in children and adolescents. *Journal of Clinical Child and Adolescent Psychology*, *37*(1), 105–130. doi:10.1080/15374410701817907

Stein, M. A., Mendelsohn, J., Obermeyer, W. H., Amromin, J., & Benca, R. (2001). Sleep and behavior problems in school-aged children. *Pediatrics*, *107*(4), E60.

Stickgold, R., & Walker, M. P. (2005). Sleep and memory: The ongoing debate. *Sleep*, *28*(10), 1225–1227.

Talamini, L. M., Bringmann, L. F., de Boer, M., & Hofman, W. F. (2013). Sleeping worries away or worrying away sleep? Physiological evidence on sleep-emotion interactions. *PloS One*, *8*(5), e62480.

Talbot, L. S., McGlinchey, E. L., Kaplan, K. A., Dahl, R. E., & Harvey, A. G. (2010). Sleep deprivation in adolescents and adults: changes in affect. *Emotion*, *10*(6), 831–841. doi:10.1037/a0020138

Van Dongen, H. P., Baynard, M. D., Maislin, G., & Dinges, D. F. (2004). Systematic interindividual differences in neurobehavioral impairment from sleep loss: Evidence of trait-like differential vulnerability. *Sleep*, *27*(3), 423–433.

Van Dongen, H. P., & Belenky, G. (2009). Individual differences in vulnerability to sleep loss in the work environment. *Industrial Health*, *47*(5), 518–526.

Vecsey, C. G., Baillie, G. S., Jaganath, D., Havekes, R., Daniels, A., Wimmer, M., ...Abel, T. (2009). Sleep deprivation impairs cAMP signalling in the hippocampus. *Nature*, *461*(7267), 1122–1125. doi:10.1038/nature08488

Walker, M. P. (2009). Sleep-dependent memory processing. In R. Stickgold, & M. Walker (eds.), *The neuroscience of sleep* (pp. 230–240). San Diego: Elsevier Academic Press.

Walker, M. P., & van der Helm, E. (2009). Overnight therapy? The role of sleep in emotional brain processing. *Psychological Bulletin*, *135*(5), 731–748. doi:10.1037/a0016570

Walkup, J. T., Albano, A. M., Piacentini, J., Birmaher, B., Compton, S. N., Sherrill, J. T., ... Kendall, P. C. (2008). Cognitive behavioral therapy, sertraline, or a combination in childhood anxiety. *The New England Journal of Medicine*, *359*(26), 2753–2766. doi:10.1056/NEJMoa0804633

Wallace, M. L., McMakin, D. L., Tan, P. Z., Rosen, D., Forbes, E. E., Ladouceur, C. D., ... Silk, J. S. (2017). The role of day-to-day emotions, sleep, and social interactions in pediatric anxiety treatment. *Behaviour Research and Therapy*, *90*, 87–95. doi:10.1016/j.brat.2016.12.012

Weiner, C. L., Elkins, R., Pincus, D., & Comer, J. (2015). Anxiety sensitivity and sleep-related problems in anxious youth. *Journal of Anxiety Disorders*, *32*, 66–72. doi:10.1016/j.janxdis.2015.03.009

Wilhelm, I., Groch, S., Preiss, A., Walitza, S., & Huber, R. (2017). Widespread reduction in sleep spindle activity in socially anxious children and adolescents. *Journal of Psychiatric Research*, *88*, 47–55. doi:10.1016/j.jpsychires.2016.12.018

Zuj, D. V., Palmer, M. A., Hsu, C. K., Nicholson, E. L., Cushing, P. J., Gray, K. E., & Felmingham, K. L. (2016). Impaired fear extinction associated with PTSD increases with hours-since-waking. *Depression and Anxiety*, *33*(3), 203–210. doi:10.1002/da.22463

10 Transdiagnostic Approaches to the Treatment of Anxiety Disorders in Children and Adolescents

Jill M. Newby and Anna C. McKinnon

Introduction

Over the past three decades, multiple evidence-based cognitive behavioral therapy (CBT) protocols have been developed for the treatment of anxiety disorders in children and adolescents. Evidence indicates that CBT is a highly effective treatment for anxiety, with approximately 60 percent of children and adolescents recovering from their anxiety disorder after completing a course of CBT (James et al., 2015). Both disorder-specific and transdiagnostic treatment protocols have been evaluated. Using the disorder-specific treatment approach to CBT, disorder-specific CBT treatment protocols that have been developed to target a single disorder (e.g., social anxiety disorder) are used to treat the patient's principal anxiety disorder (i.e., the psychiatric disorder interfering most with the patient's life). Transdiagnostic CBT protocols, on the other hand, aim to treat multiple disorders and presenting problems within the one protocol by targeting the shared vulnerabilities, overlapping symptoms, and common cognitive (e.g., overestimating the probability and cost of feared outcomes), emotional, and behavioral (e.g., situational avoidance) maintaining processes that cut across diagnostic categories (McEvoy, Nathan, & Norton, 2009). Transdiagnostic CBT interventions offer an innovative and efficient treatment option for children and adolescents with anxiety disorders, and their comorbidities (e.g., depression).

This chapter provides an overview of recent innovations in transdiagnostic CBT interventions for anxiety disorders in children and adolescents aged 7 to 17 years delivered in face-to-face clinical settings. In this chapter, we define transdiagnostic treatments, summarize the main transdiagnostic CBT protocols for anxiety disorders in children and adolescents, and provide an overview of the evidence on the efficacy of these interventions, as well as predictors, moderators, and mediators of outcomes. Our review focuses primarily on the transdiagnostic treatment of separation anxiety disorder (SAD), generalized anxiety disorder (GAD), social anxiety disorder (SoAD), panic disorder and agoraphobia, and specific phobias and anxiety comorbid with depression, but not primary diagnoses of post-traumatic stress disorder (PTSD) or obsessive-compulsive disorder (OCD) as the majority of CBT protocols for PTSD and OCD follow the disorder-specific treatment approach (see those chapters in the PTSD and OCD sections of this volume).

Overview of the Issue – The Need for Innovation

The development of disorder-specific CBT protocols has led to significant advancements in the treatment of anxiety disorders across the lifespan. However, the ever-growing number of disorder-specific CBT manuals, and multiple evidence-based treatment manuals available for any one single diagnosis (e.g., social anxiety disorder), presents a major barrier to clinician training, and the dissemination of evidence-based CBT interventions. In addition, there are high rates of comorbidity among the anxiety disorders, and between anxiety disorders and other disorders (e.g., externalizing and mood disorders), with up to 80 percent of children presenting to an anxiety disorder treatment service fulfilling criteria for more than one anxiety disorder (Kendall, Brady, & Verduin, 2001). Disorder-specific treatments allow little flexibility to treat comorbid disorders, and clinicians sometimes perceive these treatment protocols as irrelevant to patients with complex and comorbid presentations.

Although there is controversy in the literature about whether disorder-specific or transdiagnostic treatments are most effective for treating anxiety disorders, transdiagnostic approaches have great potential to overcome some of the limitations of the disorder-specific approach (Ollendick, Fraire, & Spence, 2013). Designing treatments that enable clinicians to target shared vulnerability factors, overlapping symptoms, and similar maintenance processes across the anxiety disorders should allow the clinician to treat multiple disorders in one protocol, rather than treating multiple anxiety diagnoses concurrently or sequentially with separate diagnosis-specific treatment manuals. The ease of implementation is also critically important for dissemination and training, as it is much simpler to train clinicians and therapists in the delivery of one manual, rather than multiple disorder-specific treatment manuals or approaches.

Description of Transdiagnostic Interventions

Transdiagnostic interventions (also called "generic CBT" or "unified treatments") have been defined as those that "apply the same underlying treatment principles across mental disorders, without tailoring the protocol to specific diagnoses" (p. 21, McEvoy et al., 2009), and therefore operate outside the traditional diagnostic boundaries of the DSM or ICD. According to Sauer-Zavala and colleagues (Sauer-Zavala et al., 2017), there are three different types of transdiagnostic interventions:

1. *Universally applied therapeutic principles:* interventions that fall from one "school" of psychotherapy (e.g., CBT), and contain strategies that are universally applied to a broad range of psychopathology.
2. *Modular treatments:* a clinician chooses from a set of discrete strategies to target their patients' presenting problems, regardless of their diagnosis.

3. *Treatments that target shared mechanisms:* interventions that target shared mechanisms that play an important role in the development and maintenance of a range of diagnoses or diagnostic categories.

In this review, we outline examples of each of the different types of transdiagnostic CBT interventions (universally applied CBT principles, modular CBT, and CBT treatments that target shared mechanisms) that have been designed to target anxiety disorders, anxiety comorbid with depression, and anxiety comorbid with other disorders (e.g., traumatic stress and externalizing disorders).

Transdiagnostic CBT for anxiety disorders typically aims to help the child to: (1) recognize anxious feelings, thoughts, and bodily sensations; (2) identify thoughts in anxiety-provoking situations, and develop alternative more helpful or balanced thoughts; and (3) develop coping skills to manage anxiety (e.g., helpful self-talk, relaxation skills). Behavioral strategies aim to help the child to: (4) confront, rather than avoid, situations they are afraid of, so they can learn to cope with feared situations and reduce anxious behaviors (see James et al., 2015). (5) Across these interventions, parents tend to be involved in different ways. For example, treatment could directly involve the parent, or parents may be present for conjoint or separate sessions, or sometimes parents are co-therapists (James et al., 2015). Family components may include helping parents learn ways to help their anxious child, helping parents learn adaptive and helpful ways to respond to their child's anxieties, and helping them to manage their own anxieties. (6) CBT is adapted according to the age, with younger children thought to respond better to behavioral strategies, rather than cognitive therapy components, which require certain cognitive abilities such as the capacity to evaluate a thought, in order to be successfully applied to the child's experiences.

Transdiagnostic Treatments for Anxiety Disorders in Children and Adolescents

Table 10.1 presents an overview of the most well-researched transdiagnostic CBT protocols for anxiety disorders in children and adolescents, with examples from each of the three types of transdiagnostic therapies outlined previously.

Transdiagnostic Component-Based CBT for Anxiety Disorders (Universally Applied Therapeutic Principles)

Transdiagnostic Component-Based CBT (T-CBT) for anxiety disorders has been the most extensively evaluated of the transdiagnostic therapies for child and adolescent anxiety disorders. These protocols are sometimes called generic, universal, or component-based CBT, as they are designed to treat a range of heterogeneous anxiety disorders and deliver specific CBT "components" (e.g., cognitive restructuring) in sessions throughout treatment. T-CBT protocols have been developed for the

Table 10.1 *Examples of Currently Available Transdiagnostic Treatment Protocols for Anxiety Disorders in Children and Youth and Overview of Key Components*

Treatment Package	Diagnoses	Delivery Format (individual, group, parent/child)	Number and Duration of Sessions	Treatment Components and Skills	Flexibility to Tailor the Intervention	References
Cool Kids Program [T-CBT] (adapted from the Coping Cat and Coping Koala)	DSM-IV Primary Anxiety Disorder (including OCD), excluding PTSD and Selective Mutism. Children ages 7–16 years.	Group, with joint parent and child sessions, and one parent-only session	10-session (2 hr per session) group program with children ($n=5$–7 per group) with mixed anxiety disorder diagnoses.	Psychoeducation, identifying anxiety, cognitive restructuring, gradual exposure, child management skills, assertiveness, and social skills training. One therapist-assisted in vivo exposure, with homework practice for remaining graded exposures.	Session-by session content is fixed, with at least one exposure hierarchy individualized to child's primary problem.	(Hudson et al., 2009)
Coping Cat [T-CBT]	DSM-III Primary Anxiety Disorder (SAD, Avoidant Disorder, Over-Anxious Disorder), excluding Specific Phobias. Children ages 9–13 years.	Individual, with parent sessions	16 sessions; first 8 sessions involve psychoeducation and introducing basic concepts, and second 8 sessions involve practicing skills, using role plays and in vivo and imaginal exposures.	Identifying anxious feelings, and somatic reactions, identifying and changing unrealistic anxious thoughts, relaxation, graded exposure to feared situations, coping strategies. Role-play and real-life exposures, supplemented with homework assignments to practice skills.	Session-by session content is fixed in sessions 1–8, but graded exposure and practice is individualized to child's specific fears.	(Beidas, Benjamin, Puleo, Edmunds, & Kendall, 2010; Kendall, 1994)

Table 10.1 (cont.)

Treatment Package	Diagnoses	Delivery Format (individual, group, parent/child)	Number and Duration of Sessions	Treatment Components and Skills	Flexibility to Tailor the Intervention	References
Modular approach to therapy for children with anxiety, depression, trauma or conduct problems (MATCH-ADTC Protocol) [Modular]	Any DSM-IV Anxiety Disorder (including PTSD & OCD), depression, trauma, adjustment disorders, conduct problems.	Individual	Designed to be flexible in duration and length: in one study, youth received M=22 sessions (SD=15.6), with average treatment length of 192 days (Chorpita et al., 2017).	33 modules that correspond to CBT and parent-management reigning among evidence-based therapies for the problems of interest. For example, exposure, problem solving, time-out, cognitive restructuring.	Therapist focuses on the initial problem area identified to be most important based on standardized assessments and top problems assessment. Flow charts specify default sequence of modules, but if interference arises, the sequence is altered with other modules used to address the new problem or interfering issue.	(Chorpita et al., 2017; Chorpita, Taylor, Francis, Moffitt, & Austin, 2004; Weisz et al., 2012)
Unified Protocol for Adolescents (UP-A) [Mechanisms]	Any DSM-IV Primary Anxiety Disorder (including OCD and PTSD), with or without comorbid depression symptoms. Children ages 7–12 and families.	Individual	8–21 individual sessions, with three 40-minute parent sessions to teach key concepts.	5 required (understanding emotions and behaviors, emotion awareness, flexible thinking, emotion exposures, and relapse prevention), and 3 supplemental modules (motivation, safety, and parenting emotional adolescent).	Flexible number of treatment sessions and delivery of supplemental modules.	(Ehrenreich-May et al., 2017)

Emotion Detectives [Mechanisms]	Any DSM-IV Primary Anxiety Disorder (including OCD and PTSD), with or without comorbid depression symptoms. Children ages 7–12 and families.	Group	15 90-minute sessions (2–4 clinicians), together with concurrent parent group.	Emotion awareness (including nonjudgmental awareness), emotion regulation, and emotion exposures, identifying thinking and cognitive reappraisal/ flexible thinking, behavioral activation, relapse prevention. Parent sessions focus on teaching key skills, and three parenting skills of independence, consistency, and empathy.	Session content in fixed order and format, but implementation of strategies individualized to individual's fears and concerns.	(Bilek & Ehrenreich-May, 2012; Ehrenreich-May & Bilek, 2012)
Group behavioral activation and exposure therapy [Mechanisms]	Primary clinical or subclinical DSM-IV anxiety disorder (GAD, SOAD, SAD) or depressive disorder. Children ages 12–14.	Group	10 weekly, 60-minute sessions, supplemented with two individual sessions (45 minutes).	Psychoeducation, functional assessment, problem solving, approach-oriented decision making, behavioral activation, exposures, relapse prevention.	Session content is in fixed order and format. Group leaders have flexibility to extend the treatment up to 15 sessions to permit additional exposure practice.	(Chu et al., 2009; Chu et al., 2016)

Table 10.1 (cont.)

Treatment Package	Diagnoses	Delivery Format (individual, group, parent/child)	Number and Duration of Sessions	Treatment Components and Skills	Flexibility to Tailor the Intervention	References
Integrated behavioral therapy for anxiety and depression [Mechanisms]	Primary DSM-IV depressive or anxiety disorder (SAD, GAD, SoAD). Children ages 8–17 years.	Individual	8 sessions delivered over 12 weeks. For parents of school age children (8–12 years), parents are encouraged to attend the entire session. For adolescents (13–17 years), parents are encouraged to attend half the session.	Psychoeducation, relaxation, goal setting, problem solving, overcoming avoidance, behavioral activation, relapse prevention.	Session content is fixed order and format.	(Weersing, Brent, Rozenman, & et al., 2017)

Note. ADNOS = anxiety disorder not otherwise specified, GAD = generalized anxiety disorder, SAD = separation anxiety disorder, SoAD = social anxiety disorder, OCD = obsessive-compulsive disorder, PTSD = post-traumatic stress disorder, T-CBT = transdiagnostic "generic" cognitive behavioral therapy (CBT) protocol, Modular CBT = modular transdiagnostic therapy protocol, Mechanisms = transdiagnostic CBT protocol targeting shared mechanisms across diagnoses.

treatment of anxiety in children and adolescents from 7 to 17 years of age and can be delivered in either group or individual sessions. In these interventions, each week a different CBT component or strategy is delivered (e.g., exposure stepladders, thought challenging) to the child. Common examples include the Coping Cat Program (Kendall, 1994) and the Cool Kids Program (see Hudson et al., 2009). In research trials, the intervention comprises an initial structured diagnostic and clinical assessment, although outside of research trials it is not always feasible to conduct lengthy diagnostic assessments. The assessment is followed by treatment sessions that include psychoeducation about anxiety, cognitive therapy tailored to the developmental stage of the child or young person, anxiety management techniques, graded exposure therapy, and relapse prevention. In these protocols, treatment goals are determined collaboratively between the parents and child, and components are used to address the young person's primary fears and problems. For example, in the Cool Kids program it is typical that at least one exposure hierarchy needs is developed around the young person's primary problem. Some T-CBT protocols include parent management training sessions and components, whereas others only include components for the child or adolescent. Skills and content are modified according to the age of the child. For example, the Coping Cat manual developed by Kendall and colleagues is recommended for children aged 7 to 13, with a modified version available for 14–17-year-olds.

The design of component-based T-CBT treatments is advantageous in that they can be applied to a range of anxiety disorders, symptoms, and problems. Delivery of these manuals is relatively standardized, and containing a fixed order and format, which means that these manuals can be implemented by less skilled clinicians. However, all components are intended to be delivered, even if they are not relevant for the child, and the duration of the protocol is often limited (6 to 10 group sessions, or up to 18 individual sessions). As such, there is limited flexibility for tailoring the protocol to treat patients with extensive, chronic, or complex comorbidities and problems.

Modular Approach to Therapy to Target Anxiety, Depression, Trauma, and Conduct (Modular Design)

Modular therapy approaches address some of the limitations of T-CBT approaches through the development of flexible manuals that can be tailored to suit the clients presenting needs. The Modular Approach to Therapy for Children with Anxiety, Depression, Trauma, and Conduct Problems (MATCH-ADTC, or MATCH) developed by Chorpita, Weisz, and colleagues (Chorpita et al., 2004) is an example of a modular transdiagnostic CBT protocol. Unlike most T-CBT interventions, which target only anxiety disorders, and deliver treatment in relatively standardized and fixed-order format, the MATCH protocol comprises a set of 33 separate modules that can be used to target anxiety disorders, as well as depression, trauma, and behavioral issues (e.g., oppositional and conduct disorder). In the MATCH protocol, the clinician identifies the initial problem area that is most important, based on standardized assessment measures and clinical interview, and an assessment of the patient's most impairing problems.

Flowcharts for the initial problem area (e.g., anxiety) specify a sequence of recommended modules. However, module delivery can be flexibly adapted during treatment to address the changing needs and problems of the patient. If problems arise (e.g., comorbid condition, additional stressors) that interfere with the delivery of the default sequence of modules, the sequence of modules is changed to systematically address the new problems. For example, if treatment initially focuses on depression, but then disruptive behavior interferes with therapy, the clinician can use modules to help the parents manage the oppositional behaviors before turning back to the depression modules once the oppositional behaviors have resolved. The number of sessions and treatment duration is flexible to ensure that the protocol allows sufficient time and flexibility to address complex presentations. Modular protocols can be applied with high fidelity, and yet allow greater flexibility in their delivery.

Treatments That Target Shared Mechanisms

The third approach to transdiagnostic CBT has been to target specific shared mechanisms that perpetuate anxiety disorders (or anxiety and depression). There are three main examples of these interventions: (1) The Unified Protocol for adolescents (and the Emotion Detectives program developed for younger children), which targets emotion awareness, tolerance, regulation, and emotion-driven behaviors. (2) Group-based behavioral activation and exposure therapy for youth anxiety and depression, which specifically targets avoidance and withdrawal behaviors. (3) Integrated behavioral therapy, which also targets maladaptive behaviors, but a broader set of behaviors including problem solving deficits and social skills deficits. We will cover each briefly as follows.

The Unified Protocol (UP) for Adolescents and Emotion Detectives Program for Children

The UP for adolescents is the developmental adaptation of Barlow and colleagues' transdiagnostic Unified Protocol for emotional disorders in adults (Ellard et al., 2010). Ehrenreich and colleagues adapted the adult UP into a group-delivered treatment program for children (Emotion Detectives) (Ehrenreich-May & Bilek, 2012) and individual therapy for adolescents (Unified Protocol for the Transdiagnostic Treatment of Emotional Disorders in Adolescents, or UP-A) (see Ehrenreich-May et al., 2017). The UP-A and Emotion Detectives program differ to the T-CBT protocols described previously in that they treat anxiety and depression, rather than anxiety disorders alone. The premise of treatment is that emotional health problems in children and adolescents arise from deficits in emotion regulation, emotion awareness, and maladaptive emotion-driven behaviors. The core treatment targets of the protocol are to improve emotion awareness and emotion regulation skills, and reduce emotional avoidance, and therefore aim to improve anxiety and depressive symptoms by targeting these mechanisms (Ehrenreich-May et al., 2017). Similar to the adult UP, the UP-A is underscored by intervention principles including:

(1) increasing understanding and awareness of emotions and emotional experiences; (2) preventing emotional avoidance, and developing tolerance of distressing emotions through exposure to distressing emotions, and other avoided situations and internal and somatic cues; (3) increasing cognitive flexibility, and understanding the link between thoughts, emotions, and sensations; (4) challenging negative thoughts, focused around antecedent appraisals (those that occur before a distressing situation); and (5) identifying and modifying maladaptive emotion-driven behaviors through activation, exposure, and other exercises. The techniques are applied to a range of emotions, including anxiety, fear, sadness, guilt, shame, and anger, and facilitate improvements in emotion awareness and regulation, as well as the reduction of avoidance (Ehrenreich-May et al., 2017). The Emotion Detectives program is designed for younger children and is underscored by similar intervention principles and targets as the UP-A, but is delivered in group sessions, with the children and their parents actively involved in the treatment. Each session begins with both parents and children together to review the previous session content and homework. Parents and children then attend separate groups, before reuniting together at the end of the session.

Group-Based Behavioral Activation and Exposure Therapy for Youth Anxiety and Depression

Chu et al. (Chu et al., 2009) developed a transdiagnostic group-based behavioral activation and exposure therapy protocol that comprises 10 weekly, one-hour group sessions, supplemented with two individual sessions, and is designed to treat anxiety, depression, or both. This protocol has distilled the most effective elements of cognitive behavioral therapy and behavioral activation (BA) into the one protocol to treat the core processes underlying anxiety and depression: avoidance and low activity or activity withdrawal. The first five sessions involve psychoeducation, functional assessment, problem solving, graded exposures, and behavioral activation. The second five sessions comprise graded exposures or engagement activities. The advantage of this protocol is that it distills the most effective ingredients from larger and longer multicomponent evidence-based treatment manuals, which makes it particularly useful for less experienced therapists or settings where there is a shorter duration of sessions or number of sessions allowed.

Integrated Brief Behavioral Therapy for Anxiety and Depression

Weersing et al. (Weersing et al., 2008) developed a brief 8-session integrated behavioral therapy for children with anxiety and depression, to be delivered in primary care over a 12-week period. This intervention includes four educational and skill building sessions, three practice sessions, and a relapse prevention/termination session. The intervention comprises mostly behavioral (rather than cognitive) strategies and places a core emphasis on engagement in activities and use of relaxation and problem-solving skills to manage stress. Treatment sessions include psychoeducation, goal setting, relaxation and coping with negative emotions, problem-solving skills, overcoming avoidance, behavioral activation, and relapse prevention.

Evidence Base for the Transdiagnostic Approaches

We outline the evidence for the three types of transdiagnostic CBT interventions (component-based CBT, modular CBT, and mechanism-based CBT) in separate sections as follows.

Component-Based Transdiagnostic CBT Protocols

To date, most studies evaluating transdiagnostic CBT-based protocols have focused on component-based CBT, and there is now strong evidence from replicated RCTs and meta-analyses demonstrating they are efficacious. In a meta-analysis specifically focusing on T-CBT, Ewing et al. (2015) evaluated the findings of 20 RCTs comparing T-CBT interventions for anxiety disorders in children and adolescents to nonactive control groups (no treatment, waiting list), and employed a structured diagnostic interview to assess outcomes[1]. They found that in the completer sample, those receiving T-CBT were 9.15 times more likely to recover from anxiety disorders compared to control groups, and in the intent-to-treat sample, recovery from anxiety disorders was 3.99 times higher in the T-CBT group compared to controls. These results are in line with a Cochrane review of CBT for anxiety disorders in children and adolescents (James et al., 2015), in which remission from any anxiety diagnosis for CBT versus waiting list controls showed an odds ratio (OR) of 7.85, and a number needed to treat (NNT) of 6.0, without differences in outcome between individual, group, and family involvement.

Overall, the findings of these studies indicate that T-CBT is effective in improving the clinical severity of anxiety disorders and achieving recovery from anxiety disorder diagnoses compared to no treatment or waiting list control groups. In individual RCTs, T-CBT has been shown to be more effective than active control groups. For example, Hudson et al. (2009) found that T-CBT was significantly more effective than an active control condition (group support and attention), with remission from the principal anxiety disorder at 68.6 percent versus 45.5 percent in the control condition (Hudson et al., 2009). Finally, T-CBT has been shown to be more cost-effective than alternative psychological treatments, including brief solution focused therapy (Creswell et al., 2017).

What Is the Efficacy of Transdiagnostic CBT Compared to Disorder-Specific CBT Protocols?

In adults, RCTs have been conducted that show comparable efficacy across disorder-specific and transdiagnostic approaches, with potentially small effects in favor of the transdiagnostic approach, although more research is needed to compare the

---

[1] The review by Ewing et al. [1] did not include modular or mechanisms-based protocols and solely focused on group and individual based T-CBT protocols for anxiety disorders.

approaches for specific disorders, and compare their efficacy for primary *and* secondary disorders and comorbidities (Newby et al., 2015). In children, there is very little high-quality data from RCTs to be able to make any strong inferences about which of the two approaches is advantageous.

In a systematic review and meta-analysis of 55 studies evaluating CBT for anxiety disorders (transdiagnostic component-based T-CBT: $n=25$, and disorder-specific CBT: $n=33$), Reynolds et al. (2012) found that overall effect sizes (ESs) for disorder-specific CBT protocols were medium to large (between-groups ES at posttreatment = 0.77), whereas the transdiagnostic CBT programs had medium ESs (between-groups ES at posttreatment = 0.53). They concluded that disorder-specific CBT approaches appeared to have somewhat larger effects than transdiagnostic CBT. However, it is difficult to draw meaningful conclusions from these findings, as their results were not based on direct head-to-head comparisons using RCT designs. While trials of T-CBT have typically included children with a range of anxiety disorders, in practice, samples typically comprised children with GAD, SAD, or SoAD. In contrast, trials of disorder-specific CBT interventions typically recruited children with PTSD, SoAD, or OCD.

To our knowledge, only one RCT has directly compared face-to-face transdiagnostic versus disorder-specific CBT in children with anxiety disorders, and one RCT has compared the efficacy of the two approaches delivered via the internet (Spence et al., 2017). In the first study of face-to-face CBT, Schneider et al. (2013) compared component-based T-CBT versus disorder-specific CBT in 64 children with separation anxiety disorder (SAD). They found response rates (no SAD diagnosis) of 87.5 percent versus 82.1 percent at 4-week follow-up, and 83.3 percent for disorder-specific CBT versus 75 percent for T-CBT, respectively; these differences were not significant, but small effects favored the family-based disorder-specific CBT condition over the T-CBT intervention, although their T-CBT condition did not include parent components, which is not typical of the delivery of most T-CBT interventions. In a separate RCT evaluating internet-delivered CBT in 125 youth (aged 8–17 years) with social anxiety disorder (SoAD), Spence et al. (2017) found that both T-CBT and disorder-specific CBT had equivalent treatment effects; and that both CBT groups were superior to the wait-list control group. However, the majority of patients still retained their diagnosis, with response rates (no SoAD diagnosis) at posttreatment of 17.1 percent in the disorder-specific CBT group, and 20.6 percent in T-CBT groups, and 51.9 percent and 47.1 percent for the disorder-specific and T-CBT groups, respectively, at 6-month follow-up.

Component-based T-CBT for the anxiety disorders has been demonstrated to be efficacious in RCTs comparing waiting list, usual care, and active control groups, and is more cost-effective compared to alternative non-CBT treatments (James et al., 2015). Most studies have trialled T-CBT in samples comprised primarily of patients with GAD, SAD, and SoAD; therefore, the generalizability of these findings to samples with primary OCD and PTSD is unknown (see relevant chapters in this volume). The meta-analytic evidence that disorder-specific CBT protocols are superior to transdiagnostic CBT protocols is inconclusive, and RCTs are needed to compare T-CBT with disorder-specific CBT protocols to determine their relative efficacy for treating the most commonly included diagnoses (GAD, SAD, and SoAD). Given that most of the research on transdiagnostic treatments has focused on component-based treatments, it is currently not possible to generalize these results to modular protocols or mechanisms-based or process-driven transdiagnostic manuals, which arguably have designs that can be more flexibly adapted to complex presentations.

Modular Protocols

The MATCH protocol (Chorpita et al., 2004) has been evaluated in several large RCTs. Importantly, these trials have been conducted in clinical settings with severe and complex patients, and substantial diversity in terms of ethnicity, educational background, and socioeconomic status. In one study, Weisz et al. (2012) compared modular versus standardized psychotherapies in children with depression, anxiety, and conduct problems in an effectiveness trial in ten outpatient clinics in the United States ($n = 174$ youths, aged 7–13 years), and found that modular treatment (the MATCH protocol) produced faster improvement than usual care and standard treatment, and the sample in that group had fewer diagnoses (mean = 1.23 diagnoses) compared to children and adolescents receiving usual care (mean =1.86 diagnoses). In the most recent large-scale cluster randomized effectiveness trial, Chorpita et al. (2017) compared the MATCH protocol to community-based treatment ($n=138$ youths aged 5–15). Community-based treatment consisted of county-supported evidence-based treatments for externalizing disorders, trauma, and depression. Chorpita et al. (2017) found that children randomized to the MATCH condition improved faster than the community-based treatment, providing further evidence supporting the efficacy of transdiagnostic interventions over standardized evidence-based therapies (EBTs) for anxiety, depression, and conduct problems. In addition, a recent study showed that clinicians themselves rated the modular protocol as more acceptable than the standardized manualized treatments (e.g., the Coping Cat, an example of the component-based T-CBT protocols for anxiety disorders), and were more likely to use the MATCH protocol after the completion of the RCT. This provides preliminary evidence that modular approaches may be more acceptable to clinicians, and therefore be useful to encourage the provision of evidence-based therapies in routine clinical practice.

Interventions Targeting Shared Mechanisms

Unified Protocol

The UP-A has been evaluated in an initial multiple baseline trial with three adolescents (Ehrenreich-May, et al., 2009), and an open trial (Trosper, Buzzella, Bennett, & Enrenreich, 2009), which showed that adolescents who underwent the UP-A intervention experienced clinically significant reductions in their principal anxiety disorder diagnosis, secondary diagnoses, and subclinical symptoms of anxiety and depression. Following on from the open trial, the UP was evaluated in an RCT ($n=51$ adolescents aged 12–17 years) compared to a waiting list control group (WLC). Ehrenreich-May et al. (Ehrenreich-May et al., 2017) found that the UP for adolescents outperformed a WLC condition on clinician, parent-, and youth-self-report measures, including clinician-rated severity of the patient's principal anxiety disorder diagnosis (effect sizes ranging from 0.77 to 1.84). Notably, differences between the groups were larger for clinician-rated measures compared to self-report measures, in line with the findings from their open trial. Unfortunately, there was no information about diagnostic recovery in this study.

The Emotion Detectives Treatment Protocol (for children) has now been evaluated in an open trial (Bilek & Ehrenreich-May, 2012) with 22 children ages 7–12, with a principal anxiety disorder and varying depressive symptoms. The findings for the pre-to posttreatment changes on clinician-rated anxiety disorder severity were large ($d=1.38$), but child-rated anxiety ($d=0.47$) and parent-reported depressive symptoms ($d=0.54$) were more modest (there was no information about recovery rates).

Together, these studies provide preliminary but promising evidence for the UP-A and Emotion Detectives treatment protocols. Further research is needed to compare these interventions with active and usual care control groups, with longer-term follow-up periods to determine their efficacy and utility in treating anxiety disorders and depression in children and adolescents.

Group-Based Behavioral Activation and Exposure Therapy for Youth Anxiety and Depression

Group-based behavioral activation and exposure therapy has been evaluated in a pilot trial ($n=5$, aged 12–14) (Chu et al., 2009) and a wait-list control RCT ($n=35$, aged 12–14 years) (Chu et al., 2016) in a racially diverse sample of adolescents aged 12–14 years, with the intervention delivered in a school setting. In the RCT, Chu and colleagues found that the group behavioral activation treatment was associated with greater posttreatment remission compared to WL (57.1 percent versus 28.6 percent) and, interestingly, resulted in higher rates of remission from the patient's secondary diagnoses (70.6 percent versus 10 percent). However, symptom outcomes were not significantly different at posttreatment, most likely due to lack of power (the waiting list control group only had 14 participants). This protocol shows promise and awaits further in RCTs with larger samples.

Integrated Behavioral Therapy

Following on from case studies, a recently published RCT compared the brief integrated behavioral therapy compared to referral to an outpatient community mental health care team (Weersing et al., 2017). The study included children and adolescents aged 8–17 for SAD, GAD, social phobia, MDD, dysthymic disorder, or minor depression (n =185 youths aged 8–17 years). Interventions were delivered in pediatric clinics. The study showed that the integrated behavioral therapy group had higher rates of clinical improvement (56.8 percent versus 28.2 percent) compared to the community referral group, greater reductions in symptoms, and better functioning. These findings now await replication.

In summary, the findings across studies have generally found broad support for the three main types of transdiagnostic interventions. Across studies, recovery rates have ranged from 56 percent to 75 percent. This indicates there is still scope to improve current interventions. Specifically, work is still needed to understand the most important components of transdiagnostic CBT and the conditions predicting response and nonresponse to these interventions.

Predictors, Moderators, and Mediators of Change

Identifying predictors and moderators of treatment response is critical to identify the children and adolescents for whom CBT will work, or not work, based on their demographic, clinical, family, or genetic and neuropsychological profile. Understanding these factors aids clinical decision making and will assist in the development of more effective and targeted interventions for youth who currently show a poor response to CBT. The search for consistent predictors and moderators of treatment response to T-CBT has failed to find consistent predictors of response to transdiagnostic CBT protocols for childhood anxiety disorders (Nilsen, Eisemann, & Kvernmo, 2013). Most evidence suggests that demographic factors (e.g., age, gender, socioeconomic status, race/ethnicity) do not influence treatment response. However, the most replicated finding is that children with a primary social anxiety disorder diagnosis have poorer response to T-CBT than children with other primary diagnoses (mostly SAD and GAD) (Compton et al., 2014; Hudson, Keers et al., 2015; Hudson, Rapee et al., 2015; Wergeland et al., 2016), a finding not unlike that observed in standard CBT for specific diagnoses. Although children with social anxiety disorder improve during T-CBT interventions, they do not improve as much as children with other primary diagnoses. There is some preliminary evidence that baseline anxiety severity, the presence of comorbid depression and externalizing disorders (Liber et al., 2010), and parental psychopathology may predict poorer outcomes following T-CBT (Liber et al., 2010), although findings have been mixed across studies. The involvement of parents has also yielded mixed findings in the literature, with some studies suggesting parental involvement in treatment predicts better outcomes, but other studies failing to find a difference (James et al., 2015).

Mediators of Change

Despite the large number of efficacy studies of T-CBT, there is surprisingly limited research exploring the mechanisms of change of T-CBT. Identifying the mechanisms of change of an intervention helps to understand how or why an intervention works, and to identify the active treatment components that facilitate this positive change. There is some preliminary evidence that decreases in negative thoughts (Muris et al., 2009) and increase in anxiety control and coping efficacy (ability to manage anxiety-provoking situations) (Kendall et al., 2016) may mediate improvements in anxiety symptoms during CBT. However, there are more mixed findings in the literature regarding the role of reductions in anxious thoughts and increases in positive self-talk in mediating improvements in transdiagnostic CBT. The mediating role of other processes (e.g., improved emotion tolerance and regulation, reduced behavioral avoidance, or increased activity engagement) have not been studied.

Clinical Case Illustration

Carly (9 years) lives at home with her parents, Richard and Susan, and her older sister Samantha (11 years). Carly presents to the clinic displaying symptoms consistent with diagnoses of separation anxiety disorder (primary) comorbid with generalized anxiety disorder (secondary) according to the DSM-5. Carly first showed signs of having an inhibited and anxious temperament at 3 years of age. Carly struggles to separate from her mother at the school drop-off in the morning and while she will attend play dates, she is reluctant to stay away from home overnight. Her worries characteristic of generalized anxiety disorder can be triggered by changes in routine (e.g., being late), hearing scary things on the news, competence with school work, and making mistakes. Susan accompanies Carly to a number of anxiety-provoking situations, providing her with hugs and reassurance, and this assists Carly to feel safe.

Carly completes a component-based transdiagnostic CBT program to treat child anxiety, responding well to treatment. She learns cognitive restructuring to modify unhelpful thoughts that she is "unable to cope without her mother" and that "something bad will happen if there is a sudden change to routine." Carly also completes two stepladders during her treatment. In the first stepladder, to address her fears that she is unable to cope without her mother being present, the goal is for Carly to attend a sleepover on her own. To address her fears about the consequences of changes to routine, the goal of the second stepladder is for Carly to be picked up 1-hour late from school one day. Steps on the ladder include a range of tasks such as walking the dog on a different route, going shopping at a different supermarket, and doing the bedtime routine in a different order. Carly's safety behavior of needing her mother present during these situations was also incorporated into this stepladder. Carly's parents learn valuable skills to stop allowing Carly to avoid anxiety-provoking situations. They also reduce the amount of attention they pay to her anxious behavior and limit the amount of reassurance provided in anxiety-provoking situations.

Challenges and Recommendations for Future Research

Dissemination

There is now a great deal of evidence showing that transdiagnostic CBT interventions are effective for the treatment of children and adolescents with anxiety disorders. Given that only one in three children who meet criteria for anxiety disorders currently receives treatment, the major challenge over the next decade will be to develop cost-effective and accessible approaches to disseminate these transdiagnostic interventions that are known to work for children and youth with anxiety (James et al., 2015). One approach that has shown to be highly successful and effective in disseminating CBT to adults with emotional disorders is delivering CBT via the internet, with clinician guidance provided by telephone, email, and/or messages via secure platforms. The literature on internet and mobile-based CBT interventions is surprisingly limited given the large number of transdiagnostic treatment trials in adults and the benefits of engaging children with technology. However, there is preliminary evidence showing that transdiagnostic internet-delivered CBT interventions for children and adolescents achieve large effect sizes (Ebert et al., 2015). RCTs of internet-delivered CBT protocols will also enable researchers and clinicians to answer key questions about the most effective ingredients of transdiagnostic therapies, mechanisms of change, comparing different treatment formats and content, and comparing alternative types of psychological therapy that are impractical and cost prohibitive to answer in face-to-face trials (see related chapter on this issue in this volume).

Identifying Predictors of Treatment Response

Given the mixed results in the literature, and the general failure to detect consistent predictors of response to treatment, future studies will need to combine the results of multiple trials to examine predictors across studies and samples. In addition, many studies exclude severe and complex cases, for example suicidal youths, or those with PTSD or OCD from their samples – whether or not transdiagnostic interventions are also effective for these individuals needs to be tested. Future studies will likely benefit from identifying a risk index, aggregating data across multiple genetic, clinical and demographic risk factors to identify those who are less likely to respond to treatment (Hudson, Keers et al., 2015; Hudson et al., 2013). Finally, mechanisms-based research exploring whether specific cognitive, emotional abilities or emotional dysregulation are predictive of treatment response is needed.

Improving Existing Treatments to Improve Outcomes

The final challenge for clinicians and researchers will be to develop innovative treatments and new components to CBT interventions to improve outcomes for the 30 to 40 percent of children who do not recover fully following CBT, and to develop alternative psychological therapies (and combined therapies with pharmacological adjuncts) for those who do not respond at all to CBT. Despite their many benefits, there have been some concerns within the child field that transdiagnostic approaches may not be efficiently fulfilling the transdiagnostic mission. In fact, some leading researchers have argued for placing a greater focus on treating specific disorders (James et al., 2015; Ollendick et al., 2013). Given evidence showing there is very little difference in outcomes for transdiagnostic versus disorder-specific CBT for children and adults, this suggests that moving toward the disorder-specific approach may not deliver the magic solution to improve outcomes for the children who do not currently respond to CBT.

There is considerable scope to develop longer-term modular transdiagnostic treatments and treatments that target mechanisms that are known to maintain the anxiety disorders. For example, emotion regulation difficulties are thought to be important longitudinal predictors of internalizing symptoms in children (Kim-Spoon, Cicchetti, & Rogosch, 2013). However, these deficits are not currently targeted within most CBT interventions, except for the UP-A, which is a relatively brief intervention. In clinical practice, many clinicians use techniques from "third-wave" acceptance and mindfulness-based interventions with children, in combination with their CBT techniques to address these emotion regulation deficits in conjunction with anxiety. However, there is a lack of research showing that combining acceptance, distress tolerance, or mindfulness techniques improves the outcomes of CBT interventions; more research is needed to determine whether these newer treatment approaches deliver positive outcomes for children and youth, and exploring the developmental differences in children's abilities to understand and apply these tools to reduce their anxiety and distress. By beginning to expand standard CBT for child anxiety to include these components, using a flexible transdiagnostic manual design, the ability of clinicians to be able to use manuals with children that have more complex presentations and high comorbidity will be enhanced.

Key Practice Points

- There are three main types of transdiagnostic CBT interventions: generic or universal CBT protocols, modular protocols, and mechanisms-focused protocols.
- Transdiagnostic CBT interventions are effective for the treatment of children and adolescents with anxiety disorders relative to wait-list and active interventions.
- There is currently little evidence to suggest the superiority of disorder-specific CBT over T-CBT in the treatment of anxiety disorders in childhood. Future research is needed on this topic.
- The MATCH CBT modular protocol is currently the only treatment protocol designed to be used with children in need of long-term treatment for multiple comorbidities.
- Children with a primary social anxiety disorder diagnosis have a poorer response to T-CBT than children with other primary diagnoses.

References

Beidas, R. S., Benjamin, C. L., Puleo, C. M., Edmunds, J. M., & Kendall, P. C. (2010). Flexible applications of the Coping Cat Program for anxious youth. *Cognitive and Behavioral Practice, 17*(2), 142–153. doi:10.1016/j.cbpra.2009.11.002

Bilek, E. L., & Ehrenreich-May, J. (2012). An open trial investigation of a transdiagnostic group treatment for children with anxiety and depressive symptoms. *Behavior Therapy, 43*(4), 887–897. doi:http://dx.doi.org/10.1016/j.beth.2012.04.007

Chorpita, B. F., Daleiden, E. L., Park, A. L., Ward, A. M., Levy, M. C., Cromley, T., ... Krull, J. L. (2017). Child STEPs in California: A cluster randomized effectiveness trial comparing modular treatment with community implemented treatment for youth with anxiety, depression, conduct problems, or traumatic stress [Press release].

Chorpita, B. F., Taylor, A. A., Francis, S. E., Moffitt, C., & Austin, A. A. (2004). Efficacy of modular cognitive behavior therapy for childhood anxiety disorders. *Behavior Therapy, 35*(2), 263–287. doi:https://doi.org/10.1016/S0005-7894(04)80039-X

Chu, B. C., Colognori, D., Weissman, A. S., & Bannon, K. (2009). An initial description and pilot of group behavioral activation therapy for anxious and depressed youth. *Cognitive and Behavioral Practice, 16*(4), 408–419. doi:https://doi.org/10.1016/j.cbpra.2009.04.003

Chu, B. C., Crocco, S. T., Esseling, P., Areizaga, M. J., Lindner, A. M., & Skriner, L. C. (2016). Transdiagnostic group behavioral activation and exposure therapy for youth anxiety and depression: Initial randomized controlled trial. *Behaviour Research and Therapy, 76*, 65–75. doi:http://dx.doi.org/10.1016/j.brat.2015.11.005

Compton, S. N., Peris, T. S., Almirall, D., Birmaher, B., Sherrill, J., Kendall, P. C., ... Albano, A. M. (2014). Predictors and moderators of treatment response in childhood anxiety disorders: Results from the CAMS trial. *J Consult Clin Psychol, 82*(2), 212–224. doi:10.1037/a0035458

Creswell, C., Violato, M., Fairbanks, H., White, E., Parkinson, M., Abitabile, G., ... Cooper, P. J. (2017). Clinical outcomes and cost-effectiveness of brief guided parent-delivered cognitive behavioural therapy and solution-focused brief therapy for treatment of childhood anxiety disorders: A randomised controlled trial. *The Lancet Psychiatry, 4*(7), 529–539. doi:10.1016/S2215-0366(17)30149-9

Ebert, D. D., Zarski, A.-C., Christensen, H., Stikkelbroek, Y., Cuijpers, P., Berking, M., & Riper, H. (2015). Internet and computer-based cognitive behavioral therapy for anxiety and depression in youth: A meta-analysis of randomized controlled outcome trials. *PloS One, 10*(3), e0119895. doi:10.1371/journal.pone.0119895

Ehrenreich-May, J., & Bilek, E. L. (2012). The development of a transdiagnostic, cognitive behavioral group intervention for childhood anxiety disorders and co-occurring depression symptoms. *Cognitive and Behavioral Practice, 19*(1), 41–55. doi: https://doi.org/10.1016/j.cbpra.2011.02.003

Ehrenreich-May, J., Rosenfield, D., Queen, A. H., Kennedy, S. M., Remmes, C. S., & Barlow, D. H. (2017). An initial waitlist-controlled trial of the unified protocol for the treatment of emotional disorders in adolescents. *Journal of Anxiety Disorders, 46*, 46–55. doi:https://doi.org/10.1016/j.janxdis.2016.10.006

Ehrenreich, J. T., Goldstein, C. R., Wright, L. R., & Barlow, D. H. (2009). Development of a unified protocol for the treatment of emotional disorders in youth. *Child & Family Behavior Therapy, 31*(1), 20–37. doi:10.1080/07317100802701228

Ellard, K. K., Fairholme, C. P., Boisseau, C. L., Farchione, T. J., & Barlow, D. H. (2010). Unified protocol for the transdiagnostic treatment of emotional disorders: Protocol development and initial outcome data. *Cognitive and Behavioral Practice, 17*(1), 88–101. doi:http://dx.doi.org/10.1016/j.cbpra.2009.06.002

Ewing, D. L., Monsen, J. J., Thompson, E. J., Cartwright-Hatton, S., & Field, A. (2015). A meta-analysis of transdiagnostic cognitive behavioural therapy in the treatment of child and young person anxiety disorders. *Behavioural and Cognitive Psychotherapy, 43*(5), 562–577. doi:10.1017/S1352465813001094

Hudson, J. L., Keers, R., Roberts, S., Coleman, J. R. I., Breen, G., Arendt, K., . . . Eley, T. C. (2015). Clinical predictors of response to cognitive-behavioral therapy in pediatric anxiety disorders: The Genes for Treatment (GxT) study. *J Am Acad Child Adolesc Psychiatry, 54*(6), 454–463. doi:10.1016/j.jaac.2015.03.018

Hudson, J. L., Lester, K. J., Lewis, C. M., Tropeano, M., Creswell, C., Collier, D. A., . . . Eley, T. C. (2013). Predicting outcomes following cognitive behaviour therapy in child anxiety disorders: The influence of genetic, demographic and clinical information. *J Child Psychol Psychiatry, 54*(10), 1086–1094. doi:10.1111/jcpp.12092

Hudson, J. L., Rapee, R. M., Deveney, C., Schniering, C. A., Lyneham, H. J., & Bovopoulos, N. (2009). Cognitive-behavioral treatment versus an active control for children and adolescents with anxiety disorders: A randomized trial. *J Am Acad Child Adolesc Psychiatry, 48*(5), 533–544. doi:10.1097/CHI.0b013e31819c2401

Hudson, J. L., Rapee, R. M., Lyneham, H. J., McLellan, L. F., Wuthrich, V. M., & Schniering, C. A. (2015). Comparing outcomes for children with different anxiety disorders following cognitive behavioural therapy. *Behaviour Research and Therapy, 72,* 30–37. doi:http://dx.doi.org/10.1016/j.brat.2015.06.007

James, A., & Wells, A. (2002). Death beliefs, superstitious beliefs and health anxiety. *Br J Clin Psychol, 41*(Pt 1), 43–53.

James, A. C., James, G., Cowdrey, F. A., Soler, A., & Choke, A. (2015). Cognitive behavioural therapy for anxiety disorders in children and adolescents. *Cochrane Database of Systematic Reviews, John Wiley & Sons, Ltd(2).* doi:10.1002/14651858.CD004690.pub4

Kendall, P. C. (1994). Treating anxiety disorders in children: Results of a randomized clinical trial. *J Consult Clin Psychol, 62*(1), 100–110.

Kendall, P. C., Brady, E. U., & Verduin, T. L. (2001). Comorbidity in childhood anxiety disorders and treatment outcome. *J Am Acad Child Adolesc Psychiatry, 40*(7), 787–794. doi:10.1097/00004583-200107000-00013

Kendall, P. C., Cummings, C. M., Villabo, M. A., Narayanan, M. K., Treadwell, K., Birmaher, B., . . . Albano, A. M. (2016). Mediators of change in the Child/Adolescent Anxiety Multimodal Treatment Study. *J Consult Clin Psychol, 84*(1), 1–14. doi:10.1037/a0039773

Kim-Spoon, J., Cicchetti, D., & Rogosch, F. A. (2013). A longitudinal study of emotion regulation, emotion liability-negativity, and internalizing symptomatology in maltreated and nonmaltreated children. *Child Development, 84*(2), 512–527. doi:10.1111/j.1467-8624.2012.01857.x

Liber, J. M., van Widenfelt, B. M., van der Leeden, A. J. M., Goedhart, A. W., Utens, E. M. W. J., & Treffers, P. D. A. (2010). The relation of severity and comorbidity to treatment outcome with cognitive behavioral therapy for childhood anxiety disorders. *Journal of Abnormal Child Psychology, 38*(5), 683–694. doi:10.1007/s10802-010-9394-1

McEvoy, P. M., Nathan, P., & Norton, P. J. (2009). Efficacy of transdiagnostic treatments: A review of published outcome studies and future research directions. *Journal of Cognitive Psychotherapy, 23*(1), 20–33. doi:10.1891/0889–8391.23.1.20

Muris, P., Mayer, B., den Adel, M., Roos, T., & van Wamelen, J. (2009). Predictors of change following cognitive-behavioral treatment of children with anxiety problems: A preliminary investigation on negative automatic thoughts and anxiety control. *Child Psychiatry and Human Development, 40*(1), 139–151. doi:10.1007/s10578-008-0116-7

Newby, J. M., McKinnon, A., Kuyken, W., Gilbody, S., & Dalgleish, T. (2015). Systematic review and meta-analysis of transdiagnostic psychological treatments for anxiety and depressive disorders in adulthood. *Clinical Psychology Review, 40*(0), 91–110. doi:http://dx.doi.org/10.1016/j.cpr.2015.06.002

Nilsen, T. S., Eisemann, M., & Kvernmo, S. (2013). Predictors and moderators of outcome in child and adolescent anxiety and depression: A systematic review of psychological treatment studies. *Eur Child Adolesc Psychiatry, 22*(2), 69–87. doi:10.1007/s00787-012-0316-3

Ollendick, T. H., Fraire, M. G., & Spence, S. H. (2013). Transdiagnostic treatments: Issues and commentary. In J. Ehrenreich-May & B. C. Chu (eds.), *Transdiagnostic treatments for children and adolescents: Principles and practice*. New York: The Guilford Press.

Reynolds, S., Wilson, C., Austin, J., & Hooper, L. (2012). Effects of psychotherapy for anxiety in children and adolescents: A meta-analytic review. *Clin Psychol Rev, 32*(4), 251–262. doi:10.1016/j.cpr.2012.01.005

Sauer-Zavala, S., Gutner, C. A., Farchione, T. J., Boettcher, H. T., Bullis, J. R., & Barlow, D. H. (2017). Current definitions of "transdiagnostic" in treatment development: A search for consensus. *Behavior Therapy, 48*(1), 128–138. doi:https://doi.org/10.1016/j.beth.2016.09.004

Schneider, S., Blatter-Meunier, J., Herren, C., In-Albon, T., Adornetto, C., Meyer, A., & Lavallee, K. L. (2013). The efficacy of a family-based cognitive-behavioral treatment for separation anxiety disorder in children aged 8–13: A randomized comparison with a general anxiety program. *J Consult Clin Psychol, 81*(5), 932–940. doi:10.1037/a0032678

Spence, S. H., Donovan, C. L., March, S., Kenardy, J. A., & Hearn, C. S. (2017). Generic versus disorder specific cognitive behavior therapy for social anxiety disorder in youth: A randomized controlled trial using internet delivery. *Behaviour Research and Therapy, 90*, 41–57. doi:http://dx.doi.org/10.1016/j.brat.2016.12.003

Weersing, V., Brent, D. A., Rozenman, M. S., & et al. (2017). Brief behavioral therapy for pediatric anxiety and depression in primary care: A randomized clinical trial. *JAMA Psychiatry, 74*(6), 571–578. doi:10.1001/jamapsychiatry.2017.0429

Weersing, V. R., Gonzalez, A., Campo, J. V., & Lucas, A. N. (2008). Brief behavioral therapy for pediatric anxiety and depression: Piloting an integrated treatment approach. *Cognitive and Behavioral Practice, 15*(2), 126–139. doi:http://dx.doi.org/10.1016/j.cbpra.2007.10.001

Weisz, J. R., Chorpita, B. F., Palinkas, L. A., Schoenwald, S. K., Miranda, J., Bearman, S. K., ... Gibbons, R. D. (2012). Testing standard and modular designs for psychotherapy treating depression, anxiety, and conduct problems in youth: A randomized effectiveness trial. *Arch Gen Psychiatry, 69*(3), 274–282. doi:10.1001/archgenpsychiatry.2011.147

Wergeland, G. J. H., Fjermestad, K. W., Marin, C. E., Bjelland, I., Haugland, B. S. M., Silverman, W. K., ... Heiervang, E. R. (2016). Predictors of treatment outcome in an effectiveness trial of cognitive behavioral therapy for children with anxiety disorders. *Behaviour Research and Therapy, 76*, 1–12. doi:http://dx.doi.org/10.1016/j.brat.2015.11.001

11 Dissemination and Implementation of Evidence-Based Programs for the Prevention and Treatment of Childhood Anxiety

Satoko Sasagawa and Cecilia A. Essau

Introduction

Childhood anxiety is among the most prevalent and well-documented mental disorders (Merikangas et al., 2009). Intervention programs have been shown to be effective in ameliorating anxiety symptoms and disorders, as well as acquiring versatile psychosocial skills (Barrett et al., 2007; Essau et al., 2012), and children around the world are benefiting from these developments (https://www.friendsresilience.org/international/ upload; Sep 6). Clearly, anxiety intervention programs have much to offer to a wide range of populations, and the quest toward better controlling them is on its way to success.

However, there is a large gap between research in anxiety treatment and real-life settings. Even in countries where evidence-based practices are at their best, dissemination and implementation (DI) of these programs still remain a goal to be achieved. Estimates suggest that it takes as long as 17 years to turn merely 14 percent of original research to the benefit of patient care (Balas & Boren, 2000). Child and adolescent anxiety research shows that less than 20 percent of the affected adolescents receive the treatment they need (Essau, 2005; Merikangas et al., 2011). This percentage is shocking in light of the fact that recovery rates at follow-up, if treated properly, reach as high as 72 percent (In-Albon & Schneider, 2007). The best programs, however efficacious, are powerless if they cannot reach those who will likely benefit from them. As many theorists emphasize (e.g., Comer & Barlow, 2014), DI needs to be accomplished as an independent, high-priority task in order for empirically based practices to be influential. This chapter aims to review the current status of DI in the field of childhood anxiety, and to draw a roadmap toward the wider diffusion of anxiety treatment and prevention.

Implementation Framework

Implementation can be defined as the effort to integrate a program or practice within a particular setting (Fixsen et al., 2005). Be it at the system, community, organization, or individual level, the process of introducing change in a given context is full of challenges. It is now widely recognized that simply developing an evidence-based, effective program is not enough for the public to receive its full fruitage. Implementation components and outcomes exist quite independently of the quality of the program or practice being implemented (Fixsen et al., 2005), and the science of implementation is indispensable in systematically facilitating utilization of evidence (Tabak et al., 2013).

A logical approach in implementing a particular intervention is to identify the facilitators and barriers within the process. In the earliest years of DI research, Rogers (1995) provided an extensive analysis of factors influencing decisions to adopt a given innovation. Five factors were identified: relative advantage, compatibility, complexity, trialability, and observability. According to this model, in order for a diffusion process to be successful, the new method must be associated with better results, in line with the values, norms, and perceived needs of the adopter, simple to use, flexible to experiment with (i.e., to fit the contextual needs of the environment), and its outcomes must be relatively easy to identify. Rogers' work was influential in the development of subsequent theoretical models that comprehensively capture the research-to-practice translation efforts.

The Consolidated Framework for Implementation Research (CFIR) proposed by Damschroder et al. (2009) is one such example. Based on an extensive review of the literature, this model categorizes key constructs pertaining to implementation into 5 major domains. The first domain relates to the characteristic of the intervention being implemented. Many of the factors identified in Rogers' 1995 model such as relative advantage, adaptability, trialability, and complexity of the intervention can be categorized here. As for the concept of adaptability, Damschroder et al. (2009) additionally proposed an important distinction between "core components," or essential and indispensable elements of the intervention, and "adaptable periphery," which are elements, structures, or systems to be tailored to meet the needs of a particular setting. Core versus adaptable periphery components can be differentiated through component analysis, which will provide important information for fidelity assessment. Other influential intervention characteristics include evidence strength and quality, and cost of intervention (e.g., investment, supply, and opportunity costs).

Along with the characteristics of the intervention itself, the CFIR incorporates contextual factors (inner and outer setting), characteristics of the participating individuals, and implementation process. As for the contextual factors, outer setting is the economic, political, and social context within which an organization resides; external policies/ incentives and patient needs/resources can be categorized here. The inner setting includes features of structural, political, and cultural contexts through which the implementation process will proceed. Structural characteristics (e.g., size and maturity), culture, and implementation climate of the organization are examples of inner setting. Individual characteristics include knowledge and beliefs about the intervention, self-efficacy, and identification with the organization. Process variables are the planning, engaging, executing, and reflecting/evaluating of the intervention. Overall, the CFIR model provides a structure that incorporates the context of intervention and offers a pragmatic framework for approaching the complex, interacting, multilevel, and transient states of implementation (Damschroder et al., 2009).

Stages of Implementation

Implementation is often conceptualized as a "stage" process (Fixsen et al., 2005). Although models differ in how each phase is defined, they share the basic idea that factors likely to influence implementation efforts function differently according to which point in time the intervention is at.

The Exploration, Preparation, Implementation, Sustainment (EPIS) framework (Aarons et al., 2011) is an example of a model that divides the process of implementation into several phases. Developed specifically for public mental health and social services settings, it is comprised of four basic phases: *E*xploration, adoption decision/*P*reparation, active *I*mplementation, and *S*ustainment. In the exploration phase, the possibility of new approaches to provide services is considered. Thereafter, the pathway to this new approach is planned. Provision of the new service comes next, and the final step is to maintain the service over time. As in the CFIR, outer and inner contexts are assumed; however, the EPIS model proposes that various aspects of the outer and inner context have divergent levels of significance during each phase, and what factor is proportionately important changes in accordance (Aarons et al., 2011). For example, organizational characteristic (inner context) is theorized to be a significant factor throughout the implementation process. At the stage of exploration, the organization's absorptive capacity, readiness for change, and receptive context are cited as influential factors. In the adoption, decision, and preparation phase, organizational size, role specialization, and the existence of knowledge and skills within the organization are important characteristics that support adoption of innovations. Upon active implementation, the organization structure (e.g., whether the organization is centralized), priorities and goals, and readiness for change have significant effects. For the sustainment of an intervention, a leadership and organizational culture that values evidence-based practices is essential. Thus, the influential features of the organization change depending on the implementation phase.

A process model that subdivides the active implementation process into initial implementation and full implementation is proposed by Fixsen et al. (2009). In this model, the recursive nature of the implementation process is emphasized, and each stage is assumed to interact with each other. In addition, core implementation drivers are identified: staff selection, pre-service and in-service training, ongoing coaching and consultation, staff evaluation, decision support systems, facilitative administrative support, and systems intervention. The newest model as presented by the National Implementation Research Network (NIRN; http://nirn.fpg.unc.edu/learn-implementation/implementation-drivers; uploaded Aug. 8) has been modified to include the dimension of leadership drivers (i.e., the role of leadership in resolving technical and adaptive issues), but the basic idea of integration and compensation remains unchanged. The interactive process between each component is integrated to maximize their influence on staff behavior and organizational culture, and a weakness in one component is compensated for by the strengths in other components (Fixsen et al., 2009).

Research on the Implementation of Programs for the Prevention and Treatment of Childhood Anxiety Disorders

In contrast to the substantial advancement of theoretical models, only a limited number of implementation studies have been conducted in the area of childhood anxiety disorders. On the individual and organizational level, school settings have been reported the most frequently as the site of implementation for empirically based treatments (e.g., Beidas et al., 2012; Masia-Warner et al., 2013). A major theme of these studies is whether school mental health providers can implement CBT interventions to children with anxiety as competently as specialized psychologists. In efficacy trials, therapist characteristics are frequently treated as confounders and are either ignored (i.e., therapist characteristics are either completely ignored [=uncontrolled]) or controlled for (i.e., included within the analysis as extraneous variables [=controlled for]). However, individual characteristics are a significant component in numerous implementation models, and research focusing on the characteristics of the service providers enables effective implementation within the organization, as well as dissemination to other intervention settings.

In the Beidas, Mychailyszyn et al. study (2012), school mental health providers (e.g., school psychologists, guidance counselors) who were trained in CBT for child anxiety were assessed for individual- and organizational-level variables associated with implementation outcomes. Pretraining attitudes toward evidence-based practice were positively correlated with improvement in adherence as rated by structured role-play. No correlations were found between attitudinal variables and change in skills and knowledge, nor were there significant relationships between organizational variables and adherence, skills, or knowledge. These findings suggest that although pretraining attitudes, to an extent, influence post-training adherence levels, it is nevertheless possible for a wide range of mental health providers to receive training in childhood anxiety treatment and gain professional skills and knowledge.

Masia-Warner et al. (2013), using a similar research protocol, evaluated the treatment fidelity of school counselors who were trained to implement a group intervention program for social anxiety. Results of independent ratings showed that while adherence was generally high among the professionals, there was considerable variance in the levels of competence. Another finding of this study was that levels of competence differed depending on the treatment component being delivered; for example, exposure sessions were more competently implemented compared to social skills training sessions. Taken together, the results of these studies suggest that while schools are a promising outlet of empirically based intervention, a training system for service providers that accommodates to individual characteristics is needed for the effective implementation of these interventions.

Neither of the above studies examined directly the influence of provider characteristics on treatment efficacy. However, Podell et al. (2013), through an analysis of a relatively large sample of anxious adolescents, found that therapist factors did influence treatment gains; therapists who were more collaborative and empathic and who followed the treatment manual and implemented the treatment in a developmentally appropriate way yielded better child outcomes. From previous models of implementation, it can be inferred that such variables predictive of treatment outcome are augmented not only through direct training and coaching but by establishing organizational context such as facilitative administration and a decision support system (e.g., Fixsen et al., 2009).

A pioneering example of community and system level implementation research is a large-scale evidence-based services initiative in Hawaii. A detailed account of this state-wide project in identifying and implementing effective treatments for child and adolescent mental health concerns is given in Nakamura et al. (2014). The program does not solely target anxiety disorders but is designed to promote the use of evidence-based approaches in general by building and maintaining a service system for providers that helps with the decision-making process and provides feedback of the intervention. As a first step to make this possible, the Empirical Basis to Services (EBS) Task Force defined the concept of evidence-based practices within its system of care (Chorpita et al., 2002), and created a ranking system that groups similar treatments together and focuses on the specific elements that are used within each treatment. Based on the accumulated information, a system to assist decision-making and provide feedback was established. In this system, patient-specific treatment outcome data were evaluated, and if there was a lack of progress, summary reports were reviewed to select another evidence-based intervention, or the integrity of the intervention was questioned to examine whether each process of the intervention was validly carried out. As a basis for this evaluation, routinized objective measurement was introduced.

The relative proportion of youth earning an "acceptable" status (rated using scores of emotional and behavioral well-being, academic performance, personal well-being, community living, caregiver functioning, and satisfaction) improved to 93 percent upon the installment of this initiative. The success in this system implementation has led to the proposal of new quality improvement strategies. For example, a series of workshops to train core treatment elements in which practitioners can attend without charge has been convened. Further, the initiative is training supervisors and examining its impact directly on therapist skills. For the public, information regarding evidence-based practices is offered via an internet website (http://helpyourkeiki.com/) to increase consumer knowledge. Assessment and feedback systems for the service providers, government committees, and state officials are being established to better reach a wide array of stakeholders.

A more recent example of a large-scale implementation project is the Children and Young People's Improving Access to Psychological Therapies (CYP IAPT). The CYP IAPT is a program delivered by NHS England (https://www.england.nhs.uk/mentalhealth/cyp/ iapt/; upload; July 30) whose mission is to transform existing Child and Adolescent mental health services (CAMHS) so children or young people and their families have improved access to evidence-based psychological services. The program targets anxiety disorders, depression, conduct problems, self-harm, and eating disorders. Initiated in 2011, the project has worked with CAMHS covering 90 percent of the 0 to 19 years of age population up until March 2017, and aims for 100 percent coverage by 2018.

The three major components of the project are (1) establishing a training system for practitioners, supervisors, and service managers/leads, (2) collaborative practice of evidence-based psychotherapies using routine patient-reported outcomes, and (3) the transformation of all child and adolescent mental health services in England, linking research evidence, patient preferences and values, and clinician observations into an improved model of care delivery (Shafran et al., 2014). The implementation process is based on the aforementioned model by Fixsen et al. (2009). Specifically, a stage model is assumed, and the program is developed on the basis of the seven core implementation components identified (i.e., site and staff selection, preservice training, supervision and coaching, workplace supervision and performance evaluation, decision support data systems, facilitative administration, and systems intervention).

As for the first component, a selected number of staff members are trained in the IAPT approach and returned to their service of origin to act as purveyors in the implementation process. The training consists of a generic module emphasizing the importance of evidence-based practice, collaborative care, and routine outcomes monitoring, and modality-specific components. Initially, cognitive behavioral therapy for anxiety and depression, and behavioral parent training for conduct problems were chosen as specific treatment modalities of treatment. Thereafter, systemic family therapy for depression, self-harm, conduct disorder, and eating disorder was added, as well as interpersonal therapy for depression and anxiety, and counseling for a range of milder problems (Scott, 2017).

In regard to the second component, collaborative practice and shared decision-making is one of the main focuses of the CYP IAPT (Fonagy & Clark, 2015). In order to make this possible, session-by-session outcome monitoring is employed. Evaluating clinical progress systematically enables the accumulation of evidence as well as sharing of outcomes between the practitioner and the patient. An extensive guide is provided on how to use the standardized set of measures, and weekly supervision is held based on the results of this data analysis (Shafran et al., 2014).

The involvement of children and young people in service delivery, design, and promotion is an indispensable part of the third component. The program aims for attitudinal change on the part of the practitioners, who play the role of a facilitator with an expertise instead of being a dominant decision-maker. Children and young people take an active role not only in treatment but in shaping and modifying the system. An example of this might be providing feedback and participating in educational programs for practitioners. Taken together, CYP IAPT has been successful in changing the culture of CAMHS to be more collaborative, less medical in focus, and more systematic in evaluating outcomes, and is currently being integrated into a larger CAMHS transformation strategy called Future in Mind (McDougall, 2017).

Dissemination

Dissemination can be defined as the targeted distribution of information and intervention materials to a specific public health audience, with the intent to spread knowledge and achieve greater use of evidence-based interventions (American Psychological Association Task Force on Evidence-Based Practice for Children and Adolescents, 2008). Within the field of mental health sciences, dissemination can be conceptualized as the delivery into practice settings of those specific mental health treatment technologies that have been developed and tested successfully in research settings and contexts (Chorpita & Regan, 2009). Outlets of dissemination include journals, workshop and other means of professional training, conferences, and social media.

A primary issue in the dissemination of evidence-based practices is the gap between efficacy and effectiveness. Treatment protocols can show good to very good outcomes in a clinical trial but may not be translated well into a real-world setting (Glasgow et al., 2003). Comorbid disorders, practitioner training, treatment fidelity, and attitude toward the treatment on the part of both the therapist and the patient are some factors that may compromise the outcomes of a particular intervention (Ringle et al., 2015; Southam-Gerow et al., 2012).

Literature on adult anxiety disorders suggests that one specific barrier in disseminating CBT for anxiety is the use of exposure therapies (Gunter & Whittal, 2010). Exposure is an active component of CBT for anxiety in most treatments, but for the patients, this poses a challenge that can result in a temporary increase of symptoms. As a result, many therapists fear harming their clients and refrain from using this procedure, thereby denying them the chance to benefit from treatment altogether. In order to avoid such misapprehension, Gunter and Wittal (2010) suggest the use of didactic instruction, supervised practice administering, and peer consultation.

As an example of a study on supervision and consultation of child CBT, Gleacher et al. (2011) report a translation-based training and consultation model utilized in New York. In this model, a 3-day in-person training and a biweekly follow-up phone consultation for up to a year is provided. Attrition rates of the 639 professionals who participated in the program over a two-year period ranged from 27.6 to 29.4 percent, which is a reasonable figure, and satisfaction levels of the participants were high. The results of this study demonstrate that large-scale dissemination without a costly in-person consultation is possible; however, treatment fidelity remains an issue to be resolved.

Studies addressing the relationship between clinical training and treatment fidelity, although limited in number, have been conducted. For example, Beidas, Edmunds et al. (2012), through an evaluation of 115 community therapists who did not have prior training in CBT for anxiety, reported that while attending a brief workshop enhances knowledge of CBT for youth, its impact on treatment adherence and therapist skill was small. On the other hand, ongoing consultation after the completion of the workshop accounted for a significant increase in adherence and skills. These results suggest that while a brief continuing education workshop may not be sufficient alone to influence therapist behavior or transport empirically supported treatments to the community, a relatively limited dosage of consultation (i.e., a mean of 7.2 hours in this study) can be effective in increasing treatment fidelity. Another feature of Beidas, Edmunds et al. (2012) was that participants were randomly assigned to 3 treatment modalities, one of which was a computer-based, self-guided training, and consultation for all groups were provided via the internet or telephone. No significant effect of group was observed, suggesting that workshop training and consultation need not be in-person, but can be administered from a remote location.

Beidas et al. (2014) took this study a step further by examining the effects of inner contextual factors on therapist fidelity. Specifically, the 115 therapists who participated in Beidas, Edmunds et al. (2012) were measured for their attitude toward evidence based-practices, perception of intra-organizational characteristics, and clinician demographics. Interestingly, therapists with more experience showed less treatment adherence, and therapists who reported more positive organizational climates at their agency were more adherent to the treatment protocol.

The fact that more experience is predictive of lower adherence is understandable in light of the fact that many veteran clinicians show ingenuity in adapting standard treatment protocols to tailor to the needs of their clients, and/or to fit the demands of their service settings. This leads to the question of whether it is detrimental to compromise treatment fidelity, or whether the intervention has more to gain from adaptation to individual situations. McHugh et al. (2009), through a critical review of literature on fidelity and outcomes, propose the use of transdiagnostic and modular treatment approaches to achieve a balance between fidelity and flexibility. Transdiagnostic treatment protocol targets the core processes underlying disorders with similar clinical characteristics. The effect sizes for these treatments are high; a recent meta-analysis reported that children in the treatment condition were 9.15 times more likely to recover from their anxiety diagnosis than children in the control group (Ewing et al., 2015). Similarly, modular treatments consist of basic treatment components and add supplemental modules as needed, thereby maximizing flexibility in the order and inclusion of particular modules (e.g., Chorpita et al., 2013). Taken together, these approaches can work toward increasing compatibility and trialability as proposed early on by Rogers (1995), and better disseminating effective treatment procedures.

Impact and Pathways to Impact

A successful implementation of evidence-based interventions should lead to a wide range of impact. As defined by the Research Councils UK (RCUK), research impact is "'the demonstrable contribution that excellent research makes to society and the economy" (http://www.esrc.ac.uk/research/impact-toolkit/what-is-impact/; upload: July 27, 2017). Research can have academic, economic, and societal impact. Academic impact includes the way in which research contributes to our understanding and advancing scientific, theory, and treatment of childhood anxiety. Economic and societal impact includes the way in which research benefits children with anxiety disorders and their families who take care of them, organizations (e.g., school), and the society at large.

Academic Impact

Accumulative amounts of research have been made into childhood anxiety in recent years, producing significant academic impact. In a literature review that examined trends in publications on childhood anxiety disorders, Muris and Broeren (2009) reported a significant increase in the frequency of publications on childhood anxiety disorders between 1982 and 2006; many of these developments are illustrated in this volume.

Approximately 50 percent of the studies were related to the *phenomenology of childhood anxiety disorders*. Specifically, as reported in recent epidemiological studies, anxiety disorders occur commonly in children and adolescents, and significantly more girls than boys are affected by these disorders. Anxiety disorders are not only common, they also comorbid frequently with other psychiatric disorders such as depression. Although anxiety disorders are transitory phenomena in most children and adolescents (Last et al., 1997), in some young people anxiety disorders tend to be chronic and are associated with significant psychosocial impairment at adulthood (e.g., Essau et al., 2014; Kessler et al., 2005a).

Etiology of Anxiety Disorders: A wide range of factors have been identified as increasing the risk of children developing an anxiety disorder, including the genetic transmission of childhood anxiety disorders (Eley & Gregory, 2004), the temperament traits "neuroticism" and "behavioral inhibition" (Craske, 1997), environmental factors such as overprotective parental rearing behaviors (Rapee, 1997), insecure attachment relationship (Warren et al., 1997), direct and indirect learning experiences (King et al., 1998), negative life events (Tiet et al., 2001), and cognitive biases (Vasey & MacLeod, 2001).

Assessment: The review by Muris and Broeren (2009) also highlights the fact that numerous questionnaires and interview schedules have been developed to classify symptoms of anxiety disorders based on the current classification systems.

Intervention: Numerous treatment outcome studies have been conducted that examined the effectiveness of interventions for childhood anxiety disorders (e.g., Kendall, 1994). Of all the available psychological and biological interventions, cognitive behavioral therapy (CBT) has been regarded as the treatment of choice for childhood anxiety disorders. The review recommends the need to do more research on the mediators and moderators of treatment that could provide insight into how various interventions could be used more effectively.

Individual Impact

CBT has significant impact on the children with anxiety disorders, with between 50 and 70 percent of these children responding positively to CBT (Barrett et al., 1996, 2001; Essau et al., 2012; Kendall et al., 1997; Seligman & Ollendick, 2011; Stallard et al., 2007) with treatment gains lasting for several years for many youth and their families (Barrett et al., 2001). Specifically, these studies have shown significant reductions in children's self-reported anxiety and clinical diagnosis following treatment (Barrett et al., 1996; Flannery-Schroeder & Kendall, 2000; Spence et al., 2000). The decrease in anxiety symptoms is likely to translate into reductions in the proportion of children meeting criteria for an anxiety disorder. Studies have also shown that anxious children who participated in CBT treatment to show significant reduction in their depressive symptoms compared to children in the control group at post and follow-up period (Dadds et al., 1997; Essau et al., 2013; Jaycox et al., 1994). Participation in CBT also led to significant improvement in the use of adaptive coping strategies (i.e., less use of cognitive avoidance problem solving) (Mendlowitz et al., 1999), self-esteem, and less pessimistic future outlook (Barrett & Turner, 2001).

Political Impact

Perhaps the most important political impact of research in the use of CBT in childhood anxiety is the UK's National Institute of Clinical Excellence's recommendation (NICE; Baker & Kleijnen, 2000) to use CBT as the first treatment of choice for childhood anxiety. These NICE guidelines were created to facilitate training in, and use of, evidence-based treatments in clinical practice in the UK such as the CYP IAPT.

Economic Impact

An anxiety disorder with an early onset (e.g., childhood-onset) is associated with significant impairment in various domains of psychosocial functioning (e.g., educational underachievement; greater financial dependency and impairment in quality of life; Woodward & Fergusson, 2001), as well as general health, physical and cognitive functioning in adulthood (Essau et al., 2014; Feehan et al., 1993; Ferdinand & Verhulst,1995; Keller et al.,1992; Lewinsohn et al., 1998; Pine et al., 1998; Reinherz et al., 1993). It also predicted a two- to- three-fold increased risk for anxiety in adulthood (Mathew et al., 2011; Pine et al., 1998; Woodward & Fergusson, 2001).

Although there are no data on the economic costs of childhood anxiety, the long-term cost of an anxiety disorder that begins early in life is expected to have a substantial economic cost on the individuals and their families, as well as to the society, as a result of these psychosocial impairments. Thus, providing evidence-based treatment (i.e., CBT) should reduce the economic costs of childhood anxiety as it helps to reduce the negative consequences of anxiety disorders in adulthood.

Conclusion

Research on the dissemination and implementation of evidence-based programs for the prevention and treatment of childhood anxiety has only just begun. Much of what we know is either based on theoretical models that provide a broad framework for behavioral change or based on research in adult anxiety disorders. DI has a multitude of factors that affect the process, and systematic analysis is inclined to become complex, as mediating and moderating effects can exist between any combination of these factors. As Greenhalgh et al. (2004) note, "Context and 'confounders' lie at the very heart of the diffusion, dissemination, and implementation of complex innovations. They are not extraneous to the object of the study; they are an integral part of it" (p. 615). Nevertheless, accumulating DI research in the field of childhood anxiety disorders is imperative, given that dissemination of prevention efforts at a young age is much more cost-effective compared to treating adults already manifesting symptoms (Farrell & Barrett, 2007).

Developmental factors are an important aspect when pursuing DI of childhood anxiety treatments. Intervention needs to take into account not only present functional characteristics, but also consider the developmental trajectory of the child receiving treatment. Temporal factors need to be considered when measuring outcome variables, as well as contextual factors that influence response to treatment. In this sense, DI efforts need be a system with continuity, and not a one-shot scheme. Preceding studies proposing DI models provide a fundamental framework in building such a sustainable system.

A promising site of DI is the school context, owing to its high accessibility; there are data that 70 to 80 percent of children who receive mental health services receive them in school, and for many children, the school system provides their only form of mental health treatment (Burns et al., 1995). School psychologists, guidance counselors, and other school mental health professionals are prospective key providers of services for youth. However, it is now known that didactic training has limited effect in augmenting therapist skills, and supervision is essential in disseminating and implementing evidence-based practices with fidelity. Even under supervision, some evidence-based practices may prove too complex for universal dissemination, and specialty care in the treatment of psychological treatments is necessary (Comer & Barlow, 2014). A pragmatic approach to disseminate empirically based interventions within schools may be to focus on transdiagnostic and modular treatments, and at the same time establish a system of referral that can provide more specialized protocols when needed.

An interesting finding regarding schools and mental health services use is presented by Paul et al. (2008), who investigated the decision making of 14- to 16-year-olds in attending child and adolescent mental health services. Four-fifths of the participants responded that information regarding child and adolescent mental health services should be given to all young people instead of just those referred, and the way that was endorsed the most to get information across was information imparted in the schools. Thus, combining large-scale implementation schemes for clinical anxiety and individual/organizational level prevention efforts at schools can be a feasible solution in reaching out to the population in need of anxiety intervention. Use of internet and telecommunication is another means that can be explored, for providing both specialized care and supervision for prospective service providers.

References

Aarons, G. A., Hurlburt, M., & Horwitz, S. M. (2011). Advancing a conceptual model of evidence-based practice implementation in public service sectors. *Administration and Policy in Mental Health, 38*, 4–23.

American Psychological Association Task Force on Evidence-Based Practice for Children and Adolescents (2008). *Disseminating evidence-based practice for children and adolescents: A systems approach to enhancing care.* Washington, DC: American Psychological Association.

Baker, M., & Kleijnen, J. (2000). The drive towards evidence-based health care. In N. Rowland & S. Goss (eds.), *Evidence-based counseling and psychological therapies: Research and applications* (pp. 13–29). New York: Routledge.

Balas, E. A., & Boren, S. A. (2000). Managing clinical knowledge for health care improvement. In Bemmel, J., & McCray, A. (eds.), *Yearbook of Medical Informatics 2000: Patient-Centered Systems* (pp. 65–70). Stuttgart, Germany: Schattauer.

Barrett, P. M., Dadds, M. R., & Rapee, R. M. (1996). Family treatment of childhood anxiety: A controlled trial. *Journal of Consulting and Clinical Psychology, 64*, 333–342.

Barrett, P. M. & Turner, C. (2001). Prevention of anxiety symptoms in primary school children: Preliminary results from a universal school-based trial. *British Journal of Clinical Psychology, 40*, 399–410.

Barrett, P. M., Farrell, L. J., Ollendick, T. H., & Dadds, M. (2006). Long-term outcomes of an Australian universal prevention trial of anxiety and depression symptoms in children and youth: An evaluation of the FRIENDS program. *Journal of Clinical Child and Adolescent Psychology, 35*, 403–411.

Beidas, R. S., Edmunds, J. M., Marcus, S. C., & Kendall, P. C. (2012). Training and consultation to promote implementation of an empirically supported treatment: A randomized trial. *Psychiatric Services, 63*, 660–665.

Beidas, R. S., Edmunds, J., Ditty, M., Watkins, J., Walsh, L., Marcus, S., & Kendall, P. (2014). Are inner context factors related to implementation outcomes in cognitive-behavioral therapy for youth anxiety? *Administration and Policy in Mental Health and Mental Health Services Research, 41*, 788–799.

Beidas, R. S., Mychailyszyn, M. P., Edmunds, J. M., Khanna, M. S., Downey, M. M., & Kendall, P. C. (2012). Training school mental health providers to deliver cognitive-behavioral therapy. *School Mental Health, 4*, 197–206.

Burns, B. J., Costello, E. J., Angold, A., Tweed, D., Stangl, D., Farmer, E. M., & Erkanli, A. (1995). Children's mental health service use across service sectors. *Health Affairs, 14*, 147–159.

Chorpita, B. F., & Regan, J. (2009). Dissemination of effective mental health treatment procedures: Maximizing the return on a significant investment. *Behaviour Research and Therapy, 47*, 990–993.

Chorpita, B. F., Weisz, J. R., Daleiden, E. L., Schoenwald, S. K., Palinkas, L. A., Miranda, J., ... Research Network on Youth Mental Health. (2013). Long-term outcomes for the Child STEPs randomized effectiveness trial: A comparison of modular and standard treatment designs with usual care. *Journal of Consulting and Clinical Psychology, 81*, 999–1009.

Chorpita, B. F., Yim, L. M., Donkervoet, J. C., Arensdorf, A., Amundsen, M. J., McGee, C., Serrano, A., Yates, A., Burns, J. A., & Morelli, P. (2002). Toward large-scale implementation of empirically supported treatments for children: A review and observations by the Hawaii Empirical Basis to Services Task Force. *Clinical Psychology: Science and Practice, 9*, 165–190.

Comer, J. S., & Barlow, D. H. (2014). The occasional case against broad dissemination and implementation: Retaining a role for specialty care in the delivery of psychological treatments. *American Psychologist, 69*, 1–18.

Craske, M. G. (1997). Fear and anxiety in children and adolescents. *Bulletin of the Menninger Clinic, 61* (Suppl.A), A4–A36.

Dadds, M. R., Spence, S.H., Holland, D.E., Barrett, P.M., & Laurens, K.R. (1997). Prevention and early intervention for anxiety disorders: A controlled trial. *Journal of Consulting and Clinical Psychology, 65*, 627–635.

Damschroder, L. J., Aron, D. C., Keith, R. E., Kirsh, S. R., Alexander, J. A., & Lowery, J. C. (2009). Fostering implementation of health services research findings into practice: A consolidated framework for advancing implementation science. *Implementation Science, 4*, 50.

Eley, T. C., & Gregory, A. M. (2004). Behavioral genetics. In T. L. Morris & J. S. March (eds.), *Anxiety disorders in children and adolescents* (pp. 71–97). New York: Guilford.

Essau, C. A., Lewinsohn, P.M., Olaya, B., & Seeley, J.R. (2014). Anxiety disorders in adolescents and psychosocial outcomes at age 30. *Journal of Affective Disorders, 163*, 125–132. http://dx.doi.org/10.1016/j.jad.2013.12.033

Essau, C. A., & Ollendick, T. H. (2013). *The Super Skills for Life program*. University of Roehampton.

Essau, C. A. (2005). Frequency and patterns of mental health services utilization among adolescents with anxiety and depressive disorders. *Depression and Anxiety, 22*, 130–137.

Essau, C. A., Conradt, J., Sasagawa, S., & Ollendick, T. H. (2012). Prevention of anxiety symptoms in children: Results from a universal school-based trial. *Behavior Therapy, 43*, 450–464.

Ewing, D. L., Monsen, J. J., Thompson, E. J., Cartwright-Hatton, S., & Field, A. (2015). A meta-analysis of transdiagnostic cognitive behavioural therapy in the treatment of child and young person anxiety disorders. *Behavioural and Cognitive Psychotherapy, 43*, 562–577.

Farrell, L. J., & Barrett, P. M. (2007). Prevention of childhood emotional disorders: Reducing the burden of suffering associated with anxiety and depression. *Child and Adolescent Mental Health, 12*, 58–65.

Feehan, M., McGee, R., & Williams, S. M (1993). Mental health disorders from age 15 to age 18 years. *Journal of the American Academy of Child and Adolescent Psychiatry, 32*, 1118–1126.

Ferdinand, R. F. & Verhulst, F. C. (1995). Psychopathology from adolescence into young adulthood: An 8-year follow-up study. *American Journal of Psychiatry, 152*, 1586–1594.

Fixsen, D. L., Blase, K. A., Naoom, S. F., & Wallace, F. (2009). Core implementation components. *Research on Social Work Practice, 19*, 531–540.

Fixsen, D. L., Naoom, S. F., Blase, K. A., Friedman, R. M., & Wallace, F. (2005). *Implementation Research: A Synthesis of the Literature*. Tampa, FL: University of South Florida, Louis de la Parte Florida Mental Health Institute, The National Implementation Research Network (FMHI Publication #231).

Flannery-Schroeder, E. C., & Kendall, P. C. (2000). Group and individual cognitive behavioural treatments for youth with anxiety disorders: A randomized clinical trial. *Cognitive Therapy and Research, 24*, 251–278.

Fonagy, P., & Clark, D. M. (2015). Update on the Improving Access to Psychological Therapies programme in England: Commentary on ... Children and Young People's Improving Access to Psychological Therapies. *British Journal of Psychiatry Bulletin, 39*, 248–251.

Glasgow, R. E., Lichtenstein, E., & Marcus, A. C. (2003). Why don't we see more translation of health promotion research to practice? Rethinking the efficacy-to-effectiveness transition. *American Journal of Public Health, 93*, 1261–1267.

Gleacher, A. A., Nadeem, E., Moy, A. J., Whited, A. L., Albano, A. M., Radigan, M., Wang, R., Chassman, J., Myrhol-Clarke, B., & Hoagwood, K. E. (2011). Statewide CBT training for clinicians and supervisors treating youth: The New York State Evidence Based Treatment Dissemination Center. *Journal of Emotional and Behavioral Disorders, 19*, 182–192.

Greenhalgh, T., Robert, G., Macfarlane, F., Bate, P., & Kyriakidou, O. (2004). Diffusion of innovations in service organizations: Systematic review and recommendations. *The Milbank Quarterly, 82*, 581–629.

Gunter, R. W., & Whittal, M. L. (2010). Dissemination of cognitive-behavioral treatments for anxiety disorders: Overcoming barriers and improving patient access. *Clinical Psychology Review, 30*, 194–202.

In-Albon, T., & Schneider, S. (2007). Psychotherapy of childhood anxiety disorders: A meta-analysis. *Psychotherapy and Psychosomatics, 76*, 15–24.

Jaycox, L. H., Reivich, K. J., Gillham, J., & Seligman, M. E. (1994). Prevention of depressive symptoms in school children. *Behaviour Research and Therapy, 32*, 801–816.

Keller, M. B., Lavori, P. W., Wunder, J., Beardslee, W. R., Schwartz, C. E., & Roth, J. (1992). Chronic course of anxiety disorders in children and adolescents. *Journal of the American Academy of Child and Adolescent Psychiatry, 31*, 595–599.

Kendall, P. C., Flannery-Schroeder, E., Panichelli-Mindel, S. M., Southam-Gerow, M., Henin, A., & Warman, M. (1997). Therapy for youths with anxiety disorders: A second randomized clinical trial. *Journal of Consulting and Clinical Psychology, 65*, 366–380.

Kendall, P. C. (1994). Treating anxiety disorders in children: Results of a randomized clinical trial. *Journal of Consulting and Clinical Psychology, 62*, 100–110. doi:10.1037/0022-006X.62.1.100.

Kessler, R. C., Berglund, P., Demler, O., Jin, R., Merikangas, K. R., & Walters, E. E. (2005). Lifetime prevalence and age-of-onset distributions of DSM-IV disorders in the national comorbidity survey replication. *Archives of General Psychiatry, 62*, 593–602. doi:10.1001/archpsyc.62.6.593.

King, N. J., Gullone, E., & Ollendick, T. H. (1998). Etiology of childhood phobias: Current status of Rachman's three pathways theory. *Behaviour Research and Therapy, 36*, 297–309. doi: 10.1016/S0005-7967(98)00015-1.

Last, C. G., Hansen, C., & Franco, N. (1997). Anxious children in adulthood: A prospective study of adjustment. *Journal of the American Academy of Child and Adolescent Psychiatry, 36*, 645–652.

Lewinsohn, P. M., Rohde, P., & Seeley, J. R. (1998). Major depressive disorder in older adolescents: Prevalence, risk factors, and clinical implications. *Clinical Psychology: Science and Practice, 18*, 765–794.

Masia-Warner, C., Brice, C., Esseling, P. G., Stewart, C. E., Mufson, L., & Herzig, K. (2013). Consultants' perceptions of school counselors' ability to implement an empirically-based intervention for adolescent social anxiety disorder. *Administration and Policy in Mental Health, 40*, 541–554.

Mathew, A. R., Pettit, J.W., Lewinsohn, P. M., Seeley, J. R., & Roberts, R. E. (2011). Comorbidity between major depressive disorder and anxiety disorders: Shared etiology or direct causation? *Psychological Medicine, 41*, 2023–2034.

McDougall, T. (2017). CAMHS transformation: Modernising therapeutic interventions and outcomes. In T. McDougall (ed.), *Children and young people's mental health: Essentials for nurses and other professionals* (pp. 36–43). London: Routledge.

McHugh, R. K., Murray, H. W., & Barlow, D. H. (2009). Balancing fidelity and adaptation in the dissemination of empirically-supported treatments: The promise of transdiagnostic interventions. *Behaviour Research and Therapy, 47*, 946–953.

Mendlowitz, S., Manassis, K., Bradley, S., et al. (1999). Cognitive behavioral group treatments in childhood anxiety disorders: The role of parental involvement. *Journal of the American Academy of Child & Adolescent Psychiatry, 38*, 1223–1229. doi:10.1097/00004583–199910000-00010

Merikangas, K. R., He, J. P., Burstein, M., Swendsen, J., Avenevoli, S., Case, B., ... Olfson, M. (2011). Service utilization for lifetime mental disorders in U.S. adolescents: Results of the National Comorbidity Survey-Adolescent Supplement (NCS-A). *Journal of the American Academy of Child and Adolescent Psychiatry, 50*, 32–45.

Merikangas, K. R., Nakamura, E. F., & Kessler, R. C. (2009). Epidemiology of mental disorders in children and adolescents. *Dialogues in Clinical Neuroscience, 11*, 7–20.

Muris, P. & Broeren, S. (2009). Twenty-five years of research on childhood anxiety disorders: Publication trends between 1982 and 2006 and a selective review of the literature. *Journal of Child and Family Studies, 18*, 388–395.

Nakamura, B. J., Slavin, L., Shimabukuro, S., & Keir, S. (2014). Building and advancing an evidence-based service system in Hawaii. In Beidas, R. S., & Kendall, P. C. (eds.), *Dissemination and implementation of evidence-based practices in child and adolescent mental health* (pp. 204–219). New York: Oxford University Press.

Novins, D. K., Green, A. E., Legha, R. K., & Aarons, G. A. (2013). Dissemination and implementation of evidence-based practices for child and adolescent mental health: A systematic review. *Journal of the American Academy of Child and Adolescent Psychiatry, 52*, 1009–1025.

Paul, M., Berriman, J. A., & Evans, J. (2008). Would I attend Child and Adolescence Mental Health Services? Fourteen to sixteen year olds decide. *Child and Adolescent Mental Health, 13*, 19–25.

Pine, D. S., Cohen, P., Gurley, D., Brook, J., & Ma, Y. (1998). The risk for early-adulthood anxiety and depressive disorders in adolescents with anxiety and depressive disorders. *Archives of General Psychiatry, 55*, 56–64.

Podell, J. L., Kendall, P. C., Gosch, E. A., Compton, S. N., March, J. S., Albano, A., ... Piacenti, J. C. (2013). Therapist factors and outcomes in CBT for anxious youth. *Professional Psychology: Research and Practice, 44*, 89–98.

Rapee, R. M. (1997). Potential role of childrearing practices in the development of anxiety and depression. *Clinical Psychology Review, 17*, 47–67. doi:10.1016/S0272-7358(96)00040-2.

Reinherz, H. Z., Giaconia, R.M., Lefkowitz, E. S., Pakiz, B., & Frost, A. K. (1993). Prevalence of psychiatric disorders in a community population of older adolescents. *Journal of the American Academy of Child and Adolescent Psychiatry, 32*, 369–377.

Research Councils UK (RCUK) (http://www.esrc.ac.uk/research/impact-toolkit/what-is-impact/; upload: July 27, 2017).

Ringle, V. A., Read, K. L., Edmunds, J. M., Brodman, D. M., Kendall, P. C., Barg, F., & Beidas, R. S. (2015). Barriers to and facilitators in the implementation of cognitive-behavioral therapy for youth anxiety in the community. *Psychiatric Services, 66*, 938–945.

Rogers, E. M. (1995). *Diffusion of innovations* (4th edn.). New York: Free Press.

Scott, S. (2017). A national approach to improving child and adolescent mental health care: The children and young people's improving access to psychological therapies program in England. In Weisz, J. R., & Kazdin, A. E. (eds.), *Evidence-based psychotherapies for children and adolescents*, 3rd edn. (pp. 415–428). New York: Guilford Press.

Seligman, L. D., & Ollendick, T. H. (2011). Cognitive behavior therapy for anxiety disorders in children and adolescents. *Psychiatric Clinics of North America, 20*, 217–238.

Shafran, R., Fonagy, P., Pugh, K., & Myles, P. (2014). Transformation of mental health services for children and young people in England. In Beidas, R. S., & Kendall, P. C. (eds.), *Dissemination and implementation of evidence-based practices in child and adolescent mental health* (pp. 158–178). New York: Oxford University Press.

Southam-Gerow, M. A., Rodriguez, A., Chorpita, B. F., & Daleiden, E. L. (2012). Dissemination and implementation of evidence based treatments for youth: Challenges and recommendations. *Professional Psychology: Research and Practice, 43*, 527–534.

Spence, S. H., Donovan, C., & Brechman-Toussaint, M. (2000). The treatment of childhood social phobia: The effectiveness of a social skills training-based, cognitive behavioural intervention, with and without parental involvement. *Journal of Child Psychology and Psychiatry, 41*, 713–726.

Stallard, P., Simpson, N., Anderson, S., Hibbert, S., & Osborn, C. (2007). The FRIENDS Emotional Health Programme: Initial Findings from a School-Based Project. *Child and Adolescent Mental Health, 12*, 32–37.

Tabak, R. G., Khoong, E. C., Chambers, D., & Brownson, R. C. (2013). Models in dissemination and implementation research: Useful public tools in public health services and systems research. *Frontiers in Public Health Services and Systems Research, 2*, Article 8, 1–8.

Tiet, Q. Q., Bird, H. R., Hoven, C. W., Moore, R., Wu, P., Wicks, J., et al. (2001). Relationship between specific adverse life events and psychiatric disorders. *Journal of Abnormal Child Psychology, 29*, 153–164. doi:10.1023/A:1005288130494.

Vasey, M. W., & MacLeod, C. (2001). Information-processing factors in childhood anxiety: A review and developmental perspective. In M. W. Vasey & M. Dadds (eds.), *The developmental psychopathology of anxiety* (pp. 253–277). New York: Oxford University Press.

Warren, S. L., Huston, L., Egeland, B., & Sroufe, L. A. (1997). Child and adolescent anxiety disorders and early attachment. *Journal of the American Academy of Child and Adolescent Psychiatry, 36*, 637–644. doi:10.1097/00004583–199705000-00014.

Woodward, L. J., & Fergusson, D. M., 2001. Life course outcomes of young people with anxiety disorders in adolescence. *Journal of the American Academy of Child and Adolescent Psychiatry, 40*, 1086–1093.

12 Innovations in the Treatment of Childhood Anxiety Disorders

Mindfulness and Self-Compassion Approaches

Marija Maric, Christopher Willard, Maja Wrzesien, and Susan M. Bögels

Introduction

The Guest House

This being human is a guest house.
Every morning a new arrival.

A joy, a depression, a meanness,
some momentary awareness comes
As an unexpected visitor.

Welcome and entertain them all!
Even if they're a crowd of sorrows,
who violently sweep your house
empty of its furniture,
still treat each guest honorably.
He may be clearing you out
for some new delight.

The dark thought, the shame, the malice,
meet them at the door laughing,
and invite them in.

Be grateful for whoever comes,
because each has been sent
as a guide from beyond.

RUMI, translated by Coleman Barks

This poem by Rumi is probably one of the most cited poems in mindfulness trainings all over the world. It represents the core of mindfulness approach meaning welcoming daily hassles with acceptance, calmness, self-compassion, and gratefulness. Mindfulness as a therapeutic method has gained great popularity in the past few decades and has been implemented in adults suffering from a wide range of problems including chronic somatic and mental conditions, but also anxiety disorders. So, the question arises whether mindfulness would also be beneficial for childhood anxiety disorders (CADs).

In this chapter, we aim to explore the potential important role of mindfulness and self-compassion approaches in childhood anxiety disorder etiology and treatment. Given the fact that mindfulness has gained popularity in youth clinical practice, and given the promising results with mindfulness in adults with anxiety disorders (Hofmann et al., 2010), and the established associations between self-compassion and anxiety symptoms in adults (Kirby et al., 2017; MacBeth & Gumley, 2012), this approach seems appropriate for further inquiry. Thus, this chapter first explores the need for mindfulness in CAD and provides definitions of mindfulness and self-compassion. It then moves forward to the description of the approach including highlighting recent initiatives to train mindfulness and self-compassion in children with CAD. Further, we review the scarce evidence base and candidate moderators and mediators of mindfulness therapy in CAD and of self-compassion. A case is described demonstrating the application of mindfulness and its possible working mechanisms. As mentioned, scientific investigations of mindfulness in CAD are almost nonexistent so a large part of this chapter is based on theory and our clinical experience with anxious youth and mindfulness. In this chapter, we hope to provide clinicians with a guide for implementing mindfulness and self-compassion in CAD, and moreover, highlight areas for future research.

Overview of the Issue and the Need for Innovation

Over six decades of research into the efficacy of interventions for CADs have taught us that the most (cost-)effective treatment for CAD is cognitive behavioral therapy (CBT; e.g., Bodden et al., 2008; Hollon & Beck, 2013). Existing CBT protocols generally include elements of cognitive restructuring and exposure activities aimed at targeting common anxiety symptoms such as fearful cognitions and avoidance of anxiety-provoking situations, respectively (e.g., Barrett, 2005; Bögels, 2008; Kendall & Hedtke, 2006). Occasionally, other techniques such as progressive muscle relaxation and social skills training are also included in the protocols (e.g., Heyne et al., 2014). Moreover, involving the parents or family in CBT for CAD has been found to be beneficial only under certain conditions (Manassis et al., 2014; Maric, Van Steensel, & Bögels, 2015) and does not appear cost-effective (Bodden et al., 2008); thus, the conclusion is that child-focused CBT is overall the best we have to offer at this time.

However, the tremendous advances in CBT research have brought to light several gaps in our knowledge. First, while CBT is effective for most children, on average about one-third of children with anxiety disorders do not respond at posttreatment (Walkup et al., 2008) or at follow-up (range 2–19 years; Gibby, Casline, & Ginsburg, 2017). Although many of these children have benefited from the treatment in terms of reduced anxiety symptoms, they still meet criteria for either their primary or other secondary anxiety disorders. Second, children with social anxiety disorder have been found to benefit less well from CBT than children with other disorders (e.g., Hudson et al., 2015), and given that social anxiety disorder is among the most prevalent and in many ways the most debilitating of the anxiety disorders (Detweiler et al., 2014), interventions that specifically improve the effectiveness of CBT for children with social anxiety disorder are needed. And third, from a scientific perspective, an interesting question is whether there are novel theories and theoretical constructs that could help explain the etiology or maintenance of anxiety disorders in children. A long tradition exists in explaining the etiology of anxiety disorders in children and adults from a cognitive-behavioral perspective, which highlights the importance of negative cognitions, avoidance of challenging situations, physiological responses, and anxious feelings, while, at the same time, other, yet to be discovered phenomena, may also be involved in the emergence and/or maintenance of CAD, such as the role of attention and self-compassion (Van Bockstaele & Bögels, 2014).

Attention problems play an important role in most anxiety disorders. Examples include attentional bias toward ambiguous or threatening stimuli in social anxiety disorders or poor concentration in generalized anxiety disorders (Bögels & Mansell, 2004; Semple & Lee, 2008). As mindfulness is defined as an ability to pay attention in a specific way, and mindfulness trainings are targeting this mindful attention, this link between anxiety disorders and attention can be a direct rationale for implementing mindfulness with anxious individuals.

Mindfulness is defined by Kabat-Zinn (1982) as awareness that arises through paying attention in a specific way: (a) on purpose, (b) in the present moment, and (c) nonjudgmentally. In a therapeutic context, it is a mental state achieved by focusing one's awareness on the present moment, *while calmly acknowledging and accepting one's feelings, thoughts, bodily sensations, and action tendencies.* Mindfulness is a quality of attention that in some ways children are born with and therefore do not need to purposely practice: babies appear very much in the here and now of their experience. For example, when walking with a toddler to some place, we may notice how the child is very much in the here and now, stopping to pay purposeful attention to whatever catches his or her interest on the way: a flower, an animal, or a sound. The toddler will also likely not be busy with what happened before or what will happen next, or what time we need to be at our destination, but present in the current experience. The toddler will also pay attention nonjudgmentally; for example, a piece of garbage may be just as interesting as a flower. Of course, the toddler may judge, such as deciding that dog poop smells bad, or that the piece of garbage tastes bad; however, she/he will *postpone* judgment until she or he has experienced it. Further, the toddler does not need to practice "beginners mind" – a quality that is highly valued in mindfulness training, defined as opening oneself to an experience as if it were the very first experience. Zen Master Shunryu Suzuki said, "In the beginner's mind there are many possibilities. In the expert's mind there are few" (Suzuki, 2011). In fact, we parents and teachers teach children quite the opposite of being mindful: "Don't stop all the time or you will be late for school," "Yuck, don't eat that or you will be sick," and "Don't pick that flower or people will be angry at you." Similarly, when a child is expressing interest in playing the piano, we give her a piano teacher, and the teacher gives the child assignments and grades and diplomas for a certain performance, and this makes the child judgmental about his piano playing. Therefore, in many ways, it makes more sense to teach mindfulness to parents, teachers, and therapists than to children!

But, children grow up in an adult world that teaches them to meet our standards rather than developing their own standards (Bögels, 2017). We inadvertently provide them endless conditional love, rather than unconditional love messages, whereby the experience of living may lead to biased appraisals of themselves, the world, and their future, at the loss of their beginners' minds and mindful awareness. Many young children develop clinically significant anxiety (Cartwright-Hatton, McNicol, & Doubleday, 2006), and as such, mindfulness training may help them deal with such anxieties and fears.

Description of the Approach and Assessment Phase

The mindfulness-based approach to treating children with anxiety disorders can take a number of forms, depending on the child, their specific diagnosis, age, their level of engagement and functioning, and existing support already in place. The primary goals of treatment include helping the child and system recognize triggers for anxiety and identify skills to use in those situations, while simultaneously working to reduce heightened physiological arousal. In the case illustration later, we describe a somewhat ideal scenario of a case; here, we will first offer some thoughts on how a mindfulness training for CAD could be shaped.

The most effective mindfulness-based therapy should begin with interviewing not only the child but also the parents/caregivers. This includes collecting data from the child and family including developmental and family history, as well as the course of the anxiety and past treatments. Because mindfulness should be practiced every day and become an integral part of the daily life, identifying symptoms and triggers of anxiety offers clinicians insight into the best ways and times to help the child integrate mindfulness skills into daily life and anxiety-provoking situations. Mindfulness-specific measures that can be used in this initial phase to assess the levels of mindfulness and self-compassion include, for example, Mindful Attention Awareness Scale for Adolescents (Brown et al., 2011) and Self-Compassion Scale (Neff, 2003). Engaging caregivers and educators will reinforce practice and progress in the child and their level of involvement will likely lead to more optimal outcomes. For families and children that might not understand anxiety or mental health issues, some basic psychoeducation by the clinician will help.

Once anxiety as a disorder and its unique course in the child is more fully understood by the child and caregivers, teaching of mindfulness practices can begin. Sessions can be with the child and caregivers together, or may involve caregivers joining in at the end of each session or at some of the sessions, or may involve separate sessions with caregivers, or without caregivers, depending on the child's age and the family's comfort and needs. To keep children engaged, mindfulness practices can be interwoven with other therapeutic activities as well.

Mindful Systems: Involving Caregivers, Teachers, and Clinicians

While the goal of a mindfulness-based treatment might be a child practicing mindfulness on his or her own to regulate anxiety and avoidance independently, the reality is that children, anxious children in particular, likely need significant clinician and systemic support and reinforcement toward that goal (Willard, 2016). A mindfulness-based approach thus may include working with caregivers, parents, clinicians, educators, and other relevant adults to help children recognize and understand the triggers of anxiety, and reinforce using mindfulness skills. This means in-session practice of mindfulness exercises, as well as out-of-session practices. This includes careful consideration with the child and system on when and how to practice mindfulness regularly, so that the exercises become readily accessible in the more challenging or triggering moments.

Following the results from research into CBT for child anxiety disorders more broadly, one could argue that given the lack of evidence that involving parents is beneficial it might be best to deliver mindfulness to the child alone. However, our experience is that the mindful parenting approach as developed by Bögels and her team (Bögels et al., 2014; Bögels, Lehtonen, & Restifo, 2010) is not primarily focused on helping the parents help their child, as is typical for parental involvement in CBT for children with anxiety disorders in general, but in developing mindfulness in the parents themselves. Children who suffer from severe anxiety disorders can have enormous impact on their families. For example, they may refuse to go to school, do not have a social life, constantly ask their parents for reassurance, force their parents to stay home, sleep in their parents' bed, or express that they do not want to live anymore. Parents often think that they have caused or, in the least, maintain their child's level of anxiety (or we therapists make them think that!), and feel guilty as a result. Parents suffer from high stress levels if their children have severe anxiety disorders, and their stress gets in the way of approaching their child mindfully, with beginner's mind. "Oh no, not again" they may think when their child refuses to go to school because of a test that day, rather than approaching the situation with an open mind. Parents who participate in a mindful parenting group training, either parallel to their children's mindfulness group training (Bögels et al., 2008; Van der Oord, Bögels, & Peijnenburg, 2012; Van de Weijer-Bergsma et al., 2012), or as a stand-alone training (Bögels & Restifo, 2014), learn to meditate in order to become aware of their own stress and their own cognitive, emotional, and behavioral responses toward the anxiety problem of their child, and how their child's anxiety may trigger their own anxiety. They learn to become more aware of what their child, they themselves, and their combined interactions need when the child and/or they themselves have high anxiety levels. Rather than responding automatically when their child is anxious, they learn to take a breathing space so that they open themselves to more possibilities of responding. Because of their own mindfulness practice, they become a model for their child in how to apply mindfulness skills in stressful situations, and they are in a better position to guide their child's mindfulness practice.

Clinicians can pay particular attention to which practices the child finds most helpful and the most fun, both of which will motivate further practice outside of the clinical hour. This phase may also involve practice through "symptom activation" and response prevention, such as discussing and visualizing moments of minor anxiety, then using mindfulness or breathing practices to regulate arousal. This can be augmented by systemic support and reinforcement. Perhaps the child can practice with family members or teachers in integrating mindfulness into their regular school day. The caregivers are regularly brought in, for example at the end of sessions, and the child is encouraged to teach the caregiver mindfulness practices and all together identify times to practice outside of treatment. The last stage of mindfulness treatment focuses on the child practicing and utilizing mindfulness skills independently and applying the practices proactively in situations of anticipated anxiety, as well as responsively when anxiety strikes.

Examples of Existing Mindfulness Programs for CAD

When integrating mindfulness into treatment for anxiety, we can bring mindfulness into a range of existing therapy models, although a lightly structured cognitive behavioral approach appears to have the strongest research support and theoretical rationale. To our knowledge, three different mindfulness programs for childhood anxiety exist. Manualized approach like Randye Semples' *Mindfulness Based Cognitive Therapy for Anxious Children* (MBCT-C) has gained considerable recognition in the recent years. It was developed for the population of children 9 through 12, although, as described on page 274, it was also implemented with younger children aged 7 to 8. Concepts and techniques for the program (Semple and colleagues, 2005; 2010) were adapted from two adult programs: Mindfulness-Based Stress Reduction (Kabat-Zinn, 1990) and Mindfulness-Based Cognitive Therapy (Segal et al., 2002). The training consisted of 6 weekly 45-minute sessions and was developed to train the children's attention by focusing on bodily sensations and perceptions. Mindfulness was integrated into breathing exercises, walking, and sensory experiences. The emphasis was on learning through experience (instead of information or theory), describing experiences and not labeling or judging them. Both in-session instructions and exercises were offered, as well as homework activities. Developmentally sensitive adaptations of the training included shorter sessions (i.e., 45 minutes), briefer, more repetitious activities, and smaller groups (up to 8 children) as opposed to adult mindfulness training, which typically involves 8 2-hr weekly group sessions with 9–15 clients. Further, group interactions in MBCT-C included games and physical activities. Parents of MBCT-C members are invited to engage in the training in the following ways: (a) psychoeducation about mindfulness; (b) attending to therapist-conducted mindfulness sessions; (c) learning about different mindfulness exercises; (d) participating in homework activities of the children; and (e) participating in post-training qualitative interviews on the merits of mindfulness.

Our group utilizes two different programs in our everyday clinical practice. The first one is an 8 weekly 2 hr session group program (with one booster session 8 weeks post-training) used at our clinic – UvA minds – to teach mindfulness skills to adolescents with internalizing problems. The aim is to teach participants to deal with the feelings of stress, somberness, and failure. The program is also directed toward teaching adolescents to cope with difficult and worrisome thoughts, and learning how to relax, sleep, and concentrate better. Each session consists of 30 minutes of Mindful and Active Physical Exercises (outdoor), 30 minutes of Yoga Exercises, and 60 minutes of practicing Mindfulness Exercises such as body scan, breathing exercises, and walk meditation. The adolescents learn to know their inner world, their thoughts, feelings, and bodily symptoms, and learn strategies of how to engage in difficult feelings and thoughts (e.g., treat thoughts as passing events in the mind, and not accurate representations of the reality). ABC (thoughts-feelings-behaviors) schemes, but also writing exercises (write for 5 minutes everything that comes into your mind) are implemented to make adolescents aware of their difficult thoughts. Homework includes 20 minutes daily practice of physical exercise, yoga, and mindfulness. As part of the standard procedure the clients are asked to fill in assessments pre- and post-training, and at 8 weeks follow-up. Assessments generally include measurements of psychopathology (Youth Self-Report; Achenbach et al., 2008), mindful attention (Mindful Attention Awareness Scale; Brown et al., 2011), self-compassion (Self-Compassion Scale; Neff, 2003), general satisfaction (Subjective Happiness Scale; Lyubomirsky & Lepper, 1999), and sleep (The Chronic Sleep Reduction Questionnaire; Dewald et al., 2012).

The second approach is one that can be used to help (anxious) children, adolescents, parents, and school personnel learn how to embody and share mindfulness skills (Willard, 2014; 2016). Materials offer a broad range of exercises that can be used with anxious youth and their families, and tips on how to best implement them in day-to-day activities. (See Table 12.1.)

What becomes clear after reviewing these approaches is that mindfulness techniques are easily combined with cognitive behavioral and other systemic approaches. In Table 12.1, we present the most commonly used mindfulness exercises in children and adolescents with anxiety symptoms or disorders. It is not that other types of mindfulness exercises cannot be found effective in fighting anxiety; it is that for these exercises some rationale exists about why they would be helpful in anxious children, and that we have experience in using them with anxious youth. The reader should be aware that this list emerged as a result of theoretical reviews and our clinical experience with mindfulness and anxious youth; so far, no research has been done on the most helpful ingredients of mindfulness treatment for youth anxiety disorders.

Self-Compassion for Children with Anxiety Disorders

Self-compassion is often considered as an integral part of mindfulness interventions. For instance, adopting a nonjudgmental and friendly attitude toward our experience, or kindness and compassion of the trainer can be seen as examples of self-compassion approaches within mindfulness trainings. According to Germer and Neff (2014, p. 48), "A common healing element found in both mindfulness and self-compassion is the gradual shift from resistance to friendship with emotional pain. However, mindfulness primarily invites the question *What are you experiencing?*

Table 12.1 *Mindfulness Exercises Commonly Used in Youth with Anxiety*

Name Exercise	Description	Rationale for CAD
Body scan	Bringing attention to different places in/on your body and just sensing how they feel	Grounding, body awareness, letting go
Breathing exercises	Breathing into the place in the body where a child feels anxiety; breath calm into the area when breathing in, breath out fear and anxiety	Awareness of effects of anxiety on the body
Single raisin exercise	Using all five senses to increase awareness of the whole experience	To approach new situations with beginners' minds rather than anxious apprehension
Various meditations – walking, sounds, looking, touch	Practicing awareness of senses	Sensory experience rather than thinking/worrying
ABC schemes: cognition and emotion	– Seeing thoughts and feelings as they really are, deciding which thoughts to give attention to, and to which no attention. – Disengaging from the thoughts, they are not the reality (e.g., thoughts as clouds or boats passing by)	
Imagination	Compassionate friend entering the room	Taking care of oneself when anxious
Poems	Rumi, "The Guesthouse" Cherokee Indian legend, "Two Wolves"	Pointing at important learning points in a playful way
Yoga	Mindful moving of the body	Feeling of control over the body, stilling the mind while focusing on the body
STOP	**S**top what you're doing; **T**ake a Breath; **O**bserve; **P**lan and proceed	
RAIN	**R**ecognize; **A**llow and accept; **I**nvestigate with kindness, **N**onidentify	
Contact	Notice three places where your body makes contact with the world	Grounding, body awareness
Diaries – thoughts, feelings		Awareness of experience, distancing from anxiety

and self-compassion asks, *What do you need?*" Recently, with the growing body of research on self-compassion showing its protective function against psychopathology in both child (e.g., Bluth et al., 2016) and adult populations (Westphal et al., 2015), researchers and practitioners have acknowledged the importance of targeting self-compassion in stand-alone interventions.

Neff (2003) defines self-compassion as including three elements: (1) self-kindness or treating oneself with care and compassion when experiencing challenges as opposed to self-judgment, (2) sense of common humanity or understanding that our struggles are part of the human experience as opposed to isolation, and (3) mindfulness or maintaining a balanced perspective when faced with difficulties as opposed to overidentification (i.e., being carried away by the dramatic storyline of the occurred difficulties). Within the child literature, the self-compassion concept has also been expressed as "social support turned inwards" (Bluth, Roberson, et al., 2016; Breines et al., 2014).

As in the case with the mindfulness approach, self-compassion exercises such as guided meditation, visualizations, or compassionate letter writing can be integrated into traditional therapies. Clinical experience shows that the introduction of self-compassion skills works best when all individuals with whom the patient interacts on a daily basis (e.g., teachers, family members) are involved and engaged in the treatment. However, it is important to note that some children might encounter difficulties in connecting with self-compassion, or can experience mental, physical, or emotional uneasiness arising during the practice. Indeed, individuals high in self-criticism (Warren et al., 2016) might experience "fear of compassion" (Gilbert et al., 2012) or "back draft" (Germer et al., 2014). This phenomenon can be defined as an intense pain that is released because the unconditional love (i.e., self-compassion) that is practiced reveals the conditions under which one was unloved in the past (Warren et al., 2016). Therefore, clinicians should be aware of this phenomenon, and apply recommended procedures provided during self-compassion training to help children deal with overwhelming emotions that might occur during the practice of self-compassion. Both self-compassion programs described as follows address this issue in their protocols.

Examples of Self-Compassion Programs

Although other therapies such as Dialectical Behavioral Therapy (Dimeff & Linehan, 2001) or self-esteem programs (McKay & Fanning, 1992) focus on the development of self-compassion skills during the therapeutic process, Mindful Self-Compassion (MSC) developed by Neff and Germer (2013) and Compassion Focused Therapy (CFT) developed by Gilbert (2009) can be identified as the two most well-known self-compassion interventions for adults. The first program targets nonclinical population and uses the meditation exercises and daily life practices such as soothing touch practice or compassionate movement exercise to develop self-compassion skills within an 8-week time period. The second program is designed to teach self-compassion in clinical population in different types of disorders by using imagery and meditation combined with psychoeducation.

Regarding child populations, recently a manualized and empirically validated version of the MSC program has been adapted for the teenage population by Bluth and colleagues (2016). This 8-week program of 1.5 hour is designed for teens from 11 to 19 years of age. The sessions contain guided meditation, art, and movement activities, and youth can learn mindful self-compassion across the following 8 themes: (a) definitions of mindfulness and self-compassion, (b) paying attention on purpose, (c) loving kindness, (d) self-compassion, (e) self-esteem/self-compassion, (f) living deeply, (g) working with difficult emotions, and (h) embracing your life with gratitude. Other recent attempts include adapting the CFT manual to the needs of adolescents from the clinical population who mainly experienced abuse and who score high on shame and self-criticism (Welford & Langmead, 2015; Welford, 2016).

Evidence Base for Innovation

To our knowledge, only two studies from the same research team have tested whether mindfulness intervention can be useful with children – and then only with children who have subclinical levels of anxiety. No studies of mindfulness in children with clinically referred anxiety disorders exist at this time, and this is for sure an important area for future research.

4.1 Evidence Base for Mindfulness Training in CAD

In the first open trial study, Semple and colleagues (2005) tested the feasibility and acceptability of 6 weeks of a mindfulness group training program in five anxious children aged 7 to 8 years old. The children received six 45-minute sessions of mindfulness training aimed at increasing attention to bodily sensations and perceptions. Teacher reports of behavioral problems (i.e., CBCL) indicated reductions in scores posttreatment for four of the five participants. Co-therapists observed enthusiasm and interest in practicing mindfulness by all children and an interest to continue to do so after the training. In the second trial, Semple and colleagues (2010) randomized 25 children aged 9 to 13 years old to a 12-session group mindfulness based cognitive therapy (described previously) or to a wait-list. Children were referred to the university clinic-based remedial reading tutoring program for significant reading difficulties and associated stress or anxiety feelings. At posttreatment and at 3-month follow-up, children in the mindfulness therapy group showed fewer attention problems (as assessed with CBCL Attention Problems scale; $d = .42$) as compared to the wait-list control; however, for other social-emotional problems or anxiety symptoms no differences were found between the two groups. Therefore, this controlled study does not provide compelling evidence for mindfulness as an effective treatment for child anxiety.

Thus, so far, the effectiveness of mindfulness training in anxious children is under researched. The two studies should be interpreted with caution because of the small sample of anxious children and the amount and type of different analyses conducted on that sample. Larger studies using more rigorous methodological principles are needed in order to understand whether mindfulness in (some) children with anxiety disorders is an effective approach or a helpful addition to CBT.

Evidence-Base for Self-Compassion Programs

So far, only a few studies shed light on the potential effectiveness of self-compassion approaches for child anxiety as well. First, the meta-analysis with adults (MacBeth & Gumley, 2012) shows a large effect size for the relationship between self-compassion and anxiety symptom reductions ($r = -.51$). The negative direction of the relationship indicates that higher levels of self-compassion are accompanied by lower levels of anxiety symptoms, which supports the importance of self-compassion in reduction of anxiety. Second, a recent meta-analysis on compassion-based interventions including 21 randomized control trials with adults (Kirby et al., 2017) shows significant moderate effect size for reduction of anxiety symptoms, with results remaining after including active control comparisons. The authors also conclude that although more research is needed, the existing studies highlight the potential benefits of compassion-based interventions, for various outcomes, including anxiety. Third, in light of the few studies that have investigated self-compassion in relation to anxiety symptoms and other psychopathologies in youth (e.g., Muris et al., 2016), the results showed that higher levels of self-compassion were associated with lower levels of psychopathology. Moreover, the results of the pilot study with the MSC protocol for teens showed (Bluth et al., 2015) that, among other outcomes, the anxiety symptoms decreased significantly after the intervention with a small to medium effect size ($g = -0.39$), and that self-compassion predicted decreases in anxiety. However, in a recent study using the same intervention protocol with 44 adolescents between 11 and 17 years old from nonclinical population (Bluth & Eisenlohr-Moul, 2017), these results were not confirmed. Indeed, only a significant decrease of perceived stress but no decrease in anxiety symptoms were observed from pre- to post-intervention or from pre- to follow-up. Finally, when taking into consideration studies in adult clinical population such as social anxiety disorder (Koszycki et al., 2016), post-traumatic stress disorder (Hirakoa et al., 2015), or generalized anxiety disorders (Hoge et al., 2013), self-compassion shows promising results and could be therefore considered as a potentially useful intervention for youth anxiety disorders.

In sum, the research on self-compassion in children and adolescents is relatively new and the results have to be interpreted with considerable caution. The studies show some preliminary support for the potential of self-compassion as a protective psychological factor, and effective intervention for anxiety disorder in youth. However, before making any firm evidence-based conclusions, more studies with both clinical and nonclinical samples with rigorous methodology are sorely needed.

Mediators and Moderators of Change

To date, there have been no studies that have systematically evaluated predictors, mediators, and moderators of mindfulness approaches to CADs in appropriately designed and powered trials. However, potential variables of interest for future research are explored here.

Potential Mediators and Moderators of Mindfulness Training Outcomes for CAD

How does mindfulness training for childhood anxiety disorders work, and through which mechanisms? As the primary target of mindfulness training is to increase mindful attention in the proposition that this would reduce psychopathology, one could argue that changes in attentional processes could be an important mediator of mindfulness training outcomes for childhood anxiety. Indeed, this hypothesis was tested, at least in a preliminary manner, in Semple et al.'s (2010) study in which pre- to post-changes in attentional problems (as assessed via CBCL Attention scale) were tested as a mediator of posttreatment behavior problems (CBCL total score). While mindfulness training was able to decrease attention problems over the course of the training, these decreases were not associated with decreases in behavior problems posttreatment. It should be noted that this test of mediation was weak on a number of grounds including a small sample ($n=20$ treatment completers) and use of a traditional data-analytic technique not suitable for small samples. The question also arises whether a subscale of the CBCL is the best assessment tool to assess changes in attention problems and whether other, perhaps experimental, assessment tools should be used.

As other authors suggest (Bögels, Lehetonen, & Restifo, 2010; Duncan, Coatsworth, & Greenberg, 2009), some parental variables such as acceptance and awareness could also be important processes underlying mindfulness training outcomes in children. It would be worthwhile to investigate whether existing and yet to be developed mindfulness trainings in children with anxiety disorders and their parents are able to positively influence these phenomena both in children as well as in their parents.

In terms of variables that determine for which anxious child the mindfulness training is the most and least effective, a few potential moderators have been explored, such as the severity of anxiety problems. In Semple et al.'s (2010) study, anecdotal evidence showed that the subset of children who reported clinically elevated levels of anxiety on a questionnaire at pretreatment showed the greatest reductions in anxiety symptoms and behavior problems. Further, the types of childhood anxiety disorders may be a potential moderator. As social anxiety disorder is associated with a whole range of attentional difficulties (attentional bias, self-focused attention, attentional avoidance; see Bögels & Mansell, 2004) and mindfulness training is primarily directed at targeting attention, it is possible that children suffering from social anxiety disorder may benefit the most from mindfulness interventions. As children with social anxiety disorder appear to do less well in

CBT (Hudson et al., 2015), there is a strong rationale for examining mindfulness as an alternative approach for them. Other child anxiety disorders in which pervasive rumination or worrying is the primary target of intervention (as in generalized anxiety disorder) may also benefit from mindfulness. Children with anxiety disorders in which lack of body awareness or bodily sensory integration may be an issue, as in illness anxiety disorder or in children with autistic spectrum disorder and comorbid anxiety disorders, may also particularly benefit from mindfulness. Additionally, children with anxiety disorders and comorbid externalizing problems such as ADHD may be another group for which mindfulness may be indicated, given the effects of mindfulness for youth with externalizing problems and their parents (e.g., Bögels et al., 2008). Finally, children with anxiety disorders and comorbid depression may specifically benefit from mindfulness, given the potential effectiveness of mindfulness in reducing self-criticism (a central feature of depression) and the potential effectiveness of mindful parenting for helping parents break the negative cycle of interaction with their depressed child, which may be maintaining childhood depression (Restifo & Bögels, 2009). Although such possibilities exist, none of these have been investigated to date and await experimental examination.

Mediators and Moderators of Self-Compassion Program Outcomes

The main goal of self-compassion approaches is decreasing psychopathology levels through targeting self-compassion in children and adults. The potential important role of self-compassion as a mediator or mechanism of self-compassion trainings has been investigated in a few studies so far.

Self-compassion practices increase the ability to deal with negative emotions in general, but also influence an enhancement in positive emotions (Warren et al., 2016). In this way practicing self-compassion can decrease rumination and emotion suppression but also increase positive psychological qualities such as happiness. Self-compassion has been addressed as a mechanism of change in mindfulness-based interventions studies; however, none of them target child anxiety disorders. For instance, Kuyken and his colleagues (2010) show that the decrease of depression symptoms after Mindfulness-Based Cognitive Therapy were mediated by both mindfulness and self-compassion. However, two other studies show that although self-compassion increased significantly after mindfulness interventions, it did not mediate the effect of intervention on anger (Keng et al., 2012) or anxiety (Bergen-Cico & Cheon, 2014). Finally, a recent study (Duarte & Pinto-Gouveia, 2017) shows that self-compassion did mediate the impact of the mindfulness intervention on burnout, depression, anxiety, stress, and satisfaction with life in adults. Still, this relatively modest number of studies provides initial support for the role of self-compassion as a potential mechanism being targeted during self-compassion interventions.

Although the research on the topic of potential moderators of self-compassion intervention is relatively new, some studies provide preliminary answers. In the recent meta-analysis of gender differences in self-compassion, Yarnell and colleagues (2015) reported that self-compassion levels are slightly lower for women than men, with the difference being larger in populations with higher levels of ethnic minorities. Thus, the authors suggest taking these differences into account during self-compassion interventions, without overemphasizing their effect. Regarding adolescent population, Bluth and colleagues (2017) addressed the issue of age and gender in a correlational study. They showed that older female adolescents have lower self-compassion levels than younger female adolescents, or males at all ages. The authors recommend early intervention especially with female adolescents in order to help prevent maladaptive behavioral and emotional trajectories. Since all anxiety disorders occur more frequently among females than males and there is an important peak in adolescence, reaching ratios of 2:1 to 3:1 (Beesdo et al., 2009), self-compassion can be considered as a potential intervention to prevent and treat anxiety disorders especially in young at risk females.

Clinical Case Illustration

In this clinical case example, we describe how a mindfulness approach based on *Growing Up Mindful* (Willard, 2016) was used with an 8-year-old boy (Toby) and his parents. Toby was referred to a private practice on the recommendation of his school counselor. Toby's anxiety had been affecting everything from his academic work to his social life as he became panicky throughout the school day, then back at home would become anxious and tearful again as he recalled the shame of struggling throughout the school day. Toby's overall functioning was high, but the anxiety was escalating and increasingly taking a toll on him, his family, and his schoolteachers as they struggled to understand and accommodate his anxiety. The bulk of treatment was done and progress made in weekly 45-minute sessions, though Toby and the therapist continue to check in about once a month.

The approach the therapist took was slightly different in this case as Toby had already had some mindfulness in school, mindful breathing as part of a classroom exercise, and there was little need for introduction or orientation to the idea of mindfulness. The therapist chose a mindfulness-based treatment based on Toby's very positive attitude toward mindfulness in school and at home. The sessions would also be less formally structured than manualized approaches such as Semple's (2005), but filling in gaps from what knowledge and practice Toby had gained in school.

After some basic intake and rapport building in the opening session, Toby spotted the therapist's "mindfulness bell," a simple metal and wood chime, on the therapist's desk immediately. *Is that a mindfulness bell?* he cautiously inquired. The therapist responded that it was, and Toby explained that his teacher sometimes taught mindfulness in school. *Will you show me?* the therapist asked him, hoping Toby could start to feel some ownership and empowerment in his practice by demonstrating mindfulness, while the therapist assessed his knowledge.

Gently and solemnly ringing the bell, Toby patiently instructed the therapist to *feel your breath go all the way in ... and feel your breath go all the way back out.* With a head start on mindfulness from his school, the therapist and Toby discussed different practices he had done (mostly just simple breath awareness) and agreed to explore more practices together. They also agreed that during the sessions that were largely focused on play and drawing, either he or the therapist could grab the bell, give it a ring, and they would have to do three mindful breaths.

But they did not stop there. Each week the therapist and Toby would learn and practice a new short and a new longer practice. For example, the next week it was the "hot chocolate breath." To open their session, the therapist and Toby held a cup in their hands as if holding an invisible mug, raised them to their mouths, and closed their eyes. They would breathe in imagining that they were smelling the delicious drink in their hands, then gently blowing out through their mouths, cooling off the imaginary beverage in front of them, as they cooled off their minds and bodies from any "hot" emotions like anxiety that had been building. At the end of the session, Toby and the therapist would typically practice something longer, usually about five to ten minutes of a guided visualization, with many cues and prompts on the therapist's part. The therapist would record these on his phone and share them with Toby's parents. We would follow up with a brief inquiry about any changes in or with his mind and body after each practice, rating for himself how helpful he found them and brainstorming times to use the various practices.

Often, one parent would join the therapist and Toby at the end of the session, Toby would teach them the short practice like the hot chocolate breath, and as a group they would brainstorm the most helpful times to practice during the week. These included before meals, homework, and at bedtime at home, and moments in the school day when things might get challenging like before independent work in math, or before unfamiliar social events. For the most part, Toby reported using practices at the suggested times to good benefit. The therapist would also send Toby's parents home with the week's recording, so they could practice as a family, trying to lower baseline levels of anxiety outside of the moments. Toby wrote simple reminders on his notebook, and sometimes carried an index card with his favorite practices with him to school, especially on days that all had determined to be most "triggering." By about the fourth week, at one school meeting the therapist attended, the family and therapist also shared Toby's favorite mindfulness practices with his teachers, so they could prompt him to access them during the busy day when they could see his anxiety rising and reinforce practices Toby found effective.

Week by week Toby learned new short practices, ranging from mindful breathing to mindful eating and mindful walking, which was described as feeling the bottoms of his feet when he walked. We continued exploring the five senses in depth with "superhero listening" trying to notice the five most distant sounds he could hear off in the distance as a way to focus the mind when it wandered to anxiety or just off the topic at school. The therapist and Toby would practice mindfully grounding themselves in the present by focusing on all the sensations of their feet on the floor, exploring temperature, texture, moisture, pressure, as they shifted thoughts from the future and past to ground themselves in their bodies as a practice to use before tests or speaking in class. These and other practices made up parts of the sessions, which were otherwise filled with game playing of UNO or checkers, drawing, and simple play with stuffed animals and Legos to build rapport, maintain trust, and keep up motivation. Toby also would review when he used mindfulness during the week, occasionally drawing elaborate comic books about events like using his mindfulness in rock climbing class and then feeling confident and calm enough to try rappelling.

With the introduction of each new short practice came discussions of when and how to use the practice outside of the sessions, and reviews afterward. Toby liked focusing on sounds before diving into schoolwork, feeling sensations in his feet during social events or when he had to speak in front of the class, and doing mindful breathing at other times like on the drive to school. However, breathing was not a favorite; rather he tended to prefer listening to sounds as his preferred method of grounding, and by week six or seven, this was the main practice he used outside of sessions. In the evenings, often with his family, he would listen to the recordings the therapist and he made together. Each week the therapist sent home with him a different and slightly longer visualization, and Toby would report back his favorites.

As Toby practiced between sessions, his ability to focus for longer gradually improved, up to eight minutes or so by week eight or nine with guidance and with others practicing around him. The confidence built momentum, and also helped him remember to use the shorter practices during more challenging moments in his day-to-life at school and home. As his parents liked to practice the recordings with him, as well as remaining willing to do short practices at the dinner table as a family, they too were able to enjoy the benefits and reinforce the importance of practice, making the therapist's job far easier.

Toby himself reported less anxiety after only a few weeks, while more objective observers like family and teachers reported more significant changes at around ten or twelve weeks. Toby reported that he could stay calm through school assessments, using practices to help him before challenging situations and in the moment when he felt his anxiety rising. Teachers also reported to parents fewer somatic complaints of stomach aches or nausea during school, and parents reported that Toby's mood had improved with fewer complaints of worry or somatic symptoms. Eventually, after about twelve sessions, the therapist and Toby shifted their meetings from weekly to monthly, even that primarily just because Toby enjoyed coming and practicing together. Toby and this therapist continue to check in monthly and review skills and progress, even almost two years later, though almost entirely at Toby's request.

In the end, treatment goals were largely met. Toby and his parents better understood his anxiety, as well as how to reduce it. Through practice, everyone around Toby learned how to help him identify and manage his triggers with exercises that were fun and practical, and that he began finding more of his own uses beyond just the most difficult moments of anxiety in his life that had brought him into treatment. What's more, the rest of the family, and even his teacher gained a useful skill for helping themselves and their kids manage mild to moderate anxiety.

Challenges and Recommendation for Future Research in This Area

So, could mindfulness also be beneficial for childhood anxiety disorders (CADs)? The answer is "yes," but our response is mainly based on theory and our limited clinical expertise with anxious youth and with applications of mindfulness techniques. As opposed to CBT that has earned the status of "well-established" in laboratory settings and is finding its way into usual clinical practice, exactly the opposite is happening with mindfulness. Given its perceived merits and the relative ease in applying mindfulness techniques in different settings, the popularity of mindfulness is growing even while researchers are in the early stages of examining what mindfulness exactly is and how it works in child populations. So the first remark we want to make is that more rigorous intervention studies (either RCTs or controlled single-case experimental designs) are needed in order to investigate the efficacy, mediators, and moderators of mindfulness training outcomes in childhood anxiety disorders. Second, assessments of the proposed mechanisms should be carefully designed and should involve both self-reports as well as experimental tasks (e.g., dot probe paradigms, emotional stroop tasks) targeting main change processes. Third, from our literature review and clinical experience, it seems that mindfulness and self-compassion approaches can best be integrated with existing cognitive-behavioral procedures for childhood anxiety disorders. The question remains for which anxious children is it most beneficial to receive mindfulness in addition to CBT? Ongoing studies such as the one conducted by our research team could help shed light on this. In this study with 130 anxious children and adolescents between 8 and 18 years with both clinical as well as subclinical anxiety levels (Telman et al., *in preparation*), therapists are provided with a range of therapy modules (e.g., cognitive therapy, exposure) based on a CBT protocol (Bögels, 2008). Besides the traditional CBT modules, a mindfulness module has been added to this treatment package. For each client the therapists personalize the therapy through use of specific module(s) and based on clinical expertise, pretreatment assessments and (in half of the cases) regular, during-treatment, client feedback.

Other interesting research questions are whether mindfulness and self-compassion practices can be used specifically to enhance the outcomes of certain CBT techniques in anxious youth such as exposure activities. Further, is there an effect of mindfulness on avoidance behavior in children with anxiety? For which anxious children is mindfulness in combination with CBT the most effective? As mindfulness is rapidly being disseminated into clinical practice, and among therapists in training and students of clinical child and adolescent psychology and psychiatry, it seems that the clinical researchers are the ones who should make a catch-up effort. Because we do not know for sure how and why mindfulness could work in anxious children, the above-noted research questions could initially be examined in a range of single-case studies prior to design and conduct of a randomized clinical trial. Interaction between research and practice is hereby an essential requirement given the rich experience of clinicians with mindfulness.

Key Practice Points

As discussed previously, developing best-practice recommendations for mindfulness in CAD has been hampered by the absence of scientific evidence about the efficacy and effectiveness of mindfulness in children with anxiety disorders. While keeping these limitations in mind, a few recommendations based on clinical experience and theory can be made. First, during the intake phase of the treatment, assessments of mindfulness, self-compassion, and other related constructs such as self-criticism should be obtained as well as a child's, family's, and school's interest and possibilities in practicing mindfulness. Second, at this point in time, it seems that mindfulness can best be implemented in a manualized manner and in combination with cognitive-behavioral strategies such as exposure. The concept of homework is especially important in mindfulness approaches as regular daily practice of mindfulness helps develop skills that children can then apply when feeling anxious.

Acknowledgments

The authors of this chapter have received funding from the European Union's Horizon 2020 research and innovation program under the Marie Sklodowska-Curie grant agreement No. 656333

References

Achenbach, T.M., Becker, A., Döpfner, M., Heiervang, E., Roessner, V., Steinhausen, H., & Rothenberger, A. (2008). Multicultural assessment of child and adolescent psychopathology with ASEBA and SDQ instruments: Research findings, applications, and future directions. *Child Psychology and Psychiatry, 49*, 251–275.

Barrett, P. (2005). *FRIENDS for Life: Group leaders' manual for children*. Caulfield South: Barrett Research Resources Pty Ltd.

Beesdo, K., Knappe, S., & Pine, D. S. (2009). Anxiety and anxiety disorders in children and adolescents: Developmental issues and implications for DSM-V. *The Psychiatric Clinics of North America, 32*, 483–524.

Bergen-Cico, D., & Cheon, S. (2014). The mediating effects of mindfulness and self-compassion on trait anxiety. *Mindfulness, 5*, 505–519.

Bluth, K., Roberson, P. N. E., Gaylord, S. A., Faurot, K. R., Grewen, K. M., Arzon, S., & Girdler, S. S. (2016). Does self-compassion protect adolescents from stress? *Journal of Child and Family Studies, 25*, 1098–1109.

Bluth, K., Campo, R., Futch, W., Gaylord, S. (2017). Age and gender differences in the associations of self-compassion and emotional well-being in a large adolescent sample. *Journal of Youth and adolescence, 46*, 840–853.

Bluth, K., Gaylord, S. A., Campo, R. A., Mullarkey, M., & Hobbs, L. (2015). Making friends with yourself: A mixed methods pilot study of a mindful self-compassion program for adolescents. *Mindfulness, 7*, 479–492.

Bluth, K., and Eisenlohr-Moul, T. (2017). Response to a mindful self-compassion intervention in teens: A within-person association of mindfulness, self-compassion, and emotional well-being outcomes. *Journal of Adolescence, 57*, 108–118.

Bodden, D. H. M., Dirksen, C.D., Bögels, S.M., Appelboom, C., Appelboom-Geerts, K. C. M. M. J., Brinkman, A.G., ... Nauta, M.H. (2008). Costs and cost-effectiveness of family CBT versus individual CBT in clinically anxious children. *Clinical Child Psychology and Psychiatry, 13*, 543–564.

Bögels, S. M. (2008). *Treatment of anxiety disorders in children and adolescents with cognitive-behavioral protocol Thinking + Doing = Daring*. Houten: Bohn Stafleu van Loghum, The Netherlands.

Bögels, S. M. (2017). *Mindful opvoeden in een druk bestaan: een praktische gids voor mindful ouderschap*. Ambo/anthos uitgevers, Amsterdam, The Netherlands.

Bögels, S. M., Hellemans, J., van Deursen, S., Römer, M., & van der Meulen, R. (2014). Mindful parenting in mental health care: effects on parental and child psychopathology, parental stress, parenting, coparenting, and marital functioning. *Mindfulness, 5*, 536–551.

Bögels, S., Hoogstad, B., van Dun, L., de Schutter, S., & Restifo, K. (2008). Mindfulness training for adolescents with externalizing disorders and their parents. *Behavioural and Cognitive Psychotherapy, 36*, 193–209.

Bögels, S. M., Lehtonen, A., & Restifo, K. (2010). Mindful parenting in mental health care. *Mindfulness, 1*, 107–120.

Bögels, S. M., & Mansell, W. (2004). Attention processes in the maintenance and treatment of social phobia: Hypervigilance, avoidance, and self-focused attention. *Clinical Psychology Review, 24*, 827–856.

Bögels, S. M., & Restifo, K. (2014). *Mindful parenting: A guide for mental health practitioners*. New York: Springer, Norton.

Breines, J. G., Thoma, M. V., Gianferante, D., Hanlin, L., Chen, X., & Rohleder, N. (2014). Self-compassion as a predictor of interleukin- 6 response to acute psychosocial stress. *Brain Behavior and Immunity, 37*, 109–114.

Brown, K. W., West, A. M., Loverich, T. M., & Biegel, G.M. (2011). Assessing adolescent mindfulness: Validation of an adapted Mindful Attention Awareness Scale in adolescent normative and psychiatric populations. *Psychological Assessment*. doi:10.1037/a0021338.

Cartwright-Hatton, S., McNicol, K., & Doubleday, E. (2006). Anxiety in a neglected population: Prevalence of anxiety disorders in pre-adolescent children. *Clinical Psychology Review, 26*, 817–833.

Detweiler, M. F., Comer, J. S., Crum, K. I., & Albano, A. M. (2014). Social anxiety in children and adolescents: Biological, developmental, and social considerations. In S. G. Hofmann, & P. M. DiBartolo (eds.), *Social anxiety: Clinical, developmental, and social perspectives*, 3rd edn. (pp. 729–751). London: Academic Press.

Dewald, J. F., Short, M. A., Gradisar, M., Oort, F. J., & Meijer, A. M. (2012). The Chronic Sleep Reduction Questionnaire (CSRQ): A cross-cultural comparison and validation in Dutch and Australian adolescents. *Journal of Sleep Research, 21*, 584–594.

Dimeff, L., & Linehan, M. (2001). Dialectical behavior therapy in a nutshell. *The California Psychologist, 34*, 10–13.

Duarte, J., Pinto-Gouveia, J. (2017). Mindfulness, self-compassion and psychological inflexibility mediate the effects of a mindfulness-based intervention in a sample of oncology nurses. *Journal of Contextual Behavioral Science, 6*, 125–133.

Duncan, L. G., Coatsworth, J. D., & Greenberg, M. T. (2009). A model of mindful parenting: Implications for parent-child relationships and prevention research. *Clinical Child and Family Psychology Review, 12*, 255–270.

Germer, C. and Neff, K. (2014). Cultivating self-compassion in trauma survivors. In J. Briere, V. Follette, J. Hopper, D. Rozelle, & D. Rome (eds.), *Transforming trauma: Integrating contemplative and Western psychological approaches*. New York: Guilford Press.

Gibby, B. A., Casline, E. P., & Ginsburg, G. S. (2017). Long-term outcomes of youth treated for an anxiety disorder: A critical review. *Clinical Child and Family Psychology Review, 20*, 201–225.

Gilbert P. (2009). Introducing compassion-focused therapy. *Advances in Psychiatry Treatment, 15*, 199–208.

Gilbert, P., McEwan, K., Gibbons, L., Chotai, S., Duarte, J., & Matos, M. (2012). Fears of compassion and happiness in relation to alexithymia, mindfulness, and self-criticism. *Psychology and Psychotherapy. Theory, Research and Practice, 85 (4)*, 374–390.

Heyne D. A., Sauter F. M., Ollendick T. H., Van Widenfelt B. M. & Westenberg P. M. (2014), Developmentally sensitive cognitive behavioral therapy for adolescent school refusal: Rationale and case illustration. *Clinical Child and Family Psychology Review, 17*, 191–215.

Hiraoka, R., Meyer, E. C., Kimbrel, N. A., et al. (2015). Self-compassion as a prospective predictor of PTSD symptom severity among trauma-exposed US Iraq and Afghanistan war veterans. *Journal of Trauma Stress, 28*, 127–133.

Hoge, E., Hölzel, B., Marques, L., et al. (2013). Mindfulness and self-compassion in generalized anxiety disorder: Examining predictors of disability. *Evidence Based Complementary and Alternative Medicine*, 576258.

Hofmann, S. G., Sawyer, A. T., Witt, A., & Oh, D. (2010). The effect of mindfulness-based therapy on anxiety and depression: A meta-analytic review. *Journal of Consulting and Clinical Psychology, 78*, 169–183.

Hollon, S., & Beck, A. (2013). Cognitive and cognitive-behavioral therapies. In M. J. Lambert (ed.), *Handbook of psychotherapy and behavior change* (pp. 393–443). Hoboken, NJ: John Wiley & Sons.

Hudson, J. L. Keers, R., Roberts S., Coleman J. R. I., Breen G., Arendt K., Bogels S., ... Eley T.C. (2015). Clinical predictors of response to Cognitive Behavioral Therapy in pediatric anxiety disorders: The Genes for Treatment (GxT) study. *Journal of the American Academy of Child and Adolescent Psychiatry, 54*, 454–463.

Kabat-Zinn, J. (1982). An out-patient program in behavioral medicine for chronic pain patients based on the practice of mindfulness meditation: Theoretical considerations and preliminary results. *General Hospital Psychiatry 4*, 33–47.

Kabat-Zinn, J. (1990). *Full catastrophe living*. New York: Bantam Doubleday Dell.

Kendall, P. C., & Hedtke, K. (2006). *Cognitive-behavioral therapy for anxious children: Therapist manual* (3rd edn.). Ardmore, PA: Workbook Publishing.

Keng, S., Smoski, M. J., Robins, C. J., Ekblad, A. G., & Brantley, J. G. (2012). Mechanisms of change in mindfulness-based stress reduction: Self-compassion and mindfulness as mediators of intervention outcomes. *Journal of Cognitive Psychotherapy, 26*, 270–280.

Kirby, J., Tellegen, C., & Steindl, S. (2017). A meta-analysis of compassion-based interventions: Current state of knowledge and future directions. *Behavior Therapy*. 10.1016/j.beth.2017.06.003.

Koszycki, D., Thake, J., Mavounza, C., Daoust, JP., Taljaard M., Bradwejn J. (2016). Preliminary investigation of a mindfulness-based intervention for social anxiety disorder that integrates compassion meditation and mindful exposure. *Journal of Alternative and Complementary Medicine, 22*, 363–374.

Kuyken, W., Watkins, E., Holden, E., White, K., Taylor, R.S., Byford, S., et al. (2010). How does mindfulness-based cognitive therapy work? *Behavior Research and Therapy, 48*, 1105–1112.

Lyubomirsky, S., & Lepper, H. S. (1999). A measure of subjective happiness: Preliminary reliability and construct validation. *Social Indicators Research, 46*, 137–155.

McKay, M., & Fanning, P. (1992). *Self-esteem: A proven program of cognitive techniques for assessing, improving, and maintaining your self-esteem* (2nd edn.). Oakland, CA: New Harbinger.

Macbeth, A., & Gumley, A. I. (2012). Exploring compassion: A meta-analysis of the association between self-compassion and psychopathology. *Clinical Psychology Review, 32*, 545–552.

Manassis K., Lee T.C., Bennett K., Zhao X.Y., Mendlowitz S., Duda S., ... Wood J.J. (2014). Types of parental involvement in CBT with anxious youth: A preliminary meta-analysis. *Journal of Consulting and Clinical Psychology, 82*, 1163–1172.

Maric, M., van Steensel, F. J. A., & Bögels, S. M. (2015). Parental involvement in CBT for anxiety-disordered youth revisited: Family CBT outperforms child CBT in the long term for children with comorbid ADHD symptoms. *Journal of Attention Disorders*, 1-9.

Muris, P., Meesters, C., Pierik, A., De Kock, B. (2016). Good for the self: Self-compassion and other self-related constructs in relation to symptoms of anxiety and depression in non-clinical youths. *Journal of Child Family Studies, 25*, 607–617.

Neff, K. (2003). The development and validation of a scale to measure self-compassion. *Self and Identity, 2*, 223–250.

Neff, K., & Germer C. (2013). A pilot study and randomized controlled trial of the mindful self-compassion program. *Journal of Clinical Psychology, 69*, 28–44.

Restifo, K., & Bögels, S. M. (2009). Family processes in the development of youth depression: Translating the evidence to treatment. *Clinical Psychology Review, 29*, 294–316.

Segal, Z. V., Williams, J. M. G., & Teasdale, J. D. (2002). *Mindfulness-based cognitive therapy for depression: A new approach to preventing relapse*. New York: Guilford Press.

Semple, R. J., & Lee, J. (2008). Treating anxiety with mindfulness: Mindfulness-based cognitive therapy for children. In L. A. Greco & S. C. Hayes (eds.), *Acceptance and mindfulness interventions for children, adolescents, and families* (pp. 94–134). Oakland, CA: Context Press/New Harbinger Publications.

Semple, R. J., Reid, E. F., & Miller, L. (2005). Treating anxiety with mindfulness: An open trial of mindfulness training for anxious children. *Journal of Cognitive Psychotherapy, 19*, 379–392.

Semple, R. J., Lee, J., Rosa, D., Miller, L. F. (2010). A randomized trial of mindfulness-based cognitive therapy for children: Promoting mindful attention to enhance social- emotional resiliency in children. *Journal of Child and Family Studies, 19*, 218–229.

Suzuki, S. (2011). *Zen mind, beginner's mind: Informal talks on Zen meditation and practice*. Boston: Shambala Publications Inc.

Telman, L. G. E., Maric, M., Miočević, M., Bögels, S.M., & Van Steensel, F.J.A. (in prep.). Feedback informed modular cognitive behavioural therapy for childhood anxiety disorders. Manuscript in preparation.

Westphal, M., Bingisser, M.-B., Feng, T., Wall, M., Blakley, E., Bingisser, R., et al. (2015). Protective benefits of mindfulness in emergency room personnel. *Journal of Affective Disorders*, *175*, 79–85.

Van Bockstaele, B., & Bögels, S. M. (2014). Mindfulness-based therapy for social anxiety disorder. In S. G. Hofmann, & P. M. DiBartolo (eds.), *Social anxiety: Clinical, developmental, and social perspectives*, (3rd edn.) (pp. 729–751). London: Academic Press.

Van der Oord, S., Bögels, S. M., & Peijnenburg, D. (2012). The effectiveness of mindfulness training for children with ADHD and mindful parenting for their parents. *Journal of Child and Family Studies*, *21*, 139–147.

Van de Weijer-Bergsma, E., Formsma, A. R., de Bruin, E. I., & Bögels, S. M. (2012). The effectiveness of mindfulness training on behavioral problems and attentional functioning in adolescents with ADHD. *Journal of Child and Family Studies*, *21*, 775–787.

Walkup, J. T., Albano, A. M., Piacentini, J., Birmaher, B., Compton, S. N., Sherrill, J. T., et al. (2008). Cognitive behavioral therapy, sertraline, or a combination in childhood anxiety. *The New England Journal of Medicine*, *359*, 2753–2766.

Warren, R., Smeets, E., & Neff, K. (2016). Self-criticism and self-compassion. Risk and resilience. *Current Psychiatry*, *15*, 19–33.

Welford, M. & Langmead, K. (2015). Compassion-based initiatives in educational settings. *Educational & Child Psychology, 32*(1), 71-80.

Welford, M. (2016). *Compassion focused therapy with youth workshop*. University of Twente, Twente, The Netherlands.

Willard, C. (2014). *Mindfulness for teen anxiety workbook*. Oakland: New Harbinger.

Willard, C. (2016). *Growing up mindful: Essential practices to help children, teens, and families find balance, calm, and resilience*. Louisville: Sounds True, Inc.

Yarnell, L. M., Stafford, R. E., Neff, K. D., Reilly, E. D., Knox, M. C., & Mullarkey, M. (2015). Meta-analysis of gender differences in self-compassion. *Self and Identity*, *14*, 499–520.

PART II

Obsessive-Compulsive Disorder

13 Phenomenology and Standard Care of OCD in Children and Adolescents

Erica L. Greenberg and Daniel A. Geller

Phenomenology

Obsessive-compulsive disorder (OCD) is defined by the *DSM-5* as the presence of "obsessions," "compulsions," or both (American Psychiatric Association, 2013). Obsessions are characterized by intrusive, unwanted, persistent thoughts, images, or urges that lead to marked distress or anxiety, or disgust. Compulsions are repetitive behaviors or mental acts that the individual feels driven to perform in response to an affect either stimulated by an obsession or to certain rigidly applied rules. The aim of a compulsion is to reduce anxiety or distress and/or prevent a dreaded situation, but the act is either excessive, or not connected realistically with what it was designed to prevent. The obsessive and compulsive symptoms are often accompanied by avoidance behaviors. To meet *DSM-5* criteria for OCD, the obsessions and/or compulsions must be time consuming (e.g., take up more than one hour per day) and lead to clinically significant impairment and/or distress. The obsessive/compulsive symptoms also cannot be better explained by another psychiatric condition, or be secondary to another medical condition or substance (American Psychiatric Association, 2013).

OCD was recently placed in a new *DSM-5* category, called Obsessive-Compulsive and Related Disorders (OCRD), in recognition of its distinction from other anxiety disorders. The OCRD section in *DSM-5* is comprised of syndromes characterized by repetitive behaviors, including Body Dysmorphic Disorder (BDD), Hoarding Disorder, Trichotillomania (TTM), and Excoriation (Skin Picking) Disorder (American Psychiatric Association, 2013). Although OCD was separated from anxiety disorders in *DSM-5*, anxiety often remains a prominent feature of the diagnosis. That said, anxiety is not required, and is overall a less stable feature in OCRDs. For example, many individuals who have OCD and/or other OCRDs will describe feelings of discomfort until they acquire "just-rightness," or feelings of disgust they seek to eliminate through compulsions or avoidance, rather than anxiety per se. OCRDs and anxiety disorders may also differ in their course, outcome, comorbidity, presumed genetics, and treatment responses.

Two "specifiers" were added to the OCD *DSM-5* diagnostic criteria. The first regards insight. The clinician now specifies whether the individual with OCD symptoms has good/fair insight – meaning there is some doubt about OCD-related beliefs; poor insight – meaning the individual believes the OCD beliefs are probably true; or absent insight/delusional beliefs – meaning the individual is completely convinced that the OCD beliefs are true. In an adult population, about 2 to 4 percent of patients are considered to have little or no insight (Van Ameringen, Patterson, & Simpson, 2014). Interestingly, the level of insight regarding any particular obsession may fluctuate over time, and can often vary with anxiety levels. Especially in youth, increased anxiety tends to correlate with worsened insight. In a pediatric population, about a third of youth could be characterized as having limited or poor insight (Storch et al., 2008). As noted by the *DSM-5*, children are not expected to be able to articulate the aims behind their compulsive acts, and often are unable to if asked. Poorer intellectual functioning, younger age, higher levels of depressive symptoms, lower levels of adaptation, and less perceived control over one's environment are all factors associated with lower insight (Lewin et al., 2010).

The other specifier in *DSM-5* relates to having a current or prior tic disorder. Many clinicians and researchers postulate that OCD with tics is a distinct condition in presentation, course, and treatment response, compared to OCD without tics. Prevalence estimates of those with OCD and comorbid tic disorders range from about 20 to 40 percent (Lewin et al., 2010).

Both insight and tic specifiers are important for treatment considerations and implications. Those with poorer insight tend to respond less well to standard OCD treatments. Similarly, individuals with OCD and comorbid tics tend to respond less well to selective serotonin reuptake inhibitor (SSRI) monotherapy, and may often require augmentation with dopaminergic agents (such as typical and/or atypical antipsychotics).

Factor analysis has been a useful tool in evaluating whether different symptom presentations in OCD have distinct clinical courses. In 2008, Bloch et al. completed a meta-analysis of factor analysis studies with over 5,000 participants, which yielded four consistent symptom factors in OCD (Bloch et al., 2008). These included *symmetry*: symmetry obsessions, and repeating, ordering, and counting compulsions; *forbidden thoughts*: aggressive, sexual, religious, and somatic obsessions, and checking compulsions; *cleaning*: contamination obsession and cleaning compulsions; and *hoarding*: hoarding obsessions and compulsions. Stewart et al. shortly thereafter demonstrated that although this four-factor model was imperfect and had limitations, it was overall adequate for use in children, adolescents, and adult age groups (Stewart et al., 2008). Since then, it has been shown that, for example, those with OCD and comorbid tics are more likely to have OCD symptoms in the symmetry and forbidden thoughts dimensions. Researchers are currently evaluating whether one's subtype corresponds to treatment response. In an early study, up to 90 percent of children and adolescents with OCD reported changes in the content and severity of their obsessions/compulsions over time (Rettew et al., 1992). However, because this study was completed prior to the development of symptom dimensions, it is not known whether the symptom instability was restricted to changes within dimensions (as is typically seen in adult studies), or across dimensions (Stewart et al., 2008). A more recent study by Fernandez de la Cruz et al. (2013) showed that within a pediatric population, shifts between one symptom dimension to another were rare, though changes within symptom dimensions were observed in ~15 to 45 percent of the subjects. They concluded that it is more the *severity* rather than the *content* of the symptoms that fluctuates over time.

Epidemiology

The lifetime prevalence of OCD in both children and adults is estimated to be around 1 to 3 percent (Stewart et al., 2004). The age of onset of OCD is bimodal, with the first peak occurring in late childhood/early adolescence, and the second peak occurring in young adulthood, around age 21. About half of all cases are thought to present during childhood/adolescence. The mean age of early-onset OCD is between 7.5 and 12.5 years and has a 3:2 male to female ratio (Geller, 2006). Within early-onset OCD, boys tend to have a slightly earlier onset than girls, with boys more often being pre-pubertal, and girls more often being peri-pubertal. Alternatively, adult-onset OCD has a more equal gender divide, with a slight female predominance.

There is some variance among researchers about what constitutes "early-onset," and as such, the defined age in studies has ranged from young childhood to late teens. This is important, because many consider "early-onset" OCD to be a distinct entity from adult-onset OCD, with more genetic loading, different likelihoods of specific subtypes, and increased comorbidities and tic disorders. Thus, more strictly defining the group in future studies will help to prevent confounding heterogeneity.

There is controversy around whether OCD is associated with higher or lower socioeconomic status (SES). A recent, large systematic review evaluating the contribution and association of certain environmental factors with OCD found inconsistent results (Brander et al., 2016). Of the 13 studies that evaluated SES, three showed an association with high SES, four showed an association with low SES, and five failed to show any association between SES and OCD (Brander et al., 2016). Interestingly, one cross sectional study from China showed that *both* low family income and higher education level independently doubled one's risk of having OCD (Lihua et al., 2014).

Etiology

OCD is a "multifactorial familial condition that involves both polygenic and environmental risk factors" (Pauls et al., 2014, p. 410). As such, the etiology of OCD is thought to be secondary to a combination of genetic, biological, and environmental risk factors. It is commonly believed that OCD is genetically complex and the result of multiple genes of small effect. Genes involved in the neurotransmitter systems (serotonin, dopamine, and glutamate), genes involved in neurodevelopment, and genes involved in immune responses have all been implicated (Sinopoli et al., 2017). No genes have met significance in genome-wide association studies (GWAS), but that is likely secondary to being underpowered to detect these genes of small effect. First-degree relatives of an individual with OCD have a 4 to 5 times greater chance of having OCD compared to first-degree relatives of someone without OCD (Mataix-

Cols et al., 2013). And of those first-degree relatives of someone with OCD, even more will have subthreshold obsessive-compulsive (OC) symptoms. One report estimated familial risk for a first-degree relative of an adult proband to be 12 percent, and the risk for a first-degree relative of a child proband to be about 25 percent (Brander et al., 2016). As such, age of onset is believed to be an important factor regarding genetic risk.

Early-onset OCD is associated with increased risk for tic disorders. In line with the theory that early-onset OCD and later onset OCD may represent somewhat distinct disorders, a recent cross-disorder genetics study suggested that OCD with comorbid tics may have a different and distinct genetic etiology compared to OCD alone (Yu et al., 2015).

Neuroimaging findings consistently implicate cortico-striato-thalamo-cortico (CSTC) circuitry (or loops) in OCD. The CTSC loops are believed to be involved in regulating executive functions, motor activity, emotions, problem solving, and cognitive tasks, including allocating attentional resources (Stahl, 2013). CSTC loops are implicated in movement disorders (e.g., Huntington's and Parkinson's), and in psychiatric disorders with primary difficulties in executive control and inhibition (e.g., OCD, TS, attention-deficit/hyperactivity disorder (ADHD)). The striatum (caudate and putamen), thalamus, anterior cingulate cortex, and orbitofrontal cortex, areas involved in habit formation, are the regions most often associated with OCD. Neurotransmitters involved in these circuits include dopamine, glutamate, serotonin, and GABA, which are all implicated in OCD, and targeted pharmacologically in the treatment of OCD. Of note, the CSTC areas that show increased activation in symptomatic OCD appear more typical after successful treatment, be it with medication or with therapy (Goodman et al., 2014).

While OCD is highly familial, most cases are still sporadic, i.e., with no first-degree family history. Heritability has been reported as 42 to 58 percent, indicating that only about half the risk for developing OCD derives from genes (Hudziak, 2004). As such, there has been considerable attention to epigenetic factors in the pre- and postnatal environment. Adverse perinatal events and other neurobiological and psychological trauma are all associated with increased risk of OCD. Adverse physiological or psychological events are hypothesized to modify expression of certain risk genes, leading to OC symptoms. One study reported that mothers of children with OCD had greater rates of illness in pregnancy requiring medical attention, and had more associated birth difficulties, including induction and/or prolonged labor, forceps delivery, and nuchal cord delivery (Geller et al., 2008). Cross-sectional studies have found that 25 to 65 percent of patients report stressful life events associated with OCD onset (Brander et al., 2016). Parents of children with OCD tend to have greater obsessive-compulsive personality traits, including perfectionism and preoccupation with details (Calvo et al., 2009).

OCD may also have infectious, autoimmune, endocrine, postpartum, trauma-related (i.e., traumatic brain injury), and postischemic etiologies. One proposed etiology of OCD symptoms currently receiving a lot of attention is PANDAS (Pediatric Autoimmune Neuropsychiatric Disorder Associated with Streptococcal Infection). PANDAS is characterized by the abrupt onset of OCD and other behavioral changes in a prepubertal youth often without any significant history of OCD and/or tic disorders. PANDAS, first described by Dr. Sue Swedo and colleagues at the NIMH in 1990, is hypothesized to be a postinfectious autoimmune disorder induced by a Group A Streptococcus (GAS) infection (Swedo et al., 1997). This theory was based on the long-established connection between OCD and a post-streptococcal neurologic disorder, Sydenham's chorea – known to be associated with sudden-onset OCD. The symptomatic course in those with PANDAS is thought to be more episodic than chronic (as seen in more typical OCD). The nosological entity of PANS (Pediatric Acute-onset Neuropsychiatric Syndromes) was created in 2010 to account for the many children who seemed to have an abrupt onset of OCD, but without a temporal link to Group A Streptococcus (Chang et al., 2013). In PANS, the cause might be infectious (e.g., mycoplasma-related), but it can also be metabolic, inflammatory and/or secondary to unknown factors. PANS is characterized by the sudden onset of OCD symptoms and/or eating restriction, along with other physical and behavioral ("ancillary") symptoms (Chang et al., 2013). However, unlike PANDAS, PANS is not associated with a sudden increase in tics, as tics have been observed to occur suddenly in a large portion of children without PANS/PANDAS symptomatology (Singer et al., 2000). Of note, the diagnoses of PANDAS and PANS have been cause for some controversy in the field given the current lack of biomarkers associated with either condition.

In a recent study, researchers found that of the patients referred to their specialty OCD clinic, about 5 percent met criteria for PANS and/or PANDAS (Jaspers-Fayer et al., 2017). With the exception of sometimes augmenting with anti-inflammatory agents (e.g., NSAIDS, steroids), antibiotics, and/or (in rare cases) immuno-modulatory treatments (e.g., IVIG), children with OCD secondary to PANS/PANDAS benefit from the same standard first-line treatments as those with more typical OCD (Chang et al., 2013). Practice guidelines for those with OCD secondary to PANDAS/PANS are being modified and updated as our understanding of PANDAS/PANS develops over time (Swedo, Frankovich, & Murphy, 2017). Whether children with PANDAS/PANS are ultimately found to have a distinct condition vs. a subtype of typical OCD is yet to be determined. New research showing increased inflammation in the brains of adults with OCD, and greater prevalence of OCD in youth with elevated rates of GAS, will continue to influence our thinking and understanding of the role of inflammation and autoimmune disorders in OCD (Attwells et al., 2017; Orlovska et al., 2017).

Neuropsychological Profile

While OCD has been associated with impairment in several neuropsychological subdomains, including planning, attention, inhibition, cognitive flexibility, memory, processing speed, and visuospatial functions, a large meta-analysis in 2015 found no specific or consistent deficits that met statistical significance (Abramovitch et al., 2015). Additionally, several studies have described abnormalities in neural activation without changes in behavioral performance, suggesting compensatory processes and/or inadequate behavioral probes (Gruner & Pittenger, 2017). Most recently, a large study with matched cases (*n*=102) and controls (*n*=161) reported underperformance in processing speed, and in visuospatial abilities and working memory during timed tasks. A direct relationship between OCD severity and working memory weaknesses was also noted (Geller et al., 2017). Although scores were still within the normative range, the measures indicated that in children with moderate-severe OCD (based on CY-BOCS scale scores), there were relative weaknesses compared to non–OCD children with similar demographic, educational, and comorbid psychiatric profiles. Because the scores fell within normal ranges, it could be easy to overlook the relative weaknesses that may still impact school performance in affected children (Geller et al., 2017).

Assessments

The gold standard for measuring OCD symptom severity is the Yale-Brown Obsessive Compulsive Scale (Y-BOCS) in adults, and the Children's Y-BOCS (CY-BOCS) in children and adolescents (Scahill et al., 1997; Goodman et al., 1989). Both scales are clinician-administered and interview-based and are designed to measure OCD severity without focusing on content or quantity of obsessive/compulsive symptoms. The wording in the CY-BOCS was adjusted to be more developmentally appropriate for children and adolescents. The scales have two components. The first, which is used to help establish diagnosis, is a detailed checklist of 50+ items commonly endorsed by those with OCD broken down by symptom category (Goodman et al., 1989). The second part characterizes and quantifies OCD severity by generating an obsessive sub-score and a compulsive sub-score based on five features of OC symptoms: time spent, interference, distress, resistance, and control. Several studies have found both the Y-BOCS and CY-BOCS to be reliable and valid, and to have high internal consistency. That said, both scales have limitations, including an overlap between resistance and control items, and a lower interrater agreement in the compulsion subscale and in younger children using the CY-BOCS (Scahill et al., 1997).

Differential Diagnosis

Diagnosing OCD in children can be especially difficult as many, if not all, children exhibit behavioral patterns and rituals as part of their normal development. For example, almost all young children will have a bedtime ritual. Many latency-aged children will develop "obsessions," or rather fixations on various collectible items, and may spend time repeatedly re-sorting them. Additionally, many children who play sports may wear a "lucky hat" or not want to change certain dirty clothing if they are on a winning streak. Ritualized behaviors are more concerning when they become more time-consuming and/or elaborate, disruptive to normal routine, bizarre or strange, create distress or frustration in the home, and/or need to be done to prevent adverse consequences (Chansky, 2000).

Some disorders are commonly misdiagnosed as OCD in children. Children may have repetitive actions and/or self-stimulatory behavior more consistent with an autism spectrum disorder (ASD) than OCD. Similarly, perseverative behaviors, restricted interests, and insistence on routines and sameness may be secondary to ASD rather than OCD. Ruminations and catastrophized worry about one's past and future may be more consistent with generalized anxiety; and frequent negative self-denying ruminations may be secondary to depression, especially in older children (Bloch & Storch, 2015). At times, it can be difficult to separate separation anxiety from OCD. Children with separation anxiety will have intense worries about leaving their caregiver and about their caregiver's health, but they would not engage in rituals to relieve anxiety or to prevent something bad from happening to the caregiver. Youth with BDD will have intrusive thoughts and compulsions, but these will be focused on a perceived flaw in their appearance or body part. Similarly, those with anorexia nervosa may engage in obsessions and compulsions related to food/eating, but the focus is on weight and/or thinness. Children with OCD will often confess thoughts of a suicidal, homicidal, sexual, or aggressive nature. Though these are typical, well-characterized symptoms of OCD, the clinician should additionally be sure to carefully screen for co-occurring mood disorders (with ego-syntonic suicidality), and/or a history of trauma, mood disorder, or conduct disorder.

Clinical Course of OCD

In children with OCD, "the clinical phenotype... is remarkably consistent at all ages with some allowances for developmental expression" (Geller, 2006, p. 365). Younger children more often have obsessions involving separation and fear of harm, compulsions without obsessions, and rituals involving family members, such as checking and reassurance seeking. Because children are often confused as to the nature of these ego-dystonic thoughts and urges, they will sometimes describe the OCD as a "voice in their head." Unless there are additional symptoms to think otherwise (e.g., disorganized thinking), one should be careful not to confuse this with psychosis. The clinician should also note that children tend to minimize their OCD symptoms, especially when compared to parental report. Youth also may show increased rates of hoarding compared to adults.

Adolescents with OCD tend to show more religious, sexual, and miscellaneous obsessions (Butwicka & Gmitrowicz, 2010). In general, children and adolescents with OCD experience pervasive slowness, increased responsibility, and pathological doubt (Masi et al., 2010).

In an early epidemiological study of OCD by Rasmussen and Eisen (1992), it was reported that about 5 to 10 percent of cases of OCD remit spontaneously (Rasmussen & Eisen, 1992). A more recent meta-analysis on long-term outcome of pediatric OCD by Stewart et al. (2004) of 521 participants from 16 studies, with follow-up periods ranging from 1 to 15.6 years, found that the persistence of pediatric OCD was lower than what had previously been expected (Stewart et al., 2004). The results painted a promising picture. OCD as a full clinical syndrome did not persist in most individuals. At the end-point, 60 percent exhibited only some symptoms of OCD, and 41 percent met clinical criteria for full remission. Factors that contributed to increased risk of persistence included younger age of onset, longer duration of illness at baseline, inpatient status, and psychiatric comorbidity. Increased family accommodation, which includes modifying typical family routines, facilitating patient avoidance, and engaging in compulsions with the child to reduce immediate distress, was also associated with worse functional impairment and poorer treatment response (Wu, McGuire, & Storch, 2016). In studies that measured psychosocial factors and function at longer-term follow-up, there were high rates of social dysfunction, single/unmarried status, and unemployment (Stewart et al., 2004).

Tic-Related OCD

As previously described, childhood onset, or "early-onset" OCD may represent a unique subtype of OCD compared to those with adult-onset. Early-onset OCD is associated with greater familial loading, increased tic disorders, male gender, and increased ADHD prevalence (Grados et al., 2001). In fact, the younger one is at age of onset, the greater the risk one has for comorbid ADHD, separation anxiety, phobias, agoraphobia, and multiple anxiety disorders (AACAP Practice Parameters, 2012).

Estimates suggest that 20 to 38 percent of youth with OCD have comorbid tics, called tic-related OCD (Lewin et al., 2010). Per a review by Neri & Cardona, 2013, obsessions in tic-related OCD were more related to sexual, violent, religious, and symmetry/evening out/arranging themes; as compared to contamination, fear of something going wrong, or fear of becoming ill in non-tic-related OCD. Compulsions in tic-related OCD were often related to checking, ordering, counting, repeating, touching, symmetry, needing to feel "just-right," and self-damage, versus cleaning and washing rituals in non-tic OCD (Neri & Cardona, 2013). Those with tic-related OCD also tend to increased prevalence of trichotillomania (Bienvenu et al., 2000).

A common symptom dimension in those with OCD and tics is "just-right" obsessions and compulsions. "Just-right" obsessions are described as thoughts or feelings about something feeling "not quite right," or incomplete. With just-right obsessions/compulsions, patients will often describe the need to "relieve discomfort," rather than reduce anxiety or prevent harm.

Comorbidity

In children and adolescents with OCD, comorbidity is the rule rather than the exception. In a 2010 study, Lewin et al. found that 85 percent of children with OCD had at least one comorbidity and up to 50 percent had multiple comorbidities (Lewin et al., 2010). As previously described, tic disorders were noted to be especially common, occurring in about 25 percent of children and about 10 percent of adolescents with OCD (Geller, 2006). ADHD was also very prevalent, occurring in 51 percent of children and 36 percent of adolescents (Geller 2006). Just as there appears to be a genetic link between OCD and tic disorders, there also appears to be a genetic link between OCD and ADHD, specifically in the pediatric population

(Geller et al., 2007). Anxiety disorders are common, especially separation anxiety disorder, which was seen in over 50 percent of children with OCD (Boileau, 2011). Thirty-nine percent of children and 62 percent of adolescents develop major depression at some point during their illness (Geller, 2006). Those with depression often have increased OCD symptom severity and OCD-related functional impairment. A study by Ivarsson in 2008 demonstrated a ~9 percent rate of oppositional defiant disorder (ODD) (Ivarsson, Melin, & Wallin, 2008). Those with disruptive behavior disorders, such as ADHD and ODD, in addition to OCD tended to also have greater internalizing problems and worse OCD severity. There has also been more research lately into the connection between OCD and PTSD and/or trauma exposure, as PTSD is also found to have an elevated prevalence in OCD (Lafleur et al., 2011). Autism traits are common in pediatric OCD even outside of those with clinical ASD diagnoses (Ivarsson & Melin, 2008). In a cross-sectional study with 813 consecutive OCD patients, sensory-related phenomena were present in 72 percent (Gomes de Alvarenga et al., 2012). Finally, rates of body-focused repetitive behaviors (TTM, excoriation disorder, severe nail biting) are elevated in those with OCD. The prevalence of TTM ranges between 4 and 36 percent and excoriation disorder ranges between 10 and 26 percent (Bienvenu et al., 2000).

Psychosocial Difficulties

In 1990 and again in 2005, the World Health Organization ranked OCD as one of the ten leading causes of disability worldwide (World Health Organization, 2005). OCD is often linked with increased functional impairment in the sufferer, increased family conflict and stress, and increased caregiver burden. Many youth with OCD have high levels of social and/or peer difficulties, and as they grow older, many have difficulties with isolation and/or unemployment (AACAP Practice Parameters, 2012). Treating OCD symptoms in children/adolescents is therefore essential to returning them to a normal developmental trajectory. Many of these children withdraw from peers, and/or refuse to spend time with other children if they are too busy completing compulsions or rituals.

In a clinically referred population of children and adolescents with OCD, almost 90 percent reported at least one significant OCD-related dysfunction, and almost 50 percent reported OCD-related problems at home, school, and/or socially (Piacentini et al., 2007). A comprehensive study by Lewin et al. showed that functional impairment in OCD was associated with low levels of insight, increased avoidance, pervasive slowness, and an excessive sense of responsibility (Lewin et al., 2010).

A multi-site study evaluating the effect of OCD on family functioning found that children and parents alike report significant impairments in family functioning, with worse impairment associated with worse OCD severity (Stewart et al., 2017). All family members also reported increased stress and anxiety, with parents additionally reporting increased sadness, and youth reporting increased frustration or anger. Of note, accommodation to the OCD most consistently predicted family impairment.

Treatment of OCD

Behavioral

There are behavioral and pharmacological treatments for OCD, and both are effective. Beginning with the work of Victor Meyer in 1966, the behavioral treatment of choice for OCD has been a specialized form of cognitive behavioral therapy (CBT), called Exposure and Response Prevention (ERP). CBT in OCD typically involves two components: "C" – cognitive restructuring or cognitive reappraisal, and "B" – behavioral intervention. ERP is predominantly behavioral and involves *exposing* the patient to symptom-specific stimuli to provoke their obsessions and the accompanying distress/anxiety, and then *preventing* their neutralizing *response* by asking them to abstain from their associated compulsion or avoidance behavior. Though the exact neural-mechanism of how ERP works remains uncertain, it relies on the premise that anxiety often attenuates after sufficient and repeated contact with a feared stimulus, i.e., a process termed habituation (Foa & Kozak, 1986). Another goal of this therapy is to help the patient learn to distinguish the OCD obsessions and compulsions as separate from their own interests and desires (i.e., externalizing the OCD). Children are often asked to give their OCD symptoms a name, such as the "OCD bug" or the "worry bully" to help with this task. The first technical CBT treatment manual for pediatric OCD was developed in 1998 by March and Mulle (March & Mulle, 1998). Since its development, numerous studies have shown both acceptability and efficacy (Abramowitz, Whiteside, & Deacon, 2006).

The cognitive therapy component for OCD focuses on reshaping maladaptive thoughts and faulty cognitions. Given the degree of cognitive distortions in OCD, some researchers/clinicians have postulated that a solely cognitive-therapy based approach to OCD could be effective. While it doesn't have the same strong evidence base as ERP, it may be a helpful alternative for those who don't respond to a more behaviorally based treatment (Williams et al., 2013). Conversely, in 2008, Bolton and Perrin eliminated the cognitive component and found that ERP alone was effective in reducing OCD symptoms (Bolton & Perrin, 2008).

Mean reductions in CY-BOCS scores with CBT range from 50 to 67 percent (Franklin et al., 2015). A meta-analysis of five randomized controlled trials (RCTs) with CBT for childhood OCD found the treatment to have an effect size of 1.45 (Watson & Rees, 2008). Though effect size may be moderated depending on whether there was an active control group, overall, the treatment is quite effective. Given its effectiveness, researchers and clinicians have been developing ways to modify the protocol for different populations (e.g., ages, OCD subtypes, more remote parts of countries) and to increase its dissemination.

In addition to individual-based CBT, there are also group-based, family-based, computer-based, and intensive CBT programs. Family-based CBT has been shown to be particularly effective for young children (ages 5–8) with OCD (Freeman et al., 2014). The goal of the family-based component is to help reduce levels of anger, blame, and guilt in the home, help the parent disengage from their child's OCD, increase the family's OCD-free interaction time, and help the family promote improvement and gains (Franklin et al., 2015). Group therapy CBT for pediatric OCD has also been shown to be effective. Web-based/telepsych-based treatment (live treatment though a web-cam) has inherent practical advantages regarding access to care and travel-related costs, and has been shown to be effective in at least one study in pediatric OCD, with 81 percent (of 16 patients) responding and 56 percent meeting remission criteria (of CY-BOCS <11) (Storch et al., 2011). A recent study examining cost-effectiveness of internet-delivered CBT for adolescents with OCD showed that compared to untreated controls (on a wait-list), those that underwent treatment demonstrated societal cost savings (Lenhard et al., 2017). A strategy to help with dissemination is a "supervision of supervisors" model, where clinicians conducting manual-guided CBT are given access to experts (Franklin et al., 2015). Intensive CBT, where the patient is treated with daily, rather than weekly sessions, has also been found to be effective, with some slight advantages seen immediately posttreatment (Storch et al., 2007).

CBT and ERP treatments are durable and remain effective at least nine months posttreatment (Franklin et al., 2015). In general, behavioral treatments for OCD have reduced relapse rates as compared to pharmacological approaches (Franklin et al., 2015). Those with lower initial OCD severity scores, less OCD-related impairment, greater insight, fewer comorbid externalizing symptoms, and lower levels of family accommodation tended to have greater levels of response to behavioral treatment. In contrast, patients with greater baseline OCD symptom severity and family psychopathology had poorer responses to CBT (Franklin et al., 2015).

Pharmacological

CBT should always be the first approach in the treatment of children and adolescents with OCD. However, patients who have CY-BOCS scores greater than 23 should additionally be evaluated for medication (AACAP Practice Parameters, 2012). Currently, serotonergic agents are the most effective pharmacologic treatment for OCD. SSRIs (selective serotonin reuptake inhibitors) are the first-line medication treatment for OCD. While the exact mechanisms of SSRIs are unknown, they are believed to exert their effect by blocking the reuptake of serotonin. This leads to increased accumulation of serotonin in the synapses (space between brain cells), and subsequent long-term changes in molecular expression of receptors / net decrease in synaptic serotonin transmission, which contributes to changes in mood and behavior. Side effects of SSRIs tend to be mild, but can include gastrointestinal, headache, sleep changes, and sexual side effects, among others. Another commonly used medication to treat OCD is clomipramine – a tricyclic antidepressant (TCA). In addition to serotonin, TCAs also block the reabsorption of norepinephrine and other chemical messengers. Clomipramine is the most serotonergic of all the TCAS. Unfortunately, clomipramine also has additional side effects, including weight gain, sedation, constipation, urinary retention, and dry mouth. In contrast to SSRIs, TCAs are also associated with risk of fatal overdose, lowered seizure threshold, and cardiac arrhythmia. FDA-approved medications in the United States for pediatric OCD include fluoxetine (SSRI), fluvoxamine (SSRI), sertraline (SSRI), and clomipramine (TCA).

Researchers have amassed more than 21 studies of medication trials over decades, and all show that serotonergic medications are effective in the short- and medium-term treatment of OCD (Geller et al., 2003). Pharmacotherapy typically leads to a 30 to 40 percent reduction in OCD symptoms (about a 6-point decrease on the CY-BOCS). A meta-analysis of all published medication RCTs in children and adolescents with OCD found an effect size of 0.46 (Geller et al., 2003). Geller et al. concluded that while clomipramine was superior to SSRIs in terms of symptom reduction, it should not be used as a first-line treatment for OCD because of its prominent side effect profile and risk of toxicity in overdose (Geller et al., 2003). The other SSRIs (fluoxetine, fluvoxamine, sertraline, and paroxetine) were all comparably effective. Although SNRIs (serotonin-norepinephrine reuptake inhibitors) have not been well-studied in treating OCD, given their similar mechanism, it is likely they would also have a positive effect on symptoms.

While research previously suggested that it might take many weeks to see clinical effects, new research shows that one might expect to see a benefit from SSRIs as early as two weeks after initiation (Varigonda, Jakubovski, & Bloch, 2016). That said, guidelines still recommend that an adequate trial of an SSRI in OCD should last no less than 10–12 weeks, with at least four weeks at the maximum tolerated dose (AACAP Practice Parameters, 2012). Bloch et al. conducted a meta-analysis that showed that higher doses of SSRIs are often associated with greater efficacy in OCD symptoms in adults (Bloch et al., 2010). While clinicians cannot directly generalize this finding to a pediatric population, titrating toward the maximum dose in child partial/nonresponder may still be a better option compared to switching to a medication with a potentially more serious side-effect profile. Optimal duration of treatment for children with OCD is unknown. Studies of SSRIs and clomipramine have shown that that treatment effect is typically maintained beyond 12 weeks. Adult studies show a 25 to 40 percent likelihood of relapse over the next six months even in those who continue pharmacotherapy (Neri & Cardona, 2013). Many clinicians and researchers recommend continuing treatment for an additional 6 to 12 months after symptom resolution or stabilization, and then slowly, over the course of weeks or months, tapering off.

While SSRIs are generally safe, effective, and well-tolerated, one needs to be extra cautious when treating a pediatric population. Compared with adolescents/young adults, prepubertal children are more likely to become "activated" (increased energy, irritability, aggression), and/or develop manic-like symptoms. Clinicians may need to balance the medication's positive effects on OCD/anxiety with the accompanying behavioral activation/disinhibition. One should also note that SSRIs come with a black box warning about suicide from the FDA. That said, there were no suicides in the RCTS for OCD involving SSRIs (Neri & Cardona, 2013), and a comprehensive analysis found no statistically significant increase of suicidal thinking or behavior in pooled pediatric OCD trials (Bridge et al., 2007). Finally, it is prudent to note that despite increasing long-term studies on SSRI use in children, researchers still have limited knowledge of what effect SSRIs (or any medication) may have on brain development.

The Pediatric OCD Treatment Study (POTS) was a landmark study in pediatric OCD. Given the effectiveness of both behavioral and pharmacological treatment in pediatric OCD, the objective of this large RCT was to evaluate the efficacy of CBT alone vs. pharmacological management alone (sertraline up to 200 mg daily) vs. CBT and pharmacological management combined vs. placebo in children and adolescents with OCD. One hundred twelve patients aged 7–17 were enrolled and were followed for 12 weeks. At the end of the 12 weeks, all three active treatments were significantly more efficacious in reducing symptoms (per CY-BOCS measure) compared to placebo (Pediatric OCD Treatment Study Team, 2004). The combined treatment group had a greater reduction in CY-BOCS score than either the CBT or sertraline groups alone. Regarding remission (defined as a CY-BOCS score less than or equal to 10), the combined group (54 percent) and the CBT group (39 percent) both outperformed the sertraline group (21 percent), which did not separate from placebo (4 percent) (Pediatric OCD Treatment Study Team, 2004). The results of POTS also suggested that using a combination of medication and CBT may help reduce the dose of sertraline required for symptom reduction. Interestingly, when children without a comorbid tic disorder were separated from those with a comorbid tic disorder, only the children without a comorbid tic disorder showed a significant reduction in symptoms with sertraline alone compared to placebo. The POTS trial resulted in the recommended guideline of starting ERP alone, or in combination with medication in children who have CY-BOCS > 23 and/or who are experiencing marked or severe distress (based on time occupied by OCD thoughts/compulsions, subjective distress, or functional limitations) (AACAP Practice Parameters, 2012).

Despite the recommendations from the POTS trial, given the dearth of CBT practitioners in the community, many primary care providers and child and adolescent psychiatrists were initiating SSRIs without initial or concurrent CBT treatment. Given that only 21 percent of patients in the sertraline-alone group had remission of symptoms, this was a serious issue, and led to the development of the POTS II RCT (Franklin et al., 2011). POTS II was designed to investigate the effectiveness of two CBT augmentation protocols in children who were partial responders to SRIs monotherapy (serotonin reuptake inhibitors – e.g., SSRIs and clomipramine). One group received medication management and OCD-specific CBT delivered by a psychologist, one group received medication management and instructions in CBT delivered by the treating MD, and the third group did not receive any CBT-based augmentation.

One hundred twenty-four 7- to 17-year-old youth with CY-BOCS >15 (despite an adequate SRI trial) were enrolled in the 12-week study. 69 percent in the psychologist-delivered CBT group had at least a 30 percent reduction in symptoms, compared to 34 percent in the CBT-instruction group, and 30 percent in the medication-only group (Franklin et al., 2011). The psychologist-delivered CBT outperformed the medication only group, whereas the group who received CBT instructions only did not. It was therefore concluded that developing ways to disseminate full CBT augmentation for pediatric OCD partial responders should be an important public health objective (Franklin et al., 2011). Secondary improvements in anxiety, inattention, hyperactivity, and quality of life were greatest in patients who received the full CBT augmentation treatment (Conelea et al., 2017)

About one-fourth to one-third of children don't experience effective treatment response with first-line treatments for OCD (Bloch & Storch, 2015). And, many of the ones who do respond continue to have residual symptoms. Per Bloch and Storch, treatment-refractory OCD is characterized by failing to have adequate symptom relief despite at least two trials of (adequately dosed) SSRIs or clomipramine, and an (adequate) course of CBT (Bloch & Storch, 2015). For patients who appear treatment-refractory, initial steps include confirming the OCD diagnosis, ensuring that the patient has had adequate medication trials, and if taking medication, ensuring that they are taking it consistently and as directed.

Numerous factors contribute to certain patients being particularly difficult to treat. Regarding CBT, the number of comorbid conditions, and comorbid ADHD and depression are associated with worse outcomes (Storch et al., 2008). Regarding medication (especially SSRIs), having comorbid tics is associated with reduced symptom improvement. Similarly, co-occurring ADHD is associated with worse OCD treatment response from SSRIs (improving if the ADHD is treated). In a study conducted by Geller et al. in 2003, the response rates of those with comorbid ADHD or tic disorder were 56 percent and 53 percent, respectively, compared to 75 percent of patients with OCD only (Geller et al., 2003). Having more comorbid conditions was also associated with a greater rate of relapse (Geller et al., 2003).

Factors associated with predicting a poorer response to treatment in general include comorbid tics, hoarding symptoms, poor insight, and increased parental accommodation (Bloch & Storch, 2015). Of note, although OCD with tics is less responsive to SSRI treatment compared to OCD symptoms without comorbid tics, it is equally responsive to CBT treatment. Hoarding, which is seen in up to 25 percent of youth with OCD, has a poor prognosis in both adults and children, and has been found to respond more poorly to both SSRI treatment and CBT (Samuels et al., 2014). Thirty to 40 percent of children with OCD have poor or limited insight, which is also associated with worse CBT and pharmacologic treatment outcomes (Bloch & Storch, 2015). Given that insight tends to improve with age, in cases of limited insight, time is often the best solution. Finally, family accommodation, although not linked with severity of OCD symptoms, is associated with worse treatment response. In cases of family accommodation, family involvement in treatment is recommended, and improvement in accommodation is associated with improvement in OCD symptoms posttreatment (Storch et al., 2010).

Clinical standards and data from smaller trials currently guide augmentation principles for partial- and/or nonresponders to first-line OCD treatments. If the individual is not already in CBT, CBT should be added. As per the POTS II trial, adding weekly CBT to a stable SRI regimen led to significantly improved response rates in 69 percent of youth (compared to 30 percent with no addition) (Franklin et al., 2011). Augmenting with intensive CBT (daily sessions for three weeks) was also shown to be quite helpful, as 80 percent of the children/adolescents improved

(Storch et al., 2010). In children/adolescents who are partial responders to a maximum SSRI dose, if there are no/minimal side effects, one could prudently increase the dose. Indeed, adult studies showed that increasing the dose of SSRI past the FDA-recommended amount resulted in increased symptom improvement (Bloch et al., 2010). In patients who have failed one to two trials of adequately dosed SSRIs, switching to clomipramine may be considered.

Augmenting SSRIs with clomipramine or antipsychotic medications is a well-studied and effective strategy in adults with treatment-refectory OCD, and is an augmentation strategy often used in children as well. Oftentimes adding a small dose of clomipramine (<75 mg) to an SSRI can be helpful (Bloch & Storch, 2015). However, one needs to be careful when adding clomipramine to SSRIs due to risk of serotonin syndrome, elongated QTc (a measure of electrical conductance of the heart), and due to enzyme-related (cytochrome P450 (CYP)) interactions. Of note, augmenting fluvoxamine with clomipramine may be particularly helpful as fluvoxamine inhibits the CYP enzyme that converts clomipramine to its (more noradrenergic) metabolite, keeping it more serotonergic and leading to a synergistic effect.

Whereas SRIs affect serotonin modulation, antipsychotics primarily affect dopamine modulation. AACAP Practice parameters for pediatric OCD recommends that for those with OCD with tics, poor insight, mood instability, and what was formerly known as "pervasive developmental disorder" (now autism spectrum disorder), augmentation with a neuroleptic (antipsychotic) should be considered (AACAP Practice Parameters, 2012). The most commonly used antipsychotic augmenting agents include aripiprazole, risperidone, haloperidol, quetiapine, and olanzapine, and they are typically used in modest/low doses. Other than haloperidol, these medications are known as "atypical antipsychotics" because they modulate both dopamine and serotonin, compared to typical antipsychotics (e.g., haloperidol), which only modulate dopamine. Atypical antipsychotics ("atypicals") have a somewhat restrictive side effect profile, including gastrointestinal symptoms, akathisia, blurred vision, fatigue/sedation, and "metabolic syndrome" – a group of factors that raise one's risk for heart disease, diabetes, and stroke, and include: large waistline, high triglyceride level, low HDL level, high blood pressure, and high fasting blood sugar. A meta-analysis with 278 adult patients conducted by Bloch et al. showed that overall, antipsychotic augmentation led to a greater treatment response compared to placebo (32 percent vs. 11 percent) (Bloch et al., 2006). Risperidone and haloperidol demonstrated strong evidence for efficacy in augmentation, whereas quetiapine and olanzapine failed to demonstrate efficacy (Bloch et al., 2006). A subsequent trial with aripiprazole showed positive efficacy in OCD symptom reduction in adults (Sayyah et al., 2012). Bloch et al. also showed that it is important to wait the full three months on a maximally tolerated SSRI dose before augmenting, as some patients continued to have a treatment response 2 to 3 months after initiation of SSRIs (Bloch et al., 2006). However, unlike SSRIs, patients who did not respond after one month with an antipsychotic were unlikely to improve. One should also be cautious about augmenting with an atypical if there is not already CBT in place, as CBT has outperformed atypical augmentation in at least one adult trial (Simpson et al., 2013).

Though many new compounds and treatment strategies have been tried, none thus far has been as effective as SRIs. Glutamate is a primary neurotransmitter in CTSC circuitry and has been implicated in pathogenesis of OCD. As such, there has been substantial research into the efficacy and tolerability of glutamate-based agents. Examples of glutamatergic agents include riluzole, memantine, topiramate, lamotrigine, and N-acetylcysteine. While riluzole was promising in uncontrolled studies, it was not better than placebo in an augmentation trial in children (Grant et al., 2014). Memantine was found to be superior in augmenting fluvoxamine compared to placebo in adults but has not been trialed in children (Stewart et al., 2010). Topiramate, a widely used antiepileptic and glutamatergic agent, showed mixed results in adult trials but has not been tested in children (Bloch & Storch, 2015). That said, topiramate has been shown to be helpful in treating tic-symptoms in children, and thus may be a potential augmenting agent given the association between tics and childhood-onset OCD. Lamotrigine, a very effective antiepileptic mood stabilizer, has been shown in at least one double-blinded RCT to substantially improve OCD (and mood) symptoms when added to an SRI in a treatment-resistant adult population (Bruno et al., 2012). N-acetylcysteine (NAC) is an amino acid, and a natural antioxidant with a very limited side effect profile. Adult studies have shown some positive effect of NAC monotherapy on OCD (and trichotillomania) symptoms; however, a pediatric study using NAC as monotherapy was negative (Bruno et al., 2012). That said, a group from Iran recently evaluated the effect of augmenting citalopram with NAC in a pediatric population and found that it improved resistance/control to compulsions better than placebo (Ghanizadeh et al., 2017). Overall findings have been mixed, but NAC may continue to play a role in the treatment of pediatric OCD treatment in the future.

D-Cycloserine (DCS), an antibiotic with glutamatergic properties, initially showed promise in augmenting OCD treatment. Early studies demonstrated enhanced extinction effects when used in combination with ERP. A pilot RCT in children even showed positive results; however, in a recent placebo-controlled RCT with 142 youth, augmentation of CBT with DCS did not improve OCD symptoms better than placebo (Storch et al., 2016). Ultimately, although no glutamatergic agents have proven sufficiently effective as to be incorporated into standard of care, given the positive studies, and their well-tolerated side effect profile, they continue to be worth considering, especially when other first-line options have failed.

Benzodiazepines are occasionally used early in OCD treatment to reduce the severe anxiety some OCD sufferers experience prior to benefiting from SRIs or CBT. However, at least in adult trials, they have not been shown to be effective for reducing OCD symptoms long-term or as an adjunctive therapy (Bloch & Storch, 2015). One needs to be especially vigilant if using benzodiazepines in children as they can lead to paradoxical disinhibition and/or activation.

There have been advancements in the role of neuro-modulatory and neurosurgical treatment options for OCD in the last few years. However, one should be extremely careful if considering using any permanent neurologic intervention in pediatric OCD given the higher rate of remission as compared to adults. In adults, ablative procedures typically include anterior cingulotomy, capsulotomy, subacute tractotomy, and limbic leucotomy. Deep brain stimulation (DBS) has shown some efficacy in adult cross-over trials and has the benefit of being reversible. Transcranial magnetic stimulation (TMS) is a noninvasive technique that involves using magnet strips (placed on the scalp) to induce electrical activity in the cortex underlying the magnets. A recent meta-analysis showed that TMS was superior to sham treatments for OCD symptoms in adults (Trevizol et al., 2016); however, again, there have been limited studies in children.

Future Directions

Now that we have reviewed the epidemiology and current treatment of OCD, what about the future? One new direction is exploring the connection between OCD symptoms and inflammation. In a recent study, researchers using PET scans demonstrated inflammation in the OCD-related CSTC circuit (Attwells et al., 2017). This finding may put into question practitioners' primary reliance on serotonergic medications and may pave the way for more immunomodulatory treatments.

Personalized medicine may also be in the future for the treatment of OCD. Determining whether a patient would benefit more strongly from medication or CBT could reduce time, money, and distress in both patients and practitioners. A recent study by Olatunji et al. showed through neuroimaging that those who had better responses to CBT for contamination-based OCD had more successful recruitment of limbic regions when exposed to threat cues (Olatunji et al., 2014).

While we need to continue researching new pharmacologic and neuro-modulatory options, we also need to augment our research into the safety and effectiveness of our current treatments in a pediatric population.

Research on CBT for pediatric OCD has blossomed over the last couple of decades. Given the "third wave" of CBT approaches, including acceptance and commitment therapy (ACT), dialectical behavior therapy (DBT), metacognitive therapy, and mindfulness-based cognitive therapy (MBCT), it will be interesting to see whether any of these therapies can successfully augment current treatments. There is some evidence that ACT can be helpful in youth with anxiety disorders, but it has not yet been tested in an OCD population (Park & Geller, 2014). Motivational interviewing, a technique that relies on exploring ambivalence and eliciting motivation for change, may be additionally beneficial to typical ERP. However, it has shown mixed results thus far (Franklin et al., 2015). Another behavioral technique, EMDR (eye movement desensitization and reprocessing), has recently shown to have comparable rates to CBT in a small RCT (Marsden et al., 2017). With technology playing such a significant role in our lives right now, app-based treatments, either with access to a live therapist or not, may be crucial to future CBT dissemination.

Franklin et al. lays out several future goals for the field of pediatric OCD research (Franklin et al., 2015). These include more trials comparing medication, CBT, the combination thereof, and in what order, comparing individual vs. family-based treatments, developing theory-driven studies, understanding the relative contributions of cognitive vs. behavioral components, developing treatments for the OCD subtypes, developing innovations to target specific comorbid factors, understanding the impact of our treatments in real-world settings, and learning to better manage partial responders or nonresponders. These ideas and more will help pave the way for future pediatric OCD-related research and treatments.

Acknowledgments

The Authors wish to acknowledge the contribution of Rachel Porth, B.A., research coordinator for the Pediatric OCD Program, for her assistance with manuscript preparation.

References

AACAP Practice Parameters. (2012). Obsessive-compulsive disorder. *Journal of the American Academy of Child & Adolescent Psychiatry.*

Abramovitch, A., Mittelman, A., Tankersley, A.P., Abramowitz, J.S., & Schweiger, A. (2015). Neuropsychological investigations in obsessive-compulsive disorder: A systematic review of methodological challenges. *Psychiatry Res., 228*(1), 112–120.

Abramowitz, J.S., Whiteside, S.P., & Deacon, B.J. (2006). The effectiveness of treatment for pediatric obsessive-compulsive disorder: A meta-analysis. *Behavior Therapy, 36,* 55–63.

American Psychiatric Association (2013). *Diagnostic and statistical manual of mental disorders (DSM-5)* (5th ed.). Washington, DC: American Psychiatric Association.

Attwells, S., Setiawan, E., Wilson, A.A., Rusjan, P.M., Mizrahi, R., Miler, L., & Meyer, J.H. (2017). Inflammation in the neurocircuitry of obsessive-compulsive disorder. *JAMA Psychiatry, 74*(8), 833–840.

Bienvenu, O.J., Samuels, J.F., Riddle, M.A., Hoehn-Saric, R., Liang, K.Y., Cullen, B.A., ... Nestadt, G. (2000) The relationship of obsessive-compulsive disorder to possible spectrum disorders: Results from a family study. *Biol Psychiatry, 48*(4), 287–293.

Bloch, M.H., Landeros-Weisenberger, A., Kelmendi, B., Coric, V., Bracken, M.B., & Leckman, J.F. (2006). A systematic review: Antipsychotic augmentation with treatment refractory obsessive-compulsive disorder. *Mol Psychiatry, 11*(7), 622–632.

Bloch, M.H., Landeros-Weisenberger, A., Rosario, M.C., Pittenger, C., & Leckman, J.F. (2008). Meta-analysis of the symptom structure of obsessive-compulsive disorder. *Am J Psychiatry, 165,* 1532–1542.

Bloch, M.H., McGuire, J., Landeros-Weisenberger, A., Leckman, J.F., & Pittenger, C. (2010). Meta-analysis of the dose-response relationship of SSRI in obsessive-compulsive disorder. *Molecular Psychiatry, 15*(8), 850–855.

Bloch, M.H., Panza, K.E., Yaffa, A., Alvarenga, P.G., Jakubovski, E., Mulqueen, J.M., ... Leckman, J.F. (2016). N-Acetylcysteine in the treatment of pediatric Tourette syndrome: Randomized, double-blind, placebo-controlled add-on trial. *J Child Adolesc Psychopharmacol., 26*(4), 327–334.

Bloch, M.H., & Storch, E.A. (2015). Assessment and management of treatment-refractory obsessive-compulsive disorder in children. *J Am Acad Child Adolesc Psychiatry, 54*(4), 251–262.

Boileau, B. (2011). A review of obsessive-compulsive disorder in children and adolescents. *Dialogues Clin Neurosci., 13*(4), 401–411.

Bolton, D., & Perrin, S. (2008). Evaluation of exposure with response-prevention for obsessive compulsive disorder in childhood and adolescence. *Journal of Behavior Therapy and Experimental Psychiatry, 39,* 11–22.

Brander, G., Pérez-Vigil, A., Larsson, H., & Mataix-Cols, D. (2016). Systematic review of environmental risk factors for obsessive-compulsive disorder: A proposed roadmap from association to causation. *Neurosci Biobehav Rev., 65,* 36–62.

Bridge, J.A., Iyengar, S., Salary, C.B., Barbe, R.P., Birmaher, B., Pincus, H.A., . . . Brent, D.A. (2007). Clinical response and risk for reported suicidal ideation and suicide attempts in pediatric antidepressant treatment: A meta-analysis of randomized controlled trials. *JAMA, 297*(15), 1683–1696.

Bruno, A., Micò, U., Pandolfo, G., Mallamace, D., Abenavoli, E., Di Nardo, F., . . . Muscatello, M.R. (2012). Lamotrigine augmentation of serotonin reuptake inhibitors in treatment-resistant obsessive-compulsive disorder: A double-blind, placebo-controlled study. *J Psychopharmacol., 26*(11), 1456–1462.

Butwicka A., & Gmitrowicz, A. (2010). Symptoms clusters in obsessive-compulsive disorder: Influence of age and age of onset. *Eur Child Adolesc Psychiatry, 19,* 365–370.

Calvo, R., Lazaro, L., Castro-Fornieles, J., Font, E., Moreno, E., & Toro, J. (2009). Obsessive-compulsive personality disorder traits and personality dimensions in parents of children with obsessive-compulsive disorder. *Eur Psychiatry, 24,* 201–206.

Chang, K., Frankovich, J., Cooperstock, M., Cunningham, M.W., Latimer, M.E., Murphy, T.K., . . . PANS Collaborative Consortium. (2015). Clinical evaluation of youth with pediatric acute-onset neuropsychiatric syndrome (PANS): Recommendations from the 2013 PANS Consensus Conference. *J Child Adolesc Psychopharmacol., 25*(1), 3–13.

Chansky, T. (2000). *Freeing your child from OCD.* Crown Publishers.

Conelea, C.A., Selles, R.R., Benito, K.G., Walther, M.M., Machan, J.T., Garcia, A.M., & Freeman, J.B. (2017). Secondary outcomes from the pediatric obsessive compulsive disorder treatment study II. *J Psychiatr Res., 92,* 94–100.

Fernandez de la Cruz, L., Micali, N., Roberts, S., Turner, C., Nakatani, E., Heyman, I., & Mataix-Cols, D. (2013). Are the symptoms of obsessive-compulsive disorder temporally stable in children/adolescents? A prospective naturalistic study. *Psychiatry Research, 209,* 196–201.

Foa, E.B., & Kozak, M.J. (1986). Emotional processing of fear: Exposure to corrective information. *Psychol Bull., 99*(1), 20–35.

Franklin, M.E., Kratz, H.E., Freeman, J.B., Ivarsson, T., Heyman, I., Sookman, D., . . . March, J. (2015). Accreditation Task Force of The Canadian Institute for Obsessive Compulsive Disorders. Cognitive-behavioral therapy for pediatric obsessive-compulsive disorder: Empirical review and clinical recommendations. *Psychiatry Res., 227*(1), 78–92.

Franklin, M.E., Sapyta, J., Freeman, J.B., Khanna, M., Compton, S., Almirall, D., . . . March, J.S. (2011). Cognitive behavior therapy augmentation of pharmacotherapy in pediatric obsessive-compulsive disorder: The pediatric OCD treatment study II (POTS II) randomized controlled trial. *Journal of the American Medical Association, 306,* 1224–1232.

Freeman, J., Sapyta, J., Garcia, A., Compton, S., Khanna, M., Flessner, C., . . . Franklin, M. (2014). Family-based treatment of early childhood obsessive-compulsive disorder:

The Pediatric Obsessive-Compulsive Disorder Treatment Study for Young Children (POTS Jr)–A randomized clinical trial. *JAMA Psychiatry, 71*(6), 689–698.

Geller, D.A. (2006). Obsessive-compulsive and spectrum disorders in children and adolescents. *Psychiat Clin N Am., 29*, 353–370.

Geller, D.A., Abramovitch, A., Mittelman, A., Stark, A., Ramsey, K., Cooperman, A., & Stewart, S.E. (2017). Neurocognitive function in paediatric obsessive-compulsive disorder. *World J Biol Psychiatry*, 1–10.

Geller, D.A., Biederman, J., Stewart, S.E., Mullin, B., Farrell, C., Wagner, K.D., ... Carpenter, D. (2003). Impact of comorbidity on treatment response to paroxetine in pediatric obsessive-compulsive disorder: Is the use of exclusion criteria empirically supported in randomized clinical trials? *J Child Adolesc Psychopharmacol., 13*, Suppl 1: S19–29.

Geller, D.A., Biederman, J., Stewart, S.E., Mullin, B., Martin, A., Spencer, T., & Faraone, S.V. (2003). Which SSRI? A meta-analysis of pharmacotherapy trials in pediatric obsessive-compulsive disorder. *Am J Psychiatry, 160*(11), 1919–1928.

Geller, D., Petty, C., Vivas, F., Johnson, J., Pauls, D., & Biederman, J. (2007). Examining the relationship between obsessive-compulsive disorder and attention-deficit/hyperactivity disorder in children and adolescents: A familial risk analysis. *Biol Psychiatry, 61*(3), 316–321.

Geller, D.A., Wieland, N., Carey, K., Vivas, F., Petty, C.R., Johnson, J., ... Biederman, J. (2008). Perinatal factors affecting expression of obsessive compulsive disorder in children and adolescents. *J Child Adoles Psychopharmacol., 18*(4), 373–379.

Ghanizadeh, A., Mohammadi, M.R., Bahraini, S., Keshavarzi, Z., Firoozabadi, A., & Alavi Shoshtari, A. (2017). Efficacy of N-Acetylcysteine augmentation on obsessive compulsive disorder: A multicenter randomized double blind placebo controlled clinical trial. *Iran J Psychiatry, 12*(2), 134–141.

Gomes de Alvarenga, P., de Mathis, M.A., Dominguez Alves, A.C., do Rosário, M.C., Fossaluza, V., Hounie, A.G., ... Rodrigues Torres, A. (2012). Clinical features of tic-related obsessive-compulsive disorder: Results from a large multicenter study. *CNS Spectr., 17*(2), 87–93.

Goodman, W.K., Grice, D.E., Lapidus, K.A., & Coffey, B.J. (2014). Obsessive-compulsive disorder. *Psychiatr Clin North Am., 37*(3), 257–267.

Goodman, W.K., Price, L.H., Rasmussen, S.A., Mazure, C., Fleischmann, R.L., Hill, C.L., ... Charney, D.S. (1989). The Yale-Brown obsessive compulsive scale. I. Development, use, and reliability. *Arch Gen Psychiatry, 46*, 1006–1011.

Grados, M.A., Riddle, M.A., Samuels, J.F., Liang, K.Y., Hoehn-Saric, R., Bienvenu, O.J., ... Nestadt, G. (2001). The familial phenotype of obsessive-compulsive disorder in relation to tic disorders: The Hopkins OCD family study. *Biological Psychiatry, 50*, 559–565.

Grant, P.J., Joseph, L.A., Farmer, C.A., Luckenbaugh, D.A., Lougee, L.C., Zarate, C.A. Jr., & Swedo, S.E. (2014). 12-week, placebo-controlled trial of add-on riluzole in the treatment of childhood-onset obsessive-compulsive disorder. *Neuropsychopharmacology, 39*(6), 1453–1459.

Gruner, P. & Pittenger, C. (2017). Cognitive inflexibility in obsessive-compulsive disorder. *Neuroscience, 345*, 243–255.

Hudziak, J.J., Van Beijsterveldt, C.E., Althoff, R.R. Stanger, C., Rettew, D.C., Nelson, E.C., ... Boomsma, D.I. (2004). Genetic and environmental contributions to the child behavior checklist obsessive-compulsive scale: A cross-cultural twin study. *Arch Gen Psychiatry, 61*, 608–616.

Ivarsson, T., & Melin, K. (2008). Autism spectrum traits in children and adolescents with obsessive-compulsive disorder (OCD). *J Anxiety Disord., 22*(6), 969–978.

Ivarsson, T., Melin, K., & Wallin, L. (2008). Categorical and dimensional aspects of co-morbidity in obsessive-compulsive disorder (OCD). *Eur Child Adolesc Psychiatry, 17*(1), 20–31.

Jaspers-Fayer, F., Han, S.H.J., Chan, E., McKenney, K., Simpson, A., Boyle, A., ... Stewart, S.E. (2017). Prevalence of acute-onset subtypes in pediatric obsessive-compulsive disorder. *J Child Adolesc Psychopharmacol. 27*(4), 332–341.

Lafleur, D.L., Petty, C., Mancuso, E., McCarthy, K., Biederman, J., Faro, A., ... Geller, D.A. (2011). Traumatic events and obsessive compulsive disorder in children and adolescents: Is there a link? *J Anxiety Disord., 25*(4), 513–519.

Lenhard, F., Ssegonja, R., Andersson, E., Feldman, I., Rück, C., Mataix-Cols, D., & Serlachius, E. (2017). Cost-effectiveness of therapist-guided internet-delivered cognitive behaviour therapy for paediatric obsessive-compulsive disorder: Results from a randomised controlled trial. *BMJ Open., 7*(5), e015246.

Lewin, A.B., Bergman, R.L., Peris, T.S., Chang, S., McCracken, J.T., & Piacentini J. (2010). Correlates of insight among youth with obsessive-compulsive disorder. *Journal of Child Psychology and Psychiatry, and Allied Disciplines, 51*(5), 603–611.

Lewin, A.B., Caporino, N., Murphy, T.K., Geffken, G.R., & Storch, E.A. (2010). Understudied clinical dimensions in pediatric obsessive compulsive disorder. *Child Psychiatry Hum Dev., 41*, 675–691.

Lewin, A.B., Chang, S., McCracken, J., McQueen, M., & Piacentini, J. (2010). Comparison of clinical features among youth with tic disorders, obsessive-compulsive disorder (OCD), and both conditions. *Psychiatry Res, 178*, 317–322.

Lihua, M., Tao, Z., SiYong, H., Suwen, W., Xiaoxuan, Y., Yichen, G., ... Yan, B. (2014). Obsessive compulsive disorder in general hospital outpatients: Prevalence, correlates, and comorbidity in Lanzhou, China. *Asia Pac Psychiatry, 6*(3), 308–318.

March, J. & Mulle, K. (1998). *OCD in children and adolescents: A cognitive-behavioral treatment manual.* New York: Guilford Press.

Marsden, Z., Lovell, K., Blore, D., Ali, S., & Delgadillo, J. (2017). A randomized controlled trial comparing EMDR and CBT for obsessive-compulsive disorder. *Clin Psychol Psychother.*

Masi, G., Millepiedi, S., Perugi, G., Pfanner, C., Berloffa, S., Pari, C., ... Akiskal, H.S. (2010). A naturalistic exploratory study of the impact of demographic, phenotypic and comorbid features in pediatric obsessive-compulsive disorder. *Psychopathology, 43*, 69–79.

Mataix-Cols, D., Boman, M., Monzani, B., Rück, C., Serlachius, E., Långström, N., & Lichtenstein, P. (2013). Population-based, multigenerational family clustering study of obsessive-compulsive disorder. *JAMA Psychiatry, 70*(7), 709–717.

Neri, V., & Cardona, F. (2013). Chapter 13 – "Clinical pharmacology of comorbid obsessive-compulsive disorder in Tourette syndrome," in D. Martino and A. E. Cavanna, (eds.), *International review of neurobiology: Advances in the neurochemistry and neuropharmacology of Tourette syndrome*, volume 112, Boston: Elsevier.

Neri V., & Cardona, F. (2013). Clinical pharmacology of comorbid obsessive-compulsive disorder in Tourette syndrome. *Int Rev Neurobiol., 112*, 391–414.

Olatunji, B.O., Ferreira-Garcia, R., Caseras, X., Fullana, M.A., Wooderson, S., Speckens, A., ... Mataix-Cols. D. (2014). Predicting response to cognitive behavioral therapy in contamination-based obsessive-compulsive disorder from functional magnetic resonance imaging. *Psychol Med.*, *44*(10), 2125–2137.

Orlovska, S., Vestergaard, C.H., Bech, B.H., Nordentoft, M., Vestergaard, M., & Benros, M.E. (2017). Association of streptococcal throat infection with mental disorders: Testing key aspects of the PANDAS hypothesis in a nationwide Study. *JAMA Psychiatry*, *74*(7), 740–746.

Park, J.M., & Geller, D.A. (2014). Novel approaches in treatment of pediatric anxiety. *F1000Prime Rep.*, *6*, 30.

Pauls, D.L., Abramovitch, A., Rauch, S.L., & Geller, D.A. (2014). Obsessive-compulsive disorder: An integrative genetic and neurobiological perspective. *Nat Rev Neurosci.*, *15*(6), 410–424.

Pediatric OCD Treatment Study Team. (2004). Cognitive-behavioral therapy, sertraline, and their combination for children and adolescents with obsessive-compulsive disorder: The pediatric OCD treatment study (POTS) randomized controlled trial. *Journal of the American Medical Association*, *292*, 1969–1976.

Piacentini, J., Peris, T.S., Bergman, R.L., Chang, S., & Jaffer, M. (2007). Functional impairment in childhood OCD: Development and psychometrics properties of the Child Obsessive-Compulsive Impact Scale-Revised (COIS-R). *J Clin Child Adolesc Psychol.*, *36*(4), 645–653.

Rasmussen, S.A., & Eisen, J.L. (1992). The epidemiology and clinical features of obsessive compulsive disorder. *Psychiatr Clin North Am*, *15*(4), 743–758.

Rettew, D.C., Swedo, S.E., Leonard, H.L., Lenane, M.C., & Rapoport, J.L. (1992). Obsessions and compulsions across time in 79 children and adolescents with obsessive-compulsive disorder. *J Am Acad Child Adolesc Psychiatry*, *31*(6), 1050–1056.

Samuels, J., Grados, M.A., Riddle, M.A., Bienvenu, O.J., Goes, F.S., Cullen, B., ... Nestadt, G. (2014). Hoarding in children and adolescents with obsessive-compulsive disorder. *J Obsessive Compuls Relat Disord*, *3*(4), 325–331.

Sayyah, M., Sayyah, M., Boostani, H., Ghaffari, S.M., & Hoseini, A. (2012). Effects of aripiprazole augmentation in treatment-resistant obsessive-compulsive disorder (a double blind clinical trial). *Depress Anxiety.* *29*(10), 850–854.

Scahill, L., Riddle, M.A., McSwiggin-Hardin, M., Ort, S.I., King, R.A., Goodman, W.K., ... Leckman, J.F. (1997). Children's Yale-Brown Obsessive Compulsive Scale: Reliability and validity. *Journal of the American Academy of Child and Adolescent Psychiatry*, *36*, 844–852.

Simpson, H.B., Foa, E.B., Liebowitz, M.R., Huppert, J.D., Cahill, S., Maher, M.J., ... Campeas, R. (2013). Cognitive-behavioral therapy vs risperidone for augmenting serotonin reuptake inhibitors in obsessive-compulsive disorder: A randomized clinical trial. *JAMA Psychiatry*, *70*(11), 1190–1199.

Singer, H.S., Giuliano, J.D., Zimmerman, A.M., & Walkup, J.T. (2000). Infection: A stimulus for tic disorders. *Pediatr Neurol*, *22*, 380–383.

Sinopoli, V.M., Burton, C.L., Kronenberg, S., & Arnold, P.D. (2017). A review of the role of serotonin system genes in obsessive-compulsive disorder. *Neurosci Biobehav Rev.*, *80*, 372–381.

Stahl, S.M. (2013). Chapter 7 Circuits in psychopharmacology. *Stahl's Essential Psychopharmacology* (4th edn.). Cambridge University Press.

Stewart, S.E., Geller, D.A., Jenike, M., Pauls, D., Shaw, D., Mullin, B., & Faraone, S.V. (2004). Long-term outcome of pediatric obsessive-compulsive disorder: A meta-analysis and qualitative review of the literature. *Acta Psychiatrica Scandinavica, 110*, 4–13.

Stewart, S.E., Hu, Y.P., Leung, A., Chan, E., Hezel, D.M., Lin, S.Y., ... Pauls, D.L. (2017). A multisite study of family functioning impairment in pediatric obsessive-compulsive disorder. *J Am Acad Child Adolesc Psychiatry, 56*(3), 241–249.e3.

Stewart, S.E., Jenike, E.A., Hezel, D.M., Stack, D.E., Dodman, N.H., Shuster, L., & Jenike, M.A. (2010). A single-blinded case-control study of memantine in severe obsessive-compulsive disorder. *Journal of Clinical Psychopharmacology, 30*(1), 34–39.

Stewart S. E., Rosario M. C., Baer L., Carter A. S., Brown T. A., Scharf J. M., ... Pauls, D.L. (2008). Four factor structure of obsessive-compulsive disorder symptoms in children, adolescents, and adults. *J. Am. Acad. Child Adolesc. Psychiatry, 47*, 763–772.

Storch, E.A., Caporino, N.E., Morgan, J.R., Lewin, A.B., Rojas, A., Brauer, L., ... Murphy, T.K. (2011). Preliminary investigation of web-camera delivered cognitive-behavioral therapy for youth with obsessive-compulsive disorder. *Psychiatry Research, 189*, 407–412.

Storch, E.A., Geffken, G.R., Merlo, L.G., Mann, G., Duke, D., Munson, M., ... Murphy, T.K. (2007). Family-based cognitive-behavioral therapy for pediatric obsessive-compulsive disorder: Comparison of intensive and weekly approaches. *Journal of the American Academy of Child & Adolescent Psychiatry, 46*, 469–478.

Storch, E.A., Larson, M.J., Muroff, J., Caporino, N., Geller, D., Reid, J.M., ... Murphy, T.K. (2010). Predictors of functional impairment in pediatric obsessive-compulsive disorder. *J Anxiety Disord., 24*, 275–283.

Storch, E.A., Lehmkuhl, H.D., Ricketts, E., Geffken, G.R., Marien, W., & Murphy, T.K. (2010). An open trial of intensive family based cognitive-behavioral therapy in youth with obsessive-compulsive disorder who are medication partial responders or nonresponders. *J Clin Child Adolesc Psychol., 39*(2), 260–268.

Storch E.A., Merlo, L.J., Larson, M.J., Geffken, G.R., Lehmkuhl, H.D., Jacob, M.L., ... Goodman, W.K. (2008). Impact of comorbidity on cognitive-behavior therapy response in pediatric obsessive-compulsive disorder. *J Am Acad Child Adolesc Psychiatry, 47*, 583–592.

Storch, E.A., Milsom, V.A., Merlo, L.J., Larson, M., Geffken, G.R., Jacob, M.L., ... Goodman, W.K. (2008). Insight in pediatric obsessive-compulsive disorder: Associations with clinical presentation. *Psychiatry Research, 160*(2), 212–220.

Storch, E.A., Wilhelm, S., Sprich, S., Henin, A., Micco, J., Small, B.J., ... Geller, D.A. (2016). Efficacy of augmentation of cognitive behavior therapy with weight-adjusted d-Cycloserine vs placebo in pediatric obsessive-compulsive disorder: A randomized clinical trial. *JAMA Psychiatry, 73*(8), 779–788.

Swedo, S.E., Frankovich, J., & Murphy, T.K. (2017). Overview of treatment of pediatric acute-onset neuropsychiatric syndrome. *Child Adolesc Psychopharmacol.*

Swedo, S.E., Leonard, H.L., Mittleman, B.B., Allen, A.J., Rapoport, J.L., Dow, S.P., ... Zabriskie J. (1997). Identification of children with pediatric autoimmune neuropsychiatric disorders associated with streptococcal infections by a marker associated with rheumatic fever. *Am J Psychiatry, 154*(1), 110–112.

Trevizol, A.P., Shiozawa, P., Cook, I.A., Sato, I.A., Kaku, C.B., Guimarães, F.B., ... Cordeiro, Q. (2016). Transcranial magnetic stimulation for obsessive-compulsive disorder: An updated systematic review and meta-analysis. *J ECT, 32*(4), 262–266.

Yu, D., Mathews, C.A., Scharf, J.M., Neale, B.M., Davis, L.K., Gamazon, E.R., ... Pauls, D.L. (2015). Cross disorder genome-wide analyses suggest a complex genetic relationship between Tourette's syndrome and OCD. *Am J Psychiatry, 172*(1), 82–93.

Van Ameringen, M., Patterson B., & Simpson W. (2014). DSM-5 obsessive-compulsive and related disorders: Clinical implications of new criteria. *Depress Anxiety, 31*(6), 487–493.

Varigonda, A.L., Jakubovski, E., & Bloch, M.H. (2016). Systematic review and meta-analysis: Early treatment responses of selective serotonin reuptake inhibitors and clomipramine in pediatric obsessive-compulsive disorder. *J Am Acad Child Adolesc Psychiatry, 55*(10), 851–859.e2.

Watson, H.J. & Rees, C.S. (2008). Meta-analysis of randomized, controlled treatment trials for pediatric obsessive-compulsive disorder. *Journal of Child Psychology and Psychiatry, 49*, 489–498.

Williams, M.T., Mugno, B., Franklin, M., & Faber, S. (2013). Symptom dimensions in obsessive-compulsive disorder: Phenomenology and treatment outcomes with exposure and ritual prevention. *Psychopathology, 46*(6), 365–376.

World Health Organization. (2005).

Wu, M.S., McGuire, J.F., & Storch, E.A. (2016). Anxiety sensitivity and family accommodation in obsessive-compulsive disorder. *J Affect Disord, 205*, 344–350.

14 Evidence-Based Assessment of Child Obsessive-Compulsive Disorder (OCD)

Recommendations for Clinical Practice and Treatment Research

Adam B. Lewin

Obsessive-compulsive disorder (OCD) in youth can be a complex differential diagnosis given a propensity for secrecy, overlap in symptoms with anxiety and tic-spectrum disorders, and relatively low-base rate. To varying degrees, symptoms may also manifest internally complicating recognition. Further, youth may underreport symptoms due to limited insight or low-subjective distress associated with symptoms, especially if they are able to avoid feared situations/stimuli. As a result, diagnosis is rarely straighforward and should involve a thoughtful differential diagnosis involving both patient and caregivers. In addition, systematic screening for common co-occurring psychiatric conditions is recommended as part of any assessment of childhood OCD. Finally, an assessment of childhood OCD should include an assessment of severity. Accordingly, this chapter will first present an overview of establishing the OCD diagnosis in youth, followed by a review of assessing common comorbidities followed by recommendations for assessing OCD severity. Finally, an overview of supplemental areas for assessment will be provided.

Diagnostic Review

Differential diagnostic assessment is central to any assessment of childhood OCD. According to DSM-5, OCD requires the presence of obsessions, compulsions, or both (DSM-5; American Psychiatric Association, 2013). Symptoms must result in impairment, occupy at least one hour per day, and interfere with an individual's adaptive functioning. Youth are not required to recognize symptoms as unreasonable, consistent with previous diagnostic criteria. Assessment generally consists of subjective and objective components. In specialized and/or research settings, structured diagnostic interviews are often employed. Advantages include reliability, consistent and systematic review of diagnostic criteria including exclusions, modular format, and typically screening for comorbid psychopathology. Some instruments may include categorization of symptoms and perfunctory metrics of clinical severity (e.g., single-item clinician ordinal rating). Disadvantages include the time burden to administer, training of providers/technicians, cost and varying ability to obtain third-party reimbursement for administration. Nevertheless, the Anxiety Disorders Interview Schedule for DSM-IV: Child and Parent Versions (ADIS-C/P; Silverman & Albano, 1996; Silverman et al., 2001) is recommended for use in research settings and clinical settings whenever feasible. (Notably, the ADIS-5, revised according to DSM-5, will be available in 2018; Albano & Silverman (in press).) Advantages to the ADIS include comprehensive review of all anxiety disorders, production of a severity rating for each condition, and strong psychometric properties. However, limitations include that the youth version updated for DSM-5 is yet to be released, there is a significant time-burden on patients and providers, and lack of screening for high-base rate comorbidities for youth with OCD (e.g., tic spectrum disorders).

The Schedule for Affective Disorders and Schizophrenia for School Aged Children (Present and Lifetime Versions; KSADS-PL; Kaufman et al., 1997) is an alternative objective diagnostic screener for most major diagnoses in youth. Having a modular format allowing users to skip out when below-threshold reports are made, the KSADS is especially useful in clinical research. Limitations include length/time to administer, lack of sensitivity in evaluating change (there is no severity scale – syndromes are classified only as: not present, subthreshold, or threshold), and raters need significant training and experience (there is a high need for clinical inference in determining follow-up questions and interpreting responses). However, the KSADS-PL screens broadly and can direct a more focused assessment for other diagnoses. Youth and caregivers are typically interviewed separately and the clinician integrates information obtained from all informants, although some users interview all parties together.

Unstructured clinical interviews remain the predominant form of diagnostic assessments in mental health settings. Typically, clinicians should progress through a review of symptoms based on (1) presenting complaints, (2) history/family history, (3) observations, and (4) as informed by the literature and clinical experience (e.g., asking about common comorbidities). In a general assessment, OCD (a low base-rate disorder) is generally screened via a few questions pertaining to the presence of symptoms, e.g., "does your child engage in ritualistic or repetitive checking behavior, such as ... " Unfortunately, this is an unreliable method: if the symptom example is not germane (OCD is highly heterogeneous – an example about checking or washing may not evoke an affirmative response from a child with distressing sexual intrusive thoughts), or queries or terms are misunderstood, or insight is poor, then false negatives may arise. Accordingly, broad-based parent- or child-reported questionnaires are useful screeners that probe for OCD symptoms and as such are recommended, especially if there is a patient/family history of OCD, obsessive-compulsive spectrum disorders, anxiety, anorexia, or tic-spectrum disorders. The Child Behavior Checklist (CBCL; Achenbach, 1994) offers broad-based screening; as well as the Screen for Child Anxiety Related Disorders (SCARD; Birmaher et al., 1997), which is a general screener for anxiety (including OCD) in youth. When a diagnosis of OCD is suspected, the diagnostic interview can be tailored to focus on assessing for OCD diagnostic criteria, core symptoms, and common comorbidities. In these cases, it is still recommended to incorporate DSM based checklists and symptom scales (e.g., checklist from the Children's Yale Brown Obsessive-Compulsive Inventory; CYBOCS; Scahill et al., 1997). This provides consistency and improves reliability in clinical interviewing as well as allowing for recording of diagnostic-based information in the patient's medical record. The Children's Florida Obsessive Compulsive Inventory (CFOCI; Storch et al., 2007) includes a screening measure for child OCD symptoms and a basic severity scale. Similarly, the American Psychiatric Association's (APA) Level 2 Repetitive Thoughts and Behavior Scale (age 11–17) is a shortened (5 item) adaptation of the CFOCI developed for OCD screening that can be useful (however, it remains an emerging measure without clear psychometric data). The Obsessive Compulsive Inventory, Child Version (OCI-CV; Foa et al., 2009) also provides a screening/symptom review for childhood OCD. In summary, clinical interviews should be supplemented with broad-based screeners for youth and parents. When OCD is suspected (e.g., based on family history, presenting complaint, likely comorbidity [tics, anxiety, other obsessive-compulsive spectrum illness], then supplementing the interview with parent and youth report OCD-related scales such as the CFOCI is recommended. Ideally, establishment of OCD severity (and obtaining an overview of symptoms) with the CYBOCS is gold-standard but this interview can require 30–60 minutes and may not be possible at the initial visit. Checklists from APA or DSM (or KSADS/ADIS) may be helpful for incorporation into an unstructured clinical interview to verify that the patient meets diagnostic status.

Differential Diagnosis/Assessment of Comorbidity

Central to the assessment of OCD in children is identification of comorbid psychiatric disorders and the differentiation of OCD from non-OCD neuropsychiatric syndromes that may present similarly to OCD (Lewin & Piacentini, 2017; Lewin, Storch et al., 2005). For example, a hallmark symptom among youth with anorexia is ritualistic eating behaviors/exercise routines; a patient with autism spectrum disorder (ASD) may "obsess" about his special interest in subway routes; a patient with Tourette may describe a compulsive need to touch someone else; and trichotillomania is sometimes characterized as "compulsive" hair-pulling. To further complicate matters, these syndromes may co-occur with OCD, complicating the differential impressions. Further, children may engage in compulsive and/or ritualistic play or prefer rigid routines (e.g., lining up blocks or toys by size or color; insisting on a specific bedtime routine). These behaviors must be interpreted with caution and in the developmental context (e.g., not abnormal for a toddler) and must consider distress, time, and impairment. Comorbidity may complicate both the presentation of OCD (e.g., types of symptoms) as well as OCD severity, impairment, school/social functioning, and response to interventions (Huppert et al., 2009; Lewin & Piacentini, 2010; March et al., 2007; Rapp, Bergman et al., 2016). Assessment of comorbidity can be conducted via a combination of (1) clinical interviews, (2) structured diagnostic interviews, and (3) broad-based rating scales (ideally provided to multiple informants).

Measures and interviews are more consistently employed in clinical research settings where reliable categorization is critical. However, many of the following tools can be easily integrated into a clinical setting – even sections of diagnostic interviews can be utilized to systematically validate diagnostic criteria. The ADIS or KSADS can be used to evaluate the presence or absence of criteria for most DSM-5 disorders. In addition, a variety of self-report measures can provide symptom and/or severity rating of commonly co-occurring conditions (e.g., anxiety, mood, disruptive behavior, tics). In child assessment, multiple informant report is important (e.g., child, one or both primary caregivers, and educators). The aforementioned CBCL and the Behavior Assessment System for Children (BASC; Reynolds & Kamphaus, 2002) provide broad-based screening of child symptoms (with age-normed parent, teacher, and youth report versions). Syndrome specific measures such as the Children's Depressive Inventory (CDI, Kovacs, 1992), the Multidimensional Anxiety Scale for Children (MASC; March et al., 1997), the Conners Parent/Teacher Rating Scales (e.g., Conners et al., 1998), and the Swanson, Nolan, and Pelham (SNAP) Questionnaire (e.g., Swanson et al., 1992) cover mood, anxiety, and ADHD/disruptive behavior, respectively. The Children's Saving Inventory (Storch, Muroff, Lewin et al., 2013) assesses hoarding symptoms in youth and the Body Dysmorphic Disorder Questionnaire (BDDQ; Phillips, Atala, & Pope, 1995) has been used as a BDD screening instrument in adolescents. Assessors of child OCD should also be familiar with the Yale Global Tic Severity Scale (YGTSS; Leckman et al., 1989), a clinician-rated semi-structured inventory used to assess frequency, intensity, complexity, strength, interference, and impairment of motor/phonic tics, as well as tic-related impairment.

Generalized Anxiety Disorder. Generalized Anxiety Disorder (GAD) is characterized by excessive worry about life events. GAD and OCD are highly comorbid, both characterized by obsessional doubts and ruminations, often described as excessive and uncontrollable (Brown et al., 1993; Taylor, Thordarson, & Sochting, 2002). In GAD, worries are typically focused on everyday/real-life worries, e.g., school, health, relationships, money, world events. Worries are not unrealistic but are excessive. Worries (or rather obsessions) associated with OCD are typically irrational or bizarre in nature (e.g., contamination, superstitious, sexual, religious, and aggressive themes). OCD related obsessions are typically more intrusive than GAD-worries and individuals often make greater efforts to resist OCD-based obsessions. Although repetitive thoughts occur with both syndromes, in OCD obsessions may be experienced as thoughts, impulses, or images. The content of OCD related obsessional thoughts is more likely to be regarded as taboo or personally unacceptable (or egodystonic). Patients with GAD may engage in rituals (e.g., checking or reassurance seeking) but typically with less intensity and distress when rituals cannot be completed.

Body Dysmorphic Disorder (BDD). Characterized by preoccupation with perceived defects in appearance, BDD can be difficult to differentiate from OCD.

Individuals with BDD obsess on minor (or imagined) physical anomalies and engage in ritualistic checking behavior related to their preoccupation with physical appearance (e.g., checking their nose). Insight is typically low, even in contrast to OCD. However, BDD is less common in childhood and can be differentiated from OCD on the focus of the preoccupation on physical appearance.

Tic Disorders. Tics are rapid sudden, non-rhythmic repetitive movements or vocalizations (Tourette syndrome presenting with at least two motor tics and one phonic/vocal tic for duration of one year or longer). There is a strong, bidirectional co-occurrence between OCD and tic disorders. As high as 60 percent of patients with Tourette syndrome meet criteria for OCD, and 20 to 38 percent of children with OCD report comorbid tics (Swedo et al., 1989). Identifying simple tics in youth with OCD is straightforward (e.g., sniffing, eye blinks, and throat clearing), which can usually be differentiated from compulsions by virtue of their brevity, simplicity, lack of purpose, and often involuntary nature (Mansueto & Keuler, 2005). Differentiating complex tics from compulsions on the other hand, among comorbid youth, can be challenging. For example, repeating a particular action until it "feels right" can be more difficult to distinguish as a complex tic or compulsion (Castellanos, 1998; Mansueto & Keuler, 2005). The symptom topography may be insufficient for determining whether a behavior is a tic or compulsion. In fact, many tic-like behaviors present as compulsions among adults with co-occurring OCD and tic disorders (e.g., repetitive counting, ordering and arranging, symmetry/evening-things-up, blinking/staring rituals, and touching-tapping-and-rubbing: Holzer et al., 1994). The symptom's antecedents (precursor triggers) however can help differentiate. Tics tend to be preceded by a physical sensation or urge (called the premonitory urge), whereas rituals in OCD are often preceded by intrusive thoughts. This premonitory urge associated with tics may be described as a "need to release," likened to the urge to sneeze or scratch. On the other hand, compulsions are often driven by affective arousal and cognitive content (fears/worries). While this differential may seem straightforward, most youth have not considered their behaviors in this manner. Further, young children may not experience (or be able to identify) a premonitory urge. Sometimes questions such as, "what would happen [or what are you concerned might happen] if you don't [tic/ritualize]?" Youth with tics seem less concerned and may report "I can't stop it" or "nothing," whereas youth with OCD may articulate some feared outcome, e.g., "my mother would die." Thus, the outcome following the behavior (tic/ritual) can also aid differentiation. For example, determining whether the symptom functions to reduce affective distress reduction (OCD) or urge-relief (tic). Also, consider the symptom (i.e., a symptom that could be considered a compulsion or a tic) in context. For example, if the child's history (and/or family history) is positive for OCD (or an anxiety disorder), and current presentation includes other clear-cut obsessions/compulsions (e.g., contamination fears/washing)? What about the case where two siblings have a history of tics, the patient has many clear simple tics, and there is no history of anxiety? The onset of complex tics typically follows the onset of simple tics – and complex tics are rarely the only tics present. Thus, if a complex behavior (e.g., touching something until it feels right) is the only symptom, in the absence of any history of simple tics (and in the context of more clear-cut OCD), this would most likely suggest OCD. However, if a child has no anxiety, a long history of tics, and a ritualistic spitting behavior (in the absence of any distress relief), this behavior may be best characterized as a tic.

Autism Spectrum Disorders. A core feature of Autism Spectrum Disorder (ASD) is restricted or stereotyped interests or behaviors. Autism complicates assessment of OCD, both in terms of symptom-overlap/differentiation and obfuscating information regarding symptoms. Identification of ASD should not prove challenging to skilled clinicians; assessment should screen for early history of language delays, poor pragmatics of language, difficulties with reciprocal social interactions, stereotyped movements/behavior, and fixed interests or preoccupations (e.g., fire hydrants; lawn sprinkler). The challenges present in differentiating specific behaviors that could be consistent with either OCD or ASD, for example obsessionality. Thought content can be helpful in differentiation (rarely do youth with OCD present with intrusive thoughts of ceiling fans or World War II). Affective experiences can be equally helpful: youth with OCD typically consider their symptoms to be egodystonic) whereas children with ASD often consider their behaviors to be egosyntonic. Their fixations are usually on subjects of considerable interest rather than on objects/situations related to possible threat and harm; and as such, youth with ASD do not report distress with preoccupations. More typically, disruption from a special interest results in distress (e.g., transitioning from reading about trains to homework) whereas in OCD, associated distress typically results if a ritual/routine is interrupted that is believed to abate a feared consequence.

Parents often struggle to differentiate ASD related fixated interests/preoccupations with obsessions. Even self-stimulating or stereotyped behavior (flapping, body rocking) associated with ASD may be reported as tics or rituals by parents. Generally, with education and examples, parents can be directed and provide helpful information in guiding assessments (this distinction should be made clear prior to administering standardized scales to improve validity and reliability). Youth with ASD however can be poor reporters, both in term of objective symptoms and impairment. Not uncommonly, youth with ASD do not find OCD symptoms disabling or disturbing, but rather find disruption of rituals and failure of parents to accommodate OCD-related demands to be problematic. Severity (and diagnostic) measures should be considered cautiously in youth with comorbid ASD; and multi-informant assessment is paramount.

Anorexia Nervosa. Anorexia is characterized by abnormally low weight, intense fear of gaining weight, and distorted perception of one's physical appearance, typically associated with food restriction, excessive exercise, or purging. Youth with anorexia typically have preoccupation with food and body weight. They are fearful of change (generally, but especially in body image) and weight gain (Lewin, Menzel, & Strober, 2013). Although obsessions and rituals are central features of anorexia nervosa, these thoughts and behaviors are limited to food and dietary behaviors (e.g., rigidity about eating, inflexibility about dietary and exercise behaviors, obsession with weight and appearance). OCD commonly occurs among adolescents with anorexia (Godart et al., 2002). However, OCD-related fears and behaviors can generally be distinguished from anorexia-specific worries and rituals (Jimenez-Murcia et al., 2007). Notably, severe weight loss can result from OCD (e.g., worries that food is dirty or somehow contaminated can lead to restriction). However, these patients do not endorse the fear of weight gain or altered perception of personal appearance that are the defining features of anorexia.

Schizophrenia Spectrum Disorders. Psychotic disorders, rare in childhood, are characterized by delusional thought content, hallucinations, and thought disorder. Overlaps between OCD and psychosis include immature magical thinking and unusual observable behaviors (Rodowski, Cagande, & Riddle, 2008). For example, a child with OCD may eat only from vacuum sealed packing due to fear of contamination whereas a child with psychosis may believe that aliens are trying to poison the food. Severe OCD in childhood can have a highly heterogeneous presentation and can mimic symptoms of schizophrenia spectrum disorders (e.g., catatonia; youth refusing to move due to fear of horrible outcomes to the point of neglecting all self-care or even eating). Although symptoms of OCD are usually egodystonic, this is not always the case, especially in younger children. The following areas can be used to facilitate differential between OCD and psychosis: examination of prevalence, insight, course, and response to treatment (Rodowski, Cagande, & Riddle, 2008). First, base-rates of OCD are considerably higher (as high as 4 percent in childhood; Zohar, 1999) whereas childhood psychotic disorders are rare (Boeing et al., 2007). Second, prepubertal onset of OCD is common; whereas the onset of schizophrenia prior to adolescence is markedly low. Third, youth with OCD typically recognize that symptoms are a product of one's own mind whereas individuals with psychotic disorders cannot; the presence of insight can aid the differential (Lewin, Bergman, Peris et al., 2010; Rodowski, Cagande, & Riddle, 2008). Fourth, broader occurrence of paranoia, long-standing histories of failing to trust others (even family members), deterioration of social relations, schizotypal behavior, withdrawal and isolation, bizarre attitudes/behavior, and other signs of disorganized thinking/formal thought disorder can be suggestive of prodromal psychosis in adolescence. OCD can be well hidden and youth may appear in certain contexts to be well-adjusted; this is not typically the case in prodromal schizophrenia. Finally, it is not uncommon for course and treatment outcomes to aid with differential diagnosis. Response to intervention (in conjunction with other evidence including symptom profile, history, course, and observation) can help distinguish between OCD and psychosis in some cases. For example, response to an SSRI after failing multiple treatments of antipsychotics (Rodowski, Cagande, & Riddle, 2008) may suggest OCD. Over times, adolescents and adults with child-onset OCD can often articulate their emerging insight that obsessive symptoms were products of one's own mind. Conversely, a patient with a history of unusually thinking and bizarre behavior may experience a shift from obsessional thoughts to delusional guilt and/or paranoid persecution (Insel & Akiskal, 1986), becoming less connected with reality with age.

Hypochondriasis. Hypochondriasis is the fear of contracting a disease or illness or of having a serious health condition. When the fear is exclusively related to having a disease or illness condition, based on the presence of a physical symptom, hypochondriasis may be the more appropriate diagnosis. In OCD, obsessions are typically future oriented, for example "if I don't tap 3 times I will get hypothyroidism."

Hoarding Disorder. Hoarding is characterized by excessive accumulation and persistent difficulty discarding of possessions regardless of their value. Previously classified as OCD, Hoarding Disorder is now considered a separate DSM-5 diagnosis. Hoarding behavior may occur within OCD however, for example, saving items because they may prevent perceived harm or collecting materials to improve "luck."

Depression. Depression is common among youth with OCD, especially with a prolonged course or the social isolation that frequently accompanies the OCD. Often the depression is secondary, described as a function of the burden of OCD (including bullying, isolation, withdrawal from activities due to fears/rituals, declines in academic/athletic performance). In other cases, the depression is longstanding with perhaps a parallel course but not clearly secondary to the onset of the OCD. It is important to differentiate these disorders when developing a treatment plan. For instance, in the case of severe depression, it might be necessary to treat the mood disorder first. In other cases, improvement in the OCD can dramatically improve mood, suggesting treatment of the OCD first. Careful assessment must also be made in cases of intrusive self-harm related thoughts. Differentiating between suicidal ideation and intrusive suicidal thoughts is complicated for the experienced clinician; and further difficulty occurs when pathological doubt is present (e.g., "I'm not sure if I want to kill myself or it is an obsession."). Clinicians are advised to conduct routine suicide risk assessments to ensure the safety of the child or adolescent in these cases where thoughts are not clearly obsessional. Of course, when thoughts are obsessions (vs. suicidal ideation), risk assessments and safety planning may further drive doubt and distress, and provide reassurance/safety contrary to the principles of exposure and response prevention – consequently strengthening the OCD. Accordingly, clinicians must assess carefully for depression vs. OCD, consulting with all treatment team members and including parents/caregivers (i.e., training other professionals and caregivers to monitor for mood/behavioral changes, agitation without reinforcing OCD). To be clear, any shift away from comprehensive risk assessment should be made by experienced exposure/response prevention therapists on a case-by-case basis, in the context to therapy (following a risk assessment/family discussion). Notably even these professionals continue to assess, albeit sometimes more subtly depending upon the child's OCD symptoms.

Attention Deficit Hyperactivity Disorder (ADHD). Differentiating ADHD from OCD is not complex. However, co-occurrence is not uncommon and overlap can complicate treatment. Youth with OCD may be mislabeled as inattentive when mental rituals are not detected and seen as distractibility or concentration problems. Academic problems may be attributed to ADHD but actually be a function of OCD ritualistic behavior preventing completion of assignments (rereading, rewriting) or distracting concentration away from the teacher (mental rituals). Assessment of functional impairments associated with OCD can assist the clinician in understanding the full spectrum of OCD symptoms and impact on daily routines. The Child Obsessive–Compulsive Impact Scale – Revised (COIS-R; Piacentini et al., 2007; see the following) can be a helpful tool in this regard.

Disruptive Behaviors. Externalizing behavior is not uncommon in youth with OCD when rituals are prevented or accommodation of OCD related behaviors is not met. Consider whether disruptive behaviors occur across contexts or only when rituals are disrupted (or exposure to fearful contexts/triggers/stimuli occurs). This is especially common among younger children with OCD (Lewin, Park et al., 2007). A three-year-old may not be able to verbalize that she's "having disturbing intrusive thoughts driving past a cemetery unless dad holds his breath." This may present as screaming, making demands to drive a different route, etc.

Emetophobia. Specific phobia of vomiting vs. OCD is a common challenging differential. Many youth with OCD engage in a number of rituals (overt or mentalistic) to avoid vomiting. Generally, emetophobia is considered OCD (vs. a phobia) when the rituals become excessive and unrealistic, when fears extend beyond vomiting (i.e., might be a sign of death), or when triggers become more broad and less logical.

In summary, a number of neuropsychiatric conditions mimic the presentation of OCD in youth and consequently parents, or practitioners less familiar with OCD in childhood, may mistake non-OCD symptoms (such as tics or stereotyped behavior) for compulsions. While standardized questionnaires and structured interviews can provide relative information about the preponderance of clinical symptoms, they alone do not protect against all errors (e.g., rating tic symptoms on a scale assessing OCD-compulsions). Consequently, unstructured clinical interviews, observation, and more in-depth clinician-patient interactions may be necessary for accurate differential diagnosis.

Assessment of OCD Severity

Empirical assessment of OCD severity is central to both clinical treatment and measurement in research. In the clinical setting, severity is among the factors (history and functions must also be considered) in determining level of treatment needed (i.e., standard vs. intensive treatments) (Lewin & Piacentini 2010; Selles & Lewin, 2017). Severity of symptoms, along with functionality, should be tracked throughout clinical care in order to best inform treatment decisions. In clinical research, need for consistent, reliable measurement that can be compared across settings is also important. One problem in OCD research is inconsistent measurement of outcomes (Lewin, DeNadai, Park et al., 2011; Storch, Lewin, DeNadai et al., 2010) complicating comparisons in response across research trials. Accordingly, the Children's Yale-Brown Obsessive Compulsive Scale (CYBOCS; Scahill et al., 1997), a clinician-rated, semi-structured inventory of pediatric OCD symptoms and severity over the previous week, is considered the gold-standard instrument. The CYBOCS is a clinician-administered semi-structured interview that should be delivered to parents/youth together or each respondent separately, with the clinician integrating discrepancies with follow-up queries and clinical judgment (n.b., interviewers should repeat questions about sexual, religious, and harm symptoms independently to maximize accuracy). The CYBOCS assesses past and current (past week) symptoms using a symptom checklist. The checklist is followed by a 10-item (40-point) severity scale on which the rater scores obsessions and compulsions in terms of their frequency, interference, distress, ability to which the child can resist symptoms, and the child's ability to control symptoms. To improve comparisons across studies and allow for consistent use in characterizing CYBOCS scores, normative data were published for 815 treatment seeking youth (Lewin, Piacentini, DeNadai et al., 2014). These data, obtained from compiling CYBOCS profiles from treatment seeking youth at several OCD child specialty centers (internal consistency alpha = .82; ICC = .98), provide the first empirical benchmarks for comparing individual CYBOCS scores to group data for youth seeking treatment for OCD. Mean severity was 24.9 (0–40 is the scale range). Logistic regression suggested that scores of 5 or less are transient, 4–13 are mild, 14–24 are moderate, 25–30 are moderate-severe, and greater than 30 severe (Lewin, Piacentini, DeNadai et al., 2014). These data replace the non-data driven heuristics utilized previously. Notably, data from both the severity and symptom checklist sections of the CYBOCS can be helpful in tracking treatment outcomes. Although the CYBOCS is not a diagnostic measure, a review of checklist items can help characterize OCD or establish symptom presence. Nevertheless, the measure should not be used alone to establish diagnosis. Notably, the CYBOCS has been used reliably in young children (under age 7) with OCD. However, questions are parent-focused and item and scale reliability can be variable (Lewin, Park, Jones et al., 2014; Cook, Freeman et al., 2015; Freeman et al., 2011).

Single-item measures are also helpful in measuring OCD severity. The Clinical Global Impression – Severity (CGI-S; Guy, 1976) is a 7-point ordinal scale that includes the following anchors of mental illness: 1, normal, not at all ill; 2, borderline ill; 3, mildly ill; 4, moderately ill; 5, markedly ill; 6, severely ill; or 7, extremely ill. The CGI can be applied to OCD severity or overall severity (or both). Advantages include ease of implementation including minimal time. However, clinical experience is generally needed to improve accuracy and reliability of this single-item measure. For example, if a rater has interacted with 10 OCD patients, his/her marker of "extreme" may be less informed than a clinician who has seen 50 patients. Accordingly, benchmarks should be provided to minimize error (e.g., criterion/justification for determining the rating, thus decreasing inherent subjectivity). Helpful exercises include – after determining one's rating – to justify in writing what one would need to see differently to increase/decrease the rating by one point.

The Global Axis of Functioning (GAF; American Psychiatric Association, 2013) provides an alternative single numeric rating (ranging from 1 [lowest] through 100 [superior]) to rate overall social, occupational, and psychological functioning. Finally, the Global Assessment Scale for Children (CGAS; Shaffer et al., 1983) is a single-item measure of global impairment and functioning over the previous month. The scale ranges from 1 (lowest) to 100 (highest) functioning. The CGI-S is recommended over the GAF given its use across child psychiatry research, facilitating comparisons. Notably, single-item ratings require training and experience for reliability (see exercises recommended in the previous paragraph). CGI-CYBOCS have positive correlations ($r=.58$, $p<.001$; Lewin, Piacentini, DeNadai et al., 2014)

Treatment Outcomes. OCD severity provides one measure of outcome. However, as noted previously, methodologies for assessing treatment outcome vary considerably within the childhood OCD literature, complicating interpretation. Whereas some studies compare percent reduction in symptoms, others describe outcomes in terms of number of responders (or remitters). To further complicate, definition and measurement of these terms vary (see Lewin et al., 2010, 2014; Rapp et al., 2016). Clinical remission has been defined as a situation in which a patient "no longer meets criteria for the disorder and has no more than minimal symptoms (Frank et al., 1991, p. 853). The CGI-S is used to indicate remission (typically scores of 1, normal or not at all ill; and 2 borderline illness). The posttreatment CYBOCS has also been used to denote remission. Cut-off scores have varied in the child OCD literature (see Lewin et al., 2011; Storch et al., 2012). Other studies report improvement on the basis of symptom reduction. This may include raw CYBOCS data or the Clinical Global Impression – Improvement (CGI-I; Guy, 1976). The CGI-I provides a clinician-rated ordinal global estimate of clinical improvement ranging from 1 (very much improved) to 7 (very much worse). Typically, children receiving CGI-I of 1 (very much improved) or 2 (much improved) are considered responders. Fortunately, informant agreement is strong when rating improvement in pediatric OCD using the CGI-I (Lewin, Peris, DeNadai et al., 2012). Some studies require multiple criteria to qualify a child categorically as a responder (e.g., 25 percent decrease in the CY-BOCS *and* CGI-I = much improved or very much improved; Cook et al., 2001; March et al., 1997). Using dichotomous outcomes for assessing both remission and responder status may be helpful in assessing group differences (e.g., between two different interventions), but provides little information on the amount of individual improvement (Lewin & Piacentini, 2010). Consequently, it is recommended to provide raw severity data in addition to categorical data (e.g., baseline and posttreatment CYBOCS scores and standard deviations in addition to percent reductions/categorical outcomes [X percent remitters]). Multiple indicators of change are also recommended, for example, reporting outcomes for both CYBOCS and CGI-S/I. Using single detection analysis to link CYBOCS scores to CGI ratings, Storch, Lewin, and colleagues found that to consider a child in clinical "remission," there should be: (a) CYBOCS scores of 14 or under (consistent with "mild severity" [Lewin, Piacentini, DeNadai et al., 2014]), or (b) 45 to 50 percent reduction in pretreatment CYBOCS (Storch, Lewin, DeNadai, & Murphy, 2010). The authors identified 25 percent reduction in CYBOCS to be optimal for detecting treatment "response." These findings were similar to a parallel study of adults with OCD (Lewin, DeNadai, Park et al., 2011).

Ancillary Areas of Assessment

There are a number of supplemental areas to consider assessing when evaluating youth with OCD. As with the preceding areas, this can be done through a clinical interview. Examples include impairment (e.g., in family, social, and academic domains); family accommodation, insight, and Pediatric acute-onset neuropsychiatric syndrome (PANS)/Pediatric autoimmune neuropsychiatric syndrome associated with streptococcus (PANDAS). Impairment is central to developing a treatment plan and monitoring recovery/improvement (Ivarsson, Melin, & Wallin, 2008; Piacentini, Bergman, Keller, & McCracken, 2003; Piacentini et al., 2007). Increasingly, psychosocial impairment is being tracked as an outcome marker (or clinical correlate) in studies of pediatric OCD (Barrett et al., 2008). Family accommodation is linked to improvement and impairment in childhood OCD. Especially in early childhood, a mechanism to produce change is focus on exposure therapy in the context of reducing family accommodation; consequently, assessment and measurement are important. Although findings are mixed with regard to the extent by which insight is associated with treatment outcome, insight may be linked to participation in therapy and can influence techniques employed in the context of cognitive-behavioral therapy for OCD. Finally, PANS/PANDAS can be suggestive of abrupt and fluctuating onset including acute exacerbations associated with significant neuropsychiatric impairment. Awareness of possible PANS/PANDAS presentations can guide referrals to physician experts as well as helping to adapt behavioral therapies in the context of flare-ups in symptoms.

Scales have been developed to supplement clinical interviews in assessing the previous domains (see Table 14.1). For impairment, the Child Obsessive–Compulsive Impact Scale – Revised (COIS-R; Piacentini et al., 2007) is recommended. The Family Accommodation Scale – Parent Report (FAS-PR; Pinto et al., 2013) was developed to assess family accommodation in youth. Unfortunately, there are no strong measures for insight in child OCD – many studies utilize an ancillary CYBOCS item (11) for this purpose. Diagnosis of PANS/PANDAS requires integration of complex assessment information, including history, course, laboratory/medical assays, and symptoms (see Murphy, Patel et al., 2015; Change et al., 2015). Criteria for PANDAS include: presence of clinically significant obsessions, compulsions and/or tics, abrupt onset of symptoms or a saw-toothed course of symptom severity, prepubertal onset, association with other neuropsychiatric symptoms (e.g., hyperactivity, intense anxiety, irritability, bedwetting/increased urinary frequency, tics, developmental regression, association with streptococcal infection). The diagnostic criteria for PANS include: Dramatic/abrupt onset of obsessive-compulsive disorder, presence of additional neuropsychiatric symptoms (must include: Anxiety, emotional liability, irritability, aggression behavioral regression sensory/motor abnormalities, bedwetting, or increased urinary frequency). Although measures exist for tracking PANS/PANDAS severity, patient screeners are not available and diagnosis should not be made without medical assessment.

Table 14.1 *Recommended Empirical Measures*

	Instrument	Type of Instrument	Strengths/Advantages	Limitations
Broad Based Instruments	Anxiety Disorders Interview Schedule for DSM-IV: Child and Parent Versions (ADIS)	Structured Clinical Interviews	- Captures OCD and most common comorbid conditions - Strong psychometric properties - Provides severity ratings - Emphasis on anxiety spectrum	- Time consuming
	Schedule for Affective Disorders and Schizophrenia for School Aged Children (Present and Lifetime Versions; KSADS-PL)	Structured Clinical Interviews	- Captures OCD and most common comorbid conditions - Includes psychotic and tic disorders - Easy opt-out when symptoms not endorsed	- Although can be streamlined, requires more clinical judgment - No severity scale
	Child Behavior Checklist (CBCL)	Parent, youth, and teacher report	- Parallel versions for multiple informants - Age and gender normed - Screens broadly - Strong psychometrics	- OCD related items but limited diagnostic utility for OCD/OC-Spectrum Disorders
	Behavior Assessment System for Children (BASC)	Parent, youth, and teacher report	Same as CBCL	Same as CBCL
	Clinical Global Impression – Severity (CGI-S)	Clinician rated single item	- Efficient - Used in most clinical trials - Good associations with CYBOCS - Can rate OCD specifically or functioning more generally	- Experience required - Risk of subjectivity increased
	Clinical Global Impression – Improvement (CGI-I)	Clinician rated single item	Same as CGI-S	Same as CGI-S

Table 14.1 (cont.)

	Instrument	Type of Instrument	Strengths/Advantages	Limitations
OCD Specific Measures	Children's Yale-Brown Obsessive Compulsive Scale (CYBOCS)	- OCD Specific Severity Scale and Symptom Checklist - Focuses on past week (severity) - Clinician administered	- Gold standard OCD measure - Normative data now available	- Not a diagnostic tool - Challenging in young children/patients with poor insight
	Children's Florida Obsessive Compulsive Inventory (CFOCI)	- Child symptom self-report	- Short/easy to administer - Severity and symptoms information obtained	- Psychometrics marginal and diagnostic accuracy untested
	Children's Obsessive–Compulsive Inventory – Revised (ChOCI-R; Shafran et al., 2003)	- Child and parent report of OCD symptoms	- Parallel parent and youth versions - easy to administer	- Discriminant validity marginal
	Family Accommodation Scale – Parent Report	- Parent report of family accommodation	- Good treatment sensitivity	- No patient version
	Child Obsessive–Compulsive Impact Scale – Revised (COIS-R)	- Parent and youth ratings of impairment	- Parallel versions for parents and youth - Sensitive to treatment response	- Different factor structures in parent/youth versions
	Obsessive–Compulsive Inventory – Child Version (OCI-CV)	- Self-report rating of OCD symptom presence and frequency	- Easy to administer - Assesses common symptoms - Sensitive to treatment	- Poor associations with CYBOCS/limited utility as severity measure
	Children's Saving Inventory	- Parent report of hoarding symptoms	- Good convergent validity - Easy to administer	- Tested mostly in an OCD population - No child report version

However, behavioral health providers can be aware of the symptoms so as to make appropriate referrals.

Summary. Evidence-based assessment, consisting of (1) a comprehensive diagnostic review and collection of detailed history, (2) meticulous screening for common comorbid conditions and differential diagnoses that might mimic OCD, (3) assessment of severity and symptoms, and (4) measurement of impairment, family accommodation, insight, and other factors that may relate to course or treatment outcome is clearly the ideal. This assessment could include measures with strong psychometric properties, integrate youth/self, parent and teacher reports, and repeat at multiple time points. In turn raters could be trained to reliability in each interview with regular calibration. Unfortunately, even in the context of funded clinical research, this model has gone by the wayside due to subject burden, expense, and impracticality. Although evidence-based assessment is indeed key to optimizing treatment (Lewin & Piacentini, 2010; Rapp et al., 2016), elements of the preceding can be integrated into an assessment that is feasible in the relevant context. For example, checklists informed by the diagnostic interviews can be incorporated into the standard 60-minute interview. The American Psychiatric Association has developed screener questionnaires that can be completed beforehand to help direct interviews and identify the need for more detailed screening. Moreover, assessment does not need to end at the first visit. Ongoing assessment of OCD can occur throughout a course of intervention. Even if the aforementioned desired battery is administered, a critical aspect of OCD assessment occurs within the context of exposure-and-response-prevention (ERP). Monitoring approach/avoidance, resistance, distress, defiance in the context of ERP; observing parental/family accommodation behavior; listening to the language patients and families use about each other (and observing their interactions) can be just as critical when attempting to optimize behavioral-therapies and guide decisions. Evidence-based assessment is not a measure, an interview, or a tool: it is an integrative, deductive process – a way of thinking and conceptualizing cases. The preceding tools facilitate a systematic, scientific approach to diagnosis and evaluation of outcomes. Medicine as a whole lacks strong, ubiquitous biomarkers and child psychiatry in particular is highly limited given the inherent subjectivity and variability-in-reporting ability of the patient. Nevertheless, following a systemic data-driven rubric to evaluation is a step in the right direction.

Key Practice Points

- Careful diagnosis should include structured diagnostic interviews and/or checklists derived from said interviews (or DSM-5 criteria).
- Assessment of common co-occurring conditions and mimicking conditions is critical.
- Severity of OCD should be assessed pretreatment and tracked throughout intervention.
- Information should be gathered from multiple informants.

- Evaluators should be trained to criteria in instruments and diagnostic interviewing and have regular supervision with OCD experts until reliable and accurate in the assessment of OCD and related illnesses.

References

Achenbach, T. M. (1994). Child behavior checklist and related instruments. In M.E. Maruish (ed.), *The use of psychological testing for treatment planning and outcome assessment* (pp. 517–549). Hillsdale, NJ: Lawrence Erlbaum Associates, Inc.

Albano A.M. and Silverman, W.K. (in press). *The anxiety disorders interview schedule for DSM-5: Child and parent versions*. Oxford University Press.

American Psychiatric Association. (2013). *Diagnostic and statistical manual of mental disorders (DSM-5)*. Washington, DC: American Psychiatric Association.

Barrett, P. M., Farrell, L., Pina, A. A., Peris, T. S., & Piacentini, J. (2008). Evidence-based psychosocial treatments for child and adolescent obsessive-compulsive disorder. *Journal of Clinical Child and Adolescent Psychology, 37*, 131–155.

Birmaher, B., Khetarpal, S., Brent, D., Cully, M., Balach, L, Kaufman, J. et al. (1997). The screen for child anxiety related emotional disorders (SCARED): Scale construction and psychometric characteristics. *J Am Acad Child Adolesc Psychiatry, 36*, 545–553.

Boeing, L., Murray, V., Pelosi, A., McCabe, R., Blackwood, D., & Wrate, R. (2007). Adolescent-onset psychosis: Prevalence, needs and service provision. *British Journal of Psychiatry, 190*, 18–26.

Brown, T. A., Moras, K., Zinbarg, R. E., & Barlow, D. H. (1993). Diagnostic and symptom distinguishability of generalized anxiety disorder and obsessive-compulsive disorder. *Behavior Therapy, 24*, 227–240.

Chang, K, Frankovich, J, Cooperstock, M, et al. (2015). Clinical evaluation of youth with pediatric acute-onset neuropsychiatric syndrome (PANS): Recommendations from the 2013 PANS Consensus Conference. *Journal of Child and Adolescent Psychopharmacology, 25*(1), 3–13. doi:10.1089/cap.2014.0084.

Conners, C. K., Sitarenios, G., Parker, J. D., & Epstein, J. N. (1998). The revised Conners' Parent Rating Scale (CPRS-R): Factor structure, reliability, and criterion validity. *Journal of Abnormal Child Psychology, 26*, 257–268.

Cook, N.E., Freeman, J.B., Garcia, A.M. et al. (2015). *J Psychopathol Behav Assess, 37*, 432. https://doi.org/10.1007/s10862-014-9465-7

Foa, E.B., Coles, M., Huppert, J.D., Pasupuleti, R.V., Franklin, M.E., & March, J. (2010). Development and validation of a child version of the obsessive compulsive inventory. *Behav Ther, 41*(1), 121–132.

Frank, E., Prien, R.F., Jarrett, R.B., Keller, M.B., Kupfer, D.J., Lavori, P.W., Rush, A.J., & Weissman, M.M. (1991). Conceptualization and rationale for consensus definitions of terms in major depressive disorder. Remission, recovery, relapse, and recurrence. *Archives of General Psychiatry, 48*, 851–855.

Freeman, J., Flessner, C. A., & Garcia, A. (2011). The children's Yale-brown obsessive compulsive scale: Reliability and validity for use among 5 to 8 year olds with obsessive-compulsive disorder. *Journal of Abnormal Child Psychology, 39*, 877–883.

Godart, N. T., Flament, M. F., Perdereau, F., & Jeammet, P. (2002). Comorbidity between eating disorders and anxiety disorders: A review. *International Journal of Eating Disorders, 32,* 253–270.

Guy, W. (1976). Clinical global impressions. In *ECDEU Assessment Manual for Psychopharmacology* (Revised DHEW Pub. (ADM). edn., pp. 218–222). Rockville, MD: National Institute for Mental Health.

Holzer, J. C., Goodman, W. K., McDougle, C. J., Baer, L., Boyarsky, B. K., Leckman, J. F., & Price, L. H. (1994). Obsessive-compulsive disorder with and without a chronic tic disorder. A comparison of symptoms in 70 patients. *British Journal of Psychiatry, 164,* 469–473.

Huppert, J. D., Simpson, H. B., Nissenson, K. J., Liebowitz, M. R., & Foa, E. B. (2009). Quality of life and functional impairment in obsessive-compulsive disorder: A comparison of patients with and without comorbidity, patients in remission, and healthy controls. *Depression and Anxiety, 26,* 39–45.

Insel, T. R. & Akiskal, H. S. (1986). Obsessive-compulsive disorder with psychotic features: A phenomenologic analysis. *American Journal of Psychiatry, 143,* 1527–1533.

Ivarsson, T., Melin, K., & Wallin, L. (2008). Categorical and dimensional aspects of co-morbidity in obsessive-compulsive disorder (OCD). *European Child and Adolescent Psychiatry, 17,* 20–31.

Kaufman, J., Birmaher, B., Brent, D., Rao, U., Flynn, C., Moreci, P., Williamson, D., & Ryan, N. (1997). Schedule for affective disorders and schizophrenia for school-age children-present and lifetime version (K-SADS-PL): Initial reliability and validity data. *Journal of the American Academy of Child and Adolescent Psychiatry, 36,* 980–988.

Kovacs, M. (1992). *Manual for Children's Depression Inventory.* Multi-Health Systems, Inc, North Tonawanda, NY.

Langley, A. K., Bergman, R. L., & Piacentini, J. C. (2002). Assessment of childhood anxiety. *International Review of Psychiatry, 14,* 101–113.

Leckman, J. F., Riddle, M. A., Hardin, M. T., Ort, S. I., Swartz, K. L., Stevenson, J., & Cohen, D. J. (1989). The Yale Global Tic Severity Scale: Initial testing of a clinician-rated scale of tic severity. *Journal of the American Academy of Child and Adolescent Psychiatry, 28,* 566–573.

Lewin, A.B., Bergman, R.L., Peris, T.S., Chang, S., McCracken, J.T., & Piacentini, J. (2010). Correlates of insight among youth with obsessive compulsive disorder. *Journal of Child Psychology and Psychiatry, 51*(5),603–611.

Lewin, A.B., De Nadai, A., Park, J., Goodman, W.K., Murphy, T.K., & Storch, E.A. (2011). Refining clinical judgment of treatment outcome in obsessive-compulsive disorder. *Psychiatry Research, 185,* 294–401.

Lewin, A.B., Menzel, J., & Strober, M. (2013). Assessment and treatment of comorbid anorexia nervosa and obsessive-compulsive disorder. In E.A. Storch & D. McKay (eds.) (pp. 337–348). *Handbook of treating variants and complications in anxiety disorders.* New York: Springer.

Lewin A.B., Park J.M., Jones A.M., Crawford E.A., DeNadai A.S., Menzel J., ... Storch E.A. (2014). Family-based exposure and response prevention therapy for preschool-aged children with obsessive-compulsive disorder: A pilot randomized controlled trial. *Behaviour Research and Therapy, 56,* 30–38.

Lewin, A.B., Peris, T.S., De Nadai, A. S., McCracken, J., & Piacentini, J. (2012). Agreement between therapists, parents, patients, and independent evaluators on clinical improvement in pediatric obsessive compulsive disorder. *Journal of Consulting and Clinical Psychology, 80*(6), 1102–1107.

Lewin, A.B., & Piacentini, J. (2010). Evidence-based assessment of child obsessive compulsive disorder: Recommendations for clinical practice and treatment research. *Child and Youth Care Forum, 39*(2), 73–89.

Lewin, A.B., Piacentini, J., De Nadai, A. S., Jones, A.M., Peris, T.S., Geffken, G.R., … Storch, E.A. (2014). Defining clinical severity in pediatric obsessive compulsive disorder. *Psychological Assessment, 26*, 679–684.

Lewin, A.B. & Piacentini, J. (2017). Obsessive-compulsive disorder in children. In B.J. Sadock, V.A. Sadock, & P. Ruiz (eds.), *Kaplan & Sadock's comprehensive textbook of psychiatry* (10th edn.). Philadelphia: Wolters Kluwer.

Lewin, A. B., Storch, E. A., Adkins, J., Murphy, T. K., & Geffken, G. R. (2005). Current directions in pediatric obsessive-compulsive disorder. *Pediatric Annals, 34*, 128–134.

Mansueto, C. S. & Keuler, D. J. (2005). Tic or compulsion? It's Tourettic OCD. *Behavioral Modification, 29*, 784–799.

March, J. S., Franklin, M. E., Leonard, H., Garcia, A., Moore, P., Freeman, J., & Foa, E. (2007). Tics moderate treatment outcome with sertraline but not cognitive-behavior therapy in pediatric obsessive-compulsive disorder. *Biological Psychiatry, 61*, 344–347.

March, J. S., Parker, J. D., Sullivan, K., Stallings, P., & Conners, C. K. (1997). The Multidimensional Anxiety Scale for Children (MASC): Factor structure, reliability, and validity. *Journal of the American Academy of Child and Adolescent Psychiatry, 36*, 554–565.

Murphy, T.K., Patel, P.D., McGuire, J.F., Kennel, A., Mutch, P.J., Parker-Athill, E.C., … Rodriguez, C.A. (2015b). Characterization of the pediatric acute-onset neuropsychiatric syndrome phenotype. *Child Adolesc Psycopharm, 25*, 14–25.

Phillips, K.A, Atala, K.D, & Pope, H.G. (1995). Diagnostic instruments for body dysmorphic disorder. *New research program and abstracts. American Psychiatric Association 148th Annual Meeting*; Miami, p. 157.

Piacentini, J., Peris, T. S., Bergman, R. L., Chang, S., & Jaffer, M. (2007). Functional impairment in childhood OCD: Development and psychometrics properties of the Child Obsessive-Compulsive Impact Scale-Revised (COIS-R). *Journal of Clinical Child and Adolescent Psychology, 36*, 645–653.

Rapp, A.M., Bergman, R.L., Piacentini, J., & McGuire, J.F. (2016). Evidence-based assessment of obsessive-compulsive disorder. *Journal of Central Nervous System Disease, 8*, 13–29.

Reynolds, C. R. & Kamphaus, R. W. (2002). *A clinician's guide to the Behavioral Assessment System for Children (BASC)*. Needham Heights, MA: Allyn & Bacon.

Rodowski, M. F., Cagande, C. C., & Riddle, M. A. (2008). Childhood obsessive-compulsive disorder presenting as schizophrenia spectrum disorders. *Journal of Child and Adolescent Psychopharmacology, 18*, 395–401.

Scahill, L, Riddle, M.A., McSwiggin-Hardin, M., et al. (1997). Children's Yale-Brown Obsessive-Compulsive Scale: Reliability and validity. *Journal of the American Academy of Child and Adolescent Psychiatry, 36*(6), 844–852.

Selles, R.R., & Lewin, A.B. (2017). Decision-making: Treatment options and levels of care. In A.B. Lewin & E.A. Storch, (eds.), *Understanding OCD: A guide for parents and professionals*. London: Kingsley Press.

Shaffer, D., Gould, M.S., Brasic, J., Ambrosini, P., Fisher, P., Bird, H., & Aluwahlia, S. (1983). A Children's Global Assessment Scale (CGAS). *Archives of General Psychiatry, 40*, 1228–1231.

Shafran, R., Frampton, I., Heyman, I., Reynolds, M., Teachman, B., & Rachman, S. (2003). The preliminary development of a new self-report measure for OCD in young people. J Adolesc., 26(1), 137–142.

Silverman, W. K. & Albano, A. M. (1996). *The Anxiety Disorders Interview Schedule for DSM-IV—Child and Parent Versions*. San Antonio, TX: Graywinds Publications.

Silverman, W. K., Saavedra, L. M., & Pina, A. A. (2001). Test-retest reliability of anxiety symptoms and diagnoses with the Anxiety Disorders Interview Schedule for DSM-IV: Child and parent versions. *Journal of the American Academy of Child and Adolescent Psychiatry, 40*, 937–944.

Storch, E. A., Muroff, J., Lewin, A. B., Geller, D., Ross, A., McCarthy, K., ... Steketee, G. (2011). Development and preliminary psychometric evaluation of the children's saving inventory. *Child Psychiatry and Human Development, 42* (2), 166–182.

Storch, E.A., Bagner, D., Merlo, L.J., et al. (2007). Florida obsessive-compulsive inventory: Development, reliability, and validity. *J Clin Psychol, 63*(9), 851–859.

Storch, E.A., Lewin, A.B., De Nadai, A.S., & Murphy, T.K. (2010). Defining treatment response and remission in obsessive-compulsive disorder: A signal detection analysis of the Children's Yale-Brown Obsessive-Compulsive Scale. *J Am Acad Child Adolesc Psychiatry, 49*(7), 708–717.

Swanson, J. M. (1992). *School-based assessments and interventions for ADD students*. Irvine, CA: K.C. Publications.

Swedo, S.E., Rapoport, J.L., Leonard, H., Lenane, M., & Cheslow, D. (1989). Obsessive-compulsive disorder in children and adolescents. Clinical phenomenology of 70 consecutive cases. *Archives of General Psychiatry, 46*, 335–341.

Taylor, S., Thordarson, D. S., & Sochting, I. (2002). Obsessive-compulsive disorder. In M.M. Antony & D. H. Barlow (eds.), *Handbook of assessment and treatment planning for psychological disorders* (pp. 182–214). New York: Guilford Press.

Zohar, A. H. (1999). The epidemiology of obsessive-compulsive disorder in children and adolescents. *Child and Adolescent Psychiatric Clinics of North America, 8*, 445–460.

15 Self-Help Treatments for Childhood Obsessive-Compulsive Disorder Including Bibliotherapy

Georgina Krebs and Cynthia Turner

Introduction

Although obsessive-compulsive disorder (OCD) was once considered to be rare in youth, epidemiological studies have since estimated prevalence rates of 0.25 to 4 percent among children and adolescents (Douglass, et al., 1995; Flament et al., 1988; Heyman et al., 2003; Zohar, 1999). The disorder is known to be highly impairing and can have devastating effects on young people's lives across multiple domains (Lack et al., 2009; Piacentini et al., 2003). Furthermore, in the absence of treatment the disorder typically follows a chronic course. In adulthood, OCD has been ranked among the top 10 most disabling illnesses by the World Health Organization (Murray & Lopez, 1996). Over the last decade, substantial evidence has accumulated for the efficacy of cognitive behavioral therapy (CBT) in treating pediatric OCD (Sánchez-Meca, et al., 2014; Watson & Rees, 2008). In line with the robust evidence base, there is international consensus that CBT is a first-line treatment for OCD in children and adolescents (Geller & March, 2012; NICE, 2005). However, data suggest that the majority of OCD sufferers fail to access CBT, and there is an urgent need to increase the availability of CBT for this population. Self-help treatments offer one promising solution to this major challenge.

This chapter will focus on reviewing evidence for self-help CBT-based interventions for children and adolescents with OCD; that is, interventions that do not require therapist input and are fully self-guided. In this chapter, we will first outline the barriers that currently exist to young people accessing CBT for OCD, and in so doing, highlight the need for innovation and the potential value of self-help interventions in meeting this need. We will then review the existing self-help materials available and the evidence for their efficacy. Given the paucity of research in this field, we will draw on evidence for self-help in adult OCD populations and consider the implications for children and adolescents. Finally, we will suggest priorities for future research and practice and highlight key practice recommendations.

Overview of the Issue: The Need for Innovation

Barriers to Accessing CBT for Youth with OCD. Studies of service utilization in pediatric OCD are sparse. However, in adult populations it is estimated that

59.5 percent of OCD sufferers worldwide do not access any treatment, making lack of treatment more common in OCD than anxiety and mood disorders (Kohn et al., 2004). The rates of CBT utilization may be even lower given that other treatments, such as pharmacotherapy, are often more widely available (Chowdhury, Frampton, & Heyman, 2004). Even when OCD sufferers do manage to access treatment, it is generally only after long delays. Studies in adult samples have reported delays of 15 to 17 years in accessing effective treatment for OCD (Hollander et al., 1997; Pinto et al., 2006). Moreover, childhood-onset OCD has been shown to be associated with equally lengthy delays in help-seeking, with Stengler and colleagues finding that those who reported onset of disorder before the age of 17 had their first professional contact on average 11.7 years after onset of their disorder (Stengler et al., 2013). These findings are disconcerting, not least because a longer duration of illness is predictive of poorer long-term outcome (Micali et al., 2010), highlighting the importance of early intervention for this disorder.

An important question is why do young people with OCD have such difficulty accessing CBT? The answer is likely to be multifaceted, with barriers occurring at many levels. OCD sufferers may be reluctant to seek help due to stigma (Goodwin et al., 2002), shame, and embarrassment about their OCD symptoms (Barton & Heyman, 2013; Marques et al., 2010), and/or poor insight (Geller et al., 2001). Individuals from ethnic minority backgrounds may be particularly hesitant to seek help due to differences in knowledge and cultural beliefs about OCD and its treatment (Fernandez de la Cruz et al., 2015; Goodwin et al., 2002). For example, a community-based survey study found that significantly more Black African parents than White British parents would seek help from the religious community (as opposed to health services) if their child had OCD (Fernandez de la Cruz et al., 2015). Inconvenience of sessions with respect to timings and location can be a deterrent to attending CBT sessions (Marques et al., 2010). In addition, parents may be reticent about accessing CBT due to the financial costs of treatment (Kataoka et al., 2002; Marques et al., 2010), including directly incurred treatment costs, the cost of travel and loss of income from time off work.

Even when families would like to access CBT for OCD, it may not be readily available. A case note review study conducted in a national, specialist OCD clinic in the United Kingdom revealed that only a minority of cases had received CBT prior to referral (Chowdhury, Frampton, & Heyman, 2004). Rates of CBT provision in the United Kingdom did not increase over a 10-year period, despite the publication of national clinical guidelines recommending CBT as a first-line treatment (Nair et al., 2015). Surprisingly, rates of other therapies (such as family therapy and psychodynamic therapy) did increase significantly over time, suggesting that there may be a shortage of CBT-trained therapists within child and adolescent mental health services. An additional problem is that even when CBT is offered, it may be delivered in a suboptimal form (Krebs et al., 2015; Valderhaug, Gotestam, & Larsson, 2004). A national survey conducted among clinicians treating pediatric OCD in Norway found that although the majority of professionals reported using CBT, only a third reported using exposure with response prevention (E/RP) techniques regularly (Valderhaug et al., 2007). This is at odds with the evidence-based

CBT protocols for OCD in youth (e.g., March & Mulle, 1998), as well as clinical guidelines (Geller & March, 2012; NICE, 2005), all of which highlight E/RP as being the key focus of treatment for pediatric OCD.

In summary, evidence suggests that good quality CBT is not readily available or accessed by children and adolescents with OCD in routine clinical practice. Barriers in accessing CBT may stem from reluctance of families to seek help, high costs and time commitment required for attending therapy, and a shortage of adequately trained therapists. Self-help treatments could therefore play a key role in disseminating CBT in this population by reducing problems associated with shame and stigma, geographical barriers, inconvenience, financial costs, and limited therapist capacity.

The Approach to Innovation

A number of different self-help methods have been developed. These methods include self-help books or bibliotherapy, developed either as a pure self-help intervention, or as an adjunct to therapist-delivered CBT, and internet-delivered CBT (iCBT). These approaches and the associated evidence for their efficacy are discussed as follows.

Self-Help Books for Youth with OCD. To date, three CBT self-help books have been written specifically for children and adolescents with OCD (Derisley et al., 2008; March & Benton, 2006; Sisemore, 2010). These books mirror the content of evidence-based, therapist-delivered CBT protocols, encompassing psychoeducation about OCD and anxiety, graded exposure with response prevention as guided by a hierarchy, and relapse prevention. *Talking Back to OCD* (March & Benton, 2006) was written for children and adolescents with OCD, whereas *Breaking Free from OCD* (Derisley et al., 2008) and *Free from OCD* (Sisemore, 2010) are primarily aimed at adolescents aged 11 to 16 years old. Each of the books include worksheets for young people to complete, which are designed to facilitate understanding of OCD and completion of E/RP tasks, and each chapter ends with a section written specifically for caregivers, in order to assist them in supporting their child through the program.

Given that these self-help books are based on validated, face-to-face CBT protocols, it is reasonable to conclude that the books are scientifically grounded and consistent with psychological theory and research. However, there is a dearth of studies directly evaluating the efficacy of self-help books in treating childhood OCD. Only one study to date has evaluated traditional bibliotherapy (bCBT) as a stand-alone treatment for OCD in youth. Robinson and colleagues evaluated the feasibility, acceptability, and efficacy of *Breaking Free from OCD* in a pilot trial (Robinson et al., 2013). After a 3-week monitoring period to assess symptom stability, eight 11- to 16-year-olds with OCD were given the self-help book. Participants were given guidelines with recommendations on which chapters to read over an 8-week period. All participants received weekly telephone calls from a therapist to monitor adherence and assess symptom severity, but importantly no treatment advice or therapeutic support was given. All eight participants completed the study, although only three read all chapters. Seven participants provided feedback on acceptability, with all 7 reporting that the book was "just right" in terms of readability and 71 percent saying that the book was "helpful" for fighting OCD. Furthermore, significant reductions in OCD symptoms were observed on a clinician-administered measure of OCD severity for the group as a whole (the Children's Yale-Brown Obsessive-Compulsive Scale) (CY-BOCS; Scahill, et al., 1997). While reductions were statistically significant, the overall degree of improvement was modest. In fact, the mean reduction in symptom severity as measured by the CY-BOCS was 18.5 percent, which is well below the 35 percent reduction that is widely accepted as the cutoff for defining treatment response (Skarphedinsson et al., 2017). Furthermore, no significant effects were observed on self- and parent-report measures of OCD. Therefore, while this pilot study provides preliminary evidence for the feasibility and acceptability of bCBT for youth with OCD, there remains room for improvement, and a need for further research to carefully evaluate the efficacy of such interventions.

Self-Help Material as an Adjunct to Therapist-Delivered CBT. Written self-help materials have also been evaluated as an adjunct to face-to-face CBT in youth with OCD. Bolton and colleagues conducted a randomized controlled trial to evaluate brief CBT combined with self-help (Bolton et al., 2011). Ninety-six children and adolescents (aged 10–18 years) were randomized to one of three conditions: full CBT (12 sessions), brief CBT (on average 5 sessions), or a wait-list control. The brief CBT package was supplemented by five self-help CBT sessions, which were presented as workbooks for the young people to complete at home in between face-to-face sessions. The content of the workbooks was designed to build on the concepts and strategies that had been introduced in the previous session, and in this sense was not providing novel information per se but instead was designed to facilitate consolidation and continued implementation of CBT techniques. As expected, both treatment groups displayed superior outcomes compared to the wait-list control group, thereby demonstrating their efficacy in reducing OCD severity. Importantly, the brief CBT plus self-help group showed equivalent outcomes to the full CBT group, suggesting that self-help may be a useful supplement to CBT, and may provide an effective way of increasing treatment capacity in services within the context of limited service-level resources.

Internet-Delivered CBT as a Pure Self-Help Intervention. In line with the general move toward utilizing technologies to deliver CBT (see Chapter 16 from this section), efforts in recent years have focused on developing web-based self-help CBT interventions for young people with OCD. A novel program was recently developed, called *OCD? Not Me!*, aimed at adolescents 12 to 18 years (Rees, Anderson, & Finlay-Jones, 2015). Unlike therapist-assisted internet CBT (iCBT) programs that have been developed for OCD (Andersson et al., 2012; Lenhard et al., 2017), *OCD? Not Me!* is fully self-guided and requires no therapist support. The program includes psychoeducation about OCD, goal-setting, constructing a hierarchy and graded E/RP. The program is interactive and responds to content provided by young people. For example, E/RP tasks are automatically ordered into a hierarchy based on the subjective anxiety ratings that a young person enters into the worksheets. A component for caregivers is included in the program, which provides psychoeducation, advice on how to support their child throughout the treatment, and strategies for reducing family accommodation of symptoms.

In a preliminary open trial, 334 youth were screened for inclusion in the study. Only participants in the target age range of 12 to 18 years, meeting inclusion criteria and completing pretest measures, were included in the analyses ($n=132$). The pretreatment mean of 11.6 (SE=3.0) on the Children's Florida Obsessive-Compulsive Inventory (C-FOCI; Storch et al., 2009) was consistent with pretreatment means reported in clinical samples of youth with OCD (e.g., Storch et al., 2009). The number of participants that commenced each stage of the program at the time the data were collected were: stage 1 ($n=116$), stage 2 ($n=67$), stage 3 ($n=27$), stage 4 ($n=16$), stage 5 ($n=14$), stage 6 ($n=12$), stage 7 ($n=11$), and stage 8 ($n=11$). Despite the relatively small number of young people completing all stages of the program, participants showed significant reductions in OCD symptoms ($p<.001$) and severity ($p<.001$) between pre- and posttest, with effect size calculations indicating a moderate effect for the changes in OCD symptoms between pre- and posttest ($d=.64$) (Rees, et al., 2016). The mean reduction in OCD symptom severity was 50 percent, as measured by the C-FOCI, suggesting clinically meaningful change. While this finding requires replication and further evaluation in the context of an RCT, the results are encouraging and suggest that online self-guided CBT could be an effective method to dramatically increase access to CBT among adolescents with OCD.

Given the very preliminary stage of research into self-help interventions for youth with OCD, the evidence pertaining to adult self-help interventions for OCD will be briefly reviewed.

The Evidence Base for Innovation

Self-Help Interventions for OCD in Adult Populations. The self-help programs available for young people with OCD are small compared with the options currently available for adults. A search on the internet book dealer *Amazon.com* reveals an impressive list of bibliotherapy materials for adults with OCD. Many of the self-help books (e.g., *Overcoming Obsessive-Compulsive Disorder: A Self-Help Guide Using Cognitive Behavioral Techniques*; Veale & Willson, 2009) have been written by clinical academics who develop and evaluate CBT programs for adult OCD. Like the self-help books written for young people with OCD, the books for adults typically represent a variation of validated face-to-face CBT packages. However, very few have been scientifically evaluated to establish efficacy in a self-help format, in either a guided (i.e., with minimal therapist support) or unguided (i.e., pure self-help) delivery format.

A small number of uncontrolled studies have demonstrated small to moderate within-group effect sizes (Hedges $g = 0.04$–0.51) for bibliotherapy in the treatment of adults with OCD (Gilliam et al., 2010; Moritz et al., 2011; Tolin et al., 2005). Three small randomized controlled trials have demonstrated the efficacy of *unguided* bCBT (Hauschildt, Schroder, & Moritz, 2016; Tolin et al., 2007; Vogel et al., 2014), again with small to moderate effect sizes (g = 0.13–0.65). Tolin and colleagues compared face-to-face CBT with bCBT in a sample of 41 adults (mean age =38.2 years, SD =13.1=) with moderately severe OCD. bCBT participants were given the book *Stop Obsessing! How to Overcome Your Obsessions and Compulsions* (Foa & Wilson, 2001), which provides instructions for self-administered E/RP, along with a written schedule of suggested chapters to read during a six-week period, but with no therapist support. Participants receiving face-to-face CBT displayed significantly greater reductions in OCD symptoms and self-reported functional impairment compared to those receiving bCBT, but importantly both conditions resulted in significant improvements. Similarly, a small but positive effect of bCBT was found by Vogel et al. (2014), who compared bCBT to therapist-delivered CBT via videoconferencing (VCT), and a wait-list control condition, in a sample of 30 adults (aged 28–40 years) with moderately severe OCD. Participants in the bCBT condition received *Mastery of Obsessive-Compulsive Disorder: A Cognitive Behavioral Approach* (Foa & Kozak, 1997) with no therapist guidance. Results showed that VCT was associated with superior outcomes compared to bCBT, but that both were superior to the wait-list condition, thereby demonstrating the efficacy of bCBT. In the third RCT, Hauschildt, Schroder, and Moritz (2016) evaluated the effectiveness of *myMCT* (*My Metacognitive Training for OCD*), a freely available self-help book drawing on cognitive and meta-cognitive models of OCD. Compared to participants receiving an education only control condition (i.e., OCD-specific written education material, but no treatment-related information), participants receiving the bCBT reported slightly greater levels of symptom improvement on self-report measures of OC symptoms and depression. Taken together, the results of these RCTs demonstrate the feasibility and potential benefit of unguided bCBT for at least some individuals with OCD. To date however, the research in this field is limited, and currently there are no studies that have investigated predictors or moderators of response to bCBT. This is in stark contrast to the broader literature pertaining to bCBT for adult anxiety and depression, where reviews have found that bCBT is significantly more effective than placebos or waiting lists, and may even be as effective as therapist delivered psychological therapy (e.g., Den Boer, Wiersma, & Van Den Bosch, 2004; Scogin et al., 1990). Hence, there remains a clear need to further evaluate the efficacy of self-help bibliotherapy for adult, as well as childhood OCD.

Far more scientific evaluation has been conducted on the use of computerized (cCBT) or iCBT self-help interventions for adults suffering with OCD. One of the earliest programs, *BT Steps* (Behavior Therapy Steps), developed by OCD researchers John Greist, Isaac Marks, and Lee Baer, was initially developed as an interactive telephone-activated voice-response computer intervention, supported by a manual (Marks et al., 1998). Interactive voice response is a technology that allows a computer to interact with the human user through the use of voice and tones input via the telephone keypad. The program provided initial psychoeducation, then guided participants through E/RP in a series of steps, with interactive voice response prompts. BT Steps was carefully evaluated, with an initial two non-comparative trials (Barchofen et al., 1999; Greist et al., 1998), followed by two randomized controlled trials, with one comparing BT Steps to therapist-delivered telephone CBT or relaxation (Greist et al., 2002), and another comparing different methods of delivery of BT Steps, one with on-demand telephone support and one with scheduled telephone support (Kenwright et al., 2005). The within-group effect size for BT Steps (ES = 0.84) was found to be high compared to relaxation (ES = 0.35), although not as high as telephone therapy (ES = 1.22); however, the self-help patients who progressed through to self-exposure achieved clinical outcomes comparable to those who received therapist-assisted exposure. BT Steps was concluded to be a time efficient and cost-effective method of making therapy more widely available to those who needed it. BT Steps evolved into an online program called OC Fighter. Meta-analytic support for BT Steps was offered by two studies, both concluding it was clinically efficacious for adult OCD (Mataix-Cols & Marks, 2006; Tumur et al., 2007). Following these impressive beginnings, cCBT for adult OCD has evolved to delivery via the internet (iCBT), and there are now a number of empirically supported iCBT interventions that have undergone careful evaluation. The technology innovations that have been developed and evaluated will be further discussed in Chapter 16 of this section.

Mediators and Moderators of Change

As noted throughout this chapter, while innovations in delivery of psychological therapy for youth with OCD have sought to make evidence-based treatment more accessible, evaluation of these innovations remains to be done in sufficient depth. Carefully designed randomized controlled trials to evaluate outcome have yet to emerge, and consequently, we have almost no knowledge of factors that may mediate or moderate change. Nonetheless, given that research with adults is more advanced than the research with young people, it is worth briefly reflecting on what we may be able to glean from the adult OCD self-help literature.

Certainly, self-help methods, including bCBT, cCBT, and iCBT, hold promise. However, even in adult studies, relatively little is known about whom these treatments may work best for as research pertaining to predictors and moderators of outcome is scarce. Neurocognitive variables may be especially important in self-help interventions given the increased initiative, comprehension, and self-regulation required (Diefenbach & Tolin, 2013). Diefenbach and Tolin (2013) compared guided bCBT treatment responders ($n=5$) and nonresponders ($n=13$) on exploratory clinical moderator variables. Responders and nonresponders did not differ from each other with regard to OCD severity, global illness severity, depression severity, reading ability, treatment expectancy, or motivation. However, the groups differed significantly on self-reported problems with attention, with nonresponders reporting significantly more severe problems with attention. This finding underscores the importance of further research to identify the relevant clinical and/or demographic variables to enable patient-treatment matching.

A crucial difference between adults and youth is the degree of familial involvement that may or may not be required in treatment. While for adults, an important question seems to be what degree of therapist involvement is required to optimize outcomes, for youth, the key questions may be what degree of therapist *and* parental (or carer) involvement is required to optimize outcomes. Furthermore, there is a question as to whether bCBT programs are outdated for youth, given that we live in a digital society and young people in particular may be more willing to engage with interactive, online programs compared to self-help books. On the other hand, there may also be merit in evolving both bCBT and iCBT models of self-help in order to maximize accessibility across different social and cultural groups.

Clinical Case Illustration

The following case will briefly illustrate how self-help methods may be utilized in treating youth with OCD.

> *Ellie was twelve years old. She had experienced the onset of OCD symptoms in the past ten months, which seemed to have been triggered by her older sister suffering from a vomiting virus. Ellie began being fastidious about washing her hands whenever she touched anything that belonged to her sister. However, this quickly extended to washing her hands whenever she touched anything that belonged to other people. While this behavior developed initially at home, Ellie was soon washing her hands at school and avoiding touching anything that belonged to others. When the teacher advised Ellie's parents that Ellie was spending the recess and lunch breaks in the bathroom washing, Ellie's parents sought help.*
>
> *Ellie was diagnosed with OCD. Her therapist recommended that an online CBT program might be helpful. Ellie was well supported by her parents and seemed highly motivated to overcome her OCD. The family agreed to an online program. Ellie and her parents spoke with the therapist about the importance of engaging with online therapy in the same way in which they might engage with a therapist in the clinic. They discussed the importance of making a regular time to complete sessions, and to find time each day to complete homework activities and to keep a record of what she was doing. Ellie was excited about getting started and when she received her login details from the therapist, Ellie commenced her first online session that evening.*
>
> *Ellie's therapist telephoned the family after two weeks. Ellie had completed the first two online chapters and had a good understanding of what OCD was all about. She understood how her fears of getting sick were being maintained by her handwashing rituals, and by avoiding touching things that belonged to others. Ellie had started to plan an exposure hierarchy and was looking forward to completing the next chapter, when she would begin to face her fears. When the therapist telephoned the family after another two weeks had passed, she learned that Ellie had already started her exposure tasks and was busy cutting back her handwashing rituals by reducing the amount of time she was taking to wash her hands, and by messing up the special rituals that she had developed in order to ensure her hands were properly free from germs. These rituals had involved counting to 19 while she carefully soaped each finger one-by-one, and*

then washed her hands and wrists right up to her forearms. When the therapist spoke to Ellie, Ellie told her that she was now only using a small amount of soap and that she was counting to 6 or below while she washed each finger. The therapist congratulated Ellie on the great progress that she had made and encouraged her to keep practicing her exposure task and messing up the handwashing rituals. Ellie told her how much she loved recording her homework on the computer and seeing her OCD symptoms reducing.

Ellie continued to engage with the online program right through until the end of the eight chapters. She had learned not only about the special rituals that OCD could trick her into using, she had also learned that OCD liked to trick her thinking about things as well. She learned that it really wasn't very likely that she would get sick by being around other people, and she was determined not to let OCD creep back into her life. Ellie and her parents reported finding the online program easy to follow and understand, they liked the examples given, and they liked being able to see the changes Ellie made each week being presented on the screen. They found the online format very convenient.

Challenges and Recommendations for Future Research

While there are clear benefits of self-help approaches to treatment of OCD, there are also challenges. Critics to self-help interventions argue that the therapist-client relationship may be critical in encouraging engagement, individualizing care, and meeting patient expectations regarding the legitimacy and quality of psychological therapy. Recent qualitative research investigating the patient experience for adults with OCD completing guided bibliotherapy (6 hours of professional support) and cCBT (1 hour of professional support) indicated that patient engagement with self-help interventions was mixed, with some perceiving limitations and some perceiving significant benefit (Knopp-Hoffer et al., 2016). The addition of professional support was widely regarded as important, lending weight to the need for flexibility in the provision of self-help interventions for OCD, and therapists being responsive to patient preferences when prescribing a modality of therapy (Knopp-Hoffer et al., 2016). Professionals delivering these self-help interventions also expressed mixed views, although generally felt that these interventions offered significant opportunity to patients and services running on limited resources (Gellaty et al., 2017).

The directions for future research are many and varied. There is a clear need to further develop and evaluate self-help programs for youth with OCD and their families, using scientifically robust methods. These programs need to consider the method of self-help (including bCBT, cCBT, iCBT, and mobile applications), the degree of involvement of family members, and the degree of guidance that needs to be given to families in order to maximize success. Research needs to consider what will optimize youth engagement with self-help methods and ensure that they remain engaged through to the completion of the program, since drop-out rates can be high and participants who complete self-help interventions are likely to achieve greater levels of clinical outcome than those who disengage (Mataix-Cols et al., 2006). It may be that some type of contingent reinforcement could be built into these programs in order to optimize compliance and engagement with the strategies presented.

A pertinent but unanswered question is: for whom is self-help most appropriate? One consideration may be symptom severity. Treatment management guidelines currently recommend self-help for those with mild symptoms (NICE, 2005). However, this recommendation is not yet empirically grounded and future studies should test the extent to which symptom severity predicts response to self-help in youth with OCD. There is some research to indicate that quite severe presentations of adult anxiety and depression may indeed be responsive to iCBT, and that significant risk can be safely managed using carefully designed protocols (Nielson et al., 2015; Titov et al., 2015).

Another consideration is patient characteristics such as gender, age, ethnicity, and even treatment history. For example, would older adolescents respond better to self-help interventions than younger adolescents, or vice versa, given the differential role that family members may play? Might self-help be particularly useful for certain ethnic groups, who may be reluctant to seek mental health services due to certain cultural beliefs (Fernandez de la Cruz et al., 2015; Goodwin et al., 2002)? There is some evidence that youth with OCD who have completed a previous trial of CBT may respond less well to iCBT than youth who have not previously completed CBT (Lenhard et al., 2016), suggesting that self-help may be more suitable for treatment-naïve patients. There seems to be a wide array of questions that could be investigated; however, given the limited number of self-help studies for youth with OCD, identification of predictors and moderators of outcome remain some way off.

Longevity of self-help interventions also requires careful consideration. Many of the cCBT or iCBT programs discussed have been developed by researchers using grant funding. However, when grant funding ceases, the issue of how to ensure that effective programs remain available to youth is a significant one. Any technology-based intervention requires maintenance and careful implementation of technology updates, requiring careful management and thoughtful decision-making. It may be that commercialization of iCBT programs requires consideration, or long-term government investment. Hill et al. (2017) present a thoughtful analysis of challenges and considerations when developing digital mental health innovations. Recommendations include collaborative working between clinicians, researchers, industry, and service users in order to successfully navigate challenges and to ensure e-therapies are engaging, acceptable, evidence-based, scalable, and sustainable. However, the translation from lab to real world is never without incident, and effectiveness trials rarely obtain outcomes equivalent to those seen as efficacy trials. Thus, carefully managed effectiveness trials will be required in the future. Evaluation by independent research groups, rather than those with commercial interests in an intervention, is also of high priority.

Conclusions

Given the prevalence of OCD in youth, the demand for CBT is likely to continue to outstrip the supply provided by trained therapists in a traditional, face-to-face format. For this reason, there is a clear need to identify models of service delivery that optimize the use of available resources, enabling the dissemination of effective treatment to those in need. Stepped-care models propose intervention at varying levels of intensity, depending on the severity and complexity of a patient's symptoms. The principle is to offer effective treatment at the least intensive and intrusive level appropriate. Self-help could potentially be integrated into stepped-care models as a "low-intensity" treatment, perhaps primarily for young people with OCD who have relatively mild and straightforward symptom presentations (NICE, 2005). In support of this suggestion, there is emerging evidence for the feasibility, acceptability, and efficacy of different versions of self-help in young people with OCD, including bCBT and iCBT. While this research is still in its infancy, it is backed by a larger body of evidence supporting the use of self-help in adults with OCD, anxiety, and depression. However, many questions remain unanswered and there is a clear need to further understand for whom self-help is appropriate and how self-help outcomes can be maximized.

Key Practice Recommendations.

- Many young people with OCD do not seek professional help for a variety of reasons.
- Self-help interventions, including bCBT and iCBT offer potential to close the treatment gap in OCD.
- Research with adults suggests that self-help approaches can be effective in reducing OCD symptom severity.
- There are a variety of self-help approaches available to offer to young people who present with OCD.
- Methods for optimizing treatment success in utilizing these methods have yet to be developed.
- Careful monitoring of engagement with self-help approaches and monitoring symptom reduction is likely to facilitate optimal outcomes.
- Ongoing outcome evaluation is essential in order to move this field forward and enable young people in urgent need of OCD treatment to benefit.

References

Andersson, E., Enander, J., Andrén, P., Hedman, E., Ljótsson, B., Hursti, T, ... Andersson, G. (2012). Internet-based cognitive behaviour therapy for obsessive–compulsive disorder: A randomized controlled trial. *Psychol Med, 42* (10), 2193–2203.

Andersson, E., Ljótsson, B., Hedman, E., Kaldo, V., Paxling, B., Andersson, G., ... Rück, C. (2011). Internet-based cognitive behavior therapy for obsessive compulsive disorder: A pilot study. *BMC Psychiatry, 11*(1), 125.

Bachofen, M., Nakagawa, A., Marks, I. M., Park, J. M., Greist, J. H., Baer, L., ... Dottl, S. L. (1999). Home self-assessment and self-treatment of obsessive-compulsive disorder using a manual and a computer-conducted telephone interview: Replication of a UK-US study. *Journal of Clinical Psychiatry, 60*(8), 545–549.

Barton, R., & Heyman, I. (2013). Obsessive–compulsive disorder in children and adolescents. *Paediatrics and Child Health, 23*(1), 18–23. doi:http://dx.doi.org/10.1016/j.paed.2012.10.002

Bolton, D., Williams, T., Perrin, S., Atkinson, L., Gallop, C., Waite, P., & Salkovskis, P. (2011). Randomized controlled trial of full and brief cognitive-behaviour therapy and wait-list for paediatric obsessive-compulsive disorder. *Journal of Child Psychology and Psychiatry, 52*(12), 1269–1278. doi: 10.1111/j.1469-7610.2011.02419.x

Chowdhury, U., Frampton, I., & Heyman, I. (2004). Clinical characteristics of young people referred to an obsessive compulsive disorder clinic in the United Kingdom. *Clinical Child Psychology and Psychiatry, 9*(3), 395–401. doi: 10.1177/1359104504043922

Derisley, J., Heyman, I., Robinson, S., & Turner, C. (2008). *Breaking free from OCD: A CBT guide for young people and their families*. London: Jessica Kingsley Publishers.

Den Boer, P. C. A. M., Wiersma, D., & Van Den Bosch, R. J. (2004). Why is self-help neglected in the treatment of emotional disorders? A metaanalysis. *Psychological Medicine, 34*, 959–971.

Diefenbach, G. J., & Tolin, D. F. (2013). The cost of illness associated with stepped care for obsessive-compulsive disorder. *Journal of Obsessive-Compulsive and Related Disorders, 2*(2), 144–148.

Douglass, H. M., Moffitt, T. E., Dar, R., McGee, R., & Silva, P. (1995). Obsessive-compulsive disorder in a birth cohort of 18-year-olds: Prevalence and predictors. *Journal of the American Academy of Child & Adolescent Psychiatry, 34*(11), 1424–1431.

Fernandez de la Cruz, L., Llorens, M., Jassi, A., Krebs, G., Vidal-Ribas, P., Radua, J., ... Mataix-Cols, D. (2015). Ethnic inequalities in the use of secondary and tertiary mental health services among patients with obsessive-compulsive disorder. *Br J Psychiatry, 207*(6), 530–535. doi: 10.1192/bjp.bp.114.154062

Flament, M. F., Whitaker, A., Rapoport, J. L., Davies, M., Berg, C. Z., Kalikow, K., ... Shaffer, D. (1988). Obsessive compulsive disorder in adolescence: An epidemiological study. *Journal of the American Academy of Child & Adolescent Psychiatry, 27*(6), 764–771.

Foa, E. B., & Wilson, R. (2001). *Stop obsessing! How to overcome your obsessions and compulsions*. New York: Bantam.

Foa, E. B., & Kozak, M. J. (1997). *Mastery of obsessive-compulsive disorder: Client workbook*. New York: Graywind Publications.

Gellatly, J., Pedley, R., Molloy, C., Butler, J., Lovell, K., & Bee, P. (2017). Low intensity interventions for obsessive-compulsive disorder (OCD): A qualitative study of mental health practitioner experiences. *BMC Psychiatry, 17*(1), 77.

Geller, D. A., Biederman, J., Faraone, S., Agranat, A., Cradock, K., Hagermoser, L., ... Coffey, B. J. (2001). Developmental aspects of obsessive compulsive disorder: Findings in children, adolescents, and adults. *The Journal of Nervous and Mental Disease, 189*(7), 471–477.

Geller, D. A., & March, J. S. (2012). Practice parameter for the assessment and treatment of children and adolescents with obsessive-compulsive disorder. *Journal of the*

American Academy of Child & Adolescent Psychiatry, 51(1), 98–113. doi:http://dx.doi.org/10.1016/j.jaac.2011.09.019

Gilliam, C. M., Diefenbach, G. J., Whiting, S. E., & Tolin, D. F. (2010). Stepped care for obsessive-compulsive disorder: An open trial. *Behaviour Research and Therapy, 48* (11), 1144-1149.

Goodwin, R., Koenen, K. C., Hellman, F., Guardino, M., & Struening, E. (2002). Helpseeking and access to mental health treatment for obsessive-compulsive disorder. *Acta Psychiatr Scand, 106*(2), 143–149.

Greist, J.H., Marks, I.M., Baer, L, Kobak, K.A., Wenzel, K.W., Hirsch, M.J., ... Clary, C.M. (2002). Behaviour therapy for obsessive compulsive disorder guided by a computer or by a clinician compared with relaxation as a control. *J Clin Psychiatry, 63*, 138–145.

Greist, J.H., Marks, I.M., Baer, L., Parkin, J.R., Manzo, P.A., Mantle, J.M., ... Forman, L. (1998). Self-treatment for OCD using a manual and a computerized telephone interview: A US-UK Study. *MD Comput, 15*, 149–157.

Hauschildt, M., Schröder, J., & Moritz, S. (2016). Randomized-controlled trial on a novel (meta-) cognitive self-help approach for obsessive-compulsive disorder ("myMCT"). *Journal of Obsessive-Compulsive and Related Disorders, 10*, 26–34.

Heyman, I., Fombonne, E., Simmons, H., Ford, T., Meltzer, H., & Goodman, R. (2003). Prevalence of obsessive-compulsive disorder in the British nationwide survey of child mental health. *International Review of Psychiatry, 15*(1–2), 178–184.

Hill, C., Martin, J. L., Thomson, S., Scott-Ram, N., Penfold, H., & Creswell, C. (2017). Navigating the challenges of digital health innovation: Considerations and solutions in developing online and smartphone-application-based interventions for mental health disorders. *The British Journal of Psychiatry, 11*(2), 65–69.

Hollander, E., Stein, D. J., Kwon, J. H., Rowland, C., Wong, C. M., Broatch, J., & Himelein, C. (1997). Psychosocial function and economic costs of obsessive-compulsive disorder. *CNS Spectrums, 2*, 16–25.

Kataoka, S. H., Zhang, L., & Wells, K. B. (2002). Unmet need for mental health care among US children: Variation by ethnicity and insurance status. *American Journal of Psychiatry, 159*(9), 1548–1555.

Kenwright, M., Marks, I.M., Graham, C., Franses, A., &, Mataix-Cols, D. (2005). Brief scheduled phone support from a clinician to enhance computer-aided self-help for obsessive-compulsive disorder: Randomised controlled trial. *J Clin Psychology 61*, 1499–1508.

Knopp-Hoffer, J., Knowles, S., Bower, P., Lovell, K., & Bee, P. E. (2016). 'One man's medicine is another man's poison': A qualitative study of user perspectives on low intensity interventions for Obsessive-Compulsive Disorder (OCD). *BMC Health Services Research, 16*(1), 188.

Kohn, R., Saxenall, S., Levavill, I., & Saracenoll, B. (2004). The treatment gap in mental health care. *Bulletin World Health Organisation, 82*(11), 858–866.

Krebs, G., Isomura, K., Lang, K., Jassi, A., Heyman, I., Diamond, H., ... Mataix-Cols, D. (2015). How resistant is 'treatment-resistant' obsessive-compulsive disorder in youth? *British Journal of Clinical Psychology, 54*(1), 63–75. doi: 10.1111/bjc.12061

Lack, C. W., Storch, E. A., Keeley, M. L., Geffken, G. R., Ricketts, E. D., Murphy, T. K., & Goodman, W. K. (2009). Quality of life in children and adolescents with obsessive-compulsive disorder: Base rates, parent–child agreement, and clinical correlates. *Social Psychiatry and Psychiatric Epidemiology, 44*(11), 935–942. doi: 10.1007/s00127-009-0013-9

Lenhard, F., Vigerland, S., Engberg, H., Hallberg, A., Thermaenius, H., & Serlachius, E. (2016). "On my own, but not alone"-Adolescents' experiences of internet-delivered cognitive behavior therapy for obsessive-compulsive disorder. *PloS One, 11*(10), e0164311.

Lenhard, F., Andersson, E., Mataix-Cols, D., Rück, C., Vigerland, S., Högström, J., ... Serlachius, E. (2017). Therapist-guided, internet-delivered cognitive-behavioral therapy for adolescents with obsessive-compulsive disorder: A randomized controlled trial. *Journal of the American Academy of Child & Adolescent Psychiatry, 56* (1), 10–19.e12. doi:http://dx.doi.org/10.1016/j.jaac.2016.09.515

Mahoney, A.E.J., Mackenzie, A., Williams, A.D., Smith, J., & Andrews, G. (2014). Internet cognitive behavioural treatment for obsessive compulsive disorder: A randomised controlled trial. *Behaviour Research and Therapy, 63*, 99–106.

March, J., & Benton, C. (2006). *Talking back to OCD: The program that helps kids and teens say "no way" – And parents say "way to go."* New York: The Guilford Press.

March, J. S., & Mulle, K. (1998). *OCD in children and adolescents: A cognitive-behavioral treatment manual.* New York: Guilford Press.

Marks, I. M., Baer, L., Greist, J. H., Park, J. M., Bachofen, M., Nakagawa, A., ... Mantle, J. M. (1998). Home self-assessment of obsessive-compulsive disorder. Use of a manual and a computer-conducted telephone interview: Two UK-US studies. *The British Journal of Psychiatry, 172*(5), 406–412.

Marques, L., LeBlanc, N. J., Weingarden, H. M., Timpano, K. R., Jenike, M., & Wilhelm, S. (2010). Barriers to treatment and service utilization in an internet sample of individuals with obsessive-compulsive symptoms. *Depress Anxiety, 27*(5), 470–475. doi: 10.1002/da.20694

Mataix-Cols, D., & Marks, I. M. (2006). Self-help with minimal therapist contact for obsessive–compulsive disorder: A review. *European Psychiatry, 21*(2), 75–80.

Micali, N., Heyman, I., Perez, M., Hilton, K., Nakatani, E., Turner, C., & Mataix-Cols, D. (2010). Long-term outcomes of obsessive–compulsive disorder: Follow-up of 142 children and adolescents. *The British Journal of Psychiatry, 197*(2), 128–134.

Moritz, S., Jelinek, L., Hauschildt, M., & Naber, D. (2010). How to treat the untreated: Effectiveness of a self-help metacognitive training program (myMCT) for obsessive-compulsive disorder. *Dialogues Clin Neurosci, 12*(2), 209–220.

Moritz, S., Wittekind, C. E., Hauschildt, M., & Timpano, K. R. (2011). Do it yourself? Self-help and online therapy for people with obsessive-compulsive disorder. *Current Opinion in Psychiatry, 24*(6), 541-548.

Murray, C. L., & Lopez, A. D. (1996). *The global burden of disease: A comprehensive assessment of mortality and disability from diseases, injuries, and risk factors in 1990 and projected to 2020.* Cambridge, MA: Harvard University Press.

Nair, A., Wong, Y. L., Barrow, F., Heyman, I., Clark, B., & Krebs, G. (2015). Has the first-line management of paediatric OCD improved following the introduction of NICE guidelines? *Arch Dis Child, 100*(4), 416–417. doi: 10.1136/archdischild-2014-307900

NICE. (2005). *Obsessive-compulsive disorder: Core interventions in the treatment of obsessive-compulsive disorder and body dysmorphic disorder.* NICE, London.

Nielssen, O., Dear, B. F., Staples, L. G., Dear, R., Ryan, K., Purtell, C., & Titov, N. (2015). Procedures for risk management and a review of crisis referrals from the MindSpot Clinic, a national service for the remote assessment and treatment of anxiety and depression. *BMC Psychiatry, 15*(1), 304.

Pearcy, C.P., Anderson, R.A., Egan, S.J., & Rees, C.S. (2016). A systematic review and meta-analysis of self-help therapeutic interventions for obsessive-compulsive disorder: Is therapeutic contact key to overall improvement? *J Behav Ther Exp Psychiatry, 51*, 74–83. doi: 10.1016/j.jbtep.2015.12.007.

Piacentini, J., Bergman, R. L., Keller, M., & McCracken, J. (2003). Functional impairment in children and adolescents with obsessive-compulsive disorder. *Journal of Child and Adolescent Psychopharmacology, 13*(2, Supplement 1), 61–69.

Pinto, A., Mancebo, M. C., Eisen, J. L., Pagano, M. E., & Rasmussen, S. A. (2006). The Brown Longitudinal Obsessive Compulsive Study: Clinical features and symptoms of the sample at intake. *The Journal of Clinical Psychiatry, 67*(5), 703–711.

Rees, C. S., & Anderson, R. A. (2016). Online obsessive-compulsive disorder treatment: Preliminary results of the "OCD? Not Me!" self-guided internet-based cognitive behavioral therapy program for young people. *JMIR mental health, 3*(3), e29. doi: 10.2196/mental.5363

Rees, C. S., Anderson, R. A., & Finlay-Jones, A. (2015). OCD? Not Me! Protocol for the development and evaluation of a web-based self-guided treatment for youth with obsessive-compulsive disorder. *BMJ Open, 5*(4). doi: 10.1136/bmjopen-2014-007486

Robinson, S., Turner, C., Heyman, I., & Farquharson, L. (2013). The feasibility and acceptability of a cognitive-behavioural self-help intervention for adolescents with obsessive-compulsive disorder. *Behav Cogn Psychother, 41*(1), 117–122. doi: 10.1017/s1352465812000562

Sánchez-Meca, J., Rosa-Alcázar, A. I., Iniesta-Sepúlveda, M., & Rosa-Alcázar, Á. (2014). Differential efficacy of cognitive-behavioral therapy and pharmacological treatments for pediatric obsessive–compulsive disorder: A meta-analysis. *Journal of Anxiety Disorders, 28*(1), 31–44. doi:http://doi.org/10.1016/j.janxdis.2013.10.007

Scahill, L., Riddle, M. A., McSwiggin-Hardin, M., & Ort, S. I. (1997). Children's Yale-Brown Obsessive Compulsive Scale: Reliability and validity. *Journal of the American Academy of Child & Adolescent Psychiatry, 36*(6), 844–852.

Scogin, F., Bynum, J., Stephens, G., & Calhoon, S. (1990). Efficacy of self-administered treatment programs: Meta-analytic review. *Professional Psychology: Research and Practice, 21*, 42–47.

Sisemore, T. A. (2010). *Free from OCD: A workbook for teens with obsessive-compulsive disorder. Instant Help*. Oakland: New Harbinger.

Skarphedinsson, G., De Nadai, A. S., Storch, E. A., Lewin, A. B., & Ivarsson, T. (2017). Defining cognitive-behavior therapy response and remission in pediatric OCD: A signal detection analysis of the Children's Yale-Brown Obsessive Compulsive Scale. *European Child & Adolescent Psychiatry, 26*(1), 47–55. doi: 10.1007/s00787-016-0863-0

Steffen, M, Wittekinda, CE., Hauschildta, M. & Timpano, KR. (2011). Do it yourself? Self-help and online therapy for people with obsessive-compulsive disorder. *Current Opinion in Psychiatry, 24*, 541–548.

Stengler, K., Olbrich, S., Heider, D., Dietrich, S., Riedel-Heller, S., & Jahn, I. (2013). Mental health treatment seeking among patients with OCD: Impact of age of onset. *Social Psychiatry and Psychiatric Epidemiology, 48*(5), 813–819. doi: 10.1007/s00127-012-0544-3

Storch, E. A., Khanna, M., Merlo, L. J., Loew, B. A., Franklin, M., Reid, J. M., ... Murphy, T. K. (2009). Children's Florida Obsessive Compulsive Inventory: Psychometric properties and feasibility of a self-report measure of obsessive–compulsive symptoms in youth. *Child Psychiatry and Human Development, 40*(3), 467–483. doi: 10.1007/s10578-009-0138-9

Titov, N., Dear, B. F., Staples, L. G., Bennett-Levy, J., Klein, B., Rapee, R. M., ... Purtell, C. (2015). MindSpot clinic: An accessible, efficient, and effective online treatment service for anxiety and depression. *Psychiatric Services, 66*(10), 1043–1050.

Tolin, D.F., Hannan, S., Maltby, N., Diefenbach, G.J., Worhunsky, P., & Brady, R.E. (2007). A randomized controlled trial of self-directed versus therapist-directed cognitive–behavioural therapy for obsessive–compulsive disorder patients with prior medication trials. *Behavior Therapy, 38*(2), 179–191.

Tolin, D. F., Diefenbach, G. J., Maltby, N., & Hannan, S. (2005). Stepped care for obsessive-compulsive disorder: A pilot study. *Cognitive and Behavioral Practice, 12*(4), 403–414.

Tumur, I., Kaltenthaler, E., Ferriter, M., Beverley, C., & Parry, G. (2007). Computerised cognitive behaviour therapy for obsessive-compulsive disorder: A systematic review. *Psychotherapy and Psychosomatics, 76*(4), 196–202.

Valderhaug, R., Gotestam, K. G., & Larsson, B. (2004). Clinicians' views on management of obsessive-compulsive disorders in children and adolescents. *Nordic Journal of Psychiatry, 58*(2), 125–132. doi: 10.1080/08039480410005503

Valderhaug, R., Larsson, B., Götestam, K. G., & Piacentini, J. (2007). An open clinical trial of cognitive-behaviour therapy in children and adolescents with obsessive–compulsive disorder administered in regular outpatient clinics. *Behaviour Research and Therapy, 45*(3), 577–589. doi:http://dx.doi.org/10.1016/j.brat.2006.04.011

Veale, D., & Willson, R. (2009). *Overcoming obsessive-compulsive disorder: A self-help guide using cognitive behavioural techniques*. London: Hachette UK.

Vogel, P. A., Solem, S., Hagen, K., Moen, E. M., Launes, G., Håland, Å. T., ... Himle, J. A. (2014). A pilot randomized controlled trial of videoconference-assisted treatment for obsessive-compulsive disorder. *Behaviour Research and Therapy, 63*, 162–168.

Watson, H. J., & Rees, C. S. (2008). Meta-analysis of randomized, controlled treatment trials for pediatric obsessive-compulsive disorder. *Journal of Child Psychology and Psychiatry, 49*(5), 489–498.

Wootton, B.M. (2016). Remote cognitive–behavior therapy for obsessive–compulsive symptoms: A meta-analysis. *Clinical Psychology Review, 43*, Feb 2016, 103–113.

Wootton, B.M., Dear, B.F., Johnston, L., Terides, M.D., & Titov, N. (2014). Self-guided internet administered treatment for obsessive–compulsive disorder: Results from two open trials. *Journal of Obsessive–Compulsive and Related Disorders, 3*(2), 102–108.

Wootton, B.M., Dear, B.F., Johnston, L., Terides, M.D., & Titov, N. (2015). Self-guided internet-delivered cognitive behavior therapy (iCBT) for obsessive–compulsive disorder: 12 Month follow-up. *Internet Interventions, 2*(3), 243–247.

Wootton, B.M., Titov, N., Dear, B.F., Spence, J., Andrews, G., Johnston, L., & Solley, K. (2011). An Internet administered treatment program for obsessive–compulsive disorder: A feasibility study. *Journal of Anxiety Disorders, 25*(8), 1102–1107.

Zohar, A. H. (1999). The epidemiology of obsessive-compulsive disorder in children and adolescents. *Child and Adolescent Psychiatric Clinics of North America, 8*(3), 445–460.

16 New Technologies to Deliver CBT for Young Children with Obsessive-Compulsive Disorder

Kristina Aspvall, Fabian Lenhard, Eva Serlachius, and David Mataix-Cols

The Need for Technological Innovation

While there is a broad evidence base and expert consensus for traditional, clinic-based CBT as the first-line treatment alternative for pediatric OCD (Geller & March, 2012; McGuire et al., 2015; National Institute for Health and Care Excellence [NICE], 2005), there are important barriers to accessing this treatment, which have limited its dissemination.

First, there are large geographic inequalities regarding the availability of high-quality assessment and treatment options for OCD (Goodwin et al., 2002; Kohn et al., 2004). Consequently, a majority of cases are not detected by the healthcare system (Wahl et al., 2010), and even if identified and correctly diagnosed, OCD cases are seldom treated with good quality, evidence-based CBT (Krebs et al., 2015; Valderhaug, Götestam, & Larsson, 2004). Second, in some healthcare systems, the lack of insurance coverage or out-of-pocket treatment costs keep patients from seeking treatment (Marques et al., 2010). Third, patients themselves may be hesitant to seek help, due to doubts about treatment being beneficial (Goodwin et al., 2002; Marques et al., 2010), shame and stigma associated with symptoms, as well as not knowing where to seek help (García-Soriano et al., 2014). Related to this issue, ethnic minorities are underrepresented in specialized OCD treatment services and are more unlikely to seek treatment for OCD (Fernández de la Cruz et al., 2016; Goodwin et al., 2002), underlining the socially unequal accessibility of effective treatments. Fourth, in some areas, large geographic and travel distances to the nearest clinic make office-based CBT unfeasible for those families that live in remote areas (Cavanagh, 2014). Perhaps unsurprisingly, several strong initiatives to develop innovative ways to deliver CBT for OCD have arisen in countries that have vast, sparsely populated areas, such as Sweden and Australia.

In addition, organizational challenges within healthcare appear to hinder the implementation and delivery of CBT (McHugh & Barlow, 2010). When implemented in regular health care, CBT appears to often be delivered with suboptimal quality (Krebs et al., 2015; Shafran et al., 2009). This could be related to the fact that traditional, office-based CBT is a relatively cost and resource intensive intervention, with usually between 12 and 14 one-hour sessions and the requirement of clinicians that are specialized in the delivery of CBT according to available treatment protocols. Due to the required time and expert resources, the traditional format of CBT may not be a feasible option in healthcare settings with limited budgets, small economic margins for patients to pay out of pocket, or in situations with restricted access to CBT-trained clinicians.

As a consequence of the existing treatment barriers, a majority of patients do not get access to CBT. International data indicate that more than half of all OCD sufferers do not get access to care, and in some regions 8 out of 10 patients do not get any treatment at all (Kohn et al., 2004). For those who receive treatment, waiting times from symptom onset to first diagnosis and treatment are often unacceptably long: 17 years as indicated by one study in adults (Pinto et al., 2006) and 3.5 years as indicated by a study in children and adolescents with OCD (Micali et al., 2010).

New therapeutic formats that apply modern information technology to psychological interventions have the potential to overcome some of those treatment barriers and to increase availability of CBT for young people with OCD. Such innovations could potentially:

1. provide a feasible and effective treatment format for patients who otherwise would not have had any access to care due to geographic distances, socioeconomic factors, and/or shame and stigma
2. be a cost-effective option for healthcare providers and patients due to reduced clinician time per patient
3. increase healthcare providers' capacity to treat more patients with the available resources, and perhaps freeing time for more complex cases that require more intensive, personalized care (Mataix-Cols & Marks, 2006)
4. support successful implementation of good quality CBT in regular care settings, as these formats often are more structured and standardized than traditional CBT, and therefore less susceptible to modifications that undermine the integrity of the intervention.

Technological Approaches to Innovation

Innovative formats of delivery of CBT have been developed, or are in the initial stages of development, within four distinct modalities: Internet-delivered CBT, video- or tele-conferencing, mobile phone applications (apps), and virtual reality. The use of terminology is relatively consistent within each field, but variations occur. For clarity, we use the following definitions:

Internet-Delivered CBT (or Internet-Based CBT, ICBT): Even if all the presented modalities from a technical perspective make use of the internet to some extent, the term ICBT usually refers to interventions that resemble interactive online courses and predominantly make use of text, visual materials, and written exercises. The treatment content is presented via a password-secured home page and can be either clinician-supported (*guided*) or without clinician support (*unguided*).

Video- or Teleconferencing: Videoconferencing interventions use web-cameras, Skype, or other technical video communication solutions for direct audiovisual communication with the therapist and non-office-based therapy sessions. Teleconferencing interventions simply require a telephone. In both cases, the treatment content and support are the same as in traditional face-to-face CBT, provided by a clinician in real time.

Mobile Phone Applications (Apps): App-based interventions deliver treatment content through mobile phone applications in the user's own smartphone, and are offered via download from the platform-specific operators, such as iTunes, Google play, or Android market.

Virtual Reality (VR): Virtual reality is defined as the use of audiovisual devices that present a virtual, data animated environment to the user, usually delivered via a head-mounted goggle with a screen in front of the eyes that presents the 3-dimensional space. The user is usually able to look and move around the virtual environment and interact with objects within it.

ICBT

Internet-delivered CBT has emerged in the late 1990s as a cross-disciplinary development of psychological intervention research and modern information technology (Andersson, 2009). The ICBT format is similar to that of an e-learning course, with psychoeducative texts, visual material, images and videos, written exercises to work with and, if clinician support is included, e-mail functionality. The development of ICBT within the pediatric OCD field has been lagging behind the adult field, where ICBT interventions have been scientifically evaluated since 2011 (Andersson et al., 2011; Wootton et al., 2011). To the best of our knowledge, the only two interventions that are currently available for the pediatric population are "OCD? Not me!", an unguided ICBT intervention developed at Curtin University in Australia (Rees, Anderson, & Finlay-Jones, 2015; Rees et al., 2016), and "BiP OCD," a clinician-guided intervention developed at the Karolinska Institutet in Sweden (Aspvall et al., 2018; Lenhard et al., 2014, 2016; Lenhard, Andersson, et al., 2017).

"OCD? Not me!" is an unguided, fully automated ICBT intervention for adolescents age 12 to 18 (Rees et al., 2015). Fully automated ICBT interventions without the requirement of clinician-support or feedback have the potential benefits of minimal costs for the healthcare provider and constant access for patients. A potential disadvantage of an entirely self-guided intervention is that patient retention may be limited, as illustrated by the adult OCD literature (Kenwright et al., 2005).

"OCD? Not me!" consists of eight stages, designed to be completed sequentially at a working pace of one module per week. The eight stages cover a range of evidence-based CBT components (Franklin & Foa, 2011), such as psychoeducation about OCD and the rationale for exposure and response prevention (ERP), goal setting, ERP exercises, family and others' accommodations to OCD, problem solving regarding setbacks and expectations, the impact of stress on OCD symptoms, as well as consolidation of strategies and relapse prevention. The program incorporates a number of interactive exercises, graphical feedback of weekly symptom measures and age-appropriate metaphors and images as means to engage and motivate the young patients to adhere to the intervention.

Alongside the adolescent content, parents and caregivers are provided with stage-by-stage content covering psychoeducation about OCD and addressing how to support the adolescent to complete each stage, as well as family and parent-specific content, such as coping strategies for family distress and family accommodation. Figure 16.1 displays some screenshots from "OCD? Not me!" and https://www.ocdnotme.com.au/ provides additional information for patients and professionals.

The "OCD? Not me!" program is currently being evaluated in an open trial. Preliminary data were recently reported from 132 adolescents with at least subclinical OCD (Rees et al., 2016). Patients were on average 14.58 years old (SD=1.94) and 73.5 percent met criteria for clinical OCD. There were significant treatment effects on self-rated OCD symptoms (moderate effect size of d=.64) and on self-rated OCD severity (large effect size of d=.89). These results should be considered preliminary, as this study is still ongoing, and only limited data are available from the last stages of the intervention (<10 percent), as many patients had yet to reach that part of the intervention.

"BiP OCD" is a clinician- and parent-supported ICBT intervention. BiP OCD was initially developed for adolescents 12 to 17 years with OCD (Lenhard et al., 2014, 2016; Lenhard, Andersson, et al., 2017) and later adapted for children 7 to 11 years (Aspvall et al., 2018). The adaptations for children included increased parental support and strategies for how to support and motivate the children to work with exposure exercises. The latest iteration of BiP OCD has integrated child and adolescent versions with age-adapted material for the two age groups, and expanded parental modules of 12 chapters. The treatment content is based on expert guidelines, with exposure and response prevention (ERP) as the main focus for the intervention (Franklin & Foa, 2011). The content is presented in consecutive chapters (see Table 16.1) that contain texts to read, films and animations to watch, as well as exercises for the patients to do on their own and together with their parents or primary caregivers. Patients log in to the treatment via a personal password-secured account. BiP OCD is divided into three different phases: 1) psychoeducation, including the circular, self-maintaining nature of obsessions and compulsions and the rationale for ERP, 2) the main part of treatment, focusing on ERP exercises as well as cognitive strategies, and 3) problem solving and relapse prevention. Patients have regular asynchronous contact with the clinician through messages (resembling email), usually several times per week, and occasionally via telephone. Such clinician support typically amounts to about 20 minutes per patient per week (Aspvall et al., 2018; Lenhard et al., 2017), which is approximately a third of the time required for regular face-to-face CBT sessions.

Parents are provided with caregiver-specific content within a separate track of the treatment that covers a range of topics, including family accommodation, parental coping strategies, and support of ERP exercises (see Table 16.1). The content in the

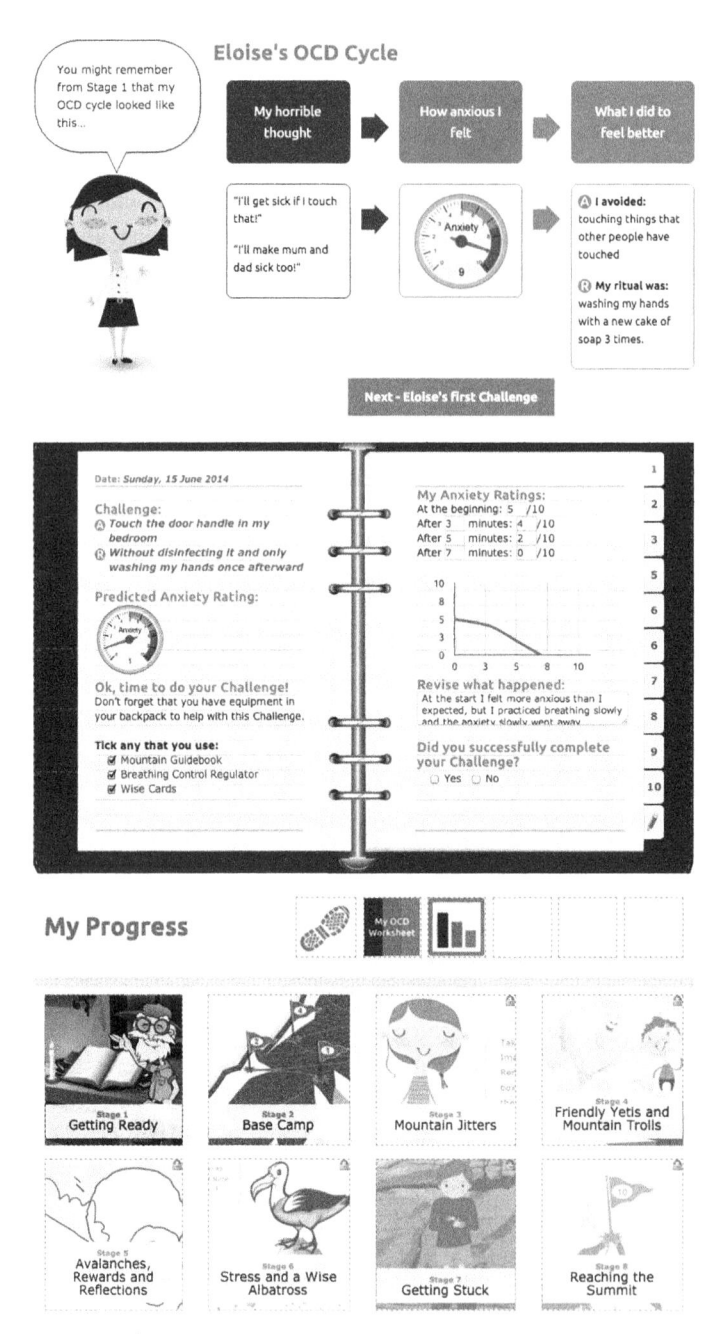

Figure 16.1 *Screenshots from "OCD? Not me!" (from top to bottom: psychoeducation regarding the OCD cycle, ERP exercise, overview of treatment progress; reproduced with permission of the author)*

child and adolescent versions of BiP OCD is similar; however, the degree of parental involvement has been adapted to the developmental needs of children and adolescents, respectively, with more parental support for children and more degrees of

Table 16.1 *Treatment Chapters and Content of BiP OCD*

Treatment Phase	Chapter	Child and Adolescent Chapters	Parent Chapters
Psychoeducation	1	Psychoeducation about OCD	Psychoeducation about OCD
	2	Psychoeducation ERP and goal formulation	Psychoeducation ERP
	3	How to do exposures?	How to do exposures?
Exposure with response prevention (ERP)	4	Testing ERP	Parental ERP coaching strategies
	5	More exposure	Barriers during treatment
	6	Family accommodation and exposure	OCD and family accommodation
	7	New steps with ERP	Motivation and parental strategies
	8	Coping with obsessions	Coping with obsessions
	9	Evaluation so far and new exposures	Evaluation so far and new exposures
	10	Reducing compulsions even further	Doing more difficult exposure
	11	Final ERP exercise	Final ERP exercises
Relapse prevention	12	Relapse prevention and lessons learned	Relapse prevention

Note: OCD = Obsessive-compulsive disorder; ERP = Exposure with response prevention

freedom for adolescents. Parents and patients are encouraged to carry out ERP exercises together and collaborate with each other regarding the treatment content in order to facilitate adherence and successful transfer of CBT skills into the everyday life of the family. Figure 16.2 displays screenshots from BiP OCD.

BiP OCD has been evaluated in several clinical trials. Results from an initial open trial with 21 adolescents with clinical OCD showed that BiP OCD was an acceptable and effective intervention, with 57 percent treatment responders at posttreatment and significant symptom reductions on clinician-rated measures (large effect size of $d=2.29$; Lenhard et al., 2014). In a subsequent randomized controlled trial, 67 adolescent OCD patients were randomized to either BiP OCD or to a wait-list. Results showed significant symptom reductions in the BiP OCD group and only minimal improvement in the wait-list, resulting in a moderate between-group effect size at posttreatment of $d=0.64$. Using strict consensus criteria (Mataix-Cols et al., 2016), 27 percent of the participants in the ICBT group were classified as responders, compared to 0 percent in the wait-list. The average clinician time to treat each patient was 17.5 minutes per week, about a third of traditional face-to-face CBT. In a third trial, the feasibility and efficacy of BiP OCD adapted for younger children with OCD (ages 7–11) was evaluated in an open trial (Aspvall et al., 2018). The results showed that ICBT also is a feasible and effective treatment for the younger age group, with significant symptom reductions after treatment (large effect size of $d=1.86$) and 64 percent treatment responders at 3-month follow-up. The average therapist time per patient was 22.0 minutes per week, including correspondence with the parents.

The cost-effectiveness of BiP OCD has been evaluated as a part of the randomized controlled trial for adolescents (Lenhard, Ssegonja, et al., 2017). When comparing the cost of healthcare use including prescription of drugs, supportive resources, school absence as well as productivity loss, the ICBT group reduced the societal cost compared to those that did not receive any treatment. This suggests that ICBT could be a cost-effective treatment for the healthcare system, but further studies are needed to establish the effect compared to regular CBT.

BiP OCD is currently being evaluated in three specialist clinics in Gothenburg, London, and Brisbane, in order to evaluate the generalizability of the clinical trial findings to regular clinical settings.

To summarize, the available data indicate promising results for both guided as well as unguided ICBT for pediatric OCD. Future studies should address the interesting question of the minimally needed amount of clinician-support to achieve effective treatment outcomes as well as aim for direct head to head comparisons of guided and unguided ICBT interventions against gold standard face-to-face CBT.

Video and Teleconferencing

In videoconferencing, the treatment is delivered remotely via web cameras, with the family having scheduled real-time sessions with a therapist (Comer et al., 2014). The treatment mimics face-to-face CBT regarding content, with the first three sessions involving psychoeducation, the main focus on exposure with response prevention in the middle sessions, and relapse prevention in the last two sessions (Comer et al., 2017; Storch et al., 2011). The treatment is adapted to the individual's symptoms and developmental level, and parental involvement in the sessions is recommended in order for parents to assist with homework assignments as well as reducing family accommodation. The therapist time is the same as in face-to-face CBT, with fourteen 60–90-minute sessions.

Another tele-health approach is to provide the treatment via the telephone (Turner et al., 2014). The procedure and method are similar to videoconferencing, with the main difference being the audio-only communication. This reduces the need of high-technology equipment for both the therapist and the patient, while still maintaining the advantages of geographical reach. Both video- and teleconferencing options greatly facilitate access to CBT but still require appointments and experienced clinicians delivering the treatment.

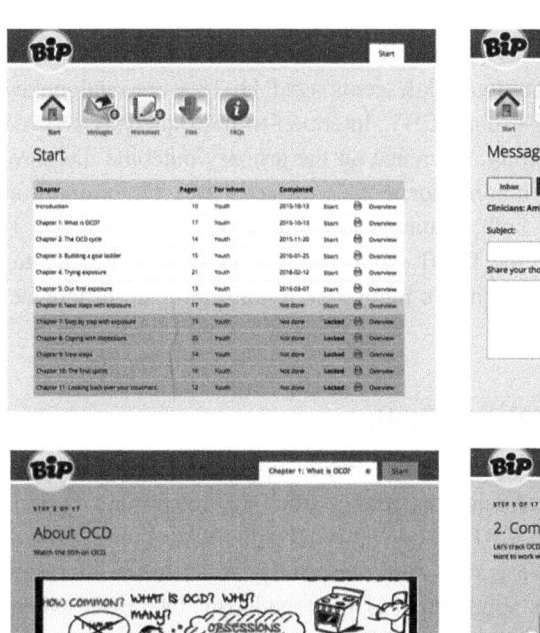

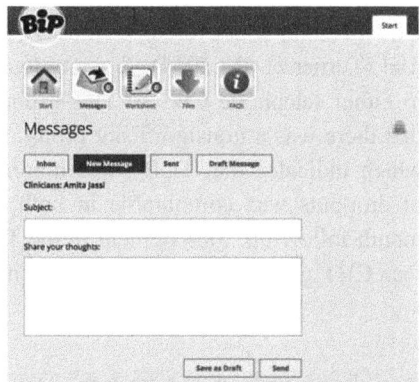

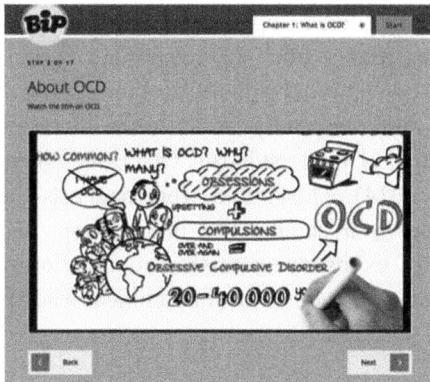

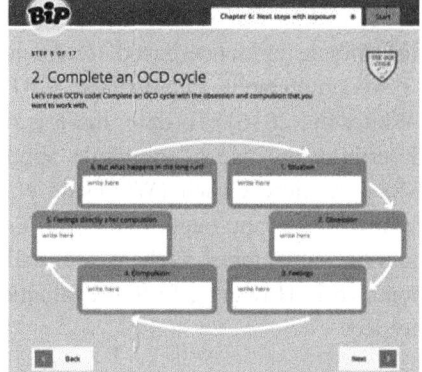

Figure 16.2 *Screenshots from BiP OCD (top right: start page with chapters, top left: e-mail functionality for communication with clinician, bottom right: psychoeducational video, bottom left: OCD cycle exercise; reproduced with permission of the author)*

Videoconferencing was evaluated in a wait-list–controlled trial including children and adolescents with OCD ($N=31$) aged 7–16 (Storch et al., 2011). Results indicated a large between-group effect size at posttreatment ($d=1.36$). Fifty-six percent of the individuals in the videoconferencing group were classified as being in remission at posttreatment, compared to 13 percent in the wait-list group, a difference that was statistically significant.

Following a small case series ($N=5$), another pilot study of early onset OCD randomized 22 children aged 4–8 to receive either family-based CBT via web camera or in the clinic (Comer et al., 2017). There was a significant decrease in symptoms in both treatment conditions. The between-group effect size was small at both posttreatment *($d=0.09$)* and 6-month follow up *($d=0.12$)*, and the responder statuses were 72.7 percent in the videoconferencing group and 60.0 percent in the clinic. There was only one participant in each group that dropped out of treatment, and remission rates were equal in both groups.

After a successful case series (*N*=10; Turner et al., 2009), telephone-delivered CBT (TCBT) was evaluated in a large-scale noninferiority randomized controlled trial (Turner et al., 2014). Seventy-two adolescents aged 11–18 were randomized to either telephone-CBT or face-to-face CBT. Intention-to-treat analysis showed that there was a nonsignificant group difference on the primary outcome measure, which indicates that TCBT was noninferior to face-to-face CBT. The proportion of dropouts was comparable in both treatment conditions (in total *N*=6). At 3-month follow-up, 58.8 percent in the TCBT group and 60.6 percent in the face-to-face CBT group were classified as being in remission, a nonsignificant difference.

Mobile Phone Applications (Apps)

The use of mobile applications has been suggested as one way to disseminate evidence-based treatment to patients from all geographic regions or to supplement face-to-face CBT as a way of enhancing the treatment (Whiteside, 2016). To date, there is only one case study (*N*=2) in the literature describing the use of a mobile application to treat pediatric OCD, the Mayo Clinic Anxiety Coach (Whiteside et al., 2014). This initial work suggests the feasibility of app-supported CBT or app as a stand-alone intervention, and possible advantages such as facilitation of exposure exercises and monitoring homework. However, further evaluation through well-controlled clinical trials is needed.

Virtual Reality

Currently there are no studies describing the use of virtual reality in treatment of pediatric OCD. There have been two papers published on virtual reality interventions for adults with OCD. In a case series, Laforest et al. (2016) used virtual reality equipment as a part of a standard CBT protocol for conducting in vitro exposure for contamination fear during the sessions. The treatment consisted of 12 sessions. It has also been described as a stand-alone treatment, where the principles of exposure and response prevention were illustrated by directing a character around in an online program during three sessions (Matthews et al., 2017).

In the case series (*N*=3) of Laforest et al. (2016), all three participants improved significantly from pre- to posttreatment, but the results were only maintained for one participant at 8-month follow-up. In the pilot study by Matthews et al. (2017), participants (*N*=78) were randomized to either virtual reality treatment or wait-list. There was a significant within-group difference at posttreatment, but no significant between-group difference. The between-group effect size was g=0.36 (95 percent CI: -0.21, 0.94).

Mediators and Moderators of Change

To the best of our knowledge, there are currently no studies that have explored mediators or moderators of change in pediatric OCD within the context of technology-delivered treatments. A study from the adult ICBT field indicated that an initial increase in obsessive beliefs at the start of treatment, perhaps contrary to expectations, is associated with better treatment outcome (Andersson et al., 2015). This might suggest that interventions should aim to initially tackle obsessive beliefs. However, replications of these findings are warranted in the pediatric OCD population.

Moreover, mechanisms of change that are specific for the field of innovative treatments in pediatric patients should be investigated further. For example, there is no empirical knowledge about whether, how much, and in which way parents should be involved in these new treatment formats. Another relationship that should be established in this novel field is the association of ERP exercise adherence, which is known to predict CBT treatment outcome in traditional face-to-face CBT (Simpson et al., 2011). There could be important differences between traditional therapist-led ERP and ERP exercises that are delivered through one of the previously presented treatment formats, which in turn could have important implications for the successful improvement of interventions. Future research should therefore prioritize the reliable measurement of such potential mediators and moderators.

Clinical Case Illustration

Simon (fictional name) is a 12-year-old boy who participated in one of the ICBT trials in Sweden. He lived in a rural area together with his parents and one younger sister. Over the last year, his OCD symptoms became more prominent and started interfering with school performance and family functioning. When they turned to their local Child and Adolescent Mental Health Service (CAMHS) unit for help, they received information about the ICBT trial and decided to apply, particularly because they could work with the treatment from home and they could spend the time doing homework assignments instead of driving two hours each way for a therapy session.

The family came for an initial assessment at the clinic to establish the diagnosis and symptom severity level. Simon had a moderately severe OCD with contamination obsessions, and extensive cleaning and washing compulsions. He avoided touching things in public places, used hand sanitizer before eating things, and asked his parents for reassurance that he would not get sick. He also had depressive symptoms secondary to the OCD. Simon had always performed well in school, had many friends, and played football three times a week, but during the last two months he had become more absent from school and football practice, and he also had started avoiding his friends due to his OCD.

After inclusion in the study, Simon and his mother received separate logins to the secure BiP OCD webpage. They were also assigned a therapist for the duration of the treatment, who was the same therapist they had met during the initial assessment. Within the first two weeks, they had completed the first three chapters including psychoeducation about OCD and the rationale for exposure with response prevention. On average, each of these chapters took about 30 minutes to complete. When they started chapter four, Simon's mother learned about parent strategies that could be helpful during the treatment and started to reinforce exposure behaviors instead of giving remarks about compulsions. Simon quickly grasped the idea behind exposure, and he worked eagerly with his exercises. He practiced touching things when going on public transport, ate food at cafés without previously cleaning his hands, and resisted asking for reassurance from his parents. At mid-treatment (week 6) his motivation decreased, and his mother had frequent contact with the therapist to problem solve how to handle the many conflicts that emerged. They discussed the treatment goals and introduced a reward system, which made Simon more eager to continue working with ERP. Simon quickly made more progress and could do more difficult exposure tasks and was reducing avoidance behaviors. During the treatment, Simon and his mother completed 10 out of the 12 chapters (including the chapter on relapse prevention). Both of them had contact with the therapist through written messages during the entire treatment.

At the posttreatment clinician assessment (week 12), Simon's symptoms had decreased to a subclinical level of severity, and at the 3-month follow-up assessment he was in remission. Simon found it very helpful to learn that he was not the only one who had OCD and to read examples about how other children had fought against their OCD. The mother expressed great satisfaction with the treatment, especially in regard to the flexible format that made it possible to work at any time, and the strategies to support her child throughout the treatment. His depressive symptoms also decreased during treatment, and his general functioning increased. The family reported that he was back in school and had a higher quality of life as a result of the decreased OCD symptoms. The therapist time was on average 20 minutes per week during the treatment, which included time spent giving feedback to both Simon and his mother. Simon was discharged from the CAMHS unit at 3-month follow-up, since he was no longer in need of treatment.

This case example demonstrates a typical patient in our ICBT trials, with a previous history of anxiety disorders, previous CBT, and living far away from a CAMHS clinic.

Challenges and Recommendations for Future Research

There is still a limited amount of research conducted on new ways to deliver CBT for children and adolescents with OCD. The research has mainly focused on self- and therapist-guided ICBT (Aspvall et al., 2018; Lenhard et al., 2014, 2017; Rees et al., 2016), teleconferencing (Turner et al., 2014), and videoconferencing (Comer et al., 2017; Storch et al., 2011), whereas systematic studies on mobile phone applications and virtual reality have been rare. While the findings are promising, the evidence to date should be regarded as preliminary. In this section, we highlight some areas that require further research before these technological innovations can become a real option for patients with OCD.

First, it will be important to establish the relative efficacy of these novel interventions, compared to standard face-to-face CBT. To date, this has been done in adolescents with insomnia (de Bruin et al., 2015), adolescents with anxiety disorders (Spence et al., 2011), and in one TCBT study in adolescents with OCD (Turner et al., 2014), with positive results. Similar studies comparing ICBT with face-to-face CBT are warranted. It is a possibility that the outcomes of ICBT trials (Lenhard et al., 2014; Lenhard, Andersson, et al., 2017; Rees et al., 2016) may be somewhat inferior to those obtained with face-to-face CBT (The Pediatric OCD Treatment Study (POTS) Team, 2004; Torp et al., 2015). If this were the case, ICBT may be more suited to use as a first-line, low-intensity intervention in a stepped-care approach, whereby uncomplicated OCD cases are first offered ICBT and nonresponders or more complex cases are offered more intensive treatment options (Mataix-Cols & Marks, 2006). Studies evaluating such a stepped-care model would be enormously informative for the field going forward.

One limitation shared by most previous ICBT studies is that the majority of participants have been self-referred patients. This may have resulted in selected patients with highly educated parents and high motivation for change. Therefore, future clinical trials should preferably be done in clinical settings, to ensure that the outcomes of ICBT and other novel treatment approaches are generalizable to the entire population of OCD patients.

Another limitation of the previous literature is that, with few exceptions (Turner et al., 2014), most studies included short follow-up periods, typically up to three months after treatment. Future studies should include longer-term follow-ups.

Another area that probably will be important in the future is the increasing emphasis on health economy analysis, to capture both the cost of OCD for the family and society at large, and the cost for treatment. This should preferably be done by comparing the cost for different treatment options, such as ICBT, face-to-face CBT, and medication. This is important for healthcare policies and decisions regarding implementation of a new treatment such as ICBT in the healthcare system.

As previously mentioned, there is limited evidence for who ICBT works for. Future research should focus on investigating moderators and mediators of outcome, to better understand treatment mechanisms and who should be offered which kind of treatment.

Another key challenge is the implementation of these innovative treatment formats in regular health care and the willingness of clinicians and decision-makers to adopt these novel approaches. The literature suggests that there are varying attitudes regarding computerized CBT dependent on clinicians' theoretical orientation, as well as concerns about the lack of human support (Vigerland et al., 2014). There might be as well technical and administrative issues, such as IT solution security and integrity of confidential patient data, the need for modified reimbursement systems, and ownership/copyright issues that pose new challenges for successful implementation.

Key Practice Points

The research into innovative ways to deliver CBT for pediatric OCD is still relatively new, but the empirical evidence for self- and therapist-guided ICBT as well as video- and teleconferencing is starting to increase and is highly promising. Clearly, however, more research is needed before these treatment modalities can be implemented in the healthcare system.

One of the main advantages of ICBT and video/teleconferencing is that it makes treatment more available for patients, especially for those who live far away from CAMHS services. ICBT in particular has a great potential to be a cost-effective treatment option since it substantially reduces the required amount of therapist time, compared to standard CBT protocols (Lenhard, Ssegonja, et al., 2017; Mataix-Cols & Marks, 2006).

To date, no study has directly compared ICBT with and without therapist support, but preliminary results from published studies may indicate that therapist-guided ICBT protocols ensure greater patient retention and therefore outcomes than entirely self-guided treatments (Lenhard, Andersson, et al., 2017; Rees et al., 2016).

An important aspect in delivering treatment online is the issue of patient safety. We want to emphasize the importance of a thorough assessment process, not only to verify that the patients meet diagnostic criteria for OCD but also to evaluate other comorbidities or risks that may interfere with the treatment or require more urgent action. During treatment, there is a need to have routine clinical assessments to monitor symptom severity, and to have a plan to handle depressive symptoms and suicidality, if needed. Continuous clinician supervision and team meetings to discuss current patients are required in the same way as in regular healthcare. In addition, there are technical requirements that need to be taken into account, for example to use double authorization to secure webpages or to use accepted software systems for videoconferencing.

As a final practice point, it is important to emphasize that these new ways to deliver CBT for pediatric OCD might not be suitable for all patients. We do not believe these options will replace standard CBT treatment or that everybody should be offered these alternatives. These new technical solutions may be best seen as a complement to, rather than a replacement for, the existing healthcare system. More research is needed to understand for whom and under which circumstances these treatment options may be best used.

References

Andersson, E., Ljótsson, B., Hedman, E., Hesser, H., Enander, J., Kaldo, V., ... Rück, C. (2015). Testing the mediating effects of obsessive beliefs in internet-based cognitive behaviour therapy for obsessive-compulsive disorder: Results from a randomized controlled trial. *Clinical Psychology & Psychotherapy, 22*(6), 722–732. https://doi.org/10.1002/cpp.1931

Andersson, E., Ljótsson, B., Hedman, E., Kaldo, V., Paxling, B. B., Andersson, G., ... Ruck, C. (2011). Internet-based cognitive behavior therapy for obsessive compulsive disorder: A pilot study. *BMC Psychiatry*, *11*(1), 125. https://doi.org/10.1186/1471-244X-11-125

Andersson, G. (2009). Using the Internet to provide cognitive behaviour therapy. *Behaviour Research and Therapy*, *47*(3), 175–180. https://doi.org/10.1016/j.brat.2009.01.010

Aspvall, K., Andrén, P., Lenhard, F., Andersson, E., Mataix-Cols, D., & Serlachius, E. (2018). Internet-delivered cognitive behavioural therapy for young children with obsessive-compulsive disorder: Development and initial evaluation of the BIP OCD Junior programme. *BJ Psych Open*, *4*(3), 106–112. doi:10.1192/bjo.2018.10

Cavanagh, K. (2014). Geographic inequity in the availability of cognitive behavioural therapy in England and Wales: A 10-year update. *Behavioural and Cognitive Psychotherapy*, *42*(4), 497–501. https://doi.org/10.1017/S1352465813000568

Comer, J. S., Furr, J. M., Cooper-Vince, C. E., Kerns, C. E., Chan, P. T., Edson, A. L., ... Freeman, J. B. (2014). Internet-delivered, family-based treatment for early-onset OCD: A preliminary case series. *Journal of Clinical Child and Adolescent Psychology*, *43*(1), 74–87. https://doi.org/10.1080/15374416.2013.855127

Comer, J. S., Furr, J. M., Kerns, C. E., Miguel, E., Coxe, S., Elkins, R. M., ... Freeman, J. B. (2017). Internet-delivered, family-based treatment for early-onset OCD: A pilot randomized trial. *Journal of Consulting and Clinical Psychology*, *85*(2), 178–186. https://doi.org/10.1037/ccp0000155

de Bruin, E. J., Bögels, S. M., Oort, F. J., & Meijer, A. M. (2015). Efficacy of cognitive behavioral therapy for insomnia in adolescents: A randomized controlled trial with internet therapy, group therapy and a waiting list condition. *Sleep*, *38*(12), 1913–1926. https://doi.org/10.5665/sleep.5240

Fernández de la Cruz, L., Kolvenbach, S., Vidal-Ribas, P., Jassi, A., Llorens, M., Patel, N., ... Mataix-Cols, D. (2016). Illness perception, help-seeking attitudes, and knowledge related to obsessive–compulsive disorder across different ethnic groups: A community survey. *Social Psychiatry and Psychiatric Epidemiology*, *51*(3), 455–464. https://doi.org/10.1007/s00127-015-1144-9

Franklin, M. E., & Foa, E. B. (2011). Treatment of obsessive compulsive disorder. *Annual Review of Clinical Psychology*, *7*, 229–243. https://doi.org/10.1146/annurev-clinpsy-032210-104533

García-Soriano, G., Rufer, M., Delsignore, A., & Weidt, S. (2014). Factors associated with non-treatment or delayed treatment seeking in OCD sufferers: A review of the literature. *Psychiatry Research*, *220*(1–2), 1–10. https://doi.org/10.1016/j.psychres.2014.07.009

Geller, D. A. D. A., & March, J. (2012). Practice parameter for the assessment and treatment of children and adolescents with obsessive-compulsive disorder. *Journal of the American Academy of Child and Adolescent Psychiatry*, *51*(1), 98–113. https://doi.org/10.1016/j.jaac.2011.09.019

Goodwin, R., Koenen, K. C., Hellman, F., Guardino, M., & Struening, E. (2002). Helpseeking and access to mental health treatment for obsessive-compulsive disorder. *Acta Psychiatrica Scandinavica*, *106*(2), 143–149. https://doi.org/10.1034/j.1600-0447.2002.01221.x

Kenwright, M., Marks, I., Graham, C., Franses, A., & Mataix-Cols, D. (2005). Brief scheduled phone support from a clinician to enhance computer-aided self-help for obsessive-compulsive disorder: Randomized controlled trial. *Journal of Clinical Psychology, 61*(12), 1499–1508. https://doi.org/10.1002/jclp.20204

Kohn, R., Saxena, S., Levav, I., & Saraceno, B. (2004). The treatment gap in mental health care. *Bulletin of the World Health Organization, 82*(11), 858–866. https://doi.org// S0042-96862004001100011

Krebs, G., Isomura, K., Lang, K., Jassi, A., Heyman, I., Diamond, H., ... Mataix-Cols, D. (2015). How resistant is "treatment-resistant" obsessive-compulsive disorder in youth? *The British Journal of Clinical Psychology / The British Psychological Society, 54*(1), 63–75. https://doi.org/10.1111/bjc.12061

Laforest, M., Bouchard, S., Bossé, J., & Mesly, O. (2016). Effectiveness of In Virtuo exposure and response prevention treatment using cognitive-behavioral therapy for obsessive-compulsive disorder: A study based on a single-case study protocol. *Frontiers in Psychiatry, 7*, 99. https://doi.org/10.3389/fpsyt.2016.00099

Lenhard, F., Andersson, E., Mataix-Cols, D., Rück, C., Vigerland, S., Högström, J., ... Serlachius, E. (2017). Therapist-guided, internet-delivered cognitive-behavioral therapy for adolescents with obsessive-compulsive disorder: A randomized controlled trial. *Journal of the American Academy of Child & Adolescent Psychiatry, 56* (1), 10–19.e2. https://doi.org/10.1016/j.jaac.2016.09.515

Lenhard, F., Ssegonja, R., Andersson, E., Feldman, I., Rück, C., Mataix-Cols, D., & Serlachius, E. (2017). Cost-effectiveness of therapist-guided Internet-delivered cognitive behavior therapy for pediatric obsessive-compulsive disorder: Results from a randomized controlled trial. *BMJ Open, 7*(5), E015246.

Lenhard, F., Vigerland, S., Andersson, E., Rück, C., Mataix-Cols, D., Thulin, U., ... Serlachius, E. (2014). Internet-delivered cognitive behavior therapy for adolescents with obsessive-compulsive disorder: An open trial. *PloS One, 9*(6), e100773. https://doi.org/10.1371/journal.pone.0100773

Lenhard, F., Vigerland, S., Engberg, H., Hallberg, A., Thermaenius, H., & Serlachius, E. (2016). "On My Own, but Not Alone" – Adolescents' experiences of internet-delivered cognitive behavior therapy for obsessive-compulsive disorder. *Plos One, 11*(10), e0164311. https://doi.org/10.1371/journal.pone.0164311

Marques, L., LeBlanc, N. J., Weingarden, H. M., Timpano, K. R., Jenike, M., & Wilhelm, S. (2010). Barriers to treatment and service utilization in an internet sample of individuals with obsessive-compulsive symptoms. *Depression and Anxiety, 27*(5), 470–475. https://doi.org/10.1002/da.20694

Mataix-Cols, D., De La Cruz, L. F., Nordsletten, A. E., Lenhard, F., Isomura, K., & Simpson, H. B. (2016). Towards an international expert consensus for defining treatment response, remission, recovery and relapse in obsessive-compulsive disorder. *World Psychiatry, 15*(1), 80–81. https://doi.org/10.1002/wps.20299

Mataix-Cols, D., & Marks, I. M. (2006). Self-help with minimal therapist contact for obsessive–compulsive disorder: A review. *European Psychiatry, 21*(2), 75–80. Retrieved from http://www.sciencedirect.com/science/article/pii/S0924933805001550

Matthews, A. J., Maunder, R., Scanlan, J. D., & Kirkby, K. C. (2017). Online computer-aided vicarious exposure for OCD symptoms: A pilot study. *Journal of Behavior Therapy and Experimental Psychiatry, 54*, 25–34. https://doi.org/10.1016/j.jbtep.2016.06.002

McGuire, J. F., Piacentini, J., Lewin, A. B., Brennan, E. A., Murphy, T. K., & Storch, E. A. (2015). A meta-analysis of cognitive behavior therapy and medication for child obsessive-compulsive disorder: Moderators of treatment efficacy, response, and remission. *Depression and Anxiety, 32*(8), 580–593. https://doi.org/10.1002/da.22389

McHugh, R. K., & Barlow, D. H. (2010). The dissemination and implementation of evidence-based psychological treatments: A review of current efforts. *American Psychologist, 65*(2), 73–84. https://doi.org/10.1037/a0018121

Micali, N., Heyman, I., Perez, M., Hilton, K., Nakatani, E., Turner, C., & Mataix-Cols, D. (2010). Long-term outcomes of obsessive-compulsive disorder: Follow-up of 142 children and adolescents. *The British Journal of Psychiatry: The Journal of Mental Science, 197*(2), 128–134. https://doi.org/10.1192/bjp.bp.109.075317

National Institute for Health and Care Excellence [NICE](2005). Obsessive-compulsive disorder: Core interventions in the treatment of obsessive-compulsive disorder and body dysmorphic disorder. NICE Guideline (CG31). *British Psychological Society.* Retrieved from http://www.nice.org.uk/guidance/cg31/resources/guidance-obsessivecompulsive-disorder-pdf

Pinto, A., Mancebo, M. C., Eisen, J. L., Pagano, M. E., & Rasmussen, S. A. (2006). The Brown Longitudinal Obsessive Compulsive Study: Clinical features and symptoms of the sample at intake. *The Journal of Clinical Psychiatry, 67*(5), 703–711. Retrieved from http://www.pubmedcentral.nih.gov/articlerender.fcgi?artid=3272757&tool=pmcentrez&rendertype=abstract

Rees, C. S., Anderson, R. A., & Finlay-Jones, A. (2015). OCD? Not Me! Protocol for the development and evaluation of a web-based self-guided treatment for youth with obsessive-compulsive disorder. *BMJ Open, 5*(4), e007486. https://doi.org/10.1136/bmjopen-2014-007486

Rees, C. S., Anderson, R. A., Kane, R. T., & Finlay-Jones, A. L. (2016). Online obsessive-compulsive disorder treatment: Preliminary results of the "OCD? Not Me!" self-guided internet-based cognitive behavioral therapy program for young people. *JMIR Mental Health, 3*(3), e29. https://doi.org/10.2196/mental.5363

Shafran, R., Clark, D. M. M., Fairburn, C. G. G., Arntz, A., Barlow, D. H. H., Ehlers, A., … Wilson, G. T. T. (2009). Mind the gap: Improving the dissemination of CBT. *Behaviour Research and Therapy, 47*(11), 902–909. https://doi.org/10.1016/j.brat.2009.07.003

Simpson, H. B., Maher, M. J., Wang, Y., Bao, Y., Foa, E. B., & Franklin, M. (2011). Patient adherence predicts outcome from cognitive behavioral therapy in obsessive-compulsive disorder. *Journal of Consulting and Clinical Psychology, 79*(2), 247–252. https://doi.org/10.1037/a0022659

Spence, S. H., Donovan, C. L., March, S., Gamble, A., Anderson, R. E., Prosser, S., & Kenardy, J. (2011). A randomized controlled trial of online versus clinic-based CBT for adolescent anxiety. *Journal of Consulting and Clinical Psychology, 79*(5), 629–642. https://doi.org/10.1037/a0024512

Storch, E. A., Caporino, N. E., Morgan, J. R., Lewin, A. B., Rojas, A., Brauer, L., … Murphy, T. K. (2011). Preliminary investigation of web-camera delivered cognitive-behavioral therapy for youth with obsessive-compulsive disorder. *Psychiatry Research, 189*(3), 407–412. https://doi.org/10.1016/j.psychres.2011.05.047

The Pediatric OCD Treatment Study (POTS) Team. (2004). Cognitive-behavior therapy, sertraline, and their combination for children and adolescents with obsessive-compulsive disorder: The Pediatric OCD Treatment Study (POTS) randomized controlled trial. *JAMA: The Journal of the American Medical Association, 292*(16), 1969–1976. https://doi.org/10.1001/jama.292.16.1969

Torp, N. C., Dahl, K., Skarphedinsson, G., Thomsen, P. H., Valderhaug, R., Weidle, B., ... Ivarsson, T. (2015). Effectiveness of cognitive behavior treatment for pediatric obsessive-compulsive disorder: Acute outcomes from the Nordic Long-term OCD Treatment Study (NordLOTS). *Behaviour Research and Therapy, 64*, 15–23. https://doi.org/10.1016/j.brat.2014.11.005

Turner, C., Heyman, I., Futh, A., & Lovell, K. (2009). A pilot study of telephone cognitive-behavioural therapy for obsessive-compulsive disorder in young people. *Behavioural and Cognitive Psychotherapy, 37*(4), 469. https://doi.org/10.1017/S1352465809990178

Turner, C. M., Mataix-cols, D., Lovell, K., Krebs, G., Lang, K., Byford, S., & Heyman, I. (2014). Telephone cognitive-behavioral therapy for adolescents with obsessive-compulsive disorder: A randomized controlled non-inferiority trial. *Journal of the American Academy of Child & Adolescent Psychiatry, 53*(12), 1298–1307.e2. https://doi.org/10.1016/j.jaac.2014.09.012

Valderhaug, R., Götestam, K., & Larsson, B. (2004). Clinicians' views on management of obsessive-compulsive disorders in children and adolescents. *Nordic Journal of Psychiatry, 58*(2), 125–132. https://doi.org/10.1080/08039480410005503

Vigerland, S., Ljótsson, B., Bergdahl Gustafsson, F., Hagert, S., Thulin, U., Andersson, G., & Serlachius, E. (2014). Attitudes towards the use of computerized cognitive behavior therapy (cCBT) with children and adolescents: A survey among Swedish mental health professionals. *Internet Interventions, 1*(3), 111–117. https://doi.org/10.1016/j.invent.2014.06.002

Wahl, K., Kordon, A., Kuelz, K. A., Voderholzer, U., Hohagen, F., & Zurowski, B. (2010). Obsessive-compulsive disorder (OCD) is still an unrecognised disorder: A study on the recognition of OCD in psychiatric outpatients. *European Psychiatry: The Journal of the Association of European Psychiatrists, 25*(7), 374–377. https://doi.org/10.1016/j.eurpsy.2009.12.003

Whiteside, S. P. H. (2016). Mobile device-based applications for childhood anxiety disorders. *Journal of Child and Adolescent Psychopharmacology, 25*(3), 246–251. https://doi.org/10.1089/cap.2015.0010

Whiteside, S. P. H., Ale, C. M., Vickers Douglas, K., Tiede, M. S., & Dammann, J. E. (2014). Case examples of enhancing pediatric OCD treatment with a smartphone application. *Clinical Case Studies, 13*(1), 80–94. https://doi.org/10.1177/1534650113504822

Wootton, B. M., Titov, N., Dear, B. F., Spence, J., Andrews, G., Johnston, L., & Solley, K. (2011). An internet administered treatment program for obsessive-compulsive disorder: A feasibility study. *Journal of Anxiety Disorders, 25*(8), 1102–1107. https://doi.org/10.1016/j.janxdis.2011.07.009

17 Interpretation and Attentional Bias Training

Elske Salemink, Lidewij Wolters, and Else de Haan

Introduction

Victor Meyer (1966) described the first effective behavioral therapeutic intervention for patients with an obsessive-compulsive disorder (OCD). This intervention, named by Meyer "the modification of expectations," is now known as exposure and response prevention (ERP). The treatment Meyer described was an in-patient treatment in which nurses effectuated the response prevention, instead of the patients themselves. Washing rituals for instance were made impossible for the patients by closing taps and removing soap. Over the years, many adjustments have been made to Meyer's intervention: the treatment became outpatient, and exposure and response prevention were not supervised by the therapist or nurse but performed by the patient alone, the so-called self-controlled exposure (Emmelkamp & Kraanen, 1977). In the late 1980s, Salkovskis and Westbrook (1989) introduced the use of cognitive interventions (cognitive therapy, CT) in OCD. Since then, the combination of these two interventions – ERP and CT – is the evidence-based treatment for OCD (see Chapter 1). Although this was initially true only for the treatment of adults, later research has shown that ERP and CT are also effective in children and adolescents (Wu, Lang, & Zhang, 2016) . However, the search for improvements or additions to treatment cannot end here. Although effective, the number of nonresponders is unacceptably high. Too many children and adolescents do not completely profit from current evidence-based treatment.

In this chapter we discuss interpretation and attentional bias training as stand-alone or as augmentation strategies to traditional CBT for children and adolescents. The study of these strategies originates in the context of anxiety in nonclinical adult subjects. Research in children and adolescents has only recently begun, first in patients with anxiety disorders and more recently in patients with OCD. Studies in youth with OCD are basically limited to one pilot study (our study), hence, we will first briefly discuss research findings in adults and nonclinical subjects, followed by research in children and adolescents.

The chapter starts with the need for innovation: a brief overview of the effectiveness of treatment and a discussion of the possibilities for improvement. Next, we discuss research on the role of cognitive biases in anxiety and OCD that are the basis for the development of cognitive bias modification strategies. Then the evidence for interpretation bias and attentional bias training is provided, followed by the role of mediators and moderators. We then present two clinical cases and end the chapter with challenges and recommendations for the future.

Overview of the Issue – The Need for Innovation

Current treatments for OCD in children and adolescents are effective but not for everybody. CBT yields a mean improvement of around 60 percent (POTS, 2004; Torp et al., 2015). The effect size for CBT has been reported as $d = 1.7$ but drops to $d = 1.2$ when controlling for nonspecific therapy factors (Sánchez-Meca et al., 2014). Furthermore, on average 60 to 70 percent of patients are improved after 14 to 16 sessions of manualized treatment. Compared to previous views of OCD as an intractable disorder, this is a significant improvement. However, it also means that 30 to 40 percent of patients do *not* improve after treatment.

For non- or partial responders, clinical guidelines recommend adding selective serotonin reuptake inhibitors (SSRIs) to CBT (Geller, March, the Aacap Committee on Quality Issues [CQI], 2012). However, this policy is not based on research findings. In the only placebo-controlled study, Skarphedinsson et al. (2014) found no additional effect of adding an SSRI for initial nonresponders to CBT. Furthermore, the use of medication entails several disadvantages, such as possible adverse effects, a heightened chance of relapse by discontinuation, and unknown effects in the long term (Geller et al., 2012). As a result, many patients and therapists have reservations about the safety and long-term benefit of medication use (Rutter et al., 2008).

This implies that the search for improvement that started with Meyer (1966) must be continued. There are several ways to continue this search: research into moderators and mediators of treatment and research into working mechanisms (Kazdin, 2007). The question whether this 30 to 40 percent of patients belongs to a separate group of patients that possibly need another form of treatment is not easy to answer. No clear picture has emerged from the many prediction studies (see for an overview Ginsburg et al., 2008). Age, sex, and duration of complaints do not appear to be significant predictors of treatment effects. Serious complaints, family factors, and comorbidity, especially autism spectrum disorder (ASD), are predictors. Severity and comorbidity with ASD predict, however, only a slower treatment response and require a longer treatment period (Wolters et al., 2016). Family factors appear to contribute both positively and negatively to the effect of treatment (Peris et al., 2012).

It has been hypothesized that cognitive changes are mediators in CBT. It is assumed that change in dysfunctional beliefs is a prerequisite for change in behavior (rituals and avoidance behavior). However, to the best of our knowledge, there are only two studies in pediatric OCD in which the role of changes in dysfunctional beliefs as a mediator is studied. In both studies, this hypothesis was not confirmed (Williams et al., 2002; Wolters et al., 2018).

Also, in adult studies, the results are equivocal. Sometimes changes in beliefs preceded changes in behavior, sometimes it was the other way around, and sometimes the changes occurred at the same time (Anholt et al., 2008; Polman et al., 2011; Rheaume & Ladouceur, 2000; Storchheim & O'Mahony, 2006).

A mediation analysis is never better than the measurement tools used to measure the possible mediator. In the previously mentioned studies, cognitions were measured with a questionnaire. It remains questionable whether a questionnaire is truly capable of measuring the appraisals and interpretations that play a role in OCD. This is well illustrated by the completion of a questionnaire by a 9-year-old boy with OCD (see Figure 17.1). At the top of the questionnaire he wrote down his age, scratched it out, wrote it down again, scratched it out, wrote, scratched and so on, until the "9" was "exactly right." But when he read the question, "I must keep working at something until it's done exactly right" in the questionnaire, he answered, "never" (Wolters, 2011).

As yet, the current studies into mediators and moderators of treatment do not (yet) give us clear clues for improving the therapy.

Whether the change of dysfunctional beliefs, appraisals, or interpretations is a mediator of treatment in OCD, we do not know. What we do know is that dysfunctional beliefs are part of the problem in maintaining symptoms. A large number of studies in both adults and children and adolescents show that cognitive bias plays a role in the mechanism and possibly also in the development of OCD (Frost & Steketee, 2002). Cognitive therapy (CT) is based on these findings. However, CT is a rational therapy with high verbal loading, which is not always adequate for all children and adolescents (and even not for all adults). An essential part of CT is so-called Socratic reasoning, in which the patient arrives at more functional cognitions by logic or rational reasoning. After such an exercise, patients sometimes say, "I know I am wrong, but I still *feel* like I am right," leaving the therapist without further arguments. For some patients, CT is not the most effective strategy to change cognitive bias. Exposure, the most effective treatment strategy for OCD (Olatunji et al., 2013), is known to change bias/cognitions as well (Jacoby & Abramowitz, 2016).

Moreover, it is questionable whether explicit change of cognitions is the most effective way of bringing about lasting changes in the outcome of the therapy. Vasey and colleagues showed that the strength of implicit associations after exposure therapy predict return of fear at one-month follow-up. This highlights that it is also important that more automatic processes such as attentional bias, interpretive bias, and implicit associations may need to be changed to reduce return of fear (Vasey et al., 2012). That brings us to the next part of this chapter: Cognitive Bias Modification (CBM), which is a method to influence cognitive bias in an implicit way. In the following, we discuss the development of CBM for OCD in children and adolescents.

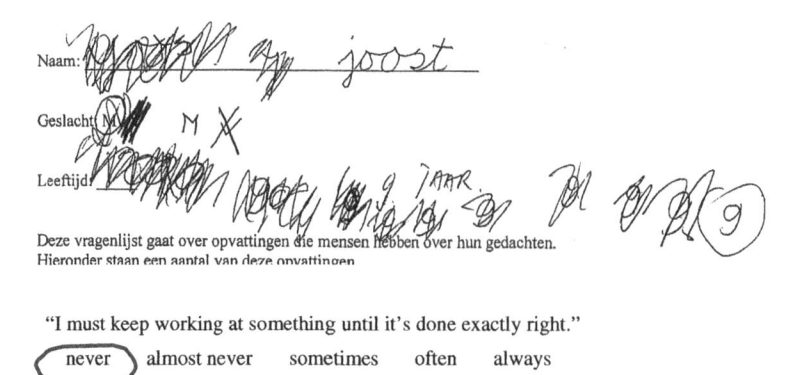

Figure 17.1 *Completion of the Top of an OCD Questionnaire and one Question by a 9-year-old Boy with OCD.*

Approach to Innovation

The most-often studied cognitive biases in anxiety and OCD are selective attention to anxious stimuli (attentional bias) and negative interpretation of ambiguous stimuli (interpretation bias). These two types of bias have been investigated extensively in adults (Amir, Foa, & Coles, 1998; Bar-Haim, 2010; Bar-Haim et al., 2007; Butler & Mathews, 1983; Mathews, Richards, & Eysenck, 1989; Mathews & MacLeod, 2005) but to a lesser extent in children and adolescents. To date, most studies have been conducted in anxiety disorders (without OCD). In the DSM-5, OCD is no longer conceptualized as an anxiety disorder, but as a disorder in which a lack of inhibition is the most prominent feature (APA, 2013). However, many scientists (especially CBT specialists) do not agree with this decision and continue to conceptualize OCD as an anxiety disorder, with solid arguments (see for instance Abramowitz, 2017). That is why we will discuss cognitive bias in OCD as well as in anxiety disorders in children and adolescents in what follows.

Attentional Bias in Anxiety Disorders

Dudeney, Sharpe, and Hunt (2015) conducted a meta-analysis of 38 studies involving 4221 children up to 18 years of age. Children that were high on trait-anxiety or were clinically anxious had a significantly stronger attentional bias toward threat related stimuli compared to control children, although the effect size was small ($d=0.21$) Also, these children had a significantly stronger attentional bias for threat-related stimuli compared to neutral stimuli, with a medium effect size ($d=0.54$). These effects are comparable but less robust than those in adults (see Bar-Haim, 2010; Bar-Haim et al., 2007). Note that also in controls a small but significant effect for threat stimuli compared to neutral stimuli was found. A number of moderators were observed: stimuli – there was evidence of an attentional bias with linguistic but not with pictorial stimuli; age – the difference between the anxious and the control group increased with age; paradigm – the effect size of the dot probe task was small ($d= 0.18$), while the Stroop task had a moderate effect size ($d= 0.44$).

Interpretation Bias in Anxiety Disorders

High-trait anxious and anxiety disordered youth have an interpretation bias toward ambiguous stimuli. Depending on the kind of anxiety disorder, they interpret information for instance in a socially anxious and threatening way (the children look at me, because they think I am stupid) or in a generalized anxious and threatening way (the siren of the ambulance means that my mother has had an accident).

In a meta-analysis of 77 studies, with 11,507 children and adolescents (mean 11.2 years of age, between 2 and 22 years), a medium effect size ($d = 0.62$) association between negative interpretation bias and anxiety was found (Stuijfzand et al., 2018). In this meta-analysis, 18 studies included a clinical sample and 57 studies included a community sample. There was significant variation between the effect sizes of the different studies however. The participants involved (clinical or community sample), comorbidity, gender, and task to assess interpretation bias did not account for this variation. Age and content specificity of the task explained part of the variation. Similar to the findings on attentional bias, with increasing age the association between negative interpretation and anxiety increased. Content specificity, that is the degree to which the task used idiographic, fear relevant stimuli turned out to be a significant moderator. The association between negative interpretation and anxiety was larger when the content of the scenario matched the anxiety subtype than when it did not match. There were very few effect sizes for children below 8 years of age, implicating that no conclusions can be drawn about the relation between interpretation bias and anxiety in young children.

Attentional Bias in OCD

Studies into attentional bias in adult OCD have reported inconsistent findings (Bradley et al., 2016). Attentional bias in children with OCD has been infrequently studied. In one study, examining attentional bias for general threat and OCD-specific threat stimuli with a dot probe task in children with OCD ($n = 58$), children with anxiety disorders ($n = 58$), and in typically developing children ($n = 58$), no evidence was found for increased selective attention for disorder-specific threat in children with OCD and other anxiety disorders compared to the community controls (Wolters et al., 2013). As children with OCD often have very specific symptoms, a lack of content specificity could (partly) explain these outcomes.

Interpretation Bias in OCD

Cognitive interpretation biases in patients with OCD are slightly different from cognitive biases in anxiety disorders. According to the cognitive theory of OCD, patients are not so much anxious about ambiguous situations, but rather about the interpretation of normally occurring intrusions (Beck & Clark, 1997; Salkovskis &

Westbrook, 1989; Williams et al., 1997). It has been established that the experience of intrusions is relatively normal, with nonclinical samples reporting the occurrence of unintentional, sudden, and threatening thoughts, such as "we will have an accident," or "my loved one will die" (Radomsky et al., 2013). Of note, is that these nonclinical individuals do not report significant distress by these intrusions. Instead, they report that they ignore them. Patients with OCD on the other hand differ in their appraisal of the intrusions and in control techniques for the intrusions. They appraise the intrusions as potentially dangerous and predicting harm, resulting in anxiety and distress. Several OCD-related dysfunctional beliefs have been identified. The Obsessive Compulsive Cognitions Working Group (OCCWG, 1997, 2003) has classified them into six domains: threat estimation (e.g., overestimation of the likelihood of negative outcomes); control of thoughts (e.g., notion that thoughts must be actively controlled); importance of thoughts (e.g., belief that intrusive thoughts are meaningful and indicative of one's character); responsibility (e.g., idea that one must be vigilant about preventing harm at all times); perfectionism (e.g., belief that one must be "perfect"); and intolerance of uncertainty (e.g., beliefs about the necessity of being certain).

Compared to the number of studies into interpretation bias in anxiety, only a few studies into interpretation bias in OCD have been performed. In a systematic review, Reynolds and Reeves (2008) reported on 11 studies, with a total of 1550 children and adolescents. Of these, only four with a total sample of 172 children and adolescents have been conducted in a clinical population. Ten out of the eleven studies suggest that the cognitive model is also applicable to children and adolescents. Cognitive constructs like thought action fusion (TAF), meta-cognitive beliefs, and responsibility assessments are all associated with OC symptoms in adolescents and children. The relationships are of moderate size. These studies all have a cross-sectional design. In the only experimental study, in which responsibility was manipulated, no relationship was found between an inflated sense of responsibility and increased ratings of distress or avoidance behavior and ritualizing (Barrett & Healy-Farrell, 2003). However, the authors note that the children were reluctant to accept responsibility in the high responsibility condition. So it is questionable whether the manipulation of responsibility was as successful as the authors indicate. The children's ratings of responsibility may have been inflated due to social desirability bias and not the experimental manipulation (Reynold & Reeves, 2008). In a later study, Reeves and Reynold (2010) showed that experimentally manipulated responsibility did have an effect on checking behavior, in nonclinical children aged 9–12 years, during a candy sorting task.

In two more recent studies, a relationship was again found between obsessive-compulsive symptoms and cognitive appraisals. In both studies cognitive biases were tested in patients and their mothers. Farrell, Waters, and Zimmer-Gembeck (2012) studied a clinical sample of children (7–11 years) and adolescents (12–17 years). Their study highlights the importance of possible effects of age, whereby age proved to be a significant moderator between cognitive bias of the child/adolescent, cognitive bias of the mother, and severity of the OCD. In children, no association was found between OCD severity and cognitive bias, whereas in adolescents a strong association was found. On the other hand, the mother's cognitive bias appeared to be associated with the symptom severity of the younger children and not with adolescents.

The study of Kadak et al. (2014) obtained less convincing results. In a group of 21 adolescents in the last class of high school, diagnosed with OCD in an epidemiological study, a difference with a non-OCD control group was found for a small number of cognitive biases (i.e., thought action fusion, morality). In addition, in some domains, there was an association between the cognitive bias of the OCD subjects and their mother, which was not true in the control group.

In conclusion, most studies provide evidence for an association between cognitive appraisals and OCD severity. However apart from the two experimental studies, the other studies are correlational in nature, or focus on differences between OCD patients and healthy controls. The next question is whether biases play a *causal* role in the development of emotional disorders, and moreover, whether biases can be directly targeted via novel interventions.

From Assessment to Treatment

Cognitive bias has been assessed by explicit methods, like questionnaires, and also by implicit, indirect methods that are capable of capturing a more automatic component of cognitive biases. To examine whether cognitive bias is not only associated with OC symptoms, but also causes them, Mathews and Mackintosh (2000) studied the question whether these implicit methods to assess cognitive interpretation bias could also be used to *change* that bias.

Their landmark study (Mathews & Mackintosh, 2000) gives not only an answer to the causality question, but is also the starting point of changing cognitive interpretation bias with implicit methods, through Cognitive Interpretation Bias Modification (CBM-I) training. Mathews and Mackintosh used a *training* paradigm that was previously used to *assess* interpretations participants made while reading short three-line stories about an ambiguous, but possibly anxiety-provoking event.

To change bias, Mathews and Mackintosh (2000) presented the same short three-line stories to a sample of participants that were recruited from a panel of community volunteers.

The stories were ambiguous in their emotional meaning, until the last word of the story. This last word resolved the ambiguity, in either a positive or a negative way. For example:

> *Your partner asks you to go to an anniversary dinner that their company is holding. You have not met any of their work colleagues. Getting ready to go, you think that the new people you will meet find you _____*
> *(friendly/boring)*

Both kinds of stories (with a positive or a negative solution of the ambiguity) were used in their studies. One group of participants read the positive solution (the positive condition) whereas the other group read the negative one. So the participants did not have a choice. They were forced to resolve the ambiguity in a positive or negative way, over and over again, as they resolved 64 of these scenarios. Mathews and Mackintosh (2000) demonstrated that interpretation could be changed by this procedure: participants in the positive condition drew more positive and fewer negative interpretations of new ambiguous situations than those in the negative condition. Participants in the negative condition also reported higher levels of state anxiety after training.

This research led to new ways to influence cognitions or interpretations with a more clinical aim: to reduce maladaptive processes in order to ultimately reduce symptoms. No rational thinking, no Socratic reasoning, rather, simply training and practicing over and over again more positive interpretations.

Since this seminal study, there have been numerous replications of Cognitive Bias Modification of Interpretations, mainly in samples of adults with anxiety disorders but also in children and adolescents. Clerkin and Teachman (2011) were the first to use this paradigm for obsessive-compulsive complaints in adults (undergraduate students). They adapted the scenarios Mathews and Mackintosh used into the typical situations that trigger OC symptoms. The scenarios were related to one of the six domains of OC symptoms described by the OCCWG (1997; 2003). As in the Mathews and Mackintosh paradigm, each scenario ended with a word that resolved the scenario in either an OC-relevant manner (negative interpretation) or in a non-OC relevant manner, a manner that contradicted the negative OC relevant interpretation (positive interpretation). For example:

> *You and a friend are having a personal discussion. You tell her that you sometimes have bizarre thoughts about hurting people you care about. Thoughts you don't really want to have.*
> *Your friend tells you this is really _____*
> *(weird/normal)*

Clerkin and Teachman examined these scenarios in a sample of undergraduate students scoring high in OC symptoms. There were two conditions, one a positive condition and the other a neutral one. In the positive condition, the ambiguity of the scenario was resolved in a non-OC relevant manner (positive condition). In the neutral condition, the participants received a non-OC relevant interpretation in 50 percent of the scenarios and a negative, OC-relevant, interpretation in 50 percent of the scenarios. The training was conducted in one session that lasted about one hour. The training had effect on interpretation bias, but the effect on OC-related emotions and the urge to neutralize was less clear (see the following for additional detail).

Based on the work of Clerkin and Teachman and in close collaboration with therapists who specialized in the treatment of pediatric OCD, we developed a CBM-I training for adolescents with OCD (Salemink, Wolters, & de Haan, 2015). We adapted the scenarios to typical adolescent situations. As in the Clerkin and Teachman study the scenarios were based on the domains described by the OCCWG (1997; 2003). An example of a training scenario is as follows:

> *You bought some roses for your mum and accidently got pricked by a thorn.*
> *You are bleeding and ask your mum to put a band-aid on it.*
> *It is _____ that this would make your mother sick.*
> *(likely/unlikely)*

We assumed that OCD patients would need more training sessions to achieve improvement, therefore we also developed new scenarios, resulting in a total of 432 scenarios. Our training consisted of eight sessions. In each session, 54 scenarios were presented, in six blocks. Patients were instructed to complete the word fragment as quickly and accurately as possible by typing the first missing letter. After each scenario a comprehension question appeared and patients were asked to press Y for yes and N for no. Feedback was presented (correct vs. incorrect answer) to reinforce the non OC-relevant interpretation. After each block the patient could take a short break. An online CBM-I program was designed, enabling adolescents to perform the training at their preferred location (at home or any other location with internet access).

In a similar vein, attentional bias modification training (ABM) has been developed. Here, participants are trained to direct their attention away from negative cues or toward positive ones. The dot probe task is typically used for this training (Lowther & Newman, 2014). This task was originally designed as an implicit measure to assess attentional bias (MacLeod, Mathews, & Tata, 1986). The dot probe task is a computerized probe detection task. In studies with children and adolescents, stimuli are faces instead of words typically used in adult research. The faces express disgust or anger or have a neutral expression. Each trial starts with a fixation cross ('+') presented in the center of the screen, and next two faces appear, one above the other. The faces are presented in disgust (or anger)-neutral or neutral-neutral pairs. Next, a target probe (E or F) is presented on one of the locations vacated by the faces. The participant has to determine where the probe appears, by a mouse-click on a predetermined button. In the training version, the probe always appears in the location of the neutral face, forcing participants to disengage the attention from threat.

To train children to direct attention toward positive stimuli, Waters et al. (2013) applied a visual search paradigm. In this paradigm angry and happy faces are presented in a 3 × 3 matrix on a screen. The faces were balanced across different positions in the matrix, angry faces appearing eight times as much as happy faces. The children were instructed to search for the happy faces. They were instructed to mouse-click on the happy faces as quickly as possible, in order to be trained to attend toward positive cues. The three-week training turned out to have a significant effect on clinician rated anxiety scores, but not on parent and child rated anxiety scores. In a more recent study with 59 clinically anxious children (6–12 years of age) (Waters et al., 2015), a visual search paradigm was supplemented with verbalization techniques to increase learning, memory consolidation, and engagement. After twelve treatment sessions in three weeks, clinician and parent rated anxiety and depression scores were significantly reduced, compared to a wait-list control group. No significant differences between the active and the control conditions were found in the analysis of child reported anxiety symptoms. In two Dutch studies, the same paradigm was used to investigate ABM as a tool for prevention or early intervention for adolescent targeting anxiety and/or depression. In both studies however, no effect of ABM on anxiety and/or depression was observed (De Voogd et al., 2014; De Voogd, Wiers, & Salemink, 2017).

Evidence-Base for Innovation

Here, the evidence base for CBM training is provided. Given that currently there is only one published study that examined CBM-I training in youth with OCD (Salemink et al., 2015), we broadened the scope. First, CBM studies focusing on anxiety in adults are presented, followed by CBM studies on anxiety in youth. Then we turn to OCD and present findings of CBM training in adults. We finish this section with results from CBM training in youth with OCD. When possible, results from meta-analyses are described.

CBM Training in Anxiety – Adults

In the context of adult anxiety, two types of CBM have been studied the most. That is, interpretive bias training (CBM-I) and attentional bias training (CBM-A; see explanation in under "Approach to Innovation" on p. 368; Description of approach). These types of training have been examined, in healthy, subclinical, and clinical samples. The first meta-analyses in 2010 (Hakamata et al.) and 2011 (Hallion & Ruscio) revealed the promise of the CBM approach. Hakamata and colleagues focused on CBM-A specifically and results revealed that this type of training had a large effect on reducing attentional bias and a medium effect on reducing anxiety (compared to a control training condition). Hallion and Ruscio combined CBM-A with CBM-I studies in their meta-analysis and concluded that, on average, there is a medium sized effect on bias; with stronger effects on interpretation than on attentional bias. Furthermore, CBM-A+I significantly reduced anxiety. There were small effects on symptoms when assessed after a stressor. While promising, these meta-analyses were also quite broad; spanning both CBM-A and I within one analysis, and also combining healthy individuals without symptoms, with studies in individuals with subclinical and clinical levels of symptoms.

With a strong increase in the number of subsequent CBM studies, more recent meta-analyses have focused more on specific procedures and specific populations enabling a more detailed analysis of CBM effectiveness. In a meta-analysis focusing specifically on CBM-I, Menne-Lothmann et al. (2014) concluded that positive CBM-I resulted in a significant increase in positive interpretations, and a significant decrease in negative mood states (no effect on stress reactivity). There was some indication that type of population moderated the effects; with better effects in more symptomatic samples (see also "Mediators and Moderators" on p. 379). Linetzky et al. (2015) specifically evaluated the clinical efficacy of CBM-A in patients with an anxiety disorder and concluded that CBM-A was associated with greater clinician-rated (but not self-reported) reductions in anxiety symptoms relative to the control training. More patients in the CBM-A conditions no longer met formal diagnostic criteria for their anxiety disorder post-training relative to patients in the control condition.

Around the same time, a broad meta-analysis in adults was published (Cristea, Kok, & Cuijpers, 2015) that again combined many aspects; CBM-A with CBM-I, single-session with multiple-sessions of training, and various populations including anxiety and depression. The overall conclusion was that CBM training had a small effect on mental health problems (see also Mogoase, David, & Koster, 2014), with significantly higher effects sizes for CBM-I than CBM-A. Importantly, there was considerable heterogeneity. Removal of outlying studies resulted in effect sizes becoming nonsignificant, resulting in a potentially more sobering conclusion regarding CBM. However, given the broad scope of the meta-analysis, the high heterogeneity does not come as a surprise.

An important question is whether we can understand the variability in CBM effectiveness. Recently, a reanalysis of the Cristea, Kok et al. (2015) meta-analysis was published (Grafton et al., 2017) that sheds light on factors that impact upon effectiveness. That is, various *procedures* (different types of training) have been employed with the intention of modifying cognitive biases (*process*). These procedures differ in their capacity to successfully modify the bias. Basically, the meta-analysis tested whether various *procedures* impact upon emotions, independent of any effect on the bias itself (e.g., the *process*). Theoretically, effects on symptoms are only expected when the bias is successfully changed (e.g., mechanism of change, see also Clarke, Notebaert, & Macleod, 2014). By distinguishing between studies in which the *process* was or was not successfully changed, the new analyses indeed revealed that only when the bias is successfully changed, are reliable effects on emotional vulnerability observed. Hence (part of) the variability in CBM effects observed in meta-analyses can be attributed to cross-study variability in whether the CBM procedures succeeded in modifying the cognitive bias.

In sum, across meta-analyses in adults, CBM training seems to be a promising new tool to reduce anxiety and emotional vulnerability, though there is great variability between studies and individuals. One aspect that proved to be relevant is whether the training was capable of modifying the bias itself. This highlights the need to develop CBM procedures that reliably change the targeted bias and also evaluate whether the CBM procedure was successful in changing the bias.

CBM Training in Anxiety – Youth

The number of studies in youth is accumulating. From a theoretical perspective, CBM training could yield stronger effects in youth, particularly in adolescents, as processing style develops during childhood and stabilizes across adolescence (see also Krebs et al., 2018). Furthermore, adolescence is also a period characterized by increased plasticity (Haller et al., 2015) and one of the meta-analyses in adults revealed stronger effects in younger participants (Mogoase et al., 2014).

To the best of our knowledge, there are two published meta-analyses that specifically examined CBM training in youth. The first is a meta-analysis with a broad scope (Cristea, Mogoase, David, & Cuijpers, 2015), including all types of CBM training and examining effects on anxiety and depression in a combined way. CBM training had a significant effect on changing bias (moderate effect size), but no significant effect on an integrated measure of mental health outcomes (combining anxiety and depression). The findings of this meta-analysis could cast doubt on the clinical utility of CBM in youth, however, as meta-analyses in adults revealed better effects for CBM-I (compared to CBM-A; Cristea, Kok, et al., 2015; Hallion & Ruscio, 2011) and better effects for anxiety (compared to depression; Hallion & Ruscio); this conclusion might be overly general. The second meta-analysis (Krebs et al., 2018) had a more focused approach: examining CBM-I effects on anxiety in youth. CBM-I training had a moderate effect on bias. That is, CBM-I significantly decreased negative interpretations and boosted positive interpretations. A small, but significant effect was observed on anxiety and also on anxiety vulnerability assessed after a stressor. Thus, in contrast to the other, more broad meta-analytic findings, this one revealed promising, albeit small, anxiolytic effects of CBM-I in youth.

CBM Training in OCD – Adults

When considering the evidence-base for CBM training in the context of adult OCD, three types of CBM paradigms have been studied, with the vast majority of studies focusing on CBM-I. We briefly discuss the findings for each type of CBM.

CBM-A. The effects of training attention away from threat was tested in undergraduate students with contamination-related symptoms (Najmi & Amir, 2010). Promising results were obtained; the training was successful in reducing attentional bias for threat, and clinically most interesting, it affected the behavioral approach of feared stimuli. That is, participants who completed the CBM-A training took more steps when approaching their feared objects than participants from the control condition. Given this finding on approaching feared stimuli, a later study examined whether CBM training (consisting of a combination of attention, interpretation, and working memory training) could affect self-directed ERP (Amir et al., 2015; Najmi & Amir, 2017). Using a multiple baseline design, it was shown that CBM can be combined with self-directed ERP (minimal therapist support), and resulted in significant reductions of OC symptoms. These are promising findings especially as the effect size was comparable to full-length ERP programs.

CBM-I. In total, there are currently nine publications concerning CBM-I training in the context of adult OC symptoms. In the first study, Clerkin and Teachman (2011) developed an OCD-relevant CBM-I training to change interpretations of intrusive thoughts. Students with elevated levels of OC symptoms were randomly allocated to either one session of CBM-I training or to a neutral training group. Results revealed that participants in the CBM-I group endorsed healthier OC-relevant interpretations and beliefs after the training. No OC symptoms were measured, but there was a nonsignificant trend for participants in the CBM-I condition to report less negative affect in response to a stressor. Subsequent studies have also examined the effects of single session CBM-I training and fairly consistently showed that the CBM-I procedure was successful in modifying interpretive bias (Beadel, Ritchey, & Teachman, 2016; Beadel, Smyth, & Teachman, 2014; Black & Grisham, 2016; Clerkin, Magee, & Parsons, 2014; Grisham et al., 2014; Williams & Grisham, 2013).

Recently, single session CBM-I training was also applied to modifying inverse reasoning (Wong & Grisham, 2017) and thought-action fusion (Siwiec et al., 2017) in the context of adult OC symptoms, increasing our understanding of the causal role of these processes in OC symptoms. In contrast to the CBM-I effects on bias, the effects on responses to a stressor were mixed and generally no effects on symptoms were observed across studies. This might be not so surprising, as only a single session of training was examined. CBM meta-analyses in anxiety indicated that more sessions of training are associated with stronger effects (Hallion & Ruscio, 2011; Menne-Lothmann et al., 2014). Such multiple-sessions of CBM-I training in adults with OCD are currently missing and crucially needed to test CBM-I's clinical utility in this context.

Approach-Avoidance CBM Training. OCD is also characterized by avoidance of fear-related stimuli. Recently, a computerized CBM training was designed that trains participants to systematically approach fear-related stimuli (Weil et al., 2017; this type of training is more often used in the field of addiction; see Wiers et al., 2013). After multiple sessions of pulling fear-related stimuli toward them, these participants reported significantly less distress caused by OC symptoms than participants in a control condition. These preliminary, pilot findings are promising, but more research is needed to evaluate the efficacy of the Approach-Avoidance CBM training in OCD.

In sum, CBM-I training is the type of CBM training most often studied in the context of adult OCD, with some studies focusing on attentional retraining and one study focusing on action tendency training. Results are promising with respect to changing the respective bias, and more mixed with respect to symptom change. Given that most studies had a more fundamental, theoretical focus and conducted a single-session of training, the clinical utility of CBM training in the context of OCD is difficult to evaluate. More research with multiple sessions of CBM (-I) training is warranted to establish the extent to which CBM training has potential clinical value in adult OCD.

CBM Training in OCD – Youth

The 13 published studies on CBM in adults with OC symptoms are in sharp contrast to the only published study on CBM in youth with OCD (Salemink et al., 2015). However, Riemann et al. (2013) tested the augmentation of "treatment as usual" with CBM-A in youth with various anxiety disorders also including OCD. On top of the standard treatment protocol, which consisted of CBT with or without medication, 42 individuals were randomly allocated to either a multi-session CBM-A training to reduce their attention to OC-related stimuli, or to a control training condition. The results were promising; significantly stronger reductions in anxiety symptoms were observed in the trained group compared to the control group. The authors also examined effects on OC symptoms, as the majority of the participants had OCD as the primary diagnosis, and here as well, the trained group experienced greater OC-symptom change than the control group. The authors argue to interpret these CBM-A findings on OC-symptoms with caution as the stimuli used were threat faces rather than OC-specific stimuli. It is unclear how reducing attention to threatening faces would affect OC symptoms.

We developed a CBM-I training for adolescents with OCD (Salemink et al., 2015). In a pilot study, we examined the added value of this CBM-I training as an adjunctive treatment to treatment as usual (that included CBT and pharmacotherapy) in adolescents with OCD. Therefore, on top of their standard treatment, half of the patients were randomly allocated to the eight-session CBM-I training ($n = 9$) or to a placebo training condition ($n = 7$). Results revealed that CBM-I training changed online interpretations during training. Adolescents who completed TAU + CBM-I were slower in making OC-related interpretations than adolescents who completed TAU + placebo training; tentatively suggesting that CBM-I delayed negative, OC-related interpretations coming to mind. With respect to clinical outcome measures, patients who completed the CBM-I training reported significantly fewer OC symptoms than patients from the placebo condition. Furthermore, clinicians rated patients from the TAU+CBM-I condition as having significantly fewer obsessive symptoms. These are promising initial findings of the clinical utility of CBM-I training in youth with OCD.

The main study limitation is the small sample size. Replication with more participants is necessary to examine the robustness of the observed effects. Another point concerns the training stimuli. One set of scenarios was developed for all patients, and this set contained interpretations covering all domains described by the OCCWG (1997; 2003). While this approach is in line with CBM-I studies in adults (e.g., Beadel et al., 2014; Clerkin & Teachman, 2011; Williams & Grisham, 2013), it is unlikely that an individual patient with OCD will endorse each of these beliefs. Indeed, many adolescents indicated that some scenarios fitted really well with their current concerns and they felt that these were the most helpful whereas other scenarios did not (see cases on p. 380). Tailoring the content of the training to the specific beliefs of a participant is an important next step in the field of CBM.

In response to this initial pilot, we have since developed new training scenarios for each of the following five domains: contamination, responsibility, unacceptable thoughts, symmetry, and perfectionism. Therapists indicate the two domains that are most relevant for each patient, and the patient then receives scenarios exclusively from these two domains. In this way, participants no longer need to complete scenarios that are irrelevant for them, and only practice interpreting relevant scenarios differently. Note that creating a CBM-I training based on misinterpretations of intrusions results in basically changing one's thoughts about one's thoughts; quite a complex and demanding approach, especially for youth. Therefore, in the second study, we also broadened the scope by including behavioral activities as well. An example is as follows:

> *Your father has to work late unexpectedly.*
> *He is not yet home, and you have to go to bed without saying "good night" to him.*
> *You are afraid that this may cause bad luck.*
> *You go to sleep anyway. Thoughts do not _____ the future.*
> *(predict)*

Finally, in this most recent study, CBM-I training was offered *before* the start of TAU, to be able to examine 1) the effects of CBM-I training on bias and OC symptoms as a pretreatment intervention and 2) the effects in combination with TAU (mainly CBT), as CBM-I pretraining might improve the effects of the evidence-based treatment. We are currently analyzing the results of this randomized controlled, multi-center trial (registered in the Dutch trial register with number NTR4275; http://www.trialregister.nl/trialreg/admin/rctview.asp?TC=4275).

Mediators and Moderators of Change

We will first discuss mediators and moderators of change in CBM in the domain of anxiety (adults and youth) and then describe these factors in the domain of OCD (adults and youth).

CBM training is based on the cognitive model of anxiety, which postulates that biased attention and interpretation play a causal role in anxiety symptoms. Changing these processes is expected to subsequently change the associated symptoms. Change in bias is thus the hypothesized mediator of change and indeed Amir et al. (2009) revealed that reduction in attentional bias mediated the effects of CBM-A training on adult anxiety. Grafton et al. (2017) provided further evidence as it was shown that only when the bias (e.g., the mediator) is successfully reduced are effects on symptoms observed. Another potential mediator is increased activity in the (dorsolateral) prefrontal cortex, and there is some evidence from neuro-imaging studies supporting this (Browning et al., 2010; Clarke et al., 2014).

Meta-analyses regarding CBM in adult anxiety have revealed various moderators of change, though there are differences across meta-analyses. Two meta-analyses indicated stronger effects after CBM-I than after CBM-A, indicating that these interventions should not be combined into one analysis, and moreover, that CBM-I might be the more promising approach (Cristea, Kok, et al., 2015; Hallion & Ruscio, 2011). With respect to age, Hakamata et al. (2010) revealed that age did not moderate training effects, while it did moderate in another meta-analysis (Mogoase et al., 2014; ranging from children to older adults). In the latter study, younger participants benefited more than older participants, tentatively suggesting that cognitive processes might be more easily changed in youth than in adults. This effect might also be related to the level of executive control, which is still developing in youth, and has been shown to moderate CBM-I training effects (Salemink & Wiers, 2012); lower cognitive control was associated with more change in the targeted bias. This suggests that training might especially be effective in individuals with less strongly developed cognitive control skills; for example, youth, but potentially also in individuals with mild intellectual disabilities (see Klein et al., 2018). Other moderators that some meta-analyses identified are symptom level (i.e., stronger effects in symptomatic samples, Menne-Lothmann et al., 2014; but not in other meta-analyses); location of training (better effects when training in the clinic or lab than at home; potentially due to online offering of training at home; Linetzky et al., 2015; Mogoase et al., 2014); and number of sessions (stronger effects with more sessions, Hallion & Ruscio, 2011, Menne-Lothmann et al., 2014, but not in Cristea, Kok, et al., 2015; Krebs et al., 2018).

In the domain of youth anxiety, both meta-analyses found no moderators of CBM training. That is, Cristea, Mogoase, et al. (2015) did not observe moderating effects of type of CBM training, number of training sessions, nor level of symptoms. Only training in a school setting seemed to improve the effects of CBM. In addition, Krebs et al. (2018) did not find moderating effects of age (child vs. adolescent), gender, or number of training trials. In addition, also baseline level of anxiety did not moderate the effects. These findings are in contrast to findings in the adult literature.

With respect to CBM training in the domain of OCD, there is less knowledge about mediators and moderators. Beadel et al. (2016) has examined whether the content of CBM-I training must match a person's fear domain to be efficacious and whether preexisting interpretive bias moderates CBM-I's efficacy. Results revealed that baseline interpretive bias did not moderate the results, while fear domain match appeared to be important.

Clinical Case Illustration

Here we present two cases to illustrate the treatment of CBT augmented with CBM-I. All adolescents received the CBM-I training where the domains were matched to their primary concerns.

Case 1: Saf

Saf is 17 years old and in his final exam year of the secondary school. Fixed routines have always been important for Saf, and for the past two years he has performed some OCD rituals. Last year the rituals took a rapid rise, particularly in periods of examinations. Saf has several routines that have to be completed following strict rules. Even a minor deviation causes a lot of stress and results in tantrums and panic. Saf has a morning routine, a bed time routine, a shower routine, and a toilet routine. He eats his meals in a fixed order, and at fixed times. Objects have to stay at fixed locations, and he often checks if important things did not get lost. He spends a lot of time checking his homework, and before he goes to sleep he checks if all doors are locked. When he cannot perform his rituals, he is afraid that something bad will happen to himself or to his parents.

Saf will be treated with CBT. Saf starts with the CBM-I training first. The training consists of 12 sessions in four weeks. Progress is monitored during the training. A CY-BOCS interview[1] is administered pre- and post-training and every training session, Saf rates interference of his OCD rituals on a visual analogue scale (VAS) ranging from 0 to 10 (10 is maximum interference). Figure 17.2 shows the VAS scores during the training. At the start of the training, Saf reports considerable interference. The situation significantly ameliorates during the CBM-I training. This progress is confirmed by the CY-BOCS. At the start of the training, Saf has a

---

[1] The *Children's Yale-Brown Obsessive Compulsive Scale* (CY-BOCS; Scahill et al., 1997) severity scale is a clinician-rated semi-structured interview evaluating the severity of OC symptoms. The total score ranges from 0 to 40. A total score of 16 or more is considered clinically significant.

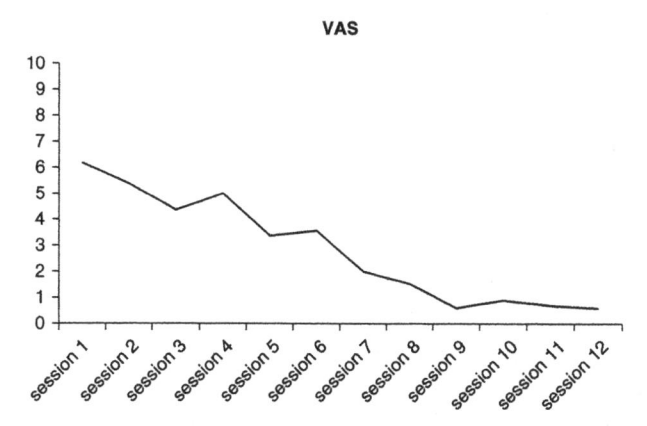

Figure 17.2 *VAS Scores of Case 1 Saf During the 12-Session CBM-I Training (pre-CBT).*

CY-BOCS total score of 34, indicating severe OCD. Post-training, Saf reports a total CY-BOCS score of 26. Although this still indicates severe OCD, a decrease of 8 points on the CY-BOCS suggests considerable improvement. Following the training, Saf starts with CBT. Progress continues and after 16 sessions CBT Saf reports a total CY-BOCS score of 2, indicating that the OCD is fully under control. No less important, Saf has passed his exams.

These results suggest that Saf has significantly benefited from the CBM training before he was able to start with regular treatment (CBT) and further benefited from the CBT. The CBM training was positively experienced by Saf. He explains that the training helped him to realize that he was not the only one with OCD and that many of his thoughts and rituals were not as strange as he used to think. Furthermore, he learned that he could ignore the obsessions and the urge to ritualize. Because this was often repeated, he remembered this message even at times when the OCD came up.

This example shows that the CBM-I training can be used during a wait-list period for regular treatment (i.e., CBT). This way, children can already benefit from this online computer training, even before treatment starts. This may lead to earlier improvement in OCD symptoms, and may increase hope and motivation for further treatment.

Case 2: Joan

Joan is an 11-year-old girl who used to be quite happy. She liked to sing and dance, and always had a lot of friends. However, in the past year she hasn't sung anymore. She looked sad and she withdrew in her room or in the bathroom more and more often. Joan often felt dirty, and although she knew that objectively this was not the case, she couldn't stand this feeling and she performed extended cleaning rituals. She spent hours and hours washing her hands until her hands were dry and sometimes even bleeding. Going to the toilet, taking a shower, and brushing her teeth were other time-consuming tasks. Nobody was allowed to enter her room, and when this rule had been violated, her mother had to thoroughly clean her room before she felt able to enter it again.

Joan found it difficult to visit the clinic to start with treatment (CBT), because this made her feel very dirty. However, she was prepared to do the online CBM-I training, which she could complete at home. At the start of the training, Joan's CYBOCS score was 26. After 12 training sessions (4 weeks), she still reported severe complaints (CY-BOCS 27). On the VAS, which she completed every training session, she also rated no progress (see Figure 17.3). After the training she started with CBT. During this treatment the CY-BOCS gradually decreased. After 16 sessions CBT, she reported a total CY-BOCS score of 15, just below the clinical cut off. CBT was successfully continued, and the CY-BOCS score further decreased.

Despite the lack of progress, Joan indicated some positive experiences with the CBM-I training. The training confirmed her idea that the cleaning rituals were in fact unnecessary. She reported that she felt more secure that she could omit the rituals, although it was not until the CBT has started that she actually stopped the rituals. Joan reported that her problems were not immediately helped by the training, however, she reported the training had changed the way she thought. She had learned that being dirty is not equivalent to being in danger. She also had some critical comments. She found that there was too much repetition in the stories, and the stories did not fully fit with her personal problems. She expected that the training would have been more effective when personalized stories had been used.

On the one hand, this case shows that not everyone may profit from the CBM-I training. On the other hand, it illustrates how the CBM-I training can provide a low threshold, first step alternative for patients that are reluctant to start with CBT. Although we found no improvement in OCD symptoms after the training, from the perspective of the patient the training had been beneficial. Joan reported that her beliefs about the OCD rituals had changed in a positive way due to the training. This may have reduced her doubt or hesitation to start CBT. After the CBM-I training, Joan was prepared to start with the CBT and perform exposure exercises. As such, the CBM-I training can be conceptualized as preparatory work for the CBT, and could be used to support this treatment. Finally, we can learn from Joan that it is important that the training scenarios fit well with a patient's personal situation.

Challenges and Recommendations for Future Research in This Area

CBM training in youth with OCD is still in its infancy. Extrapolating from the initial studies and integrating it with insights from CBM training in adults with OCD, and the broader domain of anxiety problems, suggest that, CBM-I training seems a promising tool. Effect sizes tend to be small, though significant, and the training has potential to augment evidence-based treatments. At the same time, there are challenges.

We applied CBM-I training first as an add-on to standard CBT (in parallel) and in a later study as a pre-therapy before the start of CBT. An alternative approach could be

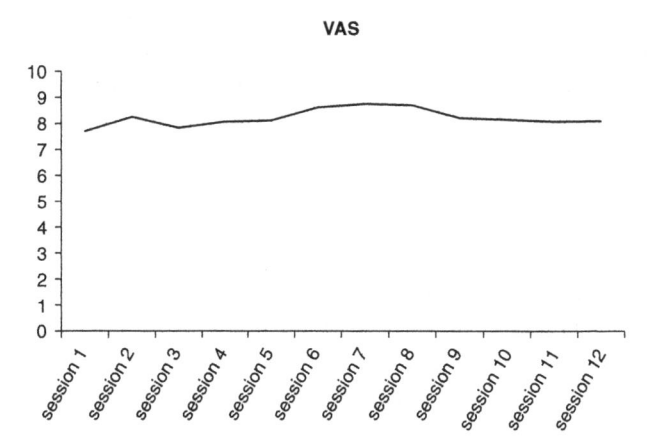

Figure 17.3 *VAS Scores of Case 2 Joan During the 12-Session CBM-I Training (pre-CBT).*

to offer CBM training after CBT as a booster intervention and to help prevent return of fear. A question for further research is to establish which approach, or combination of approaches, is most effective. Each might have the capacity to improve the effect of standard CBT. The add-on variant can intensify standard therapy, while the advantage of CBM as pre-therapy is the possibility to shorten waiting lists. Furthermore, a pretreatment CBM training could act as preparatory work for the following CBT, which might facilitate exposure and response prevention. Offering CBM after treatment could potentially prolong the effects of CBT and prevent return of symptoms.

Given the computerized nature of CBM training, it has the unique possibility to be completed online and providing the possibility to train any time during the day. A future goal may be to create an app-based training, which would enable training on one's smartphone and thus training whenever and wherever. This may also offer the opportunity to train in situations where the OCD is actually triggered. Further studies are needed to examine whether training in presence of OCD triggers and strong emotions may lead to better training effects (e.g., Kuckertz et al., 2014).

However, CBM-I need not be limited to computers or online administration. Lau, Pettit, and Creswell (2013) developed CBM-I like bedtime stories read by a parent to the child. They assumed that benign interpretation could be more easily trained through CBM-I, if training packages were administered by parents. In a first study in young nonclinical children (aged 7–11 years), three consecutive evenings of reading these bedtime stories to the child, resulted in more positive interpretations and fewer social anxiety symptoms in these children compared to a control group.

Currently, a "one-size-fits-all" approach is the standard method of delivering training. One set of stimuli is developed, and each participant gets the same set. As there are many differences between participants with the same diagnosis, and matching training to one's domain of concern improves training effects (Beadel et al., 2016), an important challenge is to move to more tailored and personalized training. We have developed a tailored CBM-I training where patients receive scenarios that match their own OCD domains. Feedback from participants has thus far been positive. The tailoring could even be brought to a next level with truly personalized and individualized scenarios by having patients develop their own scenarios as part of their treatment. To ensure the best match of scenarios with individuals' symptoms, patients could develop their own scenarios, together with their therapist, that address misinterpretations and dysfunctional behaviors. Developing such scenarios requires analyzing one's thoughts and behaviors and formulating healthier thoughts, interpretations, and more functional behavior, which can be therapeutic interventions in itself. As a next step, these individual stories could then be part of one's own CBM-I training. We recently designed such an approach. We tested this personalized CBM-I with a patient for whom the standard CBT did not work:

Case 3: Louella

Louella is a 15-year-old girl. She lives with her parents and two younger brothers in a small village. Louella has to do a lot of things that she doesn't really want to do. She arranges her books, clothes, and other objects in her room until it feels perfectly right. She also arranges the toiletries in the bathroom and the kitchenware repeatedly. Her schoolwork also takes a lot of time too, because she has to write neatly, and when she feels that is not good enough she has to start from the beginning. If she doesn't perform these compulsions, she has the feeling that something will go wrong, though she doesn't know what exactly.

CBT proves to be difficult. Despite good intentions, Louella finds it hard to perform the ERP exercises at home. After four months of therapy with minimal progress, the therapist discusses with Louella and her parents the option to add a personalized CBM-I training, allowing Louella to train with stories that perfectly fit with her OC symptoms. Louella is enthusiastic about this idea. The therapist and Louella jointly start writing scenarios for the CBM-I training. At that time, Louella still had severe complaints (CY-BOCS score of 27).

For the following months, part of each treatment session was spent on developing scenarios for the training. In the meantime, Louella starts with the standard (not-personalized) CBM-I training. Three months later, the personalized scenarios are completed. Louella has made considerable improvement by that time. The OCD complaints almost disappeared (CY-BOCS 7), Louella goes to school, finishes her school work in a reasonable time, and sees her friends regularly. However, she still wants to complete the personalized CBM-I training. One month later, when she has finished this training, the treatment is successfully completed.

Although we cannot conclude with certainty that the CBM-I training has contributed to the turning point in treatment, we can learn from the experiences of Louella and her therapist. In the evaluation, Louella rates both forms of the CBM-I training as meaningful. She describes the effect of the CBM-I trainings as follows: "The training has helped me, because I had to think in a different way intentionally, which I would normally not do. I learned how to deal with certain situations and to think in a different way. The personalized stories have helped me even more, because it was easier to understand the situations and to apply the tips in daily life. I could use these thoughts effectively in real life."

In sum, CBM training seems a promising approach, but research in youth with OCD is really at an early stage. More research is warranted to examine CBM's clinical potential, but also examine mediators and moderators of change. There clearly is room for exciting clinical research in the domain of youth OCD.

Key Practice Points

- For patients, CBM-training has potential as an add-on (and not a substitute) to CBT.
- CBM training could be provided as a pretreatment during the wait-list period or parallel to CBT treatment.
- Change in the targeted bias seems important for emotional change to occur.
- Matching training content to the patient's current concerns seems important.
- Initial promising findings in youth with OCD require replication and future research is necessary to examine CBM's effectiveness for mild or subclinical symptoms (prevention approach).

References

Abramowitz, J.J. (2017). Presidential address: Are the obsessive-compulsive related disorders related to obsessive-compulsive disorder? A critical look at DSM-5 new category. *Behavior Therapy.* doi: 10.1016/j.beth,2017.06.002

Amir, N., Beard, C., Burns, M., & Bomyea, J. (2009). Attention modification program in individuals with generalized anxiety disorder. *Journal of Abnormal Psychology, 118*, 28–33.

Amir, N., Foa, E.B., & Coles, M.E. (1998). Negative interpretation bias in social phobia. *Behaviour Research and Therapy, 36*, 945–957.

Amir, N., Kuckertz, J. M., Najmi, S., & Conley, S. L. (2015). Preliminary evidence for the enhancement of self-conducted exposures for OCD using cognitive bias modification. *Cognitive Therapy and Research, 39*, 424–440.

Anholt, G.E., Kempe, P., de Haan, E., van Oppen P., Cath, D.C., Smit, J.H., & van Balkom, A. J.L.M. (2008). Cognitive versus behavior therapy: Processes of change in the treatment of obsessive-compulsive disorder. *Psychotherapy and Psychosomatics, 77*, 38–42, doi: 10.1159/000110058

APA (2013). *Diagnostic and statistical manual of mental disorders* (5th ed.). Arlington VA: American Psychiatric Association. Bar-Haim, Y. (2010). Research Review: attention bias modification (ABM): A novel treatment for anxiety disorders. *The Journal of Child Psychology and Psychiatry, 51*, 859–870.

Bar-Haim, Y., Lamy, D., Pergamin, L., Bakermans-Kranenburg, M. J., & Van Ijzendoorn, M. H. (2007). Threat-related attentional bias in anxious and nonanxious individuals: A meta-analytic study. *Psychological Bulletin, 133*, 1–24.

Barret, P.M, & Healy-Farrel, L. (2003). Perceived responsibility in juvenile obsessive compulsive disorder: An experimental manipulation. *Journal of Clinical Child and Adolescent Psychiatry, 32*, 430–441.

Beadel, J. R., Ritchey, F. C., & Teachman, B. A. (2016). Role of fear domain match and baseline bias in interpretation training for contamination fear. *Journal of Experimental Psychopathology, 7*, 49–71.

Beadel, J. R., Smyth, F.L., & Teachman, B. A. (2014). Change processes during cognitive bias modification for obsessive compulsive beliefs. *Cognitive Therapy and Research, 38*, 103–119. doi:10.1007/s10608-013-9576-6.

Beck, A. T., & Clark, D. A. (1997). An information processing model of anxiety: Automatic and strategic processes. *Behaviour Research and Therapy, 35*, 49–58. doi:10.1016/S0005-7967(96)00069-1.

Black, M. J., & Grisham, J. R. (2016). Imagery versus verbal interpretive cognitive bias modification for compulsive checking. *Behaviour Research and Therapy, 83*, 45–52. doi:10.1016/j.brat.2016.05.009.

Bradley, M.C., Hanna, D. Wilson, P. Scott, G., Quin, P. & Dyer, K.F.W. (2016). Obsessive-compulsive symptoms and attentional bias: An eye-tracking methodology. *Journal of Behavior Therapy & Experimental Psychiatry 50*, 303–308.

Browning, M., Holmes, E. A., Murphy, S. E., Goodwin, G. M., & Harmer, C. J. (2010). Lateral prefrontal cortex mediates the cognitive modification of attentional bias. *Biological Psychiatry, 67*, 919–925.

Butler, G. & Mathews, A. (1983). Cognitive processes in anxiety. *Advances in Behaviour Research and Therapy, 5*, 51–62.

Clarke, P. J., Browning, M., Hammond, G., Notebaert, L., & MacLeod, C. (2014). The causal role of the dorsolateral prefrontal cortex in the modification of attentional bias: Evidence from transcranial direct current stimulation. *Biological Psychiatry, 76*, 946–952.

Clarke, P. J., Notebaert, L., & MacLeod, C. (2014). Absence of evidence or evidence of absence: Reflecting on therapeutic implementations of attentional bias modification. *BMC Psychiatry, 14*, 8.

Clerkin, E. M., Magee, J. C., & Parsons, E. M. (2014). Evaluating change in beliefs about the importance/control of thoughts as a mediator of CBM-I and responses to an ICT stressor. *Journal of Obsessive-Compulsive and Related Disorders, 3*, 311–318.

Clerkin, E.M., & Teachman, B.A. (2011). Training interpretation biases among individuals with symptoms of obsessive compulsive disorder. *Journal of Behavior Therapy and Experimental Psychiatry, 42*, 337–342.

Cristea, I. A., Kok, R. N., & Cuijpers, P. (2015). Efficacy of cognitive bias modification interventions in anxiety and depression: Meta-analysis. *The British Journal of Psychiatry, 206*, 7–16.

Cristea, I. A., Mogoaşe, C., David, D., & Cuijpers, P. (2015). Practitioner Review: Cognitive bias modification for mental health problems in children and adolescents: A meta-analysis. *Journal of Child Psychology and Psychiatry, 56*, 723–734. doi:10.1111/jcpp.12383.

Dudeney, J., Louise Sharpe, L., & Hunt, C. (2015). Attentional bias towards threatening stimuli in children with anxiety: A meta-analysis. *Clinical Psychology Review, 40*, 66–75.

Emmelkamp, P.M.G. & Kraanen, J. (1977). Therapist controlled exposure *in vivo* versus self-controlled exposure *in vivo*: A comparison with obsessive-compulsive patients. *Behaviour Research and Therapy, 15*, 441–444.

Farrell, L.J., Waters & Zimmer-Gembeck, M.J. (2012). Cognitive biases and obsessive-Compulsive symptoms in children: Examining the role of maternal cognitive bias and child age. *Behavior Therapy, 43*, 593–605.

Frost, R. O., & Steketee, G. (2002). *Cognitive approaches to obsessions and compulsions: Theory, assessment, and treatment.* Amsterdam, Netherlands: Pergamon/Elsevier Science Inc.

Geller, D.A., March, J., the Aacap Committee on Quality Issues (CQI). (2012). Practice parameters for the assessment and treatment of children and adolescents with obsessive compulsive disorder. *Journal of the American Academy of Child and Adolescent Psychiatry, 51*, 98–112.

Ginsburg, G.S., Newman Kingery, J., Drake, K.L., & Grados, M.A. (2008). Predictors of treatment response in pediatric obsessive-compulsive disorder. *Journal of the American Academy of Child and Adolescent Psychiatry, 47*, 868–878.

Grafton, B., Macleod, C., Rudaizky, D., Holmes, E., Salemink, E., Fox, E., & Notebaert, L. (2017). Confusing procedures with process when appraising the impact of Cognitive Bias Modification (CBM) on emotional vulnerability. *British Journal of Psychiatry, 211*, 266–271. doi: 10.1192/bjp.bp.115.176123.

Grisham, J. R., Becker, L., Williams, A. D., Whitton, A. E., & Makkar, S. R. (2014). Using cognitive bias modification to deflate responsibility in compulsive checkers. *Cognitive Therapy and Research, 38*, 505–517. doi:10.1007/s10608-014-9621-0.

Hakamata, Y., Lissek, S., Bar-Haim, Y., Britton, J. C., Fox, N. A., Leibenluft, E., . . . Pine, D. S. (2010). Attention bias modification treatment: a meta-analysis toward the establishment of novel treatment for anxiety. *Biological Psychiatry, 68*, 982–990.

Haller, S. P., Cohen Kadosh, K., Scerif, G., & Lau, J. Y. (2015). Social anxiety disorder in adolescence: How developmental cognitive neuroscience findings may shape understanding and interventions for psychopathology. *Developmental Cognitive Neuroscience, 13*, 11–20. doi: 10.10167/j dcn.2015.02002

Hallion, L. S., & Ruscio, A. M. (2011). A meta-analysis of the effect of cognitive bias modification on anxiety and depression. *Psychological Bulletin, 137*, 940–995.

Jacoby, R.J., &, Jonathan S. Abramowitz, J.S. (2016). Inhibitory learning approaches to exposure therapy: A critical review and translation to obsessive- compulsive disorder. *Clinical Psychology Review 49*, 28–40.

Kadak, M.T., Balsak, F., Besiroglu, L., & Çelik, C. (2014). Relationships between cognitive appraisals of adolescents with OCD and their mothers. *Comprehensive Psychiatry, 55*, 598–603.

Kazdin, A.E. (2007). Mediators and mechanisms of change in psychotherapy research. *Annual Review of Clinical Psychology, 3*, 1–27.

Klein, A.M., Salemink, E., de Hullu, E., Houtkamp, E., Papa, M. & van der Molen. (2018). Cognitive bias modification reduces social anxiety symptoms in socially anxious adolescents with mild intellectual disabilities: A randomized controlled trial. *Journal of Autism and Developmental Disorders, 48*, 3116–3126

Krebs, G., Pile, V., Grant, S., Degli Esposti, M., Montgomery, P., & Lau, J. Y. (2018). Research review: Cognitive bias modification of interpretations in youth and its effect on anxiety: A meta-analysis. *Journal of Child Psychology and Psychiatry, 59*, 831–844. doi: 10.1111/jcpp.12809.

Kuckertz, J. M., Gildebrant, E., Liliequist, B., Karlström, P., Väppling, C., Bodlund, O., . . . Carlbring, P. (2014). Moderation and mediation of the effect of attention training in social anxiety disorder. *Behaviour Research and Therapy, 53*, 30–40.

Lau, J.Y.F., Pettit, E., & Creswell, C. (2013). Reducing children's social anxiety symptoms: Exploring a novel parent-administered cognitive bias modification training intervention. *Behaviour Research and Therapy, 51*, 333–337. doi:10.1016/j.brat.2013.03.008.

Linetzky, M., Pergamin-Hight, L., Pine, D. S., & Bar-Haim, Y. (2015). Quantitative evaluation of the clinical efficacy of attention bias modification treatment for anxiety disorders. *Depression and Anxiety, 32*, 383–391.

Lowther, H. & Newman, E. (2014). Attention bias modification (ABM) as a treatment for child and adolescent anxiety: A systematic review. *Journal of Affective Disorders, 168*, 125–135. http://dx.doi.org/10.1016/j.jad.2014.06.051.

MacLeod C, Mathews A, Tata P. (1986). Attentional bias in emotional disorders. *Journal of Abnormal Psychology. 111*, 107–123.

Mathews, A. & Mackintosh, B. (2000). Induced emotional interpretation bias and anxiety. *Journal of Abnormal Psychology, 10*, 602–615.

Mathews, A., & MacLeod, C. (2005). Cognitive vulnerability to emotional disorders. *Annual Review of Clinical Psychology, 1*, 167–195. doi:10.1146/annurev.clinpsy.1.102803.143916.

Mathews, A., Richards, A., & Eysenck, M. (1989). Interpretation of homophones related to threat in anxiety states. *Journal of Abnormal Psychology, 98*, 31–34.

Menne-Lothmann, C., Viechtbauer, W., Höhn, P., Kasanova, Z., Haller, S. P., Drukker, M.,... & Lau, J. Y. F. (2014). How to boost positive interpretations? A meta-analysis of the effectiveness of cognitive bias modification for interpretation. *PloS One, 9*. doi:10.1371/journal.pone.0100925.

Meyer, V. (1966). Modification of expectations in cases with obsessional rituals. *Behaviour Research & Therapy, 4*, 273–280.

Mogoase, C, David, D. & Koster, E.H. (2014). Clinical efficacy of attentional bias modification procedures: An updated meta-analysis. *Journal of Clinical Psychology, 70*, 1133–1157. doi: 10.1002/jclp.22081.

Najmi, S., & Amir, N. (2010). The effect of attention training on a behavioral test of contamination fears in individuals with subclinical obsessive-compulsive symptoms. *Journal of Abnormal Psychology, 119*, 136–142.

Najmi, S., & Amir, N. (2017). Enhancement of self-conducted exposure for OCD using cognitive bias modification: A case study. *Journal of Clinical Psychology, 73*, 536–546. doi:10.1002/jclp.22451.

Obsessive Compulsive Cognitions Working Group (OCCWG). (1997). Cognitive assessment of obsessive-compulsive disorder. *Behaviour Research and Therapy, 35*, 667–681.

Obsessive Compulsive Cognitions Working Group (OCCWG). (2003). Psychometric validation of the obsessive beliefs questionnaire and the interpretation of intrusions inventory: Part I. *Behaviour Research and Therapy, 41*, 863–878.

Olatunji, B. O., Davis, M. L., Powers, M. B., & Smits, J. A. J. (2013). Cognitive-behavioral therapy for obsessive-compulsive disorder: A meta-analysis of treatment outcome and moderators. *Journal of Psychiatric Research, 47*, 33–41 doi.org/10.1016/j.jpsychires.2012.08.020.

Pediatric OCD Treatment Study Team (POTS). (2004). Cognitive behavior therapy, sertraline and their combination for children and adolescents with obsessive compulsive disorder: The Pediatric OCD Treatment Study (POTS) randomized controlled trial. *JAMA, 292*, 1969–1976.

Peris, T.S., Sugar, C.A., Bergman, R.L., Chang, S., Langley, A., & Piacentini, J. (2012). Family factors predict treatment outcome for pediatric obsessive compulsive disorder. *Journal of Consulting and Clinical Psychology, 80*, 255–263.

Polman, A., Bouman, T.K., van Geert, P.L.C., de Jong, P.J., & den Boer, J.A. (2011). Dysfunctional beliefs in the process of change of cognitive treatment in obsessive compulsive checkers. *Clinical Psychology & Psychotherapy, 18*, 256–273.

Radomsky, A.S., Alcolado, G.M., Abramowitz, J.S., Alonso, P., Belloch, A., Bouvard, M., . . . & Wong, W. (2013). Part 1- You can run but you can't hide: Intrusive thoughts on six continents. *Journal of Obsessive-Compulsive and Related Disorders, 3*, 269–279. doi.org/10.1016/j.jocrd.2013.09.002i.

Reeves, J., Reynolds, S., Coker, S. & Wilson, C. (2010). An experimental manipulation of responsibility in children: A test of the inflated responsibility model of obsessive compulsive disorder. *Journal of Behaviour Therapy and Experimental Psychiatry, 41*, 228–233.

Reynolds, S., & Reeves, J. (2008). Do cognitive models of obsessive compulsive disorder apply to children and adolescents? *Behavioural and Cognitive Psychotherapy, 36*, 463–471.

Rheaume, J., & Ladouceur, R. (2000). Cognitive and behavioural treatments of checking behaviours: An examination individual cognitive change. *Clinical Psychology and Psychotherapy, 7*, 118–127.

Riemann, B. C., Kuckertz, J. M., Rozenman, M., Weersing, V. R., & Amir, N. (2013). Augmentation of youth cognitive behavioral and pharmacological interventions with attention modification: A preliminary investigation. *Depression and Anxiety, 30*, 822–828.

Rutter, M., Bishop, D., Pine, D., Scott, S., Stevenson, J., Taylor, & Thapar, A. (2008). *Rutter's Child and Adolescent Psychiatry.* Oxford: Blackwell.

Salemink, E., Wolters, L., & de Haan, E. (2015). Augmentation of treatment as usual with online Cognitive Bias Modification of Interpretation training in adolescents with obsessive compulsive disorder: A pilot study. *Journal of Behavior Therapy and Experimental Psychiatry, 49*, 112–119. doi:10.1016/j.jbtep.2015.02.003

Salemink, E., & Wiers, R. W. (2012). Adolescent threat-related interpretive bias and its modification: The moderating role of regulatory control. *Behaviour Research and Therapy, 50*, 40–46.

Salkovskis, P.M. & Westbrook, D. (1989). Behaviour therapy and obsessional ruminations: Can *failure be turned into* success? *Behaviour Research and Therapy, 27*, 149–160.

Sánchez-Meca, J., Rosa-Alcázar, A.I., Iniesta-Sepúlveda, M., & Rosa-Alcázar, A. (2014). Differential efficacy of cognitive-behavioral therapy and pharmacological treatments for pediatric obsessive–compulsive disorder: A meta-analysis. *Journal of Anxiety Disorders, 28*, 31–44.

Scahill, L., Riddle, M. A., McSwiggin-Hardin, M., Ort, S. I., King, R. A., Goodman, W. K., et al. (1997). Children's Yale-Brown Obsessive Compulsive Scale: Reliability and validity. *Journal of the American Academy of Child & Adolescent Psychiatry, 36*, 844–852.

Siwiec, S. G., Davine, T. P., Kresser, R. C., Rohde, M. M., & Lee, H.-J. (2017). Modifying thought-action fusion via a single-session computerized interpretation training. *Journal of Obsessive-Compulsive and Related Disorders, 12*, 15–22. doi:http://dx.doi.org/10.1016/j.jocrd.2016.11.005.

Skarphedinsson, G., Weidle, B., Thomsen, P.H., Dahl, K., Torp, N.C., Nissen, . . . Ivarsson, T. (2014). Continued cognitive-behavior therapy versus sertraline for children and adolescents with obsessive–compulsive disorder that were non-responders to cognitive-behavior therapy: A randomized controlled trial. *European Child and Adolescent Psychiatry, 24*, 591–602. doi: 10.10007/s00787-014–0613-0.

Storchheim, L.E., & O'Mahoney, J.E. (2006). Compulsive behaviours and levels of belief in obsessive-compulsive disorder: A case-series analysis of their interrelationships. *Clinical Psychology and Psychotherapy, 13*, 64–79.

Stuijfzand, S., Creswell, C., Field, A.P., Pearcey, S., & Dodd, H. (2017). Research Review: Is anxiety associated with negative interpretations of ambiguity in children and adolescents? A systematic review and meta-analysis. *Journal of Child Psychology and Psychiatry, 59*, 1127–1142. doi: 10.1111/jcpp.12822.

Torp, N.C., Dahl, K., Skarphedinsson, G. Thomsen, P.H.,Valderhau, R., Weidle, B.. Ivarsson, T. (2015). Effectiveness of cognitive behavior treatment for pediatric obsessive-compulsive disorder: Acute outcomes from the Nordic Long-term OCD Treatment Study (NordLOTS). *Behaviour Research and Therapy, 64*, 15–23.

Vasey, M.W., Harbaugh, C.N., Buffington, A.G., Jones, C.R., & Fazio, R.H. (2012). Predicting return of fear following exposure therapy with an implicit measure of attitudes. *Behaviour Research and Therapy 50*, 767–774. http://dx.doi.org/10.1016/j.brat.2012.08.007.

de Voogd, E. L., Wiers, R. W., Prins, P. J. M., & Salemink, E. (2014). Visual search attentional bias modification reduced social anxiety in adolescents. *Journal of Behavior Therapy and Experimental Psychiatry, 45*, 252–259. doi: 10.1016/j.jbtep.2013.11.006.

de Voogd, E.L., Wiers, R.W., & Salemink, E. (2017). Online visual search attentional bias modification for adolescents with heightened anxiety and depressive symptoms: a randomized controlled trial. *Behaviour Research and Therapy, 92*, 57–67. doi: 10.1016/j.brat.2017.02.006.

Waters, A.M., Pittaway, M., Mogg, K., Bradley, B., & Pine, D. (2013). Attention training towards positive stimuli in clinically anxious children. *Developmental Cognitive Neuroscience, 4*, 77–84.

Waters, A. M., Zimmer-Gembeck, M. J., Craske, M. G., Pine, D. S., Bradley, B. P., & Mogg, K. (2015). Look for good and never give up: A novel attention training treatment for childhood anxiety disorders. *Behaviour Research and Therapy, 73*, 111–123.

Weil, R., Feist, A., Moritz, S., & Wittekind, C. E. (2017). Approaching contamination-related stimuli with an implicit Approach-Avoidance Task: Can it reduce OCD symptoms? An online pilot study. *Journal of Behavior Therapy and Experimental Psychiatry*.

Wiers, R. W., Gladwin, T. E., Hofmann, W., Salemink, E., & Ridderinkhof, K. R. (2013), 57, 180–188. Cognitive bias modification and cognitive control training in addiction and related psychopathology: Mechanisms, clinical perspectives, and ways forward. *Clinical Psychological Science, 1*, 192–212.

Williams, A. D., & Grisham, J. R. (2013). Cognitive Bias Modification (CBM) of obsessive compulsive beliefs. *BioMed Central Psychiatry, 13*, 256.

Williams, J.M.G., Watts, F.N., MacLeod, C., & Mathews, A. (1997). *Cognitive psychology and emotional disorders.* Oxford: John Wiley & Sons.

Williams, T.I., Salkovskis, P.M., Forrester, E.A., & Allsopp, M.A. (2002). Changes in symptoms of OCD and appraisals of responsibility during cognitive behavioural treatment: A pilot study. *Behavioural and Cognitive Psychotherapy, 30*, 69–78.

Wolters, L.H. (2011, September). Mechanisms of change in CBT for children and adolescents with OCD. In: E. de Haan (Chair). *Treating anxiety and OCD in children and adolescents: Psychological and neurobiological mechanisms of change.* Symposium conducted at the European Association for Behavioural and Cognitive Therapies (EABCT) Annual Conference, Reykjavik.

Wolters, L.H., de Haan, E., Hogendoorn, S.M., Boer, F., & Prins, P.J.M. (2016). Severe pediatric OCD and co-morbid autistic symptoms: Effectiveness of cognitive behavioral monotherapy. *Journal of Obsessive-Compulsive and Related Disorders, 10,* 69–77. doi:10.1016/j.jocrd.2016.06.002

Wolters, L.H. Prins, P.J.M., Garst, G.J.A., Hogendoorn, S.M., Boer, F., Vervoort, L., & de Haan, E. (2018). Mediating mechanisms in cognitive behavioral therapy for childhood OCD: The role of dysfunctional beliefs. *Child Psychiatry & Human Development.* Doi.org/10.1007/s10578-018-0830-8

Wolters, L.H., Vervoort, L., Hogendoorn, S.M., Prins, P.J.M., Boer, F., & de Haan, E. (2013). Selective attention for threat: No evidence of increased bias in children and adolescents with OCD. In L.H. Wolters, *Towards improving treatment for childhood OCD: Analyzing mediating mechanisms & non-response.* Thesis, University of Amsterdam, the Netherlands.

Wong, S. F., & Grisham, J. R. (2017). Causal role for inverse reasoning on obsessive-compulsive symptoms: Preliminary evidence from a cognitive bias modification for interpretation bias study. *Journal of Behavior Therapy and Experimental Psychiatry, 57,* 143–155. doi:https://doi.org/10.1016/j.jbtep.2017.06.001.

Wu, Y., Lang, Z., & Zhang, H. (2016). Efficacy of cognitive behavioral therapy in pediatric obsessive-compulsive disorder: A meta-analysis. *Medical Science Monitor, 22,* 1646–1653.

18 Innovations in Treating OCD
Brief, Intensive Treatments

Katelyn M. Dyason, Lara J. Farrell, and Allison M. Waters

Introduction

Cognitive behavioral therapy (CBT) with exposure and response prevention (E/RP) is currently recommended as the first-line psychological treatment for pediatric obsessive-compulsive disorder (OCD; Geller & March, 2012). This treatment is highly effective for the majority of children; however, there are a significant minority (~40 percent) who fail to achieve remission of symptoms following treatment. Of even greater concern, the majority of children and youth with OCD simply do not have access to these evidence-based treatments, for a wide variety of reasons. Geographical location of services, high costs associated with expert CBT, lack of trained clinicians, suboptimal therapist delivery of CBT, and therapist / patient preferences for alternative treatments are all obstacles to accessing evidence-based CBT (Goisman et al., 1993; Marques et al., 2010; Nair et al., 2015; Valderhaug et al., 2007). Moreover, given that standard CBT typically involves 12 to 20 weekly sessions of clinic-based therapy, scheduling of routine CBT can be difficult for families to manage with competing work / school and co-curricular activities. In order to meet population demands for effective, evidence-based treatment of OCD, and to provide faster symptomatic relief for an often debilitating disorder, alternative delivery of CBT is needed. This chapter therefore focuses on providing a background, rationale, and review of the extant literature base for intensive CBT for pediatric OCD. The approach will be illustrated with a clinical case example, and we will then highlight key practice points for clinicians and discuss the need for further research.

The Need for Innovation in Treatment Delivery

Affecting 2 to 3 percent of youth over the course of their childhood and adolescence (Rapoport et al., 2000), pediatric OCD is often debilitating across multiple domains of functioning, including family/home life, school, and social relationships (Piacentini et al., 2003). Commonly reported affected areas of functioning include difficulty concentrating on schoolwork, doing homework, getting ready for bed at night, and doing household chores (Piacentini et al., 2003). Sadly, the longer children suffer from OCD before receiving treatment, the more likely their OCD will persist, as either subclinical or clinical OCD (Stewart et al., 2004). Taken together, there is a strong need to intervene early in treating OCD in children and adolescents in order to provide relief, prevent disruptions to normal development, and in order to support good prognostic outcomes.

The current evidence base for pediatric OCD recommends cognitive behavioral therapy (CBT) with exposure and response-prevention (E/RP) as the first-line treatment (Carr, 2016; Geller & March, 2012; Öst et al., 2016). CBT for OCD involves psychoeducation, E/RP, cognitive coping skills, relapse prevention, and family support including reduction of family involvement in and accommodation to OCD symptoms. E/RP is the essential ingredient in effective CBT for OCD, involving exposure (E) to thoughts, images, situations, etc. where obsessions are triggered, preferably in vivo, and preventing the response (RP) of the usually accompanying compulsion (Carr, 2016; Gryczkowski & Whiteside, 2014). E/RP is conducted in a hierarchical stepped fashion, whereby the child tackles increasingly more distressing tasks over time, building coping skills and distress tolerance without overwhelming the child.

Additionally, psychopharmacological treatment with selective serotonin reuptake inhibitors (SSRIs) are recommended as an adjunct treatment to CBT should a child not respond to psychological treatments, or if symptoms are particularly severe (Carr, 2016; Gryczkowski & Whiteside, 2014), although there is limited empirical evidence that adjunct psychopharmacology provides any extra benefits than CBT alone for moderate-severe OCD (Öst et al., 2016). CBT has significantly greater response and remission rates and lower attrition rates than pharmacological treatments alone, placebo treatments, and wait-list controls (Öst et al., 2016). Within CBT studies, E/RP combined with cognitive therapy produces greater response rates than just E/RP alone (Öst et al., 2016). This being said, CBT with E/RP is not effective for all clients, or might not be as optimally effective as it could be for some clients, so there is a need to improve the effectiveness of this treatment.

As thoughtfully noted by Storch (2014), the best way to provide more effective treatment outcomes might be to make use of our current knowledge about the core components that make CBT effective, such as E/RP, rather than investing in the development of entirely new interventions. One way that treatment has been found to be more effective is by combining exposures to tackle multiple obsessions and compulsions within one exposure task (Kircanski & Peris, 2015). Another way to increase the efficacy of our treatments might be to concentrate E/RP by removing diluting elements (Storch, 2014) and providing E/RP more intensively (Farrell & Milliner, 2014; Farrell, Sluis, & Waters, 2016). Indeed, there is some preliminary evidence that very lengthy treatment (perhaps with many diluting elements) may produce smaller effect sizes than shorter or regular length treatments (Öst et al., 2016).

Typical psychological treatment for OCD lasts 12 to 20 sessions, conducted for one hour per week (Gryczkowski & Whiteside, 2014). This is a substantial time commitment for many families, especially those who have to travel to receive specialized CBT, such as families living in rural/remote areas or areas where there are no local providers of CBT for OCD. Compared to regular length treatment, intensive treatment may reduce this burden on families by requiring fewer occasions of travel, which also reduces the total amount of time spent traveling and accommodation and associated costs and requires less disruption to the family's usual routine. Some families even take an "OCD-holiday" and attend intensive treatments over a week or two, combining time away as a family with OCD treatment.

Intensive treatments provide additional benefit in that they may also provide much faster symptom relief, reducing the distress children and their families experience and restoring their normal functioning quicker. Intensive treatments may also be able to reduce duration of wait-lists, allowing more children to access treatment in a timely manner: a pertinent concern given the need for early intervention to improve overall outcomes for children with OCD (Stewart et al., 2004).

Intensive Treatments: Two Approaches

Increased Session Frequency. Two alternatives have been examined in order to make treatment more intensive: either increasing the frequency of sessions or making the sessions of a greater duration but fewer in frequency. Currently, the only randomized controlled trial of intensive CBT for pediatric OCD follows the first format. Storch et al. (2007) randomized 40 children (aged 7–17 years) to receive 14 sessions of 90-min duration of CBT delivered either daily over a period of three weeks, or delivered weekly over 12 weeks. Immediately following treatment, children receiving intensive CBT had lower overall global severity, and more children who were considered as responders or remitters (they no longer met criteria for a diagnosis of OCD). Three months following treatment, these initial findings in favor of intensive treatment had disappeared, with overall efficacy equivalent between the two treatment conditions, indicating that intensive treatment was as effective as weekly treatment but produced more rapid gains. Furthermore, in a subsequent study, intensive CBT was found to be effective at reducing symptom severity for 80 percent of children who were nonresponders or only partial-responders to an initial medication trial (Storch et al., 2010). Indeed, findings indicated that 56.6 percent of children no longer met criteria to receive a diagnosis of OCD after receiving intensive treatment, and 53.3 percent no longer met criteria 3 months after finishing treatment (Storch et al., 2010).

In a more concentrated approach to treatment, Whiteside, Brown, and Abramowitz (2008) further condensed CBT into 5 days, whereby sessions were of standard length (i.e., 1–1.5 hours) but two sessions were conducted per day. Using a case series design, two of three adolescents experienced substantial improvement over the course of treatment, and the remaining adolescent experienced improvement by the 3-month follow-up. In a larger pilot study of the same approach with 16 children and adolescents, the 5-day intensive treatment was found to be effective with significant reductions in Children's Yale-Brown Obsessive Compulsive Scale (CY-BOCS; Scahill et al., 1997) obsessions, compulsions, and total scores immediately following treatment, and furthermore, continued improvements were noted following conclusion of treatment with 10 out of 12 youth meeting criteria for clinically significant change (Whiteside & Jacobsen, 2010). In a subsequent controlled baseline study ($N = 22$), Whiteside et al. (2014) found that OCD remained stable across baseline monitoring (prior to treatment), but symptoms declined from pre- to posttreatment, and continued to decline at the 3-month follow-up.

Collectively, these results highlight the preliminary efficacy of intensive treatment for pediatric OCD by increasing the frequency of CBT sessions. This approach improves access for clients living in rural or remote locations, who would otherwise be unable to access treatment (Whiteside & Jacobsen, 2010). While this approach to CBT certainly increases accessibility to treatment, and expedites symptom relief, the approach still requires a substantive time and cost commitment, particularly for out of town clients who would need to relocate for at least a week or more to access treatment. The alternative approach to intensifying treatment for OCD is to reduce the overall number of sessions but increase the duration of sessions in order to deliver a brief, high intensity dose of CBT, which may provide even greater time and cost savings, as well as arguably enhance the dose and quality of the ERP being delivered within session.

Brief, High Intensity CBT. Similar to standard, weekly CBT, brief, high intensity CBT involves within session, therapist assisted E/RP; however, unlike standard weekly CBT whereby E/RP practice is constrained to usually less than 1 hour of therapy time, brief CBT allows for up to three hours of concentrated, continuous E/RP in any one session. Based on learning theory, Bouton (1993) demonstrated that original feared associations (CS-US pairings) that characterize anxiety can be inhibited by newly formed CS-non-US pairings that occur during E/RP – the clinical analogue of extinction training. Although fear memories are not erased from memory, they are inhibited by these newly acquired pairings. Craske et al. (2012) recently suggested that for exposure therapy to be maximally effective, it should be delivered in sessions that are close in proximity and involve multiple opportunities for the new pairings to be formed. Thus, brief, high intensity CBT involves several therapeutic conditions that might maximize exposure therapy outcomes (Ollendick, Öst, & Farrell, 2018).

Furthermore, within regular length sessions, E/RP is potentially more effective when it creates variability in distress. Kircanski and Peris (2015) found that decreased distress within E/RP sessions did not predict final treatment outcome, but rather, increased variability in distress (both significant increases and decreases in distress) predicted greater improvements in symptoms regardless of the temporal sequencing of whether increases were followed by decreases. Children who experienced a higher level of distress than expected also had greater improvements in symptoms in treatment. Kircanski and Peris (2015) suggest that this might be an important mechanism whereby children learn that they can tolerate a range of emotional states and that they can indeed tolerate more distress than they previously thought possible. Treatment sessions that are longer in length than the traditional one-hour therapy session may provide even greater opportunity for such variability in distress, with significant increases and decreases in distress over an extended session allowing for greater learning opportunities.

The second, novel approach to intensifying treatment is adapted from the one-session treatments (OSTs) that have been shown to be effective for pediatric specific phobias (Ollendick et al., 2009, 2015; Öst et al., 2001) whereby CBT with exposure therapy is conducted over one, prolonged three-hour session of exposure. Not only does a longer session allow for more increases and decreases in distress, it also allows for a greater percentage of treatment to be spent on E/RP. In a standard one-hour session, typically only 30 minutes might be dedicated to E/RP, with the remaining time taken up with opening and closing the session with reviewing psychoeducation, homework, and discussing challenges and learning. While a longer treatment session may still contain all of these elements, a substantively greater proportion of time can be dedicated to E/RP. Therefore, this second approach may fulfill Storch's (2014) recommendation for enhancing treatment outcomes via emphasizing the therapeutic ingredients that produce change (i.e., exposure therapy) while also providing other advantages and efficiencies such as reduced wait-lists, faster relief of symptoms, and increased accessibility for rural or remote families.

Our team recently conducted a controlled, multiple-baseline pilot trial to evaluate brief, high intensity CBT with E/RP for children and youth with OCD (Farrell & Milliner, 2014; Farrell, Oar, et al., 2016). After completing all initial assessments, 10 children and adolescents were randomly assigned to either a 1- or 2-week baseline condition. Following baseline monitoring, the participants then completed a one-hour psychoeducation session, followed by two intensive E/RP treatment sessions of 3.5 hours each, followed by four weekly brief e-therapy (Skype) maintenance sessions to monitor symptoms and support ongoing ERP at home. Parents and/or families were actively involved in the psychoeducation session, at the end of each intensive treatment session and in all e-therapy sessions. Participants improved on all primary outcome measures from pretreatment to posttreatment and 6-month follow-up. Eight of the children achieved reliable change on CY-BOCS (Scahill et al., 1997) total score following treatment, and seven of these maintained their reliable change at 6 months; with one further child improving by the 6-month follow-up. This pilot study therefore highlights that intensive treatment through increased duration of sessions can also be an effective approach to treatment for pediatric OCD.

Description of Brief, High Intensity CBT with E/RP: A Clinical Case Illustration

Brief, high intensity CBT for pediatric OCD (e.g., Farrell, Sluis, & Waters, 2016) is structured to begin with a 1-hour psychoeducation session (which can be conducted via e-therapy or phone for those patients out of town), followed by two intensive sessions of 3.5 hours E/RP treatment, at least one of which is conducted in the family's home (i.e., Farrell et al., 2016). It is recommended that maintenance of initial treatment gains be supported via either weekly brief phone calls or e-therapy sessions, or via a booster treatment session one month following completion of treatment. To illustrate this intensive treatment approach, we describe the case of Jessica (a pseudonym).

Jessica was a 12-year-old girl who presented to the OCD Busters research trial at Griffith University, Queensland. Jessica's main obsessions were related to feeling "just right," being responsible for something bad happening and about being a good person. Specifically, she obsessed that if she did not do things "evenly" something bad would happen in the world, such as nuclear war, which would cause her unbearable discomfort. Sometimes, she reported feeling intense discomfort without the associated worries that something bad would happen. She also worried that people would think that she was a bad person, that she was disgusting, or that she would offend people and hurt their feelings. She reported that these obsessions were almost constantly on her mind throughout the day.

These obsessions led her to complete various compulsions to alleviate her distress. Her main "evening up" compulsions were touching the opposite side of objects once she had touched one side, doing activities with two hands to avoid the need to even up, tapping her body, spinning when walking through doorways, swapping the food between both sides of her mouth when chewing, avoiding touching uneven things (e.g., cracks in the pavement), and repeating activities until she felt she had evened her body up. While completing some of these evening up routines, Jessica had to hold a positive thought in her head (e.g., "I want there to be world peace") or she believed that she could cause a bad event to happen. If she had a "bad" thought while completing an activity, she would have to repeat the activity with a positive thought in her head. Because she was thinking about trying to stop bad events from happening, bad thoughts would enter her mind frequently (e.g., "Climate change is going to cause the world to end"). She also checked with her parents, at least once a day, and sometimes her friends, whether any negative world events had occurred or were likely to happen, or whether the world was going to end.

Unfortunately, completing these compulsions only minimized her anxiety for brief periods before she would become uncomfortable or anxious again. In fact, she found that the more she completed the compulsions, the more frequent the obsessive thoughts would become, and as such, the more she would feel compelled to think good thoughts to keep out the bad thoughts. For several years, Jessica's parents recognized that Jessica had an anxious temperament and provided her with daily reassurance about bad events happening, but Jessica largely managed to keep her "evening up" compulsions hidden from her family and friends.

Prior to the presentation to our clinic, Jessica was learning about climate change in science class at school and became so distressed about this topic that she was sent to see the school counselor. After assessing Jessica, the school counselor suspected that Jessica might have OCD as Jessica reported that she had to complete certain rituals to stop bad things from happening (like climate change). The school counselor began E/RP with Jessica for half an hour once a week. After two months, Jessica's OCD had only minimally improved: her distress about bad events happening was somewhat reduced, but the frequency of the obsessions and compulsions had remained unchanged, and she was struggling to concentrate at school. The school counselor recognized that Jessica likely needed more intensive treatment than could be provided at school. As Jessica lived in a semi-rural area, there was a lack of specialized OCD treatment providers available, so Jessica's school counselor referred her to intensive treatment at the OCD Busters Program at Griffith University. As the program was offered intensively, this reduced the burden of ongoing travel on Jessica and her family.

Pretreatment Assessment. Prior to entry into the program, Jessica's mother completed the Anxiety Disorders Interview Schedule for DSM-IV – parent version (ADIS-P; Silverman & Albano, 1996) in a phone interview, which highlighted that Jessica met criteria for both obsessive-compulsive disorder and generalized anxiety disorder; these were considered to be comorbid primary diagnoses and both were assigned a clinician severity rating (CSR) of 6 out of a possible 8.

Jessica then attended an in-person session at the clinic where she was introduced to the program and completed the pretreatment CY-BOCS assessment of her OCD severity (Scahill et al., 1997). Jessica scored 15 on obsessions and 16 on compulsions, which placed her total score in the severe range. Jessica reported that her three most distressing obsessions were: (1) having to feel "just right," (2) being a good person, and (3) being responsible for something bad happening. On a scale of 0 (not at all bad) to 8 (very, very bad), Jessica reported that these obsessions had been 7, 5, and 7 in the past week, respectively. Jessica reported that her three most annoying compulsions were: (1) evening up (retouching, balancing, making thing symmetrical), (2) checking her mobile phone, and (3) seeking reassurance from her family (and sometimes friends). On the same 0 to 8 scale, Jessica reported these compulsions had been 7, 7, and 5 in the past week, respectively. Jessica's mother rated the same obsessions as 5, 5, and 6, and the compulsions as 6, 6, and 6, respectively.

Treatment: Family Psychoeducation Session. Jessica and both of her parents attended the initial psychoeducation session in-person at the clinic. The session ran for approximately an hour with the goal to provide education about OCD, the approach to treatment and the purpose of E/RP. Specifically, the session included the following components:

- *Externalizing OCD:* This component involved assisting Jessica and her parents to see OCD symptoms as part of a neurobehavioral disorder, and as separate from her, in order for Jessica to cultivate detachment from the symptoms of OCD to facilitate readiness to fight OCD symptoms. To externalize OCD, Jessica gave OCD the nickname of Jeff (the name of an annoying, bully from a novel Jessica had been reading) and drew a picture of what she imagined Jeff looked like in her head. Externalizing OCD is an important component of CBT for OCD, as it assists the child and family to ally together, in order to fight the symptoms of OCD, rather than getting angry and frustrated at the child (see March & Mulle, 1998). This was important to help Jessica's family understand that Jessica was not responsible for her compulsions, and to recognize that becoming angry with Jessica for performing her compulsions was unhelpful as it only made Jessica angry and sad, and as a result, weaker to fight Jeff. Jessica realized that the things that Jeff was telling her were not her thoughts or intentions, but rather intrusions; and the things he was making her do were not things she actually wanted to do, but things Jeff wanted to do.

- *Learning about the OCD cycle:* First, Jessica and her family learnt about the many faces (i.e., symptom clusters) of OCD. Jessica identified that the main faces that Jeff was showing her were fear of harm, getting things "just right," fear of something terrible happening, and morality fears. Next Jessica and her family learnt about the cycle of OCD. For Jessica this was described as a cycle whereby situations trigger *obsessions* or urges, such as the scenario of learning about climate change, which triggered obsessions for Jessica that she was *causing* climate change. These obsessions were thought to cause Jessica to feel anxious and drive her to perform *compulsions* in order to neutralize these feelings or prevent something bad from happening, such as evening up. The reinforcing nature of compulsions, via reduction of anxiety, was discussed with the family in order to highlight the problematic role of compulsions (and family accommodation) in perpetuating the cycle of obsessions, fears, and subsequent avoidance and ritualizing.
- *Causes of OCD:* OCD was described as a neurobehavioral disorder, which affects Jessica's thoughts, feelings, and behaviors. Jessica learnt that there is no one cause of OCD, but she learnt about multiple factors that may make it more likely for someone to develop OCD (e.g., family history of OCD, stressful life events, dysregulated circuitry in the brain). She also learnt that treatments for OCD (medication and/or psychotherapy) are the same no matter what the cause, and that treatment works by correcting behavioral and cognitive patterns that are part of the dysfunctional cycle of OCD.
- *Introduction to Exposure and Response Prevention:* This component of education builds upon the information Jessica had learnt about the cycle of OCD and about the maintaining factors of OCD. Jessica learnt that to break the cycle of OCD, she would gradually begin exposure to situations that would trigger her obsessions, and then she would prevent herself from engaging in compulsions. She learnt that gradually, her anxiety would reduce even if she did not complete the compulsion/s (via the process of habituation) and furthermore, that through the process of E/RP she would learn that (a) she could indeed tolerate the transitory distress that obsessions trigger without doing her rituals, and (b) that nothing bad happens despite not completing rituals. The family were informed that E/RP would be therapist assisted; that E/RP would occur in a gradual and stepped approach, beginning with easier steps and increasing to more challenging tasks; and most importantly, that E/RP would need to be practiced at home in-between sessions and for a number of weeks following the brief, intensive treatment.
- *Family Accommodation:* Jessica and her family learnt about how most families can unintentionally make OCD worse, even though they want to help their child, through accommodating to OCD demands. Jessica and her family identified that they were accommodating to OCD because they provided her with constant reassurance and information about world events and bad things happening, and they also completed many actions for her so that she did not have to even up (e.g.,

returning the TV remote to the coffee table). The family was educated about how family accommodation (just like compulsions) reduce anxiety, and therefore reinforce the need for Jessica to seek further assistance from them in the future. The family was asked to monitor the many ways that OCD tricks them into accommodating to Jessica's OCD, and was informed that during treatment they would be asked to gradually withdraw such accommodation – but only when given permission by Jessica, such that the process would be gradual and in her control.

- *Homework:* As homework, Jessica and her family decided on a "menu" of rewards, which Jessica would earn through completing E/RP tasks after she began her E/RP sessions. Jessica also monitored the faces of OCD that she encountered throughout the week, and the situations in which Jeff appeared in order to continue to improve her awareness of symptoms, and aid in developing an E/RP hierarchy.

Treatment: E/RP Session 1. Jessica and her mother attended the first treatment session at the clinic, which lasted 3.5 hours. Initially, any change in symptoms over the past week was discussed, followed by a review of psychoeducation and the rationale for intensive E/RP approach. Jessica then discussed the many faces of Jeff (her OCD), and she identified which areas she would like to work on first: evening up and offending people. Jessica thought of Bossing Back self-talk that she could say to Jeff when he started bothering her (e.g., "get lost Jeff, you're a liar!").

Jessica began her evening up exposures by placing herself in situations where she would normally even up (e.g., touching a wall with her left hand), and then she avoided the evening up behavior (e.g., touching the wall with her right hand). As she repeated numerous tasks of a similar nature, her anxiety and discomfort began to decrease and she felt less of an urge to ritualize. Jessica then worked on offending people by completing tasks that might offend her parents or her therapist. These tasks were more distressing for Jessica than the evening up tasks, but she was able to offend people in a silly way, and the anxiety associated with this decreased over time. For example, the therapist identified a number of minimally offensive comments she could say to Jessica and her mother, and then wrote them on the whiteboard, and then said them directly to Jessica and her mother (e.g., "I am surprised your hand writing isn't neater"; "you tend to run late for appointments don't you?"). Jessica was then encouraged to do the same exercises with her mother, the therapist, and then identify similar comments / thoughts about various friends. Finally, her progress in session was reviewed and she chose E/RP homework tasks that she thought she could work on during the week to earn points that she could exchange for rewards from her reward menu. These tasks included various examples of making herself feel uneven, without evening up (e.g., eating on one side of her mouth; wearing one sock around the house; eating with only one hand) and various E/RP tasks aimed at eliciting obsessions of fear of offending someone (e.g., on occasion not answering her friend properly; criticizing a meal prepared by her mother or father; not smiling at her teacher when her teacher spoke to her) without engaging in reassurance seeking behaviors afterwards.

Treatment: E/RP Session 2. The second intensive treatment session was conducted at Jessica's home one week later, with her father, in order to aid in generalizing the strategies between settings. Jessica was eager to report her progress in not evening up throughout the week, and how many points she had earned. She chose to build on her progress with evening up and to try more challenging evening up tasks, where she began by not evening up in situations that she found more challenging (e.g., walking through doorways, stepping on cracks with one foot). By midway through the session, she reported becoming bored with the challenges and, with the encouragement of her therapist, began saying bad thoughts while doing these actions. While her bad thoughts started off mildly (e.g., "my friend might not like me for one day"), she was able to increase the intensity of the thoughts (e.g., "my dad is going to die") while preventing compulsions (e.g., thinking good thoughts, evening up) until her distress decreased naturally.

She then continued to work on worries about offending people through completing a "roast battle" with her father and therapist. This initially made her very distressed and she consistently apologized, but with practice her distress began to diminish and she was even able to have fun and laugh during the exposure exercise. Finally, she also tried completing actions while thinking bad thoughts about the future; which initially she found too distressing to describe the thoughts out loud, but she set this as a homework task for herself that she wanted to be able to complete with practice (including making voice recordings of such thoughts).

Posttreatment Assessment. One week after completing the second E/RP session, Jessica completed a brief assessment over the phone, which also served the purpose of checking in that Jessica had begun her home practice and addressed any issues that had arisen that week. Immediately after finishing treatment, Jessica still met criteria for OCD according to her mother's report; however, this had become only just at the clinical level, with a CSR of 4. Jessica's score on the CY-BOCS also dropped to 8 for obsessions and 8 for compulsions, placing her in the moderate range, down from the severe range. Jessica's target obsessions and compulsions had also decreased substantially in severity in the last week. Her obsession of feeling just right had decreased to 3; of worrying about being a good person had decreased to 1; and being responsible for bad things happening had reduced to 1. Her compulsion of evening up had decreased to 3; her compulsion of checking her phone decreased to 1; and seeking reassurance from family was also reduced and rated as 1.

Home Practice. After completing her final E/RP session, Jessica began four weeks of home practice E/RP, monitored by a weekly brief check-in (via phone) with her parents. Throughout the week, Jessica completed her own E/RP tasks and earned a point for every task that she achieved. At her weekly check-in with her parents, Jessica summed her points and could exchange them for rewards, if she chose.

Treatment: Booster Session. After four weeks of home practice, Jessica and her parents returned for a 2-hour booster session. Jessica was noticeably happier than at previous sessions, and made jokes throughout the session. She reported that she felt like herself and had more time for doing the things that she wanted to do, as Jeff

(OCD) was so much weaker. At this final session, after reviewing her progress and difficulties that had arisen since treatment, Jessica completed more E/RP tasks, such as watching a news video about nuclear war, while engaging in activities whereby she would be uneven. These tasks elicited only minimal distress and Jessica did not need to complete any compulsions throughout the session to reduce her anxiety.

Final Assessment. After completing the booster session, Jessica was reassessed and no longer met criteria for OCD according to her mother's report, with only minimal symptoms reported and a CSR of 2 on the ADIS-P interview. Jessica's score on the CY-BOCS also dropped to 5 for obsessions and 3 for compulsions, placing her within subclinical range. Jessica's target obsessions and compulsions had also decreased substantially in severity. She and her mother both rated all three target obsessions and compulsions as 1 out of a possible 8, with the exception of the obsession of being a good person and the compulsion of checking her phone, which were both 0.

Challenges and Recommendations for Future Research

Brief, high intensity E/RP provides a number of potential advantages over standard, one-hour weekly CBT sessions in treating pediatric OCD, including faster relief from symptoms, increased access to care, and importantly, efficiencies in terms of both time and potential costs. Given the highly debilitating nature of OCD for the child, as well as the profoundly negative impact that OCD can have on the entire family through family accommodation and parental distress, providing efficient and effective early intervention is particularly important. If OCD can be treated within a few sessions, rather than treatment that occurs over many months, then impairments may be reduced, functioning improved, and a child's sense of general competence repaired, circumventing cascading problems that frequently occur when illness is prolonged. Despite promising outcomes from pilot studies and preliminary trials of intensive treatments for pediatric OCD, larger scale randomized controlled trials are needed in order to determine the relative efficacy of these treatments, and the possible immediate and longer-term advantages that this approach may provide. Moreover, such studies would allow for the important investigation of predictors and moderators of treatment response, which would inform clinical guidelines and more personalized approaches to care.

Currently, it is not yet known whether the delivery of exposure therapy in a prolonged session format provides enhanced outcomes over shorter duration sessions. Given that preliminary work by Kircanski and Peris (2015) found that increased variability in distress within session was associated with superior outcomes, longer sessions of more concentrated E/RP may indeed facilitate this process. Understanding the mechanisms associated with emotional variability and superior therapeutic outcomes remains an important focus for future research. For example, research exploring whether emotional variability leads to greater violation of threat expectancies, or alternatively enhanced coping efficacy, and moreover, whether such processes are enhanced in high intensity treatments may inform therapeutic advances. Developing novel approaches to assess and monitor such mechanisms throughout therapy currently provides a challenge for researchers, yet is one approach that may lead to further progress in enhancing exposure therapy outcomes.

Despite the potential advantages of brief, high intensity approaches, there remain a number of challenges to be considered before larger scale implementation of such an approach occurs. In Australia, while the federal government provides patient rebates for psychological therapies under the Better Access Scheme for Mental Health services (www.health.gov.au), currently patients can only claim for a maximum of one, one-hour session per day. Thus, families would be financially disadvantaged by accessing a treatment offered in a concentrated approach such as the one described here. In other countries there may also be similar restrictions by insurance providers on rebates for extended sessions. Along similar lines, scheduling three-hour-long sessions might provide a challenge for some practitioners in certain contexts (i.e., schools, hospitals). Despite these challenges, it has been our experience that brief, high intensity sessions are well tolerated by children with OCD (even among children as young as 6 years of age), and are rated as highly accepted, and effective by both children and parents alike.

Key Practice Points

Exposure therapy with response prevention remains the most well-validated and effective intervention for children and youth with OCD. Brief, high intensity E/RP may provide more efficient and favorable outcomes for children and youth, and their families. Providing families with a range of modalities for accessing evidence-based CBT ultimately provides consumers with greater flexibility and choice in services. When traditional, weekly CBT fails to achieve a favorable response, a more concentrated, high intensity approach may be another effective alternative, with ongoing, protracted weekly sessions, or pharmacological augmentation strategies. In delivering brief, high intensity CBT for OCD we recommend a number of key practice points.

- Prior to commencing brief, high intensity CBT, ensure a thorough evidence-based assessment of OCD symptoms and severity, family accommodation, and co-occurring mental health disorders. Following assessment, ensure a family psychoeducation session to educate the family about OCD, the principles of E/RP, and the nature of the intensive approach. In particular, highlight the importance of between-session E/RP practice, and ongoing E/RP practice following the initial intensive treatment. Brief, high intensity CBT is viewed as a "kick-start" to bossing back OCD, which will require ongoing E/RP practice.
- Provide families with support during the phase following therapy – usually for a period of one month to support generalization of strategies at home and across contexts. Therapists might provide brief weekly check-in calls, or alternatively, schedule a booster session three weeks following the brief treatment.

- Whenever possible, provide E/RP sessions across contexts to facilitate optimal outcomes. Given that OCD symptomatology is frequently much more pronounced in the home setting, we recommend at least one high intensity (3-hour) session to be conducted within the home.
- Involve parents in treatment whenever possible, and flexibly determine the amount of time parents are involved in the within-session E/RP depending on the child's age and the nature of the family context. For example, parents of younger children may spend one-third to one-half of the session time in session; whereas parents of adolescents might only spend the last half an hour with the therapist. The amount of time parents spend in session also varies depending on the degree of family accommodation and amount of family distress/conflict associated with OCD. Ensure all parents understand the nature of OCD and over the course of therapy, become proficient in supporting their child in E/RP practice at home. Furthermore, ensure the child and family agree on a gradual (but eventually complete) reduction of family accommodation throughout the treatment to ensure successful outcomes.
- Although treatment is brief, therapists are advised not to rush E/RP in session one. Take time for reviewing psychoeducation material at the commencement of the first intensive E/RP session, develop fear hierarchies collaboratively with the child, and take E/RP steps slow and gradual to begin with. This approach facilitates early E/RP success, enhanced therapeutic rapport and trust, and mastery of strategies. A slow and steady start to E/RP will facilitate more rapid progress over the following sessions.
- Novice therapists, or those with less experience in delivering CBT for pediatric OCD, should seek consultation and supervision by expertly trained CBT therapists when in doubt.

References

Bouton, M. E. (1993). Context, time, and memory retrieval in the interference paradigms of Pavlovian learning. *Psychological Bulletin, 114*(1), 80.

Carr, A. (2016). Chapter 18: Repetition Problems. *The handbook of child and adolescent clinical psychology* (3rd edn.). Oxon, UK: Routledge.

Craske, M. G., Liao, B., Brown, L., & Vervliet, B. (2012). Role of inhibition in exposure therapy. *Journal of Experimental Psychopathology, 3*(3), 322–345. doi: 10.5127/jep.026511

Farrell, L. J., & Milliner, E. (2014). Intensive cognitive behavioural treatment for obsessive compulsive disorder in children and adolescents. *Psychopathology Review, 1*(1), 182–188. doi: 10.5127/pr.034113

Farrell, L. J., Oar, E. L., Waters, A. M., McConnell, H., Tiralongo, E., Garbharran, V., & Ollendick, T. (2016). Brief intensive CBT for pediatric OCD with E-therapy maintenance. *Journal of Anxiety Disorders, 42*, 85–94. doi: 10.1016/j.janxdis.2016.06.005

Farrell, L. J., Sluis, R., & Waters, A. M. (2016). Intensive treatment of pediatric OCD: The case of Sarah. *Journal of Clinical Psychology: In Session, 72*(11), 1174–1190. doi: 10.1002/jclp.22397

Geller, D. A., & March, J. (2012). Practice parameter for the assessment and treatment of children and adolescents with obsessive-compulsive disorder. *Journal of the American Academy of Child & Adolescent Psychiatry*, *51*(1), 98–113. doi: 10.1016/j.jaac.2011.09.019

Goisman, R. M., Rogers, M. P., Steketee, G. S., Warshaw, M. G., Cuneo, P., & Keller, M. B. (1993). Utilization of behavioral methods in a multicenter anxiety disorders study. *The Journal of Clinical Psychiatry*, *54*(6), 213–218.

Gryczkowski, M. R., & Whiteside, S. P. H. (2014). Pediatric obsessive-compulsive disorder. In E. A. Storch & D. McKay (eds.), *Obsessive-compulsive disorder and its spectrum: A life-span approach*. Washington, DC: American Psychological Association.

Kircanski, K., & Peris, T. S. (2015). Exposure and response prevention process predicts treatment outcome in youth with OCD. *Journal of Abnormal Child Psychology*, *43*, 543–552. doi: 10.1007/s10802-014-9917-2

Marques, L., LeBlanc, N. J., Weingarden, H. M., Timpano, K. R., Jenike, M., & Wilhelm, S. (2010). Barriers to treatment and service utilization in an internet sample of individuals with obsessive–compulsive symptoms. *Depression and Anxiety*, *27*(5), 470–475.

Nair, A., Wong, Y. L., Barrow, F., Heyman, I., Clark, B., & Krebs, G. (2015). Has the first-line management of paediatric OCD improved following the introduction of NICE guidelines? *Archives of Disease in Childhood*, *100*(4), 416–417.

Ollendick, T. H., Öst, L. G., & Farrell, L. J. (2018). Innovations in the psychosocial treatment of youth with anxiety disorders: Implications for a stepped care approach. *Evidence-Based Mental Health*, *21*(3), 112–115.

Ollendick, T. H., Ost, L. G., Reuterskiold, L., Costa, N., Cederlund, R., Sirbu, C., ... Jarrett, M. A. (2009). One-session treatment of specific phobias in youth: A randomized clinical trial in the United States and Sweden. *Journal of Consulting and Clinical Psychology*, *77*(3), 504–516. doi: 10.1037/a0015158

Ollendick, T. H., Halldorsdottir, T., Fraire, M. G., Austin, K. E., Noguchi, R. J. P., Lewis, K. M., ... Whitmore, M. J. (2015). Specific phobias in youth: A randomized controlled trail comparing one-session treatment to a parent-augmented one-session treatment. *Behavior Therapy*, *46*, 141–155.

Öst, L. G., Riise, E. N., Wergeland, G. J., Hansen, B., & Kvale, G. (2016). Cognitive behavioral and pharmacological treatments of OCD in children: A systematic review and meta-analysis. *Journal of Anxiety Disorders*, *43*, 58–69. doi: 10.1016/j.janxdis.2016.08.003

Öst, L. G., Svensson, L., Hellström, K., & Lindwall, R. (2001). One session treatment of specific phobias in youths: A randomized clinical trial. *Journal of Consulting and Clinical Psychology*, *69*, 814–824. doi: 10.1037/0022-006x.69.5.814

Piacentini, J., Bergman, R. L., Keller, M., & McCracken, J. (2003). Functional impairment in children and adolescents with obsessive-compulsive disorder. *Journal of Child and Adolescent Psychopharmacology*, *13*(S1), S61–S69.

Rapoport, J. L., Inoff-Germain, G., Weissman, M. M., Greenwald, S., Narrow, W. E., Jensen, P. S.,... Canino, G. (2000). Childhood obsessive-compulsive disorder in the NIMH MECA study: Parent versus child identification of cases. *Journal of Anxiety Disorders*, *14*(6), 535–548. doi: 10.1016/S0887-6185(00)00048-7

Scahill, L., Riddle, M. A., McSwiggin-Hardin, M., Ort, S. I., King, R. A., Goodman, W. K., ... Leckman, J. F. (1997). Children's Yale-Brown Obsessive

Compulsive Scale: Reliability and Validity. *Journal of the American Academy of Child & Adolescent Psychiatry, 36,* 844–852.

Silverman, W. K., & Albano, A. M. (1996). *The Anxiety Disorders Interview Schedule for DSM-IV-Child and Parent Versions.* London: Oxford University Press.

Stewart, S. E., Geller, D. A., Jenike, M., Pauls, D., Shaw, D., & Faraone, S. V. (2004). Long-term outcome of pediatric obsessive-compulsive disorder: A meta-analysis and qualitative review of the literature. *Acta Psychiatrica Scandinavica, 110,* 4–13.

Storch, E. A. (2014). Can we improve psychosocial treatments for child anxiety? *Depression and Anxiety, 31*(7), 539–541. doi: 10.1002/da.22283

Storch, E. A., Geffken, G. R., Merlo, L. J., Mann, G., Duke, D., Munson, M.,... Goodman, W. K. (2007). Family-based cognitive-behavioral therapy for pediatric obsessive-compulsive disorder: Comparison of intensive and weekly approaches. *Journal of the American Academy of Child & Adolescent Psychiatry, 46*(4), 469–478. doi: 10.1097/chi.0b013e31803062e7

Storch, E. A., Lehmkuhl, H. D., Ricketts, E., Geffken, G. R., Marien, W., & Murphy, T. K. (2010). An open trial of intensive family based cognitive-behavioral therapy in youth with obsessive-compulsive disorder who are medication partial responders or nonresponders. *Journal of Clinical Child & Adolescent Psychology, 39*(2), 260–268. doi: 10.1080/15374410903532676

Valderhaug, R., Larsson, B., Götestam, K. G., & Piacentini, J. (2007). An open clinical trial of cognitive-behaviour therapy in children and adolescents with obsessive-compulsive disorder administered in regular outpatient clinics. *Behavior Research and Therapy, 45,* 577–589. doi: 10.1016/j.brat.2006.04.011

Whiteside, S. P., Brown, A. M., & Abramowitz, J. S. (2008). Five-day intensive treatment for adolescent OCD: A case series. *Journal of Anxiety Disorders, 22*(3), 495–504. doi: 10.1016/j.janxdis.2007.05.001

Whiteside, S. P., & Jacobsen, A. B. (2010). An uncontrolled examination of a 5-day intensive treatment for pediatric OCD. *Behavior Therapy, 41,* 414–422. doi:10.1016/j.beth.2009.11.003

Whiteside, S. P., McKay, D., De Nadai, A. S., Tiede, M. S., Ale, C. M., & Storch, E. A. (2014). A baseline controlled examination of a 5-day intensive treatment for pediatric obsessive-compulsive disorder. *Psychiatry Research, 220*(1–2), 441–446. doi: 10.1016/j.psychres.2014.07.006

19 Pharmacologic-Augmented Treatments

Sophie C. Schneider and Eric A. Storch

Introduction

Despite strong evidence supporting the efficacy of cognitive behavioral therapy (CBT) for pediatric obsessive-compulsive disorder (OCD), a substantial number of young people do not experience remission from OCD following CBT (Öst et al., 2016). The clinical guidelines of the American Academy of Child and Adolescent Psychiatry AACAP; (Geller, March, & AACAP Committee on Quality Issues, 2012) recommend augmenting CBT with pharmacologic treatment if there is incomplete response to CBT, or if client characteristics are likely to interfere with CBT delivery. The following chapter will provide an overview of the recommendations for pharmacologic treatment of pediatric OCD and the current evidence base for the pharmacologic augmentation of CBT for pediatric OCD. It will then discuss potential innovations for traditional augmentation approaches and provide an overview of novel augmentation strategies using cognitive enhancers of learning and exposure therapy outcomes. Finally, it will outline some of the key directions for future research.

Overview of Pharmacologic Augmentation of CBT

Recommendations for Pharmacologic Monotherapy

The recommended pharmacologic treatment for pediatric OCD involves selective serotonin reuptake inhibitors (SSRIs; Geller, March, & AACAP Committee on Quality Issues, 2012); specifically, fluvoxamine, sertraline, fluoxetine, and paroxetine, all of which have been well studied in pediatric OCD (Bloch & Storch, 2015; Ivarsson et al., 2015). A meta-analysis found that, across 14 studies of pediatric OCD, there was a moderate advantage of short-term (8 to 14 week duration) SSRI monotherapy over placebo (Hedge's $g = 0.43$) in OCD symptom reduction (Ivarsson et al., 2015). Treatment response, defined as a minimum of 25 percent reduction in symptom severity, was significantly higher for those receiving SSRI medication compared to placebo (53.4 percent vs. 34.7 percent). However, meta-analyses (McGuire et al., 2015; Öst et al., 2016) also indicate that overall SSRI treatment effects are smaller than CBT monotherapy, which is associated with a large effect on OCD symptom reduction compared to both active (e.g., relaxation training) or non-active (e.g., wait-list) control conditions ($g = 1.28$), and further, that response to treatment occurs in in 69.6 percent of cases. Finally, results also indicated that SSRIs are less likely to produce overall remission of OCD, relative to CBT (24.1 percent vs. 52.7 percent).

Clinical Management of SSRIs

SSRI treatment should begin at a low dose, building up slowly over time in order to minimize side effects while maximizing therapeutic benefit (Bloch & Storch, 2015; Varigonda, Jakubovski, & Bloch, 2016). An adequate medication trial should include at least 10 weeks of treatment, with dosage increasing as needed until the maximum recommended or maximum tolerated dose is delivered for several weeks (Geller March, & AACAP Committee on Quality Issues, 2012). Typically reported side effects of SSRIs include sleep disturbance, dizziness, gastrointestinal symptoms, sedation, and sexual dysfunction (Stewart & Stachon, 2014). In a study of 47 youth with OCD treated with CBT plus sertraline or placebo, the most commonly reported adverse events in the CBT plus sertraline group were headache (52 percent), insomnia (35 percent), diarrhea (32 percent), decreased appetite (29 percent), and sore throat (23 percent; Storch et al., 2013). Interestingly, the CBT plus placebo group also reported a significant number of such adverse events, though the sertraline group reported around twice the rate of decreased appetite, diarrhea, and exacerbated behavior problems compared to the placebo group.

Although many SSRI side effects are minor and/or transient, youth receiving SSRI treatment should be closely monitored for activation syndrome (also known as behavioral activation). Activation syndrome involves a range of symptoms including irritability, akathisia (motor agitation), disinhibition, mania, and self-harm (Goodman, Murphy, & Storch, 2007; Reid et al., 2015). In one study of 56 youth with OCD, poorer treatment response was associated with increased symptoms of irritability, akathisia, and disinhibition, but not with symptoms of mania or suicidal ideation (Reid et al., 2015). When activation syndrome symptoms emerge, they should prompt a medication review, as it may be helpful to reduce the SSRI dose, or delay planned dose increases. The relationship between SSRI use in youth and suicide risk has been the subject of much attention, particularly after a study of 4,582 subjects in pediatric SSRI clinical trials found that SSRIs were associated with a 1.66 risk ratio for suicidality compared to placebo, and that in 100 youth treated with SSRIs, 1 to 3 patients may have an increase of suicidality (Hammad, Laughren, & Racoosin, 2006). However, it should be noted that of the 24 included clinical trials, 16 were focused on the treatment of major depressive disorder, and only 4 focused on OCD. A more recent review of 14 studies treating pediatric OCD (including 1136 youth aged 6 to 18 years) with SSRIs or clomipramine (a tricyclic antidepressant with nonselective serotonin reuptake inhibiting effects) found no incidents of serious adverse events, that is, life threatening or potentially disabling outcomes (Ivarsson et al., 2015). Regardless, it is recommended that the initiation of SSRIs be closely monitored by a psychiatrist who can perform regular monitoring of OCD symptoms and side effects and adjust dosage in order to minimize side effects while maximizing treatment benefits. This is particularly important when youth are prescribed multiple pharmacologic agents; in one study there was a 77 percent higher risk of parent-reported side effects when SSRIs were combined with another pharmacologic agent, compared to when SSRIs were used alone (Hilt et al., 2014).

Current treatment guidelines are to continue the use of SSRIs for 6 to 12 months after dose stabilization (Geller, March, & AACAP Committee on Quality Issues, 2012). However, little is known about the long-term effects of SSRI use in youth as most pediatric treatment trials have only evaluated the effects of SSRIs over a few months (Ivarsson et al., 2015). As the course of OCD may be more episodic in youth than in adults, it is unclear how long youth should remain on medication, and what the risk of relapse is when medication is discontinued (Bloch & Storch, 2015). Where discontinuation is required or recommended, medication should be slowly tapered down to minimize side effects, and close monitoring provided for risk of relapse (Bloch & Storch, 2015).

Strategies for Augmenting CBT with SSRIs

Since CBT and SSRIs are both efficacious when used as a monotherapy, they are often combined in order to achieve additional therapeutic benefits. According to current clinical guidelines, the optimum method for combining CBT and SSRI treatment will depend on the needs and circumstances of the individual (Geller, March, & AACAP Committee on Quality Issues, 2012; Stewart & Stachon, 2014). A particularly important factor in treatment decisions is the current severity of the OCD symptoms. The gold standard for assessment of youth OCD is the Children's Yale Brown Obsessive Compulsive Scale (CY-BOCS; Scahill et al., 1997), which assesses the nature and severity of OCD symptoms. CY-BOCS severity is assessed by 10 items measuring distress, interference, resistance, control, and the time occupied by OCD symptoms, with each item scored from 0 to 4. A CY-BOCS total severity score of less than 5 indicates slight or doubtful symptoms, a score of 5 to 13 indicates mild symptoms with little functional impairment, 14 to 24 suggests moderate symptoms requiring effort to function, 25 to 30 indicates moderate-severe symptoms with limited functioning, and a score of 30 or above indicates severe symptoms with assistance needed to function (Lewin, Piacentini, et al., 2014). In cases where the OCD is of mild to moderate severity and there are no other complicating factors (such as comorbid depression or family dysfunction), treatment should begin with CBT alone, and SSRIs would be added only if there was insufficient treatment response to an initial and adequate dose of CBT (including exposure and response prevention). In those with moderate to severe OCD, concurrent treatment with CBT and SSRIs is recommended. Beginning treatment with SSRI monotherapy is recommended only in cases where a client is unable to engage in CBT, which may be the case for clients who do not have access to expert CBT, or for clients affected by complicating characteristics such as comorbid depression, poor insight, low motivation, or high family dysfunction. It is recommended in these cases that

CBT would then be added when the individual is well enough or prepared to engage with therapy.

There are currently only a limited number of studies that have specifically evaluated different approaches for combining CBT and SSRIs, thus the AACAP clinical guidelines (Geller, March, & AACAP Committee on Quality Issues, 2012) are largely based on clinical expertise and consensus. In a small study of 10 youth who were previously noncompliant with behavior therapy, Neziroglu et al. (2000) found that combined SSRI and behavior therapy was more effective than SSRI alone. The Pediatric OCD Treatment Study (POTS) Team (2004) studied 112 youth in a randomized, controlled multi-center study, and found that combined CBT and SSRI treatment was superior to either CBT or SSRI monotherapy, which did not differ significantly from each other. However, the outcomes of the CBT and SSRI monotherapy conditions differed significantly between two of the largest study sites, such that combined therapy was similarly effective to CBT alone at one of the sites. The second POTS study (POTS II) focused on 124 youth with OCD who were partial responders to SSRIs, and found that combined SSRI management plus a full course of CBT was superior both to ongoing SSRI management alone, and to SSRI management plus a brief, psychiatrist-delivered "instructions in CBT" program (Franklin et al., 2011). Finally, Storch et al. (2013) found that the addition of an SSRI to CBT was not more effective than placebo plus CBT in 47 youth with OCD. Although the differing designs of these studies make direct comparisons of outcome difficult, a meta-analysis by Ivarsson et al. (2015) found that pooled across a range of studies, combined treatments were superior to SSRI monotherapy, but there was no significant difference between combined treatment and CBT monotherapy. Further, Skarphedinsson et al. (2015) provided continued treatment to 50 youth who had failed to respond to a course of CBT, and found that approximately 50 percent of youth improved regardless of whether they received further CBT, or switched to SSRI treatment. Taken together these findings challenge the largely accepted recommendation that SSRIs are required in those who fail to respond to an initial course of CBT.

Conclusions about the efficacy of combined treatments compared to CBT monotherapy must be made with caution, as there are few combined treatment studies in pediatric OCD. Further, these studies did not specifically evaluate the AACAP recommendations for how and when to combine treatments (Geller, March, & AACAP Committee on Quality Issues, 2012). That is, there has been no published study comparing combined treatment to CBT alone in those with severe OCD, and no evaluation of the effect of different methods of combining SSRI and CBT. More precisely, information is lacking on how best to combine CBT with SSRIs; for example, it is unclear whether both interventions should begin simultaneously, or if SSRIs should be started first with the intention of achieving symptomatic reduction prior to beginning CBT (Storch et al., 2013). As SSRI side effects of irritability, akathisia, and disinhibition may be associated with poorer response to combined treatment (Reid et al., 2015), outcomes for combined treatment may be dependent on how the different therapies interact. Thus, at present, treatment recommendations primarily rely on clinical judgment to decide when and how to augment CBT with SSRIs.

The Approach to Innovation

As the evidence to guide best practice pharmacologic augmentation of CBT is limited, there is a wide scope for innovation and improvements to clinical practice. Such innovations can be broadly divided into two approaches to CBT augmentation, namely traditional augmentation strategies and novel augmentation strategies.

Traditional Augmentation Strategies

What can be termed the "traditional" approach to the pharmacologic augmentation of CBT involves the addition of a pharmacologic agent that directly reduces the symptoms of OCD. The best example of this is the addition of SSRIs to CBT, but this could also involve other agents that directly reduce OCD symptoms. Research across anxiety disorders suggests that traditional combined therapies deliver inconsistent benefits, with modest benefits at best (Otto, McHugh, & Kantak, 2010). This does not mean that such treatments should not be used; instead, it is important to determine who will benefit from a combined treatment approach, and how best to deliver this treatment. A range of research directions are available that may help to address these challenges.

Identifying Predictors and Moderators of Treatment Outcome. There is increasing interest in identifying individual pretreatment factors that are associated with treatment response. Such variables may be associated with response to treatment regardless of treatment type (predictors) or may be associated with differing effects across treatment conditions (moderators). If particular characteristics were known to be associated with treatment outcome, they may help to guide families toward the most effective treatment for them. Despite the interest in the identification of predictors and moderators, recent meta-analyses and reviews (Caporino & Storch, 2016; McGuire et al., 2015; Öst et al., 2016) indicate few consistent findings in pediatric OCD trials. This may reflect differences in study methodology, as well as the limited number of studies to date that have directly evaluated predictors of response.

Moderators of pediatric OCD treatment outcome have been explored in two meta-analyses. Öst et al. (2016) found that treatment effect size was positively associated with higher OCD severity and a higher percentage of participants with a comorbid anxiety disorder, both in CBT and pharmacotherapy studies. McGuire et al. (2015) found a positive association between CBT effect size and higher frequency of participants with comorbid tic disorders or anxiety disorders, but this effect was not observed for SSRI studies. A review of potential moderators and predictors of outcome also identified family accommodation and parent-reported externalizing symptoms as potentially important pretreatment variables (Caporino & Storch, 2016). Across OCD treatment modalities, participant characteristics such as age, sex, race, and socioeconomic background are rarely associated with treatment outcome.

The only combined CBT and SSRI study to examine multiple potential predictors was the first POTS trial. Garcia et al. (2010) found that across treatment conditions, improvement was positively predicted by lower baseline levels of OCD severity, functional impairment, externalizing symptoms, and family accommodation, and by higher levels of insight. Interestingly, the POTS study also indicated that tic disorders and a family history of OCD may moderate treatment outcome. Across the whole POTS sample, combined treatment was the most effective, followed by CBT, then SSRI, then placebo treatment. In those with tic disorders, SSRI treatment was no more effective than placebo, but combined treatment remained superior to CBT alone (March et al., 2007). In contrast, there were no significant pairwise differences across treatment conditions in youth with family history of OCD (parent or sibling), but treatment effects were attenuated more strongly in CBT than in other treatment conditions (Garcia et al., 2010). Together, these results suggest that combined therapy and CBT monotherapy may be recommended in those with comorbid tic disorders, but that combined therapy or SSRI monotherapy may be recommended in those with a family history of OCD.

Studies of predictors and moderators of pediatric OCD treatment outcome have produced interesting findings, and potentially valuable directions for future research. However, further research is needed before these findings can be clearly applied as clinical guidelines. It would be particularly valuable to evaluate variables identified in the AACAP guidelines (Geller, March, & AACAP Committee on Quality Issues, 2012) as requiring combined treatment; these include severe OCD, family dysfunction and accommodation, and comorbidity with depression, externalizing disorders, and other disorders that may interfere with therapy.

Treatment Preferences and Expectancies

The issue of attitudes toward different treatment modalities is often not considered or examined within research trials. This may be unsurprising given the importance of random group allocation to many research studies. Nevertheless, attitudes toward treatments are likely to be very important in routine clinical settings. Individuals are unlikely to engage with a treatment if they find it unacceptable, or if they have poor expectations of success.

A study that surveyed parents seeking treatment for a child with OCD indicated that CBT monotherapy was the most preferred treatment (68 percent), followed by combined CBT and SSRI (32 percent), with only 1 percent preferring SSRI monotherapy (Lewin et al., 2014). Preference for CBT monotherapy was especially high for parents of younger children and children who had not previously taken medication, and 70 percent of parents were concerned about potential negative effects of medication. These findings are in sharp contrast to the limited availability of expert

CBT in the community (Franklin et al., 2015), suggesting that many young people may not have access to a preferred course of treatment.

As parents are the primary decision-makers regarding treatment, it is clearly important to ensure that they agree with the therapist about planned treatment. Interestingly, Lewin et al. (2011) found that greater posttreatment OCD symptom improvement was significantly associated with child and therapist positive expectancies about CBT, but not with parental expectancies of outcome. Higher child expectancies were associated with greater homework compliance, and lower rates of treatment drop-out. Interestingly, the factors associated with expectancies differed across reporter; parental expectancies were negatively associated with parents' own OCD symptoms, child depressive symptoms, and child-reported OCD interference; child expectancies were negatively associated with the number of comorbid diagnoses, depression symptoms, externalizing symptoms, parent- and child-rated OCD interference, and positively associated with perceived control; and therapist expectancies were negatively associated with child depressive and externalizing symptoms, child-reported OCD interference, and positively associated with child perceived control (Lewin et al., 2011). This indicates that it may be valuable to identify factors associated with negative treatment expectancies, so that these can be addressed early in treatment. Expectancies about treatment outcome are also thought to be important in the success of pharmacologic treatment programs (Rief et al., 2016). Therapists should thus evaluate and consider parent and child attitudes when deciding between treatment options. Regardless of the treatment selected, it is important to maximize positive expectancies of treatment in all parties involved in the therapeutic process (Rief et al., 2016) in order to improve engagement, compliance, and outcomes associated with the treatment.

Rapid Identification of Response to SSRIs

Clinical guidelines report that it may take up to 12 weeks to see the full effects of an SSRI on OCD symptoms (Geller, March, & AACAP Committee on Quality Issues, 2012). However, a meta-analysis examining session-by-session symptom change in SSRI monotherapy trials reported that over 85 percent of the benefit of SSRIs over placebo occurred in the first two weeks of treatment, with minimal differences observed after the sixth week of treatment (Varigonda et al., 2016). Although it is too early to recommend changing clinical practice based on one study, if response or nonresponse to a course of SSRIs can be predicted within just a few weeks, this could greatly reduce the duration of ineffective medication trials, and lead to alternative approaches of management and therefore more rapid improvements in OCD symptomology.

Identifying Problematic Side Effects

As noted previously, side effects are commonly associated with SSRI treatment of OCD. Although these symptoms are often minor, some side effects may have the potential to interfere with the effects of CBT (Reid et al., 2015). Therefore, it is crucial to identify clinically significant side effects as soon as possible, and to manage the medication dose appropriately. Within combined treatment studies, psychologists are likely to have the most frequent clinical contact, so close relationships between psychologists and psychiatrists may be beneficial in identifying problematic side effects as quickly as possible.

When assessing side effects, clinicians typically rely on periodic symptom reports from parents and children. Although these are undoubtedly valuable, parents are likely to lack information about symptoms experienced during school hours and overnight, and young people may find it difficult to accurately recall their symptoms. It can also be difficult to accurately recall symptoms over periods of days or weeks. Recent studies have thus explored the use of objective measures of clinically relevant SSRI side effects. For example, Bussing et al. (2015) examined whether a watch-like actigraph that measures the frequency and intensity of motion could be used as a measure of activation syndrome symptoms. The study found that changes in parent-reported activation symptoms corresponded with increases in actigraph-measured daytime and nighttime activity. If used in clinical practice, such a device could be useful for early detection of changes in physiological activity, and potentially, to monitor sleep quality. A system that provides high-quality objective information about common medication side effects could result in quicker identification of adverse reactions to common medications. As drop-out from medication studies can be due to side effects (Reid et al., 2015), this could also improve retention of families in treatment. If the utility of the actigraph approach is validated in other clinical populations, future applications could involve the use of smartphone and commercial activity trackers for data capture (Bussing et al., 2015), and potentially, automatic data analysis and clinician notification of activation syndrome symptoms.

Biomarkers of SSRI Response

Biomarkers refer to individual biological characteristics that can predict response to a particular treatment. The identification of valid biomarkers of treatment response could thus help to select between treatments, or to fine-tune how a treatment is delivered in a more personalized approach. Exploratory pediatric OCD studies have examined the volume of specific brain regions such as the amygdala, frontal and cingulate regions, the concentration of neurotransmitters in brain regions implicated in OCD like glutamate in the caudate nucleus, and genetic profiles relating to neurotransmitter systems or drug metabolism (Grabb & Gobburu, 2016).

An example of how biomarkers may be used clinically is that individuals differ on how quickly they metabolize particular pharmacologic agents (Maron & Nutt, 2015), and so will achieve different levels of neurotransmitter change at equivalent SSRI dosages. As gradual dose increases are generally recommended for young people (Geller, March, & AACAP Committee on Quality Issues, 2012), some youth will experience effects more rapidly than others, and slow responders could experience long periods of ineffective medication when doses are gradually increased. If drug-specific metabolic profiles are identified, this could help to decrease the duration of ineffective treatment and achieve symptomatic changes more quickly. At present, biomarker research is at a relatively early stage and cannot be used to guide clinical practice (Grabb & Gobburu, 2016). However, biomarkers remain a topic of great interest given the potential for improving treatment selection and delivery.

Alternative Pharmacologic Agents

Clomipramine, a tricyclic antidepressant with nonselective serotonin reuptake inhibition properties, was the earliest approved pharmacologic treatment for OCD in pediatric populations (Geller, March, & AACAP Committee on Quality Issues, 2012). When used as a monotherapy, it has a similar or greater treatment effect than SSRIs (Ivarsson et al., 2015). It can also be combined with an SSRI to enhance the serotonergic effects of the medications, especially in the instance of SSRI nonresponse. However, clomipramine should be used with caution due to the greater frequency of reported side effects, and the potential for serious side effects including seizures, cardiac events, and fatal overdose (Bloch & Storch, 2015).

The most common non-SSRI pharmacologic agents explored for OCD are the atypical neuroleptics, also known as antipsychotics (Geller, March, & AACAP Committee on Quality Issues, 2012). These affect both the dopamine and serotonin systems, and are generally used in combination with SSRIs for those with very severe or treatment-resistant OCD. However, a meta-analysis of antipsychotic augmentation of SSRI in 12 studies involving 391 adults with OCD only provided clear support for one antipsychotic, risperidone (Dold et al., 2013). A subsequent larger trial found no advantage of risperidone over placebo (Simpson, Foa, Liebowitz, & et al., 2013). In pediatric OCD, some positive results have been reported for SSRI augmentation with risperidone and aripiprazole (Masi et al., 2010; Thomsen, 2004), but there is a lack of high-quality randomized controlled trials to guide clinical practice. Due to the potential for serious side effects with atypical neuroleptics (Bloch & Storch, 2015), these should be used with caution in pediatric OCD.

In recent years, there has been particular interest in the role of the glutamate system in understanding the biological mechanisms of OCD. Although the evidence for this association is mixed, some adult studies have found an association between OCD and glutamate-related genes and high glutamate levels in a subset of individuals with OCD (Pittenger, 2015a). In youth receiving CBT, lower pretreatment brain glutamate signaling predicted greater posttreatment OCD symptom improvement, and glutamate signaling dropped over the course of treatment (O'Neill et al., 2017). A number of glutamatergic agents have been studied for the management of OCD, including ketamine, memantine, glycine, D-cycloserine (DCS), riluzole, N-acetylcysteine, and anticonvulsants (Pittenger, 2015b). Increasing interest in the role of glutamate in OCD has led to many small and uncontrolled studies, typically in adult samples. Although there are some promising results, especially in those who have failed to respond to treatment, further high-quality research is needed before glutamatergic agents can be recommended for routine clinical use in any age group.

Although a range of other pharmacologic agents (e.g., stimulants, St John's Wort, and opiates) have been examined for the treatment of pediatric OCD, there is currently insufficient evidence to recommend their use as part of standard clinical care (Geller, March, & AACAP Committee on Quality Issues, 2012). Further, there are few high-quality studies comparing SSRI monotherapy to SSRI with additional pharmacologic agents (such as clomipramine) in pediatric OCD, and no study that examines outcomes when alternative pharmacologic treatments are combined with CBT. In sum, the modest effects of SSRI monotherapy provide encouragement for continued use in the management of some cases of OCD, but evaluation of alternate pharmacologic treatments is certainly warranted.

The Interaction between CBT and Pharmacotherapy

The assumption underlying the use of combined treatment is that the benefits of CBT and SSRI monotherapies should be additive, that is, combining SSRIs with CBT should produce a greater treatment effect than either modality alone (Pontoski & Heimberg, 2010). Although equivocal findings in pediatric OCD may be a function of the limited research, studies across a range of anxiety disorders have also found that augmenting CBT with pharmacotherapy produces inconsistent results, and an overall modest benefit at best compared to CBT monotherapy (Graham, Callaghan, & Richardson, 2014; Otto et al., 2010). This does not mean that there is no potential benefit to pharmacologic augmentation; instead, there is a growing recognition that pharmacologic agents may in fact interact with CBT (Graham et al., 2014). This means that augmenting CBT with SSRIs may lead to improved outcomes for some, no additional benefit for others, and potentially, to poorer response in some.

Uncertainty as to the mechanisms of treatment effects has prompted a return to basic science, such as exploring the neural mechanisms of disorder processes and of treatment response (Rief et al., 2016). Such studies have provided some insights into the relationship between CBT and SSRIs, suggesting that the range of effects of SSRIs on the brain may enhance some neural processes important for CBT, while suppressing others (Graham et al., 2014). For example, pharmacologic agents like SSRIs may interfere with the processes of fear extinction by suppressing cortisol (Otto et al., 2010). In effect, the use of SSRIs during CBT has the potential to reduce the effectiveness of the CBT itself if certain core processes are disrupted. Importantly, the interaction between pharmacology and CBT may also vary as a function of the sequencing of the therapies, and of individual attributions for success (Pontoski & Heimberg, 2010). It is also possible that relapse or return of fear after treatment may be affected by interactions between SSRI and CBT (Otto et al., 2010).

Given that SSRI augmentation of CBT is often recommended for pediatric OCD (Geller, March, & AACAP Committee on Quality Issues, 2012) and that many youth with OCD are already taking SSRIs by the time they begin CBT (Storch et al., 2016), it is crucial to better understand the interactions between treatments. It appears likely that SSRI augmentation is only of benefit to some individuals; thus, it must be a research priority to understand when such treatments are of benefit, and how best to combine treatments to maximize outcomes. Although research investigating potential interactions between CBT and pharmacologic agents is in the early stages, recent findings reflect an increasingly sophisticated understanding of the neural mechanisms of effect for both treatments. Such research has also led to alternative augmentation strategies with novel pharmacologic agents.

Novel Augmentation Strategies

The equivocal outcomes of traditional pharmacologic augmentation of CBT may be related, in part, to the varied effects of such medications on the brain. Thus, novel augmentation strategies have been developed that use cognitive enhancers; pharmacologic agents that enhance specific cognitive processes important to CBT, instead of reducing OCD symptoms directly (Singewald et al., 2015). In particular, there is great interest in enhancing the outcomes of extinction learning processes that underlie exposure therapy by boosting emotional learning and the consolidation of such learning (McGuire, Lewin, & Storch, 2014). This is a prime example of translational research, where findings from animal models of fear extinction have guided the identification of novel pharmacologic agents with potential clinical applications (Davis et al., 2006). For a comprehensive overview of how pharmacotherapy can target the neural processes of fear extinction, see Singewald et al. (2015). Potential cognitive enhancers include DCS, brain-derived neurotrophic factor, glucocorticoids and cortisol, yohimbine hydrochloride, among many others.

Illustration of a Novel Augmentation of CBT: DCS

DCS as a Cognitive Enhancer

DCS is the most thoroughly investigated cognitive enhancer to date, as it has been used for many years as an antibiotic treatment for tuberculosis, and as such, there is ample data to support its safety (Sulkowski et al., 2014). Furthermore, given that DCS is inexpensive to administer and is associated with few side effects, it constitutes a good target for cognitive enhancement research that may be particularly acceptable both to families and clinicians.

DCS is a partial agonist of the glycine binding site of the N-methyl-D-aspartate (NMDA) glutamate receptor, which is involved in fear extinction (McGuire et al., 2014). Rodent studies indicated that when administered close to the time of extinction learning (the laboratory analogue of exposure therapy), DCS facilitated the extinction of fear, increased the generalization of extinction, and reduced the reinstatement of learned fear that can occur following extinction (Davis et al., 2006). Thus, DCS may produce faster extinction learning, which may generalize more easily to other contexts, and may help to protect against relapse of fear.

Early clinical trials using DCS to augment CBT for anxiety disorders in adults reported moderate effect sizes in favor of DCS over placebo (Norberg, Krystal, & Tolin, 2008). This led to strong interest in the use of DCS as a cognitive enhancer across a range of disorders in adults, including OCD, specific phobias, social anxiety disorder, panic disorder, post-traumatic stress disorder, substance use disorders, and eating disorders (Otto et al., 2016). However, due to the potential for developmental differences in the neural mechanisms of fear learning (Kim & Richardson, 2010), pediatric outcomes must be examined directly, rather than relying on adult research.

Efficacy of DCS for Pediatric OCD

To date, four studies have examined DCS augmentation of CBT relative to placebo in pediatric OCD. The first two studies showed some promise for the use of DCS. Storch et al. (2010) administered DCS or placebo to 30 youth immediately prior to seven out of ten CBT sessions, and found a moderate but nonsignificant effect of DCS ($d = .31–.47$). Farrell et al. (2013) gave DCS or placebo to 17 youth one hour before five of nine CBT sessions, and found a significant interaction effect of DCS over placebo, from the posttreatment to the one-month follow-up assessment, whereby youth who received DCS evidenced greater improvements. In contrast, two recent studies do not support added benefits of DCS. Mataix-Cols et al. (2014) administered DCS or placebo to 27 youth with OCD immediately after each of 10 CBT sessions, and found no advantage of DCS at any time point. The authors noted that administering DCS after the exposure session could have clinical benefit in cases where the exposure tasks were not successful, and animal research supported the efficacy of post-exposure DCS administration. However, as the authors did not compare pre- and post-session administration of DCS, it is not possible to determine whether the timing of the dose influenced the results. The largest study to date was conducted by Storch et al. (2016), who administered DCS or placebo to 142 youth with OCD one hour before seven of 10 CBT sessions. This study found no overall benefit of DCS over placebo, although the researchers noted that the high efficacy of CBT may have led to ceiling effects for the DCS intervention. The cumulative findings of these four studies are consistent with the wider DCS research, whereby early research indicated significant benefits of DCS (Norberg et al., 2008); however, more recent studies, some with much larger samples, have found no overall effect (Ori et al., 2015).

Several recent meta-analyses have been conducted to synthesize these inconsistent findings across child and adult research. Mataix-Cols et al. (2017) conducted an individual participant data meta-analysis of DCS augmentation of exposure-based CBT in OCD, anxiety, and post-traumatic stress disorder. They found that DCS yielded a small significant effect at posttreatment, but not at follow-up. In contrast, a meta-analysis of OCD studies by Gu et al. (2017) found no overall effect of DCS on OCD severity at posttreatment, but suggested that study design differences like timing, dose, and number of sessions may influence study findings. Bürkner et al. (2017) conducted a meta-analysis of DCS augmentation of behavior therapy for OCD and anxiety, and found a very small effect of DCS. Although results of individual studies and meta-analyses remain mixed, this does not indicate that DCS has no place as an augmentation of CBT. Rather, these studies highlight the need to understand the underlying mechanisms of cognitive enhancers, identify moderators of outcome to allow treatment personalization, and extend research into the cognitive enhancement of CBT.

Lessons from DCS Research

DCS outcome studies indicate that dose timing may be particularly important when using a cognitive enhancer. This is because DCS is used acutely in order to consolidate learning around the time of exposure. It is usually administered 1 to 2 hours prior to exposure in order to reach peak blood levels during and immediately after the exposure task (Hofmann et al., 2015). Mataix-Cols et al. (2014) proposed that post-session administration of DCS should be clinically effective, but this has yet to be conclusively demonstrated in human subjects. Thus, it appears that doses delivered after exposure may lead to suboptimal concentrations of DCS available to augment the exposure session. The importance of dose timing is in contrast to SSRIs, which are used for their chronic effects over a much longer time.

Another important consideration is how often to use cognitive enhancers. Unlike SSRIs, which are used chronically for months or years and take many weeks to produce clinical effects, DCS has very acute effects and rapidly loses efficacy with increased dosing, possibly due to desensitization of targeted receptors (Singewald et al., 2015). Thus, DCS is only suitable for short-term use, and the number of sessions using DCS should be carefully planned, and exposure optimized in the augmented sessions.

Findings from DCS studies have suggested that the effect of cognitive enhancers may vary according to the characteristics of the exposure tasks. Specifically, a study of adults with height phobia found that DCS only provided a benefit when "good" exposure occurred, that is, when fear substantially reduced at the end of an exposure session (Smits et al., 2013). Conversely, when exposure was less successful, DCS may actually enhance the original fear memory (Hofmann et al., 2015). Thus, DCS may promote any emotional learning that occurs during exposure therapy, making good exposure better, and bad exposure worse. The clinical implication is that cognitive enhancers should only be used when exposure tasks are highly likely to lead to successful reduction of fear. However, despite the suggestion of specificity of DCS enhancement in adult studies, a study of 50 youth with anxiety disorders found no evidence that outcomes of DCS augmentation were associated either with the strength of child-reported fear reduction following exposure, with differences in child-reported experienced versus anticipatory anxiety, or with clinician evaluation of exposure success (Rapee et al., 2016). Thus, further research is required to evaluate the relationship between exposure quality and the effects of cognitive enhancers.

Another finding from DCS research is that cognitive enhancers may be ineffective unless there is a strong emotional response to the exposure task (Otto et al., 2016). The use of cognitive enhancers may thus be indicated only for high steps on a fear hierarchy, or for intensive treatment sessions. This finding is also interesting in light of the suggestion that SSRI use may interfere with the augmentation effects of DCS during exposure (Andersson et al., 2015). Although this finding was not replicated in the largest trial of DCS for pediatric OCD (Storch et al., 2016), it indicates the need to consider interactions between multiple pharmacologic agents in order to understand the complex interplay between CBT, neuronal systems, and pharmacologic agents.

Overall, research studies indicate that DCS does not provide consistent benefits to CBT when CBT is already highly efficacious. However, it has been proposed that DCS may speed the response to exposure, such that fewer sessions may be required (Chasson et al., 2010). Given the limited availability of highly trained CBT therapists, an intervention that reduces the amount of in-session exposure needed for successful CBT may reduce the time taken to treat clients and potentially reduce the cost of CBT. Further, experiencing successful exposure earlier in treatment may help to encourage further exposure tasks, and potentially even reduce dropout. However, pediatric trials that examined mid-treatment effects of DCS relative to placebo did not find support for earlier therapeutic benefits associated with DCS (Mataix-Cols et al., 2014; Storch et al., 2016). Alternately, it has been proposed that DCS may be used to "rescue"' treatment in those who are not responding to CBT at the expected rate (Otto et al., 2016). In their DCS study, Farrell et al. (2013) specifically recruited young people who had failed to respond to a previous course of CBT, and reported a significant advantage of DCS over placebo at the one-month follow-up. Thus, it may be that DCS is not needed when exposure sessions are highly effective but may be of benefit when an individual fails to respond fully to CBT.

Summary of DCS Findings

Although the evidence for the use of DCS is mixed, research on cognitive enhancers represents an impressive advance in the use of translational neuroscience to guide clinical practice. Use of short-term cognitive enhancers may provide a method of CBT augmentation that is safe, efficient, and therefore more acceptable to families than chronic SSRI use. Further research on DCS and other cognitive enhancers is needed to determine efficacy, moderators of outcome, clinical utility, and the long-term impact of their use.

Challenges and Recommendations for Future Research

Currently, research on the pharmacologic augmentation of CBT for pediatric OCD is relatively limited in comparison to that of psychosocial interventions. Traditional augmentation strategies, where CBT is augmented with SSRIs, have yielded inconsistent and often underwhelming results (Ivarsson et al., 2015). Research on the neural mechanisms of CBT and SSRIs has led to a better understanding of each process, and of the potential interactions between multiple treatments. Although the use of cognitive enhancers has been described as one of the most exciting developments in treatment research in recent years (Rapee et al., 2016), DCS has not demonstrated consistent advantages in pediatric OCD studies of varying designs (Mataix-Cols et al., 2014; Storch et al., 2016). However, it should be noted that research into all types of pharmacologic augmentation of CBT is in its early stages, and as such, there is much to learn about how these treatments work, both individually and in combination.

Moreover, much of the recent research on the neural processes of CBT has come from adult samples. However, animal research indicates substantial developmental differences in the neural underpinnings of fear and fear extinction (Kim & Richardson, 2010); therefore, it is essential to evaluate such processes directly in children and adolescents. Unfortunately, there is little research on new pharmacologic agents for pediatric mental health disorders, possibly in part due to additional challenges in drug testing in this age group, including sensitivity to side effects, potential for developmental differences across pediatric samples, and enhanced placebo response obscuring medication outcomes (Grabb & Gobburu, 2016). Future directions for pharmacologic augmentation of CBT for pediatric OCD are thus likely to involve refinement in our use of existing pharmacologic agents, and their integration with CBT.

It is clear that it is not sufficient to combine our best monotherapies and expect to see additive benefits for all individuals. Instead, there is an increasing focus on understanding individual differences in response to both CBT and SSRI treatments, alone and in combination (Graham et al., 2014). Given that a large number of youth receive SSRIs prior to beginning CBT, it is also important to know whether this may actually interfere with CBT outcomes (Otto et al., 2010), and if so, how this can be overcome. The ongoing identification of predictors and moderators of treatment response is crucial, especially when deciding whether pharmacologic augmentation of CBT is required. Such predictors may include aspects of OCD or comorbid disorder presentation, family-level variables, or biological markers. Future research into pediatric OCD interventions should also consider enhancing nonspecific mechanisms of improvement such as positive treatment expectancies, addressing difficulties in past treatment, enriching the social environment, and increasing levels of physical activity (Rief et al., 2016). The identification of valid predictors of treatment outcome will have great utility in assisting clinicians to select the most appropriate treatment for each individual.

Key Practice Points

Although CBT and SSRIs are both efficacious when used as monotherapies, there is limited research to guide when and how to augment CBT with pharmacologic agents. Currently, the only recommended first-line medication for pediatric OCD is SSRIs (Geller, March, & AACAP Committee on Quality Issues, 2012). The limited number of studies that have combined CBT with SSRIs have reported inconsistent findings, and a meta-analysis concluded that combined treatment was more efficacious than SSRIs alone, but not different to CBT alone (Ivarsson et al., 2015).

However, these studies did not specifically test the AACAP recommendations for the use of combined therapy, namely, that it be used in preference to CBT monotherapy when OCD is moderate to severe, or where CBT engagement may be compromised by comorbid disorders like depression or externalizing disorders, family dysfunction, or other factors (Geller, March, & AACAP Committee on Quality Issues, 2012). Therefore, decisions about when to augment CBT with SSRIs are still primarily guided by a child's initial treatment response, clinical expertise and family preferences.

When augmenting CBT with SSRIs, it is important to conduct an adequate medication trial, typically lasting for at least 10 weeks, with close monitoring of symptomatic change and side effects (Geller, March, & AACAP Committee on Quality Issues, 2012). It is particularly important to monitor for the emergence of activation syndrome and suicidality, as such symptoms can be highly distressing and also interfere with CBT outcome (Reid et al., 2015). There is limited information to guide the optimum sequencing when combining medication and CBT; however, as SSRIs can take several weeks to produce symptomatic change, the best results may be observed when an adequate SSRI trial is delivered prior to beginning CBT (Storch et al., 2013), although it is unclear for whom this approach is most effective.

Although there are few studies of combined treatment outcomes in pediatric OCD, research across a number of anxiety disorders has revealed that the augmentation of CBT with SSRIs does not simply lead to additive benefits (Otto et al., 2010). Instead, these treatments appear to interact with each other, producing benefits for some, but not for others. Such issues are compounded in pediatric research, as there may be developmental differences in the neural systems underpinning OCD, in medication response, and in the effects of chronic medication use (Grabb & Gobburu, 2016; Kim & Richardson, 2010). As the augmentation of CBT with SSRIs is a part of standard clinical practice (Geller, March, & AACAP Committee on Quality Issues, 2012), it is vital to evaluate recommendations for when and how to augment CBT with pharmacotherapy, and determine who is most likely to benefit from such approaches.

Research on cognitive enhancers represents an exciting new wave of pharmacologic augmentation research informed by translational neuroscience, particularly from animal models of fear extinction (Davis et al., 2006). Despite promising results from early studies, recent studies of the efficacy of DCS have revealed inconsistent findings (Ori et al., 2015). Importantly, preliminary research suggests that DCS may enhance both positive and negative emotional learning experiences, and therefore, more research is needed to inform how best to use DCS for maximum benefit. At present, there is insufficient evidence to recommend the use of DCS or other cognitive enhancers as part of routine clinical practice. However, research indicates the potential utility of cognitive enhancers in the selective enhancement of CBT.

Although the pharmacologic augmentation of CBT for pediatric OCD is a common sense strategy based on combining two existing efficacious treatments, research has revealed that these treatments may interact in nuanced ways that we are only beginning to appreciate. There is increasing interest in understanding the neural processes of these treatments, and in predicting who will benefit from augmented CBT. Ideally, such research will lead to the personalization of interventions based on valid markers of treatment response, which could include aspects of the disorder presentation, biological characteristics, demographic features, and environmental factors. However, until further treatment outcome research is available, decisions regarding the pharmacologic augmentation of CBT must be guided by existing recommendations (Geller, March, & AACAP Committee on Quality Issues, 2012), family preferences for treatment, and expert clinical judgment.

References

Andersson, E., Hedman, E., Enander, J. M., Radu Djurfeldt, D., Ljotsson, B., Cervenka, S., ... Ruck, C. (2015). D-cycloserine vs placebo as adjunct to cognitive behavioral therapy for obsessive-compulsive disorder and interaction with antidepressants: A randomized clinical trial. *JAMA Psychiatry, 72*(7), 659–667. doi:10.1001/jamapsychiatry.2015.0546

Bloch, M. H., & Storch, E. A. (2015). Assessment and management of treatment-refractory obsessive-compulsive disorder in children. *Journal of the American Academy of Child and Adolescent Psychiatry, 54*(4), 251–262. doi:10.1016/j.jaac.2015.01.011

Bürkner, P.-C., Bittner, N., Holling, H., & Buhlmann, U. (2017). D-cycloserine augmentation of behavior therapy for anxiety and obsessive-compulsive disorders: A meta-analysis. *PloS One, 12*(3), e0173660. doi:10.1371/journal.pone.0173660

Bussing, R., Reid, A. M., McNamara, J. P. H., Meyer, J. M., Guzick, A. G., Mason, D. M., ... Murphy, T. K. (2015). A pilot study of actigraphy as an objective measure of SSRI activation symptoms: Results from a randomized placebo controlled psychopharmacological treatment study. *Psychiatry Research, 225*(3), 440–445. doi:10.1016/j.psychres.2014.11.070

Caporino, N. E., & Storch, E. A. (2016). Personalizing the treatment of pediatric obsessive-compulsive disorder: Evidence for predictors and moderators of treatment outcomes. *Current Behavioral Neuroscience Reports, 3*(1), 73–85. doi:10.1007/s40473-016-0066-5

Chasson, G. S., Buhlmann, U., Tolin, D. F., Rao, S. R., Reese, H. E., Rowley, T., ... Wilhelm, S. (2010). Need for speed: Evaluating slopes of OCD recovery in behavior therapy enhanced with d-cycloserine. *Behaviour Research and Therapy, 48*(7), 675–679. doi:10.1016/j.brat.2010.03.007

Davis, M., Ressler, K., Rothbaum, B. O., & Richardson, R. (2006). Effects of D-Cycloserine on extinction: Translation from preclinical to clinical work. *Biological Psychiatry, 60*(4), 369–375. doi:10.1016/j.biopsych.2006.03.084

Dold, M., Aigner, M., Lanzenberger, R., & Kasper, S. (2013). Antipsychotic augmentation of serotonin reuptake inhibitors in treatment-resistant obsessive-compulsive disorder: A meta-analysis of double-blind, randomized, placebo-controlled trials. *International Journal of Neuropsychopharmacology, 16*(3), 557–574. doi:10.1017/s1461145712000740

Farrell, L. J., Waters, A. M., Boschen, M. J., Hattingh, L., McConnell, H., Milliner, E. L., ... Storch, E. A. (2013). Difficult-to-treat pediatric obsessive-compulsive disorder: Feasibility and preliminary results of a randomized pilot trial of d-cycloserine-augmented behavior therapy. *Depression and Anxiety, 30*(8), 723–731. doi:10.1002/da.22132

Franklin, M. E., Kratz, H. E., Freeman, J. B., Ivarsson, T., Heyman, I., Sookman, D., ... March, J. (2015). Cognitive-behavioral therapy for pediatric obsessive-compulsive disorder: Empirical review and clinical recommendations. *Psychiatry Research*, *227*(1), 78–92. doi:10.1016/j.psychres.2015.02.009

Franklin, M. E., Sapyta, J., Freeman, J. B., Khanna, M., Compton, S., Almirall, D., ... March, J. S. (2011). Cognitive-behavior therapy augmentation of pharmacotherapy in pediatric obsessive compulsive disorder: The pediatric OCD treatment study II (POTS II) randomized, controlled trial. *JAMA*, *306*(11), 1224–1232. doi:10.1001/jama.2011.1344

Garcia, A. M., Sapyta, J. J., Moore, P. S., Freeman, J. B., Franklin, M. E., March, J. S., & Foa, E. B. (2010). Predictors and moderators of treatment outcome in the pediatric obsessive compulsive treatment study (POTS I). *Journal of the American Academy of Child and Adolescent Psychiatry*, *49*(10), 1024–1033. doi:10.1016/j.jaac.2010.06.013

Geller, D. A., March, J., & AACAP Committee on Quality Issues. (2012). Practice parameter for the assessment and treatment of children and adolescents with obsessive-compulsive disorder. *Journal of the American Academy of Child and Adolescent Psychiatry*, *51*(1), 98–113. doi:10.1016/j.jaac.2011.09.019

Goodman, W. K., Murphy, T. K., & Storch, E. A. (2007). Risk of adverse behavioral effects with pediatric use of antidepressants. *Psychopharmacology*, *191*(1), 87–96. doi:10.1007/s00213-006-0642-6

Grabb, M. C., & Gobburu, J. V. S. (2017). Challenges in developing drugs for pediatric CNS disorders: A focus on psychopharmacology. *Progress in Neurobiology*, *152*, 38–57. doi:10.1016/j.pneurobio.2016.05.003

Graham, B. M., Callaghan, B. L., & Richardson, R. (2014). Bridging the gap: Lessons we have learnt from the merging of psychology and psychiatry for the optimisation of treatments for emotional disorders. *Behaviour Research and Therapy*, *62*, 3–16. doi:10.1016/j.brat.2014.07.012

Gu, W., Storch, E. A., Zhao, Q., Xu, T., & Wang, Z. (2017). Effects of D-cycloserine augmentation on cognitive behavioral therapy in patients with obsessive-compulsive disorder: A systematic review and meta-analysis. *Journal of Obsessive-Compulsive and Related Disorders*, *13*, 24–29. doi:10.1016/j.jocrd.2017.03.001

Hammad, T. A., Laughren, T., & Racoosin, J. (2006). Suicidality in pediatric patients treated with antidepressant drugs. *Archives of General Psychiatry*, *63*(3), 332–339. doi:10.1001/archpsyc.63.3.332

Hilt, R. J., Chaudhari, M., Bell, J. F., Wolf, C., Koprowicz, K., & King, B. H. (2014). Side effects from use of one or more psychiatric medications in a population-based sample of children and adolescents. *Journal of Child and Adolescent Psychopharmacology*, *24*(2), 83–89. doi:10.1089/cap.2013.0036

Hofmann, S. G., Otto, M. W., Pollack, M. H., & Smits, J. A. (2015). d-Cycloserine augmentation of cognitive behavioral therapy for anxiety disorders: An update. *Current Psychiatry Reports*, *17*(1), 532. doi:10.1007/s11920-014-0532-2

Ivarsson, T., Skarphedinsson, G., Kornør, H., Axelsdottir, B., Biedilæ, S., Heyman, I., ... March, J. (2015). The place of and evidence for serotonin reuptake inhibitors (SRIs) for obsessive compulsive disorder (OCD) in children and adolescents: Views based on a systematic review and meta-analysis. *Psychiatry Research*, *227*(1), 93–103. doi:10.1016/j.psychres.2015.01.015

Kim, J. H., & Richardson, R. (2010). New findings on extinction of conditioned fear early in development: Theoretical and clinical implications. *Biological Psychiatry, 67*(4), 297–303. doi:10.1016/j.biopsych.2009.09.003

Lewin, A. B., McGuire, J. F., Murphy, T. K., & Storch, E. A. (2014). Editorial perspective: The importance of considering parent's preferences when planning treatment for their children – the case of childhood obsessive-compulsive disorder. *Journal of Child Psychology and Psychiatry, 55*(12), 1314–1316. doi:10.1111/jcpp.12344

Lewin, A. B., Peris, T. S., Lindsey Bergman, R., McCracken, J. T., & Piacentini, J. (2011). The role of treatment expectancy in youth receiving exposure-based CBT for obsessive compulsive disorder. *Behaviour Research and Therapy, 49*(9), 536–543. doi:10.1016/j.brat.2011.06.001

Lewin, A. B., Piacentini, J., De Nadai, A. S., Jones, A. M., Peris, T. S., Geffken, G. R., ... Storch, E. A. (2014). Defining clinical severity in pediatric obsessive-compulsive disorder. *Psychological Assessment, 26*(2), 679–684. doi:10.1037/a0035174

March, J. S., Franklin, M. E., Leonard, H., Garcia, A., Moore, P., Freeman, J., & Foa, E. (2007). Tics moderate treatment outcome with sertraline but not cognitive-behavior therapy in pediatric obsessive-compulsive disorder. *Biological Psychiatry, 61*(3), 344–347. doi:10.1016/j.biopsych.2006.09.035

Maron, E., & Nutt, D. (2015). Biological predictors of pharmacological therapy in anxiety disorders. *Dialogues in Clinical Neuroscience, 17*(3), 305–317.

Masi, G., Pfanner, C., Millepiedi, S., & Berloffa, S. (2010). Aripiprazole augmentation in 39 adolescents with medication-resistant obsessive-compulsive disorder. *Journal of Clinical Psychopharmacology, 30*(6), 688–693. doi:10.1097/JCP.0b013e3181fab7b1

Mataix-Cols, D., Fernandez de la Cruz, L., Monzani, B., Rosenfield, D., Andersson, E., Pérez-Vigil, A., ... the DCS Anxiety Consortium. (2017). D-cycloserine augmentation of exposure-based cognitive behavior therapy for anxiety, obsessive-compulsive, and posttraumatic stress disorders: A systematic review and meta-analysis of individual participant data. *JAMA Psychiatry, 74*(5), 501–510. doi:10.1001/jamapsychiatry.2016.3955

Mataix-Cols, D., Turner, C. M., Monzani, B., Isomura, K., Murphy, C., Krebs, G., & Heyman, I. (2014). Cognitive-behavioural therapy with post-session D-cycloserine augmentation for paediatric obsessive-compulsive disorder: Pilot randomised controlled trial. *British Journal of Psychiatry, 204*(1), 77–78. doi:10.1192/bjp.bp.113.126284

McGuire, J. F., Lewin, A. B., & Storch, E. A. (2014). Enhancing exposure therapy for anxiety disorders, obsessive compulsive disorder, and posttraumatic stress disorder. *Expert Review of Neurotherapeutics, 14*(8), 893–910. doi:10.1586/14737175.2014.934677

McGuire, J. F., Piacentini, J., Lewin, A. B., Brennan, E. A., Murphy, T. K., & Storch, E. A. (2015). A meta-analysis of cognitive behavior therapy and medication for child obsessive–compulsive disorder: Moderators of treatment efficacy, response, and remission. *Depression and Anxiety, 32*(8), 580–593. doi:10.1002/da.22389

Neziroglu, F., Yaryura-Tobias, J. A., Walz, J., & McKay, D. (2000). The effect of fluvoxamine and behavior therapy on children and adolescents with obsessive-compulsive disorder. *Journal of Child and Adolescent Psychopharmacology, 10*(4), 295–306. doi:10.1089/cap.2000.10.295

Norberg, M. M., Krystal, J. H., & Tolin, D. F. (2008). A meta-analysis of d-cycloserine and the facilitation of fear extinction and exposure therapy. *Biological Psychiatry, 63*(12), 1118–1126. doi:10.1016/j.biopsych.2008.01.012

O'Neill, J., Piacentini, J., Chang, S., Ly, R., Lai, T. M., Armstrong, C. C., ... Nurmi, E. L. (2017). Glutamate in pediatric obsessive-compulsive disorder and response to cognitive-behavioral therapy: Randomized clinical trial. *Neuropsychopharmacology, 42*, 2414–2422. doi:10.1038/npp.2017.77

Ori, R., Amos, T., Bergman, H., Soares-Weiser, K., Ipser, J. C., & Stein, D. J. (2015). Augmentation of cognitive and behavioural therapies (CBT) with d-cycloserine for anxiety and related disorders. *Cochrane Database of Systematic Reviews* (5), Cd007803. doi:10.1002/14651858.CD007803.pub2

Öst, L.-G., Riise, E. N., Wergeland, G. J., Hansen, B., & Kvale, G. (2016). Cognitive behavioral and pharmacological treatments of OCD in children: A systematic review and meta-analysis. *Journal of Anxiety Disorders, 43*, 58–69. doi:10.1016/j.janxdis.2016.08.003

Otto, M. W., Kredlow, M. A., Smits, J. A. J., Hofmann, S. G., Tolin, D. F., de Kleine, R. A., ... Pollack, M. H. (2016). Enhancement of psychosocial treatment with d-cycloserine: Models, moderators, and future directions. *Biological Psychiatry, 80*(4), 274–283. doi:10.1016/j.biopsych.2015.09.007

Otto, M. W., McHugh, R. K., & Kantak, K. M. (2010). Combined pharmacotherapy and cognitive-behavioral therapy for anxiety disorders: Medication effects, glucocorticoids, and attenuated treatment outcomes. [Clinical psychology : a publication of the Division of Clinical Psychology of the American Psychological Association]. *Clinical Psychology, 17*(2), 91–103. doi:10.1111/j.1468–2850.2010.01198.x

Pittenger, C. (2015a). Glutamate modulators in the treatment of obsessive-compulsive disorder. *Psychiatric Annals, 45*(6), 308–315. doi:10.3928/00485713-20150602-06

Pittenger, C. (2015b). Glutamatergic agents for OCD and related disorders. *Current Treatment Options in Psychiatry, 2*(3), 271–283. doi:10.1007/s40501-015-0051-8

Pontoski, K. E., & Heimberg, R. G. (2010). The myth of the superiority of concurrent combined treatments for anxiety disorders. *Clinical Psychology: Science and Practice, 17*(2), 107–111. doi:10.1111/j.1468–2850.2010.01200.x

Rapee, R. M., Jones, M. P., Hudson, J. L., Mahli, G. S., Lyneham, H. J., & Schneider, S. C. (2016). d-Cycloserine does not enhance the effects of in-vivo exposure among young people with broad-based anxiety disorders. *Behaviour Research and Therapy, 87*, 225–231. doi:10.1016/j.brat.2016.10.004

Reid, A. M., McNamara, J. P. H., Murphy, T. K., Guzick, A. G., Storch, E. A., Geffken, G. R., & Bussing, R. (2015). Side-effects of SSRIs disrupt multimodal treatment for pediatric OCD in a randomized-controlled trial. *Journal of Psychiatric Research, 71*, 140–147. doi:10.1016/j.jpsychires.2015.10.006

Rief, W., Barsky, A. J., Bingel, U., Doering, B. K., Schwarting, R., Wöhr, M., & Schweiger, U. (2016). Rethinking psychopharmacotherapy: The role of treatment context and brain plasticity in antidepressant and antipsychotic interventions. *Neuroscience and Biobehavioral Reviews, 60*, 51–64. doi:10.1016/j.neubiorev.2015.11.008

Scahill, L., Riddle, M. A., McSwiggin-Hardin, M., Ort, S. I., King, R. A., Goodman, W. K., ... Leckman, J. F. (1997). Children's Yale-Brown Obsessive Compulsive Scale: Reliability and validity. *Journal of the American Academy of Child and Adolescent Psychiatry, 36*(6), 844–852. doi:10.1097/00004583-199706000-00023

Simpson, H., Foa, E. B., Liebowitz, M. R., & et al. (2013). Cognitive-behavioral therapy vs risperidone for augmenting serotonin reuptake inhibitors in obsessive-compulsive disorder: A randomized clinical trial. *JAMA Psychiatry, 70*(11), 1190–1199. doi:10.1001/jamapsychiatry.2013.1932

Singewald, N., Schmuckermair, C., Whittle, N., Holmes, A., & Ressler, K. J. (2015). Pharmacology of cognitive enhancers for exposure-based therapy of fear, anxiety and trauma-related disorders. *Pharmacology and Therapeutics, 149*, 150–190. doi:10.1016/j.pharmthera.2014.12.004

Skarphedinsson, G., Weidle, B., Thomsen, P. H., Dahl, K., Torp, N. C., Nissen, J. B.,... Ivarsson, T. (2015). Continued cognitive-behavior therapy versus sertraline for children and adolescents with obsessive–compulsive disorder that were nonresponders to cognitive-behavior therapy: A randomized controlled trial. *European Child and Adolescent Psychiatry, 24*(5), 591–602. doi:10.1007/s00787-014-0613-0

Smits, J. A. J., Rosenfield, D., Otto, M. W., Powers, M. B., Hofmann, S. G., Telch, M. J.,... Tart, C. D. (2013). D-Cycloserine enhancement of fear extinction is specific to successful exposure sessions: Evidence from the treatment of height phobia. *Biological Psychiatry, 73*(11), 1054–1058. doi:10.1016/j.biopsych.2012.12.009

Stewart, S. E., & Stachon, A. C. (2014). Pharmacotherapy for obsessive-compulsive and related disorders among children and adolescents. In E. A. Storch & D. E. McKay (eds.), *Obsessive-compulsive disorder and its spectrum: A life-span approach* (pp. 293–316). Washington, DC: American Psychological Association.

Storch, E. A., Bussing, R., Small, B. J., Geffken, G. R., McNamara, J. P., Rahman, O.,... Murphy, T. K. (2013). Randomized, placebo-controlled trial of cognitive-behavioral therapy alone or combined with sertraline in the treatment of pediatric obsessive–compulsive disorder. *Behaviour Research and Therapy, 51*(12), 823–829. doi:10.1016/j.brat.2013.09.007

Storch, E. A., McKay, D., Reid, J., Geller, D., Goodman, W., Lewin, A., & Murphy, T. (2010). D-Cycloserine augmentation of cognitive-behavioral therapy: Directions for pilot research in pediatric obsessive-compulsive disorder. *Child and Youth Care Forum, 39*(2), 101–112. doi:10.1007/s10566-010-9094-6

Storch, E. A., Wilhelm, S., Sprich, S., Henin, A., Micco, J., Small, B. J.,... Geller, D. A. (2016). Efficacy of augmentation of cognitive behavior therapy with weight-adjusted d-cycloserine vs placebo in pediatric obsessive-compulsive disorder: A randomized clinical trial. *JAMA Psychiatry, 73*(8), 779–788. doi:10.1001/jamapsychiatry.2016.1128

Sulkowski, M. L., Geller, D. A., Lewin, A. B., Murphy, T. K., Mittelman, A., Brown, A., & Storch, E. A. (2014). The future of D-Cycloserine and other cognitive modifiers in obsessive-compulsive and related disorders. *Current Psychiatry Reviews, 10*(4), 317–324. doi:10.2174/1573400510666140619224942

The Pediatric OCD Treatment Study (POTS) Team. (2004). Cognitive-behavior therapy, sertraline, and their combination for children and adolescents with obsessive-compulsive disorder: The pediatric OCD treatment study (POTS) randomized controlled trial. *JAMA, 292*(16), 1969–1976. doi:10.1001/jama.292.16.1969

Thomsen, P. H. (2004). Risperidone augmentation in the treatment of severe adolescent OCD in SSRI-refractory cases: A case-series. *Annals of Clinical Psychiatry, 16*(4), 201–207. doi:10.3109/10401230490522016

Varigonda, A. L., Jakubovski, E., & Bloch, M. H. (2016). Systematic review and meta-analysis: Early treatment responses of selective serotonin reuptake inhibitors and clomipramine in pediatric obsessive-compulsive disorder. *Journal of the American Academy of Child and Adolescent Psychiatry, 55*(10), 851–859. doi:10.1016/j.jaac.2016.07.768

20 Enhanced Family Approaches in Childhood OCD

Jeffrey J. Sapyta and Colleen M. Cowperthwait

Introduction

Obsessive-compulsive disorder (OCD) is a serious psychological condition, with childhood prevalence estimated to be between 1 percent and 3 percent (Rapoport et al., 2000). The debilitating nature of obsessions and compulsions for children and their families often results in significant disruption of normal development and across all functional domains (Piacentini et al., 2003).

For the past 20 years, there have been tremendous advances in the treatment of pediatric OCD, and CBT with an emphasis on exposure and response prevention has been demonstrated to be the monotherapy of choice (Storch, Mariaskin, & Murphy, 2009). During its development, pediatric CBT for OCD has transformed from a primarily individual approach with caregivers coming in for brief check-ins (e.g., March & Mule, 1998) into a treatment involving parents and other caregivers more actively in most sessions (Freeman, Sapyta et al., 2014; Lewin et al., 2014; Piacentini et al., 2011). These various approaches have independently increased family involvement in reducing accommodation, enhancing family communication, and improving emotional regulation skills for all family members. Reviews of protocols that include family-based CBT elements for pediatric OCD indicate that treatment effects are large, as well as indicate that protocols that target family accommodation directly have a significantly positive impact on child functioning (Anderson et al., 2015; Thompson-Hollands et al., 2014).

In this chapter, we provide evidence and clinical guidelines for improving outcomes for pediatric OCD by implementing CBT including both exposure and response prevention (ERP) and extensive family elements. To justify these recommendations, we will first review the pediatric OCD treatment literature and how the addition of family elements can significantly improve outcomes. We will also review factors that can mediate or moderate treatment outcomes in pediatric OCD treatment. Finally, we will provide a case example illustrating the application of these approaches in families and provide recommendations regarding treatment structure and various models of family-based CBT for youth with OCD.

Family Context Crucial for Understanding and Addressing OCD

The impact of family members on the maintenance of OCD across the lifespan is well known (Abramowtiz et al., 2013; Farrell & Barrett, 2007). OCD symptoms in youth OCD often elicit the direct involvement of caregivers and other loved ones (Peris et al., 2008; Storch, Geffken, Merlo, Jacob, et al., 2007), ranging from direct participation in rituals to criticism of the youth engaging in rituals (Przeworski et al., 2012). Several family-related components have been identified as key targets of any family-based intervention.

Family Accommodation. One of the most studied family factors relevant to OCD is family accommodation. Family accommodation are all actions taken by family members to reduce the expression of youth OCD symptoms. This often is manifested as either yielding family priorities to achieve successful avoidance of OCD-related triggers or facilitating the completion of compulsions if a child is already upset (Storch, Geffken, Merlo, Jacob, et al., 2007; Peris et al., 2008). Family accommodation is powerfully ubiquitous in families with OCD, with some studies reporting over 97 percent of reporters acknowledging almost daily accommodation to symptoms (Flessner et al., 2011; Stewart et al., 2008). By the time families seek therapy, accommodation of OCD is often highly ingrained, since it's often the primary way families have been ostensibly keeping OCD-related distress under control. Families reporting higher levels of OCD accommodation before treatment tend to fare worse, even when controlling for baseline severity (Amir, Freshman, & Foa, 2000). Although ostensibly pragmatic and well-intentioned, family accommodation can exacerbate symptoms by reinforcing avoidance and compulsive behavior.

Caregiver Distress. Although family accommodation to OCD is typically viewed as a reaction to the child's distress, there is mounting evidence suggesting that OCD manifestations in children also directly negatively impact other family members. OCD places a strain on families and a burden on individual family members, and is associated with significant anxiety, depression, and distress among close family members of individuals with OCD (Steketee et al., 1998). In an interesting study involving adults, romantic partners of OCD patients demonstrate greater emotional arousal when conversing about their loved ones' OCD symptoms than a comparison group of romantic partners with anorexia nervosa (Fischer et al., 2017). Parents and relatives of individuals with OCD can also show poor coping skills, which exacerbates family stress in the presence of OCD symptoms (Barrett, Shortt, & Healy, 2002; Chambless et al., 2001). Youth with OCD who also have a first-degree relative with OCD (e.g., parent) have a stark attenuation of CBT-treatment response unless augmented with medication (Garcia et al., 2010). Caregivers may harbor untreated OCD themselves, which can attenuate parent treatment engagement without direct attention to the parent's symptoms. Finally, due to the strain that OCD places on families, relatives living with individuals with OCD often have negative feelings about the patients, particularly when relatives believe that patients are able but unwilling to control their behavior (Chambless et al., 2001).

Family Communication Dynamics. Along with the aforementioned family accommodation patterns typically found in homes with an individual with OCD, how family members interact reflexively to any salient distress is also important. *Expressed emotion* (EE) is a concept drawn from research into family factors important in mood and schizophrenia, and it refers to the observed style of behaviors family members exhibit when they respond to an episode of a psychiatric disorder. It has been a useful construct for operationalizing the bidirectional nature of negative affective exchanges between family members when one is feeling acute distress. The EE construct has evolved over time and is primarily defined as behaviors related to excessive *hostile criticism* (blame, explicit hostility toward family member) and emotional *overinvolvement* (overprotectiveness, conspicuous self-sacrifice, exaggerated emotional responses toward the child) that generate parent-child interactions that are both negatively arousing to family members and interfere with engaging in prosocial behavior management strategies (Peris & Miklowitz, 2015).

Conceptualizing maladaptive family dynamics by way of EE is relevant, as maladaptive parent-child interactions can be better described and targeted under this framework. For example, parents of anxious youth tend to display less warmth and are more reactive to their children's distress than parents of non-anxious youth (Hudson, Comer, & Kendall, 2008). Parents of children with OCD have also been shown to display less confidence in their child's abilities, less problem solving and less promotion of independence in a family discussion task relative to mother-child dyads when a child has anxiety, or externalizing problems (Barrett, Shortt, & Healy, 2002). Moreover, parents of anxious children have been observed to intervene sooner and provide more limited opportunities for child-directed control when problem solving (Krohne & Hock, 1991; Chorpita, Brown, & Barlow, 1998). It's important to highlight that parental responses to child distress are very likely shaped over time by bids from the child, especially given the finding that children with OCD often manifest elevated disruptive behaviors and rage that can make tolerating the child's distress even more difficult (Lebowitz, Omer, & Leckman, 2011). Identifying and mapping these relevant communications and rearing behaviors is crucial, in order to help the family with behavioral alternatives that facilitate reducing distress more effectively and promote greater independent coping with the child.

Common Elements of Family-Based CBT for Pediatric OCD

Given the role of family behaviors in maintaining or worsening OCD symptoms and the deleterious impact of OCD on family functioning, families should be actively involved in the treatment of OCD in youth (Anderson et al., 2015). Including relevant caregivers in treatment for youth with OCD is important because of the family's role in the maintenance of symptoms and direct impact they can provide to shape future behavior that's more consistent with goals and values for both the youth with OCD and the family (Lebowitz, 2013; Merlo et al., 2010; Twohig et al., 2015). Family-based approaches tend to converge on several common treatment modules. These include provision of psychoeducation to child and relevant family members, standard exposure and response prevention tasks, orientation to parenting skills (e.g., tolerance of personal distress, differential attention, modeling, scaffolding child's autonomy when they engage in skills), problem solving, addressing problematic family processes (e.g., family accommodation, expressed emotion), and relapse prevention.

Functional Assessment. Across formats of treatment for youth with OCD, the first step in implementing family approaches is a careful assessment of family functioning and parental coping skills, in addition to OCD symptoms and youth coping skills (Peris & Miklowitz, 2015). This should include a functional assessment of the behavioral patterns that contribute to the maintenance of problematic behaviors and OCD symptoms, considering all factors within the patient, relevant caregivers, and interpersonally between family members (Marien et al., 2009). Such an assessment models a non-blaming stance, externalizes OCD-related communication patterns from ego-syntonic family activities, helps develop a synthesized view of adaptive and maladaptive family behavioral patterns, and identifies the transactional nature of family interactions and youth OCD symptoms (Steketee et al., 1998).

Determining Family-Based Format. Assessment of family members' responses to OCD symptoms, in addition to youth OCD symptoms, helps determine psychoeducational content for family members and the extent to which family members should participate in ERP sessions, and scaffold homework assignments. The amount of parent involvement is flexible, and is titrated based on both clinical and developmental considerations (Renshaw, Steketee, & Chambless, 2005; Thompson-Hollands et al., 2014). A rule-of-thumb we have used in our clinic for parent involvement is the following: for a typical 10-year-old, the ratio involvement of caregivers to identified patient in session time will be about 50/50 and will vary more or less from that age (e.g., parent involvement increases as child age decreases from 10). Although parent involvement in ERP-driven child sessions will typically wane as a child gets older, parents of older adolescents could be involved extensively if their compulsions demand routine caregiver involvement or they are not functioning significantly in age appropriate activities (e.g., going to school regularly). For many families, CBT sessions can proceed with each session being divided between time for the family, parent-, and child-only portions. Others may proceed with separate child- and parent-only sessions each week.

Based on functional assessment, targets in the psychoeducation phase of treatment could include providing a neurobiological framework to explain youth's behavior and symptoms of OCD, increasing understanding of the transactional nature of family interactions and behavioral responses that reinforce or accommodate OCD, and family vulnerabilities and impact of family stress on individuals and family functioning (Peris & Miklowitz, 2015; Steketee et al., 1998).

Addressing Family Accommodation. Based on the functional assessment of adaptive and maladaptive family behavioral patterns in response to OCD, targets in the behavioral phase of treatment include specifically targeting family accommodation of OCD. The functional assessment should flesh out both the child's and parent's experience of distress in episodes where accommodation occurred. Family members can vary dramatically in how and why they engage in family accommodation. For example, some have acknowledged that they are intervening due to the difficulty of seeing their child struggle. Yet, others can report they feel more connected to their child when they are patiently explaining why they don't need to fear their obsessions, especially if it's on a topic whereby they are particularly passionate or knowledgeable (e.g., related to their faith or vocation). The therapist should be careful about understanding the relationship between accommodation and the parent's values, before establishing a strong stance on reducing or eliminating behaviors that may be reinforcing OCD.

Regardless of the various approach and avoidance factors for each family member, the clinician then aims to reconcile each family member's impact on accommodation pattern to the inevitable reinforcement of OCD. Now with the knowledge of the underlying factors informing the accommodation patterns of the family, the therapist can provide effective alternatives the parents can use that can truly help their child feel better while communicating in a way that promotes child autonomy. Some of these effective alternatives include; in the moment differential attention (e.g., positive attention for adaptive coping behaviors, planned ignoring for reassurance seeking), and scaffolding help in a fashion that encourages the child to increase use of individual coping tools while parents scale back efforts to intervene inappropriately. Consistent with the promotion of child autonomy, the child should be involved in choosing how to gradually reduce accommodation patterns. For example, children can be involved in generating alternative ways family members can interact with OCD more flexibly in specific contexts. Children could also collaborate with caregivers about an "accommodation budget," where parents agree to engage in reassurance for a finite amount of times daily – perhaps linking bonus rewards/points if a child does not use all of her budgeted bids for accommodation.

Modeling Emotion Regulation and Distress Tolerance. Given the relationship between poor coping skills among family members of individuals with OCD, family approaches to treating OCD in youth should include training in emotion regulation and distress tolerance for all relevant family members (Barrett, Healy-Farrell, & March, 2004; Chambless et al., 2001; Choate-Summers et al., 2008; Freeman et al., 2003; Lebowitz, 2013; Peris & Piacentini, 2013). To this end, contemporary family-based treatment for OCD includes parent training in positive coping, including adaptive problem solving (Barrett et al., 2004; Choate-Summers et al., 2008). Due to the reactivity of youth with OCD, parents will be more effective in delivering prompts and corrections neutrally if they are prepared to proactively anticipate negative affect from the child and tolerate the distress it will elicit (Peris & Milklowitz, 2015). Family-based treatments might also include emotion regulation training for parents, specifically emotion labeling and monitoring, training in sleep hygiene and relaxation, mindfulness meditation, and self-soothe strategies (Stewart et al., 2017). These interventions are helpful in order to decrease parents' own stress and model effective coping to their children, as well as provide parents tools with which to tolerate their own distress associated with watching youth in distress without accommodating OCD (Lebowitz, 2013; Peris & Miklowitz, 2015; Peris & Piacentini, 2013). Parents will also be able to model to the child how to address personal distress in a proactive, independent fashion.

Improving Effective Critical Communication. Although high EE is generally associated with poorer treatment outcomes among adults with OCD, family-member *nonhostile* criticism, for example, family members expressing dissatisfaction with specific OCD behavior without expressing personal rejection, is actually associated with *improved* patient outcomes in treatment (Chambless & Steketee, 1999). Given these findings, enhanced family-based treatment for OCD might include teaching effective communication and conflict resolution strategies, with the goal to reduce hostility and increase positive feedback and support (Freeman et al., 2003; Steketee et al., 1998). A key goal is to provide parents tools to express concerns that are more effective, tolerable to themselves, and less stressful for the child to experience. Examples of communication interventions include providing written communication to youth with OCD in order to reduce the likelihood of arguments, increasing warmth, mixing criticism with praise, delivering critical feedback in specific and constructive ways, expressing hope and optimism toward the youth, providing encouragement to completion of tasks, and modeling brainstorming and positive problem solving (Anderson et al., 2015; Kircanski & Peris, 2015; Lebowitz, 2013; Peris & Miklowitz, 2015; Piacentini et al., 2011; Schlup, Farrell, & Barrett, 2011).

Improving Family Reinforcements. In addition to reducing conflict-laden communication, family members may be taught to serve as cheerleaders and skills coaches for youth with OCD (Choate-Summers et al., 2008; Comer et al., 2014; Lenhard et al., 2014; Lewin et al., 2014; Renshaw et al., 2005). Employing parents to help youth understand treatment, provide effective reward programs to increase motivation to complete exposure assignments and carry out home practice tasks, and review coping strategies enhances generalization of skills and learning (Benito et al., 2012; Choate-Summers et al., 2008; Marien et al., 2009; Storch et al., 2011; Thompson-Hollands et al., 2014).

As treatment progresses and symptoms/functioning begin to change, the therapist should routinely check-in about the families' impressions of improvement, agreement on treatment tasks/goals, and ongoing motivation to change. Particularly in families where the child is responding to ERP elements well, families may wish to focus on further improving family communication and reinforcements on topics not related to OCD. Naturally, practicing family-based skills on other sources of distress can improve rapport and overall functioning, as well as facilitate generalization of skills to later OCD targets.

Evidence Base for Family-Based Innovations in OCD

The nature and extent of family involvement in CBT treatment is flexible, and varies widely based on both clinical and developmental considerations (Barrett et al., 2008; Barrett, Healy-Farrell, & March, 2004; Bolton & Perrin, 2008; Bolton et al., 2011; Piacentini et al., 2002). Other formats of treatment for youth with OCD include family therapy (Lewin et al., 2014; Storch, Geffken, Merlo, Mann, et al., 2007), youth-only group (Thienemann et al., 2001), multifamily groups (Martin & Thienemann, 2005), and parent-only therapy (Lebowitz, 2013). Although many of these formats have shown promise and demonstrated positive outcomes, individual (with some family involvement) and family exposure-based therapy for youth with OCD have demonstrated effectiveness across research groups, and, according to expert consensus, are considered "first line" treatments for youth with OCD (Barrett et al., 2008; Freeman, Garcia et al., 2014).

Recent work has reviewed attempts to enhance exposure-based therapy with increased parent involvement and a greater emphasis on family-based elements with promising results. A recent meta-analytic review of family-based interventions for OCD demonstrates large effects (i.e., *Cohen's d* = 1.68), and family interventions in this review that directly target family accommodation were found to be a significant, positive moderator of child functioning despite not finding similar differences in symptom improvement (Reynolds et al., 2013; Thompson-Hollands et al., 2014). Clinic samples with families exhibiting strong expressed emotion and other treatment interfering characteristics (e.g., high conflict, poor cohesion) had a weighted effect size difference of 0.65 favoring a family-based OCD intervention over standard exposure-based therapy (Peris and Piacentini, 2013). Given the nature of the communication dynamics in families with a child with OCD, therapists should devote further focus on effective family communication and reducing accommodation directly among family members.

Despite these promising results, simply including parents in more sessions does not always improve outcomes. A recent randomized control trial not included in the aforementioned meta-analysis tested different formats of a CBT manual focusing on both cognitive techniques as well as exposure and response prevention (Derisley et al., 2008). Families of adolescents were then randomized to either a format that included a parent substantively involved in only 3 sessions versus the parent being involved in all sessions extensively (e.g., helped child complete diaries, support their child in behavior experiments). Despite the significant difference between formats, there were no differences found in symptom reduction at end of treatment or a 6-month follow-up (Reynolds et al., 2013).

Given these discrepant findings, future research should investigate how parents can ideally be involved with their child's treatment to enhance outcomes at different developmental ages. For example, it would be interesting to test whether an increase in parent involvement is most effective in a format emphasizing child-focused tasks (helping a child develop hierarchies, in vivo exposure) or emphasizing parent-focused treatment tasks (parent emotion regulation, communication training, problem solving, personal accommodation to OCD). These findings may be further moderated by a child's age, as it would be expected that a parent's salient involvement in treatment tasks should be reduced as a child reaches mid- to late-adolescence.

Predictors and Moderators of Response in Pediatric OCD

Although the average effect of family-based OCD treatment is robust, a portion of patients either do not respond well or terminate prematurely (Garcia et al., 2010; Olatunji et al., 2013). As a result, there is great interest in understanding factors that may predict treatment response. Although several studies have investigated possible predictors and moderators in pediatric OCD treatment, efficacy trials remain underpowered to adequately address these questions and completely insufficient to determine mediators (Kraemer, Frank, & Kupfer, 2006). Although determining who may benefit from specific treatments is important, it would be wise to consider these findings with caution.

OCD treatment predictors indicate specifically *which* patients are likely to benefit from treatment. These can include both open-label studies and randomized control trials. Predictive factors specific to the patient have been replicated across different research groups (Garcia et al., 2010; Ginsburg et al., 2008; Storch et al., 2008); the most consistent predictors in youth include baseline OCD severity, insight, comorbid externalizing disorder, and OCD-related functional impairment. Specific to family processes, factors such as continued family accommodation, and deleterious family dynamics (high conflict/blame, poor cohesion) have been predictive of attenuated symptom improvement (Garcia et al., 2010; Keeley et al., 2008; Peris & Piacentini, 2013). Studies focusing on adult OCD patients indicate similar findings; family members presenting with high expressed emotion are associated with poor treatment adherence and outcomes and families expressing more warmth and empathy typically have improved outcomes (Chambless & Steketee, 1999).

Pediatric OCD treatment moderators indicate *which patients in a specific treatment* are more likely to benefit from a treatment. Naturally, these require studies with multiple active treatment groups or meta-analyses that can aggregate studies that compare active treatments to a control comparison. Few studies have had the proper design to look adequately at moderators (Garcia et al., 2010; Turner et al., 2018). The only CBT-related moderator identified is highly relevant to the discussion of family-based treatment. The original POTS study, which had much less family-based elements than contemporary treatments, identified that children with a first degree relative with OCD (sibling, parent) had a six-fold decrease in the effect size of CBT monotherapy. This reduction in effect made CBT monotherapy no more beneficial than pill placebo, and the efficacy of CBT when combined with an SRI was significantly attenuated (Garcia et al., 2010). Although it's unknown whether the attenuation of CBT efficacy could be explained by genetic or the direct influence of their first-degree relative, it's likely that engaging with these family members about their own OCD could help better understand the functional underpinnings of the identified patient's symptoms and family accommodation.

Clinical Case Illustration: "Cynthia"

Cynthia is a 16-year-old Latina female with obsessions about being exposed to bedbugs, and compulsions including ritualized bathing, cleaning her clothing and personal items, scanning upholstered furniture before sitting in it, and superstitious checking rituals at bedtime. These symptoms have been present since early adolescence and have been significantly impairing. Cynthia has never attended a sleepover, because she's both concerned about the possibility of encountering bedbugs and embarrassed about performing scanning and rituals in front of her friends. The family plans vacations around avoiding hotels and staying with extended family whose homes Cynthia deems "safe."

She presented to our clinic following an emergency room visit for suicidal communications in the context of OCD symptoms. As the first session began Cynthia was guarded, and parents appeared somewhat righteously indignant, reporting Cynthia needs to "shape up" and "quit causing chaos in the family." In the first session, a functional assessment of the behavioral patterns and family factors that have historically maintained OCD was conducted and prompted a discussion of the suicidal communication that landed Cynthia in the emergency room. Cynthia reported that, late one evening, she experienced highly upsetting obsessive thoughts related to the cleanliness of her recently laundered clothes and the likelihood that her dirty clothes hamper and washer/dryer could be harboring bedbugs. Her father initially empathized with Cynthia's concerns and agreed to take her to the laundromat in the morning. Cynthia repeatedly insisted that her parents take her to the laundromat immediately that night and she became more visibly upset. When her father refused to take her to the laundromat immediately, Cynthia began screaming and crying and accusing her parents of ignoring her feelings. Her mother responded by calling Cynthia "manipulative and abusive." Cynthia became dysphoric and hopeless, and expressed that she wished she were dead.

After completing the behavioral analysis and consulting with Cynthia's psychiatrist, it was decided to proceed with twice weekly family-based CBT: one individual session with Cynthia per week focused primarily on ERP principles and only including parents for brief check-ins, and one family session per week with Cynthia, her mother, and her father focused primarily on family expectations/privileges, family communication training, and some parent-only time for parent management training.

Treatment targets for Cynthia in individual therapy included decreasing frequency and severity of obsessive thoughts and decreasing time spent engaging in ritualized behavior, decreasing suicidal ideation and communications, and increasing her ability to independently self-soothe and problem solve in the context of high intensity emotion. Treatment targets involving the parents in adjunctive family therapy included decreasing child's reliance on parents for urgent participation in compulsions (excessive reassurance, discussing logical alternatives to bedbug infestations, excessive accommodation of cleaning clothes outside of home), increasing parents' modeling of their own use of emotional regulation and behavioral activation skills, appropriately scaffolding to support Cynthia's developing emotion regulation and problem solving skills of her own, and increasing positive communication and pleasant family interactions.

Family-based CBT for Cynthia followed a manualized, family-based treatment of early childhood OCD protocol (e.g., Freeman et al., 2003) adapted and developmentally tailored for adolescence. Psychoeducation about the neurobiological framework of OCD and family patterns that maintain OCD and exacerbate family distress was provided to both Cynthia and her parents. An exposure hierarchy was created with Cynthia individually, and exposure tasks were completed in session with therapist assistance. Her parents were informed about upcoming home exposure tasks and given guidance about appropriate monitoring of home practice and effective cheerleading and reinforcement of Cynthia's home practice with desired increased privileges (e.g., extended curfew with friends, increased time with device on weekends). Family therapy sessions focused on improving family communication through decreased use of judgmental or antagonistic language (e.g., Cynthia's suicidal communications and escalating demands for accommodation, parents' labeling Cynthia as "manipulative"), increased use of warm verbal validation and motivational/cheerleading language, and increased relationship-enhancing, non-obsessional family pleasant events. For example, in one family session after a particularly distressing week, Cynthia created a list of validating and reinforcing statements that each of her parents could use when she is distressed, and her mother agreed to weekly "mother-daughter dinner dates" to increase opportunities for non-OCD, non-family therapy related pleasant interactions.

The whole family benefited greatly from treatment. Through engaging in planned exposures at home, Cynthia dramatically reduced time spent bathing, doing laundry, and engaging in superstitious rituals. Decreased ritualizing helped Cynthia increase the time she spent on homework and sleep. She also decreased avoidance behaviors outside her home, which dramatically increased her opportunity to engage in enjoyable activities. She actually graduated from treatment when she got a part in a play and chose to attend play practice after school rather than therapy. She was able to wear costumes and sit on furniture on set with ease, greatly improving her mood and sense of mastery. Cynthia's parents learned to gradually and consistently decrease family habits that had been catering to Cynthia's OCD-related demands. This included anticipating contexts where conflict often came up (e.g., prior to bed during the latter half of the school week) and proactively scheduling coping activities (e.g., increased sleep and exercise, using relaxation techniques ahead of tough conversations). They also learned to warmly acknowledge and validate Cynthia's experience of anxiety, without trying to urgently make Cynthia's distress go away. By the end of treatment, they reported that learning to validate Cynthia's experience without feeling responsible for problem solving or "getting her out of it" was the single most helpful skill they'd acquired. They reported that they felt "free" and that this freedom allowed them to "just be parents," which significantly increased pleasant family interactions.

Challenges and Recommendations for Future Research

Pediatric OCD treatment has undergone significant advancements in the past two decades. Exposure-based CBT treatment for OCD remains the first treatment of choice but may be enhanced by actively assessing family involvement and addressing ubiquitous OCD-related processes such as family accommodation and the distress experienced by all family members. Future research should investigate how parents can ideally be involved with their child's treatment to enhance outcomes in respective treatment tasks across different developmental ages. Future work should also continue to expand the research base to other promising formats that can involve families (e.g., internet-delivered treatment), and alternative psychotherapies (e.g., motivational interviewing, family therapy, parent training) that can facilitate children and families who are ambivalent about actively engaging in exposure work (Freeman, Garcia et al., 2014).

Key Practice Points

- Pediatric obsessive-compulsive disorder (OCD) exposure-based treatment can be significantly enhanced with additions of family-based elements.
- Families are routinely involved in the maintenance of OCD. OCD in children frequently elicits distress in family members and as such, results in shaping family behavior to be accommodating of the child's compulsions or avoidant of obsession triggers.
- The entrenchment of OCD in family habits over time can elicit bidirectional exchanges of negative affect, leading to high expressed emotion and other maladaptive communication strategies in affected family members.
- Family-based elements often include an added emphasis of parent-centered skills, which are flexibly included in treatment based on a functional analysis of symptoms (enhancing distress tolerance, scaffolding assistance to the child that doesn't reinforce OCD).
- Family-based elements often include an added emphasis on improving communication between family members (improving warmth and assertiveness when communicating, reducing urgent accommodation of OCD symptoms, improving reward systems).

References

Abramowitz, J. S., Baucom, D. H., Wheaton, M. G., Boeding, S., Fabricant, L. E., Paprocki, C., & Fischer, M. S. (2013). Enhancing exposure and response prevention for OCD: A couple-based approach. *Behavior Modification, 37*(2), 189–210. doi: 10.1177/0145445512444596

Amir, N., Freshman, M., & Foa, E. B. (2000). Family distress and involvement in relatives of obsessive-compulsive disorder patients. *Journal of Anxiety Disorders, 14*(3), 209–217. doi: 10.1016/S0887-6185(99)00032-8

Anderson, L. M., Freeman, J. B., Franklin, M. E., & Sapyta, J. J. (2015). Family-based treatment of pediatric obsessive-compulsive disorder: Clinical considerations and application. *Child and Adolescent Psychiatric Clinics of North America, 24*(3), 535–555. doi:10.1016/j.chc.2015.02.003

Barrett, P. M., Farrell, L., Pina, A. A., Peris, T. S., & Piacentini, J. (2008). Evidence-based psychosocial treatments for child and adolescent obsessive-compulsive disorder. *Journal of Clinical Child & Adolescent Psychology, 37*(1), 131–155. doi:10.1080/15374410701817956

Barrett, P. M., Healy-Farrell, L., & March, J. S. (2004). Cognitive-behavioral family treatment of childhood obsessive-compulsive disorder: A controlled trial. *Journal of the American Academy of Child and Adolescent Psychiatry, 43*(1), 46–62. doi:10.1097/01.CHI.0000096367.43887.13

Barrett, P. M., Shortt, A., & Healy, L. (2002). Do parent and child behaviours differentiate families whose children have obsessive-compulsive disorder from other clinic and non-clinic families? *Journal of Child Psychology and Psychiatry, 43*(5), 597–607. doi:10.1111/1469-7610.00049

Benito, K. G., Conelea, C., Garcia, A. M., & Freeman, J. B. (2012). CBT specific process in exposure-based treatments: Initial examination in a pediatric OCD sample. *Journal of Obsessive-Compulsive and Related Disorders, 1*, 77–84. doi:10.1016/j.jocrd.2012.01.001

Bolton, D., & Perrin, S. (2008). Evaluation of exposure with response-prevention for obsessive compulsive disorder in childhood and adolescence. *Journal of Behavior Therapy and Experimental Psychiatry, 39*(1), 11–22. doi: 10.1016/j.jbtep.2006.11.002

Bolton, D., Williams, T., Perrin, S., Atkinson, L., Gallop, C., Waite, P., & Salkovskis, P. (2011). Randomized controlled trial of full and brief cognitive-behaviour therapy and wait-list for paediatric obsessive-compulsive disorder. *Journal of Child Psychology and Psychiatry, 52*(12), 1269–1278. doi:10.1111/j.1469-7610.2011.02419.x

Chambless, D. L., Bryan, A. D., Aiken, L. S., Steketee, G., & Hooley, J. M. (2001). Predicting expressed emotion: A study with families of obsessive–compulsive and agoraphobic outpatients. *Journal of Family Psychology, 15*(2), 225–240. doi:10.1037/0893-3200.15.2.225

Chambless, D. L., & Steketee, G. (1999). Expressed emotion and behavior therapy outcome: A prospective study with obsessive-compulsive and agoraphobic outpatients. *Journal of Consulting and Clinical Psychology, 67*(5), 658–665. doi:10.1037/0022-006X.67.5.658

Choate-Summers, M. L., Freeman, J. B., Garcia, A. M., Coyne, L., Przeworski, A., & Leonard, H. L. (2008). Clinical considerations when tailoring cognitive behavioral treatment for young children with obsessive compulsive disorder. *Education and Treatment of Children, 31*(3), 395–416. doi:10.1353/etc.0.0004

Chorpita, B. F., Brown, T. A., & Barlow, D. H. (1998). Perceived control as a mediator of family environment in etiological models of childhood anxiety. *Behavior Therapy, 29*(3), 457–476. doi: 10.1016/S0005-7894(98)80043-9

Comer, J. S., Furr, J. M., Cooper-Vince, C. E., Kerns, C. E., Chan, P. T., Khanna, M.,... Freeman, J. B. (2014). Internet-delivered, family-based treatment for early-onset OCD: A preliminary case series. *Journal of Clinical Child & Adolescent Psychology, 43*(1), 74–87. doi:10.1080/15374416.2013.855127

Derisley, J., Heyman, I., Robinson, S., & Turner, C. (2008). Breaking free from OCD: A CBT guide for young people and their families. *London: Jessica Kingsley Publishers.* doi:10.1111/j.1475-3588.2009.00530_5.x

Farrell, L.J. & Barrett, P. M. (2007). The function of the family in childhood obsessive-compulsive disorder: Family interactions and accommodation. In T. Murphy & E.

Storch (eds.), *Handbook of child and adolescent obsessive-compulsive disorder*, pp. 313–332. Mahwah, NJ: Lawrence Erlbaum Associates Publisher.

Fischer, M. S., Baucom, D. H., Baucom, B. R., Abramowitz, J. S., Kirby, J. S., & Bulik, C. M. (2017). Disorder-specific patterns of emotion coregulation in couples: Comparing obsessive compulsive disorder and anorexia nervosa. *Journal of Family Psychology, 31*(3), 304. doi: 10.1037/fam0000251

Flessner, C. A., Freeman, J. B., Sapyta, J., Garcia, A., Franklin, M. E., March, J. S., & Foa, E. (2011). Predictors of parental accommodation in pediatric obsessive-compulsive disorder: Findings from the Pediatric Obsessive-Compulsive Disorder Treatment Study (POTS) trial. *Journal of the American Academy of Child & Adolescent Psychiatry, 50*(7), 716–725. doi: 10.1016/j.jaac.2011.03.019

Freeman, J., Garcia, A., Frank, H., Benito, K., Conelea, C., Walther, M., & Edmunds, J. (2014). Evidence base update for psychosocial treatments for pediatric obsessive-compulsive disorder. *Journal of Clinical Child & Adolescent Psychology, 43*(1), 7–26. doi:10.1080/15374416.2013.804386

Freeman, J., Garcia, A., Fucci, C., Karitani, M., Miller, L., & Leonard, H. L. (2003). Family-based treatment of early-onset obsessive-compulsive disorder. *Journal of Child and Adolescent Psychopharmacology, 13(Suppl. 1)*, S71–S80. doi:10.1089/104454603322126368

Freeman, J., Sapyta, J. J., Garcia, A., Compton, S. N., Khanna, M., Flessner, C.,... Franklin, M. E. (2014). Family-based treatment of early childhood obsessive-compulsive disorder: The Pediatric Obsessive-Compulsive Disorder Treatment Study for Young Children (POTS Jr)—A randomized clinical trial. *JAMA Psychiatry, 71*(6), 689–698. doi:10.1001/jamapsychiatry.2014.170

Garcia, A. M., Sapyta, J. J., Moore, P. S., Freeman, J. B., Franklin, M. E., March, J. S., & Foa, E. B. (2010). Predictors and moderators of treatment outcome in the Pediatric Obsessive Compulsive Treatment Study (POTS I). *Journal of the American Academy of Child and Adolescent Psychiatry, 49*(10), 1024–1033; quiz 1086. doi: 10.1016/j.jaac.2010.06.013

Ginsburg, G. S., Kingery, J. N., Drake, K. L., & Grados, M. A. (2008). Predictors of treatment response in pediatric obsessive-compulsive disorder. *Journal of the American Academy of Child & Adolescent Psychiatry, 47*(8), 868–878. doi: 10.1097/CHI.0b013e3181799ebd

Hudson, J. L., Comer, J. S., & Kendall, P. C. (2008). Parental responses to positive and negative emotions in anxious and nonanxious children. *Journal of Clinical Child & Adolescent Psychology, 37*(2), 303–313. doi: 10.1080/15374410801955839

Keeley, M. L., Storch, E. A., Merlo, L. J., & Geffken, G. R. (2008). Clinical predictors of response to cognitive-behavioral therapy for obsessive-compulsive disorder. *Clinical Psychology Review, 28*(1), 118–130. doi: 10.1016/j.cpr.2007.04.003

Kircanski, K., & Peris, T. S. (2015). Exposure and response prevention process predicts treatment outcome in youth with OCD. *Journal of Abnormal Child Psychology, 43*, 543–552. doi:10.1007/s10802-014-9917-2

Kraemer, H., Frank, E., & Kupfer, D. (2006). Moderators of treatment outcomes. *JAMA, 296*, 1286–1289. doi: 10.1001/jama.296.10.1286.

Krohne, H. W., & Hock, M. (1991). Relationships between restrictive mother-child interactions and anxiety of the child. *Anxiety Research, 4*(2), 109–124. doi: 10.1080/08917779108248768

Lebowitz, E. R. (2013). Parent-based treatment for childhood and adolescent OCD. *Journal of Obsessive-Compulsive and Related Disorders, 2*, 425–431. doi:10.1016/j.jocrd.2013.08.004

Lebowitz, E. R., Omer, H., & Leckman J. F. (2011). Coercive and disruptive behaviors in pediatric obsessive-compulsive disorder. *Depression and Anxiety, 28*(10), 899–905. doi: 10.1002/da.20858

Lenhard, F., Vigerland, S., Andersson, E., Rück, C., Mataix-Cols, D., Thulin, U.,... Serlachius, E. (2014). Internet-delivered cognitive behavior therapy for adolescents with obsessive-compulsive disorder: An open trial. *PloS One, 9*(6), 1–11. doi:10.1371/journal.pone.0100773

Lewin, A. B., Park, J. M., Jones, A. M., Crawford, E. A., De Nadai, A. S., Menzel, J.,... Storch, E. A. (2014). Family-based exposure and response prevention therapy for preschool-aged children with obsessive-compulsive disorder: A pilot randomized controlled trial. *Behaviour Research and Therapy, 56*, 30–38. doi:10.1016/j.brat.2014.02.001

March, J.S., & Mulle, K. (1998). *OCD in children and adolescents: A cognitive-behavioral treatment manual.* New York: Guilford Press.

Marien, W. E., Storch, E. A., Geffken, G. R., & Murphy, T. K. (2009). Intensive family-based cognitive-behavioral therapy for pediatric obsessive-compulsive disorder: Applications for treatment of medication partial- or nonresponders. *Cognitive and Behavioral Practice, 16*(3), 304–316. doi:10.1016/j.cbpra.2008.12.006

Martin, J. L., & Thienemann, M. (2005). Group cognitive-behavior therapy with family involvement for middle-school-age children with obsessive-compulsive disorder: A pilot study. *Child Psychiatry and Human Development, 36*(1), 113–127. doi:10.1007/s10578-005-3496-y

Merlo, L. J., Storch, E. A., Lehmkuhl, H. D., Jacob, M. L., Murphy, T. K., Goodman, W. K., & Geffken, G. R. (2010). Cognitive behavioral therapy plus motivational interviewing improves outcome for pediatric obsessive-compulsive disorder: A preliminary study. *Cognitive Behaviour Therapy, 39*(1), 24–27. doi:10.1080/16506070902831773

Olatunji, B. O., Davis, M. L., Powers, M. B., & Smits, J. A. (2013). Cognitive-behavioral therapy for obsessive-compulsive disorder: A meta-analysis of treatment outcome and moderators. *Journal of Psychiatric Research, 47*(1), 33–41. doi: 0.1016/j.jpsychires.2012.08.020

Peris, T. S., Bergman, R. L., Langley, A., Chang, S., McCracken, J. T., & Piacentini, J. (2008). Correlates of accommodation of pediatric obsessive-compulsive disorder: Parent, child, and family characteristics. *Journal of the American Academy of Child and Adolescent Psychiatry, 47*(10), 1173–1181. doi:10.1097/CHI.0b013e3181825a91

Peris, T. S., & Miklowitz, D. J. (2015). Parental expressed emotion and youth psychopathology: New directions for an old construct. *Child Psychiatry and Human Development, 46*, 863–873. doi:10.1007/s10578-014-0526-7

Peris, T. S., & Piacentini, J. (2013). Optimizing treatment for complex cases of childhood obsessive compulsive disorder: A preliminary trial. *Journal of Clinical Child & Adolescent Psychology, 42*(1), 1–8. doi:10.1080/15374416.2012.673162

Piacentini, J., Bergman, R. L., Keller, M., & McCracken, J. (2003). Functional impairment in children and adolescents with obsessive-compulsive disorder. *Journal of Child and Adolescent Psychopharmacology, 13*(Suppl 1), S61–S69. doi: 10.1089/104454603322126359

Piacentini, J., Bergman, R. L., Chang, S., Langley, A., Peris, T., Wood, J. J., & McCracken, J. (2011). Controlled comparison of family cognitive behavioral therapy and psychoeducation/relaxation training for child obsessive-compulsive disorder. *Journal of the American Academy of Child and Adolescent Psychiatry, 50*(11), 1149–1161. doi:10.1016/j.jaac.2011.08.003

Piacentini J., Bergman, R.L., Jacobs, C., McCracken, J., & Kretchman, J. (2002). Open trial of cognitive behavior therapy for childhood obsessive–compulsive disorder. *Journal of Anxiety Disorders, 16*, 207–219. doi: 10.1016/S0887-6185(02)00096-8

Przeworski, A., Zoellner, L. A., Franklin, M. E., Garcia, A., Freeman, J., March, J. S., & Foa, E. B. (2012). Maternal and child expressed emotion as predictors of treatment response in pediatric obsessive-compulsive disorder. *Child Psychiatry and Human Development, 43*, 337–353. doi:10.1007/s10578-011-0268-8

Rapoport, J. L., Inoff-Germain, G., Weissman, M. M., Greenwald, S., Narrow, W. E., Jensen, P. S.,... & Canino, G. (2000). Childhood obsessive–compulsive disorder in the NIMH MECA Study: Parent versus child identification of cases. *Journal of Anxiety Disorders, 14*(6), 535–548. doi: 10.1016/S0887-6185(00)00048-7

Renshaw, K. D., Steketee, G., & Chambless, D. L. (2005). Involving family members in the treatment of OCD. *Cognitive Behaviour Therapy, 34*(3), 164–175. doi:10.1080/16506070510043732

Reynolds, S.A., Clark, S., Smith, H., Langdon, P.E., Payne, R., Bowers, G., ... McIlwham, H. (2013). Randomized controlled trial of parent-enhanced CBT compared with individual CBT for obsessive-compulsive disorder in young people. *Journal of Consulting and Clinical Psychology, 81*(6), 1021–1026. doi: 10.1037/a0034429

Schlup, B., Farrell, L., & Barrett, P. M. (2011). Mother-child interactions and childhood OCD: Effects of CBT on mother and child observed behaviors. *Child & Family Behavior Therapy, 33*(4), 322–336. doi:10.1080/07317107.2011.623920

Steketee, G., van Noppen, B., Lam, J., & Shapiro, L. (1998). Expressed emotion in families and the treatment of obsessive compulsive disorder. *In Session: Psychotherapy in Practice, 4*(3), 73–91. doi:10.1002/(SICI)1520–6572(199823)4:3%3C73::AID-SESS6%3E3.0.CO;2–9

Stewart, S. E., Hu, Y.-P., Leung, A., Chan, E., Hezel, D. M., Lin, S. Y.,... Pauls, D. L. (2017). A multisite study of family functioning impairment in pediatric obsessive-compulsive disorder. *Journal of the American Academy of Child and Adolescent Psychiatry, 56*(3), 241–249. doi:10.1016/j.jaac.2016.12.012

Stewart, S.E., Beresin, C., Haddad, S., Egan Stack, D., Fama, J., & Jenike, M. (2008). Predictors of family accommodation in obsessive-compulsive disorder. *Annals of Clinical Psychiatry, 20*(2), 65–70. doi: 10.1080/10401230802017043

Storch, E. A., Caporino, N. E., Morgan, J. R., Lewin, A. B., Rojas, A., Brauer, L.,... Murphy, T. K. (2011). Preliminary investigation of web-camera delivered cognitive-behavioral therapy for youth with obsessive-compulsive disorder. *Psychiatry Research, 189*, 407–412. doi:10.1016/j.psychres.2011.05.047

Storch, E. A., Geffken, G. R., Merlo, L. J., Jacob, M. L., Murphy, T. K., Goodman, W. K.,... Grabill, K. (2007). Family accommodation in pediatric obsessive-compulsive disorder. *Journal of Clinical Child & Adolescent Psychology, 36*(2), 207–216. doi:10.1080/15374410701277929

Storch, E. A., Geffken, G. R., Merlo, L. J., Mann, G., Duke, D., Munson, M.,... Goodman, W. K. (2007). Family-based cognitive-behavioral therapy for pediatric obsessive-compulsive disorder: Comparison of intensive and weekly approaches. *Journal of the American Academy of Child and Adolescent Psychiatry, 46*(4), 469–478. doi:10.1097/chi.0b013e31803062e7

Storch, E. A., Mariaskin, A., & Murphy, T. K. (2009). Psychotherapy for obsessive-compulsive disorder. *Current Psychiatry Reports, 11*(4), 296–301. doi: 10.1007/s11920-009-0043-8

Storch, E. A., Merlo, L. J., Larson, M. J., Geffken, G. R., Lehmkuhl, H. D., Jacob, M. L., ... Goodman, W. K. (2008). Impact of comorbidity on cognitive-behavioral therapy response in pediatric obsessive-compulsive disorder. *Journal of the American Academy of Child & Adolescent Psychiatry, 47*(5), 583–592. doi: 10.1097/CHI.0b013e31816774b1

Thienemann, M., Martin, J., Cregger, B., Thompson, H. B., & Dyer-Friedman, J. (2001). Manual-driven group cognitive-behavioral therapy for adolescents with obsessive-compulsive disorder: A pilot study. *Journal of the American Academy of Child and Adolescent Psychiatry, 40*(11), 1254–1260. doi:10.1097/00004583-200111000-00004

Thompson-Hollands, J., Edson, A., Tompson, M. C., & Comer, J. S. (2014). Family involvement in the psychological treatment of obsessive-compulsive disorder: A meta-analysis. *Journal of Family Psychology, 28*(3), 287–298. doi:10.1037/a0036709

Turner, C., O'Gorman, B., Nair, A., & O'Kearney, R. (2018). Moderators and predictors of response to cognitive behaviour therapy for pediatric obsessive-compulsive disorder: A systematic review. *Psychiatry Research, 261*, 50–60. doi: 10.1016/j.psychres.2017.12.034

Twohig, M. P., Abramowitz, J. S., Bluett, E. J., Fabricant, L. E., Jacoby, R. J., Morrison, K. L., ... Smith, B. M. (2015). Exposure therapy for OCD from an acceptance and commitment therapy (ACT) framework. *Journal of Obsessive-Compulsive and Related Disorders, 6*, 167–173. doi:10.1016/j.jocrd.2014.12.007

21 Treatments for Obsessive-Compulsive Disorder and Comorbid Disorders

Tord Ivarsson and Bernhard Weidle

Introduction

Obsessive-compulsive disorder is commonly associated with other comorbid problems and disorders (D. A. Geller et al., 2003; Ivarsson, Melin, & Wallin, 2008). These disorders may vary in expression, from milder symptoms, without rendering clinical implications, to severe disorders being major obstacles for treatment. The latter may need treatment in their own right before treatment for OCD, and/or may require adaptations to the OCD treatment. Thus, the clinician needs to take comorbidities into account and to evaluate them as needed. The common comorbid disorders can be roughly grouped into neuropsychiatric disorders (e.g., attention-deficit hyperactivity disorder, autism spectrum disorder, and Tourette's syndrome), affective disorders (e.g., depression), and anxiety disorders (e.g., specific phobias, generalized anxiety disorder). Prevalence estimates of comorbid conditions across studies vary (see each subsection following), and both differences across samples and ascertainment methods may be causes for these discrepancies. Still, all studies come up with a similar figure for the presence of any type of comorbidity, with estimates suggesting that only approximately 1 out of 4 to 5 patients have OCD alone. Why is it the case that OCD is associated with such high rates of comorbidity? In fact, in this respect OCD is very similar to autism (Mattila et al., 2010), and thus, one answer may be related to underlying developmental vulnerabilities.

OCD: A Developmental Disorder?

First, the high prevalence of developmental disorders in pediatric OCD (more than 40 percent in our clinical study) could imply that OCD itself may have similar underlying mechanisms. Particularly the high prevalence of autistic symptoms and disorders, as well as tic disorders and ADHD, points toward broad developmental deficits associated with OCD. Secondly, in imaging and neuropsychological studies, the presence of brain anomalies (e.g., error signaling and response inhibition problems), as well as cognitive inflexibility is an indication that this may be the case (Britton et al., 2010; Huyser et al., 2009). However, findings so far have been inconsistent (Abramovitch, Abramowitz, et al., 2015; Geller et al.,

2017). The possibility that OCD is a developmental disorder of the goal-directed system has been suggested (Geller et al., 1998, 2001; Huyser et al., 2009; Ivarsson et al., 2017). However, this notion needs to be confirmed in empirical studies. Nevertheless, clinicians need to consider co-occurring developmental deviations.

Do comorbidities matter? Some of these co-occurring symptoms do not reach diagnostic levels, but may still affect the quality of life and the ability to collaborate in treatment, e.g., attention difficulties or externalizing behaviors. On the other hand, many other problems that reach a diagnostic level, e.g., other internalizing or externalizing problems, do not affect treatment outcome once confounding factors and multi-collinearity have been taken into account (Torp et al., 2015; Weidle et al., 2014). In the coming sections, we will discuss these different groups of comorbidity one by one considering what the clinician needs to be aware of for each comorbidity.

A complicating matter is that different types of comorbidity may have a differential impact on the outcome of different treatments (i.e., CBT and SSRI). Thus, a clinician may improve the chances of remission for the patient by considering the match between the treatment that is to be offered and the comorbidities: that is, CBT, SSRI only or combination treatment may be preferable depending on the kind of comorbidity that is present and on the OCD presentation itself. Interestingly, CBT may be the treatment that is least sensitive to the influence of comorbidity (Storch, Bjorgvinsson, et al., 2010). However, the impact of comorbid disorders varies; for example comorbid tics or anxiety disorders may have less impact, while other forms of comorbidity, for example ADHD, may have greater impact (Storch et al., 2008). On the other hand, these findings differ across samples (Farrell et al., 2012; Højgaard et al., 2017; Torp et al., 2015). Pharmacological treatments (i.e., serotonin reuptake inhibiting (SRI) medications), which have a reliable although moderate effect (Ivarsson et al., 2015), in general do not seem to be affected by comorbid disorders (Ginsburg et al., 2008), albeit reports of an attenuated effect on SSRI from comorbid ADHD and from tics have been reported (Geller et al., 2003; March et al., 2007). Here as well, contrasting findings do occur in the literature (Skarphedinsson et al., 2015).

Ascertainment Issues

A clinician, whether psychotherapist or psychopharmacologist, needs valid and reliable methods in order to gain insight into comorbid problems. The gold standard is semi-structured interviews (e.g., Children's schedule for affective disorders and schizophrenia (KSADS; Kaufman et al., 1997) and the Anxiety disorders interview schedule (ADIS; Silverman, Saavedra, & Pina, 2001)). There are several studies showing validity and reliability of the KSADS and ADIS in different cultures (Jarbin et al., 2017; Kaufman et al., 1997; Silverman et al., 2001). Although more resource-demanding than parent- and self-ratings of symptoms, they cannot be replaced by them, in terms of determining a clinical diagnosis of OCD, and comorbidity profiles (Ivarsson et al., 2017). In short, child reports and parent reports contribute in diverse ways to the final diagnosis, and discrepancies need to be carefully considered to establish a reliable diagnostic work-up. Broadband scales like the Achenbach System of Empirically Based Assessment (ASEBA), allowing for both self-, parent-, and teacher ratings (Achenbach, 2002) that are psychometrically validated and used across cultures, are also useful to screen for comorbid symptoms. These scales are valuable aids, but do not include the systematic comparison of parental and child reports across diagnostic criteria that a semi-structured interview provides. Still, these scales are far better than merely using unstructured clinical interviews, which are notoriously unreliable (Rettew et al., 2009). In situations with limited resources such broadband scales can be used for screening, allowing the clinician to reserve semi-structured interviews for cases where indications for comorbidity are present. However, we do recommend that a semi-structured interview like the KSADS or ADIS should be part of the diagnostic work-up in all cases, as the costs for ineffective treatments that may be initiated without careful diagnostic formulations are so much higher. Moreover, patients that fail their OCD treatment because of comorbidity may lose their belief in prescribed treatments, resulting in even higher costs. Using a semi-structured interview increases also the likelihood that symptoms are allocated to the right disorder, e.g., that the presence of attention problems are part of a pervasive disorder like ADHD rather than being the consequence of obsessive ruminations (Guzick et al., 2017), a distinction that demands careful questioning.

Comorbid ADHD

ADHD is one of the three most common comorbidities in OCD. More than 50 studies, mainly of pediatric OCD, report prevalence rates ranging from 10 to 50 percent, with a few outliers reporting prevalence rates up to 60 percent (Abramovitch et al., 2015). The reported differences depend on assessment methods, age, and whether the prevalence is derived from a clinical or a population sample. In addition, attention deficit symptoms on a subclinical level seem to be a part of the total symptom burden (Ivarsson et al., 2008). However, the notion of ADHD as a frequent comorbidity of OCD has been challenged. It has been suggested that inflated rates of ADHD-OCD co-occurrence may be mediated by the presence of tic disorders or impaired neuronal maturational processes in pediatric OCD, leading to possibly transient ADHD-like symptoms, which may be misdiagnosed as ADHD (Abramovitch, Dar, et al., 2015). Support for this viewpoint comes from a recent treatment study that found a decline of ADHD symptoms following successful OCD treatment, regardless of treatment modality, i.e., CBT-E/RP alone or in combination with SSRIs (Guzick et al., 2017). This controversy is not only of scientific interest, because conceptualization of comorbidity and sequencing of treatment may moderate treatment outcome. A qualitative review (Halldorsdottir & Ollendick, 2014) exploring the influence of comorbid ADHD on CBT found evidence that youth with co-occurring ADHD and anxiety disorders (specifically, in the two studies of pediatric OCD) had worse outcomes than their counterparts without ADHD.

Therefore, careful assessment of comorbid ADHD symptoms in OCD cases is of utmost importance in order to avoid misdiagnosing OCD symptoms as ADHD, especially in the presence of comorbid tic disorders. On the other hand, it is equally important not to overlook genuine ADHD comorbidity, because this might be the most impairing factor in tic disorders and an obstacle to effective treatment of OCD.

Patients with comorbid ADHD have problems in executive functioning (Hosenbocus & Chahal, 2012), compromising goal-directed behavior, which is essential for compliance with the demands of a successful CBT course. Patients with OCD and ADHD may therefore benefit from treatment for ADHD prior to OCD treatment, improving their ability to cooperate with the CBT demands. However, scientific evidence for this notion is scarce (King, Dowling, & Leow, 2017). More research on comorbid OCD and ADHD, including outcome of different treatment options, is much needed. Currently, the US practice parameter (Geller & March, 2012) recommends to first treat OCD in patients with comorbid OCD and ADHD. Conversely, we argue that this recommendation should be refined. Provided appropriate assessment of ADHD, the disorder with the most pervasive effect on executive function, i.e., ADHD, should be treated first. Given the advantages of CBT over SSRI treatment regarding effect size and patient preference as outlined previously in this book, the first line treatment option should be providing optimal conditions for a successful course of CBT. Pharmacological treatment of comorbid ADHD before CBT/SSRI for OCD allows not only evaluating the effect of drugs on ADHD symptoms, but also on OCD symptoms, which may decrease as well. On the other hand, when OCD onset clearly precedes ADHD-like symptoms, or the ADHD diagnosis is less certain, targeting OCD symptoms first could be the better option, because attention problems might improve following OCD treatment (Guzick et al., 2017). In all cases the treatments need to be coordinated, ensuring that CBT for the OCD begins when adequate compliance and sufficiently scaffolded executive functioning in the child is established, i.e., when the child can cooperate and comply with the treatment demands.

There is a long-standing belief that stimulant medication, especially methylphenidate, may exacerbate or even provoke obsessions and compulsions and anxiety symptoms. However, the evidence is sparse and based on industrial drug labeling and a few single case descriptions (see, for example, Jhanda, Singla, & Grover, 2016). Methylphenidate and dexamphetamine are often used interchangeably in ADHD treatment, but have differing effects on dopaminergic and serotonergic metabolism. Joffe, Swinson, and Levitt (1991) compared methylphenidate, dextroamphetamine, and placebo in 11 patients with primary OCD. Dextroamphetamine but not methylphenidate had a significantly greater anti-obsessive-compulsive effect compared to placebo. Insel et al. (1983) reported significant improvement of obsessional symptoms following administration of d-amphetamine compared with placebo in 12 patients with severe chronic OCD. Interestingly the improvement of OCD was correlated with improved performance on an attention task. A recent meta-analysis identifying 23 studies involving 2959 children with ADHD suggested that treatment with stimulants reduced the risk of anxiety compared with placebo, possibly as a secondary effect of improved control of ADHD symptoms (Coughlin et al.,

2015). Worsening of anxiety symptoms during stimulant medication is more likely to occur coincidentally, rather than being a side effect of stimulants (Coughlin et al., 2015). Nevertheless, if present, this problem could probably be addressed and solved with CBT and ERP exercises as it otherwise may lead to discontinuation of a potentially helpful stimulant treatment.

In the presence of ADHD symptoms, treatment for OCD needs to be adapted to the patient's shorter attention span, impulsivity, and reduced stamina. Halldorsdottir and Ollendick (2014) recommend modifications of CBT including highly structured sessions, explicit expectations for the child's involvement in the therapy, engaging and interactive activities during sessions, providing reduced information in multiple ways, and to adjust the content and duration of the sessions to the attention span of the child. Such adjustments might include shorter treatment sessions, breaks with pleasurable activities during sessions, predictable treatment sessions, focusing only on the most important goals, i.e., motivating and preparing the child for exposure exercises. In addition, checking whether the content was understood is crucial, as well as assuring that homework exercises will be performed. To this end the help of technical devices, for example smartphone alerts, or involving parents to a greater extent in supervising exposure exercises, is essential. However, these adaptations of CBT need to be empirically tested.

A promising novel development are groups for youth with ADHD based on CBT techniques with focus on improving self-organizing skills, which have proved to be effective in adults (Solanto et al., 2010). Similar CBT-based group therapies are currently under evaluation in children and adolescents when medication is not tolerated or insufficient to improve functioning (Antshel & Olszewski, 2014). For cases with ADHD and comorbid OCD, sequenced or combined CBT formats targeting both ADHD and OCD should be developed and studied. A pilot study (Farrell et al., 2012) evaluated the effectiveness of group CBT for OCD in a pediatric sample, consisting of complex comorbidity: 86 percent had a secondary and 74 percent a tertiary psychiatric diagnosis. Encouragingly, group CBT for OCD was found to be largely effective for these young people with a variety of comorbid conditions. However, the youth with comorbid ADHD were less likely to achieve remission at 6-months follow-up, suggesting a stronger dose of CBT, or an augmented CBT protocol may be warranted for these youth with comorbid ADHD.

Comorbid Autism Spectrum Disorders

Subclinical autistic symptoms are common (10 to 17 percent) in children with OCD (Arildskov et al., 2015), also when compared to controls (Weidle et al., 2012). Of children and adolescents treated for OCD, 8 to 21 percent fulfilled the diagnostic criteria for an Autism Spectrum Disorder (ASD) (Griffiths et al., 2017; Ivarsson & Melin, 2008). The opposite case is even more likely, with a meta-analysis of prevalence studies determining an OCD prevalence of 17 percent in individuals with ASD < 18 years of age (van Steensel, Bogels, & Perrin, 2011). Previously, obsessive-compulsive symptoms were often regarded either as a part of the repetitive behavior immanent to ASD, or considered impossible or at least difficult to both assess and to treat. However, compulsions and obsessions are found to add significantly to the burden of impairment in ASD (Russell et al., 2005). Successfully treated OCD can markedly improve functioning and quality of life in affected individuals. Therefore, OCD symptoms should be assessed, distinguished from repetitive behaviors and special interests, and appropriately treated. Consequently, CBT for OCD has been adapted to the needs of individuals with ASD with initial sporadic case reports of successful treatment courses (Lehmkuhl et al., 2008; Reaven & Hepburn, 2003). The first randomized treatment study with adolescents and young adults with comorbid ASD and OCD compared CBT relative to anxiety management (Russell et al., 2013). Both treatments resulted in a significant reduction of OCD symptoms, assessed with the YBOCS. The CBT group had more responders to the treatment, but between-group differences were not significant. A second controlled trial (Murray et al., 2015) assessed outcomes for individually tailored, protocol driven CBT for OCD among 22 young people with comorbid OCD and ASD compared to matched controls with OCD, but no ASD. Both groups responded to treatment; however, the OCD + ASD group achieved overall smaller decreases in symptoms and lower remission rates at posttreatment than the OCD only group. The first and to date only review focusing on the effectiveness of CBT for individuals with ASD and OCD exclusively (Kose, Fox, & Storch, 2017), identified a total of eleven studies including three randomized control trials (RCTs), one case controlled study, two single subject experimental designs, and five case studies. However, one of the three evaluated RCTs included children with OCD and autistic symptoms without defined comorbid ASD diagnoses (Wolters et al., 2016). Eight other controlled trials, including four with a group session format, examined the use of CBT- based approaches for mainly non-OCD anxiety disorders in ASD in children and adolescents, all of which found that CBT was superior to control conditions (Sukhodolsky et al., 2013). Selles et al. (2015) recently highlighted the problem of poor maintenance of CBT gains for anxiety in youth with ASD. At posttreatment evaluation 10–26 months following treatment, treatment gains were on average well-maintained, but a considerable group of participants experienced symptom relapse. Five participants (16 percent) in this study had OCD.

A diagnosis of OCD should be based on the same criteria as in children without ASD including impairment in daily life functioning. However, OCD like symptoms, such as rigidity, repetitive and ritualized patterns of behavior, preoccupation with details, and a near-obsessive focus on restricted areas of interests, are part of the clinical presentation of ASD. Literal interpretation of facts immanent to ASD could be misinterpreted as obsessions (e.g., about toxicity of the environment or nutrition principles). Unlike compulsions, repetitive behavior and rigidity rituals in ASD are driven by the need for sameness and perceived as pleasant and not performed to avoid anxiety or disgust. In addition, rigidity is a more stable and continuous trait of the child's personality, while OCD symptoms typically develop with a point of onset, although sometimes insidious.

Treatment of OCD in children with ASD or subsyndromal traits may need to be adjusted to the patients' communication style and deficits, their areas of interest, impairment in executive and social functioning, and their perception of the environment. Modifications of standard CBT protocols for OCD in ASD are available (Kose et al., 2017; Krebs, Murray, & Jassi, 2016) and commonly include the following adjustments:

- Communication needs to be succinct, clear, and precise, with a focus on the essential messages and a clear expression of treatment goals. Metaphors and implicit messages may be interpreted literally and should be avoided or explained.
- Motivational factors should be assessed and promoted. For children with OCD without ASD, incentives to cooperate in treatment are mostly social, i.e., to overcome OCD so that the child can spend more time with friends. Because of the lack of social motivation, social goals should be substituted by other rewards for the child with ASD, for example, avoiding stress when accidentally in contact with germs, or fuss from parents, or gaining more time for their special interest, when OCD is conquered.
- Extended and repeated psychoeducation to enhance insight into the irrational nature of their obsessions should be provided. Poor insight is frequently due to impaired ability for introspection, literal perception of language (e.g., exaggerated alerts of danger in the media), and impaired social judgment.
- Clear structure for the sessions, and visual support (working schedules, symptom mapping, homework assignment, etc.) may enhance compliance to treatment.
- Greater parents' involvement is recommended to foster generalization of training gains to real life situations and to maintain motivation, to encourage ERP-exercises, and to supervise and monitor homework assignments.

Repetitive behavior and rigidity may overlap with OCD symptoms and constitute a serious obstacle for compliance with exposure treatment. In these very complex situations, pharmacological treatment of ASD symptoms may be of value. Risperidone and aripiprazole are the two best-studied medications for ASD and found to be beneficial to reduce challenging and repetitive behavior, although the evidence base for medication is weak (McPheeters et al., 2011). SSRIs have shown some benefit in a few studies, but in general there is no evidence to support the use of SSRIs to treat autism in children (Williams et al., 2013). The atypical antipsychotics that are found to be most beneficial in ASD are the same that are recommended as augmentation strategy for SSRI refractory OCD (see chapter 19, Pharmacologic-Augmented Treatments). Therefore, in children with OCD and ASD who are not able to comply with the demands of exposure therapy or have only insufficient effect from CBT and an SSRI trial, there might be an additional benefit of these compounds both to augment weak SSRI response and to reduce rigidity and repetitive behavior. Of novel formats for CBT delivery, concentrated exposure and response prevention (ERP) seems to be promising for comorbid OCD and ASD. An intensive ERP regimen (range 24–80 daily sessions) for OCD in 11 adolescents with ASD, modified and adjusted in accordance with evidence-based findings for the needs of this population, was found to yield a response rate of 78 percent (Iniesta-Sepulveda et al., 2017). Continued efforts to modifying CBT protocols for OCD in ASD youth including their empirical evaluation are mandatory to improve outcomes in this especially vulnerable group.

Comorbid Disruptive Behavioral Disorders

Disruptive behavior disorders are reported with a prevalence between 9 and 53 percent in pediatric OCD (Ivarsson et al., 2008; Storch, Lewin, et al., 2010). Both clinical and subclinical oppositional defiant disorder (ODD) and conduct disorder (CD) are associated with increased severity of OCD symptoms and poorer treatment outcome (Storch, Lewin, et al., 2010; Torp et al., 2015). Explosive outbursts representing a failure to control aggressive impulses are classified as an independent disorder, named Intermittent Explosive Disorder (IED) in the DSM-5 chapter of Disruptive, Impulse-Control, and Conduct Disorders (American Psychiatric Association, 2013). However, the DSM-5 criteria for IED require that the recurrent outbursts cannot be explained by another mental disorder. Although disruptive behavior in OCD can represent true comorbidity, in many cases, the disruptive behaviors are motivated by the preexisting OCD. Few studies have tried to differentiate between OCD-related anger outbursts and non-OCD related comorbid disruptive disorders. Lebowitz, Omer, and Leckman (2011) compared disruptive behaviors of children with and without OCD, based on parental reports. The two groups showed different patterns of disruptive behaviors, although overlapping to some extent. This suggests that children with OCD may exhibit more specific OCD-related disruptive behaviors, different from classical aggressive symptoms. Storch et al. (2012) found a high prevalence of rage attacks in a sample of children 6–16 years with OCD, also without comorbid disruptive behavior disorders. Rage attacks were frequently associated with a disruption of OCD-related behaviors often involving limit-setting situations. The authors conceptualized a coercive cycle of parent-child interaction, like that seen between caregivers and youth with disruptive behavior disorders. For example, when a child performs compulsions like washing with exaggerated soap consumption and parents try to stop this behavior with reprimands, the child may react with extreme anger. Consequently, parents may try to avoid the unpleasant anger outbursts by not interfering with compulsions, and thus, the child's behavior is inadvertently reinforced by learning that expressing rage causes parents to accept the compulsive behavior. Consecutively, increased accommodation behavior by the parents may contribute to worsening of OCD symptoms.

There is other evidence supporting the observation that rage attacks are frequent in pediatric OCD and in general related to OCD and not to a comorbid disruptive disorder. Krebs et al. (2013) used the item "temper outbursts" from the conduct subscale of the Strengths and Difficulties Questionnaire (Goodman, 2001) to estimate temper outbursts in a large specialist OCD clinical sample and in a nonclinical community sample. Roughly 30 to 40 percent of young people with OCD reported temper outbursts both in the clinical and community samples, while other disruptive behaviors were found to be uncommon. Interestingly, temper outbursts were particularly related to co-occurrent depressed mood. Clinically most important, temper outbursts as well as depressive symptoms improved with CBT for OCD and did not impede OCD treatment response. This lends support to the concept of a different mechanism of aggression in ODD/CD and OCD. In ODD/CD, the child refuses to recognize authority mainly with the goal to engage in self-directed pleasurable activities, while in OCD aggressive behavior usually is provoked by authorities interfering with the need to perform rituals. Therefore, a comprehensive assessment including in-depth interview with both the child and parent is needed for differential diagnosis. When aggressive behavior is motivated by the need to conduct rituals without interference by others, reframing and directing anger against OCD and not parents is a helpful technique, usually embedded in CBT. On the other hand, the presence of true comorbid ODD/CD is associated with elevated levels of aggression, negativity, and hostility challenging the therapeutic alliance. A possible solution is a stepwise treatment plan, i.e., first to treat the comorbid ODD or CD, for example with Parent Management Training (PMT) (Sukhodolsky et al., 2013), allowing for building an alliance subsequently. Sukhodolsky et al. (2013) evaluated six sessions of PMT for the ODD, followed by twelve sessions of ERP for the OCD, while controls received twelve sessions of ERP for the OCD only. Those who received the combination did better than the controls. The study needs to be replicated however using a bigger sample.

Treatment for ODD before OCD might establish a base for subsequent CBT, but for those who do not respond to this approach, drug treatment can be considered, e.g., in patients with elevated levels of aggression and high parental accommodation. The pharmacological intervention against disruptive behaviors are atypical antipsychotics, usually Risperidone and Aripiprazole, which may be beneficial, albeit the documentation is weak (Pringsheim et al., 2015).

Comorbid Tics/Tourette's disorder

Tic disorders are the most prevalent comorbid disorders in OCD, occurring in about a third of patients. In populations with Tourette's syndrome (TS), OCD symptoms range from 11 to 80 percent (Robertson, 2000). The onset of OCD, when associated with TS, is on average two years later than the onset of tics (Leckman, 2002). Patients with tic-related OCD report more aggressive, religious, and sexual obsessions as well as checking, counting, ordering, touching, and symmetry-compulsions than patients with non-tic-related OCD do (Leckman et al., 1994; Worbe et al., 2010), findings that have been confirmed in children and adolescents (Masi et al., 2005). Studies of the influence of comorbid tic disorders on OCD treatment outcome have shown inconsistent results. For CBT outcome, comorbid TS seems to have negligible impact (Himle et al., 2003; Piacentini et al., 2002). In the NordLOTS sample, those with OCD and comorbid tics (30 percent of participants) had more OCD-related impairment and more comorbidity (ODD, autism spectrum disorder, social anxiety, and ADHD), but showed no difference in terms of OCD severity or response to CBT compared to those with non-tic related OCD (Højgaard et al., 2017). However, among CBT nonresponders, sertraline was superior to continued CBT in patients with comorbid TS (Skarphedinsson et al., 2015), a finding that needs to be replicated. Benett et al. (2015) compared outcomes of CBT for pediatric patients with OCD and a tic disorder with a matched group of children with OCD and no tics at posttreatment and at 3- or 6-month follow-up. In both groups response rates were high with 72 percent of responders posttreatment and about 80 percent at follow-up. In drug trials, however, comorbid tics have been associated with poorer treatment response (Ginsburg et al., 2008; March et al., 2007).

The differentiation between tics and compulsions is clinically important, as there exist effective treatment options for both conditions. In addition, response to treatment might diverge in medication trials. The distinction can be difficult in cases with repetition rituals and "just right" perceptions, because of the similarity and overlap of symptoms. In a clinical context, a careful assessment of the antecedents of the phenomenon is central. Compulsions are anteceded by cognitions (anxiety provoking thoughts or preoccupations) in most cases and are goal-directed, while tics are anteceded by physical sensations, usually described as a premonitory urge, in the whole or in parts of the body. In cases where a differentiation is very difficult or impossible, a practical approach could be to classify the behavior in the context of, and according to the prevalence and the degree of the symptoms. If the repetitive movement or action is rare or isolated and the child has no other tics, it is clinically appropriate to regard the disorder as OCD. Likewise, when the child has many other tics and only a few compulsions the behavior could be regarded as a tic. However, as mentioned, a considerable number of children are presenting with both conditions, or developing the other comorbid condition after a previous period with only one of them.

Behavioral Intervention for Tics

Treatment for tics other than psychoeducation is considered as necessary, when tics are causing functional impairment or significant discomfort. Behavioral interventions aimed to reduce tics are recommended as first line treatment in clinical guidelines (Murphy et al., 2013; Verdellen et al., 2011). Comprehensive Behavioral Intervention for Tics (CBIT) is a treatment package where the central component, Habit Reversal Training (HRT), consisting of training in tic awareness and competing response, is extended with relaxation training, functional interventions, and social support (Piacentini et al., 2002). The effectiveness of behavioral treatments for tic disorders has been evaluated to date in six reviews. The most recently published review (McGuire et al., 2014) identified eight RCTs comprising 438 participants. A random effects meta-analysis found a medium to large effect size for behavioral therapy relative to comparison conditions including awareness training, wait-list, or nondirective therapy. When examining comorbidity, no significant association was identified between the percent of study participants with OCD and effect size. However, a small negative association between the percent of study participants with ADHD and effect size was identified, suggesting that these patients may need other or concomitant treatment. A recent paper provides an overview of systematic reviews and meta analyses of both pharmacological and behavioral interventions for tic disorders (Yang et al., 2016).

Exposure and Response Prevention (ERP) versus CBIT/HRT

ERP has been applied successfully and is currently considered to be an efficacious treatment for TS, although long-term effects need to be determined (Frank & Cavanna, 2013) and the vast majority of studies of behavioral treatment for tics evaluated HRT. Verdellen and colleagues (2004) assessed treatment outcome of ERP compared with HRT. Both treatment strategies resulted in significant reduction of tics without differences between treatment conditions. The common denominator for both interventions is to interrupt the stimulus-response sequences, which maintain the behavior. HRT usually targets one tic at a time and the method is practiced at specific times of the day, whereas in ERP the patient is asked to suppress all occurring tics during several times of the day. In case of multiple and highly variable tics, ERP has been recommended. However, it can be easier to motivate kids for HRT, where the competing response technique offers a tool to fight against tics, other than to simply resist the urge. Altogether, patient preference and therapist expertise might be the key factor for treatment choice. If none of the behavioral interventions, despite being delivered adequately, have been effective, the addition of a pharmacological compound should be considered (Verdellen et al., 2011).

Sequencing of Treatment for OCD with Comorbid TS

None of the mentioned CBT studies targeting comorbid tics and OCD have described modifications of CBT to adjust for the presence of tics. In all studies CBT is delivered in the same format to young people with or without tics, providing little evidence to guide treatment choices. However, as a rule of thumb the main treatment strategy may be chosen based on the prevalence of symptoms and degree of impairment. For example, if OCD-symptoms are dominating the clinical presentation, ERP should be offered. Accordingly, when tics are dominant and constitute the impairing symptoms, HRT should be offered. If the child fails with the ERP technique, it is crucial to differentiate between OCD-symptoms and tics. If not, it will deprive the child from the experience of having defeated OCD, maintaining cognitions that some of the "OCD-symptoms" might be invincible, or at least more difficult to overcome. Probably, it is more helpful to establish a cognition that the child has succeeded and defeated OCD, but that tics are a different foe, which needs a different strategy, namely HRT (or the addition of pharmacologic therapy). In children with TS as the primary disorder, the presence of comorbid compulsions that often are more impairing than tics could be overlooked, preventing the child from an effective course of ERP. In addition to the practical considerations listed previously, the developmental aspects of both disorders should inform all therapeutic interventions. Tics have the greatest effect on a patient's self-esteem and peer and family relationships from age 7 to 12 years, with an exacerbation period between age 10 and 13 years and a possible remission from age 16 to 20 years (Leckman, 2002). To have the natural course of TS in mind and adjusting therapeutic interventions accordingly is essential.

In cases where treatment for tics is required and behavioral interventions failed or were not available, pharmacological treatment for tics should be added. Typical antipsychotics, such as haloperidol and pimozide, are effective (Murphy et al., 2013), but replaced by second generation antipsychotics, because of their unfortunate side effect profile. The most extensively used and studied atypical antipsychotic is risperidone, while aripiprazole is considered as promising therapy; Clonidine and guanfacine are considered as first-line treatment in cases of comorbid ADHD (Roessner et al., 2011; Yang et al., 2016). Atypical antipsychotics can be used as augmentation strategy for SSRI refractory OCD (see Chapter 19: Pharmacologic-Augmented Treatments). Although there is still limited evidence to support the use of antipsychotic augmentation for OCD symptoms in youths with tic-related OCD, there might be a synergistic benefit of using both an SSRI and an atypical antipsychotic in that they target both the tics and OCD in the treatment.

Deep Brain Stimulation

Deep brain stimulation (DBS) is a surgical technique with stereotactically guided implantation of electrodes at selected targets, mainly globus pallidus internus and thalamus especially for patients with TS only, and patients with comorbid obsessive-compulsive symptoms, anxiety, and depression. The first systematic review (Piedad, Rickards, & Cavanna, 2012) assessed 43 studies including 99 participants, concluding that DBS is a promising treatment option for patients with severe impairment related to tics, who did not respond to pharmacological and behavioral interventions. A recent review from the Tourette Syndrome Association International Deep Brain Stimulation Database and Registry Study Group (Schrock et al., 2015) provides an overview of all reported cases of TS DBS including recommendations for selection, assessment, and management of potential TS DBS cases. Interestingly the study group recommended to remove the previously suggested 25-year-old age limit, with the specification that a multidisciplinary team approach for screening and a consultation of a local ethics committee is employed for consideration of cases involving persons younger than 18 years of age. However, there are still many caveats. Optimal target selection is under debate (Hashemiyoon, Kuhn, & Visser-Vandewalle, 2017), and some studies have shown a higher risk for post-DBS complications in TS patients, both topics in need of comprehensive investigation. Though still evolving, DBS seems to emerge as a promising approach for complex cases of treatment refractory and very severely affected patients.

Comorbid Affective Disorders

The prevalence of depression varies across the different studies, with rates between 10 and 73 percent (Heyman et al., 2001; Ivarsson et al., 2008). Some of this variance may be due to different severities, leading to different estimates of a disorder. In some cases, depression may be a separate disorder with a course mainly determined by other than OCD-related factors. However, usually depression is separate but follows the nature and course of the OCD-syndrome (Storch, Lewin, et al., 2012). In many cases depressive symptoms occur without the presence of a depressive syndrome, usually denoted by the term "demoralization," i.e., the subject feels helpless, hopeless, and saddened by the symptoms, impairment, and quality of life. See Golubchic et al. (2013) for an example in OCD. When depression is at clinical levels, Storch and collaborators (2012) showed that both OCD-related and other factors increased the risk of depression. Results from that study found that depression occurred more often in older than younger patients, and more often among girls than boys. With regard to OCD-related factors, patients with more severe OCD and greater levels of impairment were more often depressed. Another factor associated with increased depression was the presence of family accommodation, i.e., that the family adapts to a great extent to the illness, something that is known to increase OCD severity (Garcia et al., 2010). Moreover, having other anxiety symptoms (e.g., generalized anxiety, social anxiety, and separation anxiety) as well increases the risk of depression. However, these risk factors are not merely an effect of having a severe psychiatric disorder such as OCD. Even when controlling for OCD severity, gender, age, and impairment, patients with both OCD and an anxiety disorder were more often depressed. Impairment seems to play a mediating role between OCD severity and depression, i.e., it is among the severely ill and impaired that depression is increased.

However, there may also be specific OCD-related factors associated with depression. In a large international sample (Højgaard et al., 2017), the symmetry/hoarding factor was more strongly associated with comorbid depression than the other OCD factors (unacceptable thoughts and contamination and cleaning). Thus, the clinician needs to be sensitive to these factors and examine the presence of depression carefully, especially when one or more of these factors are present. Ratings of depression, using self-report inventories before and following treatment, are recommended (Storch, Lewin, et al., 2012) so that obstacles to treatment and residual depression can be detected.

Does Depression as a Comorbid Problem Matter? Should It Be Treated in Its Own Right?

There are indeed indications that depressive symptoms (but not a diagnosed disorder) lead to worse CBT outcome (Garcia et al., 2010; Torp et al., 2015). First, extant data show that OCD-treatment (i.e., CBT with ERP) as the first-line treatment (see Chapter 13) must be pursued so that impairment is reduced significantly, i.e., remission must be the goal, not only treatment response in the depressed OCD-patient (Storch, Lewin, et al., 2012). It is to be presumed, although explicit data are lacking, that at least mild to moderate depression is alleviated as well. It is, however, not known whether ERP needs to be adapted to that form of comorbidity (Storch, Lewin, et al., 2012), for example, if CBT techniques directed toward depression are needed, at least during some phase of the treatment. For patients with moderate-severe depression, it seems probable from depression studies (see Cox et al., 2012 for a review) that depression needs to be targeted, often with an SSRI or combined treatment (e.g., an SSRI plus CBT). Data from a review and meta-analysis of naturalistic outcome studies showed that an affective disorder at follow-up increased the risk of persistent OCD (Stewart et al., 2004). Micali (2010) observed in a long-term follow-up that "emotional" symptoms (some of them affective) at baseline had little consequences for the OCD long-term outcome. Similarly, Bloch (2009) found that an affective disorder in childhood did not affect adult outcome, though depression was much more common in those who did not remit from the OCD. In conclusion, the long-term outcome studies do not show that comorbid depression in childhood is a serious problem. However, most studies are fairly small and have great variation in length of follow-up, increasing the uncertainty of the findings.

Comorbid Anxiety Disorders

As described previously, comorbid anxiety disorders are very common, both at subclinical and at clinical levels, so that almost half of the patients (45 percent) have a comorbid anxiety disorder (Ivarsson et al., 2008). In contrast to ADHD and DBD, it does not seem as though comorbid anxiety disorders have strong effects on OCD treatment outcome, at least not on CBT (Storch et al., 2008). Stewart (2004) also reported that childhood anxiety disorders do not affect the long-term outcomes for children with OCD. In conclusion, it does not seem like a childhood anxiety disorder has any major impact on neither CBT, nor SSRI outcome. If a patient with OCD has a clinically significant anxiety disorder that does not improve following CBT and/or SSRI treatment for OCD, we argue that the anxiety disorder requires to be targeted in its own right. Current meta-analyses and reviews state that for mild-moderate anxiety, CBT like the Coping Cat program may be beneficial (James et al., 2015; Reynolds et al., 2012). In cases with moderate to severe anxiety, an SSRI may need to be added (Strawn et al., 2015).

Case Example

"Marc" was an 11-year-old boy when he was referred to the clinic by his family's general practitioner for assessment and treatment of OCD. The parents reported a history of normal pregnancy and uncomplicated delivery and neonatal period. Psychomotor development including developmental milestones was described to be within the normal range. There was no family history of OCD. The age of onset for OCD symptoms was at about 8 years, starting with fear of germs, exaggerated hand washing, and avoidance of touching "dirty" surfaces. The parents described a variety of OCD symptoms and avoidance behavior: He had preoccupations about various chemicals (e.g., fuel, perfume, silicone), and excessive seeking reassurance by parents that these substances would not harm him. He avoided public restrooms and bathrooms in other private homes, preventing him from staying overnight with friends. He had time-consuming toilet rituals, such as sitting on the toilet for up to two hours and using up to 30 pieces of toilet paper to assure that he was clean. In addition, he had a variety of medically unexplained somatic symptoms and complaints as nausea, headache, abdominal pain, and sense of general weakness, often interfering with school attendance. He was afraid of needles and injections, resulting in his withdrawal from the ordinary vaccination program.

Assessment with the Children's Yale-Brown Obsessive-Compulsive Scale (CY-BOCS) (Scahill et al., 1997) and the Schedule for Affective Disorders and Schizophrenia for School Aged Children (K-SADS-PL) (Kaufman et al., 1997) indicated that he met the criteria for OCD. Initial CY-BOCS total score was 32, indicating severe OCD (obsessions score 15 and compulsions scores 17). K-SADS-PL indicated specific syringe phobia and symptoms of other anxiety disorders, especially separation anxiety, but below the clinical range. He was treated with standard CBT consisting of 14 weekly sessions of individual CBT with E/RP, followed by shorter sessions with one or both parents joining in. Posttreatment assessment showed improvement, but still impairing OCD, characterized by CY-BOCS total score of 21 points. After an additional sequence with 14 weekly sessions of individual CBT with E/RP, CY-BOCS total score was stagnant (22 points). Treatment plan was then changed to a course with sertraline, starting with a low dose of 25 mg daily, gradually increased to 175 mg. A maximum dose of 200 mg was tried for a few days, but because of persistent nausea reduced back to 175 mg. He experienced a limited improvement, but at follow up, 18 months after sertraline treatment started, total CY-BOCS score was 19. Sub-threshold anxiety symptoms, somatic complaints, and tendency to school refusal had remained unchanged. At this point treatment strategy was reanalyzed and sertraline was gradually discontinued, because effect, if any, was only temporal. Persisting deficits in executive functioning exemplified by his lacking ability to do effective exposure exercises, even in the presence of insight, led to reassessment of potentially overlooked comorbidity, namely ADHD. A comprehensive assessment concluded with the diagnosis of ADHD, primarily inattentive type, acknowledging that inattentive symptoms were overshadowed by his OCD in the previous assessments. Consecutively, treatment with methylphenidate depot was found to improve his executive functions substantially. Following this, his attendance to school improved, he arrived at school on time, did homework chores with much less procrastination, was socially more active, and psychosomatic complaints faded out. Follow-up after 24 months showed complete remission of OCD symptoms (CY-BOCS total score 0).

Conclusions

In general, if comorbid disorders present with OCD, and if they would likely impede treatment of OCD, they may need to be treated before addressing OCD to improve the final outcome (Storch et al., 2008). New formats of delivering CBT that are currently under development and scientific evaluation, for example, Brief Intensive Treatments (Chapter 6) and new technologies including Web-CBT, Mobile

Apps & Virtual Reality (Chapter 4) may well have the potential to improve treatment outcomes in different subgroups of OCD, including when comorbidity occurs. For example, could children with OCD and comorbid ADHD comply more easily with a brief, but intensive exposure program demanding sustained executive functioning to a much lesser degree than traditional CBT formats? The same line of argument applies to children with OCD and comorbid ASD, who might be able to relate better and to benefit more from technology-delivered CBT programs. However, the evidence base for adaptions of these novel developments to different comorbidity subgroups by now is more or less nonexistent. Adaptations of the CBT technique or sequencing of treatments may also be necessary when disruptive behavior complicates treatment. Even if comorbid depression and anxiety disorders seldom are a serious problem, we suggest thorough assessment and to treat and to monitor these conditions as recommended.

Key Practice Points

- Assessing comorbid conditions in OCD is important: they are frequent and have implications for treatment outcome.
- Thorough assessment of comorbidities and their impact contributes to determining which disorder to treat first, considering modular approaches may be appropriate.
- In case of CBT failure, comorbidity should be reassessed, because OCD symptoms may have overshadowed comorbid conditions.

References

Abramovitch, A., Abramowitz, J. S., Mittelman, A., Stark, A., Ramsey, K., & Geller, D. A. (2015). Research Review: Neuropsychological test performance in pediatric obsessive-compulsive disorder–a meta-analysis. *Journal of Child Psychology and Psychiatry and Allied Disciplines*, 56(8), 837–847. doi:10.1111/jcpp.12414

Abramovitch, A., Dar, R., Mittelman, A., & Wilhelm, S. (2015). Comorbidity between attention deficit/hyperactivity disorder and obsessive-compulsive disorder across the lifespan: A systematic and critical review. *Harvard Review of Psychiatry*, 23(4), 245–262. doi:10.1097/HRP.0000000000000050

Achenbach, T. M. (2002). Ten-year comparisons of problems and competencies for national samples of youth: Self, parent and teacher reports. *Journal of Emotional and Behavioral Disorders*, 10(4), 194–203.

American Psychiatric Association. (2013). *Diagnostic and statistical manual of mental disorders (DSM-5)* (5th edn.). Washington, DC: American Psychiatric Publishing.

Antshel, K. M., & Olszewski, A. K. (2014). Cognitive behavioral therapy for adolescents with ADHD. *Child and Adolescent Psychiatric Clinics of North America*, 23(4), 825–842. doi:10.1016/j.chc.2014.05.001

Arildskov, T. W., Hojgaard, D. R., Skarphedinsson, G., Thomsen, P. H., Ivarsson, T., Weidle, B.,... Hybel, K. A. (2015). Subclinical autism spectrum symptoms in pediatric obsessive-compulsive disorder. *European Child and Adolescent Psychiatry*, 1–13. doi:10.1007/s00787-015-0782-5

Bennett, S., Stark, D., Shafran, R., Heyman, I., & Krebs, G. (2015). Evaluation of cognitive behaviour therapy for paediatric obsessive-compulsive disorder in the context of tic disorders. *Journal of Behavior Therapy and Experimental Psychiatry, 49*(Pt B), 223–229. doi:10.1016/j.jbtep.2015.03.004

Bloch, M. H., Craiglow, B. G., Landeros-Weisenberger, A., Dombrowski, P. A., Panza, K. E., Peterson, B. S., & Leckman, J. F. (2009). Predictors of early adult outcomes in pediatric-onset obsessive-compulsive disorder. *Pediatrics, 124*(4), 1085–1093. doi:10.1542/peds.2009-0015

Britton, J. C., Rauch, S. L., Rosso, I. M., Killgore, W. D., Price, L. M., Ragan, J.,... Stewart, S. E. (2010). Cognitive inflexibility and frontal-cortical activation in pediatric obsessive-compulsive disorder. *Journal of the American Academy of Child and Adolescent Psychiatry, 49*(9), 944–953. doi:10.1016/j.jaac.2010.05.006

Coughlin, C. G., Cohen, S. C., Mulqueen, J. M., Ferracioli-Oda, E., Stuckelman, Z. D., & Bloch, M. H. (2015). Meta-analysis: Reduced risk of anxiety with psychostimulant treatment in children with attention-deficit/hyperactivity disorder. *J Child Adolesc Psychopharmacol, 25*(8), 611–617. doi:10.1089/cap.2015.0075

Cox, G. R., Callahan, P., Churchill, R., Hunot, V., Merry, S. N., Parker, A. G., & Hetrick, S. E. (2012). Psychological therapies versus antidepressant medication, alone and in combination for depression in children and adolescents. *Cochrane Database Syst Rev, 11*, CD008324. doi:10.1002/14651858.CD008324.pub2

Farrell, L., Waters, A., Milliner, E., & Ollendick, T. (2012). Comorbidity and treatment response in pediatric obsessive-compulsive disorder: A pilot study of group cognitive-behavioral treatment. *Psychiatry Research, 199*(2), 115–123. doi:10.1016/j.psychres.2012.04.035

Frank, M., & Cavanna, A. E. (2013). Behavioural treatments for Tourette syndrome: An evidence-based review. *Behavioural Neurology, 27*(1), 105–117. doi:10.3233/BEN-120309

Garcia, A. M., Sapyta, J. J., Moore, P. S., Freeman, J. B., Franklin, M. E., March, J. S., & Foa, E. B. (2010). Predictors and moderators of treatment outcome in the Pediatric Obsessive Compulsive Treatment Study (POTS I). *Journal of the American Academy of Child and Adolescent Psychiatry, 49*(10), 1024–1033. doi:10.1016/j.jaac.2010.06.013

Geller, D., Biederman, J., Jones, J., Park, K., Schwartz, S., Shapiro, S., & Coffey, B. (1998). Is juvenile obsessive-compulsive disorder a developmental subtype of the disorder? A review of the pediatric literature. *Journal of the American Academy of Child and Adolescent Psychiatry, 37*(4), 420–427. doi:10.1097/00004583-199804000-00020

Geller, D. A., Abramovitch, A., Mittelman, A., Stark, A., Ramsey, K., Cooperman, A.,... Stewart, S. E. (2017). Neurocognitive function in paediatric obsessive-compulsive disorder. *World J Biol Psychiatry*, 1–10. doi:10.1080/15622975.2017.1282173

Geller, D. A., Biederman, J., Faraone, S., Agranat, A., Cradock, K., Hagermoser, L.,... Coffey, B. J. (2001). Developmental aspects of obsessive compulsive disorder: Findings in children, adolescents, and adults. *Journal of Nervous and Mental Disease, 189*(7), 471–477.

Geller, D. A., Biederman, J., Stewart, S. E., Mullin, B., Farrell, C., Wagner, K. D.,... Carpenter, D. (2003). Impact of comorbidity on treatment response to paroxetine in pediatric obsessive-compulsive disorder: Is the use of exclusion criteria empirically supported in randomized clinical trials? *J Child Adolesc Psychopharmacol, 13 Suppl 1*, S19–29. doi:10.1089/104454603322126313

Geller, D. A., & March, J. (2012). Practice parameter for the assessment and treatment of children and adolescents with obsessive-compulsive disorder. *Journal of the American Academy of Child and Adolescent Psychiatry, 51*(1), 98–113. doi:10.1016/j.jaac.2011.09.019

Ginsburg, G. S., Kingery, J. N., Drake, K. L., & Grados, M. A. (2008). Predictors of treatment response in pediatric obsessive-compulsive disorder. *Journal of the American Academy of Child and Adolescent Psychiatry, 47*(8), 868–878. doi:10.1097/CHI.0b013e3181799ebd

Golubchik, P., Kodesh, A., & Weizman, A. (2013). Attention-deficit/hyperactivity disorder and comorbid subsyndromal depression: What is the impact of methylphenidate on mood? *Clinical Neuropharmacology, 36*(5), 141–145. doi:10.1097/WNF.0b013e31829eb204

Griffiths, D. L., Farrell, L. J., Waters, A. M., & White, S. W. (2017). Clinical correlates of obsessive compulsive disorder and comorbid autism spectrum disorder in youth. *Journal of Obsessive-Compulsive and Related Disorders, 14*, 90–98. doi:10.1016/j.jocrd.2017.06.006

Guzick, A. G., McNamara, J. P. H., Reid, A. M., Balkhi, A. M., Storch, E. A., Murphy, T. K.,... Geffken, G. R. (2017). The link between ADHD-like inattention and obsessions and compulsions during treatment of youth with OCD. *Journal of Obsessive-Compulsive and Related Disorders, 12*, 1–8. doi:10.1016/j.jocrd.2016.11.004

Halldorsdottir, T., & Ollendick, T. H. (2014). Comorbid ADHD: Implications for the treatment of anxiety disorders in children and adolescents. *Cogn Behav Pract, 21*(3), 310–322. doi:10.1016/j.cbpra.2013.08.003

Hashemiyoon, R., Kuhn, J., & Visser-Vandewalle, V. (2017). Putting the pieces together in Gilles de la Tourette Syndrome: Exploring the link between clinical observations and the biological basis of dysfunction. *Brain Topography, 30*(1), 3–29. doi:10.1007/s10548-016-0525-z

Heyman, I., Fombonne, E., Simmons, H., Ford, T., Meltzer, H., & Goodman, R. (2001). Prevalence of obsessive-compulsive disorder in the British nationwide survey of child mental health. *The British Journal of Psychiatry: The Journal of Mental Science, 179*(4), 324–329. doi:10.1192/bjp.179.4.324

Himle, J. A., Fischer, D. J., Van Etten, M. L., Janeck, A. S., & Hanna, G. L. (2003). Group behavioral therapy for adolescents with tic-related and non-tic-related obsessive-compulsive disorder. *Depression and Anxiety, 17*(2), 73–77. doi:10.1002/da.10088

Højgaard, D. R. M. A., Skarphedinsson, G., Nissen, J. B., Hybel, K. A., Ivarsson, T., & Thomsen, P. H. (2017). Pediatric obsessive-compulsive disorder with tic symptoms: clinical presentation and treatment outcome. *European Child & Adolescent Psychiatry, 26*(6), 681–689. doi:10.1007/s00787-016-0936-0

Hosenbocus, S., & Chahal, R. (2012). A review of executive function deficits and pharmacological management in children and adolescents. *J Can Acad Child Adolesc Psychiatry, 21*(3), 223–229.

Huyser, C., Veltman, D. J., de Haan, E., & Boer, F. (2009). Paediatric obsessive-compulsive disorder, a neurodevelopmental disorder?: Evidence from neuroimaging. *Neuroscience and Biobehavioral Reviews, 33*(6), 818–830.

Iniesta-Sepulveda, M., Nadeau, J. M., Ramos, A., Kay, B., Riemann, B. C., & Storch, E. A. (2017). An initial case series of intensive cognitive-behavioral therapy for obsessive-compulsive disorder in adolescents with autism spectrum disorder. *Child Psychiatry and Human Development.* doi:10.1007/s10578-017-0724-1

Insel, T. R., Hamilton, J. A., Guttmacher, L. B., & Murphy, D. L. (1983). D-amphetamine in obsessive-compulsive disorder. *Psychopharmacology, 80*(3), 231–235.

Ivarsson, T., & Melin, K. (2008). Autism spectrum traits in children and adolescents with obsessive-compulsive disorder (OCD). *Journal of Anxiety Disorders, 22*(6), 969–978. doi:10.1016/j.janxdis.2007.10.003

Ivarsson, T., Melin, K., & Wallin, L. (2008). Categorical and dimensional aspects of co-morbidity in obsessive-compulsive disorder (OCD). *European Child & Adolescent Psychiatry, 17*(1), 20–31. doi:10.1007/s00787-007-0626-z

Ivarsson, T., Skarphedinsson, G., Andersson, M., & Jarbin, H. (2017). The validity of the SCARED-R scale and sub-scales (accepted). *Child Psychiatry and Human Development.* doi:10.1007/s10578-017-0746-8

Ivarsson, T., Skarphedinsson, G., Kornør, H., Axelsdottir, B., Biedilae, S., Heyman, I.,... March, J. (2015). The place of and evidence for serotonin reuptake inhibitors (SRIs) for obsessive compulsive disorder (OCD) in children and adolescents: Views based on a systematic review and meta-analysis. *Psychiatry Research, 227*(1), 93–103. doi:10.1016/j.psychres.2015.01.015

Ivarsson, T., Weidle, B., Skarphedinsson, G., & Valderhaug, R. (2017). Neurobiological and neurodevelopmental perspectives on OCD and their clinical implications. In *The Wiley handbook of obsessive compulsive disorders* (pp. 283–310). Hoboken, NJ: John Wiley & Sons.

James, A. C., James, G., Cowdrey, F. A., Soler, A., & Choke, A. (2015). Cognitive behavioural therapy for anxiety disorders in children and adolescents. *Cochrane Database Syst Rev, 2*, CD004690. doi:10.1002/14651858.CD004690.pub4

Jarbin, H., Andersson, M., Rastam, M., & Ivarsson, T. (2017). Predictive validity of the K-SADS-PL 2009 version in school-aged and adolescent outpatients. *Nord J Psychiatry, 71*(4), 270–276. doi:10.1080/08039488.2016.1276622

Jhanda, S., Singla, N., & Grover, S. (2016). Methylphenidate-induced obsessive-compulsive symptoms: A case report and review of literature. *J Pediatr Neurosci, 11*(4), 316–318. doi:10.4103/1817-1745.199461

Joffe, R. T., Swinson, R. P., & Levitt, A. J. (1991). Acute psychostimulant challenge in primary obsessive-compulsive disorder. *J Clin Psychopharmacol, 11*(4), 237–241.

Kaufman, J., Birmaher, B., Brent, D., Rao, U., Flynn, C., Moreci, P.,... Ryan, N. (1997). Schedule for affective disorders and schizophrenia for school-age children-Present and lifetime version (K-SADS-PL): Initial reliability and validity data. *Journal of the American Academy of Child and Adolescent Psychiatry, 36*(7), 980–988. doi:10.1097/00004583-199707000-00021

King, J., Dowling, N., & Leow, F. (2017). Methylphenidate in the treatment of an adolescent female with obsessive-compulsive disorder and attention deficit hyperactivity disorder: A case report. *Australas Psychiatry, 25*(2), 178–180. doi:10.1177/1039856216671664

Kose, L. K., Fox, L., & Storch, E. A. (2017). Effectiveness of cognitive behavioral therapy for individuals with autism spectrum disorders and comorbid obsessive-compulsive disorder: A review of the research. *Journal of Developmental and Physical Disabilities.* doi:10.1007/s10882-017-9559-8

Krebs, G., Bolhuis, K., Heyman, I., Mataix-Cols, D., Turner, C., & Stringaris, A. (2013). Temper outbursts in paediatric obsessive-compulsive disorder and their association with depressed mood and treatment outcome. *Journal of Child Psychology and Psychiatry and Allied Disciplines, 54*(3), 313–322. doi:10.1111/j.1469-7610.2012.02605.x

Krebs, G., Murray, K., & Jassi, A. (2016). Modified cognitive behavior therapy for severe, treatment-resistant obsessive-compulsive disorder in an adolescent with autism spectrum disorder. *Journal of Clinical Psychology, 72*(11), 1162–1173. doi:10.1002/jclp.22396

Lebowitz, E. R., Omer, H., & Leckman, J. F. (2011). Coercive and disruptive behaviors in pediatric obsessive-compulsive disorder. *Depression and Anxiety, 28*(10), 899–905. doi:10.1002/da.20858

Leckman, J. F. (2002). Tourette's syndrome. *Lancet, 360*(9345), 1577–1586. doi:10.1016/S0140-6736(02)11526-1

Leckman, J. F., Grice, D. E., Barr, L. C., de Vries, A. L., Martin, C., Cohen, D. J.,... Rasmussen, S. A. (1994). Tic-related vs. non-tic-related obsessive compulsive disorder. *Anxiety, 1*(5), 208–215.

Lehmkuhl, H., Storch, E., Bodfish, J., & Geffken, G. (2008). Brief report: Exposure and response prevention for obsessive compulsive disorder in a 12-year-old with autism. *Journal of Autism and Developmental Disorders, 38*(5), 977–981. doi:10.1007/s10803-007-0457-2

March, J. S., Franklin, M. E., Leonard, H., Garcia, A., Moore, P., Freeman, J., & Foa, E. (2007). Tics moderate treatment outcome with sertraline but not cognitive-behavior therapy in pediatric obsessive-compulsive disorder. *Biol.Psychiatry, 61*(3), 344–347.

Masi, G., Millepiedi, S., Mucci, M., Bertini, N., Milantoni, L., & Arcangeli, F. (2005). A naturalistic study of referred children and adolescents with obsessive-compulsive disorder. *J Am Acad Child Adolesc.Psychiatry, 44*(7), 673–681.

Mattila, M. L., Hurtig, T., Haapsamo, H., Jussila, K., Kuusikko-Gauffin, S., Kielinen, M.,... Moilanen, I. (2010). Comorbid psychiatric disorders associated with Asperger syndrome/high-functioning autism: A community- and clinic-based study. *Journal of Autism and Developmental Disorders, 40*(9), 1080–1093. doi:10.1007/s10803-010-0958-2

McGuire, J. F., Piacentini, J., Brennan, E. A., Lewin, A. B., Murphy, T. K., Small, B. J., & Storch, E. A. (2014). A meta-analysis of behavior therapy for Tourette Syndrome. *Journal of Psychiatric Research, 50*, 106–112. doi:10.1016/j.jpsychires.2013.12.009

McPheeters, M. L., Warren, Z., Sathe, N., Bruzek, J. L., Krishnaswami, S., Jerome, R. N., & Veenstra-Vanderweele, J. (2011). A systematic review of medical treatments for children with autism spectrum disorders. *Pediatrics, 127*(5), e1312-1321. doi:10.1542/peds.2011-0427

Micali, N., Heyman, I., Perez, M., Hilton, K., Nakatani, E., Turner, C., & Mataix-Cols, D. (2010). Long-term outcomes of obsessive-compulsive disorder: Follow-up of 142 children and adolescents. *British Journal of Psychiatry, 197*(2), 128–134. doi:10.1192/bjp.bp.109.075317

Murphy, T. K., Lewin, A. B., Storch, E. A., Stock, S., American Academy of, C., & Adolescent Psychiatry Committee on Quality, I. (2013). Practice parameter for the assessment and treatment of children and adolescents with tic disorders. *Journal of the American Academy of Child and Adolescent Psychiatry, 52*(12), 1341–1359. doi:10.1016/j.jaac.2013.09.015

Murray, K., Jassi, A., Mataix-Cols, D., Barrow, F., & Krebs, G. (2015). Outcomes of cognitive behaviour therapy for obsessive-compulsive disorder in young people with and without autism spectrum disorders: A case controlled study. *Psychiatry Research, 228*(1), 8–13. doi:10.1016/j.psychres.2015.03.012

Piacentini, J., Bergman, R. L., Jacobs, C., McCracken, J. T., & Kretchman, J. (2002). Open trial of cognitive behavior therapy for childhood obsessive-compulsive disorder. *Journal of Anxiety Disorders, 16*(2), 207–219.

Piedad, J. C., Rickards, H. E., & Cavanna, A. E. (2012). What patients with gilles de la tourette syndrome should be treated with deep brain stimulation and what is the best target? *Neurosurgery, 71*(1), 173–192. doi:10.1227/NEU.0b013e3182535a00

Pringsheim, T., Hirsch, L., Gardner, D., & Gorman, D. A. (2015). The pharmacological management of oppositional behaviour, conduct problems, and aggression in children and adolescents with attention-deficit hyperactivity disorder, oppositional defiant disorder, and conduct disorder: A systematic review and meta-analysis. Part 2: Antipsychotics and traditional mood stabilizers. *Can J Psychiatry, 60*(2), 52–61. doi:10.1177/070674371506000203

Reaven, J., & Hepburn, S. (2003). Cognitive-behavioral treatment of obsessive-compulsive disorder in a child with Asperger syndrome: A case report. *Autism, 7*(2), 145–164.

Rettew, D. C., Lynch, A. D., Achenbach, T. M., Dumenci, L., & Ivanova, M. Y. (2009). Meta-analyses of agreement between diagnoses made from clinical evaluations and standardized diagnostic interviews. *Int J Methods Psychiatr Res, 18*(3), 169–184. doi:10.1002/mpr.289

Reynolds, S., Wilson, C., Austin, J., & Hooper, L. (2012). Effects of psychotherapy for anxiety in children and adolescents: A meta-analytic review. *Clinical Psychology Review, 32*(4), 251–262. doi:10.1016/j.cpr.2012.01.005

Robertson, M. M. (2000). Tourette syndrome, associated conditions and the complexities of treatment. *Brain, 123* (Pt 3), 425–462.

Roessner, V., Plessen, K. J., Rothenberger, A., Ludolph, A. G., Rizzo, R., Skov, L.,... Group, E. G. (2011). European clinical guidelines for Tourette syndrome and other tic disorders. Part II: pharmacological treatment. *European Child and Adolescent Psychiatry, 20*(4), 173–196. doi:10.1007/s00787-011-0163-7

Russell, A. J., Jassi, A., Fullana, M. A., Mack, H., Johnston, K., Heyman, I.,... Mataix-Cols, D. (2013). Cognitive behavior therapy for comorbid obsessive-compulsive disorder in high-functioning autism spectrum disorders: A randomized controlled trial. *Depression and Anxiety, 30*(8), 697–708. doi:10.1002/da.22053

Russell, A. J., Mataix-Cols, D., Anson, M., & Murphy, D. G. (2005). Obsessions and compulsions in Asperger syndrome and high-functioning autism. *The British Journal of Psychiatry: The Journal of Mental Science, 186*, 525–528. doi:10.1192/bjp.186.6.525

Scahill, L., Riddle, M. A., McSwiggin-Hardin, M., Ort, S. I., King, R. A., Goodman, W. K.,... Leckman, J. F. (1997). Children's Yale-Brown Obsessive Compulsive Scale: Reliability and validity. *Journal of the American Academy of Child and Adolescent Psychiatry, 36*(6), 844–852. doi:10.1097/00004583-199706000-00023

Schrock, L. E., Mink, J. W., Woods, D. W., Porta, M., Servello, D., Visser-Vandewalle, V.,... Registry Study, G. (2015). Tourette syndrome deep brain stimulation: A review and updated recommendations. *Movement Disorders: Official Journal of the Movement Disorder Society, 30*(4), 448–471. doi:10.1002/mds.26094

Selles, R. R., Arnold, E. B., Phares, V., Lewin, A. B., Murphy, T. K., & Storch, E. A. (2015). Cognitive-behavioral therapy for anxiety in youth with an autism spectrum disorder: A follow-up study. *Autism: The International Journal of Research and Practice, 19*(5), 613–621. doi:10.1177/1362361314537912

Silverman, W. K., Saavedra, L. M., & Pina, A. A. (2001). Test-retest reliability of anxiety symptoms and diagnoses with the Anxiety Disorders Interview Schedule for DSM-IV: Child and parent versions. *Journal of the American Academy of Child and Adolescent Psychiatry, 40*(8), 937–944. doi:10.1097/00004583-200108000-00016

Skarphedinsson, G., Compton, S., Thomsen, P. H., Weidle, B., Dahl, K., Nissen, J. B.,... Ivarsson, T. (2015). Tics moderate sertraline, but not cognitive-behavior therapy response in pediatric obsessive-compulsive disorder patients who do not respond to cognitive-behavior therapy. *J Child Adolesc Psychopharmacol, 25*(5), 432–439. doi:10.1089/cap.2014.0167

Solanto, M. V., Marks, D. J., Wasserstein, J., Mitchell, K., Abikoff, H., Alvir, J. M., & Kofman, M. D. (2010). Efficacy of meta-cognitive therapy for adult ADHD. *Am J Psychiatry, 167*(8), 958–968. doi:10.1176/appi.ajp.2009.09081123

Stewart, S. E., Geller, D. A., Jenike, M., Pauls, D., Shaw, D., Mullin, B., & Faraone, S. V. (2004). Long-term outcome of pediatric obsessive-compulsive disorder: A meta-analysis and qualitative review of the literature. *Acta Psychiatrica Scandinavica, 110*(1), 4–13.

Storch, E. A., Bjorgvinsson, T., Riemann, B., Lewin, A. B., Morales, M. J., & Murphy, T. K. (2010). Factors associated with poor response in cognitive-behavioral therapy for pediatric obsessive-compulsive disorder. *Bulletin of the Menninger Clinic, 74*(2), 167–185. doi:10.1521/bumc.2010.74.2.167

Storch, E. A., Jones, A. M., Lack, C. W., Ale, C. M., Sulkowski, M. L., Lewin, A. B.,... Murphy, T. K. (2012). Rage attacks in pediatric obsessive-compulsive disorder: Phenomenology and clinical correlates. *Journal of the American Academy of Child and Adolescent Psychiatry, 51*(6), 582–592. doi:10.1016/j.jaac.2012.02.016

Storch, E. A., Lewin, A. B., Geffken, G. R., Morgan, J. R., & Murphy, T. K. (2010). The role of comorbid disruptive behavior in the clinical expression of pediatric obsessive-compulsive disorder. *Behaviour Research and Therapy, 48*(12), 1204–1210. doi:10.1016/j.brat.2010.09.004

Storch, E. A., Lewin, A. B., Larson, M. J., Geffken, G. R., Murphy, T. K., & Geller, D. A. (2012). Depression in youth with obsessive-compulsive disorder: Clinical phenomenology and correlates. *Psychiatry Research, 196*(1), 83–89. doi:10.1016/j.psychres.2011.10.013

Storch, E. A., Merlo, L. J., Larson, M. J., Geffken, G. R., Lehmkuhl, H. D., Jacob, M. L.,... Goodman, W. K. (2008). Impact of comorbidity on cognitive-behavioral therapy response in pediatric obsessive-compulsive disorder. *Journal of the American Academy of Child and Adolescent Psychiatry, 47*(5), 583–592.

Strawn, J. R., Welge, J. A., Wehry, A. M., Keeshin, B., & Rynn, M. A. (2015). Efficacy and tolerability of antidepressants in pediatric anxiety disorders: A systematic review and meta-analysis. *Depression and Anxiety, 32*(3), 149–157. doi:10.1002/da.22329

Sukhodolsky, D. G., Bloch, M. H., Panza, K. E., & Reichow, B. (2013). Cognitive-behavioral therapy for anxiety in children with high-functioning autism: A meta-analysis. *Pediatrics, 132*(5), e1341-1350. doi:10.1542/peds.2013-1193

Sukhodolsky, D. G., Gorman, B. S., Scahill, L., Findley, D., & McGuire, J. (2013). Exposure and response prevention with or without parent management training for children with obsessive-compulsive disorder complicated by disruptive behavior: A multiple-baseline across-responses design study. *Journal of Anxiety Disorders, 27*(3), 298–305. doi:10.1016/j.janxdis.2013.01.005

Torp, N. C., Dahl, K., Skarphedinsson, G., Compton, S., Thomsen, P. H., Weidle, B., ... Ivarsson, T. (2015). Predictors associated with improved cognitive-behavioral therapy outcome in pediatric obsessive-compulsive disorder. *Journal of the American Academy of Child and Adolescent Psychiatry, 54*(3), 200–207 e201. doi:10.1016/j.jaac.2014.12.007

van Steensel, F. J., Bogels, S. M., & Perrin, S. (2011). Anxiety disorders in children and adolescents with autistic spectrum disorders: A meta-analysis. *Clinical Child and Family Psychology Review, 14*(3), 302–317. doi:10.1007/s10567-011-0097-0

Verdellen, C., van de Griendt, J., Hartmann, A., Murphy, T., & Group, E. G. (2011). European clinical guidelines for Tourette syndrome and other tic disorders. Part III: Behavioural and psychosocial interventions. *European Child & Adolescent Psychiatry, 20*(4), 197–207. doi:10.1007/s00787-011-0167-3

Verdellen, C. W., Keijsers, G. P., Cath, D. C., & Hoogduin, C. A. (2004). Exposure with response prevention versus habit reversal in Tourette's syndrome: A controlled study. *Behaviour Research and Therapy, 42*(5), 501–511. doi:10.1016/S0005-7967(03)00154-2

Weidle, B., Jozefiak, T., Ivarsson, T., & Thomsen, P. (2014). Quality of life in children with OCD with and without comorbidity. *Health Qual Life Outcomes, 12*(1), 152. doi:10.1186/s12955-014-0152-x

Weidle, B., Melin, K., Drotz, E., Jozefiak, T., & Ivarsson, T. (2012). Preschool and current autistic symptoms in children and adolescents with obsessive-compulsive disorder (OCD). *Journal of Obsessive-Compulsive and Related Disorders, 1*(3), 168–174. doi:10.1016/j.jocrd.2012.04.002

Williams, K., Brignell, A., Randall, M., Silove, N., & Hazell, P. (2013). Selective serotonin reuptake inhibitors (SSRIs) for autism spectrum disorders (ASD). *Cochrane Database Syst Rev, 8*(8), CD004677. doi:10.1002/14651858.CD004677.pub3

Wolters, L. H., de Haan, E., Hogendoorn, S. M., Boer, F., & Prins, P. J. M. (2016). Severe pediatric obsessive compulsive disorder and co-morbid autistic symptoms: Effectiveness of cognitive behavioral therapy. *Journal of Obsessive-Compulsive and Related Disorders, 10*, 69–77. doi:10.1016/j.jocrd.2016.06.002

Worbe, Y., Mallet, L., Golmard, J. L., Behar, C., Durif, F., Jalenques, I., ... Hartmann, A. (2010). Repetitive behaviours in patients with Gilles de la Tourette syndrome: Tics, compulsions, or both? *PLoS One, 5*(9), e12959. doi:10.1371/journal.pone.0012959

Yang, C., Hao, Z., Zhu, C., Guo, Q., Mu, D., & Zhang, L. (2016). Interventions for tic disorders: An overview of systematic reviews and meta analyses. *Neuroscience and Biobehavioral Reviews, 63*, 239–255. doi:10.1016/j.neubiorev.2015.12.013

22 Transdiagnostic Approaches

Yolanda E. Murphy, Anna Luke, and
Christopher A. Flessner

Introduction

Pediatric obsessive-compulsive disorder (OCD) is a debilitating disorder that is highly heterogeneous in presentation and course. Symptoms are highly variable across several established clusters, with themes of symmetry/ordering, religious/forbidden thoughts, contamination/cleaning, doubts about harm/checking, and collecting/hoarding (Williams et al., 2014; Alvarenga et al., 2015). These symptom dimensions are associated with distinct differences in familial components, neurological substrates, comorbidity patterns, and treatment outcome (Leckman, Bloch, & King, 2009; Ivarsson & Valdergaug, 2006). Age of onset also varies and appears to be bimodal, with a mean age of onset of 10 years of age for children and 21 years of age for adults. Despite differences in clinical presentation, one known aspect of pediatric OCD is that comorbid psychiatric disorders are the rule rather than the exception. In addition to being associated with increased OCD symptom severity and poorer treatment response, comorbid symptoms further complicate the presentation and hinder treatment of an already heterogeneous disorder. The purpose of this chapter is to highlight the use of transdiagnostic treatments to target OCD and comorbid disorders. Additionally, relevant clinical research on mediators and moderators of treatment change for transdiagnostic interventions are discussed.

Overview of the Issue

Pediatric OCD is highly comorbid with other psychological disorders, with research estimates suggesting that up to 80 percent of youth with OCD have at least one comorbid disorder (Lewin et al., 2010; Storch et al., 2008), with most studies reporting multiple comorbid conditions (Marcks et al., 2011). At a diagnostic level, the Diagnostic and Statistical Manual of Mental Disorders-Fifth Edition (DSM-V) recognizes 14 other disorders that broadly share OCD symptoms (e.g., Body Dysmorphic Disorder, Trichotillomania) and thus must be considered by clinicians (Gillan, Fineberg, & Robbins, 2017). For children in particular, the age at which comorbidities first develop may impact the clinical profile and further development of this already highly heterogeneous disorder (de Mathis et al., 2013). Thus, comorbidities present both diagnostic- and treatment-specific challenges, as well as impact individuals on a more global level of overall burden, all of which are associated with protracted illness (Mancebo et al., 2014).

Patterns of Comorbidity in Pediatric OCD. Research demonstrates a well-established relationship between childhood OCD and tic disorders (TD), including Tourette syndrome and chronic motor/vocal tics. Research supports a bidirectional association between these disorders, with an estimated 40 to 50 percent of children with TD meeting the criteria for an OCD diagnosis (Kostek et al., 2016; Lebowitz et al., 2012), and an estimated 20 to 38 percent of children with OCD reporting comorbid tics (Lewin & Piacentini., 2010). Adults with comorbid OCD and TD are more likely to endorse symptoms of violent/sexual thoughts and imagery, and endorse higher rates of psychiatric disorders such as Attention Deficit Hyperactive Disorder (ADHD), trichotillomania, and body dysmorphic disorder (Bennett et al., 2015). There has been comparatively less research within pediatric populations and therefore evidence is less conclusive. Evidence for differences in obsessional content and additional comorbidities is mixed, with most studies finding no difference in OCD severity in those with and without comorbid TD (Bennett et al., 2015). However, compared to children without comorbid TD, those with dual diagnoses are more likely to have an earlier age of onset of OCD symptoms, have greater impairments in psychological function, and endorse worse overall quality of life (Lebowitz et al., 2012; Pringsheim, 2017). Notably, high prevalence rate and bidirectional overlap between OCD and TDs have led to the addition of a "tic-related specifier" to OCD in the DSM-V, leading some to believe that co-occurring OCD and TD may be a specific subtype of OCD.

Although younger and older children have similar rates of comorbidities, the specific cluster of other common comorbidities differs by age. ADHD and Oppositional Defiant Disorder (ODD) are among the most common comorbid diagnoses found within younger populations (i.e., before the age of 12; Boileau, 2011; Bennett et al., 2015), with estimates ranging from 15 to 51 percent (Farrell et al., 2006; Geller et al., 2001). Both ADHD and ODD are associated with increased OCD symptom severity, as well as attenuated treatment response and remission rates (Farrell et al., 2012; Kameg et al., 2015). For example, the interruption of compulsive rituals by others can lead to increased distress that may evolve into behavioral disturbances among most children, yet may be exacerbated among youths with ODD (Barton & Heyman, 2013). Furthermore, it is possible that ADHD interferes with treatment due to inattentiveness to relevant concepts and executive functioning deficits that impede with independent planning needed in therapy, such as homework assignments (Storch et al., 2008).

Similarly, greater levels of comorbid anxiety are associated with greater impairment in pediatric OCD and are highly prevalent among youths 10 years of age and older (Micali et al., 2010; Skriner et al., 2016). It is possible that up to 55 percent of youth with OCD meet criteria for an anxiety diagnosis, further complicating the clinical profile of OCD (Bennett et al., 2015; Fineberg et al., 2013). In pediatric samples, both increased levels of anxiety and OCD symptom severity are associated with attrition in treatment studies (Aderka et al., 2011; Knopp et al., 2013). What is more, clients with comorbid anxiety may be more likely to exhibit avoidance tendencies that block adherence to exposure treatment (Jakubovski et al., 2013). Previous research among youths has also found comorbid internalizing symptoms to be a predictor of negative cognitive behavioral therapy (CBT) outcomes, such that children with higher levels of symptoms had poorer outcomes than those with lower levels (Torp et al., 2015). Conversely, several studies have found that comorbid anxiety disorders are associated with a larger treatment effect size, with the robust response possibly linked to more fear-based symptomology in children (Öst et al., 2016).

Lastly, high rates of comorbidity between OCD and autism spectrum disorder (ASD) and autistic traits have been found in clinical youth samples (Griffiths et al., in press; Farrell et al., 2012; Lewin et al., 2010). Prevalence rates from epidemiological studies vary widely, from 8 to 81 percent (Stone & Chen, 2016). This may be due in part to the difficulty in distinguishing OCD from ASD, given their shared characteristics of stereotyped behaviors and rigid interests (Reaven & Hepburn, 2003) that result in repetitive acts and cognitive preoccupations. Unsurprisingly, the compounded symptoms of comorbid OCD and ASD symptoms may elicit considerable distress (Wu, Rudy, & Storch, 2014), with dual diagnoses linked to increased psychosocial impairment and worsened response to CBT compared to those with a singular OCD diagnosis (Griffiths et al., 2017; Krebs & Heyman, 2014; Murray et al., 2015).

Traditional versus Transdiagnostic Approaches to Treatment. In traditional therapy, therapists typically rank order treatment goals at the start of their intervention, and then work sequentially targeting one problem at a time (Barlow, Allen, & Choate, 2004). Although this approach is evidence-based, it is also associated with a number of problems for both clients with multiple clinical problems and their therapists. For example, within the context of pediatric OCD, comorbidities may lead to shifting symptom profiles over time, as well as exacerbating functional impairment (Chu, 2012). Increased comorbidity of OCD with other disorders may also confound clinicians' ability to accurately evaluate and identify OCD specific symptoms. Consequently, clinicians can face challenges choosing the appropriate disorder-specific treatment protocol and intervention targets, thus delaying treatment of comorbid disorders (Clark & Taylor, 2009). In addition to having a known negative effect on treatment outcome, targeting comorbidities independently or sequentially presents additional problems for therapies such as Exposure with Response Prevention (ERP; Abramowitz, 2004). For example, a child with OCD and a comorbid disruptive disorder may be unmotivated and resistant to therapy tasks (e.g., confronting exposure stimuli), and may exhibit disruptive behaviors (e.g., temper tantrums) that impede the therapist's ability to conduct exposures (Storch et al., 2008). Thus, it may better serve the child to choose an integrative approach that targets both OCD and ODD symptoms simultaneously. In addition to complications of comorbid conditions, some disorder-specific protocols may be unable to address external factors known to influence the maintenance of OCD (Storch et al., 2010). For example, CBT treatments that do not specifically address family-based components may be impeded by the effects of family accommodation, which are antithetical to the goals of CBT (Francazio et al., 2016). Given the limitations of disorder-specific treatments in addressing the complicating factors of comorbidities, there is increasing interest in the development and use of more unified treatments that are integrated or modifiable in order to address multiple disorders.

In contrast to traditional treatments, transdiagnostic treatments are defined as intervention protocols that employ the same core treatment principles for use beyond a specific diagnosis (i.e., without tailoring the protocol to specific disorder; McEvoy, Nathan, & Norton, 2009). Strong transdiagnostic treatments must be flexible enough to address multiple psychiatric symptoms, as well as be conceptually matched to treatment goals (Ehrenreich-May & Chu, 2013). A strong streamlined protocol that targets underlying mechanistic factors may allow for reduction in treatment length and cost, as well as minimize training time and case formulation for multiple psychiatric illnesses (Cougle, 2012). The following sections will highlight two such treatments and how they might be applied to pediatric OCD. Notably, transdiagnostic treatments are a relatively new area, particularly for OCD, and even more so for pediatric OCD. As such, this chapter will draw evidence from the adult OCD literature as needed to illustrate the approach.

Description of Approaches to Innovation

Cognitive Remediation Therapy (CRT)

Cognitive Remediation Therapy is a broad term referring to various cognitive and skill-building exercises intended to improve cognitive impairments and rigid, maladaptive thinking styles found in several disorders. In OCD, evidence suggests that the repetitive, automated behaviors may be a result of impairments in executive functioning (Grant et al., 2016). Deficits in visuo-spatial memory, set-shifting, and cognitive inflexibility are among those that OCD shares with other disorders, and are associated with abnormalities in the fronto-striatal brain structure (Shin et al., 2014; Grant et al., 2016). CRT was originally developed for the treatment of cognitive deficits in individuals with traumatic brain injury, but has since been extended as a transdiagnostic treatment of psychological disorders with cognitive impairments. As such, CRT may represent a plausible alternative for the transdiagnostic treatments of children with OCD and related disorders.

The delivery and content of CRT exercises, while highly variable, are based on core aspects incorporating training of flexibility, cognitive exercises, and real-life situation exercises. Specific modules are broken down into cognitive exercises and practical skills. Cognitive restorative exercises involve the repetitive completion of attention and memory tasks, such as those targeting sensory representations of environmental stimuli (e.g., block design) that are aimed at improving cognitive functioning (Medalia & Bowie, 2016). To improve client awareness of cognitive biases and inflexibility, neurocognitive exercises are often paired with strategy-based, metacognition components that encourage clients to "think about thinking [styles]" and replace maladaptive information processing strategies with more efficient ones (Tchanturia & Davies, 2010). Task emphasis and intervention modules can be individualized based upon relevant disorder-specific impairments, such as deficits in goal-directed behavior, planning, and set-shifting/cognitive flexibility commonly found in OCD (Gillan, Fineberg, & Robbins, 2017; van den Heuvel et al., 2005). For example, Buhlmann et al. (2006) developed an intervention to improve visual-spatial memory in adults with OCD using recall tasks of complex geometric figures. Participants were taught adaptive skills such as prioritizing drawing basic meaningful units before details. Visual-spatial exercises such as this aim to enhance a client's awareness of object location and improve learning and recall strategies. Neurocognitive exercises can also be delivered via a computer, an approach that has also been used with adults with hoarding disorder (DiMauro et al., 2014). Both neuro- and meta-cognitive methods can be delivered as an adjunctive or stand-alone treatment for various comorbid disorders.

Modified Exposure and Response Prevention (ERP)

ERP is a therapist-guided set of behavioral techniques addressing obsessions and compulsions concurrently. Pathological fear responses of obsessions and compulsions are reduced through (a) prolonged, systemic exposure to feared stimuli and situations, and (b) voluntary prevention of carrying out maladaptive compulsive or safety-seeking behaviors done to avoid or reduce stress (Abramowitz & Jacoby, 2014). Preventing compulsive rituals allows the client to learn that the intrusive thoughts, images, or situations are not high-risk, and that the anxiety will go away even if the ritual is not performed. This in turn reduces fear and other negative reactions previously used to alleviate obsession-generated anxiety (Abramowitz & Jacoby, 2014; Zohar, 2012). Briefly, traditional ERP for pediatric OCD typically includes psychoeducation for the parent and child (i.e., information about OCD and ERP implementation), compilation of the child's anxiety provoking situations, development of a fear hierarchy, and implementation of exposures with response prevention. While ERP can incorporate the established components from other therapies to address clinical comorbidities (e.g., cognitive restructuring), the behavioral components of ERP are typically considered the active ingredient for reduction of OCD symptoms (Lombroso & Scahill, 2008).

In contrast to traditional versions of ERP, transdiagnostic versions target shared psychological processes that underlie certain classes of disorders and thus serve as maintaining factors for comorbid symptoms. These processes may be cognitive-affective thinking styles (such as thought action fusion) or broad personality traits, such as perfectionism. Both thought-action fusion and perfectionism are known risk factors for OCD, anxiety disorders, and eating disorders (Coughtry et al., 2017; Gutner et al., 2016). Perfectionism, in particular, is a well-established transdiagnostic risk factor for psychopathology and comorbidities in general (Hood & Antony, 2016), as well as in OCD-related disorders such as hoarding disorder, body dysmorphic disorder, and trichotillomania (Pinto et al., 2017). In OCD, perfectionism can be frequently seen in the client's need for certainty that can lead to doubting/

checking or for things to be "just right" (McKay & Mancusi, 2015). Elevated levels of perfectionism have been shown to impede ERP treatment response in both children and adults with OCD (Egan, Wade, & Shafran, 2011). Given its role in multiple psychiatric disorders, several treatments have been created specifically targeting the personality dimensions, such as CBT for perfectionism (CBT-P; Egan et al., 2014). CBT-P protocols are intended to fundamentally change a client's viewpoints through changing broad behaviors and situations and teaching the client to respond more flexibly.

Although no such protocol exists for pediatric OCD, it has been noted that CBT-P and ERP contain many similarities and are thus likely compatible (Pinto et al., 2017). For example, a CBT-P for eating disorders protocol developed by Fairburn, Cooper, and Shafran (2003) consists of four key elements that could easily be adapted for OCD symptoms: "(1) identifying perfectionism as a problem and establishing its maintaining mechanisms (e.g., repeated performance checking and avoidance); (2) conducting behavioral experiments to challenge perfectionism-related beliefs (e.g., reducing the frequency of checking behavior, exposure to avoided situations); (3) cognitive-behavioral methods to address the individual's personal standards, rigidity, and self-criticism; (4) broadening the individual's self-evaluation by adopting alternative ways of thinking and behaving" (Pinto et al., 2017). Such targets from CBT-P could be modified to specifically target OCD fears surrounding uncertainty/doubting, incompleteness, or just not right fears (Pinto et al., 2017). Additionally, interventions targeting perfectionism in adults provide evidence for the reduction of symptoms across a range of disorders (Egan et al., 2011).

ERP for OCD can also be modified within a transdiagnostic context by focusing on maintaining repetitive behaviors seen across disorders. For example, Verdellen and colleagues (2008) applied a modified version of ERP to young adults with tics. Participants completed training sessions in which they were asked to refrain from engaging in tics for as long as possible. The therapist kept track of how long the tic was able to be suppressed. If a tic occurred, the therapist encouraged the participant to increase their effort. In the exposure response sessions, participants attempted to suppress tics and impulses for 2 consecutive hours. Participants were asked to focus on the internal and sensory experiences, as well as corresponding body sensations, while being encouraged by the therapist to continue refraining from the tic behavior. When the urge to perform the tic abated, ERP was then applied to other relevant sensations and urges.

ERP has also been tailored with family-based modifications for comorbidities such as anxiety, ODD, and ADHD (Ale & Krackow, 2011). Children with OCD often exhibit disruptive or coercive behaviors such as verbal/physical aggression, nagging, and "emotional blackmail," such as accusing the parent of not caring if they refuse to accommodate the obsessional behavior (Lebowitz, Panza, & Bloch, 2016). Thus, modifying ERP for parental involvement may improve treatment outcome (Taboas et al., 2015) and reduce comorbid anxiety symptoms. Treatment strategies for more coercive behavior include skills training to improve attention and positive feedback for appropriate behavior, setting consistent limits and expectations, and setting time-outs for negative behavior (Forehand, Jones, & Parent, 2013). An example of traditional ERP modified to include family-based involvement may be found in the core components of Cognitive Behavioral Family-Based Treatment (CBFT) – an intervention developed for young children with OCD by Freeman and colleagues (2003). CBFT decreases the focus on cognitive components to some ERP-based protocols and, in its place, significantly increases the role of intervention techniques designed to target the family's involvement in the client's OCD and related symptoms. Parents are trained as ERP instructors for their children. The authors note that asking parents to tolerate their own distress (that may arise while assisting their children with distressing exposures or homework) also serves as its own "exposure" function for parents (Freeman et al., 2008).

Similar work has been applied in preschool children, targeting OCD and associated behavioral problems (Ginsburg et al., 2011). Within this treatment protocol, an emphasis is placed upon reducing anxiety-enhancing parenting behaviors, increasing knowledge of effective problem-solving skills, and improving behavioral strategies for dealing with problematic behaviors. As with CBFT, children are exposed to feared stimuli with the aid of the parents while clinicians provide modeling and feedback to parents; however, the authors also incorporate behavioral strategies for targeting oppositional behaviors (i.e., ignoring bad behaviors, communicating commands effectively, encouraging via parent-child interaction tasks). Thus, in some instances, CBFT may be used as an effective manner by which to target both OCD-related, other anxiety-, and oppositional behaviors in youths. An interpretation of possible applications for pediatric OCD can be found in the case illustration described as follows.

Evidence Base for Innovation

Cognitive Remediation Therapy (CRT)

To date, cognitive remediation has received no empirical investigation among children with OCD and only two studies have investigated the use of cognitive remediation among adults with OCD. In one such study, Park and colleagues (2006) administered 5 weeks of cognitive training aimed at executive functioning processes often impaired with OCD (i.e., organization and memory). Fifteen participants were randomly selected to receive CRT and 15 participants were randomly assigned to a control condition. Participants in the training received nine, 60-minute sessions (twice a week) during which they were taught visual organizational strategies and everyday problem-solving skills. Participants in the control condition received no treatment aside from medications already taken at the start of the study. Posttreatment findings indicated that participants in the CRT group demonstrated greater symptom improvement (with notably greater alleviation from obsessions compared to compulsions) and memory improvement compared to the control group (as indicated by scores on the Yale Brown-Obsessive Compulsive Scale and Rey-Osterrieth Complex Figure Test, respectively). Findings of cognitive improvement are similarly indicated in Buhlman's 2006 study, in which researchers developed a

CRT intervention to improve visual-spatial memory in adults with OCD using recall tasks of complex geometric figures. Though specific changes in OCD symptoms were not assessed, findings did indicate that participants who received CRT demonstrated improved organizational skills compared to those who did not receive training.

Cognitive remediation has also been preliminarily assessed within hoarding disorder to improve cognitive function. Though a disorder now distinct from OCD (i.e., hoarding disorder is not characterized by key OCD symptoms such as intrusive/ unwanted thoughts), compulsive hoarding has historically been considered a subtype of OCD and may manifest as an OCD-related symptom (e.g., an individual's obsessions and compulsions may contribute to hoarding behaviors; Mataix-Cols et al., 2010). In a 2014 pilot study, DiMauro and colleagues assigned 17 participants with hoarding disorder to either a cognitive remediation trial or relaxation training. Participants in the cognitive remediation trial received eight weeks of computerized cognitive exercises designed to improve attention, while participants in relaxation training received eight weeks of meditation and stress reduction exercises. Though neither group demonstrated significant improvements in hoarding symptoms, results did indicate that cognitive remediation was highly feasible (i.e., high attendance for sessions, high ratings of participant satisfaction, no treatment drop-out) and participants who received this treatment demonstrated greater improvements in attention compared to those who received relaxation training. From this, the authors suggest that CRT may be a beneficial adjunct to CBT for hoarding disorder (e.g., alleviating attention deficits that may improve CBT response and/or engagement); however, additional research is necessary (e.g., replication, randomized control trial with CRT as an adjunct).

Interestingly, though research examining CRT within adult populations with OCD is scarce, and not existent for youths, the findings from the adult literature discussed previously mirror previous research demonstrating the efficacy of CRT for other disorders characterized by cognitive difficulties similar to those found among children with OCD (e.g., anorexia nervosa, schizophrenia, and ADHD; Dahlgren & Stedal, 2017; O'Connell, 2006; Wykes et al., 2007). This prior work, both within and outside the field of OCD research, suggests that CRT (particularly for organizational strategies and attention) may hold promise as a feasible and potentially efficacious intervention for improving symptoms and cognitive deficits in patients with OCD and comorbidities; however, additional research is clearly warranted and this is particularly true within youth populations.

Modifying Exposure and Response Prevention (ERP)

As discussed previously, transdiagnostic versions of ERP may be adapted to target shared psychological processes (e.g., perfectionism) underlying comorbidities. Though such interventions have yet to be assessed in an OCD transdiagnostic context, burgeoning research in distinct disorders demonstrates promising results. For example, literature assessing the effects of cognitive behavioral therapies for perfectionism across various disorders (e.g., eating disorders, anxiety, depression) demonstrates efficacy within both child and adult samples – though child studies are relatively scarce (Fairburn et al., 2003; Morris & Lomax, 2014; Steele et al., 2013). Similar to CRT however, no research has assessed these interventions among children with OCD and only one study to date has assessed CBT for perfectionism (i.e., CBT-P) in adult OCD. In this study, Sadri and colleagues (2017) conducted a pilot intervention comparing the effects of an eight-week group CBT-P to an eight-week wait-list. Results indicated that CBT-P was associated with improvements in perfectionism and OCD severity; however, changes were not considered to be clinically significant and drop-out rates throughout the intervention were high. This suggests that while CBT-P may have some benefit for OCD, additional research is clearly necessary. Such investigation may focus on improving intervention feasibility (e.g., increasing use of motivation strategies, beginning with individual rather than group therapy), integrating additional components targeting OCD symptoms to improve treatment efficacy (e.g., augmenting cognitive strategies with traditional ERP), and expanding intervention scope to child samples.

Further modifications to ERP may also address cross cutting domains such as family risk factors (e.g., CBFT). Available research – though limited – suggests that these modifications are efficacious (Freeman et al., 2003; Freeman et al., 2014). For example, Ginsburg's (2011) study assessed CBFT among seven young children with OCD. Within this study, CBFT consisted of 12 alternating sessions of ERP and parent intervention aimed at modifying family risk factors for OCD (e.g., reduction in anxiety enhancing parenting behaviors, behavioral strategies). Results indicated that family-based ERP was feasible (i.e., high levels of treatment satisfaction) and successful in reducing both OCD symptoms (i.e., six out of seven children identified as treatment responders, with a 33 to 66 percent reduction in CYBOCS scores) and parental accommodation. Improvements were maintained at a one-month follow-up.

Similarly, in a comorbid context, Ale and Krackow (2011) examined family modifications to ERP for the concurrent treatment of OCD and ODD. In this study, authors administered a 16-session protocol integrating ERP and behavioral parent training to a 6-year-old child with comorbid OCD and ODD and his mother. The authors' case conceptualization indicated that the child's OCD and ODD were related in that his undesirable behaviors (e.g., tantrums, noncompliance, aggression) stemmed from an inability to avoid anxiety inducing experiences and his mother's permissive parenting. Integrated treatment included core components of ERP (e.g., gradual exposure using fear hierarchies) and parent training (e.g., teaching the mother to implement token-economies, time out). Interestingly, although these components targeted their specific disorders, they also facilitated treatment of the comorbidity as well. For example, in one exposure task the child became frustrated and threw a pencil at his mother. Pulling from parent training skills his mother appropriately placed him in time out for his aggressive behavior, yet continued with ongoing exposures. Assessment at the 3½-month follow-up indicated a decrease in anxiety, obsessions, and compulsions, as well as a decrease in externalizing symptoms. Although limited by the general dearth of research within this area, these studies suggest that CBFT (i.e., family-based ERP) may be a feasible and efficacious approach for OCD comorbidities highlighted by strong familiar risk factors and warrants further research.

Beyond family-based treatment, ERP has also been assessed for repetitive behaviors, such as those seen in tic disorders, albeit in only one study. Verdellen and colleagues (2004) examined the treatment efficacy of ERP versus habit reversal therapy, an evidence-based therapeutic approach utilized frequently among patients with tic disorders, in 43 young adults with Tourette's syndrome. Results indicated that participants in both treatments demonstrated significant improvements (as indicated by scores received on the Yale Global Tic Severity Scale and tic frequency registrations). Although clearly requiring replication, this suggests that among young adults, ERP may be a viable transdiagnostic option for clients presenting with not only OCD but also other disorders characterized by compulsive or ritualized behaviors. Furthermore, this approach may be particularly beneficial for clients presenting with tic-related OCD. Thus, future research specifically within child populations is needed.

Mediators and Moderators of Change

Given scant research assessing the transdiagnostic treatment of children with OCD and comorbidities, it is perhaps unsurprising that no research exists examining mechanisms of change in these treatments (i.e., mediators and moderators). Therefore, to initiate identification of these mechanisms, clinicians and researchers are strongly advised to consider the underlying theory at the core of the previously discussed interventions, as well as existing research in which these mechanisms are investigated for disorder specific treatments. For example, theory underlying CRT posits that cognitive exercises will improve cognitive deficits noted in various psychological disorders (by strengthening and refining neural circuits), in turn alleviating a risk or maintaining factor of the pathology. Similarly, researchers hypothesize that remediation tasks (such as those designed to improve planning) may also improve clients' real life coping skills (i.e., ability to cope with and manage response to environmental stressors), subsequently leading to improvements in overall functioning; Wykes & Spaulding, 2011). Based on such theory, mediators of a pediatric transdiagnostic CRT may include improvements in client cognitive functioning and coping skills. Though initial studies examining CRT across various disorders indicate improvements in cognitive/executive functioning and disorder symptoms subsequent to remediation intervention, such findings are mixed and warrant further replication within research protocols seeking to utilize CRT within a pediatric OCD (and related comorbidity) context (Eack et al., 2011; Urben et al., 2012). Further, in a review of CRT for schizophrenia, Wykes and Spaulding (2011) concluded that therapist expertise may moderate remediation effects (i.e., therapists with lower levels of training demonstrated less beneficial effects). This may suggest that, for CRT, therapist expertise that is either nonspecific (e.g., ability to increase therapy motivation, engagement) or specific to CRT (e.g., ability to administer appropriate remediation skills) is an integral component of change. Considering the limitations of this finding (i.e., findings based on one form of remediation therapy with an adult sample), additional research with children and within an OCD-related context is warranted.

With respect to modified ERP, mediators may include mechanisms currently identified for traditional ERP (e.g., client and treatment factors including adaptive client development of cognitive and behavioral coping behaviors, therapy variables such as cognitive strategies and extent of exposures administered; Chu et al., 2015), as well as mediators associated with specific integrated components. For example, mediators of change for family-based ERP integrating behavioral parenting may include both traditional ERP mediators and mediators of behavioral parent training (e.g., changes in parenting behavior; Forehand et al., 2014). In a similar fashion, moderators of transdiagnostic treatments, particularly modified ERP, may also include moderators related to traditional ERP (e.g., disorder severity, level of insight, family accommodation, comorbidity, and parental anxiety; Flessner et al., 2011; Garcia et al., 2010), and moderators related to added components (e.g., moderators of behavioral training, habit reversal therapy). Clinicians and researchers may also wish to consider the moderating role of therapy specific variables (e.g., number/lengths of sessions, therapeutic alliance, therapist experience) in relation to treatment outcome.

Clinical Case Illustration

As noted previously, evidence for the transdiagnostic treatment for youths with OCD and related problems is currently nonexistent. As such, the following case illustration demonstrates an example of modified ERP for within a hypothetical therapeutic context.

Max is an 8-year-old Caucasian boy brought to a pediatric psychology outpatient clinic by his mother at the beginning of his summer break. Max lived at home with his stay-at-home mother, his older sister, and his father, who worked long hours during the week. At the beginning of the school year, Max became increasingly worried about dirt and becoming "contaminated." At the time of initial intake, he insisted upon carrying liquid sanitizer with him at all times and required his mother to regularly (i.e., multiple times each day) clean surfaces at home. Max's teacher expressed concern at the frequency of his hand-washing at the classroom sink, as well as his disruptive behavior when other children touched his desk. Max refused to wear any of his "outside" clothing into his room at home and showered twice a day for excessive amounts of time. His family reported that Max becomes extremely distressed if his mother does not wash his towels or common surfaces after each use, and throws tantrums until one of his parents complies with this requirement. Max reported feeling nervous that he would make his family members sick from germs and reported frequent nightmares in which his family became deathly ill. Max's mother reported that his sister had become very frustrated with his cleaning demands concerning their shared bathroom. Max was unable to touch public tables or surfaces without distress, and as a result, Max's parents stopped going to restaurants for family dinners. In addition to germ-related fears, Max reported feeling constantly worried that something bad would happen to his mother. For example, Max began to dissolve into tears and worry whenever his mother left the house, and insisted that she remain near him during playdates, which became infrequent. At the start of summer break, Max's mother reported spending a large portion of her day cleaning and reassuring Max, which she described as the impetus behind seeking services. The therapist believed that Max had a primary diagnosis of OCD, as well as separation anxiety disorder. The following illustration is an example of how modified ERP could be used to address Max's comorbid symptoms. Based on previous family-based interventions, the therapist decided on a 12-session Modified ERP treatment (Ginsburg et al., 2011). Sessions would alternate between joint ERP sessions with Max and his mother and individual sessions focusing on specific behavioral strategies targeted at Max's mother.

Case Conceptualization. Max experienced distress stemming from perfectionistic tendencies, as evidenced by his obsessions and compulsions around cleaning. Additionally, Max experienced behavioral avoidance as manifested in both OCD and separation anxiety symptoms, seen in his inability to a) experience negative affect without attempting to decrease distress without compulsions and b) be left alone. Both comorbid disorders were perpetuated by his parents' reinforcing behaviors, which possibly worsened Max's symptom severity by limiting his opportunities to disconfirm his fears surrounding cleanliness and loneliness. Transdiagnostic targets were thus chosen as a means of reducing parent-child dyad anxiety/accommodation and behavioral avoidance, improving negative affect tolerance, and altering Max's perfectionistic thinking style via family-based ERP.

Treatment. During the first sessions, the therapist obtained baseline measures and a functional assessment of Max's obsessions (fear triggers), his cognitive explanation for obsessional fears, and his subsequent compulsive rituals. Max, his mother, and the therapist worked together to generate treatment goals. Max wanted to be able to shower and clean less, to feel comfortable touching other surfaces, and to worry less about his mother. In a joint session, the therapist explained the symptoms and causes of OCD in a developmentally appropriate manner to Max, before providing his mother with psychoeducation on the symptoms and maintaining factors of OCD and separation anxiety. The therapist had Max's mother describe the ways that she and her husband responded to his various obsessions in order to identify and target parental accommodation. All three then worked together to devise an exposure task list of hierarchical fears, which included both OCD symptoms (e.g., touching dirty tables) and separation anxiety fears (e.g., mother leaving during a playdate). The therapist explained the concept of subjective units of distress using a fear thermometer for each thought, which was used as an anchor point to gauge how Max ranked various distressing situations, as well as to track acute and long-term changes in his anxiety.

Modified ERP: After exposures were discussed and approved, Max was confronted with his feared triggers or stimuli and asked to refrain from any compulsory or safety behaviors such as washing his hands. ERP was delivered via gradual exposure, which involved systematically introducing fear-eliciting situations to the patient, beginning with moderately fearful situations until progressing to the most feared. Parent role: After initial sessions, the therapist began to instruct and guide Max's mother on how to oversee exposures, providing encouragement and feedback throughout. During each exposure, the therapist checked in with Max to ask what his fear thermometer ratings were (i.e., subjective units of distress, 0 to 10). At the end of each session, the therapist, Max, and his mother discussed homework assignments. After several sessions of ERP, Max and his mother were asked to carry out ERP techniques between sessions, taking several hours to practice the same exposure tactics but in different contexts outside of therapy. In session, the therapist coached Max and his mother on how to implement self-guided exposures around their house (e.g., working with Max on his contamination fear by guiding him through the house touching all of the "dirty" surfaces).

Parent Sessions: During parent sessions, the therapist met alone with Max's mother to discuss Max's progress and subsequent plans for therapy. Sessions focused on reducing negative parent–child interactions, as well as setting boundaries for Max's behaviors and responding appropriately to disruptive behavior. The therapist conducted role-plays in which the mother practiced appropriate responses to compliant (i.e., attending to Max's positive behavior when he did not take two showers) and noncompliant (i.e., ignoring Max's temper tantrum when she would not wash towels) behaviors. After meeting separately with the therapist, Max's mother rejoined Max so that the therapist could observe the parent-child interactions with feedback. Max's mother was also given homework assignments of identifying and ignoring 2 disruptive behaviors (crying when towels were not washed and refusing to eat off the family plates) that she would ignore between sessions.

This case of comorbid OCD and separation anxiety illustrates the utility in choosing treatment that can target comorbidities or other clinically relevant barriers to treatment, such as family functioning. Transdiagnostic treatments such as those discussed previously target pathological processes thought to be shared with multiple psychological disorders.

Challenges and Recommendations for Future Research

Review of transdiagnostic treatments for youths with OCD and comorbidities indicates several critical challenges. Perhaps most evident of these challenges are the limited number of transdiagnostic interventions available to clinicians and the similarly scant research assessing and evaluating these treatments. As such, though the interventions discussed herein appear promising for the young client, limited availability and research may rightfully decrease the likelihood that clinicians utilize transdiagnostic interventions for children with OCD. Therefore, it is recommended that future research further examine the efficacy of these interventions (e.g., replication studies, comparing transdiagnostic interventions to treatment as usual).

Similarly, our review of OCD comorbidities and available transdiagnostic treatments indicates that only a fraction of comorbidities are actually targeted by current transdiagnostic options. For example, although also comorbid with OCD, autism symptoms have yet to be targeted in a pediatric transdiagnostic OCD treatment. As alluded to previously, this challenge may be addressed through additional research identifying core components (e.g., change mechanisms) across treatments. Identification of these components may facilitate subsequent development of new transdiagnostic approaches, such as the development of new approaches based on overlapping treatment components or the application of current transdiagnostic options for the treatment of additional disorders. Furthermore, identifying these components, particularly among child samples, may indicate critical ways in which youth treatments should differ from adult treatments (e.g., treatments may contain different mediators and moderators depending on sample age). This may be particularly important for child interventions as a majority of child treatments are often adapted from adult protocols and thus may require developmental modifications (e.g., CRT for OCD children).

Further addressing the issue of limited treatment options, it may also be useful for researchers to examine additional transdiagnostic treatments used with common OCD comorbidities. For example, the Unified Protocol for the Transdiagnostic Treatment of Emotional Disorders for Children and Adolescents and Emotion Detectives Treatment Program are two cognitive behavioral interventions designed for the transdiagnostic treatment of emotional disorders (e.g., anxiety, depression; Bilek & Ehrenreich-May, 2012; Ehrenreich et al., 2008). Though also intended for the treatment of OCD, few children with OCD have actually been included in research with these interventions (e.g., research including one OCD child out of 22 children; Bilek & Ehreneich-May, 2012). Thus, it is currently impossible to discern whether such treatments are useful for concurrent OCD and emotion-based comorbidities. However, given the emotional aspects of OCD (e.g., symptoms associated with poor emotion regulation; Fergus & Bardeen, 2014) and preliminary efficacy of these treatments with emotion-based comorbidities (e.g., anxiety, depression; Ehrenreich-May et al., 2017), future research may consider further examining the utility of these treatments with OCD.

In addition to future research developing and assessing transdiagnostic treatments, it is also important that research further identify conditions under which transdiagnostic treatments are actually most appropriate for children with OCD. Theoretically, though transdiagnostic approaches hold potential benefits for client and clinician, no research to date identifies optimal context for these treatments. It is plausible that there are situations or clients in which treatment as usual (e.g., addressing symptoms sequentially rather than concurrently) or therapy enhancements are necessary for maximum symptom improvement (e.g., disorders that are too dissimilar may require use of disorder specific treatments; some symptoms may require inclusion of medications). For example, some research suggests that behavioral treatment of OCD may be adversely affected by comorbid PTSD, particularly when symptoms are intricately related (e.g., OCD symptoms as a result of traumatic experiences; Gershuny et al., 2002). In this scenario, treatment exposures may worsen PTSD symptoms. Though additional research may be able to appropriately modify ERP to address related PTSD symptoms, it is also plausible that treatment as usual may be the best option for these symptoms. Therefore, in child research and clinical settings it will be important to not only identify symptoms that are successfully treated with transdiagnostic approaches, but also symptoms that are optimally treated with other approaches.

Key Practice Points

There are several key points to consider in therapists' transdiagnostic approach to OCD and comorbidities. First, similar to any therapy context, it is essential that clinicians administer a comprehensive assessment of client symptoms, perhaps providing increased attention to those symptoms commonly comorbid with pediatric OCD, and subsequently develop an informed case conceptualization. This step will increase the likelihood that all client symptoms are recognized and will further inform the clinician's decision as to the most appropriate form of treatment for their client. After identifying symptoms and formulating a working case conceptualization, clinicians should consider available treatments and empirical evidence for such treatments. To this end, clinicians should initially consider whether a transdiagnostic approach is appropriate for the client (e.g., can the comorbidities be treated using a transdiagnostic approach or would it be more beneficial to address symptoms sequentially). Given the lack of clear evidence supporting the efficacy of transdiagnostic interventions for pediatric OCD, clinicians should carefully evaluate available data, as well as pros and cons of employing a less supported approach. If clinicians opt to use a transdiagnostic intervention, they will need to use considerable clinical judgment in determining what transdiagnostic approach is most appropriate for their client and may need to consider developing their own theory-based approach (e.g., for comorbidities in which formal transdiagnostic approaches are unavailable). Throughout this process (particularly given no research assessing moderators or optimal settings of transdiagnostic treatment) clinicians should remain flexible, monitor client progress frequently (for OCD as well as all comorbid symptoms), and consider potential modifications as necessary (e.g., consider the need for medication as well as further modifications to treatment components based on relevant comorbidities).

References

Abramowitz, J. S. (2004). Treatment of obsessive-compulsive disorder in patients who have comorbid major depression. *Journal of Clinical Psychology, 60*(11), 1133–1141.

Abramowitz, J. S., & Jacoby, R. J. (2014). The use and misuse of exposure therapy for obsessive-compulsive and related disorders. *Current Psychiatry Reviews, 10*(4), 277–283.

Abramowitz, J. S., Storch, E. A., Keeley, M., & Cordell, E. (2007). Obsessive-compulsive disorder with comorbid major depression: What is the role of cognitive factors?. *Behaviour Research and Therapy*, *45*(10), 2257–2267.

Aderka, I. M., Foa, E. B., Applebaum, E., Shafran, N., & Gilboa-Schechtman, E. (2011). Direction of influence between posttraumatic and depressive symptoms during prolonged exposure therapy among children and adolescents. *Journal of Consulting and Clinical Psychology*, *79*(3), 421.

Ale, C.M. & Krackow, E. (2011). Concurrent treatment of early childhood OCD and ODD: A case illustration. *Clinical Case Studies*, *10*(4), 312–323.

Alvarenga, P. G., Cesar, R. C., Leckman, J. F., Moriyama, T. S., Torres, A. R., Bloch, M. H., ... Miguel, E. C. (2015). Obsessive-compulsive symptom dimensions in a population-based, cross-sectional sample of school-aged children. *Journal of Psychiatric Research*, *62*, 108–114.

Austern, D., Farber, T., & Marinchak, J. (2013). Considerations for modifying exposure and response prevention: The cases of Mr. H and Angela. *Pragmatic Case Studies in Psychotherapy*, *9*(1), 98–106.

Barlow, D. H., Allen, L. B., & Choate, M. L. (2004). Toward a unified treatment for emotional disorders. *Behavior Therapy*, *35*(2), 205–230.

Barton, R., & Heyman, I. (2013) Obsessive-compulsive disorder in children and adolescents. *Paediatrics and Child Health (United Kingdom)*, *23*(1), 23.

Bennett, S. Stark, D. Shafran, R. Heyman, I. & Krebs, G. (2015). Evaluation of cognitive behaviour therapy for paediatric obsessive-compulsive disorder in the context of tic disorders. *Journal of Behavior Therapy and Experimental Psychiatry*, *49*, 223–229.

Bilek, E. L., & Ehrenreich-May, J. (2012). An open trial investigation of a transdiagnostic group treatment for children with anxiety and depressive symptoms. *Behavior Therapy*, *43*(4), 887–897.

Boileau, B. (2011). A review of obsessive-compulsive disorder in children and adolescents. *Dialogues in Clinical Neuroscience*, *13*(4), 401.

Buhlmann, U., Deckersbach, T., Engelhard, I., Cook, L.M., Rauch, S. L., Kathmann, N., ... Savage, C.R. (2006). Cognitive retraining for organizational impairment in obsessive–compulsive disorder. *Psychiatry Research*, *144*, 109–116.

Choate-Summers, M. L., Freeman, J. B., Garcia, A. M., Coyne, L., Przeworski, A., & Leonard, H. L. (2008). Clinical considerations when tailoring cognitive behavioral treatment for young children with obsessive compulsive disorder. *Education and Treatment of Children*, *31*(3), 395–416.

Chu, B. C. (2012). Translating transdiagnostic approaches to children and adolescents. *Cognitive and Behavioral Practice*, *19*(1), 1-4.

Chu, B.C., Colognori, D.B., Yang, G., Xie, M., Bergman, R.L., & Piacentini, J. (2015). Mediators of exposure therapy for obsessive-compulsive disorder: Specificity and temporal sequence of client and treatment factors. *Behavior Therapy*, *46*(3), 395–408.

Clark, D. A., & Taylor, S. (2009). The transdiagnostic perspective on cognitive-behavioral therapy for anxiety and depression: New wine for old wineskins?. *Journal of Cognitive Psychotherapy*, *23*(1), 60–66.

Coughtrey, A., Shafran, R., Bennett, S., Kothari, R., & Wade, T. (2017). Mental contamination: Relationship with psychopathology and transdiagnostic processes. *Journal of Obsessive-Compulsive and Related Disorders*, *17*, 39–45.

Cougle, J. R. (2012). What makes a quality therapy? A consideration of parsimony, ease, and efficiency. *Behavior Therapy*, *43*(3), 468–481.

Dahlgren, C.L. & Stedal, K. (2017). Cognitive remediation therapy for adolescents with anorexia nervosa – treatment satisfaction and the perception of change. *Behavioral Sciences*, *7*(2), 23.

de Mathis, M. A., Diniz, J. B., Hounie, A. G., Shavitt, R. G., Fossaluza, V., Ferrão, Y., ... Miguel, E. C. (2013). Trajectory in obsessive-compulsive disorder comorbidities. *European Neuropsychopharmacology*, *23*(7), 594–601.

DiMauro, J., Genova, M., Tolin, D. F., & Kurtz, M. M. (2014). Cognitive remediation for neuropsychological impairment in hoarding disorder: A pilot study. *Journal of Obsessive-Compulsive and Related Disorders*, *3*(2), 132–138.

Eack, S.M., Pogue-Geile, M.F., Greenwald, D.P., Hogarty, S.S., & Keshavan, M.S. (2011). Mechanisms of functional improvement in a 2-year trial of cognitive enhancement therapy for early schizophrenia. *Psychological Medicine*, *41*, 1253–1261.

Egan, S. J., Wade, T. D., & Shafran, R. (2011). Perfectionism as a transdiagnostic process: A clinical review. *Clinical Psychology Review*, *31*(2), 203–212.

Egan, S. J., Wade, T. D., Shafran, R., & Antony, M. M. (2014). *Cognitive-behavioral treatment of perfectionism*. New York: Guilford Publications.

Ehrenreich-May, J., & Chu, B. C. (eds.). (2013). *Transdiagnostic treatments for children and adolescents: Principles and practice*. New York: Guilford Publications.

Ehrenreich-May J., Rosenfield, D., Queen, A.H., Kennedy, S.M., Remmes, C.S., & Barlow, D.H. (2017). An initial waitlist-controlled trial of the unified protocol for the treatment of emotional disorders in adolescents. *Journal of Anxiety Disorders*, *46*, 46–55.

Fairburn, C. G., Cooper, Z., & Shafran, R. (2003). Cognitive behavior therapy for eating disorders: A "transdiagnostic" theory and treatment. *Behaviour Research and Therapy*, *41*, 509–528.

Farrell, L., Barrett, P., & Piacentini, J. (2006). Obsessive–compulsive disorder across the developmental trajectory: Clinical correlates in children, adolescents and adults. *Behaviour Change*, *23*(2), 103–120.

Farrell, L., Waters, A., Milliner, E., & Ollendick, T. (2012). Comorbidity and treatment response in pediatric obsessive-compulsive disorder: A pilot study of group cognitive-behavioral treatment. *Psychiatry Research*, *199*(2), 115–123.

Fergus, T. A. & Bardeen, J.R. (2014). Emotion regulation and obsessive-compulsive symptoms: A further examination of associations. *Journal of Obsessive-Compulsive and Related Disorders*, *3*, 243–248.

Fineberg, N. A., Reghunandanan, S., Brown, A., & Pampaloni, I. (2013). Pharmacotherapy of obsessive-compulsive disorder: Evidence-based treatment and beyond. *Australian & New Zealand Journal of Psychiatry*, *47*(2), 121–141.

Flessner, C.A., Freeman, J.B., Sapyta, J., Garcia, A., Franklin, M.E., March, J.S., & Foa, E. (2011). Predictors of parental accommodation in pediatric obsessive-compulsive disorder: Findings from the pediatric obsessive-compulsive disorder treatment study (POTS) trial. *Journal of the American Academy of Child & Adolescent Psychiatry*, *50*(7), 716–725.

Forehand, R., Jones, D. J., & Parent, J. (2013). Behavioral parenting interventions for child disruptive behaviors and anxiety: What's different and what's the same. *Clinical Psychology Review*, *33*(1), 133–145.

Forehand, R., Lafko, N., Parent, J., & Burt, K.B. (2014). Is parenting the mediator of change in behavioral parent training for externalizing problem of youth? *Clinical Psychology Review*, *34*(8), 608–619.

Francazio, S. K., Flessner, C. A., Boisseau, C. L., Sibrava, N. J., Mancebo, M. C., Eisen, J. L., & Rasmussen, S. A. (2016). Parental accommodation predicts symptom severity at long-term follow-up in children with obsessive–compulsive disorder: A preliminary investigation. *Journal of Child and Family Studies, 25*(8), 2562–2570.

Freeman, J. B., Garcia, A. M., Coyne, L., Ale, C., Przeworski, A., Himle, M., ... Leonard, H. L. (2008). Early childhood OCD: Preliminary findings from a family-based cognitive-behavioral approach. *Journal of the American Academy of Child & Adolescent Psychiatry, 47*(5), 593–602.

Freeman, J. B., Garcia, A. M., Fucci, C., Karitani, M., Miller, L., & Leonard, H. L. (2003). Family-based treatment of early-onset obsessive-compulsive disorder. *Journal of Child and Adolescent Psychopharmacology, 13*(2,Supplement 1), 71–80.

Freeman, J., Sapyta, J., Garcia, A., Compton, S., Khanna, M., Flessner, C., ... Franklin, M. (2014). Family-based treatment of early childhood obsessive-compulsive disorder. The pediatric obsessive-compulsive disorder treatment study for young children (POTS Jr) – a randomized clinical trial. *JAMA Psychiatry, 71*(6), 689–698.

Garcia, A.M., Sapyta, J.J., Moore, P.S., Freeman, J.B., Franklin, M.E., March, J.S., & Foa, E. B. (2010). Predictors and moderators of treatment outcome in the pediatric obsessive compulsive treatment study (POTS I). *Journal of the American Academy of Child & Adolescent Psychiatry, 49*(10), 1024–1033.

Geller, D. A., Biederman, J., Faraone, S., Agranat, A., Cradock, K., Hagermoser, L., ... Coffey, B. J. (2001). Developmental aspects of obsessive compulsive disorder: findings in children, adolescents, and adults. *The Journal of Nervous and Mental Disease, 189*(7), 471–477.

Gershuny, B.S., Baer, L., Jenike, M.A., Minichiello, W.E., & Wilhelm, S. (2002). Comorbid posttraumatic stress disorder: Impact on treatment outcome for obsessive-compulsive disorder. *The American Journal of Psychiatry, 159*, 852–854.

Gillan, C. M, Fineberg, N.A.,& Robbins, T.W. (2017). A trans-diagnostic perspective on obsessive-compulsive disorder. *Psychological Medicine, 47*(9), 1528–1548.

Ginsburg, G. S., Burstein, M., Becker, K. D., & Drake, K. L. (2011). Treatment of obsessive compulsive disorder in young children: An intervention model and case series. *Child & Family Behavior Therapy, 33*(2), 97–122.

Grant, J. E., Fineberg, N., van Ameringen, M., Cath, D., Visser, H., Carmi, L., & van Balkom, A. J. (2016). New treatment models for compulsive disorders. *European Neuropsychopharmacology, 26*(5), 877–884.

Griffiths, D. L., Farrell, L. J., Waters, A. M., & White, S. W. (in press). ASD traits among youth with obsessive–compulsive disorder. *Child Psychiatry and Human Development*.

Griffiths, D. L., Farrell, L. J., Waters, A. M., & White, S. W. (2017). Clinical correlates of obsessive compulsive disorder and comorbid autism spectrum disorder in youth. *Journal of Obsessive-Compulsive and Related Disorders, 14*, 90–98.

Gutner, C. A., Galovski, T., Bovin, M. J., & Schnurr, P. P. (2016). Emergence of transdiagnostic treatments for PTSD and posttraumatic distress. *Current Psychiatry Reports, 18*(10), 95.

Hood, H. K., & Antony, M. M. (2016). Treatment of perfectionism-related obsessive-compulsive disorder. In *Clinical handbook of obsessive-compulsive and related disorders* (pp. 85–97). New York: Springer International Publishing.

Ivarsson, T., & Valderhaug, R. (2006). Symptom patterns in children and adolescents with obsessive–compulsive disorder (OCD). *Behaviour Research and Therapy, 44*(8), 1105–1116.

Jakubovski, E., Diniz, J. B., Valerio, C., Fossaluza, V., Belotto-Silva, C., Gorenstein, C., & Shavitt, R. G. (2013). Clinical predictors of long-term outcome in obsessive-compulsive disorder. *Depression and Anxiety, 30*(8), 763–772.

Kameg, K. M., Richardson, L., & Szpak, J. L. (2015). Pediatric obsessive-compulsive disorder: An update for advanced practice psychiatric nurses. *J Child Adolesc Psychiatr Nurs, 28*(2), 84–91.

Knopp, J., Knowles, S., Bee, P., Lovell, K., & Bower, P. (2013). A systematic review of predictors and moderators of response to psychological therapies in OCD: Do we have enough empirical evidence to target treatment?. *Clinical Psychology Review, 33*(8), 1067–1081.

Kostek, N. T., Garcia-Delgar, B., Rojas, A., Luber, M., & Coffey, B. J. (2016). Approaches to the diagnosis and treatment of OCD with comorbid tic disorders. *Current Treatment Options in Psychiatry, 3*(3), 253–265.

Krebs, G., & Heyman, I. (2014). Obsessive-compulsive disorder in children and adolescents. *Archives of Disease in Childhood*, archdischild-2014.

Lebowitz, E. R., Motlagh, M. G., Katsovich, L., King, R. A., Lombroso, P. J., Grantz, H., ... & Coffey, B. J. (2012). Tourette syndrome in youth with and without obsessive compulsive disorder and attention deficit hyperactivity disorder. *European Child & Adolescent Psychiatry*, 1–7.

Lebowitz, E. R., Panza, K. E., & Bloch, M. H. (2016). Family accommodation in obsessive-compulsive and anxiety disorders: a five-year update. *Expert Review of Neurotherapeutics, 16*(1), 45–53.

Leckman, J. F., Bloch, M. H., & King, R. A. (2009). Symptom dimensions and subtypes of obsessive-compulsive disorder: A developmental perspective. *Dialogues in Clinical Neuroscience, 11*(1), 21.

Lewin, A. B., Chang, S., McCracken, J., McQueen, M., & Piacentini, J. (2010). Comparison of clinical features among youth with tic disorders, obsessive–compulsive disorder (OCD), and both conditions. *Psychiatry Research, 178*(2), 317–322.

Lewin, A. B., & Piacentini, J. (2010, April). Evidence-based assessment of child obsessive compulsive disorder: Recommendations for clinical practice and treatment research. In *Child & Youth Care Forum, 39*(2), 73–89, Springer US.

Lombroso, P. J., & Scahill, L. (2008). Tourette syndrome and obsessive–compulsive disorder. *Brain and Development, 30*(4), 231–237.

Mancebo, M. C., Boisseau, C. L., Garnaat, S. L., Eisen, J. L., Greenberg, B. D., Sibrava, N. J., ...& Rasmussen, S. A. (2014). Long-term course of pediatric obsessive–compulsive disorder: 3 years of prospective follow-up. *Compr Psychiatry, 55*(7), 1498–1504.

Marcks, B. A., Weisberg, R. B., Dyck, I., & Keller, M. B. (2011). Longitudinal course of obsessive-compulsive disorder in patients with anxiety disorders: A 15-year prospective follow-up study. *Compr Psychiatry, 52*(6), 670–677.

Mataix-Cols, D., Frost, R.O., Pertusa, A., Clark, L.A., Saxena, S., Leckman, J.F.,... Wilhelm, S. (2010). Hoarding disorder: A new diagnosis for DSM-V? *Depression and Anxiety, 27*(6), 556–572.

McEvoy, P. M., Nathan, P., & Norton, P. J. (2009). Efficacy of transdiagnostic treatments: A review of published outcome studies and future research directions. *Journal of Cognitive Psychotherapy, 23*(1), 20–33.

McKay, D., & Mancusi, L. (2015). Treatment of "not-just-right experiences" in childhood obsessive-compulsive disorder. *Clinical handbook of obsessive-compulsive and related disorders: A case-based approach to treating pediatric and adult populations.* New York: Springer.

Medalia, A., & Bowie, C. R. (eds.). (2016). *Cognitive remediation to improve functional outcomes.* New York: Oxford University Press.

Micali, N., Heyman, I., Perez, M., Hilton, K., Nakatani, E., Turner, C., & Mataix-Cols, D. (2010). Long-term outcomes of obsessive–compulsive disorder: Follow-up of 142 children and adolescents. *The British Journal of Psychiatry, 197*(2), 128–134.

Morris, L. & Lomax, C. (2014). Review: Assessment, development, and treatment of childhood perfectionism a systematic review. *Child and Adolescent Mental Health, 19*(4), 225–234.

Murray, K., Jassi, A., Mataix-Cols, D., Barrow, F., & Krebs, G. (2015). Outcomes of cognitive behaviour therapy for obsessive–compulsive disorder in young people with and without autism spectrum disorders: A case controlled study. *Psychiatry Research, 228*(1), 8–13.

O'Connell, R.G., Bellgrove, M.A., Dockree, P.M., & Robertson, I. (2006). Cognitive remediation in ADHD: Effects of periodic non-contingent alerts on sustained attention response. *Neuropsychological Rehabilitation, 16*(6), 653–665.

Öst, L. G., Riise, E. N., Wergeland, G. J., Hansen, B., & Kvale, G. (2016). Cognitive behavioral and pharmacological treatments of OCD in children: A systematic review and meta-analysis. *Journal of Anxiety Disorders, 43*, 58–69.

Park, H. S., Shin, Y.-W., Ha, T. H., Shin, M. S., Kim, Y. Y., Lee, Y. H., et al. (2006). Effect of cognitive training focusing on organizational strategies in patients with obsessive-compulsive disorder. *Psychiatry and Clinical Neurosciences, 60*, 718–726.

Pinto, A., Dargani, N., Wheaton, M. G., Cervoni, C., Rees, C. S., & Egan, S. J. (2017). Perfectionism in obsessive-compulsive disorder and related disorders: What should treating clinicians know? *Journal of Obsessive-Compulsive and Related Disorders, 12*, 102–108.

Pringsheim, T. (2017). Tic severity and treatment in children: The effect of comorbid attention deficit hyperactivity disorder and obsessive compulsive behaviors. *Child Psychiatry & Human Development, 48*(6), 1–7.

Reaven, J. & Hepburn, S. (2003). Cognitive-behavioral treatment of obsessive-compulsive disorder in a child with Asperger syndrome. *Autism, 7*(2), 145–164.

Sadri, K., Anderson, R.A., McEvoy, P.M., Kane, R.T., & Egan, S.J. (2017). A pilot investigation of cognitive behavioural therapy for clinical perfectionism in obsessive-compulsive disorder. *Behavioural and Cognitive Psychotherapy, 45*, 312–320.

Shafran, R., Cooper, Z., & Fairburn, C. G. (2002). Clinical perfectionism: A cognitive–behavioural analysis. *Behaviour Research and Therapy, 40*(7), 773–791.

Shin, N. Y., Lee, T. Y., Kim, E., & Kwon, J. S. (2014). Cognitive functioning in obsessive-compulsive disorder: A meta-analysis. *Psychological Medicine, 44*(6), 1121–1130.

Skriner, L. C., Freeman, J., Garcia, A., Benito, K., Sapyta, J., & Franklin, M. (2016). Characteristics of young children with obsessive–compulsive disorder: Baseline features from the POTS Jr. sample. *Child Psychiatry Hum Dev., 47*(1), 83–93.

Steele, A.L., Waite, S., Egan, S.J., Finnigan, J., Handley, A., & Wade, T.D. (2013). Psycho education and group cognitive-behavioural therapy for clinical perfectionism: A case-series evaluation. *Behavioural and Cognitive Psychotherapy, 41*, 129–143.

Stone, W. S., & Chen, G. (2016). Comorbidity of autism spectrum and obsessive-compulsive disorders. *North American Journal of Medicine and Science, 8*(3).

Storch, E. A., Björgvinsson, T., Riemann, B., Lewin, A. B., Morales, M. J., & Murphy, T. K. (2010). Factors associated with poor response in cognitive-behavioral therapy for pediatric obsessive-compulsive 189 disorder. *Bulletin of the Menninger Clinic, 74*(2), 167–185.

Storch, E. A., Merlo, L. J., Larson, M. J., Geffken, G. R., Lehmkuhl, H. D., Jacob, M. L., ... Goodman, W. K. (2008). Impact of comorbidity on cognitive-behavioral therapy response in pediatric obsessive-compulsive disorder. *J Am Acad Child Adolesc Psychiatry, 47*(5), 583–592.

Taboas, W. R., McKay, D., Whiteside, S. P., & Storch, E. A. (2015). Parental involvement in youth anxiety treatment: Conceptual bases, controversies, and recommendations for intervention. *Journal of Anxiety Disorders, 30*, 16–18.

Tchanturia, K., & Hambrook, D. (2010). Cognitive remediation therapy for anorexia nervosa. In C. M. Grilo & J. E. Mitchell (eds.), *Treatment of eating disorders* (pp. 130–150). New York: Guilford Press.

Torp, N. C., Dahl, K., Skarphedinsson, G., Compton, S., Thomsen, P. H., Weidle, B., ... & Ivarsson, T. (2015). Predictors associated with improved cognitive-behavioral therapy outcome in pediatric obsessive-compulsive disorder. *Journal of the American Academy of Child & Adolescent Psychiatry, 54*(3), 200–207.

Urben, Sebastien, Pihet, S., Jaugey, L., Halfon, O., & Holzer, L. (2012). Computer-assisted cognitive remediation in adolescents with psychosis or at risk for psychosis: A 6 month follow-up. *Acta Neuropsychiatrica, 24*, 328–335.

van den Heuvel, O. A., Veltman, D. J., Groenewegen, H. J., Cath, D. C., van Balkom, A. J., van Hartskamp, J., ... van Dyck, R. (2005). Frontal-striatal dysfunction during planning in obsessive-compulsive disorder. *Archives of General Psychiatry, 62*(3), 301–309.

Verdellen, C. W., Hoogduin, C. A., Kato, B. S., Keijsers, G. P., Cath, D. C., & Hoijtink, H. B. (2008). Habituation of premonitory sensations during exposure and response prevention treatment in Tourette's syndrome. *Behavior Modification, 32*(2), 215–227.

Verdellen, C. W. J., Keijsers, G. P. J., Cath, D. C., & Hoogduin, C. A. L. (2004). Exposure with response prevention versus habit reversal in Tourette's syndrome: A controlled study. *Behaviour Research and Therapy, 42*(5), 501–511.

Williams, M. T., Farris, S. G., Turkheimer, E. N., Franklin, M. E., Simpson, H. B., Liebowitz, M., & Foa, E. B. (2014). The impact of symptom dimensions on outcome for exposure and ritual prevention therapy in obsessive-compulsive disorder. *Journal of Anxiety Disorders, 28*(6), 553–558.

Wu, M. S., Rudy, B. M., & Storch, E. A. (2014). Obsessions, compulsions, and repetitive behavior: Autism and/or OCD. In *Handbook of autism and anxiety* (pp. 107–120). New York: Springer International Publishing.

Wykes, T., Newton, E., Landau, S., Rice, C., Thompson, N., Frangou, S. (2007). Cognitive remediation therapy (CRT) for young early onset patients with schizophrenia: An exploratory randomized controlled trial. *Schizophrenia Research, 94*(1–3), 221–230.

Wykes, T., & Spaulding, W.D. (2011). Thinking about the future cognitive remediation therapy–what works and could we do better? *Schizophrenia Bulletin, 37*, S80–S90.

Zohar, J. (ed.). (2012). *Obsessive compulsive disorder: Current science and clinical practice.* Hoboken, NJ: John Wiley & Sons.

23 Pediatric OCD

Dissemination and Implementation

Martin E. Franklin, Jordan A. Katz, Bradley C. Riemann, and Simone Budzyn

Introduction

Obsessive-compulsive disorder (OCD) is a complex condition associated with significant morbidity, comorbidity, and functional impairment across the developmental spectrum, and pediatric onset appears to be the norm. As far as treatment efficacy is concerned, cognitive behavioral therapies (CBT) developed for pediatric OCD have typically yielded substantial and durable symptom reduction and improvements in functioning (for reviews see Abramowitz et al., 2005; Barrett et al., 2008; Franklin et al., 2015; Watson & Rees, 2008). As would be expected, the efficacy trials in pediatric OCD that have been conducted in the last twenty years intentionally employed design elements that emphasized internal validity. These design choices, such as careful sample selection, use of manualized interventions, and random assignment to condition, allowed for isolation of the treatment signal, yet gave short shrift to external validity and generalizability beyond the academic medical context in which most of the seminal studies were conducted. This may well be a scientific necessity, as it is important to establish a treatment's efficacy before testing the limits of its generalizability. Nevertheless, such design choices leave questions about treatment transportability to more clinical settings unanswered, and thus necessitate the study of generalizability more explicitly using study design elements that emphasize external validity.

Fortunately, such advances have been made recently in pediatric OCD with respect to the examination of CBT's effectiveness within more diverse patient samples, with a wider range of therapist expertise than typically available in efficacy randomized controlled trials (RCTs), greater psychiatric comorbidity, and in more clinical as opposed to research settings. On the whole, these data have supported the generalizability of CBT: it appears that robust and durable outcomes can be achieved even in those CBT studies that emphasized external validity. These findings now set the stage for even larger and more ambitious efforts to make this form of treatment more readily available to youth all over the world who struggle with OCD.

In our view, the move from studying patient outcomes in academic clinics closely associated with the examination of efficacy toward clinical settings where patient samples, therapists, treatment approach, and treatment context all vary requires careful consideration. Foremost among these considerations is the creation of a common treatment culture built firmly upon an empirically informed understanding of OCD psychopathology and CBT theory, even if some of the more pedantic aspects of presenting research findings require modification to meet the training audience's interests, expertise, and more clinically focused professional needs. Developing a comprehensive understanding of the fundamentals of theory promotes the artful application of the clinical procedures in practice with OCD and should continue to be emphasized, even in these more clinical settings. Investigating whether and how positive results can be realized in clinical settings wherein CBT expertise for pediatric OCD is less available than in tightly controlled clinical trials is a matter of great public health importance, since it is already clear that there is a paucity of such expertise in most clinical and community settings.

In terms of precedent in the adult OCD literature, evidence from effectiveness research with adult patients treated by supervised interns and junior level clinical faculty indicated that these patients achieved clinically meaningful and statistically significant symptom reductions on average following intensive CBT that were comparable to those achieved by patients of highly experienced clinicians (Franklin et al., 2000, 2003). Moreover, such positive outcomes appear to be achievable with very severe patients with complex prior treatment histories and substantial depressive comorbidity treated in intensive outpatient or even residential settings (e.g., Abramowitz et al., 2000). As is the case with virtually every psychiatric disorder that occurs across the developmental spectrum, with the possible exception of ADHD, the efficacy and then effectiveness literatures in adult OCD was built first, followed by age-downward extension of protocols validated with adults for use with adolescents and children. Thus, although there is less guidance available from the less extensive pediatric OCD treatment outcome literature than is the case for adult treatment, there is sufficient evidence to support CBT's efficacy and to indicate that next stage efforts should commence to disseminate it more broadly for youth suffering from this condition.

Notably, most of the randomized controlled trials evaluating the efficacy of CBT for pediatric OCD actually employed clinicians with a range of clinical expertise, all of whom had the benefit of supervision from expert-level clinicians with years of experience in CBT (e.g., Freeman et al., 2014; Piacentini et al., 2011). Thus, the evidence base for CBT in pediatric OCD is built upon the assumption that master clinicians with decades of experience are not required as treatment providers in order to achieve excellent patient outcomes, and that clinicians with less experience can provide effective treatment through learning and applying the skills taught by experts (Franklin et al., 2013). This is fortunate, since the paucity of CBT expertise at any level is an ongoing problem for families of youth with OCD who seek CBT beyond the academic centers that typically develop and test these protocols.

Review of the CBT Outcome Literature

Definition of terms

Before launching into an extensive discussion of the literature, it is important first to define the terms we will use to differentiate the various types of treatment outcome studies conducted thus far. Efficacy trials, which we only touch upon here briefly, focus primarily on detecting a signal from a carefully defined set of treatment procedures. In order to do so, it is crucial to carefully define and limit the sampling frame, employ a control and/or comparison group, clearly designate methods and outcome measures, and use accepted statistical methods to compare the groups at pre- and posttreatment to determine if the data support the conclusion that the treatment caused observed changes in symptoms and functioning. Internal validity is prioritized in efficacy work, and sometimes is achieved at the expense of external validity, a point not lost on critics of randomized controlled trials as the primary means of establishing if a treatment works (see Westen et al., 2004).

Effectiveness research grew out of efforts to address the concerns raised by RCT critics and is focused more on generalizability of findings to clinical settings and practice (e.g., Persons & Silbershatz, 1998). For example, the sampling frame in effectiveness studies is often more flexible so as to allow "real" patients to enter the trials, treatment may be delivered in a more clinically flexible manner without careful efforts to promote adherence to manuals, and comparison groups are also seen as less crucial to the mission since efficacy is not so much the question as generalizability to clinical settings. A good example of the progression from efficacy to effectiveness can be seen in work done in adult OCD: carefully controlled randomized trials were employed to establish the efficacy of CBT for OCD (e.g., Foa et al., 1992, 2005; Marks et al., 1980), which were then followed on by a series of studies examining effectiveness of CBT for OCD in outpatient clinics (Franklin et al., 2000; Warren & Thomas, 2001). These effectiveness trials were characterized by a wide variety of therapist experience levels (Franklin et al., 2003) and treatment visit schedules (Abramowitz et al., 2003), and were conducted intentionally with greater flexibility with respect to inclusion of patients with psychiatric comorbidity and concomitant pharmacotherapy (Abramowitz et al., 2000; Franklin et al., 2002). Collectively these studies established that CBT was an efficacious treatment that could be delivered in weekly sessions or more intensively, and that good outcomes could also be achieved outside the carefully controlled context of randomized clinical trials. What these studies did not address, however, is how best to extend the use of these methods into routine clinical practice.

More recent efforts have been made in the field to extend even beyond effectiveness studies under the flagship of the emerging field known as implementation science, which has been defined as "the scientific study of methods to promote the systematic uptake of clinical research findings and other evidence-based practices into routine practice" (Beidas et al., 2012). In implementation science, the process by which clinical agencies train, incorporate, implement, and maintain adherence to the protocols is the focus of study rather than clinical outcomes per se, and thus practitioner variables such as knowledge prior to training, knowledge after training, and behavior in the clinic after training are primary dependent variables. Beidas and colleagues (2012), for example, found that ongoing supervision after workshop attendance was associated with greater change in therapist behavior in treatment delivery than was workshop attendance alone. Other studies in this area have focused more on changing the climate in community clinical agencies so that dissemination can be promoted, supported, and maintained (see Glisson et al., 2012, 2016a, 2016b). The low base rate of OCD in community settings makes OCD-specific work in clinical agencies especially challenging. As has been the case with pediatric anxiety and mood disorders encountered in clinical settings more broadly, the use of transdiagnostic protocols in such agencies is one way to get around the low base rate issue (e.g., Chorpita et al., 2015; Weisz et al., 2012), but as yet there is no evidence that OCD will respond to a transdiagnostic protocol. Indeed, given the nuances of the clinical presentation of OCD, as well as its treatment, it is not necessarily a foregone conclusion that OCD would respond comparably to other disorders treated with such methods. These caveats notwithstanding, there is certainly room for further study of whether OCD can be treated effectively using transdiagnostic protocols or if the clinical subtleties of the disorder itself and its treatment require that the interventionist, or at least the clinical supervisor, have more subspecialty expertise (for an example in pediatric OCD see Valderhaug et al., 2007).

As follows, we review the studies we do have in pediatric OCD, where the bulk of the work has focused on efficacy and effectiveness, with a handful of studies now explicitly attempting to bridge the gap between examining patient outcomes (efficacy and effectiveness) and examining the processes and methods that best promote therapist learning and agency acceptance of empirically supported interventions.

Efficacy. An earlier chapter in this volume reviewed the efficacy literature in detail, and hence we will not belabor these findings here. Suffice it to say that we now have almost twenty randomized controlled trials that support the use of CBT for pediatric OCD in comparison to a wide variety of control groups. The evidence is generally strong for CBT's efficacy, has been generated out of multiple labs around the world, and is largely consistent across trials. What we still lack in the pediatric OCD efficacy literature, however, is a sufficiently large database comprised of studies that have tested the same or at least slightly different treatment regimens. Replication is the hallmark of good science, and unfortunately the pediatric OCD literature is seriously lacking in replication studies. For example, there are very few randomized studies that have examined the relative and/or combined efficacy of CBT and any form of pharmacotherapy (e.g., Asbahr et al., 2005; De Haan et al., 1998) and in fact only one trial, the POTS I study (Pediatric OCD Treatment Study Team (POTS), 2004), meets even minimal methodological standards regarding sample size and the use of a no-treatment control group to account for the passage of time and repeated assessment. We also do not have any carefully controlled studies of treatment sequencing, i.e., a placebo-controlled medication trial followed by a randomized controlled trial of CBT for medication partial and nonresponders, and thus we must interpolate across the empirical gaps when discussing the common clinical scenario with patients who have already undergone a trial of a medication of established efficacy. The effectiveness literature fills in some of these gaps, as will be discussed as follows, but there is still work on efficacy yet to be done. We vigorously encourage investigators to try to find creative ways to work together, for example, to take on another issue in the field that looms as a barrier to our understanding of which treatments work best for which patients, namely a large-scale efficacy study to examine response to treatment by OCD subtype such as those with feared consequences versus those with "Not Just Right" OCD or incompleteness. The search for the Holy Grail of neurobiological mechanisms (Insel, 2014; Insel & Cuthbert, 2015) drove the funding in the United States and hence moved the field away from efficacy research across disorders (Deacon, 2013), and thus some of these suggested avenues for developing the pediatric OCD efficacy database further may best be pursued within international collaborations in which the intellectual interests of clinical scientists and pressing patient needs set the agenda rather than agency priorities.

Effectiveness. One of the observations made by the POTS investigative team in completing the POTS I trial was that it was becoming more and more challenging by the late 1990s and early 2000s to find children and adolescents with OCD who had not been previously exposed to pharmacotherapy. Indeed, despite growing evidence for the efficacy of CBT both then and since, most pediatric OCD patients treated in the community receive monotherapy with a serotonin reuptake inhibitor (SRI) as their first-line treatment. However, even adequate trials of these medications leave the great majority of patients with clinically significant residual symptoms (Freeman et al., 2009), and thus the chances for remission or excellent response are lower with medication alone – for example, POTS I indicated that the rate of excellent response (posttreatment CY-BOCS total < 10) in children treated with sertraline only was just 21 percent, meaning that four out of five youth who participated in a carefully monitored, adequate medication trial still had significant residual symptoms at posttreatment. These observations led the investigative team to design POTS II (Franklin et al., 2011), a next phase research trial with efficacy and effectiveness design elements included to address the issue of treatment augmentation (adding an additional treatment to a current treatment) as well as treatment transportability (developing a treatment in a research setting specifically for use in community clinical settings). The relative efficacy of three conditions was examined over the course of 12 weeks: (1) 7 sessions of medication management (MM) provided by a study psychiatrist (MM only); (2) 7 MM sessions plus 14 sessions of OCD-specific CBT as delivered by a study psychologist (MM+CBT); and (3) 7 sessions of MM plus instructions in CBT delivered by the study psychiatrist assigned to provide MM (MM+I-CBT). In terms of effectiveness elements of the trial, the POTS team chose to recruit patients who were already on an SRI rather than using a "home-grown" sample of treatment-naïve patients whom would then be put on a specific medication regimen by the treatment team. The rationale for this design decision was driven in part by practical factors (e.g., having to incur the costs of the initial pharmacotherapy trial on a limited study budget) but also by a desire to enhance generalizability of findings to clinical practice, where psychiatrists and even pediatricians conduct pharmacotherapy treatments more flexibly than would be done in the context of an efficacy study. A total of 124 children and adolescents ages 7–17 were recruited at three sites (Penn, Duke, & Brown); inclusion criteria required that patients already were taking an adequate dose of a serotonergic medication (either a selective SRI or clomipramine) for OCD and yet still were experiencing clinically significant OCD symptoms. Findings indicated that MM+CBT was superior to MM alone and to MM+I-CBT, which, contrary to study hypotheses, failed to separate statistically from one another (69 percent response for MM+CBT versus 34 percent for MM+I-CBT and 30 percent for MM alone, where response was defined as a 30 percent reduction in baseline CY-BOCS score). POTS II thus provided further evidence for the efficacy of combined treatment, in this case administered sequentially rather than simultaneously, and also highlighted the potential need for using the "full dose" of CBT in order to achieve optimal outcomes. It also is notable that results on the continuous CY-BOCS outcomes for MM+CBT were somewhat attenuated relative to what was achieved with combined treatment (CBT + sertraline) in POTS I, which could reflect sampling difference, sequencing effects, or the possible influence of partial response to an initial treatment on subsequent outcomes. The findings obtained in POTS II were highly convergent with those from an adult augmentation trial (Simpson et al., 2008) in which MM+CBT augmentation outcomes were less robust than what had been reported in the literature for CBT or combined treatment administered simultaneously.

Asbahr and colleagues (2005) conducted a smaller effectiveness study in which they randomized 40 patients ages 9–17 inclusive to one of two active conditions: pharmacotherapy with sertraline or group-based CBT. Similar to de Haan et al. (1998), the study design could not support confident conclusions regarding medication effects per se because of the absence of a placebo control group. However, it did afford another opportunity to compare medication alone to a group format for CBT, a version of which had already been found efficacious for children and adolescents with OCD in Barrett et al.'s (2004) seminal efficacy trial. Moreover, because the study was conducted in Brazil, it also provided an opportunity to translate and back-translate manuals and measures that could prove helpful in dissemination efforts thereafter. Asbahr and colleagues based their group intervention on the CBT manual of March and Mulle (1998), which is the same protocol evaluated and ultimately validated in POTS I and POTS II. Findings indicated that both forms of treatments were associated with significant symptom reduction on OCD measures (including the CY-BOCS), but only sertraline was associated with a reduction in depressive symptoms as well. The absence of a group by time interaction at posttreatment on OCD measures led to the conclusion that group CBT and SER were comparable in terms of acute efficacy. Of note, however, the percent reductions reported on the CY-BOCS for the group protocol used in Asbahr et al. (2005) were less robust than those reported by Barrett et al. (2004), indicating some variability in response that cannot be isolated easily because of differences in the flexibility of sampling procedures, manuals used, therapist background, training and supervision, and the type of clinical setting.

In another efficacy trial that blended in effectiveness design elements, Williams et al. (2010) attempted to examine the effects of cognitive as opposed to behavioral techniques and explanations but did so in a decidedly clinical context. Williams et al. (2010) presented a cognitive rationale for treatment that emphasized the importance of cognitions related to exaggerated responsibility. Exposure exercises were included in the protocol, but their rationale involved attempting to test what happens to OCD-related cognitions and emotions. Moreover, therapists did not emphasize the importance of habituation and did not wait for anxiety to dissipate even in the context of exposure exercises. This greater focus on identifying and changing misconceptions to carry out compulsions differentiated the rationale from the more commonly used behavioral explanations that involve resisting impulses to engage in rituals. Twenty-one youth with OCD (ages 9–18) were randomized to either 10 one-hour sessions of CBT or a 12-week wait-list and were evaluated by blind assessors six months posttreatment. At posttreatment, the group who received cognitive therapy demonstrated significantly more improvement on the CY-BOCS than the wait-list group (48 percent vs. 7 percent reduction). In an immediate treatment-delayed comparison design, the wait-list group was treated using the same cognitive protocol and made similar gains, with no significant differences between the groups noted at 6-month follow-up (60 percent symptom reduction from baseline to 6-month follow-up in CBT group versus 52 percent reduction in wait-list+CBT group). Although differences were evident on the primary measure, no significant differences were reported at posttreatment between the groups on secondary analyses that comprised self-report measures of OCD, anxiety, depression, and OCD-related cognitions. Perhaps the key aspect of the study involved its setting: patients were treated by therapists who were not OCD experts in an outpatient clinical setting as opposed to an academic context, which lends further credibility to the potential for dissemination of this protocol despite the more complex rationale for treatment as compared to the relatively straightforward theoretical model and rationale typically used for exposure plus response prevention. This is especially important given that behavioral protocols are generally put forth as easier for training purposes than are cognitive therapies, yet therapists in this clinical context were able to implement the treatment successfully despite not identifying as being strictly cognitive therapists themselves.

Out of recognition that CBT for pediatric OCD often does not reach most patients who need help, Storch et al. (2011) conducted a trial designed to address the limited availability of CBT by adapting an evidence-based treatment protocol for real-time delivery over web-video camera (webcam). Advantages of this approach include reducing the cost and burden of services; increasing the types of settings in which CBT can be delivered (e.g., home, community agencies, school); increasing privacy and relative anonymity, thereby possibly reducing individual barriers/stigma associated with treatment; and potentially improving treatment quality by conducting exposures in naturalistic settings. Thirty-one youth with OCD (ages 7–16) were randomly assigned to 14 sessions of web-CBT (W-CBT) or a 4-week truncated wait-list control WL). W-CBT followed the protocol in POTS, in which participants received 14 60- to 90-minute sessions of family-based CBT over 12 weeks, with adaptations made in order for sessions to be conducted over webcam (e.g., handouts e-mailed before sessions, completed homework assignments read aloud to therapist, parents instructed on coaching child through within-session exposures conducted out of therapist's view). When controlling for baseline group differences (i.e., severity of OCD symptoms was higher in the W-CBT group), W-CBT was superior to WL on all primary outcome measures with large effect sizes. Thirteen of 16 youth (81 percent) in the W-CBT arm were treatment responders (defined as at least 30 percent reduction in CY-BOCS and a 1 or 2 on CGI-I), versus only two of 15 (13 percent) youth in the WL group. Although therapists reported some difficulty adjusting to this treatment modality (e.g., building the therapeutic alliance, reading visual cues of anxiety), parents generally reported high satisfaction with the treatment approach. Despite its limitations (e.g., small sample size, brief wait-list control), this study suggests that web-based delivery is a promising strategy for improving the reach of CBT into those communities for select patients in which access to in-person CBT is limited geographically or for other practical reasons (e.g., family scheduling difficulties). This small trial thus sets the stage for larger effectiveness studies to follow that can aim at making CBT more practical and readily available to patients beyond the context of the academic medical settings in which most of these protocols were developed and validated.

Valderhaug and colleagues (2007) conducted a small open trial in which the effectiveness of CBT was examined in community clinics in Norway using a novel supervision method, namely a "supervision of supervisors" approach. Twenty-eight youth ages 8–17 inclusive participated in the trial, which was a test of the manual developed by Piacentini, Langley, and Roblek (2007), which was delivered by community clinicians as part of their regular patient flow. The developers provided remote supervision of the clinical supervisors, which constituted a step away from the closer supervision procedures that characterize randomized controlled trials. The acute and long-term outcomes in this open study (60 percent CY-BOCS reduction at posttreatment and 69 percent at follow-up) compared favorably to outcomes achieved in randomized controlled trials, and provided pilot data for the much larger Nordic Long-term OCD Treatment Study (NordLOTS; Ivarsson et al., 2010; Torp et al., 2015a) study described as follows.

The multinational (Norway, Sweden, and Denmark) NordLOTS study currently represents the largest published trial involving pediatric OCD patients exposed to CBT, as all 269 participants received open label CBT (14 weekly sessions) in Phase 1 (Torp et al., 2015a). At the end of Phase 1, 50 eligible participants classified as nonresponsive to CBT were then randomized to receive sertraline or continued CBT for 16 more weeks (Skarphedinsson, Weidle, & Ivarsson, 2015). The Phase 1 outcomes were especially notable given a range of sites from research-oriented to purely clinical, which had no bearing on posttreatment outcomes. Moreover, the percentage reduction on the CY-BOCS (53 percent) and the percentage of the sample classified as responders (73 percent; CY-BOCS < 15) and remitters (49 percent; CY-BOCS < 10) were robust and compared favorably with findings from the large-scale efficacy studies conducted around the world. Attrition was also low during Phase 1 (10 percent), again attesting to the robustness of the protocol even outside the research context. A difference between clinical strategies for nonresponders was not identified in Phase 2, although the study's aims were compromised to an extent by the success of Phase 1: with a larger than anticipated responder rate, there were fewer nonresponders to randomize in Phase 2, thus providing insufficient statistical power for hypothesis testing. Nevertheless, inspection of the Phase 2 outcomes by condition suggests that low power was not entirely responsible for the absence of a statistically significant difference between the two conditions: 50 percent of the continued CBT group met criteria for response, in comparison to 45 percent in the sertraline group. Thus, both strategies appear to be useful in the clinical management of nonresponse, even in an effectiveness context.

In that same vein, Farrell and colleagues (2010) conducted an effectiveness study in Australia in which they delivered CBT in an outpatient, community-based specialist clinic in which they treated 33 youth with OCD. Here again the setting is most notable, in that the therapists were OCD-novice clinicians trained in a more generalist model, who were supervised by experts working in a community clinic, and hence the transportability of the treatment to such settings and clinicians was the focus of this study. The percentage change on the CY-BOCS (61 percent) and the responder rate (absence of an OCD diagnosis at posttreatment: 63 percent) were very encouraging, and compared well with the effect sizes achieved in a number of published trials on CBT for pediatric OCD. The absence of a control group does limit the extent to which the treatment itself can be said to account for symptom change, but there is already a strong evidence base attesting to efficacy in general, and the substantive contribution of this paper to the literature should not be underestimated as a result.

Another effectiveness trial was conducted by Leonard et al. (2016), who focused more on issues pertaining to the sampling frame. In that study, 172 residential patients received multimodal treatment that included intensive CBT (approximately 26.5 hours per week for multiple weeks), medication management, and additional cognitive-behavioral interventions (e.g., behavioral activation strategies for patients with comorbid depression). What set this study apart was the residential setting and, perhaps to be expected given the treatment context, patient complexity: psychiatric comorbidity was the norm, with 92 percent of participants meeting diagnostic criteria for at least two DSM disorders besides OCD. In addition, CBT was provided by bachelor's level clinicians supervised by a licensed psychologist, which lends further credence to conceptualizing this study through the effectiveness lens. Findings provided empirical support for this multimodal approach: 79 percent met study response criteria (CY-BOCS change > 25 percent) at posttreatment, 41 percent met criteria for excellent response (CY-BOCS < 10), and 64 percent met criteria for clinically significant change relative to baseline (Jacobson & Truax, 1991). Of those participants available for follow-up (mean follow-up time = 1.5 years posttreatment), 89 percent still maintained their responder status at that time point. The specific effects of CBT cannot be isolated given the multimodal approach, but such an approach is characteristic of clinical treatment for the severe and complex presentations of patients in this sample, hence increasing external validity of these findings to those treated in a residential milieu.

Moderators and predictors. Although there are many viable candidates for prediction or moderation of CBT response, there is as yet an insufficient empirical foundation upon which to make confident and empirically informed judgments about which patients will and which will not respond fully to this form of treatment, or any treatment for that matter. Ultimately, it will be of great benefit to be able to use patient, therapist, intervention, and associated contextual factors to make such predictions, but such endeavors are compromised by having an insufficient number of clinical outcome studies available and by sample sizes recruited specifically to permit hypothesis testing for primary aims regarding treatment efficacy rather than prediction or moderation. Because of their sample sizes, NordLOTS and the large-scale effectiveness study by Leonard and colleagues (2016) may provide the best opportunities thus far to examine key questions that still plague the field, most notably which patients under which conditions receiving which treatments are most (or least) likely to respond? Building the evidence base upon which to make such recommendations is one of the most important goals facing our field in the next decade, and those opportunities will require large-scale collaborations to help offset the issues inherent in studying a low base-rate disorder. There is potential methodological advantage that may aid in developing such collaborations, which is the reliance upon a virtually universal measure of treatment outcome in pediatric OCD, the Children's Yale-Brown Obsessive Compulsive Scale (CY-BOCS; Scahill et al., 1997). In other fields, such as social anxiety disorder, in which myriad measures are used, even summarizing the extant literature quickly descends into a veritable Tower of Babel because of reliance on so many different instruments to measure treatment outcome. In pediatric OCD this is not the case, and thus the possibility of cross-site data sharing and collaborative science remains within reach. One of our goals in writing this chapter is to vigorously encourage such efforts, since increasing sample size will improve our precision in identifying signals for prediction of treatment outcome in general or, more importantly, moderation of treatment outcome by condition. Discovery of moderators may then lead us to mediators, i.e., the underlying mechanisms by which the moderators exert their influence, which in turn can promote improved understanding of OCD psychopathology and treatment development efforts aimed at the mediators thus discovered.

Some progress has been made in identifying factors that could inform clinical judgment regarding treatment selection. Ginsburg and colleagues (2008) reviewed the data on prediction or moderation of outcome in pediatric OCD and identified baseline OCD symptom severity and family psychopathology as predictors of poorer response to CBT. In the POTS I trial, the presence of comorbid tic symptoms served as a moderator of pharmacotherapy response, i.e., predicted poorer outcome to sertraline alone but not to the treatment conditions that included CBT (CBT alone or the combination of CBT with sertraline; March et al., 2007). The NordLOTS trial confirmed that CBT outcomes in Phase 1 were not affected by the presence of concomitant tics (Hojgaard et al., 2017). Collectively these findings suggest that CBT should be delivered to treat youth with OCD regardless of their tic status or the setting in which treatment will be provided. Notably, despite the large sample size, the only predictor of CBT response that survived in the multivariate analysis was patient age, such that younger patients tended to have more robust outcomes (Torp et al., 2015b). A comprehensive examination of the POTS I dataset published after Ginsburg and colleagues' systematic review (Garcia et al., 2010) identified several predictors of response to all treatments, and included some of the usual suspects: lower OCD symptom severity, less OCD-related impairment, greater insight, fewer comorbid externalizing symptoms, and lower levels of family accommodation were associated with better outcomes. With respect to predicting response to specific treatments, only a family history of OCD emerged as a moderator: although family history did attenuate outcome at least somewhat across all treatment conditions, those with a family history had a six-fold decrease in effect size for CBT monotherapy compared to those without such a history. The mechanism by which this moderation occurred has yet to be elucidated, although examination of family variables in another RCT may prove helpful in thinking about how this effect may have been realized. Peris and colleagues (2008) examined data from Piacentini et al.'s (2011) RCT and found that families with lower levels of parental blame and family conflict as well as higher levels of family cohesion at baseline were more likely to have a child who responded to CBT. These observations led this investigative team to modify the family component of their treatment to focus more specifically on reducing accommodation, which is a prime example of how studying moderators can illuminate new directions in the effort to improve our treatments. What these data tell us in general about pediatric OCD is that family environment and family history of OCD are important considerations to take into account clinically when treating OCD.

What's Next? Proposed Studies of Dissemination and Implementation

The efficacy of CBT for pediatric OCD is now well-established, and significant strides have been made recently into exploring its effectiveness in more clinical contexts as well. Next stage research into the effectiveness of this treatment must now move more vigorously (and rigorously) toward dissemination. Models of how to achieve good clinical outcomes have been tested initially. For example, the supervision of supervisors model examined by Valderhaug and colleagues (2007). Moving forward, larger, randomized studies constitute the next step in establishing CBT for pediatric OCD as a treatment that can be delivered outside the academic context without significant decline in response rates, symptom reduction, and functional improvement. From an implementation science perspective, one could think about randomization of clinics or perhaps even therapists within clinics to treatment by trained (but not yet expert) clinicians who either have or do not have access to regular expert supervision. Because transportability to more clinical settings does not necessarily guarantee sustainability after access to expert training and ongoing consultation are removed, subsequent trials could then involve fading expert supervision to determine whether the treatment could be sustained successfully within the participating clinics without academic partnership in treatment implementation. Precedent has already been set in pediatric anxiety disorder treatment more broadly speaking whereby Beidas and colleagues (2012) demonstrated the utility of ongoing access to consultation in terms of affecting therapist behavior change. Such trials would allow researchers to examine patient, therapist, supervisor, and setting variables that are associated with effective and durable patient outcomes, which could then spawn next stage studies devoted to remediating modifiable factors known to compromise treatment. On a smaller scale this has already been done around the issue of family accommodation (for a review see Peris & Piacentini, 2014).

An emphasis placed in implementation science is on viewing the process as bidirectional, in that the clinical settings and agencies encouraging their therapists to participate in training in empirically supported treatments also have valuable information to share with the trainers with respect to aspects of treatment that may be more or less feasible or preferred by the clients seen in their settings. For example, patients in community settings may attend fewer treatment appointments than those willing to be randomized in clinical efficacy trials, which may then encourage treatment procedure modifications for therapists to use the most powerful procedures earlier, such as exposure plus response prevention.

Stepped care studies might also be incorporated into trials in which treatments with the least expensive and onerous treatments available (e.g., online OCD programs, bibliotherapy) could be attempted prior to referral to participating clinical sites. As was the intent in NordLOTS, patients who fail to respond to the initial interventions could then be sent on to expert sites for more intensive care developed ideographically based on therapists' and supervisors' clinical judgment regarding individual patients' reasons for nonresponse (e.g., between session noncompliance, family accommodation, family history of OCD). Such efforts could help make treatments more widely available, reduce wait times at subspecialty clinics, and thereby reduce illness burden for patients and families seeking CBT for OCD.

Summary and Conclusions

CBT for pediatric OCD has blossomed in the last twenty years into an empirically supported treatment for this disabling condition, with randomized studies from around the world attesting to its efficacy relative to various comparison conditions and to active medications. As has been demonstrated with adults suffering from OCD, the effects of CBT for children and adolescents appear to be both robust and durable, with follow-up studies indicating that CBT's effects last for up to nine months after treatment has ended. Intensive treatment regimens are efficacious and effective, although weekly treatment for approximately 12–14 weeks appears to be sufficient for most patients. With respect to making clinical judgments regarding whether a more intensive form of CBT is needed for a given patient, future studies now need to examine whether symptom severity, comorbidity, readiness for change, and case complexity (e.g., family problems) necessitate the more intensive approaches, and whether treatment setting differentially influences outcome and retention. The degree of family involvement in treatment and the degree to which this involvement needs to target specific family predictors of poorer response (e.g., accommodation) also remains an issue in need of more study. What is clear developmentally, however, is that the treatment of very young children likely requires a family-based approach, and the first multi-site, large-scale RCT of this protocol provided encouraging news with respect to the efficacy of this approach (Freeman et al., 2014). Dissemination of this treatment for young children, validated in POTS Jr. (Freeman et al., 2014), is another priority for the field. Some of this work has begun in earnest (e.g., Comer et al., 2017), and will be especially important to extend further given the lack of expertise available in the community to provide psychotherapy services for *any* conditions that affect young children.

Although it is clear that CBT involving ERP is an efficacious and effective treatment both alone and in combination with pharmacotherapy, these same data also suggest that response to treatment is neither universal nor complete. More work needs to be done to isolate the elements of patient presentation and treatment delivery that underlie successful immediate and long-term outcomes. For example, in adult OCD, Simpson et al. (2011) found a strong relationship between session adherence and CBT outcome, findings that are now strongly emphasized in clinical work with this population. Dissemination of these key factors will likely result in more patients being offered an effective treatment in clinical practice settings (Krebs & Heyman, 2010). Examination of moderators and predictors of treatment response, especially in more diverse and clinically focused settings, will help the field move forward in terms of treatment development efforts as the mediators of such effects are better understood. These data will help investigators discover and then emphasize the core elements of treatment in order to promote optimal treatment outcomes beyond the academic medical context.

Key Practice Points

Treatment of OCD in youth should involve CBT either with or without concomitant pharmacotherapy. The visit schedule can range from weekly to intensive (daily) sessions, and residential options have been found effective for more severe patients for whom complex psychiatric comorbidity is the norm. Assessment of all patients should include a detailed screen of OCD symptoms as well as the common anxiety and depressive disorders that frequently co-occur. At this point it is safe to say that treatment should be guided by one of the validated CBT manuals, and need not necessarily be delivered by subspecialty expert OCD therapists provided that supervision is available. The extent to which treatment effectiveness generalizes to clinical settings that do not have access to expert supervision remains to be discovered. Web-based CBT appears to be effective, and this approach may help make treatment more readily available to patients living in communities in which a paucity of expertise remains.

References

Abramowitz, J.S, Foa, E. B, & Franklin, M. E. (2003). Exposure and ritual prevention for obsessive-compulsive disorder: Effects of intensive versus twice-weekly sessions. *Journal of Consulting & Clinical Psychology, 71*, 394–398.

Abramowitz, J. S., Franklin, M. E., Street, G. P., Kozak, M. J., & Foa, E. B. (2000). Effects of comorbid depression on response to treatment for obsessive–compulsive disorder. *Behavior Therapy, 31*, 517–528.

Abramowitz, J. S., Whiteside, S. P. & Deacon, R. J. (2005). The effectiveness of treatment for pediatric obsessive-compulsive disorder: A meta-analysis. *Behavior Therapy, 36*, 55–63.

Asbahr, F. R., Castillo, A. R., Ito, L. M., Latorre, M. R. D. O., Moriera, M. N., & Lotufo-Neto, F. (2005). Group cognitive–behavioral therapy versus sertraline for the treatment of children and adolescents with obsessive–compulsive disorder. *Journal of the American Academy of Child & Adolescent Psychiatry, 44*, 1128–1136.

Barrett, P. M., Farrell, L., Pina, A., Peris, T. S., & Piacentini, J. (2008). Evidence-based psychosocial treatments for child and adolescent obsessive-compulsive disorder. *Journal of Clinical Child & Adolescent Psychology, 37*, 131–155.

Barrett, P., Healy-Farrell, L., & March, J.S. (2004). Cognitive-behavioral family treatment of childhood obsessive-compulsive disorder: A controlled trial. *Journal of the American Academy of Child and Adolescent Psychiatry, 43*, 46–62.

Beidas, R. S., Edmunds, J. M., Marcus, S. C., & Kendall, P. C. (2012). Training and consultation to promote implementation of an empirically supported treatment: A randomized trial. *Psychiatric Services, 63*, 660–665.

Chorpita, B., F., Park, A., Tsai, K., Korathu-Larson, P., Higa-McMillan, C., Nakamura, B. J., ... Krull, J. (2015). Therapist satisfaction across different treatment designs in the child STEPS randomized effectiveness trial. *Journal of Consulting and Clinical Psychology, 83*, 709–718.

Comer, J. S., Furr, J. M., Kerns, C. E., Miguel, E., Coxe, S., Elkins, R. M., ... Freeman, J. B. (2017). Internet-delivered, family-based treatment for early-onset OCD: A pilot randomized trial. *Journal of Consulting and Clinical Psychology, 85*, 178–186.

Deacon, B. J. (2013). The biomedical model of mental disorder: A critical analysis of its validity, utility, and effect on psychotherapy research. *Clinical Psychology Review, 33*, 846–861.

de Haan, E., Hoodgum, K. A. L., Buitelaar, J. K., & Keijsers, G. (1998). Behavior therapy versus clomipramine in obsessive–compulsive disorders in children and adolescents. *Journal of the American Academy of Child & Adolescent Psychiatry, 37*, 1022–1029.

Farrell, L. J., Schlup, B., & Boshcen, M. J. (2010). Cognitive-behavioral treatment of childhood obsessive-compulsive disorder in community-based clinical practice: Clinical significance and benchmarking against efficacy. *Behaviour Research & Therapy, 48*, 409–417.

Foa, E. B., Kozak, M. J., Steketee, G., & McCarthy, P. R. (1992). Treatment of depressive and obsessive–compulsive symptoms in OCD by imipramine and behavior therapy. *British Journal of Clinical Psychology, 31*, 279–292.

Foa, E. B., Liebowitz, M. R., Kozak, M. J., Davies, S., Campeas, R., Franklin, M. E., ... Tu, X. (2005). Randomized, placebo-controlled trial of exposure and ritual prevention, clomipramine, and their combination in the treatment of obsessive-compulsive disorder. *The American Journal of Psychiatry, 162*, 151–161.

Franklin, M. E., Abramowitz, J. S., Bux, D. A., Zoellner, L. A., & Feeny, N. C. (2002). Cognitive-behavioral therapy with and without medication in the treatment of obsessive compulsive disorder. *Professional Psychology: Research and Practice, 33*, 162–168.

Franklin, M. E., Abramowitz, J. S., Furr, J., Kalsy, S., & Riggs, D. S. (2003). A naturalistic examination of therapist experience and outcome of exposure and ritual prevention for OCD. *Psychotherapy Research, 13*, 153–167.

Franklin, M. E., Abramowitz, J. S., Kozak, M. J., Levitt, J. T., & Foa, E. B. (2000). Effectiveness of exposure and ritual prevention for obsessive-compulsive disorder: Randomized compared with nonrandomized samples. *Journal of Consulting and Clinical Psychology, 68*, 594–602.

Franklin, M. E., Dingfelder, H. E., Coogan, C. G., Garcia, A. M., Sapyta, J. J., & Freeman, J. (2013). Cognitive behavioral therapy for pediatric obsessive compulsive disorder: Development of expert-level competence and implications for dissemination. *Journal of Anxiety Disorders, 27*, 745–753.

Franklin, M. E., Kratz, H. E., Freeman, J. B., Ivarsson, T., Heyman, I., Sookman, D., & March, J. (2015). Cognitive-behavioral therapy for pediatric obsessive-compulsive disorder: Empirical review and clinical recommendations. *Psychiatry Research, 227*, 78–92.

Franklin, M.E., Sapyta, J., Freeman, J.B., Khanna, M., Compton, S., ... March, J.S. (2011). Cognitive behavior therapy augmentation of pharmacotherapy in pediatric obsessive compulsive disorder: The pediatric OCD treatment study II randomized controlled trial. *Journal of the American Medical Association, 306*, 1224–1232.

Freeman, J. B., Choate-Summers, M., Garcia, A. M., Moore, P. S., Sapyta, J. J., Khanna, M. S., ... Franklin, M. E. (2009). The pediatric obsessive-compulsive disorder treatment study II: Rationale, design and methods. *Child and Adolescent Psychiatry and Mental Health, 3*. doi:http://dx.doi.org/10.1186/1753-2000-3-4

Freeman, J., Sapyta, J., Garcia, A., Compton, S., Khanna, M., Flessner, C., ... Franklin, M. (2014). Family-based treatment of early childhood obsessive-compulsive disorder: The pediatric obsessive-compulsive disorder treatment study for young children (POTS Jr.) – A randomized clinical trial. *JAMA Psychiatry, 71*, 689–698.

Garcia, A. M., Sapyta, J. J., Moore, P. S., Freeman, J. B., Franklin, M. E., March, J. S., & Foa, E. B. (2010). Predictors and moderators of treatment outcome in the Pediatric Obsessive Compulsive Treatment Study (POTS I). *Journal of the American Academy of Child and Adolescent Psychiatry, 49*, 1024–1033.

Ginsburg, G. S., Kingery, J. N., Drake, K. L., & Grados, M. A. (2008). Predictors of treatment response in pediatric obsessive-compulsive disorder. *Journal of the American Academy of Child and Adolescent Psychiatry, 47*, 868–878.

Glisson, C., Hemmelgarn, A., Green, P., Dukes, D., Atkinson, S., & Williams, N. J. (2012). Randomized trial of the availability, responsiveness, and continuity (ARC) organizational intervention with community-based mental health programs and clinicians serving youth. *Journal of the American Academy of Child and Adolescent Psychiatry, 51*, 780–787.

Glisson, C., Williams, N. J., Hemmelgarn, A., Proctor, E., & Green, P. (2016a). Aligning organizational priorities with ARC to improve mental health service outcomes. *Journal of Consulting and Clinical Psychology, 84*, 713–725.

Glisson, C., Williams, N. J., Hemmelgarn, A., Proctor, E., & Green, P. (2016b). Increasing clinicians' EBT exploration and preparation behavior in youth mental health services by changing organizational culture with ARC. *Behavior Research and Therapy, 76*, 40–46.

Hojgaard, D. M. A., Skarphedinsson, G., Nissen, J. B., Hybel, K. A., Ivarsson, T., & Thomsen, P. H. (2017). Pediatric obsessive-compulsive disorder with tic symptoms: Clinical presentation and treatment outcome. *European Child & Adolescent Psychiatry, 26*, 681–689.

Insel, T. R. (2014). The NIMH research domain criteria (RDoC) project: Precision medicine for psychiatry. *The American Journal of Psychiatry, 171*, 395–397.

Insel, T. R., & Cuthbert, B. N. (2015). Brain disorders? Precisely: Precision medicine comes to psychiatry. *Science, 348*, 499–500.

Ivarsson, T., Thomsen, P. H., Dahl, K., Valderhaug, R., Weidle, B., Nissen, J. B., ... Melin, K. (2010). The rationale and some features of the nordic long-term OCD treatment study (NordLOTS) in childhood and adolescence. *Child & Youth Care Forum, 39*, 91–99.

Jacobson, N. S., & Truax, P. (1991). Clinical significance: A statistical approach to defining meaningful change in psychotherapy research. *Journal of Consulting and Clinical Psychology, 59*, 12–19.

Krebs, G., & Heyman, I. (2010). Treatment-resistant obsessive-compulsive disorder in young people: Assessment and treatment strategies. *Child and Adolescent Mental Health, 15*, 2–11. doi:10.1111/j.1475-3588.2009.00548.x

Leonard, R. C., Franklin, M. E., Wetterneck, C. T., Riemann, B. C., Simpson, H. B., Kinnear, K., ... Lake, P. M. (2016). Residential treatment outcomes for adolescents with obsessive-compulsive disorder. *Psychotherapy Research, 26*, 727–736.

March, J. S., Franklin, M. E., Leonard, H., Garcia, A., Moore, P., Freeman, J., et al. (2007). Tics moderate treatment outcome with sertraline but not cognitive-behavior therapy in pediatric obsessive-compulsive disorder. *Biological Psychiatry, 61*, 344–347.

March, J. S., & Mulle, K. (1998). *OCD in children and adolescents: A cognitive-behavioral treatment manual*. New York: Guilford Press.

Marks, I. M., Stern, R. S., Mawson, D., Cobb, J., & McDonald, R. (1980). Clomipramine and exposure for obsessive-compulsive rituals: I. *British Journal of Psychiatry, 136*, 1–25.

Pediatric OCD Treatment Study Team (POTS) (2004). Cognitive-behavioral therapy, sertraline, and their combination for children and adolescents with obsessive-compulsive disorder: The Pediatric OCD Treatment Study (POTS) randomized controlled trial. *Journal of the American Medical Association, 292*, 1969–1976. doi:10.1001/jama.292.16.1969

Peris, T.A., Bergman, R.L., Langley, A., Chang, S., McCracken, J.T., Piacentini, J. (2008). Correlates of accommodation of pediatric obsessive-compulsive disorder: Parent, child and family characteristics. *Journal of the American Academy of Child and Adolescent Psychiatry, 47*, 1173–1181.

Peris, T. S., & Piacentini, J. (2014). Addressing barriers to change in the treatment of childhood obsessive compulsive disorder. *Journal of Rational-Emotive & Cognitive-Behavior Therapy, 32*, 31–43.

Persons, J. B., & Silberschatz, G. (1998). Are results of randomized controlled trials useful to psychotherapists? *Journal of Consulting and Clinical Psychology, 66*, 126–135.

Piacentini, J., Bergman, L., Chang, S., Langley, A., Peris, T., Wood, J. J., & McCracken, J. (2011). Controlled comparison of family cognitive behavioral therapy and psychoeducation/relaxation training for child obsessive-compulsive disorder. *Journal of the American Academy of Child and Adolescent Psychiatry, 50*, 1149–1161.

Piacentini, J., Langley, A., & Roblek, T. (2007). *Cognitive-behavioral treatment of childhood OCD: It's only a false alarm, therapist guide*. New York: Oxford University Press.

Scahill, L., Riddle, M. A., McSwiggin-Hardin, M., Ort, S. I., King, R. A., Goodman, W. K., ... Leckman, J. F. (1997). Children's Yale-Brown Obsessive

Compulsive Scale: Reliability and validity. *Journal of the American Academy of Child & Adolescent Psychiatry, 36*, 844–852.

Simpson, H., Foa, E., Liebowitz, M., Ledley, D., Huppert, J., Cahill, S., et al. (2008). A randomized, controlled trial of cognitive-behavioral therapy for augmenting pharmacotherapy in obsessive-compulsive disorder. *American Journal of Psychiatry, 165*, 621–630.

Simpson, H. B., Maher, M. J., Wang, Y., Bao, Y., Foa, E. B., & Franklin, M. (2011). Patient adherence predicts outcome from cognitive-behavioral therapy in obsessive-compulsive disorder. *Journal of Consulting and Clinical Psychology, 79*, 247–252.

Skarphedinsson, G., Weidle, B., & Ivarsson, T. (2015). Sertraline treatment of nonresponders to extended cognitive-behavior therapy in pediatric obsessive-compulsive disorder. *Journal of Child and Adolescent Psychopharmacology, 25*(7), 574–579. http://doi.org/10.1089/cap.2015.0041

Storch, E. A., Caporino, N. E., Morgan, J. R., Lewin, A. B., Rojas, A., Brauer, L., ... Murphy, T. K. (2011). Preliminary investigation of web-camera delivered cognitive-behavioral therapy for youth with obsessive-compulsive disorder. *Psychiatry Research, 189*, 407–412.

Torp, N. C., Dahl, K., Skarphedinsson, G., Thomsen, P. H., Valderhaug, R., Weidle, B., ... Ivarsson, T. (2015a). Effectiveness of cognitive behavior treatment for pediatric obsessive-compulsive disorder: Acute outcomes from the nordic long-term OCD treatment study (NORDLOTS). *Behaviour Research and Therapy, 64*, 15–23.

Torp, N. C., Dahl, K., Skarphedinsson, G., Thomsen, P. H., Valderhaug, R., Weidle, B., ... Ivarsson, T. (2015b). Predictors associated with improved cognitive-behavioral therapy outcome in pediatric obsessive-compulsive disorder. *Journal of the American Academy of Child and Adolescent Psychiatry, 54*, 200–207.

Valderhaug, R., Larsson, B., Gotestam, K. G., & Piacentini, J. (2007). An open clinical trial of cognitive-behaviour therapy in children and adolescents with obsessive-compulsive disorder administered in regular outpatient clinics. *Behaviour Research & Therapy, 45*, 577–589.

Warren, R., & Thomas, J. C. (2001). Cognitive–behavior therapy of obsessive–compulsive disorder in private practice: An effectiveness study. *Journal of Anxiety Disorders, 15*, 277–285.

Watson, H.J. & Rees, C.S. (2008). Meta-analysis of randomized, controlled trials for pediatric obsessive-compulsive disorder. *Journal of Child Psychology and Psychiatry, 49*, 489–498.

Weisz, J. R., Chorpita, B. F., Palinkas, L. A., Schoenwald, S. K., Miranda, J., Bearman, S. K., ... Gibbons, R. D. (2012). Testing standard and modular designs for psychotherapy treating depression, anxiety, and conduct problems in youth: A randomized effectiveness trial. *Archives of General Psychiatry, 69*, 274–282.

Westen, D., Novotny, C. M., & Thompson-Brenner, H. (2004). The empirical status of empirically supported psychotherapies: Assumptions, findings, and reporting in controlled clinical trials. *Psychological Bulletin, 130*, 631–663.

Williams, T. I., Salkovskis, P. M., Forrester, L., Turner, S., White, H., & Allsopp, M. A. (2010). A randomised controlled trial of cognitive behavioural treatment for obsessive compulsive disorder in children and adolescents. *European Children and Adolescent Psychiatry, 19*, 449–456.

24 New Wave Therapies for Pediatric OCD

R. Lindsey Bergman and Michelle Rozenman

In prior chapters, evidence-based psychosocial interventions (i.e., cognitive behavior therapy [CBT]/exposure response prevention [ERP] for pediatric OCD were discussed in detail. As experts attempt to improve pediatric OCD treatment response, newer "third wave" psychotherapy approaches have been developed and tested for OCD and related conditions. These new therapies have demonstrated preliminary support for the treatment of adults with a variety of psychiatric conditions. While third wave approaches may still emphasize behavior change, several of them also broadly emphasize development of skills to notice and accept thoughts and feelings without necessarily attempting to change their content or respond to them behaviorally. A description of the full list of interventions that fall under new wave therapies is outside of the scope of this chapter (see Hofmann, Sawyer, & Fang, 2010; Kahl, Winter, & Schweiger, 2012; Öst, 2008 for reviews). However, three types of new wave interventions – mindfulness-based interventions, Acceptance and Commitment Therapy (ACT), and Dialectical Behavior Therapy (DBT) – have shown some promise in treating adults with OCD and related conditions, with a few studies being conducted with youth. Following, we briefly describe and review the extant research on ACT and DBT and how these may be relevant to pediatric OCD intervention. We then turn specifically to mindfulness-based intervention for the remainder of this chapter, as mindfulness may be especially suited to conceptualizations and treatment of OCD. We outline challenges and directions for future research in this area, and end by providing key practice points for clinicians who may wish to begin incorporating aspects of mindfulness intervention into their ERP practice with children and adolescents suffering from OCD.

A Need for Innovation of Pediatric OCD Interventions

As described in previous chapters, approximately two-thirds of OCD sufferers report a chronic symptom course, with symptoms often requiring long-term management (Visser et al., 2014). While the evidence suggests that CBT and selective serotonin reuptake inhibitors (SSRIs) are currently the recommended approaches for treating pediatric OCD (Geller et al., 2012), approximately half of youth who receive these interventions remain in the impaired range at posttreatment (March et al., 2004). Moreover, parents of youth with OCD report a preference of behavioral intervention over pharmacotherapy, and parents of young children generally do not rate pharmacotherapy as an acceptable intervention approach (Lewin et al., 2014). Together, these data indicate that not all families are open to all available evidence-based approaches and, even with receipt of gold-standard intervention, a substantial proportion of youth will not experience symptom relief. Thus, there remains substantial room for improvement of psychosocial interventions for youth with OCD.

New Wave Therapies: Approach to Innovation and Evidence Base

In the last two decades, psychopathology intervention researchers have begun to develop and test a group of interventions, labeled "new wave" or "third wave" (Hayes et al., 2004), for a variety of health and mental health problems in adults and, more recently, in youth. While these new wave therapies are quite heterogeneous, they have some common features that distinguish them from those of traditional CBT models. Most broadly, these interventions do not focus on attempts to alter or challenge the content of cognitions. Instead, to the extent that cognition is emphasized, a goal of these interventions is to develop skills in order to accept thoughts rather than struggle with (i.e., attempt to change) them. The traditional CBT approach places emphasis on maladaptive cognitions that are believed to trigger anxiety and require modification during the treatment of anxiety. Intervention researchers have challenged traditional CBT for its lack of evidence to support this model of cognitive change (Longmore & Worrell, 2007). These new wave approaches highlight noticing thoughts without attempting to challenge or modify them; this, in turn, is proposed to increase one's ability to tolerate emotional distress related to unwanted thoughts.

It should be noted that the third wave interventions are not clearly a strict departure from CBT models either in theory or in practice. In fact, some researchers consider these third wave approaches an extension of CBT (Hofmann et al., 2010). Indeed, the few clinical trials that have conducted head-to-head comparisons in adult psychiatric patients have found that new wave approaches result in comparable treatment response to CBT or behavior therapy at posttreatment, although in some trials the third wave approach appears to result in continued improvements over long-term follow-up (Arch et al., 2012; Clarke et al., 2014). Based on the research evidence, described further as follows, and our clinical experiences, we currently view these new wave therapies as augmentation or alternative strategies to addressing OCD in youth.

Although each of the third wave approaches uses some techniques consistent with traditional CBT models (e.g., problem solving, eliminating avoidance), each third wave therapy also includes some distinct techniques based on the intervention's broad goals and perspective on managing mental health symptoms. In this chapter, we focus on three third wave interventions that have demonstrated preliminary support in addressing OCD and related conditions: ACT, DBT, and mindfulness-based approaches, including Mindfulness-Based Stress Reduction (MBSR) and

Mindfulness-Based Cognitive Therapy (MBCT). One skill set common to all of these intervention approaches is mindfulness, or "the awareness that emerges through paying attention on purpose, in the present moment, and nonjudgmentally" (Kabat-Zinn, 2003). Said differently, mindfulness is a means with which to attend to "thoughts and feelings in the present moment without making any judgments as to their meaning or value" (Hannan & Tolin, 2005). Such an approach may be particularly relevant to the treatment of OCD, as a core diagnostic feature of OCD is an overemphasis on thoughts as negative, intolerable, or dangerous. Broadly, the third wave approaches, and specifically the mindfulness components of these interventions may teach individuals with OCD to perceive their thoughts as nonpermanent mental experiences, rather than focusing on changing distress associated with the thoughts. In the remainder of this section, we describe the broad treatment goals and techniques of ACT, DBT, and mindfulness-based approaches, including the extant evidence base for use of these approaches with OCD and related disorders.

Acceptance and Commitment Therapy (ACT) is a third wave approach to psychotherapy that embraces several strategies (including mindfulness) to promote psychological flexibility and the pursuit of personal goals that are in line with one's values. With regard to psychological flexibility, this treatment target is defined as enhancing the capacity to make contact with experience in the present moment, and based on what is possible in that moment, persisting in or changing behavior in the pursuit of goals and values (Blackledge et al., 2005). In regard to pursuing personal goals, behavior change is a specific goal inasmuch as current behavior is not in line with one's personal commitments and values. That is, symptom reduction is not targeted per se; rather the emphasis is on replacing actions that are counter to one's committed values and life choices with actions that reflect those goals. With regard to OCD, a lack of cognitive flexibility and a focus on thoughts as dangerous and upsetting has been demonstrated to lead to avoidance in both adults and children (Abramowitz, Lackey, & Wheaton, 2009; Briggs & Price, 2009). ACT's focus on increasing psychological flexibility may address these core difficulties related to the role of cognition (i.e., obsessions) in OCD.

Treatment techniques in ACT include but are not limited to: acceptance of inner experiences (i.e., thoughts and feelings), being present and attending to internal experiences and external events as they occur without judging those experiences and events (i.e., mindfulness), and defusion, or viewing cognition as an ongoing process rather than a causal event. Together, these processes are proposed to improve psychological flexibility in order to pursue one's goals and values. Similar to CBT, ACT may use behavioral interventions such as exposure, problem solving, and role-play to increase pursuit of personal goals. However, in contrast to traditional cognitive restructuring in CBT (which has the goal of changing the content of cognitions), ACT views thoughts as mental states that should be observed and accepted rather than modified or avoided.

Studies of ACT as an intervention for pediatric OCD are limited, with only two published trials. A small open trial of ACT involving three adolescents diagnosed with OCD (Armstrong, Morrison, & Twohig, 2013) suggested feasibility of ACT with adolescent OCD patients, acceptability of the intervention to youths and parents, and very preliminary data supporting symptom reduction (40 percent mean reduction in self-reported compulsions from pre-to-posttreatment). Moreover, symptom reduction was maintained at 3-month follow-up. In this treatment trial, typical ACT treatment elements were applied to OCD symptoms, including but not limited to the use of metaphors to explain the concepts of defusion, acceptance, and responsibility to personal values. Neither in-session nor out-of-session exposures to feared stimuli (i.e., the content of obsessions) were included in the intervention, but treatment did include assignments for participants to engage in "behavioral commitments" that were periods of time during which participants agreed to refrain from engaging in compulsive behaviors. A second small open trial ($N=3$) using a multiple baseline design was conducted with school-aged children with OCD (Barney et al., 2017). In this study, both parents and children participated in all sessions, led by a school psychologist, with parents conceptualized as an at-home support for treatment facilitation. Their results also provide preliminary support for OCD symptom reduction (47 percent average self-reported symptom reduction across participants), as well as for improvements in psychological flexibility, an ACT treatment target.

Given this limited literature in pediatric OCD, a review of the evidence base for ACT in adult OCD and related conditions is warranted. First, it should be noted that meta-analytic findings across anxiety and OC-spectrum disorders suggest that ACT is equally as effective as CBT (Bluett et al., 2014). With regard to specific trials, ACT has been tested in adults with OCD, as well as in those with hair pulling disorder (trichotillomania). Open trials provided early evidence for ACT as a stand-alone treatment for adults with OCD (Twohig, Hayes, & Masuda, 2006) and skin picking (Twohig et al., 2006), as well as an adjunctive intervention for adults with hair pulling disorder (Crosby et al., 2012; Twohig & Woods, 2004). Subsequent randomized trials provided additional support that ACT results in greater OCD symptom reduction and greater maintenance of treatment gains over 3-month follow-up than progressive muscle relaxation in adults (Twohig et al., 2010). Importantly, similar to pediatric studies, in Twohig et al.'s (2010) treatment trial, participants were instructed to confront feared stimuli using ACT skills during daily life but did not participate in exposure exercises during sessions. Prolonged contact with the feared stimuli in attempts to reduce anxiety or distress related to the stimuli was not a goal as it is with CBT or exposure and response prevention (ERP). However, the ACT model is not inconsistent with exposure-based treatment, and the exclusion of exposures in ACT trials for OCD has been primarily a methodological strategy at this early stage of investigation (Dehlin, Morrison, & Twohig, 2013). That is, investigators excluded exposures so as to better isolate the specific effects of the ACT treatment without also capturing effects that might have been due to exposures. Given the established efficacy of exposures in the treatment of OCD, unless otherwise contraindicated, the clinical treatment of OCD using ACT is likely maximized when exposures are also included. For specific recommendations on the application of ACT to OCD based on the extant adult literature, see (Twohig, Morrison, & Bluett, 2014; Twohig, 2009; Twohig et al., 2015).

Dialectical Behavior Therapy (DBT) is a third wave intervention initially developed to treat borderline personality disorder (Linehan, 2015) that has since been applied to other psychiatric conditions. The focus of DBT is on dialectics, or reconciling between acceptance and change to improve emotion regulation. DBT teaches mindfulness and emotion regulation skills alongside more traditional CBT skills to target cognitions, emotions, and behaviors. To our knowledge, there are no published trials of DBT for OCD, and it is unclear how a stand-alone DBT protocol might apply to pediatric OCD. However, there is a rationale for applying DBT to OCD-related disorders (e.g., hair pulling disorder, skin picking disorder): an associated feature of these conditions is the experience of negative affect before pulling/picking (Shusterman et al., 2009; Snorrason, Smári, & Ólafsson, 2010), which the DBT framework and skills may be able to address. DBT has been preliminarily tested as an adjunctive intervention to cognitive behavioral therapy in both adults (Keuthen et al., 2010, 2012) and adolescents (Welch & Kim, 2012) with hair pulling disorder, with promising results. We do caution that DBT in its original format is a multifaceted intervention that includes several intervention modalities and skills to address safety, skill practice, and social functioning (e.g., emergency phone coaching, multifamily group, clinician process group about patients) for some conditions (i.e., borderline personality disorder). Therefore, we advise clinicians interested in DBT to obtain formal training in this third wave intervention.

Following formal DBT training, we began to utilize some DBT distress tolerance skills as a supplement to ERP and mindfulness practice (described further as follows) with OCD-affected youth. In particular, we teach our pediatric patients physical grounding strategies such as digging their heels into the floor, noticing the feeling of one's body in their chair, feet in their shoes, hands on their lap, and grabbing onto their chair to feel the temperature and texture of the chair. We also often use mental grounding activities, such as describing the environment in detail using all senses or describing an everyday event (e.g., making a peanut butter and jelly sandwich). It should be noted that these strategies might also be called mindfulness strategies, as we typically ask youths to view the exercise with curiosity, noticing both their thoughts and the environment. Thus, while we have drawn these distress tolerance strategies from our formal DBT training, these skills are not inconsistent with experiential mindfulness practice in mindfulness-based interventions.

We also use a modified version of DBT's behavior chains for use with children and adolescents with OCD who experience emotional outbursts and/or aggressive behavior. Behavior chains in DBT are focused on a patient's problem behavior, most often self-injury in the traditional DBT model. In our practice, we teach patients behavior chains when they frequently tantrum (e.g., yell, scream, act aggressively toward parents); often, but not always, this behavior occurs when youth are triggered by and/or when parents decline to provide accommodations or reassurance related to their OCD symptoms. Youth are asked to identify the problem behavior (typically the height of the conflict or youth's verbal or physical aggression), the specific event or obsession that precipitated the problem behavior, and then draw a detailed "timeline" of the chain of events (i.e., youth's thoughts, feelings, and behaviors) that led up to the problem behavior, as well as its consequences. Youths then identify points in the timeline during which they might have done something differently to avoid the problem behavior. While youths are first taught and complete timelines following the problem behavior, our expectation for youths is that they begin to become more aware of the problem behavior and eventually take breaks from situations in which the problem behavior might emerge in order to proactively complete behavior chains and distress tolerance skills. Said differently, our ultimate goal is that eventually youths are able to disengage from situations in which they might engage in the problem behavior and complete a behavior chain instead.

Mindfulness-Based Approaches to Treating OCD

As described previously, mindfulness has been defined as "the awareness that emerges through paying attention on purpose, in the present moment, and nonjudgmentally to the unfolding of experience moment by moment" (Kabat-Zinn, 2003) or "the process by which one attends to their thoughts and feelings in the present moment without making any judgments as to their meaning or value" (Hannan & Tolin, 2005). Mindfulness-based stress reduction (MBSR) was established in 1979 by Jon Kabat Zinn and since been used successfully to treat or augment treatment for a wide variety of medical (diabetes, heart disease, asthma, hypertension, fibromyalgia) and psychological (depression, anxiety, stress disorders) difficulties. Mindfulness-based cognitive therapy (MBCT) combines traditional cognitive therapy with mindfulness techniques and was developed to prevent relapse among adults treated for major depression.

Both MBSR and MBCT are typically delivered in a group format and include education about mindfulness, as well as practice of formal mindful meditation exercises to be conducted both in session and at home. Formal mindfulness exercises include focusing, sustaining, and switching attention, accepting the present moment experience (e.g., sensations in the body, "I have an upsetting thought right now"), and redirecting attention when it wanders or when one judges or attempts to modify their internal experience. Experiential mindfulness exercises often use the breath as an "anchor" for attention when the mind wanders or for thoughts and feelings that are difficult to experience. Sound, touch, and taste may also be used as anchors, depending on the particular exercise. For children, it is typically recommended that mindfulness practice includes concrete activities such as movement or touch, and that the formal meditation component be brief. Following mindfulness exercises, participants typically discuss and share their experience with other members during group intervention. All mindfulness interventions have in common the concept of decentering, or the perspective that thoughts are mental events that do not necessarily reflect an individual or reality. In addition to formal mindfulness practice, or meditation, mindfulness is also practiced in an informal or "everyday" way such that individuals are encouraged to be more present while engaging in daily activities.

The developers of MBCT and MBSR programs have cautioned that mindfulness instructors must have extensive experience with their own mindfulness practices before attempting to use the program with clients. Therefore, it may be difficult for clinicians with primary expertise in OCD to begin implementing these full protocols in their clinical practice.

Central to OCD is a difficulty tolerating distress related to disturbing intrusive thoughts (i.e., obsessions), leading to subsequent attempts to suppress those unwanted thoughts, or engage in compulsions in attempts to relieve distress associated with the thoughts. Both suppression and compulsions inevitably lead to cycles of increased avoidance, fear, and OCD symptoms (Abramowitz, 2017).

The rationale for use of mindfulness in OCD is that mindfulness teaches individuals to view their thoughts as subjective, impermanent experiences that do not necessarily reflect reality, and do not need to be suppressed or otherwise modified. In turn, the individual may be able to develop tolerance of obsessions and mitigate the OCD cycle. This is in stark contrast to cognitive restructuring techniques in traditional CBT for OCD, which may inadvertently perpetuate the notion that thoughts are dangerous and should be modified. Consistent with a mindfulness-based and decentering approach, in our clinical practice, we often incorporate language that reflects the impermanent, ever-changing nature of, and nonjudgmental attitude about thoughts, including: "thoughts are just thoughts" and "no thought or feeling lasts forever."

In the absence of an evidence base to suggest an alternate practice, in our clinical treatment of pediatric OCD, we use mindfulness to augment ERP (see case example that follows). This involves familiarizing youth with the principles of mindfulness and conducting brief mindfulness exercises in between ERP activities. In group format with parents and pediatric OCD patients, we discuss the incorporation of a mindful view of internal experience (e.g., thoughts) into daily life, with the hope that they may begin to view obsessions in a decentered way.

Evidence Base

While the adult mindfulness literature is ever-growing, only two studies have used mindfulness (MBCT) for treatment and prevention of anxiety disorders in youth (Biegel et al., 2009; Semple, Reid, & Miller, 2005), with positive results. However, neither of these studies included youth with OCD. There is also some support for mindfulness intervention leading to anxiety symptom reduction in typically developing youths (Lee et al., 2008). Increasingly, clinicians are obtaining training in mindfulness-based approaches for youth anxiety disorders yet, to our knowledge, child OCD researchers have not yet begun to assess mindfulness for the treatment of pediatric OCD or to examine potential mechanisms.

Over the last 20 years, evidence has been accumulating that mindfulness may be an effective component in the treatment for adults with OCD. Most recently, MBCT has been demonstrated as efficacious and well-tolerated in an open trial targeting residual OCD symptoms following a trial of CBT (Sguazzin et al., 2017). Other studies have demonstrated the usefulness of mindfulness techniques (versus distraction) in decreasing both anxiety and the urge to neutralize distressing thoughts among adults with OCD (Wahl et al., 2013); as well as the effectiveness of mindfulness strategies at reducing OCD symptoms in nonclinical populations (Hanstede, Gidron, & Nyklíček, 2008); and finally, among clinically diagnosed individuals (Hertenstein et al., 2012; Liu, Han, & Xu, 2011; Madani et al., 2013). Although the extant evidence seems to suggest that mindfulness-based strategies are acceptable and helpful for adult OCD, randomized controlled trials are required to obtain evidence regarding the effectiveness of mindfulness as compared to other treatments known to be effective (e.g., exposure and response prevention).

Mindfulness: Underlying Mechanisms

As mentioned previously, mindfulness-based interventions have demonstrated positive psychiatric outcomes among adult and youth populations. To our knowledge, no studies have examined neurobiological underpinnings and/or mechanisms of change for mindfulness in youth or adults with OCD. However, the broader mindfulness literature proposes some mediators of psychiatric symptom change that may be relevant. These are briefly reviewed here, although we should note that the research literature is at an early stage in this area. In order to demonstrate mechanisms of OCD symptom change in youth, randomized clinical trials of mindfulness-based intervention would need to incorporate neuroimaging and/or identify temporal precedence of mindfulness change preceding symptom change. It should also be noted that the mechanisms underlying mindfulness in adults may be distinct from those in youth given neurobiological and neurocognitive development in the former age group.

In healthy controls and adult psychiatric patients, several underlying mechanisms have been posited to underlie the efficacy of mindfulness. Preliminary findings indicate that the mechanism of action underlying mindfulness involves increased tolerance to emotionally valenced stimuli (Arch & Craske, 2006; Lee & Orsillo, 2014) and improved emotional regulation and acceptance of emotional states (Menezes et al., 2013). Studies using fMRI to investigate neural mechanisms suggest that, in typical adults, mindfulness meditation increases activation in higher-order cortical regions while subsequently down-regulating areas involved in emotional processing (e.g., amygdala; Lutz et al., 2013; Zeidan et al., 2013). These results suggest that mindfulness may increase an individual's ability to manage negative cognition, regulate emotional arousal, and tolerate distress. Furthermore, there is considerable overlap in the brain regions involved in fear extinction and those that show structural and functional changes following mindfulness training (Tang, Holzel, & Posner, 2015). Identification of mechanisms by which mindfulness may lead to symptom relief is an active area of investigation, but at this time there is no empirical consensus about which of these putative mechanisms might be responsible for positive psychiatric outcome and/or how they may interact with one another.

Illustration of Incorporating Mindfulness into ERP

As noted previously, in our clinical practice, we utilize mindfulness to augment ERP for pediatric OCD. As group intervention is part of our treatment modality, we most often conduct group mindfulness exercises with several patients at once, although we also sometimes ask patients to practice mindfulness with their therapist individually. Mindfulness is conducted before or after each ERP session. This involves a basic three-to-five-minute guided meditation (e.g., breath meditation, body scan, sound meditation) or some other experiential activity (e.g., savoring meditation, movement or walking meditation). We then follow with a group discussion of the benefits of mindfulness, individual patient experiences during the exercise including whether they were able to redirect attention back to the exercise when they became distracted, and the connection between mindfulness and OCD treatment for each participant. Finally, youth are often assigned to practice at home the same mindfulness exercise that they completed in session.

Case Illustration

"Max" was a 14-year-old boy with OCD symptoms focused on fears that his 11-year-old sister was contaminated. He engaged in very frequent mental compulsions (counting, repeating phrases in his head) that interfered with his functioning in every domain of daily life (school, family life, social, etc.). Max received intensive ERP treatment and was also on SSRI medication. During daily treatment, Max participated in mindfulness exercises and learned about the basic premise of mindfulness; that is, being in the present moment, without trying to change his thoughts or feelings, and instead view them with curiosity and awareness rather than judgment. He recognized the relevance to OCD in that he previously attempted to change his obsessive thoughts (by doing compulsions) and judged them as "bad" and in need of eradication. He occasionally listened to brief guided mindfulness exercises at home that were assigned but found it difficult to do so, saying that he "couldn't focus" at home. We then introduced a commonly used mindfulness exercise utilizing an acronym, S.T.O.P., which coaches the individual to Stop, Take a breath, Observe [what is going on around them at the moment and in their body/thoughts] and then Proceed [with whatever activity the individual was supposed to be doing at that time]. Max practiced STOP at various times throughout the treatment day when he was prompted by his phone alarm. After practice in session, we then asked Max to set his alarm to prompt him to use STOP at home as well. This practice proved helpful to Max, as did repeated practice of brief mindfulness meditation exercises consisting of focus on breath or sounds and practice redirecting attention back to these anchors when his thoughts drifted elsewhere. Over time, Max verbalized that the mindfulness practices helped him "fight" OCD by increasing his awareness that he was experiencing distressing thoughts and "creating space" for him between the thoughts and compulsions that sometimes helped him to resist the compulsions. He also said, "I have noticed that OCD-related thoughts are no different than regular thoughts. They're just thoughts."

In a small (*N*=19; Bergman, Rozenman, & Piacentini, 2014) open trial of youth with severe OCD receiving ERP augmented with mindfulness as described previously, youths provided very positive feedback regarding their experiences with mindfulness. The majority of youths reported that their ability to be mindful had increased over time and, importantly, 56 percent of them reported that practicing mindfulness helped them change their awareness of intrusive thoughts. Youths also provided comments about the experiential mindfulness practices, including: "It is easier to bring my attention back to the present moment when my mind wanders" and "Accepting obsessive thoughts and not resisting, allows [the thoughts] to go away and I don't do compulsions." These qualitative data provide some evidence that youths ages 9 to 17 in our practice are able to understand and relate mindfulness concepts to their symptoms. Additionally, anecdotal information from parents of these children and adolescents indicates that youths often use mindfulness concepts in response to experience of obsessions in their daily lives.

Challenges and Recommendations for Future Research

As with all novel interventions, and as discussed previously, the new wave therapies have not been extensively studied in samples of OCD-affected adults, with even fewer trials in youth. Research in this area faces several challenges with regard to empirical research findings and clinical considerations. First, third wave approaches have not yet demonstrated sufficient support (due to the few extant trials) to deem them efficacious for OCD-related disorders (e.g., Öst, 2008). As the field continues to test the efficacy and effectiveness of these new wave therapies, it will be important to answer questions about how new wave approaches compare to traditional ERP/CBT for OCD and the efficacy of these approaches as stand-alone versus augmentation. Future work might also test moderators of treatment response, or whether certain youth or family characteristics or OCD symptom clusters might be better addressed with third wave, rather than ERP/CBT, intervention. Finally, given the developing brain, it will be important to assess whether the neural mechanisms proposed to underlie new wave therapies that have been identified in adult trials also apply to pediatric patients (Kalra & Swedo, 2009).

There are also challenges for the practicing clinician who may be interested in incorporating mindfulness or other third wave approaches into their treatment of children and adolescents with OCD. First, while manuals, programs, and apps have been developed for young children and adolescents, little has been done to explore how cognitive development may impact learning abstract concepts core to mindfulness, such as meta-cognition. Consultation with experts and additional pilot work with youth of all ages may result in guidelines for how to introduce and reflect upon experiential mindfulness exercises depending on the child or adolescent's cognitive development and abstract thinking skills. Next, our pediatric patients often have misconceptions that mindfulness is meant to modify their internal state (e.g., feel less anxious, feel more relaxed). While some may report reductions in anxiety or feelings of relaxation after an experiential mindfulness exercise (e.g., focus on the breath), it is good to keep again in mind that the aim of mindfulness is to observe internal states and external experiences nonjudgmentally without attempting to modify them. This may become especially difficult if a patient begins to use mindfulness as a compulsion (e.g., "I have to do mindfulness when I have an obsession so that I feel better"). Similarly, while mindfulness may be used during early or very difficult exposures in order to titrate the child's level of distress, our perspective is that ultimately the child should be able to use mindfulness concepts (e.g., "I notice that I'm very distressed, but I also know that no feeling lasts forever") without specifically engaging in experiential practice in attempts to downregulate distress.

We recommend that interested clinicians obtain formal mindfulness training and consult with mindfulness practitioners to ensure that they teach and use skills appropriately with their patients. ACT and DBT have more formalized training curriculums available by experts in the field. Clinicians practicing CBT need to take care to ensure that patients are not given contradictory instructions. Specifically, it would be confusing to youngsters if they were simultaneously instructed to challenge irrational thoughts (central to CBT) vs accept them (central to mindfulness). For this reason, and because there is evidence that self-directed mindfulness had no effect on OCD symptoms in adults (Cludius et al., 2015) it is not recommended that clinicians direct youth to initiate mindfulness practice outside of the treatment setting. For additional recommendations regarding incorporation of mindfulness into ERP, see Fairfax (2008).

Key Practice Points

- New wave, or third wave, therapy approaches that have demonstrated preliminary support for the treatment of OCD and related conditions in adults include: mindfulness-based interventions, Acceptance and Commitment Therapy (ACT), and Dialectical Behavior Therapy (DBT).
- Distinct from traditional CBT, these third wave therapies emphasize acceptance of thoughts (i.e., thoughts do not need to be changed or challenged). However, new wave therapies also use techniques consistent with traditional CBT, such as problem solving and promotion of approach behavior, to replace avoidance of feared situations.
- Mindfulness skills include focusing, sustaining, and switching attention, accepting the present moment experience, and redirecting attention when it wanders or when one judges or attempts to modify their internal experience. A common theme in mindfulness is that thoughts are mental events that do not necessarily reflect an individual or reality. In regard to OCD, obsessions can be viewed as impermanent experiences that do not necessarily reflect reality, will dissipate on their own (i.e., no thought lasts forever), and do not need to be suppressed or otherwise modified.
- Given the sparsity of research on new wave approaches in pediatric OCD samples, it is recommended that mindfulness be used to augment exposure-based practice, but not replace it. Also, clinicians practicing CBT should be careful not to give contradictory

instructions to patients (i.e., simultaneous instructions to challenge irrational thoughts as in CBT and instructions to accept irrational thoughts as in mindfulness).
- Interested clinicians should obtain formal mindfulness training and consult with mindfulness practitioners to ensure that they teach and use skills appropriately with their patients. ACT and DBT have more formalized training curriculums available by experts in the field.
- For children, formal mindfulness practice should include brief, experiential activities (e.g., touch, movement) before or after each ERP session. Youth should also be encouraged to be more present and use mindfulness skills in their daily life activities.
- While some may report that they feel relaxed or less anxious after mindfulness practice, mindfulness exercises are not for relaxation. Formal mindfulness practice instructs one to observe their internal states and external experiences nonjudgmentally without attempting to modify them.

References

Abramowitz, J. S., Lackey, G. R., & Wheaton, M. G. (2009). Obsessive-compulsive symptoms: The contribution of obsessional beliefs and experiential avoidance. *Journal of Anxiety Disorders, 23*(2), 160–166. http://doi.org/10.1016/j.janxdis.2008.06.003

Abramowitz, J. S. (2017). Presidential address: Are the obsessive-compulsive related disorders related to obsessive-compulsive disorder? A critical look at DSM-5's new category. *Behavior Therapy, 49*(1), 1–11.

Arch, J. J., & Craske, M. G. (2006). Mechanisms of mindfulness: Emotion regulation following a focused breathing induction. *Behaviour Research and Therapy, 44* (12), 1849–1858. http://doi.org/10.1016/j.brat.2005.12.007

Arch, J. J., Eifert, G. H., Davies, C., Vilardaga, J. C. P., Rose, R. D., & Craske, M. G. (2012). Randomized clinical trial of cognitive behavioral therapy (CBT) versus acceptance and commitment therapy (ACT) for mixed anxiety disorders. *Journal of Consulting and Clinical Psychology, 80*(5), 750–765. http://doi.org/10.1037/a0028310

Armstrong, A. B., Morrison, K. L., & Twohig, M. P. (2013). A preliminary investigation of acceptance and commitment therapy for adolescent obsessive-compulsive disorder. *Journal of Cognitive Psychotherapy, 27*(2), 175–190. http://doi.org/10.1891/0889-8391.27.2.175

Barney, J. Y., Field, C. E., Morrison, K. L., & Twohig, M. P. (2017). Treatment of pediatric obsessive compulsive disorder utilizing parent facilitated acceptance and commitment therapy. *Psychology in the Schools, 54*(1), 88–100. http://doi.org/10.1002/pits.21984

Bergman, R. L., Rozenman, M., & Piacentini, J. (2014). *Improving tolerance of intrusive thoughts: A pilot trial of mindfulness meditation in pediatric OCD*. Paper presented at the Association for Behavioral and Cognitive Therapies.

Biegel, G. M., Brown, K. W., Shapiro, S. L., & Schubert, C. M. (2009). Mindfulness-based stress reduction for the treatment of adolescent psychiatric outpatients: A randomized clinical trial. *Journal of Consulting and Clinical Psychology, 77*(5), 855–866. http://doi.org/10.1037/a0016241

Blackledge, J. T., & Barnes-Holmes, D. (2005). Core processes in acceptance and commitment therapy. In *Acceptance and commitment therapy – Contemporary theory research and practice*, J. T. Blackledge, Joseph Ciarrochi, & Frank P. Deane, eds. (pp. 41–58). Bowen Hills, Queensland, Australia: Australian Academic Press. Retrieved from https://contextualscience.org/files/Blackledge_Barnes-Holmes_2009.pdf

Bluett, E. J., Homan, K. J., Morrison, K. L., Levin, M. E., & Twohig, M. P. (2014). Acceptance and commitment therapy for anxiety and OCD spectrum disorders: An empirical review. *Journal of Anxiety Disorders, 28*(6), 612–624. http://doi.org/10.1016/j.janxdis.2014.06.008

Briggs, E. S., & Price, I. R. (2009). The relationship between adverse childhood experience and obsessive-compulsive symptoms and beliefs: The role of anxiety, depression, and experiential avoidance. *Journal of Anxiety Disorders, 23*(8), 1037–1046. http://doi.org/10.1016/j.janxdis.2009.07.004

Clarke, S., Kingston, J., James, K., Bolderston, H., & Remington, B. (2014). Acceptance and commitment therapy group for treatment-resistant participants: A randomized controlled trial. *Journal of Contextual Behavioral Science, 3*(3), 179–188. http://doi.org/10.1016/j.jcbs.2014.04.005

Cludius, B., Hottenrott, B., Alsleben, H., Peter, U., Schröder, J., & Moritz, S. (2015). Mindfulness for OCD? No evidence for a direct effect of a self-help treatment approach. *Journal of Obsessive-Compulsive and Related Disorders, 6*, 59–65. http://doi.org/10.1016/j.jocrd.2015.05.003

Crosby, J. M., Dehlin, J. P., Mitchell, P. R., & Twohig, M. P. (2012). Acceptance and commitment therapy and habit reversal training for the treatment of trichotillomania. *Cognitive and Behavioral Practice, 19*(4), 595–605. http://doi.org/10.1016/j.cbpra.2012.02.002

Dehlin, J. P., Morrison, K. L., & Twohig, M. P. (2013). Acceptance and commitment therapy as a treatment for scrupulosity in obsessive compulsive disorder. *Behavior Modification, 37*(3), 409–430. http://doi.org/10.1177/0145445512475134

Fairfax, H. (2008). The use of mindfulness in obsessive compulsive disorder: Suggestions for its application and integration in existing treatment. *Clinical Psychology and Psychotherapy, 15*(1), 53–59. http://doi.org/10.1002/cpp.557

Geller, D. A., March, J., Psychiatry, A. A. of C. and A., Flament, M., Whitaker, A., Rapoport J., ... Tolin, D. F. (2012). Practice parameter for the assessment and treatment of children and adolescents with obsessive-compulsive disorder. *Journal of the American Academy of Child & Adolescent Psychiatry, 51*(1), 98–113. http://doi.org/10.1016/j.jaac.2011.09.019

Hannan, S. E., & Tolin, D. F. (2005). Acceptance and mindfulness-based behavior therapy for obsessive-compulsive disorder. In *Acceptance and mindfulness-based approaches to anxiety: Conceptualization and treatment*, S. M. Orsillo & L. Roemer, eds. (pp. 271–299). New York: Springer Science+Business Media. http://doi.org/http://dx.doi.org/10.1007/0–387-25989–9_11

Hanstede, M., Gidron, Y., & Nykliček, I. (2008). The effects of a mindfulness intervention on obsessive-compulsive symptoms in a non-clinical student population. *The Journal of Nervous and Mental Disease, 196*(10), 776–779. http://doi.org/10.1097/NMD.0b013e31818786b8

Hayes, S. C., Masuda, A., Bissett, R., Luoma, J., & Guerrero, L. F. (2004). DBT, FAP, and ACT: How empirically oriented are the new behavior therapy technologies? *Behavior Therapy, 35*(1), 35–54. http://doi.org/10.1016/S0005-7894(04)80003–0

Hertenstein, E., Rose, N., Voderholzer, U., Heidenreich, T., Nissen, C., Thiel, N., ... Külz, A. K. (2012). Mindfulness-based cognitive therapy in obsessive-compulsive disorder – A qualitative study on patients' experiences. *BMC Psychiatry, 12*(1), 185. http://doi.org/10.1186/1471-244X-12-185

Hofmann, S. G., Sawyer, A. T., & Fang, A. (2010). The empirical status of the "New Wave" of CBT. *Psychiatric Clinics of North America, 33*(3), 701–710 . http://doi.org/10.1016/j.psc.2010.04.006

Kabat-Zinn, J. (2003). Mindfulness-based interventions in context: Past, present, and future. *Clinical Psychology: Science and Practice, 10*(2), 144–156. http://doi.org/10.1093/clipsy/bpg016

Kahl, K. G., Winter, L., & Schweiger, U. (2012). The third wave of cognitive behavioural therapies: What is new and what is effective? *Current Opinion in Psychiatry, 25*(6), 522–528. http://doi.org/10.1097/YCO.0b013e328358e531

Kalra, S. K., & Swedo, S. E. (2009). Children with obsessive-compulsive disorder: Are they just "little adults"? *The Journal of Clinical Investigation, 119*(4), 737–746. http://doi.org/10.1172/JCI37563

Keuthen, N. J., Rothbaum, B. O., Fama, J., Altenburger, E., Falkenstein, M. J., Sprich, S. E., ... Welch, S. S. (2012). DBT-enhanced cognitive-behavioral treatment for trichotillomania: A randomized controlled trial. *Journal of Behavioral Addictions, 1*(3), 106–114. http://doi.org/10.1556/JBA.1.2012.003

Keuthen, N. J., Rothbaum, B. O., Welch, S. S., Taylor, C., Falkenstein, M., Heekin, M., ... Jenike, M. A. (2010). Pilot trial of dialectical behavior therapy-enhanced habit reversal for trichotillomania. *Depression and Anxiety, 27*(10), 953–959. http://doi.org/10.1002/da.20732

Lee, J. K., & Orsillo, S. M. (2014). Investigating cognitive flexibility as a potential mechanism of mindfulness in generalized anxiety disorder. *Journal of Behavior Therapy and Experimental Psychiatry, 45*(1), 208–216. http://doi.org/10.1016/j.jbtep.2013.10.008

Lee, J., Semple, R. J., Rosa, D., & Miller, L. (2008). Mindfulness-based cognitive therapy for children: Results of a pilot study. *Journal of Cognitive Psychotherapy, 22*(1), 15–28. http://doi.org/10.1891/0889.8391.22.1.15

Lewin, A. B., McGuire, J. F., Murphy, T. K., & Storch, E. A. (2014). The importance of considering parent's preferences when planning treatment for their children – the case of childhood obsessive-compulsive disorder. *Journal of Child Psychology and Psychiatry, 55*(12), 1314–1316. http://doi.org/10.1111/jcpp.12344

Linehan, M. M. (2015). *DBT skills training manual*, 2nd edn. New York: Guilford Press. Retrieved from http://ovidsp.ovid.com/ovidweb.cgi?T=JS&PAGE=reference&D=psyc11&NEWS=N&AN=2015-05780-000

Liu, X.-H., Han, K.-L., & Xu, W. (2011). Effectiveness of mindfulness-based cognitive behavioral therapy on patients with obsessive-compulsive disorder. Retrieved September 26, 2017, from http://psycnet.apa.org/record/2012–00306-007

Longmore, R. J., & Worrell, M. (2007). Do we need to challenge thoughts in cognitive behavior therapy? *Clinical Psychology Review, 27*(2), 173–187. http://doi.org/10.1016/j.cpr.2006.08.001

Lutz, J., Herwig, U., Opialla, S., Hittmeyer, A., Jäncke, L., Rufer, M., ... Brühl, A. B. (2013). Mindfulness and emotion regulation-an fMRI study. *Social Cognitive and Affective Neuroscience, 9*(6), 776–785. http://doi.org/10.1093/scan/nst043

Madani, A., Kananifar, N., Hamid Atashpour, S., & Hussain Bin Habil, M. (2013). The effects of mindfulness group training on the rate of obsessive-compulsive disorder symptoms on the women in Isfahan City (Iran). *International Medical Journal, 20*(1), 13–17.

March, J. S., Foa, E., Gammon, P., Chrisman, A., Curry, J., Fitzgerald, D., ... Team, P. (2004). Cognitive-behavior therapy, sertraline, and their combination for children and adolescents with obsessive-compulsive disorder – The Pediatric OCD Treatment Study (POTS) randomized controlled trial. *JAMA-Journal of the American Medical Association, 292*(16), 1969–1976. http://doi.org/10.1001/jama.292.16.1969

Menezes, C. B., de Paula Couto, M. C., Buratto, L. G., Erthal, F., Pereira, M. G., & Bizarro, L. (2013). The improvement of emotion and attention regulation after a 6-week training of focused meditation: A randomized controlled trial. *Evidence-Based Complementary and Alternative Medicine, 2013*, 1–11. http://doi.org/10.1155/2013/984678

Öst, L. G. (2008). Efficacy of the third wave of behavioral therapies: A systematic review and meta-analysis. *Behaviour Research and Therapy, 46*(3), 296–321. http://doi.org/10.1016/j.brat.2007.12.005

Semple, R. J., Reid, E. F. G., & Miller, L. (2005). Treating anxiety with mindfulness: An open trial of mindfulness training for anxious children. *Journal of Cognitive Psychotherapy, 19*(4), 379–392. http://doi.org/10.1891/jcop.2005.19.4.379

Sguazzin, C. M. G., Key, B. L., Rowa, K., Bieling, P. J., & McCabe, R. E. (2017). Mindfulness-based cognitive therapy for residual symptoms in obsessive-compulsive disorder: A qualitative analysis. *Mindfulness, 8*(1), 190–203. http://doi.org/10.1007/s12671-016-0592-y

Shusterman, A., Feld, L., Baer, L., & Keuthen, N. (2009). Affective regulation in trichotillomania: Evidence from a large-scale internet survey. *Behaviour Research and Therapy, 47*(8), 637–644. http://doi.org/10.1016/j.brat.2009.04.004

Snorrason, Í., Smári, J., & Ólafsson, R. P. (2010). Emotion regulation in pathological skin picking: Findings from a non-treatment seeking sample. *Journal of Behavior Therapy and Experimental Psychiatry, 41*(3), 238–245. http://doi.org/10.1016/j.jbtep.2010.01.009

Tang, Y.-Y., Holzel, B. K., & Posner, M. I. (2015). Traits and states in mindfulness meditation. *Nature Reviews Neuroscience, 17*(1), 59–59. http://doi.org/10.1038/nrn.2015.7

Twohig, M. P. (2009). The application of acceptance and commitment therapy to obsessive-compulsive disorder. *Cognitive and Behavioral Practice, 16*(1), 18–28. http://doi.org/10.1016/j.cbpra.2008.02.008

Twohig, M. P., Abramowitz, J. S., Bluett, E. J., Fabricant, L. E., Jacoby, R. J., Morrison, K. L., ... Smith, B. M. (2015). Exposure therapy for OCD from an acceptance and commitment therapy (ACT) framework. *Journal of Obsessive-Compulsive and Related Disorders, 6*, 167–173. http://doi.org/10.1016/j.jocrd.2014.12.007

Twohig, M. P., Hayes, S. C., & Masuda, A. (2006). A preliminary investigation of acceptance and commitment therapy as a treatment for chronic skin picking. *Behaviour Research and Therapy, 44*(10), 1513–1522. https://doi.org/10.1016/j.brat.2005.10.002

Twohig, M. P., Hayes, S. C., Plumb, J. C., Pruitt, L. D., Collins, A. B., Hazlett-Stevens, H., & Woidneck, M. R. (2010). A randomized clinical trial of acceptance and commitment therapy versus progressive relaxation training for obsessive-compulsive disorder.

Journal of Consulting and Clinical Psychology, 78(5), 705–716. http://doi.org/10.1037/a0020508

Twohig, M.P., Morrisson, K.L., & Bluett, E.J. (2014). Acceptance and commitment therapy for obsessive compulsive disorder and obsessive compulsive spectrum disorders: A review. *Current Psychiatry Reviews, 10*(4), 296–307. http://dx.doi.org/10.2174/1573400510666140714172145

Twohig, M. P., & Woods, D. W. (2004). A preliminary investigation of acceptance and commitment therapy and habit reversal as a treatment for trichotillomania. *Behavior Therapy, 35*(4), 803–820. http://doi.org/10.1016/S0005-7894(04)80021-2

Visser, H. A., van Oppen, P., van Megen, H. J., Eikelenboom, M., & van Balkom, A. J. (2014). Obsessive-compulsive disorder; chronic versus non-chronic symptoms. *Journal of Affective Disorders, 152–154*, 169–174. http://doi.org/10.1016/j.jad.2013.09.004

Wahl, K., Huelle, J. O., Zurowski, B., & Kordon, A. (2013). Managing obsessive thoughts during brief exposure: An experimental study comparing mindfulness-based strategies and distraction in obsessive–compulsive disorder. *Cognitive Therapy and Research, 37*(4), 752–761. http://doi.org/10.1007/s10608-012-9503-2

Welch, S. S., & Kim, J. (2012). DBT-enhanced cognitive behavioral therapy for adolescent trichotillomania: An adolescent case study. *Cognitive and Behavioral Practice, 19*(3), 483–493. http://doi.org/10.1016/j.cbpra.2011.11.002

Zeidan, F., Martucci, K. T., Kraft, R. A., McHaffie, J. G., & Coghill, R. C. (2013). Neural correlates of mindfulness meditation-related anxiety relief. *Social Cognitive and Affective Neuroscience, 9*(6), 751–759. http://doi.org/10.1093/scan/nst041

PART III

Post-Traumatic Stress Disorder

25 Trauma-Focused Cognitive Behavioral Therapy

An Evidence-Based Approach for Helping Children Overcome the Impact of Child Abuse and Trauma

Melissa K. Runyon, Elizabeth Risch, and Esther Deblinger

Introduction

Exposure to one or more potentially traumatic events (PTEs) in childhood is an unfortunately common experience, with nearly 60 percent of children in the United States reporting at least one form of victimization (e.g., sexual abuse, physical assault) in a one-year time period. Some children are quite resilient, experiencing minimal or only acute difficulties and recovering naturally over time, whereas others may suffer episodic and/or chronic psychosocial difficulties across the life-span (Bryant, Salmon, Sinclair, & Davidson, 2007; Cloitre et al., 2009; Kendall-Tackett, Williams, & Finkelhor, 1993). Early effective evidence-based interventions may help to disrupt the potentially lifelong negative effects of childhood trauma. Four evidence-based therapy models identified under the child trauma section of the California Clearinghouse of Evidence-based Programs for Child Welfare (CEBC) website have either met the requirements for the Supported by Research Evidence category (i.e., Child-Parent Psychotherapy – Lieberman, Van Horn, & Ghosh Ippen, 2005) or have met the more rigorous requirements for the Well-Supported by Research Evidence category (i.e., eye movement desensitization and reprocessing – Shapiro, 2001; prolonged exposure for adolescents – Foa, Chrestman, & Gilboa-Schechtman, 2008; and trauma-focused cognitive behavioral therapy (TF-CBT) – Cohen, Deblinger, Mannarino, & Steer, 2004, 2016). According to Morina, Koerssen, and Pollet (2016), TF-CBT (Cohen, Mannarino, & Deblinger, 2016; Deblinger, Cohen, Mannarino, Runyon, & Heflin, 2015) has more research support demonstrating the model's effectiveness for helping children overcome the impact of trauma than any other treatment available with more than 20 randomized trials being completed to date (Cohen, Mannarino, & Deblinger, 2016). Given the strong record of empirical support for TF-CBT, the present chapter includes a summary of supporting research; a review of predictors, moderators, and mediators associated with treatment outcomes; a clinical description of the model; and a case study illustrating the practical implementation of TF-CBT.

Importance of Evidence-Based Therapies to Help Children Overcome Trauma

According to a meta-analysis, approximately 16 percent of youth develop PTSD after exposure to a traumatic event (Alisic et al., 2014). The current *Diagnostic and Statistical Manual of Mental Disorders* (DSM-5) delineates PTSD as encompassed in four symptom clusters, namely re-experiencing, avoidance, negative cognitions and mood, and hyperarousal (American Psychological Association, 2013). Re-experiencing of the trauma involves overwhelming emotional and/or physiological distress in relation to memories or reminders of the event. In response to this overwhelming distress, youth may seek to avoid reminders of the traumatic event, as well as their own thoughts and feelings related to the event. Avoidance is a common maintenance factor in fear-related disorders (Foa & Rothbaum, 1998; Pineles, Mostoufi, Ready, Street, Griffin et al., 2011). Further, avoidance limits a youth's intentional processing and meaning making of their experiences and may increasingly undermine their developmental trajectory. The negative cognitions and mood symptoms account for the development of inaccurate and/or unhealthy beliefs about the world, the self, and others. For youth who experience interpersonal traumas, overgeneralized and negative beliefs about relationships, others, and one's self can develop, such as believing people cannot be trusted or that one is a bad kid. Youth are more likely to experience increased negatively valenced emotions and may have difficulty experiencing positive emotions. The final symptoms cluster, hyperarousal, includes a number of behavioral symptoms (i.e., sleep and concentration difficulties) arising from an overactive, easily stimulated sympathetic nervous system.

Youth may exhibit a continuum of PTSD symptoms ranging from post-traumatic stress symptoms (PTS) that do not meet full PTSD criteria to more complex trauma reactions. Other youth may exhibit symptoms of anxiety, depression, disruptive behavior, or substance use disorders after trauma exposure. Complex trauma describes a core set of impairments resulting from traumatic experiences occurring in an interpersonal context, repeatedly, and typically over a prolonged period of time (e.g., incest or witnessing chronic domestic violence in the home). The domains impacted in complex trauma are emotional and behavioral dysregulation, relationships and attachment, dissociation, cognition and thinking, and self-concept. Complex trauma has not been established as a formal diagnosis in the DSM-5, and there is continued debate and research on the unique symptom profile (Kliethermes, Schacht, & Drewry, 2014). However, the ICD recognizes the diagnosis of complex trauma, and the findings of a national survey of agencies in the National Child Traumatic Stress Network suggest that 78 percent of youth receiving mental health treatment in the community have a complex trauma history (Spinazzola et al., 2005). Thus, further understanding of unique difficulties and treatment needs of youth experiencing complex trauma will have implications for trauma-focused treatment.

PTS reactions may be chronic if left untreated, resulting in both mental and physical health impairments in adulthood. The Adverse Childhood Experiences (ACEs) study (Felitti et al., 1998) has demonstrated a longitudinal relationship between childhood adversity (e.g., abuse, separation from caregivers) and chronic mental and physical health conditions. A higher number of ACEs increases the likelihood an individual will suffer from diseases, such as chronic obstructive pulmonary disorder, cardiac disease, cancer, depression, and alcoholism and substance use in later life (Felitti et al., 1998). The societal financial costs of child maltreatment are substantial, with the lifetime financial burden for new fatal and nonfatal child maltreatment cases in 2008 being an estimated $124 billion in the United States (Xiangming, Brown, Florencea, & Mercya, 2012).

Increased awareness of the prevalence of trauma and acknowledgment of the impact on individual and societal functioning has resulted in a movement toward the development of trauma-informed systems (e.g., child-serving systems, including social services, public education, and health care) that offer support to and address the needs of children who experience trauma. This allows for individuals interacting with children to view their emotional and behavioral presentation through a trauma-informed lens leading to a better conceptualization and understanding of their presenting problems. One of the treatment approaches frequently embedded in these trauma-informed systems is TF-CBT, a model that has earned the Substance Abuse and Mental Health Administration's (SAMHSA) highest rating for empirical support and has been widely disseminated, both nationally and internationally.

TF-CBT Practice Components

TF-CBT is a short-term (12–16 ninety-minute sessions) cognitive behavioral therapy model that also incorporates concepts from attachment, humanistic, and family systems theory. The treatment approach incorporates psycho-education, skill building, and trauma narration and processing. Within a given session, the therapist may spend varying amounts of time with the child, the caregiver(s), and the whole family to best accomplish the treatment goals. TF-CBT has been applied across many settings (residential, outpatient, home based), with single, multiple, and complex trauma types, and in diverse populations (Cohen, Mannarino, & Deblinger, 2016).

The essential components of TF-CBT are represented by the acronym PRACTICE: Psycho-education and parenting (P), Relaxation (R), Affect regulation (A), Cognitive coping (C), Trauma narration and processing (T), In vivo mastery (I), Conjoint sessions (C), and Enhancing safety and future development (E). The inclusion of various treatment components in therapy sequentially follows the acronym, with appropriate clinical caveats. For example, when safety risks are present, the "Enhancing safety" component including the development of a safety plan, is moved to the start of treatment. Similarly, the "Parenting" component is often a focus throughout the entire course of treatment, and "Conjoint" sessions may be initiated early in treatment to provide caregivers with opportunities to practice the parenting skills with their children while the therapist observes. In general, there is flexibility and overlap of components within and across individual treatment sessions.

Treatment is provided in three phases, stabilization (PRAC), trauma narrative and processing (T), and consolidation (ICE). The explicit and intentional focus on the youth's trauma is initiated in the assessment and included in each component of TF-CBT. Progress through the components of TF-CBT is facilitated by the inclusion of gradual exposure to the traumatic memories in each session. In this way, most youth increasingly become less avoidant of initiating the trauma narration process as the treatment progresses.

In the first phase of treatment, psycho-education initiates the treatment process by providing information that promotes a healthy understanding of the youth's traumatic experiences. When secrecy and isolation are associated with childhood traumatic experiences, such as in the case of sexual abuse and other interpersonal violence, youth often develop feelings of self-blame, guilt, shame, and a sense of being different from peers. Thus, families are taught general facts about the traumas experienced (e.g., how common is domestic violence), traumatic stress responses (e.g., PTS symptoms, how a child feels after family fighting), and the process of recovery (e.g., treatment description, time frame). Through the process of psycho-education, the young person is exposed to the discussion of the experienced traumatic events in general terms. Further, conjoint activities facilitate discussions about trauma in a safe and supportive environment to increase comfort in discussing the topic.

As mentioned earlier, the parenting component is often a consistent focus over the course of treatment sessions. Broadly, goals within the parenting component are fostering a trauma-informed perspective and parenting style and are providing developmentally appropriate behavior management strategies. It is essential that parenting work be provided in a manner that is supportive and collaborative with the caregivers. Caregivers participate in a parallel process of TF-CBT, learning PRAC skills to cope with their own emotional reactions to their children's trauma, so they can serve as good coping models and reinforce their children's use of effective coping skills through praise and positive reinforcement. Later this parallel learning also helps caregivers cope with their own emotional reactions to the trauma(s) and when clinically appropriate it prepares them to respond in a positive, supportive manner when children share their trauma narratives with the caregiver.

Relaxation provides a skill to manage distress in both the youth's and the caregiver's daily lives (related to trauma memories and everyday stressors) and within session to manage distress during gradual exposure. Families are taught the physiological impacts of stress and trauma, including the fight-flight-freeze response. Specific relaxation techniques taught may vary and include focused breathing, progressive muscle relaxation, imagery, and naturally relaxing activities. An important focus is aiding families to identify trauma reminders and use relaxation to reduce distress. Thus, relaxation techniques are taught early in treatment and practiced regularly both at home and in the sessions.

In the affect regulation component, families learn to identify and communicate their feelings and develop methods for managing distress. Youth often lack awareness and language for their internal states; thus, this is taught in sessions and practiced with support of caregivers in the home environment. Often a version of a "Feel Better Plan" or coping skills toolbox is developed with a family to encourage use of healthy coping techniques (e.g., diaphragmatic breathing, mindfulness, guided imagery, assertive expression of emotions) or activities when a child is experiencing high levels of distress.

Teaching the connections between thoughts, feelings, and behaviors is central in the cognitive coping component. Families learn and practice applying cognitive theory to their day-to-day lives, as well as how trauma may impact one's thinking. Cognitive coping skills, such as catching and challenging cognitive distortions and positive self-talk may be taught for managing day-to-day stress. Teaching youth to identify and challenge daily unhelpful thoughts is a precursor for the cognitive processing of trauma-related thoughts and beliefs, which is encouraged only after youth have completed their trauma narrative. Caregivers, on the other hand, may be encouraged to use cognitive coping skills in relation to distressing trauma-related thoughts at this stage of treatment.

The middle phase of treatment focuses on trauma narration and processing. During this phase, youth are engaged in narration of specific traumatic memories through a gradual process that eventually includes their most feared memories. Additionally, the cognitive processing of the traumatic memories allows for correction of unhealthy beliefs and placement of the event(s) in the context of the youth's present life and future. A final focus and often a final narrative chapter reflect the youth's improvement, growth, and future plans for life. During trauma narration with the youth, the therapist also meets individually with the caregiver(s) to prepare for the upcoming conjoint sharing of the youth's trauma experiences when clinically appropriate.

In the final phase, treatment focuses on helping the child integrate and consolidate skills, addressing any remaining avoidant behaviors through in vivo mastery, participating in conjoint sessions to create open communication relating to the traumatic experiences with caregivers, and developing skills for enhancing safety and the child's future development. More specifically, in vivo mastery targets any non-harmful real-life stimuli that trigger fear or avoidant responses. For example, a youth abused near train tracks may develop a fear reaction to trains and train sounds. A fear hierarchy is established with the youth to guide an exposure and desensitization plan. Caregivers are integral in the implementation of the plan as they will be responsible for encouraging non-avoidance behaviors during in vivo exposure activities outside of sessions.

Conjoint trauma-processing sessions entail the youth sharing of their trauma experiences with the caregiver(s), caregiver(s) involvement in validation of youth and corrective processing of dysfunctional beliefs, and celebration of all the youth has accomplished. Safety, as mentioned, is imbued throughout all trauma-focused therapy sessions, as creating an emotionally and physically safe environment is essential to treating trauma survivors. Thus, safety skills training and concerns may be a focus at both the onset and end of treatment depending on the presenting concerns. The focus of safety sessions is tailored to the unique concerns of the family. Personal safety skills training may include the development of healthy boundaries and relationships, teaching and monitoring private parts rules, creation of safety plans for potentially high-risk and unsafe environments, and/or providing sexual health education.

Summary of Evidence Base Supporting TF-CBT

Several independent research studies examining trauma-focused CBT-based therapies for children who experience child sexual abuse (CSA) were conducted in the early 1990s and provided strong support for the therapy model currently known as TF-CBT. In their first randomized controlled trial (RCT), Deblinger, Lippmann, and Steer (1996) compared a 12-session CBT protocol provided to the child alone, the parent alone, or the child and parent combined to treatment as usual (TAU) in a community sample of children and adolescents (aged 7 to 13 years) who had developed PTSD after being sexually abused. Treatment effects on PTSD symptoms, depression, externalizing behavior problems, and parenting practices were evaluated via pre- and post-assessments. It was found that the CBT interventions with the child alone and with the combination of child and parent were superior in reducing PTSD symptoms when compared to TAU. Those participants where only the parents received treatment did not report a significant decrease in PTSD symptoms when compared to those who received TAU. Further, the parent alone and the child and parent combined conditions were better in improving parenting practices, as well as reducing externalizing behaviors and child depression. A subsequent assessment of the youth participating in this trial showed that these treatment gains were largely maintained at a two-year follow-up (Deblinger, Steer, & Lippmann, 1999). Around the same time of this study, Cohen and Mannarino (1996a) conducted a randomized trial that examined a 12-session CBT treatment for preschoolers who had a history of CSA and found significant improvements in externalizing behaviors, inappropriate sexual behaviors, and internalizing symptoms compared to those children who received nondirective supportive therapy (NST), with these gains being maintained at one-year follow-up (Cohen & Mannarino, 1997). Another study by Cohen and Mannarino (1998a) replicated these findings in children aged 7 to 14 years impacted by sexual abuse by demonstrating the superiority of trauma-focused CBT compared to NST for reducing depressive symptoms and improving social competence. Further, examination of trauma-focused CBT provided in a group format demonstrated increased efficacy in both caregiver and child outcomes as compared to a supportive group (Deblinger, Stauffer, & Steer, 2001).

These initial findings led to the first multisite evaluation of the current TF-CBT protocol (Cohen et al., 2006; Cohen, Mannarino, & Deblinger, 2016; Deblinger et al., 2015). In this large RCT including 229 children and adolescents (aged 8 to 14 years), TF-CBT was found to be superior to client-centered therapy for reducing PTSD, depression, behavior problems, shame, and abuse-related attributions. In addition, caregivers demonstrated benefits of reduced depression and abuse-related emotional distress and improved parenting practices and support for their child (Cohen et al., 2004). These gains were maintained at 6- and 12-month follow-ups (Deblinger, Mannarino, Cohen, & Steer, 2006). Further, while this study focused primarily on CSA, youth in the sample experienced on average 3.66 trauma types (e.g., physical abuse, exposure to domestic violence, bullying, natural disaster), demonstrating the effectiveness of TF-CBT with poly-victimization.

Expanding the evidence base for various trauma types and settings, a pilot study (n=39) demonstrated that a modified version of TF-CBT was effective in reducing PTSD symptoms and traumatic grief in youth (aged 6 to 17 years) who had experienced a traumatic loss of a family member (Cohen, Mannarino, & Staron, 2006). More recently, an abbreviated (8-session) version of TF-CBT was found superior to community treatment in a RCT (n=124) for children (aged 7 to 14 years) exposed to intimate partner violence and their non-offending caregivers (Cohen, Mannarino, & Iyenger, 2011).

The treatment developers have further examined TF-CBT for effectiveness of key components, treatment length, and its application in combination with psychotropic medication. A dismantling study (Deblinger, Mannarino, Cohen, Runyon, & Steer, 2011) varied treatment length (8 vs. 16 sessions) and written trauma narratives (present vs. absent) in TF-CBT. Findings demonstrated that all TF-CBT conditions were effective in reducing PTSD symptoms; however, specific findings may guide tailoring treatment to client presentation. Specifically, abuse-related fear and distress in both youth and caregivers responded well to the 8-session intervention with a trauma narrative, whereas parenting practices were most improved and the largest decreases in externalizing behavior problems were found among families participating in the 16 sessions with no trauma narrative condition (Deblinger et al., 2011). The positive results documented in this study were maintained at 6- and 12-month follow-up (Mannarino, Cohen, Deblinger, Runyon, & Steer, 2012). A RCT comparing TF-CBT with or without addition of sertraline, a selective serotonin reuptake inhibitor, found no significant, additive benefit of medication in reducing PTSD symptoms over and above the effects of the psychological intervention (Cohen, Mannarino, Perel, & Staron, 2007).

Investigations in other clinics across the United States and the rest of the world have replicated the positive outcomes associated with TF-CBT that were documented in the research conducted by its developers. In an early RCT conducted in Australia (King et al., 2000), 36 youth who had experienced sexual abuse (aged 5 to 17 years) received individual CBT, family CBT, or a wait-list control condition. Children in both trauma-focused CBT conditions reported significantly fewer PTSD symptoms compared to those on the wait-list. Inclusion of family members in treatment was important as that group showed the greatest reduction in anxiety symptoms at 3-month follow-up (King et al., 2000). Allen and Hoskowitz (2016) also carried out a study involving 260 youth (aged 3 to 12 years) with a history of sexual abuse who received TF-CBT from community therapists trained in this method. Greater improvements were associated with a greater use of the structured CBT techniques, while poorer outcomes were associated with the use of more play/experiential techniques. Several investigations have documented the efficacy of TF-CBT for helping children in foster care overcome the impact of trauma. A seminal, quasi-experimental study conducted by Lyons, Weiner, and Schneider (2006) documented significant larger reductions in trauma symptoms, placement disruptions, and episodes of running away from foster care homes for those foster children (aged 3 to 18 years) who had received TF-CBT as compared to TAU. A more recent RCT reported on foster caregivers of 46 children (aged 5 to 16 years) who had received TF-CBT plus engagement strategy offered over the phone or in-person or standard TF-CBT. Significantly more children and caregivers attended the initial session and completed TF-CBT in the TF-CBT plus engagement condition when compared to those in the standard TF-CBT condition. Children in both conditions reported significant reductions in trauma symptoms at posttreatment (Dorsey et al., 2014); however, fewer children accessed treatment in the standard condition. In addition to the short-term positive outcomes associated with TF-CBT for both children and caregivers, the early identification and treatment of traumatized youth with TF-CBT may result in a long-term cost savings as well (Greer, Grasso, Cohen, & Webb, 2014).

Research documenting the positive outcomes for families participating in TF-CBT has also been replicated in several studies conducted in Europe. In a RCT conducted by Goldbeck, Muche, Sachser, Tutus, and Rosner (2016) in eight German outpatient clinics, youth (aged 7 to 17 years), presenting with PTS symptoms were assigned to 12 sessions of TF-CBT or a wait-list control condition. TF-CBT was associated with significantly greater reductions of PTS symptoms and other emotional and behavioral problems. A similar RCT evaluating TF-CBT in Norway demonstrated that traumatized youth (aged 10 to 18 years) who received TF-CBT had significantly greater reductions in PTS symptoms, depression, general mental health problems, and functional impairments than those receiving TAU (Jensen et al., 2014). In another investigation conducted in the Netherlands, Diehle, Opmeer, Boer, Mannarino, and Lindauer (2015) randomly assigned children (aged 8 to 18 years) to 8 sessions of TF-CBT or EMDR. TF-CBT and EMDR were both associated with significant pre- to posttreatment improvements in PTS symptoms, and there was no difference in length of treatment between the two conditions. While both TF-CBT and EMDR were associated with reductions in children's trauma symptoms, an equal dose of TF-CBT was also associated with significant reductions in children's depression and hyperactive symptoms demonstrating that TF-CBT was somewhat more effective in producing symptom improvements across multiple domains of functioning.

Several studies examining the efficacy TF-CBT have been conducted in non-Western countries, especially on the African continent. In one study, children (aged 5 to 16 years) presenting with trauma-related symptoms to five community sites in Lusaka, Zambia, were randomly assigned to 10 to 16 sessions of TF-CBT or regular community services. At follow-up, there were significantly greater improvements in PTS symptoms and daily functioning for those receiving TF-CBT from lay counselors as compared to those receiving community services (Murray et al., 2015). Two randomized, controlled studies also examined outcomes associated with TF-CBT for youth who had been exposed to trauma in the Democratic Republic of Congo. In the first study, 12- to 17-year-old girls who were victims of sexual abuse and on average had experienced as many as 11 other traumatic experiences were randomly assigned to a 15-session TF-CBT group or a wait-list control group. The results demonstrated that compared to a wait-list control condition, TF-CBT led to significantly greater improvements in scores of scales measuring PTS symptoms, depression, anxiety, conduct problems, and prosocial behavior (O'Callaghan, McMullen, Shannon, Rafferty, & Black, 2013). The second study involved boys (aged 13 to 17 years) who were former child soldiers exposed to numerous traumatic experiences including the atrocities of this war-torn nation. Compared to the wait-list control group, the TF-CBT group demonstrated significantly greater improvements in all areas (McMullen, O'Callaghan, Shannon, Black, & Eskin, 2013). Another study examined child outcomes associated with a 12-session group TF-CBT Traumatic Grief protocol for 58 orphaned children (aged 5 to 18 years) in Tanzania. After participation in group TF-CBT delivered by lay counselors, significant improvements in grief, PTS, and depressive symptoms and behavior problems were reported and maintained at 3- and 12-month follow-up. Finally, research has also demonstrated reductions in PTSD symptoms for youth in Japan and Canada after their participation in TF-CBT, further highlighting TF-CBT's applicability and efficacy across various countries and cultures (Kameoka et al., 2015; Konanur, Muller, Cinamon, Thornback, & Zorzella, 2015).

Predictors, Moderators, and Mediators Associated with TF-CBT Treatment Outcomes

Early TF-CBT clinical trials not only supported the model's efficacy in treating child trauma as compared to wait-lists and other available treatments (see for a review, Morina et al., 2016), but these studies and subsequent studies also identified predictors of optimal treatment outcomes for participating youth. Early research examining the model demonstrated the importance of caregiver involvement and caregiver support for optimal outcomes for traumatized youth (Cohen & Mannarino, 1996b; Deblinger et al., 1996). For example, Deblinger and colleagues (1996) reported significant improvements in PTS symptoms when treating the child alone. However, parental involvement in treatment was critical to the significant improvements seen with respect to behavior problems, child depression, and parenting practices. Further evidence supported the important role of the parent in the child's recovery when Cohen and Mannarino (1996b) reported that parental abuse-related emotional distress was significantly correlated with treatment outcomes for preschool children receiving TF-CBT or NST. The best predictor of treatment outcomes at 6- and 12-month follow-up was parental support.

Caregiver support plays an important role in youth's ability to process traumatic events and replace unproductive thoughts with healthy ones during the trauma narration and processing phase. In a study examining the relationship between in-session caregiver behavior and children's symptomology (Yasinski et al., 2016), caregivers' emotional processing during the trauma narrative and processing phase predicted decreases in both internalizing and externalizing symptoms for children.

At follow-up, caregiver support predicted lower internalizing symptoms for children while caregiver avoidance of abuse-related material and blame of the child was associated with increases in internalizing and externalizing symptoms. Caregiver blame and avoidance had a negative impact on the child's emotional processing of the traumatic events (Yasinski et al., 2016). Recent studies have shown that caregiver mental health diagnosis and emotional symptoms may predict early dropout from TF-CBT, thereby possibly attenuating the treatment response (Wamser-Nanney & Steinzor, 2017; Lai, Tiwari, Self-Brown, Cronholm, & Kinnish, 2017). These findings highlight the importance of involving a non-offending caregiver in TF-CBT, as well as the parallel process of teaching the caregivers PRAC skills to manage their abuse-related emotions and thoughts in order to enhance their ability to support their children and serve as positive coping models (Cohen & Mannarino, 1996b, 1998b).

Therapeutic alliance, a common element of all therapies, also predicts optimal outcomes for youth in TF-CBT. In a study conducted in Norway (Ormhaug, Jensen, Wentzel-Larsen, & Shirk, 2014), the association between the quality of the therapeutic alliance and treatment outcome was examined in traumatized youth (aged 10 to 18 years) who were randomly assigned to TF-CBT or TAU. Results demonstrated that youth receiving TF-CBT reported significantly lower PTS symptoms compared to those receiving TAU, with therapeutic alliance serving as an important predictor of reductions in PTS and other symptoms for only those receiving TF-CBT. These findings highlight the importance of the therapeutic alliance for the successful delivery and outcome of TF-CBT (Cohen, Mannarino, & Deblinger, 2016; Deblinger et al., 2015). In a structured EBT such as TF-CBT, therapists ask children and their caregivers to engage in PRACTICE assignments both in therapy and at home, as well as to engage in recounting details of highly aversive experiences and share related intimate thoughts and feelings. A strong therapeutic alliance likely encourages youth cooperation with these assignments as well as the gradual exposure process that requires a sense of safety and trust in the therapist and the treatment approach.

As a part of an effectiveness trial conducted by Webb, Hayes, Grasso, Laurenceau, & Deblinger (2014), predictors of outcomes associated with TF-CBT were examined for 81 children (aged 6 to 15) who received an average of 10 treatment sessions (Ready et al., 2015). Ready et al. (2015) coded accommodation (adaptive/productive trauma-related thoughts about self, others, or the world) and overgeneralization (maladaptive/unproductive trauma-related thoughts about self, others, and the world) in youth during trauma narration and processing sessions. As expected, higher levels of overgeneralization predicted less improvement in internalizing symptoms at posttreatment and increases in externalizing symptoms at 12-month follow-up. Whereas, more accommodation predicted decreased internalizing symptoms. Accommodation also moderated the negative impact of overgeneralization on internalizing and externalizing symptoms. In a related study, Hayes et al. (2017) examined how accommodation and overgeneralization were associated with unproductive versus constructive processing of traumatic events during trauma narration and processing. Sessions during this phase of TF-CBT were coded for indicators of unproductive processing (overgeneralization, rumination, avoidance) and constructive processing (de-centering ability to gain insight and distance oneself from trauma-related material to promote cognitive processing and change), accommodation of corrective information), as well as levels of negative emotion. Higher levels of rumination, less de-centering, and more negative emotion were associated with overgeneralization, while less avoidance and more de-centering were associated with accommodation that might allow for processing and cognitive change. De-centering also predicted improvement in posttreatment externalizing symptoms. These findings highlight the importance of cognitive change replacing unproductive trauma-related beliefs with adaptive/productive thoughts in the processes of treating PTSD and other behavioral difficulties.

Studies examining TF-CBT have examined moderating and mediating variables. According to Papakostas and Fava (2008), moderators of treatment outcome involve factors present at the initiation of treatment that influence the likelihood of a particular outcome occurring following treatment. In contrast, mediators of treatment outcome (sometimes referred to as correlates) are measurable *changes* that occur over the course of treatment and correlate with treatment outcome. A study seeking to triage youth in treatment examined pretreatment characteristics (potential moderators) in relationship to early treatment response (defined as subclinical symptom level at session four) and found that approximately 32 percent to 45 percent (per parent or self-report, respectively) of children could be defined as early treatment responders. Children with lower pretreatment symptom level, fewer traumas, younger age, and non-White ethnicity were more likely to be early treatment responders (Wamser-Nanney, Scheeringa, & Weems, 2014). Notably, these symptom reductions were achieved prior to engaging in trauma narration and processing, replicating the improvements found in the abbreviated conditions in a previously conducted dismantling study (Deblinger et al., 2011).

Before engaging in trauma narration and processing, therapists prepare youth by teaching them PRAC skills, which aid them in self-regulation and management of painful emotions both in and outside the therapy sessions. Interestingly, Sharma-Patel and Brown (2016) examined whether self-blame and emotional dysregulation mediate and/or moderate treatment outcomes, including PTS, depressive symptoms, and conduct problem, for youth who completed trauma-focused treatment. Caregivers and youth completed assessment measures at pretreatment, mid-treatment prior to beginning the trauma narration and processing, and again at posttreatment. Changes in self-blame, but not in emotional regulation, at mid-treatment was a partial mediator of conduct problems. Emotional dysregulation moderates improvements in PTS symptoms and conduct problems at posttreatment. Specifically, youngsters with higher levels of emotional dysregulation reported reductions in posttreatment PTS symptoms, while youngsters with low levels of emotional dysregulation demonstrated improvements in PTS symptoms at mid- and posttreatment. As such, emotional regulation and self-blame, which are important targets of TF-CBT, appear to impact the treatment response.

TF-CBT Case Illustration

Beckham, a 13-year-old boy, was referred for TF-CBT after being sexually abused on multiple occasions by his paternal uncle. In addition to a history of CSA, Beckham witnessed extensive domestic violence between his biological parents that resulted in his mother seeking care at the local emergency room due to broken bones on at least two occasions. Beckham sustained injuries ranging from mild bruises to severe cuts and abrasions while intervening to protect his mother from his father's assaultive behavior. He was also the target of severe physical abuse (PA) and emotional abuse by his father. As a result, Beckham was placed in foster care and experienced placement changes on three separate occasions over a period of 6 months when his respective foster parents complained of his aggressive and noncompliant behaviors, until his placement with Ms. Roberts, his current pre-adoptive mother.

Beckham is an intelligent student who is capable of doing well academically, but his emotional and behavioral reactions to his traumatic past interfere with his functioning in school and several other important domains. Despite his history of multiple, complex traumas, Beckham is capable of forming relationships and has maintained some friendships that are important to him. He also reports a desire to have a forever family, though he remains skeptical about the reality of this possibility.

Beckham was also referred for a medical examination to diagnose and treat the impact of his CSA when it was revealed that he had not received an exam as part of the initial investigation. The child abuse pediatrician who conducted the examination assessed for any physical injury and sexually transmitted infections and took a complete medical history during which Beckham disclosed the CSA experiences by his uncle. Beckham's uncle was charged and arrested for multiple counts of sexual assault of a minor and endangering the welfare of a minor. Beckham has had no contact with his father for more than two years since his father's incarceration on a drug charge. Child Protective Services records indicate that Beckham's father was substantiated for child physical abuse of Beckham at ages 6 and 9. Beckham was waiting for his mother at the child protection office visitation room when he received notification that his mother overdosed and died.

During his initial therapy assessment, Beckham disclosed that the CSA began with his uncle hugging him a lot, which made Beckham feel loved, yet uncomfortable at times. He reported that he did not recall any hugs or affection from his parents. He added that he feels angry, like he's going to explode, when Ms. Roberts hugs him. In response to a trauma history inventory, Beckham also disclosed that he had frequently witnessed violence between his parents and that his father beat him with his fist and objects (such as a belt and bat), and that his father frequently called him names, such as stupid and cursed at him. Beckham stated that he had difficulty concentrating at school and sleeping because thoughts of his uncle touching him, his dad hurting his mother, and the day the case worker told him his mother died were always popping into his mind.

Ms. Roberts revealed that Beckham was a loving child who was very kind and helpful to others at times, but that his mood changed to rage with the "flip of a switch." She stated that she never knew what was going to set him off. She indicated that she recently noticed he was somewhat irritable and withdrawn at home, and there had been a few incidents where he had minor physical altercations with peers at school. She described Beckham as distant and having difficulty forming relationships with others. Ms. Roberts became tearful and stated that although she loved Beckham, she feared he was permanently damaged and would never be able to truly bond with and love her or anyone else. After all, "how could a child overcome what Beckham has experienced," she proclaimed.

Based on his responses to standardized assessment measures, Beckham met criteria for PTSD; had mild depressive symptoms; and reported negative cognitions about himself, the world, and others, and he described himself as often angry. Ms. Roberts reported a mild level of depression herself, significant parenting distress, and significant behavior problems for Beckham. She described him as thoughtful toward her at times, but uncooperative and aggressive toward others.

During the initial phase of TF-CBT, the stabilization and skill-building phase, the PRAC components were presented to Beckham and Ms. Roberts in individual sessions. During these sessions, the therapist offered psycho-education about trauma-related reactions to normalize Beckham's responses; provided basic information about the prevalence, impact, and dynamics of sexual abuse, physical abuse, and domestic violence; and gave treatment expectations including the documented efficacy of TF-CBT. The therapist instilled hope by emphasizing that Beckham had two things associated with the best possible outcome for a youth exposed to trauma: a supportive caregiver and his participation in effective treatment.

Coping skills were then introduced to help Beckham and his caregiver cope with general life stressors as well as trauma reminders and the associated thoughts, feelings, and behaviors that those reminders elicited. Given Beckham's emotional liability and dysregulation, the therapist spent three additional sessions focusing on PRAC skills, until in-session observation as well as reports by Ms. Roberts and Beckham demonstrated some increased ability to exercise self-control and regulate his emotional reactions. He enjoyed yoga poses and controlled deep breathing and indicated these skills helped him remain slightly more focused and calm.

Noting that Beckham was somewhat avoidant of discussing the abuse, domestic violence, and loss of his mother, the therapist initially encouraged him to share a positive narrative about making the winning shot in the final game of a local basketball tournament. Next, he was gently encouraged to provide a similar narrative (i.e., baseline trauma narrative) about the traumatic experiences that resulted in his being removed from his biological mother's care. Beckham responded by disclosing that his father had hurt him and his mother really bad and that "She's [mom] dead now." He spontaneously added, "Everybody hurts me and leaves me. I guess it's my fault for being such a bad kid all the time. You know, even my uncle did sexual stuff to me and my mom killed herself." The therapist reflected back Beckham's statements about his traumatic experiences in an effort to acknowledge the abuse and trauma and to validate his feelings. In subsequent sessions, the therapist would continue to gently encourage Beckham to talk about the abuse, violence, and loss of a loved one in general terms, as this was considered as lower-level gradual exposure that served to increase comfort and a sense of mastery over discussing trauma-related material. The development of a trauma narrative was purposely not mentioned in the initial phase, as the therapist did not wish to increase Beckham's tension and anxiety. In addition to the lower-level exposure exercises to desensitize Beckham and decrease his anxiety, the therapist focused on psycho-education and skill-building activities to help Beckham feel less alone and cope with daily life stressors. This work also helped to gradually prepare Beckham for the trauma narration and processing component during the middle phase of treatment.

Given the critical role of parenting in TF-CBT for reducing undesirable behaviors, Ms. Roberts was reminded of the importance of providing a great deal of structure, clear limits, and positive feedback to children after they have experienced traumatic events to enhance their sense of safety, security, and confidence. The therapist emphasized the benefits of specific praise and positive reinforcement as powerful tools for increasing Beckham's positive, prosocial behaviors. Ms. Roberts was also encouraged to pay special attention and to praise Beckham when he was using PRAC skills to regulate his emotions. Ms. Roberts was instructed to praise Beckham every time he engaged in yoga and deep breathing to stay focused and regulated, as well as every time he was kind; expressed his anger in a calm, appropriate manner; or interacted in a positive way with peers or adults. Ms. Roberts also learned reflective listening, so she could help Beckham to feel heard when he expressed feelings or thoughts in appropriate ways. The therapist reviewed parent-child interactions to help Ms. Roberts identify trauma reminders that seemed to underlie Beckham's intense emotional reactions to seemingly innocuous statements or even positive gestures (e.g., hugs) on her part. Early in treatment due to safety concerns, Beckham and Ms. Roberts negotiated a behavioral contract where Beckham was expected to be kind to others (no aggressive behavior toward others). The contract outlined negative consequences for aggressive behavior and rewards for prosocial behavior that were agreed upon by Beckham and Ms. Roberts.

Next, Beckham and Ms. Roberts participated in coping skills practice activities focused on relaxation, affective expression and modulation, and cognitive coping. Emotional regulation skills were particularly important to Beckham given his emotional liability and how easily he became dysregulated. The therapist helped Beckham identify a range of emotions by examining the feelings that were underneath his surface reaction of anger, including feeling abandoned, alone, betrayed, sad, scared, damaged, shameful, unloved, and worthless. There was a noticeable decrease in Beckham's aggression toward others as he practiced removing himself from situations and using deep breathing and yoga with self-talk to handle anger-provoking situations in a calm manner. Both Ms. Roberts and the therapist gave Beckham praise and positive feedback to encourage the use of adaptive coping skills.

Ms. Roberts had a lot of negative beliefs about Beckham and his ability to overcome the impact of trauma and to develop long-term, healthy relationships. After teaching Ms. Roberts the interrelationship between thoughts, feelings, bodily sensations, and behavior, the therapist elicited a number of dysfunctional thoughts Ms. Roberts had about Beckham. These thoughts included: "Beckham will be just like his father (violent/aggressive toward others." "Beckham will never be able to recover from all of the horrible things he's experienced." "He will never have a close relationship with anyone." and "Why isn't my love and attention enough to help him change?" These thoughts were related to a number of distressing emotions, such as hopelessness, helplessness, sadness, frustration, and failure. Over time, the therapist used Socratic questioning to challenge Ms. Roberts's distortions, such as "Do you think most children who have experience adversity bounce back?" "What do you see in Beckham's behavior that suggests that he is quite resilient?" "What positive qualities has he inherited from his parent(s) and what qualities has he learned from you?" and "How do you think you are influencing his future?" Ms. Roberts began to identify many kind and positive traits that Beckham displayed in conjunction with many strengths he possessed that demonstrated that the trauma did not define who he was as a person and hence would not affect his entire life. This contradictory evidence was used to help Ms. Roberts challenge her distortions and identify more productive replacement thoughts.

The therapist used a card game with questions related to sexual abuse, physical abuse, and violence to continue psycho-education (Deblinger, Neubauer, Runyon, & Baker, 2006). Beckham read several therapeutic books about boys who were sexually abused (Satullo & Bradway, 1987) and had been exposed to domestic violence and physical abuse by a parent. Beckham and his therapist also reviewed a website with a list of celebrities who had experienced sexual abuse and violence. These activities served as lower-level gradual exposure exercises and prepared Beckham to progress to trauma narration and processing. Beckham and Ms. Roberts were well prepared before participating in brief conjoint sessions where Beckham demonstrated to Ms. Roberts the coping skills he was learning. Together they practiced yoga poses and deep breathing and shared some very positive, warm moments while exchanging specific praise with each other. These experiences seemed to help Beckham develop greater feelings of control and mastery.

During the trauma narration and processing phase, the therapist and Beckham reviewed his coping skills toolkit and discussed how deep breathing, yoga, and other strategies could be used to enhance his comfort and sense of control and mastery throughout the process. Beckham was encouraged to use the subjective units of distress scale (SUDS) to make his therapist aware of the intensity of his feelings during the narration of his traumatic experiences, so the sessions could be gradually paced and provide opportunity to use skills to decrease his distress levels. Beckham and his therapist engaged in positive rituals (e.g., listening to music for 5 minutes together) before ending the weekly sessions. Due to his extensive trauma history, Beckham was invited to develop a timeline that listed the multiple traumas, as well as the positive events he experienced over the course of his life. While reviewing his timeline, Beckham asked the therapist why everyone was always leaving him. He quickly followed by saying that he was a "bad kid," so bad that his mom killed herself to get away from him, his Dad had beaten him, and Ms. Roberts would probably also leave. He also added that he didn't remember a time when he felt safe. The distress associated with these thoughts was acknowledged with compassion, and the importance of identifying the events that led to these beliefs through trauma narration was highlighted.

The therapist encouraged Beckham to create a trauma narrative as a means to improve his sleep and concentration at school and reduce the disturbing, recurring thoughts of trauma and loss. He was reluctant but agreed once the therapist explained that he would potentially help the therapist understand how these types of experiences affected other kids, so she could be of help to them as well. Subsequently, Beckham wrote a brief introductory chapter that included a description of his current family, as well as his favorite activities. To increase his sense of control, Beckham was given two choices for each chapter of his narrative. Examples of choices were general information about abuse and trauma, positive interactions with his dad and uncle and/or the first or last episode of abuse. The therapist also paid particular attention to eliciting experiences that reflected themes related to his feelings of loss, abandonment, safety concerns, and being bad, worthless, and unlovable. As therapy continued, the therapist gave Beckham choices each session focusing on experiences that reflected these themes. During each session, he was encouraged to add chapters ultimately including the scariest and worst incidents of sexual abuse and domestic violence to ensure the therapist was accessing all of Beckham's most negative cognitions that were contributing to his symptoms. Each chapter was carefully recorded and read back to Beckham as part of the gradual exposure process. Next, the therapist reviewed the chapter line-by-line and inquired about Beckham's thoughts, feelings, and bodily sensations. Each time, he reported feeling relief and his SUDS scores over time reflected less anxiety.

Beckham expressed many unhelpful cognitions, including "Everyone leaves me because I'm an unlovable and bad kid." "All people will eventually hurt me." and "The world is not a safe place." Psycho-education, Socratic questioning, and best friend role plays were used to help Beckham process his experiences, while also identifying, challenging, and replacing dysfunctional thoughts with healthy, productive ones that were incorporated into his narrative. After Beckham had processed his entire narrative, he added a positive ending to his book by writing a final chapter about what he learned in therapy, his new family, and positive feelings about his family, friends, and expectations for the future. Over the course of treatment, the therapist determined that the sharing of the trauma narrative would bring Beckham and Ms. Roberts closer. Thus, both Beckham and Ms. Roberts were carefully prepared for this conjoint session for optimal therapeutic outcomes. As Beckham completed the chapters, the therapist shared the chapters with Ms. Roberts individually to gradually assist her in coping with hearing about the traumas Beckham had experienced.

The final phase of TF-CBT focused on the consolidation of skills, trauma-focused conjoint sessions, and final therapeutic activities that enhance safety and future development. During the conjoint session, Beckham shared his trauma narrative with Ms. Roberts while pausing between chapters so she could reflect back some of his words, acknowledge his feelings, and praise his ability to write and describe his experiences in detail. Ms. Roberts praised Beckham for all of his hard work in therapy and for trusting her enough to share his experiences, thoughts, and feelings with her. Beckham was offered education about healthy sexuality, healthy relationships, dating, and dating violence. In both individual and conjoint sessions, Beckham practiced safety skills and problem solving through role-plays that depicted potentially violent or uncomfortable situations.

At the end of therapy, the therapist assisted Beckham in navigating the grief process related to the loss of his mother by incorporating additional traumatic grief components (Cohen, Mannarino, & Deblinger, 2006, 2016) from TF-CBT. First, she offered psycho-education about the stages of grief and read a book together with Beckham about a child who lost his mother. To say goodbye, Beckham wrote a farewell letter to his mother. Beckham and Ms. Roberts planned a symbolic funeral service that they held at his mother's grave since he was unable to attend her burial. Beckham created a journal including positive memories about his mother along with photos of her and him that had been retrieved from his mother's house after her death. Beckham talked about not having his mom attend his graduation and wedding and participate in his children's lives. The therapist helped him identify other people that could fulfill these roles in his life, and Ms. Roberts was identified as his primary person.

After this session, the family completed standardized assessment measures, which revealed improvements with respect to PTSD and depressive symptoms and aggressive behaviors. The therapist noted improvements in Ms. Roberts's parenting skills as well as enhanced parent-child interactions. In fact, Ms. Roberts began to express more enthusiasm and confidence about the adoption process and expressed greater appreciation for Beckham's strengths in overcoming his traumatic experiences and traumas. A graduation celebration was finally planned that involved a review of therapy progress and sharing of favorite snacks, graduation certificates, and music.

Emerging Innovations, Challenges, and Recommendations for Future Research

TF-CBT is an evidence-based treatment that continues to evolve in response to research. Thus far, research has both replicated earlier findings with diverse populations and settings and helped to identify factors that appear to be associated with varied treatment needs in terms of length, intensity, and focus of treatment. In addition, recent research is attempting to vary efforts to increase access to TF-CBT, acknowledging that the standard provision of outpatient mental health is insufficient to address the overwhelming therapeutic needs resulting from childhood trauma. Toward this end, Salloum and colleagues tested a stepped-care provision of TF-CBT, in which families attended only three in-person therapy sessions and completed parent-led home activities, followed by a second evaluation to determine if additional treatment was needed. The study provided preliminary support for effectiveness and family receptiveness to a stepped-care TF-CBT (Salloum, Dorsey, Swaidan, & Storch, 2015; Salloum, Small et al., 2015; Salloum, Wang et al. 2015). These studies indicate that for some youth, abbreviated or parent-facilitated treatment may be both clinically effective and cost-effective.

Another focus of TF-CBT research has been on the dissemination of training in this model of treatment. Cohen, Mannarino, Jankowski et al. (2016) examined methods of training therapists to implement TF-CBT with youth in residential settings by comparing treatment outcomes between therapists trained via web-based training courses and those who received web-based training plus face-to-face training and bimonthly phone consultation. The findings of this investigation demonstrated that significantly more therapists who participated in face-to-face training and phone consultation conducted trauma screenings, completed treatment, and more frequently implemented treatment with fidelity as compared to therapists randomly assigned to the other condition. Other research efforts have also begun to examine the ongoing sustainability of TF-CBT implementation practices beyond the training period. Research examining TF-CBT supervision in terms of the potential benefits of incorporating symptom and fidelity monitoring, with and without behavior rehearsal (in which the clinician practices a TF-CBT component for an upcoming session, with supervisor feedback) is currently underway (see Dorsey et al., 2013), and the results may have important implications for supervision practices across evidence-based interventions.

Integration of technology into the provision of TF-CBT seeks to address barriers of both therapist fidelity and client engagement by means of standardized and engaging software. For example, the TF-CBT Triangle of Life smartphone application was developed to help youth learn and apply cognitive coping skills. Additional computer programs and apps have been developed to support therapists' efforts to teach other effective coping and parenting skills to TF-CBT clients. In fact, an initial feasibility pilot project demonstrated the potential value of technological innovations in enhancing the implementation of TF-CBT with youth and their caregivers, and further research on technology-assisted TF-CBT treatment is underway (Ruggerio et al., 2017).

Another area of developing research concerns the measurement of physiological and neurological correlates of treatment response. In this vein, MRI findings have been examined within a sample of adolescent girls with PTSD who participated in TF-CBT. Adolescents with greater amygdala activity to both threat and neutral stimuli at pretreatment showed less improvement in PTSD symptoms compared to adolescents with greater discriminatory amygdala response to threat versus neutral stimuli (Cisler et al., 2015). In a second analysis conducted on the data of this sample, findings showed self-reported emotional regulation improvement and PTSD symptom reduction paired with greater changes in inhibition of amygdala to frontal cortex (Cisler et al., 2016). While research documents the negative effects of trauma and abuse on brain development, future research examining the potential benefits of therapy on brain development is encouraged as such studies may have important implications that highlight the plasticity of the brain in terms of healing.

Key Practice Components of TF-CBT

Research has indicated that the support and emotional well-being of a caregiver is associated with positive outcomes for children (Cohen & Mannarino, 1996b, 1998b). In addition, it has been documented that the caregivers' participation in treatment is critical for change in terms of children's behaviors (Deblinger et al., 1996). Parenting guidance is regarded as a critical component of TF-CBT for optimal outcomes related to trauma recovery (Cohen & Mannarino, 1998b; Deblinger et al., 1996). Thus, the research on caregiver engagement and involvement, cited earlier, is of great importance and should continue to be pursued to enhance treatment fidelity and positive outcomes for children and adolescents.

All of the TF-CBT PRACTICE components are conceptualized as equally important to the therapeutic process (Cohen, Mannarino, & Deplinger, 2006). However, the trauma narration and processing component, which involves gradually encouraging children to write about their traumatic experiences has been examined more closely in terms of its impact on outcomes in a randomized trial (Deblinger et al., 2011). The results of a multisite clinical trial demonstrated that TF-CBT produced significant symptom improvements among participants as well as enhanced reports of parenting practices and children's personal safety skill knowledge across all four TF-CBT treatment conditions regardless of the number of TF-CBT sessions (8 vs. 16) or whether a trauma narrative was written. Interestingly, the eight-session TF-CBT condition that included the trauma narration component seemed to be the most effective and efficient means of ameliorating parental abuse–specific distress and children's levels of abuse-related fear and general anxiety. Despite these and other positive outcomes with respect to TF-CBT in general, therapists new to the model sometimes express concern about encouraging a child to discuss their traumatic experiences due to a fear of interfering with the development of the therapeutic relationship and potentially "re-traumatizing" the child. To our knowledge, no findings have supported such concerns. Moreover, it should be noted that when children have been asked what was most helpful in the therapy process, the majority of children assigned to TF-CBT have reported that talking about the abusive experiences endured was the most helpful aspect of TF-CBT (Deblinger et al., 2006, 2011). More recently, Dittmann and Jensen (2014) replicated the previous findings when they interviewed adolescents who experienced an array of traumatic events about their experiences with TF-CBT. One theme identified across interviews was that while it was most difficult to talk about the traumas, discussing the traumas was the most helpful aspect of their TF-CBT experience.

In terms of concerns about interfering with the development of the therapeutic relationship, recent research has examined the influence of the therapeutic alliance outcomes among children and caregivers impacted by trauma. In fact, the results of a RCT conducted by Ormaug et al. (2014) found that the therapeutic alliance affected outcomes significantly more among those families randomly assigned to TF-CBT as compared to those assigned to TAU. These results highlight the value of research with respect to the therapeutic alliance as well as the importance of clinically attending to the therapist-client relationship in the context of treatment.

Though there is still much to be learned about the impact and treatment of childhood trauma, it is gratifying to know that clinicians and researchers share the desire to pose important questions to the field to ensure that interventions produce optimal outcomes for children and adolescents who have faced adversity. As a result, research, training, and clinical efforts all will likely continue to contribute to the field's advancements in important ways.

References

Alisic, E., Zalta, A. K., vanWesel, F., Larsen, S. E., Hafstad, G. S., Hassanpour, K., & Smid, M. G. (2014). Rates of posttraumatic stress disorder in trauma-exposed children and adolescents: A meta-analysis. *British Journal of Psychiatry, 204*, 335–340. doi: 10.1192/bjp.bp.113.131227

Allen, B., & Hoskowitz, N. A. (2016). Structured trauma-focused CBT and unstructured play/experiential techniques in the treatment of sexually abused children: A field study with practicing clinicians. *Child Maltreatment, 22*(2), 112–120. doi:10.1177/1077559516681866

American Psychiatric Association. (2013). *Diagnostic and statistical manual of mental disorders: DSM-5*. Washington, DC: American Psychiatric Association.

Bryant, R. A., Salmon, K., Sinclair, E., & Davidson, P. (2007). The relationship between acute stress disorder and posttraumatic stress disorder in injured children. *Journal of Traumatic Stress, 20*(6), 1075–1079. doi:10.1002/jts.20282

Cisler, J. M., Sigel, B. A., Kramer, T. L., Smitherman, S., Vanderzee, K., Pemberton, J., & Kilts, C. D. (2015). Amygdala response predicts trajectory of symptom reduction during trauma-focused cognitive-behavioral therapy among adolescent girls with PTSD. *Journal of Psychiatric Research, 71*, 33–40. doi:10.1016/j.jpsychires.2015.09.011

Cisler, J. M., Sigel, B. A., Steele, J. S., Smitherman, S., Vanderzee, K., Pemberton, J., … Kilts, C. D. (2016). Changes in functional connectivity of the amygdala during cognitive reappraisal predict symptom reduction during trauma-focused cognitive-behavioral therapy among adolescent girls with post-traumatic stress disorder. *Psychological Medicine, 46*(14), 3013–3023.

Cloitre, M., Stolback, B. C., Herman, J. L., van der Kolk, B., Pynoos, R., Wang, J., & Petkova, E. (2009). A developmental approach to complex PTSD: Childhood and adult cumulative trauma as predictors of symptom complexity. *Journal of Traumatic Stress, 22*(5), 399–408. doi:10.1002/jts.20444

Cohen, J. A., Deblinger, E., Mannarino, A. M., & Steer, R. (2004). A multisite, RCT for children with sexual abuse-related PTSD symptoms. *Journal of the American Academy of Child and Adolescent Psychiatry, 43*(4), 393–402. doi:10.1097/00004583-2004040000-00005

Cohen, J. A., & Mannarino, A. P. (1996a). A treatment outcome study for sexually abused preschool children: Initial findings. *Journal of the American Academy of Child & Adolescent Psychiatry, 35*(1), 42–50. doi:10.1097/00004583-199601000-00011

Cohen, J. A., & Mannarino, A. P. (1996b). Factors that mediate treatment outcome of sexually abused preschool children. *Journal of the American Academy of Child & Adolescent Psychiatry, 35*(10), 1402–1410. doi:10.1097/00004583-199610000-00028

Cohen, J. A., & Mannarino, A. P. (1997). A treatment study for sexually abused preschool children: Outcome during a one-year follow-up. *Journal of the American Academy of Child & Adolescent Psychiatry, 36*(9), 1228–1235. doi:10.1097/00004583-199709000-00015

Cohen, J. A., & Mannarino, A. P. (1998a). Factors that mediate treatment outcome of sexually abused preschool children: Six- and 12-month follow-up. *Journal of the American Academy of Child & Adolescent Psychiatry, 37*(1), 44–51. doi:10.1097/00004583-199801000-00016

Cohen, J. A., & Mannarino, A. P. (1998b). Interventions for sexually abused children: Initial treatment outcome findings. *Child Maltreatment*, *3*(1), 17–26. doi:10.1177/1077559598003001002

Cohen, J. A., Mannarino, A. P., & Deblinger, E. (2006). *Treating trauma and traumatic grief in children and adolescents*. New York, NY: The Guilford Press.

Cohen, J. A., Mannarino, A. P., & Deblinger, E. (2016). *Treating trauma and traumatic grief in children and adolescents* (2nd ed.). New York: The Guilford Press.

Cohen, J. A., Mannarino, A. P., & Iyenger, S. (2011). Community treatment of posttraumatic stress disorder for children exposed to intimate partner violence: A RCT. *Archives of Pediatrics & Adolescent Medicine*, *165*(1), 16–21. doi:10.1001/archpediatrics.2010.247

Cohen, J. A., Mannarino, A. P., Jankowski, K., Rosenberg, S., Kodya, S., & Wolford II, G. L. (2016). A randomized implementation study of trauma-focused cognitive behavior therapy for adjudicated teens in residential treatment facilities. *Child Maltreatment*, *21*(2), 156–167. doi:10.1177/1077559515624775

Cohen, J. A., Mannarino, A. P., Perel, J. M., & Staron, V. (2007). A pilot RCT of combined trauma-focused CBT and sertraline for childhood PTSD symptoms. *Journal of the American Academy of Child & Adolescent Psychiatry*, *46*, 811–819. doi:10.1097/chi.0b013e3180547105

Cohen, J. A., Mannarino, A. P., & Staron, V. R. (2006). A pilot study of modified cognitive-behavior therapy or child traumatic grief (CBT-CTG). *Journal of the American Academy of Child & Adolescent Psychiatry*, *45*, 1465–1473. doi: 10.1097/01.chi.0000237705.43260.2c

Deblinger, E., Lippmann, J., & Steer, R. (1996). Sexually abused children suffering from posttraumatic stress symptoms: Initial treatment outcome findings. *Child Maltreatment*, *1*(4), 310–321. doi:10.1177/1077559596001004003

Deblinger, E., Mannarino, A. P., Cohen, J. A., Runyon, M. K., & Heflin, A. H. (2015). *Child sexual abuse: A primer for treating children, adolescents, and their nonoffending caregivers* (2nd edn.). New York: Oxford University Press.

Deblinger, E., Mannarino, A. P., Cohen, J. A., Runyon, M. K., & Steer, R. A. (2011). Trauma-focused cognitive behavior therapy for children: Impact of the trauma narrative component and treatment length. *Depression and Anxiety*, *28*, 67–75. doi: 10.1002/da.20744

Deblinger, E., Mannarino, A. P., Cohen, J. A., & Steer, R. A. (2006). Follow-up study of a multisite, randomized, controlled trial for children with sexual abuse-related PTSD symptoms: Examining predictors of treatment response. *Journal of the American Academy of Child & Adolescent Psychiatry*, *45*(12). doi: 10.1097/01.chi.0000240839.56114.bb

Deblinger, E., Neubauer, F., Runyon, M. K., & Baker, D. (2006). *What do you know? A therapeutic card game about child sexual and physical abuse and domestic violence*. Stratford, NJ: CARES Institute.

Deblinger, E., Stauffer, L., & Steer, R. (2001). Comparative efficacies of supportive and cognitive behavioral group therapies for children who were sexually abused and their nonoffending mothers. *Child Maltreatment*, *6*(4), 332–343. doi: 10.1177/1077559501006004006

Deblinger, E., Steer, R. A., & Lippmann, J. (1999). Two-year follow-up study of cognitive behavior therapy for sexually abused children suffering from post-traumatic stress symptoms. *Child Abuse & Neglect*, *23*(12), 1371–1378. doi:10.1016/S0145-2134(99)00091-5

Diehle, J., Opmeer, B. C., Boer, F., Mannarino, A. P., & Lindauer, R. J. L. (2015). Trauma-focused cognitive behavioral therapy or eye movement desensitization and reprocessing: What works in children with posttraumatic stress symptoms? A RCT. *European Child & Adolescent Psychiatry*, *24*(2), 227–236. doi:10.1007/s00787-014-0572-5

Dittmann, I., & Jensen, T. K. (2014). Giving a vice to traumatized youth-experiences with trauma-focused cognitive behavioral therapy. *Child Abuse & Neglect*, *38*, 1221–1230. doi:10.1016/j.chiabu.2013.11.008

Dorsey, S., Pullmann, M., Berliner, L., Koschmann, E. F., McKay, M., & Deblinger, E. (2014). Engaging foster parents in treatment: A randomized trial of supplementing trauma-focused cognitive behavioral therapy with evidence-based engagement strategies. *Child Abuse & Neglect*, *38*(9), 1508–1520. doi:10.1016/j.chiabu.2014.03.020

Dorsey, S., Pullmann, M. D., Deblinger, E., Berliner, L., Kerns, S. E., ... Garland, A. F. (2013). Improving practice in community-based settings: A randomized trial of supervision – study protocol. *Implementation Science*, *8*(89). doi: 10.1186/1748-5908-8-89

Felitti, V. J., Anda, R. F., Nordenberg, D., Williamson, D. F., Spitz, A. M., Edwards, V., ... Marks, J. S. (1998). Relationship of childhood abuse and household dysfunction to many of the leading causes of death in adults: The adverse childhood experiences (ACE) study. *American Journal of Preventative Medicine*, *14*, 245–258.

Foa, E. B., Chrestman, K., & Gilboa-Schechtman, E. (2008). *Prolonged exposure manual for children and adolescents suffering from PTSD*. New York: Oxford University Press.

Foa E. B., & Rothbaum, B. O. (1998). *Treating the trauma of rape: Cognitive–behavioral therapy for PTSD*. New York: The Guilford Press.

Goldbeck, L., Muche, R., Sachser, C., Tutus, D., & Rosner, R. (2016). Effectiveness of trauma-focused cognitive behavioral therapy for children and adolescents: A RCT in eight German mental health clinics. *Psychotherapy and Psychomatics* *85*(3), 159–170. doi:10.1159/000442824

Greer, D., Grasso, D. J., Cohen, A., & Webb, C. (2014). Trauma-focused treatment in a state system of care: Is it worth the cost? *Administration and Policy in Mental Health and Mental Health Services Research*, *41*(3), 317–323. doi: 10.1007/s10488-013-0468-6

Hayes, A. M., Yasinski, C., Grasso, D., Ready, C. B., Alpert, E., McCauley, T., ... Deblinger, E. (2017). Constructive and unproductive processing of traumatic experiences in trauma-focused cognitive-behavioral therapy for youth. *Behavior Therapy*, *48*, 166–181. doi:10.1016/j.beth.2016.06.004

Jensen, T. K., Holt, T., Ormhaug, S. M., Egeland, K., Granly, L., Hoaas, L. C., ... Wentzel-Larsen, T. (2014). A randomized effectiveness study comparing trauma-focused cognitive behavioral therapy with therapy as usual for youth. *Journal of Clinical Child & Adolescent Psychology*, *43*(3), 356–369. doi:10.1080/15374416.2013.822307

Kameoka, S., Yagi, J., Arai, Y., Nosaka, S., Saito, A., Miyake, W., ... Asukai, N. (2015). Feasibility of trauma-focused cognitive behavioral therapy for traumatized children in Japan: A pilot study. *International Journal of Mental Health Systems*, *9*(26), (Open Access). http://dx.doi.org/10.1186/s13033-015-0021-y

Kendall-Tackett, K., Williams, L., & Finkelhor, D. (1993). Impact of sexual abuse on children: A review and synthesis of recent empirical studies. *Psychological Bulletin, 113*, 164–180. doi:10.1027//0033-2909.113.1.164

King, N. J, Tange, B. J., Mullen, P., Myerson, N., Heyne, D., Rollings, S., ... Ollendick, T. H. (2000). Treating sexually abused children with posttraumatic stress symptoms: A randomized clinical trial. *Journal of the American Academy of Child & Adolescent Psychiatry, 39*, 1347–1355. doi:10.1097/00004583-200011000-00008

Kliethermes, M., Schacht, M., & Drewry, K. (2014). Complex trauma. *Child and Adolescent Psychiatric Clinics of North America, 23*(2), 339–361. doi: 10.1016/j.chc.2013.12.009

Konanur, S., Muller, R. T., Cinamon, J. S., Thornback, K., & Zorzella, P. M. (2015). Effectiveness of trauma-focused cognitive behavioral therapy in a community-based program. *Child Abuse & Neglect, 50*, 159–170. doi:10.1016/j.chiabu.2015.07.013

Lai, B., Tiwari, A., Self-Brown, S., Cronholm, P., & Kinnish, K. (2017). Patterns of caregiver factors predicting participation in trauma-focused cognitive behavioral therapy. *Journal of Child and Adolescent Trauma* (online). doi:10.1007/s40653-017-0177-5

Lieberman, A. F., Van Horn, P., & Ghosh Ippen, C. (2005). Toward evidence-based treatment: Child-parent psychotherapy with preschoolers exposed to marital violence. *Journal of the American Academy of Child and Adolescent Psychiatry, 44*(12), 1241–1248.

Lyons, J. S., Weiner, D. A., & Schneider, A. (2006). *A field trial of three evidence based practices for trauma with children in state custody.* Report to the Illinois Department of Children and Family Services. Evanston, IL: Mental Health Resources Services and Policy Program, Northwestern University.

Mannarino, A. P., Cohen, J. A., Deblinger, E., Runyon, M. K., & Steer, R. A. (2012). Trauma-focused cognitive behavior therapy for children: Sustained impact of treatment 6–12 months later. *Child Maltreatment, 17*(3), 231–241.

McMullen, J., O'Callaghan, P., Shannon, C., Black, A., & Eskin, J. (2013). Group trauma-focused cognitive-behavioural therapy with former child soldiers and other war-affected boys in the DR Congo: A RCT. *Journal of Child Psychology and Psychiatry, 54*(11), 1231–1241. doi:10.1111/jcpp.12094

Morina, M., Koerssen, R., & Pollet, T. V. (2016). Interventions for children and adolescents with posttraumatic stress disorder: A meta-analysis of comparative outcome studies. *Clinical Psychology, 47*, 41–54.

Murray, L. K., Skavenski, S., Kane, J. C., Mayeya, J., Dorsey, S., Cohen, J. A., ... Bolton, P. A. (2015). Effectiveness of trauma-focused cognitive behavioral therapy among trauma-affected children in Lusaka, Zambia – A randomized clinical trial. *JAMA Pediatrics, 169*(8), 761–769. doi:10.1001/jamapediatrics.2015.0580

O'Callaghan, P., McMullen, J., Shannon, C., Rafferty, H., & Black, A. (2013). A RCT of trauma-focused cognitive behavioral therapy for sexually exploited, war-affected Congolese girls. *Journal of the American Academy of Child & Adolescent Psychiatry, 52*(4), 359–369. doi:10.1016/j.jaac.2013.01.013

Ormaug, S. M., Jensen, T. K., Wentzel-Larsen, T., & Shirk, S. R. (2014). The therapeutic alliance in treatment of traumatized youths: Relation to outcome in a randomized clinical trial. *American Psychological Association, 82*(1), 52–64. doi:10.1037/a0033884

Papakostas, G. I., & Fava, M. (2008). Predictors, moderators, and mediators (correlates) of treatment outcome in major depressive disorder. *Dialogues in Clinical Neuroscience, 10*(4), 439–451.

Pineles, S. L., Mostoufi, S. M., Ready, C. B., Street, A. E., Griffin, M. G., & Resick, P. A. (2011). Trauma reactivity, avoidant coping, and PTSD symptoms: A moderating relationship? *Journal of Abnormal Psychology, 120*(1), 240–246. doi: 10.1037/a0022123

Ready, C. B., Hayes, A. M., Yasinski, C. W., Webb, C., Gallop, R., Deblinger, E., & Laurenceau, J. P. (2015). Overgeneralized beliefs, accommodation, and treatment outcome in youth receiving trauma-focused cognitive behavioral therapy for childhood trauma. *Behavior Therapy, 46*, 671–688. doi:10.1016/j.beth.2015.03.004

Ruggerio, K. J., Saunders, B. E., Davidson, T. M., Lesky Cook, D., & Hanson, R. (2017). Leveraging technology to address the quality chasm in children's evidence-based psychotherapy. *Psychiatric Services, 63*(7), 650–652. doi:10.1176/appi.ps.201600548'

Salloum, A., Dorsey, C. S., Swaidan, V. R., & Storch, E. A. (2015). Parents' and children's perception of parent-led trauma-focused cognitive behavioral therapy. *Child Abuse & Neglect, 40*(2), 12–23. doi:10.1016/j.chiabu.2014.11.018

Salloum, A., Small, B. J., Robst, J., Scheeringa, M. S., Cohen, J. A., & Storch, E. A. (2015). Stepped and standard care for childhood trauma: A pilot randomized clinical trial. *Research on Social Work Practice (Online First)*, 1–11. doi:10.1177/1049731515601898

Salloum, A., Wang, W., Robst, J., Murphy, T. K., Scheeringa, M. S., Cohen, J. A., & Storch, E. A. (2015). Stepped care versus standard trauma-focused cognitive behavioral therapy for young children. *Journal of Child Psychology and Psychiatry, 57*(5), 614–622. doi:10.1111/jcpp.12471

Satullo, J., & Bradway, R. (1987). *It happens to boys too.* Pittsfield, MA: Center for Berkshires Press.

Shapiro, F. (2001). *Eye movement desensitization and reprocessing: Basic principles, protocols, and procedures* (2nd edn.). New York: The Guilford Press.

Sharma-Patel, K., & Brown, E. J. (2016). Emotion regulation and self-blame as mediators and moderators of trauma-specific treatment. *Psychology of Violence (APA), 6*(3), 400–409. doi:10.1037/vio0000044

Spinazzola, J., Ford, J. T., Zucker, M., van der Kolk, B. A., Silva, S., Smith, F. S., & Blaustein, M. (2005). Complex trauma exposure, outcomes, and intervention among children and adolescents. *Psychiatric Annals, 35*(5), 433–439.

Wamser-Nanney, R. & Steinzor, C. E. (2017). Factors related to attrition from trauma-focused cognitive behavioral therapy. *Child Abuse & Neglect, 66*, 73–83. doi:10.1016/j.chiabu.2016.11.031

Wamser-Nanney, R., Scheeringa, M. S., & Weems, C. F. (2014). Early treatment response in children and adolescents receiving CBT for trauma. *Journal of Pediatric Psychology, 41*(1), 1–11. doi:10.1093/

Webb, C., Hayes, A. M., Grasso, D., Laurenceau, J-P., & Deblinger E. (2014). Trauma-focused cognitive behavioral therapy for youth: Effectiveness in a community setting. *Psychological Trauma: Theory, Research, Practice, and Policy 6*(5), 555–562. doi.org/10.1037/a0037364

Xiangming, F., Brown, D. S., Florencea, C. S., & Mercya, J. A. (2012). The economic burden of child maltreatment in the United States and implications for prevention. *Child Abuse and Neglect, 36*(2), 156–165. doi:10.1016/j.chiabu.2011.10.006

Yasinski, C., Hayes, A. M., Ready, C. B., Cummings, J. A., Berman, I. S., McCauley, T., & Deblinger, E. (2016). In-session caregiver behavior predicts symptom change in youth receiving trauma-focused cognitive behavioral therapy (TF-CBT). *Journal of Consulting and Clinical Psychology, 84*(12), 1066–1077. doi:10.1037/ccp0000147

26 Advances in the Assessment of PTSD in Children and Young People

David Trickey and Richard Meiser-Stedman

Introduction

Since 1980, when post-traumatic stress disorder (PTSD) was first defined in the *Diagnostic and Statistical Manual of Mental Disorders*, 3rd edn. (DSM-III: American Psychiatric Association, 1980), there have been important advances in the diagnostic definition, understanding, assessment, and treatment of PTSD in children and young people. The changes in the definition of PTSD have been far-reaching, and the two major diagnostic systems (DSM and the International Classification of Diseases – ICD – published by the World Health Organisation) have become increasingly diverse. However, symptoms of re-experiencing of the traumatic event(s) and avoidance have been constant elements throughout all iterations. Theoretical advances have led to the development of differing theories that seek to explain the occurrence of PTSD (e.g., Brewin, Gregory, Lipton, & Burgess, 2010; Ehlers & Clark, 2000; Elbert & Schauer, 2002; Foa, Steketee, & Rothbaum, 1989; Stickgold, 2002), and a variety of interventions have been produced to ameliorate the symptoms of PTSD in children and young people, some of which have empirical support (e.g., De Roos et al., 2017; Deblinger, Steer, & Lippmann, 1999; Ruf et al., 2010; Smith et al., 2007).

It is crucial that assessment techniques advance at a similar pace to these other developments to ensure that they are as accurate as possible; only then can assessment inform the development of useful models, ensure that children and young people receive the appropriate intervention, and confirm the effectiveness of such interventions.

A brief overview of commonly used measures is shown in Table 26.1. However, it is worth noting that similar lists that are occasionally updated are also available (National Center for PTSD, 2017; National Child Traumatic Stress Network, 2017).

Advances in Diagnostic Classification Systems

The current DSM-5 (American Psychiatric Association, 2013) defines the qualifying event for PTSD as "exposure to actual or threatened death, serious injury, or sexual violence"; the classification then requires symptoms of intrusions (one symptom required from a list of five), avoidance (one symptom from a list of two),

Table 26.1 *Measures for Use with Traumatized Children and Young People*
Structured Interviews for Diagnosis

Clinician Administered PTSD Scale for Children and Adolescents (CAPS-CA-5)

Age range:	7–18
Respondent:	Child / young person
Number of items:	30 items
Published psychometric properties:	DSM-5 version currently being validated, but it is based on validated DSM-IV version (Steinberg et al., 2004)
Availability:	www.ptsd.va.gov/professional/assessment/child/caps-ca.asp (free)

Child PTSD Symptom Scale – Interview Version for DSM-5 (CPSS-5-I)

Age range:	8–18
Respondent:	Child / young person
Number of items:	27 items
Published psychometric properties:	Validity and reliability (Foa et al., 2018)
Availability:	foa@mail.med.upenn.edu (free)

PTSD Module of Anxiety Disorders Interview Schedule for DSM-IV – Child Version (ADIS for DSM-IV:C)

Age range:	7–16
Respondent:	Separate interview schedules for child / young person or caregiver
Number of items:	Caregiver schedule: 27 (including 9 trauma history items)
Child / young person schedule:	29 (including 10 trauma history items) 29 (including 10 trauma history items)
Published psychometric properties:	
Availability:	https://global.oup.com/ (payment required)

Diagnostic Infant and Preschool Assessment (DIPA)

Age range:	1–6
Respondent:	Caregiver
Number of items:	34 (including 13 trauma history items)
Published psychometric properties:	Reliability and validity (DSM-IV; Scheeringa & Haslett, 2010)
Availability:	http://medicine.tulane.edu/departments/psychiatry/research/dr-scheeringas-lab/manuals-measures-trainings (free)

Children's PTSD Inventory
(CPTSDI)

Age range:	6–18
Respondent:	Child / young person
Number of items:	50
Published psychometric properties:	Reliability (Saigh et al., 2000)
	Validity (DSM-IV PTSD; Yasik et al., 2001)
Availability:	www.pearsonclinical.co.uk (payment required)

Symptom Questionnaires

Children's Revised Impact of Event Scale
(CRIES-8 and CRIES-13)

Age range:	8–18
Respondent:	Child / young person
Number of items:	8 (CRIES-8)
	13 (CRIES-13)
Published psychometric properties:	Reliability, validity, clinical thresholds (DSM-IV): 17+ (CRIES-8) and 30+ (CRIES 13) (Perrin et al., 2005)
Availability:	www.childrenandwar.org (free)

Child PTSD Symptom Scale – Self-Report Version for DSM-5
(CPSS-5-SR)

Age range:	8–18
Respondent:	Child / young person
Number of items:	27
Published psychometric properties:	Reliability, validity, clinical threshold 31 (Foa et al., 2018)
Availability:	foa@mail.med.upenn.edu (free)

UCLA PTSD Reaction Index for DSM-5 (Children/Adolescent)
(UCLA PTSD RI)

Age range:	7–18
Respondent:	Child / young person or caregiver
Number of items:	55 (including 23 trauma history items)
Published psychometric properties:	Reliability, validity, clinical threshold of 35 (Rolon-Arroyo et al., 2017)
Availability:	www.reactionindex.com (payment required)

UCLA DSM-5 PTSD Reaction Index for Young Children (UCLA PTSD RI YC)

Age range:	0–6
Respondent:	Caregiver
Number of items:	96 (including 22 trauma history items)
Published psychometric properties:	DSM-5 version currently being validated
Availability:	www.reactionindex.com (payment required)

Child Trauma Screening Questionnaire (CTSQ)

Age range:	6–18
Respondent:	Child / young person
Number of items:	10
Published psychometric properties:	Reliability, validity, clinical threshold of 5 (DSM-IV; Kenardy, Spence, & Macleod, 2006)
Availability:	j.kenardy@uq.edu.au (free)

Other Questionnaires

Child Post Traumatic Cognitions Inventory (CPTCI)

Age range:	6–18
Respondent:	Child / young person
Number of items:	25 (short form: 10)
Published psychometric properties:	Reliability and validity (McKinnon et al., 2016)
Availability:	www.childrenandwar.org (free)

Trauma Memory Quality Questionnaire (TMQQ)

Age range:	10–18
Respondent:	Child / young person
Number of items:	14
Published psychometric properties:	Validity (Meiser-Stedman et al., 2007)
Availability:	www.childrenandwar.org (free)

changes in cognitions and mood (two symptoms from a list of seven), and arousal and reactivity (two symptoms from a list of six).

There are some marked differences with the previous DSM-IV version (American Psychiatric Association, 2000); therefore, measures that are specifically based upon, and validated with, DSM-IV criteria cannot be assumed to be valid for the DSM-5 criteria. To date, only two DSM-IV measures have been updated to be consistent with DSM-5 and have produced data on their validity and reliability. The Child PTSD Symptom Scale (CPSS; Foa, Johnson, Feeny, & Treadwell, 2001) has an interview version, a self-report version, and a brief screening version all consistent with DSM-5 and have all been validated (Foa, Asnaani, Zang, Capaldi, & Yeh, 2018). The UCLA PTSD Reaction Index (Steinberg, Brymer, Decker, & Pynoos, 2004) has also been updated and validated for DSM-5 (Rolon-Arroyo et al., 2017; Steinberg et al., 2004) and provides a version for use with a child or young person, and a version for use with a caregiver.

The recent 11th edition of the International Classification of Diseases (ICD-11) has now produced more simplified criteria for PTSD requiring one symptom of re-experiencing of the traumatic event in the present, one symptom of avoidance, and one symptom of perceptions of heightened threat (Maercker et al., 2013).

These two differing systems will inevitably lead to discrepancies in which children and young people fulfil diagnostic criteria. Danzi and LaGreca (2016) found in two separate samples of children and young people exposed to hurricanes that the agreement between ICD-11 and DSM-5 systems was poor, with fewer than half of the children fulfilling both sets of criteria. Obviously, the disparate developments in the diagnostic systems regarding the classification of PTSD also have repercussions for the assessment of the disorder.

PTSD in Young Children

There are some differences in the way that PTSD presents in children of various ages and developmental levels (Salmon & Bryant, 2002). For example, the core symptoms of intrusions and avoidance may be less apparent in children younger than age 7 (Fletcher, 1996), and younger children may be more likely to show their reactions to traumatic events through behavioral symptoms and traumatic play (Scheeringa, Zeanah, Myers, & Putnam, 2003). It is therefore crucial to take these developmental differences into account when assessing the impact of traumatic events on younger children. Accordingly, DSM-5 provides a separate classification of PTSD in children age 6 and younger (American Psychiatric Association, 2013). The classification combines the symptom subgroups of avoidance and changes in cognitions, and it acknowledges that intrusive memories may not be experienced as distressing and may appear in the child's play. Recognizing that the classification is largely based on information provided by the caregivers, the requirement of only one symptom from a combined avoidance and change in cognitions symptom cluster is wholly appropriate. In keeping with the developmental level of the age group, symptoms of reckless behavior and self-harm were eliminated, while temper tantrums have been added.

Relatedly, a number of studies support the inclusion of alternative, developmentally sensitive criteria that acknowledge the differences in presentation in young children and recognize the importance of combining child self-report with the report of caregivers (Meiser-Stedman, Smith, Glucksman, Yule, & Dalgleish, 2008; Meiser-Stedman, Smith, Yule, Glucksman, & Dalgleish, 2017; Scheeringa, Wright, Hunt, & Zeanah, 2006). Nevertheless, once children are able to provide their own report, their opinions are a crucial part of the classification process; relying on parents alone for youth aged 7–10 years would result in significantly lower rates of PTSD, and raises the question of whether our current methods of assessing PTSD in preschoolers are underestimating the prevalence of very young children. Long-term follow-up research of young children exposed to trauma may be necessary to accurately confirm whether clinical symptoms of PTSD are genuinely absent.

Complex PTSD

ICD-11 has now defined a new diagnosis of Complex PTSD, which will consist of the core symptoms of PTSD mentioned earlier and additional difficulties in three domains: affect (such as heightened emotional reactivity, violent outbursts, reckless or self-destructive behavior, and dissociation), self-concept (such as persistent beliefs about oneself as being diminished, defeated, or worthless and feelings of shame or guilt), and relational functioning (such as difficulties feeling close to others, avoiding or deriding social engagement, and difficulties sustaining relationships; Maercker et al., 2013). This diagnostic development obviously requires assessments to advance accordingly and at present there are limited options for assessing Complex PTSD in children and young people. There is a self-report questionnaire that assesses the symptoms of ICD-11–defined PTSD and Complex PTSD in adults (Karatzias et al., 2017), but this measure is yet to be robustly evaluated, and there is currently no published equivalent for use with children and young people.

Until there are further advances and an equivalent, psychometrically sound instrument is developed for youth, clinicians and researchers seeking to assess children and adolescents for Complex PTSD systematically will have to rely on using data from different questionnaires. For example, one study examining the existence of complex PTSD retrospectively in a sample of treatment-seeking traumatized children and young people combined individual items from three assessment tools to examine the presence of symptoms of PTSD and Complex PTSD (Sachser, Keller, & Goldbeck, 2017). These authors used the Clinician-Administered PTSD Scale for Children and Adolescents (CAPS-CA; Weathers, Keane, & Davidson, 2001) to assess for the core ICD-11 PTSD symptoms and three symptoms of ICD-11 Complex PTSD (violent outbursts, guilt, and feeling disconnected from others); one item from the UCLA PTSD Reaction Index (Steinberg & Beyerlein, 2013) to assess the Complex PTSD symptom of not feeling close to others, and two items from the Child Post-traumatic Cognitions Scale (Meiser-Stedman et al., 2009) to assess Complex PTSD symptoms of feeling worthless and being overly sensitive. The existence of a Complex PTSD group (40.6 percent of the overall sample) that endorsed many of these symptoms as well as the "core" symptoms of PTSD was supported by a latent class analysis. The other, larger group of clients only reported the core PTSD symptoms with any frequency.

Advances in Use of Assessment

Diagnosis

Regardless of which classification system is being used, a comprehensive assessment of PTSD will need to assess which of the criteria are met. This requires a detailed assessment of the traumatic event, or events, as well as the symptoms. A good assessment takes data gathered from a variety of sources and informants and weaves them together, making sense of any apparent contradictions. Such a thorough assessment can be assisted by systematic, standardized, psychometrically robust instruments such as questionnaires and semi-structured interviews.

Using questionnaires or semi-structured interviews can provide a focused approach that ensures that relevant areas are covered in the assessment, so that the relevant diagnostic algorithm can be applied. This can be particularly helpful given that avoidance is a hallmark symptom of PTSD and the structure of the interview can help clinicians to not be sidetracked by the child's or young person's avoidance.

Such measures can also produce a quantitative evaluation of symptoms resulting in a numerical score. Many measures, particularly the self-report questionnaires, have "cut-off" scores that indicate a particular likelihood that the child or young person fulfils the criteria for PTSD. Using a simple cut-off score on a scale can offer a useful indication of what a score means and can provide a useful benchmark to help evaluate interventions by comparing how many children and young people are above the cut off before and after an intervention. But using self-report questionnaires as the only source of data could result in many children and young people either being wrongly identified as having PTSD or not being identified with PTSD when they should have been. Some research indicates that use of self-report questionnaires alone may lead to up to 31 percent of children and young people with PTSD (as diagnosed by a more robust measure) not being identified (e.g., Stallard, Velleman, & Baldwin, 1999). To accurately and robustly diagnose PTSD, it is necessary to assess symptoms and ensure that they comply with a specific algorithm or profile. This requires a careful and comprehensive assessment and not simply completing a short questionnaire.

Differential Diagnosis and Co-Occurring Diagnoses. As theoretical understanding of psychological disorders advances, increasingly specific models are being proposed, leading to more specific therapeutic interventions contingent on the diagnosis or diagnoses. Accurate differential diagnosis is therefore crucial to ensure that distressed children and young people do not get misdiagnosed and thereby offered inappropriate interventions (such as antidepressants intended for the treatment of depressed mood or psycho-stimulants intended for the treatment of restless behavior and concentration difficulties of a child or young person who actually has PTSD).

Furthermore, PTSD very often co-occurs with other psychological problems (e.g., Fletcher, 1996), so comprehensive assessment is crucial to ensure that the child or young person is not denied effective interventions for other disorders because the clinician assumed that all of their symptoms were explained by a diagnosis of PTSD. Assessment of PTSD in particular may be prone to some specific difficulties because the diversity of PTSD symptoms means that it may easily be confused with other diagnoses. For example, persistent negative emotional state, markedly diminished interest or participation in significant activities, feelings of detachment from others, persistent inability to experience positive emotions, problems with concentration and sleep disturbance are all symptoms of DSM-5 PTSD, and yet all of them could easily be accounted for by a depressive disorder. In a similar vein, the hyperarousal and concentration problems of PTSD could be mistaken for the hyperactivity and attention deficits found in DSM-5 attention deficit/hyperactivity disorder (ADHD).

This means that assessments of traumatized children and young people must be careful, comprehensive and as precise as possible to avoid significant adverse consequences. Differential diagnosis can be assisted by clinicians taking the time to gather an account of the child or young person's history of potentially traumatic events, together with careful consideration of when the symptoms began in relation to the events. Intrusive vivid memories are a core symptom of PTSD and should also be given special attention for the purpose of distinguishing the child or young person's difficulties.

Specific Assessment of the Nature of Memories. One symptom that is diagnostic of PTSD and not other disorders is the intrusive nature of the memory. Although DSM-5 lists a number of ways in which the memory may intrude, and other symptom measures may assess the frequency or severity of intrusive memories, it can sometimes be helpful to examine systematically the quality or nature of the memories of the event to consider the extent to which they are characteristic of trauma memories. The Trauma Memory Quality Questionnaire may be of particular use in this regard; this short 11-item self-report instrument has been validated on children and young people aged 10 and above and has been shown to be related to severity of symptoms of PTSD, as well as to PTSD diagnostic status (Meiser-Stedman, Smith, Yule, & Dalgleish, 2007). Understanding the quality of memories for events, rather than just frequency of intrusions may help to differentiate between PTSD and other disorders (e.g., ADHD or generalized anxiety disorder).

Symptom Monitoring

Research indicates that if clinicians have access to information about how their clients have responded to routine measures of symptoms, then therapy is more effective. Furthermore, this effect is larger, the more that the therapist refers to the information (Bickman, Kelley, Breda, de Andrade, & Riemer, 2011). Even outside of actual therapy, symptom monitoring may have a simple positive impact in and of itself on symptoms of PTSD (Smith et al., 2007). Systematically quantifying levels of symptoms regularly throughout the course of therapy can help identify whether there has been improvement or deterioration, which is crucial to keeping therapy moving in the right direction. If a measure indicates that symptoms are deteriorating, this can be discussed with the client to determine if it is an accurate reflection of their experience; if it is, then efforts can be made to understand why this may be the case and whether therapy should be adjusted accordingly. Research has found that some children and young people make sudden gains when receiving therapy (Aderka, Appelbaum-Namdar, Shafran, & Gilboa-Schechtman, 2011). Routine, systematic use of a measure of symptoms will help identify and quantify these sudden gains, enabling clinicians and their clients to reflect upon what may have caused them, which may help make the remaining therapy more efficient.

However, using symptom-monitoring questionnaires is likely to be most effective if the clinician has some knowledge of how these instruments operate. They should at the very least have some awareness of how to interpret the scores generated by the measure and be aware of the fact that these assessments are only proxy measures of psychological distress and functioning, so the score from a questionnaire is likely to fluctuate to a certain degree even if actual symptoms are stable. It is therefore useful to know how much change in a score is necessary to represent a meaningful change in actual symptom levels.

The 8-item version of the Children's Revised Impact of Event Scale (CRIES-8) may be particularly useful for symptom monitoring over the course of therapy because at 8 items it is short and therefore time efficient. Other self-report questionnaires and some semi-structured interviews have been updated to take into account new DSM-5 criteria, whereas the CRIES-8 simply focuses on the systematic assessment of the two core groups of symptoms (i.e., intrusions or re-experiencing and avoidance) that have remained fundamental to the classification of PTSD regardless of version or system. There is, however, a suggested cut-off score of 17; scores 17 or higher indicate a high likelihood of DSM-IV PTSD (Perrin et al., 2005). Regardless of how this measure operates in relation to DSM-5 or ICD-11 PTSD criteria, this cut-off point does at least provide some understanding of how high a score needs to be to be considered pathological.

For example, Figure 26.1 shows the scores on the CRIES-8 throughout a short course of trauma-focused cognitive behavior therapy for a 14-year-old girl who had developed PTSD after being exposed to a violent physical assault. The therapy consisted of a total of 8 sessions including assessment and discharge. It is obvious in the graph that the initial score at assessment of 26 is well above the suggested cut-off point and as such indicates a relatively high level of symptoms and a high probability of fulfilling the diagnostic criteria for PTSD. By the second session, the score had *increased* to 28. It can be difficult to know whether small increases are genuinely indicative of worsening symptoms (and equally whether small decreases are genuinely indicative of improvement in symptoms). The Reliable Change Criterion for whatever measure is being used can help determine whether an observed change in the score is within the amount of change that could be expected simply as a result of using the measure repeatedly (for a user-friendly guide to the

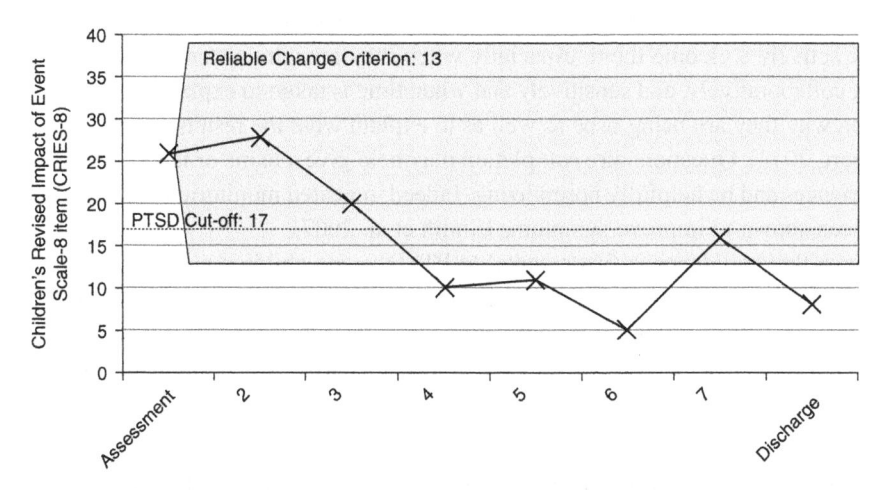

Figure 26.1 *Session by Session Symptom Tracking Using the CRIES-8*

development and use of reliable change, see Fugard, 2014). In this example, the Reliable Change Criterion for the CRIES is 13, meaning that the increase of 2 points (from session 1 to session 2) is well within expected fluctuation of the measure. In addition to using statistics to help clinicians understand changes in scores, it is also important to ask the client about their experiences of change throughout therapy. For example: "the questionnaire shows a slightly higher score since your last session, but even if things had not changed we would expect the score to go up and down more than this amount, so I'm just wondering what you think? Do you think that generally your symptoms remain fairly stable, or do you feel like your symptoms have become worse?" The second session consisted of explaining the rationale for trauma-focused work and some preliminary mapping out of the event.

By the third session, the score had dropped eight points to a score of 20. Although this is encouraging, the total is still well above the clinical cut-off and would therefore be considered a high score, and the amount of change would still not be considered beyond normal fluctuation. This session consisted largely of detailed trauma-focused work.

By the fourth session, the score had fallen below the cut-off point and the total change now exceeded the reliable change criterion. In the seventh session, the score had risen (following an event during the previous week that was highly reminiscent of the original traumatic event). Having tracked the scores from week to week, it was obvious to the client, as well as the therapist, that the trauma-focused work although challenging, had been helpful and as such, the client was keen to return to that work in the expectation that it would lead to a decrease in her symptoms.

Avoidance and Acceptability of Questionnaires

Some clinicians are concerned that questionnaires or other assessment tools may impede the therapeutic relationship or the therapeutic process. Although of course some children and young people may see questionnaires as overly burdensome, many actively welcome them, especially when they are administered unapologetically, collaboratively, and sensitively and when time is taken to explain to the young person why they are being used as well as to explain what the results mean (Law & Wolpert, 2014). Questionnaire completion may help give a name or label to difficult experiences and be helpfully normalizing. Indeed, repeated monitoring of symptoms has been shown to improve symptoms (Smith et al. 2007).

Given that avoidance is fundamental to PTSD, some children and young people may find it impossible to answer a direct question about their symptoms, whereas they may feel more comfortable completing a questionnaire either individually or in a conversation with the clinician that allows the focus to be on the questionnaire rather than on themselves.

Screening Large Numbers of Children and Young People Following Potentially Traumatic Events

Following incidents that are experienced by large numbers of people, such as natural disasters or terrorist attacks, it may not be feasible to assess individuals carefully and comprehensively. In such situations, when the numbers who witnessed the event are high but available resources limited, it may be more realistic to provide a briefer assessment to detect clinically significant PTSD symptoms (as opposed to making an actual diagnosis) and thereby identify those who would warrant further assessment, and if appropriate intervention.

The choice of measure or measures used in such a screening approach will depend on many factors such as the type of event, the characteristics of the population exposed, and the nature of the services available to those who are identified as needing additional assessment or intervention. If the purpose of such an approach is to identify those who require specific support or intervention as opposed to those who recover spontaneously, then the timing of the screening requires careful consideration. Findings from research repeatedly show that following various potentially traumatic events, traumatic symptoms are common but will remit in many children and young people without specific intervention (De Young & Kenardy, 2013; La Greca et al., 2013; Le Brocque, Hendrikz, & Kenardy, 2010). One meta-analysis indicates that more than 50 percent of children and young people initially reporting symptom levels above the threshold for the measure used will spontaneously recover, but that the improvement three to six months after the event is more modest (Hiller et al., 2016). Therefore, screening *early* (e.g., within the first month) would identify large numbers of children and young people with symptoms, many of whom will improve without specific interventions. Screening *later* (e.g., at six months) will identify much smaller numbers, although these will be unlikely to improve without additional help. At the same time, this also means that these very distressed children, young people, and their families will have had to wait for the intervention that could have helped even early on (e.g., Meiser-Stedman, Smith, McKinnon et al., 2017). In practice, some flexibility is warranted; in many contexts, intervention immediately following screening may not be feasible, either for resource reasons or the nature of the recovery environment. For example, the young person may be relocated, recovering from extensive physical injuries, or their caregivers may not be able to facilitate early access to treatment. It is important to make sure that families know that intervention is available and that they are given repeated opportunities to access such support.

Facilitating Discussions and Enhancing Support

Assessment tools such as self-report questionnaires provide much more than quantitative information. If completed in collaboration with the child or young person, and where appropriate their caregiver, they provide an opportunity for discussion about the client's symptoms but also about the similarities and differences between the client's and their caregiver's reports. When done sensitively, such discussions can improve communication and enhance the support available to the child or young person outside of therapy sessions. For example, the Child and Family Traumatic Stress Intervention uses questionnaires as a therapeutic intervention not simply as an assessment tool and has been proven to reduce the development of PTSD (Berkowitz, Stover, & Marans, 2011).

Assessing Trauma History

Abundant evidence shows that adverse childhood experiences (ACEs) have a significant and long-lasting impact on the mental and physical health of individuals, and that many individuals have experienced multiple potentially traumatic events (e.g., Gilbert et al., 2015). This means that when assessing a child or young person who has experienced a potentially traumatic event, it may be important to ascertain what other negative events they have experienced. Assessing the trauma history enables the clinician to understand better the context of specific events and what assumptions and beliefs the child or young person may have brought to specific events. Assessment of such histories should not be restricted to extreme events but should include questioning about a variety of difficult events that may have had a lasting impact on the young person and should use specific closed questions rather than open-ended ones as research indicates this is likely to elicit more information about past events (Frissa et al., 2016; McDonald, Borntrager, & Rostad, 2014).

Given the difficulties of differential diagnosis, and the fact that the presence of a potentially traumatic event is a requirement for a diagnosis of PTSD, it may be important to assess systematically and specifically for histories of potentially traumatic events in all children and young people being assessed for psychological difficulties, especially for those problems that are most likely to be confused for PTSD such as ADHD and anxiety problems. Even in assessments of PTSD, it is important to clarify the link between potentially traumatic events and the specific development of symptoms rather than make assumptions based on limited information. If not directly responsible for the PTSD symptoms, preceding traumatic events may have set the scene for the reaction to a subsequent event, and it is also possible that subsequent events may have an impact on reactions to previous events.

Guiding the Focus of an Intervention

In addition to monitoring the symptoms themselves, a systematic assessment of factors that maintain or perpetuate the difficulties is important, partly because this can lead to a fuller understanding of the problems, but more importantly because modification of these factors can reduce symptoms (Smith et al., 2013). The meaning made of the event is considered by some evidence-based approaches to be central in the development and treatment of PTSD (Meiser-Stedman, 2002; Nixon et al., 2010). The Child Post-Traumatic Cognitions Inventory (CPTCI; Meiser-Stedman et al., 2009) is a 25-item questionnaire that was developed for use with 6- to 18-year-olds to systematically evaluate the child or young person's view of themselves and the world since the traumatic event or events. This questionnaire not only helps explore how the traumatic event has changed the child or young person's cognitions; it can also lead to fruitful and focused discussions: using the simple questions and answers as a starting point, clinicians can follow up with further gentle, curious inquiry. Sometimes in therapy, cognitive change occurs simply by giving the child or young person the opportunity to explore their thoughts, which begins with being able to reflect upon and label the meaning of the event (Trickey, 2013). If time is limited, or if there are concerns about using questionnaires, then there is a short version (CPTCI-S), consisting of 10 questions, which has been found to have excellent psychometric properties (McKinnon et al., 2016). Cut-off points of 46–48 and 16–18 on the CPTCI and the CPTCI-S, respectively, have been found to be related to the likely classification of PTSD. This does not mean that either version of the CPTCI is diagnostic as such, but it does confirm the strength of the relationship between appraisals as measured on this instrument and PTSD symptoms and gives an idea of what is a "toxic" amount of negative appraisal. This supports the rationale for focusing on such appraisals within treatment.

Providing Feedback to Therapist on the Therapeutic Process

Research supports the importance of the therapeutic alliance with the child or young person for positive outcome from therapy (Ormhaug, Jensen, Wentzel-Larsen, & Shirk, 2014). Given that therapy for PTSD may involve approaching things that the child or young person is actively avoiding, a strong therapeutic alliance may be even more crucial to successful therapy than it is for other types of psychological problems. Therefore, it can be useful to routinely seek feedback on the quality of the alliance using a measure specifically designed for this purpose, such as the Session Rating Scale (Low, Miller, & Squire, 2014). Many of the tools produce a numerical value representing the child's or young person's view of the quality of the therapeutic alliance, or how therapy is progressing. This score may be of particular interest during therapy when it is higher or lower than usual and enables the therapist to identify individual sessions that according to the child's or young person's view were of particular value or considered to be of less value.

In addition, the use of such tools can give a useful message to the child or young person that the therapist is specifically, genuinely, and routinely interested in their view of therapy, which makes it a more collaborative venture and may separate it from other interactions they have with adults. Often, more useful than the actual scores obtained are the discussions about what the child or young person finds helpful and why. Sometimes such feedback can initially be somewhat guarded, as many children and young people are not used to being asked for their view on such interactions, and they may take a while to realize that the inquiry is a genuine one.

Advances in Approaches to Assessment

Choice of Respondents

As noted earlier, avoidance is a fundamental aspect of PTSD, regardless of which diagnostic system is being used. This means that it is useful to integrate reports from different respondents when assessing a traumatized child or young person, to ensure that as little relevant information as possible is withheld from the clinician conducting the assessment. The younger the child, the more the assessment is likely to rely on reports of the adults around them such as caregivers and teachers. However, children and young people may attempt to hide their difficulties from their caregivers to try to protect them from further distress. It was for this reason that the Clinical Practice Guideline for PTSD published by the National Institute for Health and Care Excellence in England and Wales specifically recommended that children and young people being assessed for PTSD should routinely be directly asked about their symptoms separately from their caregivers (NICE, 2018).

Indeed, a meta-analysis has quantified the discrepant reporting of symptoms between caregiver and child or young person, finding that if only caregivers are asked about a child's or young person's symptoms, the rate of PTSD found is less than a third of that found if the child or young person is asked (Alisic et al., 2014). This indicates that failing to ask children and young people themselves about their symptoms is likely to lead to substantial underestimation of PTSD and subsequently not being offered the appropriate intervention that would decrease their distress and increase their functioning.

Electronic Formats

Recent technological advances now make it possible for children, young people, and their caregivers to complete questionnaire assessments electronically on computers, tablets, or phones. This can make the collection, analysis, interpretation, and scoring more efficient as well as reducing human error in calculating scores (Patalay, Hayes, Deighton, & Wolpert, 2016). However, there is a dearth of research evaluating equivalence across different formats for assessment of mental health difficulties in children and young people. Two studies that do exist have demonstrated a difference between paper and electronic formats. Young people completing the Me and My School self-report questionnaire (Deighton et al., 2013) produced a lower total score when completing the paper version compared to completing the electronic version (Patalay, Deighton, Fonagy, & Wolpert, 2015), whereas young people completing the self-report version of the Strength and Difficulties Questionnaire (Goodman, 2001) scored higher on the hyperactivity subscale (and thereby also higher on the total problems score) but lower on the impact score if completing a paper version compared to the electronic version (Patalay et al., 2016). This might be because children and young people are more comfortable disclosing certain information in different formats (Suler, 2004). Given that avoidance is so central to PTSD, this may be a particular issue with the assessment of PTSD. Further research specific to measures of PTSD in children and young people is required before clinicians can assume that scores obtained from different formats are equivalent; therefore, clinicians must be cautious when interpreting scores from one format using research based on another format.

Key Practice Points

Children and young people who have PTSD will be by definition avoidant and may take longer than other children and young people to be prepared to share details of the event and of their symptoms. Some may never be prepared to be open with a professional. An assessment that is rushed, too short, too blunt, or does not invest the time required to make a child or young person feel sufficiently at ease risks failing to identify many children and young people who have been traumatized by events and are struggling with difficulties that may well respond to the appropriate intervention. But if done in a sensitive compassionate, focused way, using suitable assessment tools, then it is usually possible to gather sufficient information from children, young people, and their caregivers to assess the impact of potentially traumatic events. It is important to gather sufficient information to differentiate PTSD from other psychological problems to avoid offering traumatized children and young people the wrong intervention.

Those administering assessments will need to make choices about which tools to use and when to use them, based on the purpose of the assessment, the clients to be assessed, the service context, and the time available. There will be times when it may be prudent to screen children and young people with a view to identifying those that require a fuller assessment.

Developmental adaptations will need to be made to assessments to take into account the age and cognitive abilities of children and young people, and where appropriate, caregivers should be involved, but gathering information directly from the child or young person is important whenever possible.

Despite the reservations of some clinicians, feedback from actual children and young people indicates that they do not mind the use of questionnaires if their purpose and results are explained to them.

References

Aderka, I. M., Appelbaum-Namdar, E., Shafran, N., & Gilboa-Schechtman, E. (2011). Sudden gains in prolonged exposure for children and adolescents with posttraumatic stress disorder. *Journal of Consulting and Clinical Psychology, 79* (4), 441.

Alisic, E., Zalta, A. K., van Wesel, F., Larsen, S. E., Hafstad, G. S., Hassanpour, K., & Smid, G. E. (2014). Rates of post-traumatic stress disorder in trauma-exposed children and adolescents: Meta-analysis. *British Journal of Psychiatry, 204,* 335–340. doi:10.1192/bjp.bp.113.131227

American Psychiatric Association. (1980). *DSM-III: Diagnostic and statistical manual of mental disorders* (3rd ed.). Washington, DC: Author.

American Psychiatric Association. (2000). *Diagnostic and statistical manual, Text Revision (DSM-IV-TR)*. Washington, DC: Author.

American Psychiatric Association. (2013). *Diagnostic and statistical manual of mental disorders: DSM-5*. Washington, DC: Author.

Berkowitz, S. J., Stover, C. S., & Marans, S. R. (2011). The child and family traumatic stress intervention: Secondary prevention for youth at risk of developing PTSD. *Journal of Child Psychology and Psychiatry, 52*(6), 676–685.

Bickman, L., Kelley, S. D., Breda, C., de Andrade, A. R., & Riemer, M. (2011). Effects of routine feedback to clinicians on mental health outcomes of youths: Results of a randomized trial. *Psychiatric Services, 62*(12), 1423–1429.

Brewin, C. R., Gregory, J. D., Lipton, M., & Burgess, N. (2010). Intrusive images in psychological disorders: Characteristics, neural mechanisms, and treatment implications. *Psychological Review, 117*(1), 210.

Danzi, B. A., & La Greca, A. M. (2016). DSM-IV, DSM-5, and ICD-11: Identifying children with posttraumatic stress disorder after disasters. *Journal of Child Psychology and Psychiatry, 57*(12), 1444–1452.

De Roos, C., Van der Oord, S., Zijlstra, B., Lucassen, S., Perrin, S., Emmelkamp, P., & De Jongh, A. (2017). EMDR versus cognitive behavioral writing therapy versus waitlist in pediatric PTSD following single-incident trauma: A multi-center randomized clinical trial. *Journal of Child Psychology and Psychiatry, 58*(11), 1219–1228.

De Young, A., & Kenardy, J. (2013). Posttraumatic stress disorder in young children. *Anxiety and Depression, 19*(20), 12.

Deblinger, E., Steer, R. A., & Lippmann, J. (1999). Two-year follow-up study of cognitive behavioral therapy for sexually abused children suffering post-traumatic stress symptoms. *Child Abuse & Neglect, 23*(12), 1371–1378.

Deighton, J., Tymms, P., Vostanis, P., Belsky, J., Fonagy, P., Brown, A., ... Wolpert, M. (2013). The development of a school-based measure of child mental health. *Journal of Psychoeducational Assessment, 31*(3), 247–257.

Ehlers, A., & Clark, D. M. (2000). A cognitive model of posttraumatic stress disorder. *Behavior Research and Therapy, 38*(4), 319–345.

Elbert, T., & Schauer, M. (2002). Psychological trauma: Burnt into memory. *Nature, 419* (6910), 883.

Fletcher, K. E. (1996). Childhood posttraumatic stress disorder. In E. J. Mash & R. A. Barkley (eds.), *Child psychopathology* (2nd edn., pp. 242–276). New York: Guildford.

Foa, E. B., Asnaani, A., Zang, Y., Capaldi, S., & Yeh, R. (2017). Psychometrics of the Child PTSD Symptom Scale for DSM-5 for trauma-exposed children and adolescents. *Journal of Clinical Child & Adolescent Psychology, 47*(1), 38–46.

Foa, E. B., Johnson, K. M., Feeny, N. C. & Treadwell, K. R. (2001). The child PTSD Symptom Scale: A Preliminary examination of its psychometric properties. *Journal of Clinical Child Psychology, 30*(3), 376–384.

Foa, E. B., Steketee, G., & Rothbaum, B. O. (1989). Behavioral/cognitive conceptualizations of post-traumatic stress disorder. *Behavior Therapy, 20*(2), 155–176.

Frissa, S., Hatch, S. L., Fear, N. T., Dorrington, S., Goodwin, L., & Hotopf, M. (2016). Challenges in the retrospective assessment of trauma: Comparing a checklist approach to a single item trauma experience screening question. *BMC Psychiatry, 16*(1), 20.

Fugard, A. (2014). A statistical interlude ... understanding uncertainty in mental health questionnaire data. In D. Law & M. Wolpert (eds.), *Guide to Using Outcomes and Feedback Tools*, pp. 77–85. CAMHS Press, Wiley Online

Gilbert, L. K., Breiding, M. J., Merrick, M. T., Thompson, W. W., Ford, D. C., Dhingra, S. S., & Parks, S. E. (2015). Childhood adversity and adult chronic disease: An update from ten states and the District of Columbia, 2010. *American Journal of Preventive Medicine, 48*(3), 345–349.

Goodman, R. (2001). Psychometric properties of the strengths and difficulties questionnaire. *Journal of the American Academy of Child Adolescent Psychiatry, 40*(11), 1337–1345. doi:10.1097/00004583-200111000-00015

Hiller, R. M., Meiser-Stedman, R., Fearon, P., Lobo, S., MacKinnon, A., Fraser, A., & Halligan, S. L. (2016). Changes in the prevalence and symptom severity of child PTSD in the year following trauma: A meta-analytic study. *Journal of Child Psychology and Psychiatry, 57*(8), 884–898.

Karatzias, T., Shevlin, M., Fyvie, C., Hyland, P., Efthymiadou, E., Wilson, D., ... Cloitre, M. (2017). Evidence of distinct profiles of posttraumatic stress disorder (PTSD) and complex posttraumatic stress disorder (CPTSD) based on the new ICD-11 trauma questionnaire (ICD-TQ). *Journal of Affective Disorders, 207*, 181–187.

Kenardy, J. A., Spence, S. H., & Macleod, A. C. (2006). Screening for posttraumatic stress disorder in children after accidental injury. *Pediatrics, 118*(3), 1002–1009.

La Greca, A. M., Lai, B. S., Llabre, M. M., Silverman, W. K., Vernberg, E. M., & Prinstein, M. J. (2013). Children's postdisaster trajectories of PTS symptoms: Predicting chronic distress. *Child & Youth Care Forum, 42*(8), 351–369.

Law, D., & Wolpert, M. (2014). *Guide to using outcomes and feedback tools with children, young people and families*. CAMHS Press, Wiley Online.

Le Brocque, R. M., Hendrikz, J., & Kenardy, J. A. (2010). The course of posttraumatic stress in children: Examination of recovery trajectories following traumatic injury. *Journal of Pediatric Psychology, 35*(6), 637–645.

Low, D., Miller, S. D., & Squire, B. (2014). Session Rating Scale (SRS) and Child Session Rating Scale (CSRS). In D. Law & M. Wolpert (eds.), *Guide to using outcomes and feedback tools* (pp. 143–151). CAMHS Press, Wiley Online

Maercker, A., Brewin, C. R., Bryant, R. A., Cloitre, M., Ommeren, M., Jones, L. M., ... Rousseau, C. (2013). Diagnosis and classification of disorders specifically associated with stress: Proposals for ICD-11. *World Psychiatry, 12*(3), 198–206.

McDonald, M. K., Borntrager, C. F., & Rostad, W. (2014). Measuring trauma: Considerations for assessing complex and non-PTSD Criterion A childhood trauma. *Journal of Trauma & Dissociation, 15*(2), 184–203.

McKinnon, A., Smith, P., Bryant, R., Salmon, K., Yule, W., Dalgleish, T., ... Meiser-Stedman, R. (2016). An update on the clinical utility of the Children's Post-Traumatic Cognitions Inventory. *Journal of Traumatic Stress, 29*(3), 253–258.

Meiser-Stedman, R. (2002). Towards a cognitive-behavioral model of PTSD in children and adolescents. *Clinical Child and Family Psychology Review, 5*(4), 217–232.

Meiser-Stedman, R., Smith, P., Bryant, R., Salmon, K., Yule, W., Dalgleish, T., & Nixon, R. D. (2009). Development and validation of the Child Post-Traumatic Cognitions Inventory (CPTCI). *Journal of Child Psychology and Psychiatry, 50*(4), 432–440. doi:10.1111/j.1469-7610.2008.01995.x

Meiser-Stedman, R., Smith, P., Glucksman, E., Yule, W., & Dalgleish, T. (2008). The posttraumatic stress disorder diagnosis in preschool- and elementary school-age children exposed to motor vehicle accidents. *American Journal of Psychiatry, 165*(10), 1326–1337.

Meiser-Stedman, R., Smith, P., Yule, W., & Dalgleish, T. (2007). The Trauma Memory Quality Questionnaire: Preliminary development and validation of a measure of trauma memory characteristics for children and adolescents. *Memory, 15*(3), 271–279. doi:10.1080/09658210701256498

Meiser-Stedman, R., Smith, P., Yule, W., Glucksman, E., & Dalgleish, T. (2017). Posttraumatic stress disorder in young children three years post-trauma: Prevalence and longitudinal predictors. *Journal of Clinical Psychiatry, 78*(3), 334.

Meiser-Stedman, R., Smith, P., McKinnon, A., Dixon, C., Trickey, D., Ehlers, A., ... Goodyer, I. (2017). Cognitive therapy as an early treatment for post-traumatic stress disorder in children and adolescents: A randomized controlled trial addressing preliminary efficacy and mechanisms of action. *Journal of Child Psychology and Psychiatry, 58*(5), 623–633.

National Center for PTSD. (2017). Child measures of trauma and PTSD. Retrieved from www.ptsd.va.gov/professional/assessment/child/index.asp

National Child Traumatic Stress Network. (2017). Measures review database. Retrieved from www.nctsn.org/resources/online-research/measures-review

NICE. (2018). The management of PTSD in adults and children in primary and secondary care. *National Clinical Practice Guideline*. Retrieved from www.nice.org.uk

Nixon, R. D., Nehmy, T. J., Ellis, A. A., Ball, S.-A., Menne, A., & McKinnon, A. C. (2010). Predictors of posttraumatic stress in children following injury: The influence of appraisals, heart rate, and morphine use. *Behavior Research and Therapy, 48*(8), 810–815.

Ormhaug, S. M., Jensen, T. K., Wentzel-Larsen, T., & Shirk, S. R. (2014). The therapeutic alliance in treatment of traumatized youths: Relation to outcome in a randomized clinical trial. *Journal of Consulting and Clinical Psychology, 82*(1), 52.

Patalay, P., Deighton, J., Fonagy, P., & Wolpert, M. (2015). Equivalence of paper and computer formats of a child self-report mental health measure. *European Journal of Psychological Assessment, 31*(1), 54–61.

Patalay, P., Hayes, D., Deighton, J., & Wolpert, M. (2016). A comparison of paper and computer administered strengths and difficulties questionnaire. *Journal of Psychopathology and Behavioral Assessment, 38*(2), 242–250.

Perrin, S., Meiser-Stedman, R., & Smith, P. (2005). The Children's Revised Impact of Event Scale (CRIES): Validity as a screening instrument for PTSD. *Behavioral and Cognitive Psychotherapy, 33*(4), 487.

Rolon-Arroyo, B., Rooney, E., Kaplow, J., Calhoun, K., Layne, C. M., Steinberg, A. M., & Pynoos, R. S. (2017, November). *Psychometric properties of the UCLA PTSD Reaction Index for DSM-5 (RI-5): Identifying clinically significant PTSD in culturally-diverse youth*. Paper presented at the International Society for Traumatic Stress Studies 33rd Annual Meeting, Chicago, Illinois.

Ruf, M., Schauer, M., Neuner, F., Catani, C., Schauer, E., & Elbert, T. (2010). Narrative exposure therapy for 7- to 16-year-olds: A randomized controlled trial with traumatized refugee children. *Journal of Traumatic Stress, 23*(4), 437–445.

Sachser, C., Keller, F., & Goldbeck, L. (2017). Complex PTSD as proposed for ICD-11: Validation of a new disorder in children and adolescents and their response to trauma-focused cognitive behavioral therapy. *Journal of Child Psychology and Psychiatry, 58*(2), 160–168.

Saigh, P. A., Yasik, A. E., Oberfield, R. A., Green, B. L., Halamandaris, P. V., Rubenstein, H., ... McHugh, M. (2000). The children's PTSD inventory: Development and Reliability. *Journal of Traumatic Stress, 13*(3), 369–380.

Salmon, K., & Bryant, R. A. (2002). Posttraumatic stress disorder in children: The influence of developmental factors. *Clinical Psychology Review, 22*(2), 163–188.

Scheeringa, M. S., & Haslett, N. (2010). The reliability and criterion validity of the Diagnostic Infant and Preschool Assessment: A new diagnostic instrument for young children. *Child Psychiatry & Human Development, 41*(3), 299–312.

Scheeringa, M. S., Wright, M. J., Hunt, J. P., & Zeanah, C. H. (2006). Factors affecting the diagnosis and prediction of PTSD symptomatology in children and adolescents. *American Journal of Psychiatry, 163*(4), 644–651.

Scheeringa, M. S., Zeanah, C. H., Myers, L., & Putnam, F. W. (2003). New findings on alternative criteria for PTSD in preschool children. *Journal of the American Academy of Child & Adolescent Psychiatry, 42*(5), 561–570.

Smith, P., Perrin, S., Dalgleish, T., Meiser-Stedman, R., Clark, D. M., & Yule, W. (2013). Treatment of posttraumatic stress disorder in children and adolescents. *Current Opinion in Psychiatry, 26*(1), 66–72.

Smith, P., Yule, W., Perrin, S., Tranah, T., Dalgleish, T., & Clark, D. M. (2007). Cognitive-behavioral therapy for PTSD in children and adolescents: A preliminary randomized controlled trial. *Journal of the American Academy of Child & Adolescent Psychiatry, 46*(8), 1051–1061.

Stallard, P., Velleman, R., & Baldwin, S. (1999). Psychological screening of children for post-traumatic stress disorder. *The Journal of Child Psychology and Psychiatry and Allied Disciplines, 40*(7), 1075–1082.

Steinberg, A. M., & Beyerlein, B. (2013). *UCLA PTSD Reaction Index: DSM-5 version*. Los Angeles, CA: The National Child Traumatic Stress Network.

Steinberg, A. M., Brymer, M. J., Decker, K. B., & Pynoos, R. S. (2004). The University of California at Los Angeles post-traumatic stress disorder reaction index. *Current Psychiatry Reports, 6*(2), 96–100.

Stickgold, R. (2002). EMDR: A putative neurobiological mechanism of action. *Journal of Clinical Psychology, 58*(1), 61–75.

Suler, J. (2004). The online disinhibition effect. *Cyberpsychology & Behavior, 7*(3), 321–326.

Trickey, D. (2013). Post-traumatic stress disorders. In P. Graham & S. Reynolds (eds.), *Cognitive behaviour therapy for children and families* (3rd edn., pp. 235–254). Cambridge: Cambridge University Press.

Weathers, F. W., Keane, T. M., & Davidson, J. R. (2001). Clinician-Administered PTSD Scale: A review of the first ten years of research. *Depression and Anxiety, 13*(3), 132–156.

Yasik, A. E., Saigh, P. A., Oberfield, R. A., Green, B., Halamandaris, P., & McHugh, M. (2001). The validity of the Children's PTSD Inventory. *Journal of Traumatic Stress, 14*(1), 81–94.

27 New Technologies to Deliver CBT (Including Web-Based CBT, Mobile Apps, and Virtual Reality)

Danielle Weiss and Meghan L. Marsac

Introduction

In recent years, greater attention has been given to child exposure to potentially traumatic events and the subsequent cognitive and emotional consequences of such exposure (Anda et al., 2006; Felitti & Anda, 1997; Felitti et al., 1998; Glaser, van Os, Portegijs, & Myin-Germeys, 2006; Hovens et al., 2010; Majer, Nater, Lin, Capuron, & Reeves, 2010). However, despite the increased recognition that millions of children experience significant symptoms of post-traumatic stress each year within the United States (prevalence rates ranging from 5 percent to 30 percent post-trauma exposure), and a number of evidence-based treatments (e.g., CBT, trauma focused cognitive behavioral therapy (TF-CBT)) that have been shown to effectively treat child PTSD symptoms, a number of barriers prevent children from obtaining the treatment that they need (Boydell et al., 2006; Cohen & Mannarino, 2015; Crawford & Simonoff, 2003; Deblinger, Steer, & Lippmann, 1999; Flink, Beirens, Butte, & Raat, 2013; Meredith et al., 2009; Merikangas et al., 2010; Murry, Heflinger, Suiter, & Brody, 2011; Price, Kassam-Adams, Alderfer, Christofferson, & Kazak, 2016; Reardon et al., 2017; Webb, Hayes, & Deblinger, 2014). Barriers can be conceptualized as structural (e.g., availability of providers, transportation, affordability) or perceptual (e.g., stigma, beliefs toward mental health diagnoses and treatment; Owens et al., 2002).

Structural Barriers

High-quality treatment with pediatric providers trained in evidence-based practices for PTSD may be difficult to find (Boydell et al., 2006; Gamm, Stone, & Pittman, 2003; Jameson & Blank, 2007; Owens et al., 2002). Even where care is readily available, many caretakers report long wait-lists when seeking mental health treatment for their child (Boydell et al., 2006; Crawford & Simonoff, 2003; Flink et al., 2013; Guzder, Yohannes, & Zelkowitz, 2013; Klasen & Goodman, 2000; Sawyer et al., 2004; Sayal, Mills, White, Merrell, & Tymms, 2015). This may be even more of a challenge for families residing in rural communities. In the United States, 19 percent of families live in rural communities (US Census, 2010). The number of psychologists per 100,000 people in rural areas is 4.2 compared to 29 per 100,000 in urban areas (Miller, Petterson, Burke, Phillips, & Green, 2014). The number of providers specializing in treating children who need trauma-specific services is even fewer (Gamm et al., 2003; Goldsmith, Wagenfeld, Manderscheid, & Stiles, 1997; Jameson & Blank, 2007; Rost, Fortney, Fischer, & Smith, 2002). Because of the limited availability of providers, children and families living in rural communities are often forced to travel far distances to seek treatment. Traveling for psychological services has additional monetary costs and may take time away from school for a child and work for their parent(s).

In addition to access, cost of care can be substantial (Girio-Herrera et al., 2013; Harwood et al., 2009; Meredith et al., 2009; Owens et al., 2002; Sawyer et al., 2004; Thurston & Phares, 2008). This can create a challenge for many families, particularly those with lower income whose health insurance does not cover services. Children without health insurance have especially high rates of unmet mental health needs relative to insured children (Kataoka, Zhang, & Wells, 2002). Even for those who do have mental health coverage, families often have to pay for a portion of services, which can be expensive. The number of sessions insurance companies are willing to cover is also often limited (Aetna, 2012; CIGNA, 2009).

Perceptual Barriers

Across cultures, many people continue to carry stigmas about mental health disorders that prevent children from receiving appropriate mental health treatment (Boydell et al., 2006; Harwood et al., 2009; Klasen & Goodman, 2000; Meredith et al., 2009; Murry et al., 2011; Pullmann et al., 2010; Reardon et al., 2017). For example, those who reside in rural areas may experience a heightened fear of social stigma and a reduced sense of confidentiality due to the nature of small, intertwined communities (Boydell et al., 2006; Pullmann et al., 2010). One study suggested that as a result of this social stigma, families residing in African American rural communities reported a preference toward family, church, and schools as sources of support over mental health services (Murry et al., 2011). While social support is often a protective factor, reliance on these supports alone may help explain the underutilization of mental health treatment among African Americans (Cuffe, Waller, Cuccaro, Pumariega, & Garrison, 1995; Murry et al., 2011). Other research has demonstrated that parents have reported fears associated with stigma such as not wanting to have their child labeled and concerns over self-fulfilling prophecy (Harwood et al., 2009; Klasen & Goodman, 2000). In addition to stigma, parents have reported relationship challenges with clinicians such as feeling that the provider is not hearing their concerns and that they are being blamed for their child's challenges (Klasen & Goodman, 2000; Reardon et al., 2017; Sayal et al., 2015). Further perceptual barriers include the absence of a trusting relationship and previous poor experiences with mental health providers (Murry et al., 2011; Reardon et al., 2017; Sayal et al., 2015).

Innovative technological approaches to delivery of trauma-based care may help address structural and perceptual barriers by offering a more affordable intervention option for families and allowing children to access interventions at home to preserve child and family anonymity, as well as reduce social stigmas (Bunnell, Davidson,

Dewey, Price, & Ruggiero, 2017; Kenardy, Cox, & Brown, 2015; Marsac et al., 2015; Shealy, Davidson, Jones, Lopez, & de Arellano, 2015).

Web and Mobile Interventions

The application of technology can facilitate treatment in several ways. Web-based or mobile-based programs have the potential to be used as either stand-alone treatment and/or additive components to in-person interventions. In addition, web-based and mobile-based technology can be used as either secondary preventive (i.e., prevent PTSD in youth exposed to a potentially traumatic events), early intervention (i.e., aimed to decrease symptoms of PTSD that emerge in the early aftermath of trauma exposure), or treatment tools (i.e., goal to treat youth with established PTSD). To date, the web- and mobile-based CBT interventions that have been developed to prevent psychological symptoms (PTSD, anxiety, depression) and/or early intervention include Coping Coach, Kids and Accidents, Bounce Back Now, MindRight, and Life Improvement for Teens (LIFT; Bunnell et al., 2017; Cox, Kenardy, & Hendrikz, 2010; Jaycox, n.d.; Kassam-Adams et al., 2015b; Kenardy et al., 2015; "MindRight," n.d.; Price, Yuen, Davidson, Hubel, & Ruggiero, 2015; Ruggiero et al., 2015). Each of these interventions is designed for primary use by children and adolescents; parents may use some interventions with their child or encourage them to utilize the intervention on their own. Only Triangle of Life has been designed to assist in the treatment of PTSD as a conjunctive intervention (Assigana et al., 2014). Currently, to our knowledge, there are no stand-alone technology-based treatments.

PTSD Prevention/Early Intervention Tools

Coping Coach (contact authors for access) is a web-based program that aims to prevent (not treat) the development of PTSD in children exposed to an acute trauma (Kassam-Adams et al., 2015b; Marsac et al., 2013, 2015). The program was created for families to use independently, without the support of a mental health professional. Coping Coach was developed by combining CBT-based program theory concepts (specifically focusing on recognizing feelings, learning the cognitive triad, recognizing and changing unhelpful thoughts to helpful thoughts, and choosing approach-based strategies to face trauma-related fears) with internet-specific behavior change models (e.g., motivation, skill building; Marsac et al., 2015; Ritterband, Thorndike, Cox, Kovatchev, & Gonder-Frederick, 2009). The intervention was developed obtaining user-based feedback. The first prototype yielded positive feedback from families but had functionality problems; thus, program technology was re-evaluated and revised resulting in a new prototype that was found to be acceptable and feasible with better functionality (Marsac et al., 2015). The second prototype was selected for further evaluation as described in the evidence-base section later in the chapter.

Level 1:
Feeling Identification

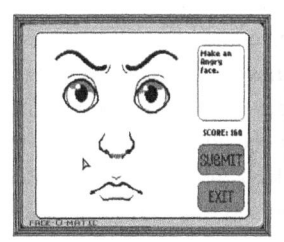

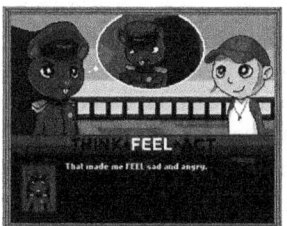

Level 2:
Cognitive Traid / Adaptive

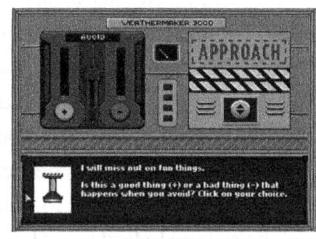

Level 3:
Approach vs. Avoidance Behaviors

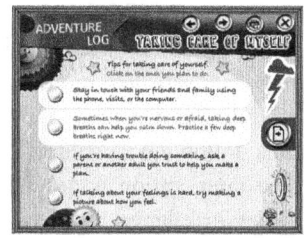

Adventure log example

Figure 27.1 *Sample Content from Coping Coach Intervention Levels and Adventure Log*

The Coping Coach intervention is structured as an interactive game following four child characters who have been exposed to traumatic events (house fire, community violence, car crash, asthma attack) and who exhibit responses consistent with post-traumatic stress symptoms (maladaptive appraisals, avoidance behaviors). Using a story-based plot line, children work their way through three levels, which are all based in cognitive behavioral principles and have social support seeking intertwined: feeling identification, the cognitive triad and appraisals, approach vs. avoidance behaviors. In addition, children complete an activity log following each level in which they apply concepts to their own scenario. To receive a full intervention "dose," children are asked to complete the entire program one time, with encouragement to play more than once. Parents are asked to encourage their child's use of the program and are provided the opportunity to play along separately (with their own login information), but the game itself is designed for child use. The activity log can be saved and shared (e.g., with a child's doctor). See Figure 27.1 for sample intervention content.

Kids and Accidents (http://kidsaccident.psy.uq.edu.au) is also a preventive/early intervention web-based tool designed to provide education (normalizing trauma reactions) and promote recovery in children after a road traffic accident (Kenardy et al., 2015). The intervention is grounded in cognitive behavioral and resiliency theories and incorporates elements on how to best respond to children after a trauma (such as validating feelings, offering the opportunity to the talk about the accident; Bisson & Cohen, 2006; Ehlers & Clark, 2000; Kenardy, Thompson, Le Brocque, & Olsson, 2008; Kumpfer, 1999; Ponsford et al., 2001). Similar to Coping Coach, this resource is not intended as a stand-alone treatment for children with significant diagnosed PTSD.

Kids and Accidents is structured as an interactive self-help web-based intervention with separate sections for children (aged 10 and younger) and adolescents (aged 11 and older). The content for children and adolescents is developmentally tailored based on age. The intervention provides children with a number of strategies framed around helping them recover emotionally from their accident. Categories include feelings (how to identify and normalize), heroes (how to identify role models), problem solving (six steps), reaching out (how to obtain social support), talk to yourself (cognitive restructuring), help (how to find more help), growing and learning (identify what they have learned from their accident experience), and identifying personal strengths. Youth can select any activity to complete in any order. See Figure 27.2 for sample intervention content.

The Bounce Back Now (contact authors for access) PTSD-specific intervention is a part of a larger series of web-based, self-help modules targeting adolescents after a natural disaster. The PTSD module was designed to screen adolescents for elevated post-traumatic stress symptoms following a natural disaster and to provide an internet-based intervention. The intervention is grounded in cognitive behavioral techniques and emphasizes behavior change by providing psycho-education and self-guided instructions on how to complete exposures to trauma stimuli, decrease avoidance, and develop adaptive coping strategies (Pynoos, 1994; Ruggiero, Morris, & Scotti, 2001; Yuen et al., 2015).

Bounce Back Now is structured as an interactive webpage for adolescents aged 12–17 years. After logging in, the user is brought to the intervention's homepage displaying the four Bounce Back Now modules: (1) stress and anxiety, (2) smoking, (3) alcohol, and (4) mood. Selecting the "stress and anxiety" icon leads to the PTSD module. After selecting this icon, the adolescent is presented with a brief screener to assess their post-traumatic stress symptoms. Adolescents who report significant symptoms are encouraged to complete the module, whereas adolescents who do not report significant symptoms are invited, but not required, to exit the module and told that they may find other modules more helpful (Yuen et al., 2015). See Figure 27.3 for sample intervention content.

MindRight (http://getmindright.org) is a text-messaging platform to help at-risk youth recover from trauma ("MindRight," 2017). The messaging platform is grounded in cognitive behavioral therapy, acceptance and commitment therapy, and mindfulness-based stress reduction. Upon signing up, youth are paired with a coach from the community (e.g., former teacher, college student) with whom they speak daily. Coaches are trained to provide empathy to urban youth exposed to violence through daily check-ins to build emotional intelligence, to normalize experiences through adaptive psycho-education, and to stabilize those with post-traumatic stress symptoms by teaching CBT coping and mindfulness techniques. Additionally, the app empowers community agencies to respond quickly to youth who are in need by enabling real-time alerts in escalated and crisis situations, screening for trauma exposure, and providing weekly reports on youths' emotional wellness ("MindRight," 2017).

Life Improvement for Teens (LIFT) is a web-based, self-paced intervention that helps teens who have been exposed to a potentially traumatic event build stress-management skills (Jaycox, n.d.). The intervention is designed for adolescents aged 12–18 years. LIFT is structured as an online course that contains interactive games to teach adolescents how to reduce distress and improve

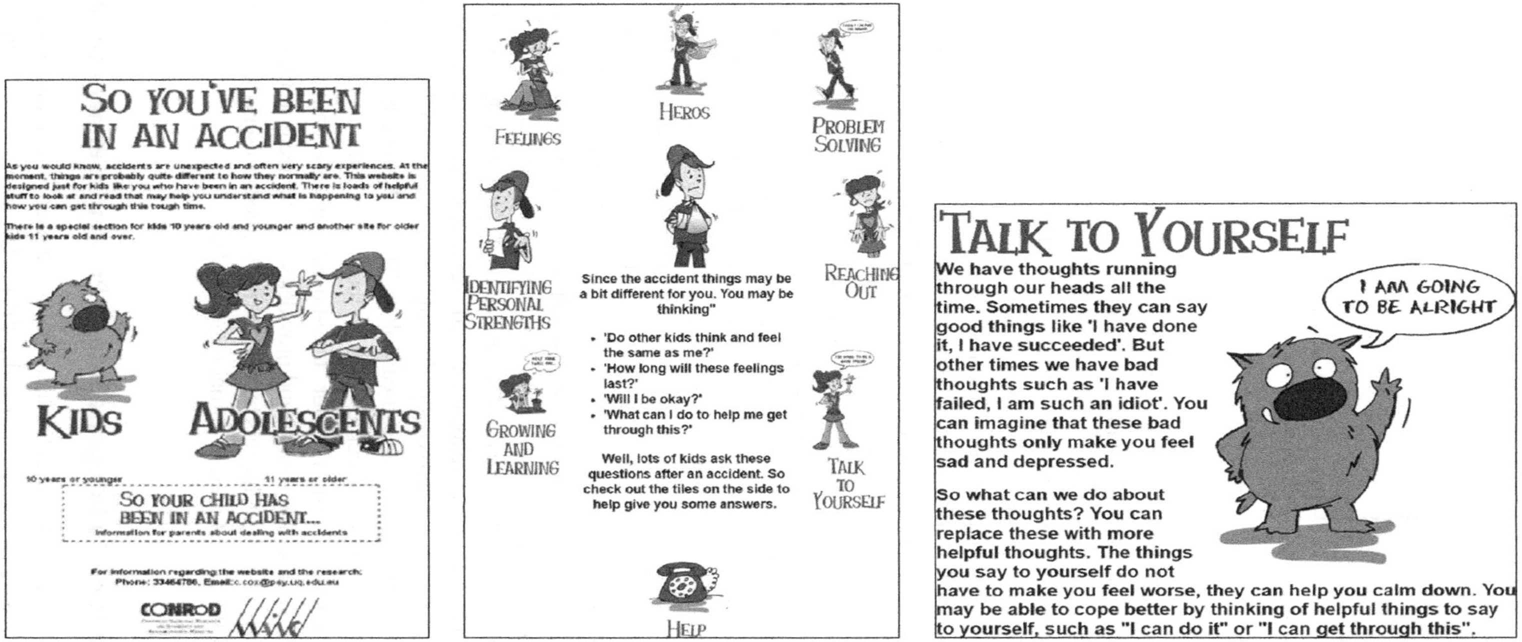

Introduction to intervention   List of intervention activities   Using cognitive restructuring / self-talk

Figure 27.2 *Sample Content from Kids and Accidents Intervention*

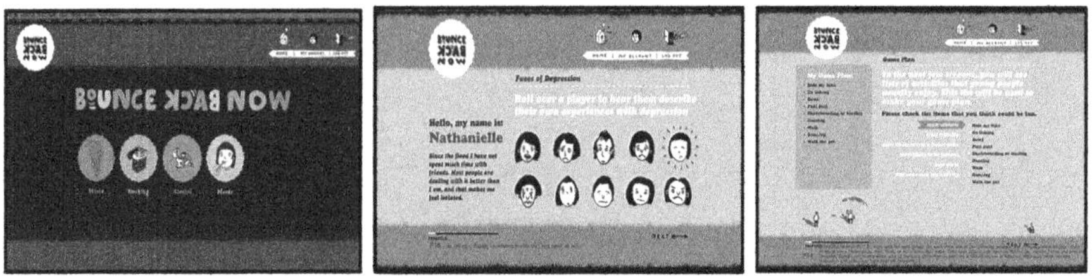

| Content choices | Mood assessment tool | Activity planning |

Figure 27.3 *Sample Content from Bounce Back Now*

adaptive coping skills. LIFT is grounded in CBT and offers teens psychoeducation regarding stress and trauma, as well as normalizing common reactions to stress. Throughout the course, adolescents learn about the cognitive triangle and how trauma and stress can affect thoughts, feelings, and actions. The intervention also assesses participants' own stress level and provides personalized reports to help players track their stress level.

Participants of LIFT work their way through seven chapters: welcome to LIFT, feelings, thoughts, facing fears, processing trauma, problem solving, and putting it all together. Chapters begin with an introduction video, describing what the course will entail and what users will learn (e.g., how to manage stress). Following this, users work their way through various activities. For example, one activity includes sorting through good stress, bad stress, and trauma. More specifically, users must choose whether to drag the statement "As she walks into the school, she thinks about her old friends and wonder if she'll be able to make new friends" into the "good stress," "bad stress," or "trauma" bucket. The intervention also includes several audio-guided demonstrations of progressive muscle relaxation, positive imagery, and steady breathing to help increase adolescent's abilities to cope with trauma and stress. Throughout the intervention, there are several check-ins to assess symptoms. For example, after relaxation demonstrations prompts may appear, "Now that you've tried some relaxation techniques, where are you on the stress thermometer? Please use the slider bar to rate your stress level on a scale of 0–10, with '0' being completely relaxed and '10' being extremely upset." Finally, the intervention also places an emphasis on goal setting. In particular, LIFT uses a SMART goals framework to help teens create self-care plans. The goals worksheet outlines what SMART goals are ("S" is for "specific," "M" is for "measurable," "A" is for "attainable," "R" is for "relevant," and "T" is for "time-bound"), gives examples of what each of these aspects of goal setting means, and provides space for teens to fill in their own SMART goals (Jaycox, n.d.). Chapters build on skills learned as users progress through the program, so LIFT is best used in chronological order.

Mobile Tools to Integrate into In-Person Treatment for PTSD

Triangle of Life was created as a tool to be used in conjunction with TF-CBT in-person treatment (Assigana et al., 2014). The application is tailored for children aged 8–12 years. The primary aims of the game are to assist and solidify skills learned during the cognitive-processing step of TF-CBT. The game was developed by combining best gaming practices (e.g., including aspects of the 100 lenses through which a game design can be viewed – game experiences based on users' different viewpoints / goals) with concepts of learning (e.g., flow for the learner) and motivation (Keller, 1987; Malone & Lepper, 1987; Mirvis, Csikszentmihalyi, & Csikzentmihaly, 1991; Schell, 2008). TF-CBT Triangle of Life can be used on any mobile device (iPhone, Android, iPad). Similarly to Coping Coach, TF-CBT Triangle of Life is structured in game-like format following a lion (player is the lion) as they interact with other animals through the Savannah, progressing through misfortunes grounded in misunderstood behaviors and maladaptive thoughts. The game was chosen to take place in the animal kingdom to avoid human biases, preconceptions, and expectations (Assigana et al., 2014). Unlike the other interventions, the Triangle of Life program was created with the specific purpose of being used in conjunction with PTSD treatment.

The application is designed as a series of mini-games. By selecting each icon (fish, monkey, owl, rhino, elephant, panther, and wolf), children work through various situations in which thoughts, feelings, and behaviors are connected. In each level, players must drag statements (e.g., "I headbutted her") to the appropriate pieces of the triangle (e.g., the "behaviors" section). After this, the child player is asked to replace each animal's negative thoughts (e.g., "Owl ignored me") with more adaptive thoughts (e.g., "Maybe Owl didn't notice Monkey because he was busy").

Evidence Base for Web and Mobile Interventions

To date, several web- and mobile-based CBT interventions have initial data to support their use for prevention of psychological symptoms (PTSD, anxiety, depression) and / or early intervention (Coping Coach, Kids and Accidents, Bounce Back Now; Bunnell et al., 2017; Cox et al., 2010; Kassam-Adams et al., 2015b; Kenardy et al., 2015; Price et al., 2015; Ruggiero et al., 2015). To our knowledge, no web or mobile interventions are currently available as stand-alone treatment for PTSD in children or have been compared to traditional face-to-face treatment. As described earlier, the Triangle of Life mobile app has been developed to be used in conjunction with TF-CBT treatment but does not have empirical support to date (Assigana et al., 2014). Other innovative programs have been created based in CBT theory, but researchers have yet to publish outcome data on effectiveness in decreasing PTSD, such as MindRight and LIFT (Jaycox, n.d.; "MindRight," 2017). The existing interventions with some empirical support are all designed to be used by children aged 7 and older. Each of these interventions is based in CBT theory and promotes social support as a key strategy for emotional recovery. Only MindRight incorporates the use of text messages as an optional part of the program and the utility of these messages is yet to be determined ("MindRight," 2017). See Table 27.1 for a summary of web-based intervention tools.

Table 27.1 Summary of Evaluations of Web-Based PTSD Interventions for Children

Intervention	Type of technology	Type of event(s)	Age	Sample size	Post-trauma time point	Primary outcome measure	Main effect on child PTSD	Other findings
Coping Coach (Kassam-Adams et al., 2015b)	Online intervention – structured as game	Acute medical event (designed for any acute trauma)	8–12	72	< 2 weeks or > 12 weeks	Child PTSD Symptom Scale (CPSS)	Yes – comparing effect sizes (medium effect sizes in favor of the immediate intervention group for between-group differences in change in PTSS severity from baseline to 6 weeks ($d = -.68$) and from baseline to 12 weeks ($d = -.55$)	Larger effect size for those at-risk Intervention timing may be flexible
Kids and Accidents (Cox et al. 2010; Kenardy et al. 2015)	Online intervention	Road traffic accidents	7–16	56	< 2 weeks	Impact of Events Scale-Revised (IES-R); Child Trauma Symptom Questionnaire	Yes – in groups w/ high initial distress ($d = 0.94$)	Decrease in anxiety ($d = .33$) and anger symptoms ($d = .30$)
Bounce Back Now (Ruggiero et al. 2015; Bunnell et al., 2017)	Online intervention	Tornado	12–17	987	5–14 months	National Survey of Adolescents (NSA) PTSD Module	Yes, trending ($B = .36$, $p = .06$)	Significant decrease depression symptoms ($B = .42$, $p = .03$)

Coping Coach

A pilot randomized clinical trial was conducted to examine the whether or not use of the Coping Coach intervention would result in decreased PTSD symptoms in children who had experienced a potentially traumatic acute medical event (Kassam-Adams et al., 2015b). Participants included 72 children (immediate intervention = 36, wait-list–control = 36) aged 8–12 who were hospitalized for an acute medical event that had occurred within the past 2 weeks. Participants completed assessments of PTSD symptoms at baseline, 6 weeks, 12 weeks, and 18 weeks post-injury. The wait-list group was given access to the intervention following their 12-week assessment. Usage during the intervention trial was tracked to help determine intervention fidelity. Thirty-five of 36 children (97 percent) in the immediate invention group initiated the Coping Coach intervention, and 19 (53 percent) completed the entire game at least one time. Of the 28 children in the wait-list group who were eligible for the intervention (e.g., who completed the 12-week assessment), 19 (68 percent) used the intervention, and 15 (54 percent) completed the entire intervention. At a 6-week follow-up, medium between-group effect sizes suggested that children who used the Coping Coach intervention had a larger decrease in PTSD symptoms from baseline to 6 weeks post-trauma. The wait-list control group also showed a larger decrease in PTSD symptoms from 12 weeks to 18 weeks post-trauma (which was their intervention period) compared to the immediate intervention group. Exploratory analyses suggested that the intervention may have been more helpful for children who started with higher PTSD symptoms (Kassam-Adams et al., 2015b). Thus, while more research is needed, the Coping Coach intervention is a promising tool for prevention / early intervention.

Kids and Accidents

Eighty-five children (44 intervention, 41 no-treatment control) participated in a randomized clinical trial of Kids and Accidents (Cox et al., 2010). All participants were between ages of 7 and 16 years and were hospitalized overnight as the result of an unintentional injury (e.g., fractured limb). Children completed a trauma symptom questionnaire at baseline (T1), 4–6 weeks post-baseline (T2), and again 6 months post-baseline (T3). Intervention usage was measured by using the Subjective Intervention Evaluation. Of the 44 children who were randomly assigned to participate and use the Kids and Accidents invention, 18 (56 percent) initiated the intervention. There were no significant differences between those who initiated intervention and those who did not with regard to outcomes and demographics. Of the 18 children who visited the Kids and Accidents website, 10 (56 percent) visited 1 time and 8 (44 percent) visited 2–3 times. Ten (56 percent) child participants reported that the intervention was helpful, and 6 (33 percent) perceived the intervention to have a positive effect on them (Cox et al., 2010). Although not statistically significant, initial analyses revealed a trend that children who used the intervention had decreased PTSD symptoms at T2 and T3, while the control group displayed increased symptom levels at both time points (Cox et al., 2010). When initial PTSD symptoms were high (75th percentile), children who received the Kids and Accidents intervention reported significantly lower PTSD symptoms at 6-month follow-up compared to those in the control group (Kenardy et al., 2015). Thus, it may be that Kids and Accidents is most helpful for those children who demonstrate significant PTSD symptoms in the early aftermath of their injury. Additional research is needed to further examine the effectiveness of this intervention.

Bounce Back Now

An address-based randomized clinical trial was conducted to examine the effectiveness of Bounce Back Now in reducing post-traumatic stress among adolescents aged 12–17 years affected by tornados (Ruggiero et al., 2015). Adolescents and their parents were enrolled and completed baseline interviews, as well as 4-month and 12-month follow-ups. Once the baseline interview was completed, families were given instruction on how to visit the web intervention. Of the 2,000 families recruited, 987 accessed the website. Upon visiting the webpage, families were randomized to receive one of three conditions: (1) the Bounce Back Now intervention ($N = 364$), (2) the Bounce Back Now intervention plus a parental mental health self-help intervention ($N = 366$), or (3) a control condition that included information such as the prevalence rates of natural disasters, including myth and fact questions, but no psycho-education, feedback, or recommendations were provided ($N = 257$). Follow-up results indicated that among those adolescents who used the intervention, 76 percent found the website easy to use and 74 percent would recommend it to others (Price et al., 2015). The most frequently cited reason for not using the intervention was being "too busy" followed by feeling that the intervention was "not relevant to current concerns" (Bunnell et al., 2017; Price et al., 2015). At the 12-month follow-up only, both PTSD symptoms and symptoms of depression were lower in the Bounce Back Now intervention group compared to the control condition. While researchers had hypothesized that adding the parental component to the intervention would help adolescents improve even further, findings actually suggested that the Bounce Back Now intervention alone had an effect that was significantly larger on PTSD and depressive symptoms in adolescents (Ruggiero et al., 2015). In a subsequent study, researchers assessed the differences in access and completion of the intervention for those in urban / suburban (N = 1,321) versus rural (N = 676) communities, both affected by a tornado (Bunnell et al., 2017). Results of this investigation demonstrated no significant differences in the rate of access or completion of the intervention based on geographic location. Additionally, among those who did not access the intervention, reasons for not participating did not significantly differ based on location. Thus, initial research on the Bounce Back Now intervention suggests that it may be a feasible and effective way to reach adolescents following natural disasters across geographic location (Bunnell et al., 2017).

MindRight and LIFT

The effectiveness of MindRight and LIFT have not yet been tested.

Triangle of Life

Qualitative data from 20 children aged 11–14 years (in a school setting) indicated that children found the game fun to play; older children (aged 13 and 14) reported that while they still enjoyed the game, they rated it as easy (Assigana et al., 2014). While TF-CBT has strong evidence supporting it as a treatment, research has yet to determine if the Triangle of Life intervention increases positive outcomes and / or treatment engagement (Cohen & Mannarino, 2015; Deblinger et al., 1999; Foa, Keane, Friedman, & Cohen, 2009; Webb et al., 2014).

Mediators and Moderators of Technology-Based Interventions

Given the current state of the research, very little is known regarding mediators and moderators of technology-based interventions. It can likely be assumed that many of the technology-based interventions would have similar mediators as those presented in CBT treatment (e.g., changes in maladaptive cognitions) since most of these interventions utilize CBT theoretical underpinnings (e.g., see Chapter 6 of this book; Smith et al., 2007). Potential moderators may include how well a child (and their parents) understand the content as presented in online or mobile programs, how comfortable they are with the technology itself, and / or whether they have regular access to the technology to complete the programs at the desired time. In addition, it may be that the design of the technology program moderates intervention effect. As mentioned earlier in several of the descriptions of technology-based interventions, following internet behavior change models and / or game development theory in designing technology-based interventions may serve to increase engagement and encourage children to obtain a higher intervention dose (e.g., Keller, 1987; Malone & Lepper, 1987; Mirvis et al., 1991; Schell, 2008). Finally, it may be that symptom severity in early proximity of the trauma may serve as a potential moderating variable (Kassam-Adams et al., 2015b; Kenardy et al., 2015). More research is needed to delineate mediators and moderators as applied to PTSD interventions that utilize technology.

Clinical Case Example

Sally is an 11-year-old girl who was injured in a motor vehicle collision two weeks ago. While her physical injuries are expected to fully resolve, Sally's mother is noting that Sally has fears about riding in cars. While this has not prevented Sally from doing the things that she needs to do (e.g., go to school), she is hesitant to take any unnecessary car rides (e.g., to go visit a friend). Sally also reported having difficulty falling asleep at night. Other PTSD symptoms related to Sally's potentially traumatic motor vehicle crash and subsequent injury are unknown. Sally's mother asks the medical team who treated Sally's physical injuries how long Sally will have these new fears and if she needs to take Sally for counseling. Sally's medical team explained that many children experience new fears in the first few weeks following an injury. Because Sally has symptoms of PTSD but limited impairment from symptoms, her medical team recommended that she start the Coping Coach intervention and return for follow-up in four weeks.

No one in Sally's family had used mental health services in the past, so Sally's mother was relieved that her doctor gave them an intervention that they could start at home. In addition, Sally loved video games and was very comfortable with web-based games. Once her mother provided her with the log-in information, Sally worked through the Coping Coach program in under an hour. Sally's mother was interested in what Sally was learning, so she used her own log-in to play through the game as well. Sally found the feelings portion of the game rather easy but was surprised to learn that other children experience fears as she did after a motor vehicle collision. Following the examples in the games, Sally was able to recognize some of her unhelpful thoughts (e.g., "I might get hurt again if I get in that car") and reframe them (e.g., "My mom will be careful on our drive to school"). Sally also learned that she was trying to avoid the car and while it might feel safer in the moment, it only got harder over time. After Sally finished the game, she shared her activity log with her mother, and they were able to talk through her feelings and fears more easily. Her mother encouraged her to play the Coping Coach game several more times. Sally would have preferred not to complete the same game with the same story lines but was compliant with her mother's encouragement. Sally and her mother saved all the activity logs to take to Sally's four-week follow-up appointment. At her follow-up appointment, Sally's symptoms were somewhat improved but still bothering her and her mother. Her medical team referred Sally for TF-CBT treatment for more intensive support and more tailored skill building.

In Sally's case, she had a supportive family member and easy access to a computer and the internet. These strengths helped her success in using Coping Coach; however, the persistence of her symptoms required a more intensive treatment approach over time. See Figure 27.4 for treatment paths and potential ways to integrate web- / mobile-based technology into management of Sally's emotional recovery.

Challenges and Recommendations for Future Research in This Area

There are a number of challenges to building, evaluating, and maintaining innovative interventions that maximize the use of current technology to prevent or treat pediatric PTSD. While a great benefit of these programs is to reduce cost for children and families, start-up costs and continued maintenance costs are high. Rapidly changing technology can present difficulties, especially if intervention developers conduct large-scale research studies prior to making interventions available; often by the time these trials are completed, technology has changed. In creating and evaluating

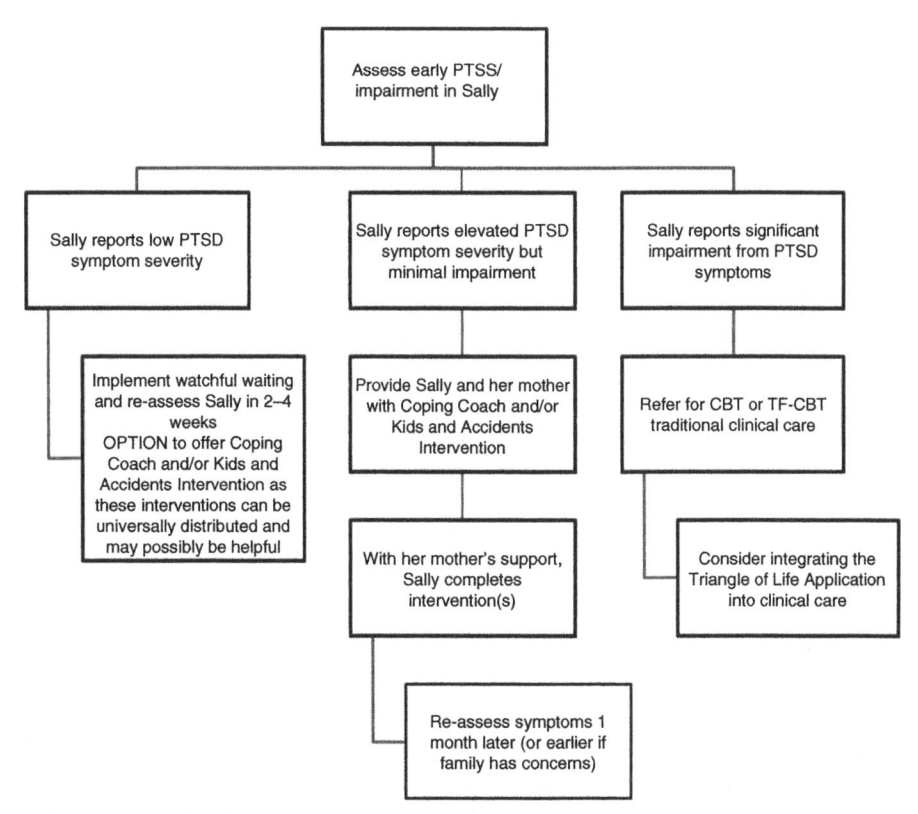

Figure 27.4 *Potential Steps to PTSD Prevention/Early Intervention/Treatment Using Web-/Mobile-Based Technology*

technology-based interventions, it may be helpful for developers to use program theory as a guide to help specify clear goals and mechanisms of change and to engage in user feedback and expert review of content early in intervention development (Kassam-Adams et al., 2015a; Winston & Jacobsohn, 2010). When mechanisms of change are clearly defined and evaluated, intervention developers can ensure that the key intervention targets remain the same even if the delivery of the targets changes to keep up with technological advancements. Future research should examine the cost effectiveness of web-based / mobile-based interventions to help advocate for funding and / or reimbursement to help with development and maintenance over time.

To our knowledge, no research to date has examined any of the interventions reviewed in this chapter as treatment tools or conjunctive treatment tools to use with PTSD treatment. In addition, there is a gap in our knowledge regarding potential mediators and / or moderators of technology-based interventions. Ethical challenges may deter the examination of stand-alone web-based / mobile-based tools as treatment for PTSD since in-person TF-CBT and CBT have consistently demonstrated positive outcomes. However, as the field stands now, many children are not receiving any treatment at all. Thus, web-based / mobile-based tools may offer a way to reach these children. Creating web-based platforms based in CBT principles and learning from current web-based preventive / early interventions as described earlier may allow for the creation of these resources. Evaluating PTSD treatment interventions in children who would not otherwise receive any care or starting treatment intervention research in conjunction with in-person (or virtual) treatment may provide a starting point to be able to better extend resources.

Key Practice Points and Recommended Resources for Practice

Technological interventions provide a unique opportunity to reach those who may not otherwise have access to mental health services following exposure to a potentially traumatic event (Bunnell et al., 2017; Kenardy et al., 2015; Marsac et al., 2015; Shealy et al., 2015). Of the interventions described in this chapter, all of those that have been tested in a randomized controlled trial (Coping Coach, Kids and Accidents, Bounce Back Now) have shown some initial effectiveness, demonstrating potential benefits for a wider range of families (Bunnell et al., 2017; Cox et al., 2010; Kassam-Adams et al., 2015b; Kenardy et al., 2015; Price et al., 2015; Ruggiero et al., 2015). Those who are at a primary point of contact with children and families after a traumatic event (e.g., emergency department providers) may want to consider offering children and parents information on preventative interventions (Coping Coach and Kids and Accidents) as a means to prevent the development of post-traumatic stress symptoms. While these interventions appear to be most effective in children with higher initial symptoms, they can be distributed broadly at minimal cost. Though additional research is needed on TF-CBT Triangle of Life, MindRight, and LIFT, their foundation in CBT techniques suggests they would likely be of benefit to children and families coping with trauma. Clinicians may consider integrating these tools into practice and examining if they help promote engagement or solidify skills at an individual level.

References

Aetna. (2012). Aetna. Retrieved August 9, 2017, from www1.aetna.com/employer-plans/document-library/states/CA-HMO-Ded-1500.pdf

Anda, R. F., Felitti, V. J., Bremner, J. D., Walker, J. D., Whitfield, C., Perry, B. D., ... Giles, W. H. (2006). The enduring effects of abuse and related adverse experiences in childhood: A convergence of evidence from neurobiology and epidemiology. *European Archives of Psychiatry and Clinical Neuroscience, 256*(3), 174–186. https://doi.org/10.1007/s00406-005-0624-4

Assigana, E., Chang, E., Cho, S., Kotecha, V., Liu, B., Turner, H., ... Stevens, S. M. (2014). TF-CBT Triangle of Life: A game to help with cognitive behavioral therapy. *Proceedings of the First ACM SIGCHI Annual Symposium on Computer-Human Interaction in Play*, 9–16. https://doi.org/10.1145/2658537.2658684

Bisson, J. I., & Cohen, J. A. (2006). Disseminating early interventions following trauma. *Journal of Traumatic Stress*. https://doi.org/10.1002/jts.20175

Boydell, K. M., Pong, R., Volpe, T., Tilleczek, K., Wilson, E., & Lemieux, S. (2006). Family perspectives on pathways to mental health care for children and youth in rural communities. *The Journal of Rural Health: Official Journal of the American Rural Health Association and the National Rural Health Care Association, 22*(2), 182–188. https://doi.org/10.1111/j.1748-0361.2006.00029.x

Bunnell, B. E., Davidson, T. M., Dewey, D., Price, M., & Ruggiero, K. J. (2017). Rural and urban/suburban families' use of a web-based mental health intervention. *Telemedicine and E-Health, 23*(5), 390–396. https://doi.org/10.1089/tmj.2016.0153

CIGNA. (2009). Summary of benefits. Retrieved August 9, 2017, from www.cigna.com/pdf/2010_IND_DEP_sob_HMO_AZ_HCR.pdf

Cohen, J. A., & Mannarino, A. P. (2015). Trauma-focused cognitive behavior therapy for traumatized children and families. *Child and Adolescent Psychiatric Clinics of North America.* https://doi.org/10.1016/j.chc.2015.02.005

Cox, C. M., Kenardy, J. A., & Hendrikz, J. K. (2010). A randomized controlled trial of a web-based early intervention for children and their parents following unintentional injury. *Journal of Pediatric Psychology, 35*(6), 581–592. https://doi.org/jsp095 [pii] \n10.1093/jpepsy/jsp095

Crawford, T., & Simonoff, E. (2003). Parental views about services for children attending schools for the emotionally and behaviourally disturbed (EBD): A qualitative analysis. *Child: Care, Health and Development, 29*(6), 481–490. https://doi.org/10.1046/j.1365-2214.2003.00368.x

Cuffe, S. P., Waller, J. L., Cuccaro, M. L., Pumariega, A. J., & Garrison, C. Z. (1995). Race and gender differences in the treatment of psychiatric disorders in young adolescents. *Journal of the American Academy of Child and Adolescent Psychiatry, 34*(11), 1536–43. https://doi.org/10.1097/00004583-199511000-00021

Deblinger, E., Steer, R. A., & Lippmann, J. (1999). Two-year follow-up study of cognitive behavioral therapy for sexually abused children suffering post-traumatic stress symptoms. *Child Abuse & Neglect, 23*(12), 1371–1378. https://doi.org/http://dx.doi.org/10.1016/S0145-2134(99)00091-5

Ehlers, A., & Clark, D. M. (2000). A cognitive model of posttraumatic stress disorder. *Behaviour Research and Therapy, 38*(4), 319–345. https://doi.org/10.1016/S0005-7967(99)00123-0

Felliti, V., & Anda, R. (1997). The Adverse Childhood Experiences (ACE) study. Atlanta, GA: Center for Disease Control and Prevention, 1–2.

Felitti, V. J., Anda, R. F., Nordenberg, D., Williamson, D. F., Spitz, A. M., Edwards, V., … Marks, J. S. (1998). Relationship of childhood abuse and household dysfunction to many of the leading causes of death in adults: The adverse childhood experiences (ACE) study. *American Journal of Preventive Medicine, 14*(4), 245–258. https://doi.org/10.1016/S0749-3797(98)00017-8

Flink, I. J. E., Beirens, T. M. J., Butte, D., & Raat, H. (2013). The role of maternal perceptions and ethnic background in the mental health help-seeking pathway of adolescent girls. *Journal of Immigrant and Minority Health, 15*(2), 292–299. https://doi.org/10.1007/s10903-012-9621-7

Foa, E. B., Keane, T. M., Friedman, M. J., & Cohen, J. A. (2009). Effective treatments for PTSD: Practice guidelines from the International Society for Traumatic Stress Studies (2nd edn.). In E. B. Foa, T. M. Keane, M. J. Friedman, & J. A. Cohen (eds.), *Effective treatments for PTSD: Practice guidelines from the International Society for Traumatic Stress Studies* (pp. xiii, 658). New York: Guildford Press. Retrieved from http://libraryproxy.griffith.edu.au/login?url=http://ovidsp.ovid.com/ovidweb.cgi?T=JS&CSC=Y&NEWS=N&PAGE=fulltext&D=psyc6&AN=2008-18599-000%5Cnhttp://hy8fy9jj4b.search.serialssolutions.com/?url_ver=Z39.88-2004&rft_val_fmt=info:ofi/fmt:kev:mtx:journal&rfr_

Gamm, L., Stone, S., & Pittman, S. (2003). Mental health and mental disorders – a rural challenge: A literature review. In L. Gamm, L. Hutchinson, B. Dabney, & A. Dorsey (eds.), *Rural Healthy People 2010: A companion document to Rural Healthy People 2010* (pp. 97–113). College Station, TX: The Texas A&M University System Health Science Center, School of Rural Public Health, Southwest Rural Health Research Center.

Girio-Herrera, E., Owens, J. S., & Langberg, J. M. (2013). Perceived barriers to help-seeking among parents of at-risk kindergarteners in rural communities. *Journal of Clinical Child and Adolescent Psychology: The Official Journal for the Society of Clinical Child and Adolescent Psychology, American Psychological Association, Division 53*, *42*(1), 68–77. https://doi.org/10.1080/15374416.2012.715365

Glaser, J. P., van Os, J., Portegijs, P. J. M., & Myin-Germeys, I. (2006). Childhood trauma and emotional reactivity to daily life stress in adult frequent attenders of general practitioners. *Journal of Psychosomatic Research*, *61*(2), 229–236. https://doi.org/10.1016/j.jpsychores.2006.04.014

Goldsmith, H. F., Wagenfeld, M. O., Manderscheid, R. W., & Stiles, D. (1997). Specialty mental health services in metropolitan and nonmetropolitan areas: 1983 and 1990. *Administration and Policy in Mental Health*, *24*(6), 475–488.

Guzder, J., Yohannes, S., & Zelkowitz, P. (2013). Helpseeking of immigrant and native born parents: A qualitative study from a Montreal child day hospital. *Journal of the Canadian Academy of Child and Adolescent Psychiatry*, *22*(4), 275–281.

Harwood, M. D., O'Brien, K. A., Carter, C. G., & Eyberg, S. M. (2009). Mental health services for preschool children in primary care: A survey of maternal attitudes and beliefs. *Journal of Pediatric Psychology*, *34*(7), 760–768. https://doi.org/10.1093/jpepsy/jsn128

Hovens, J. G. F. M., Wiersma, J. E., Giltay, E. J., Van Oppen, P., Spinhoven, P., Penninx, B. W. J. H., & Zitman, F. G. (2010). Childhood life events and childhood trauma in adult patients with depressive, anxiety and comorbid disorders vs. controls. *Acta Psychiatrica Scandinavica*, *122*(1), 66–74. https://doi.org/10.1111/j.1600-0447.2009.01491.x

Jameson, J. P., & Blank, M. B. (2007). The role of clinical psychology in rural mental health services: Defining problems and developing solutions. *Clinical Psychology: Science and Practice*. https://doi.org/10.1111/j.1468-2850.2007.00089.x

Jaycox, L. (n.d.). Life Improvement For Teens (LIFT). Retrieved January 12, 2016, from www.3cisd.com/LIFT-case-study

Kassam-Adams, N., Marsac, M. L., Kohser, K. L., Kenardy, J. A., March, S., & Winston, F. K. (2015a). A new method for assessing content validity in model-based creation and iteration of eHealth interventions. *Journal of Medical Internet Research*, *17*(4), e95. https://doi.org/10.2196/jmir.3811

Kassam-Adams, N., Marsac, M. L., Kohser, K. L., Kenardy, J., March, S., & Winston, F. K. (2015b). Pilot randomized controlled trial of a novel web-based intervention to prevent posttraumatic stress in children following medical events. *Journal of Pediatric Psychology*, *41*, jsv057-. https://doi.org/10.1093/jpepsy/jsv057

Kataoka, S. H., Zhang, L., & Wells, K. B. (2002). Unmet need for mental health care among U.S. children: Variation by ethnicity and insurance status. *American Journal of Psychiatry, 159*(9), 1548–1555. https://doi.org/10.1176/appi.ajp.159.9.1548

Keller, J. M. (1987). Development and use of the ARCS model of motivational design. *Journal of Instructional Development, 10*(1932), 2–10. https://doi.org/10.1002/pfi.4160260802

Kenardy, J., Thompson, K., Le Brocque, R., & Olsson, K. (2008). Information-provision intervention for children and their parents following pediatric accidental injury. *European Child and Adolescent Psychiatry, 17*(5), 316–325. https://doi.org/10.1007/s00787-007-0673-5

Kenardy, Cox, & Brown, F. L. (2015). A web-based early intervention can prevent long-term pts reactions in children with high initial distress following accidental injury. *Journal of Traumatic Stress, 28*(4), 366–369. https://doi.org/10.1002/jts.22025

Klasen, H., & Goodman, R. (2000). Parents and GPs at cross-purposes over hyperactivity: A qualitative study of possible barriers to treatment. *British Journal of General Practice, 50*(452), 199–202.

Kumpfer, K. L. (1999). Factor and processes contributing to resilience: The resilience framework. *Resilience and Development: Positive Life Adaptations*, 179–224. https://doi.org/10.1007/b108350

Majer, M., Nater, U. M., Lin, J.-M. S., Capuron, L., & Reeves, W. C. (2010). Association of childhood trauma with cognitive function in healthy adults: A pilot study. *BMC Neurology, 10*, 61. https://doi.org/10.1186/1471-2377-10-61

Malone, T. W., & Lepper, M. R. (1987). Making learning fun: A taxonomy of intrinsic motivations for learning. In R. Snow & M. J. Farr (eds.), *Aptitude learning and instruction* (pp. 223–253). Hillsdale, NJ: Erlbaum. https://doi.org/10.1016/S0037-6337(09)70509-1

Marsac, M. L., Kohser, K. L., Winston, F. K., Kenardy, J., March, S., & Kassam-Adams, N. (2013). Using a web-based game to prevent posttraumatic stress in children following medical events: Design of a randomized controlled trial. *European Journal of Psychotraumatology, 4*(SUPPL.), 1–10. https://doi.org/10.3402/ejpt.v4i0.21311

Marsac, M. L., Winston, F. K., Hildenbrand, A. K., Kohser, K. L., March, S., Kenardy, J., & Kassam-Adams, N. (2015). Systematic, theoretically-grounded development and feasibility testing of an innovative, preventive web-based game for children exposed to acute trauma. *Clinical Practice in Pediatric Psychology, 3*(1), 12–24. https://doi.org/10.1037/cpp0000080

Meredith, L. S., Stein, B. D., Paddock, S. M., Jaycox, L. H., Quinn, V. P., Chandra, A., & Burnam, A. (2009). Perceived barriers to treatment for adolescent depression. *Medical Care, 47*(6), 677–685. https://doi.org/10.1097/MLR.0b013e318190d46b

Merikangas, K. R., He, J.-P., Burstein, M., Swanson, S. A., Avenevoli, S., Cui, L., ... Swendsen, J. (2010). Lifetime prevalence of mental disorders in U.S. adolescents: Results from the National Comorbidity Survey Replication – Adolescent Supplement (NCS-A). *Journal of the American Academy of Child and Adolescent Psychiatry, 49*(10), 980–989. https://doi.org/10.1016/j.jaac.2010.05.017

Miller, B. F., Petterson, S., Burke, B. T., Phillips, R. L., & Green, L. a. (2014). Proximity of providers: Colocating behavioral health and primary care and the prospects for an integrated workforce. *The American Psychologist, 69*(4), 443–451. https://doi.org/10.1037/a0036093

MindRight. (2017). Retrieved from http://getmindright.org/

Mirvis, P. H., Csikszentmihalyi, M., & Csikzentmihaly, M. (1991). Flow: The psychology of optimal experience. *Academy of Management Review*, *16*(3), 636–640. https://doi.org/10.5465/AMR.1991.4279513

Murry, V. M., Heflinger, C. A., Suiter, S. V., & Brody, G. H. (2011). Examining perceptions about mental health care and help-seeking among rural African American families of adolescents. *Journal of Youth and Adolescence*, *40*(9), 1118–1131. https://doi.org/10.1007/s10964-010-9627-1

Owens, P. L., Hoagwood, K., Horwitz, S. M., Leaf, P. J., Poduska, J. M., Kellam, S. G., & Ialongo, N. S. (2002). Barriers to children's mental health services. *Journal of the American Academy of Child and Adolescent Psychiatry*, *41*(6), 731–738. https://doi.org/10.1097/00004583-200206000-00013

Ponsford, J., Willmott, C., Rothwell, A., Cameron, P., Ayton, G., Nelms, R., . . . Ng, K. (2001). Impact of early intervention on outcome after mild traumatic brain injury in children. *Pediatrics*, *108*(6), 1297–1303. https://doi.org/10.1542/peds.108.6.1297

Price, M., Yuen, E. K., Davidson, T. M., Hubel, G., & Ruggiero, K. J. (2015). Access and completion of a web-based treatment in a population-based sample of tornado-affected adolescents. *Psychological Services*, *12*(3), 283–290. https://doi.org/10.1037/ser0000017

Price, J., Kassam-Adams, N., Alderfer, M. A., Christofferson, J., & Kazak, A. E. (2016). Systematic review: A reevaluation and update of the integrative (trajectory) model of pediatric medical traumatic stress. *Journal of Pediatric Psychology*, *41*(1), 86–97. https://doi.org/10.1093/jpepsy/jsv074

Pullmann, M. D., Vanhooser, S., Hoffman, C., & Heflinger, C. A. (2010). Barriers to and supports of family participation in a rural system of care for children with serious emotional problems. *Community Mental Health Journal*, *46*(3), 211–220. https://doi.org/10.1007/s10597-009-9208-5

Pynoos, R. S. (1994). Traumatic stress and developmental psychopathology in children and adolescents. In R. S. Pynoos (ed.), *Posttraumatic stress disorder: A clinical review* (pp. 65–98). Baltimore: The Sidran Press.

Reardon, T., Harvey, K., Baranowska, M., O'Brien, D., Smith, L., & Creswell, C. (2017). What do parents perceive are the barriers and facilitators to accessing psychological treatment for mental health problems in children and adolescents? A systematic review of qualitative and quantitative studies. *European Child & Adolescent Psychiatry*, *26*, 623–647. https://doi.org/10.1007/s00787-016-0930-6

Ritterband, L., Thorndike, F., Cox, D., Kovatchev, B., & Gonder-Frederick, L. (2009). A behavior change model for internet interventions. *Annals of Behavioral Medicine*, *38*(1), 18–27. https://doi.org/10.1007/s12160-009-9133-4.A

Rost, K., Fortney, J., Fischer, E., & Smith, J. (2002). Use, quality, and outcomes of care for mental health: The rural perspective. *Medical Care Research and Review*, *59*(3), 231–265. https://doi.org/10.1177/1077558702059003001

Ruggiero, K. J., Morris, T. L., & Scotti, J. R. (2001). Treatment for children with posttraumatic stress disorder: Current status and future directions. *Clinical Psychology – Science and Practice*, *8*(2), 210–227. https://doi.org/10.1093/clipsy/8.2.210

Ruggiero, K. J., Price, M., Adams, Z., Stauffacher, K., McCauley, J., Danielson, C. M. . . . Resnick, H. S. (2015). Web intervention for adolescents affected by disaster: Population-based randomized controlled trial. *Journal of the American Academy of Child and Adolescent Psychiatry*, *54*(9), 709–717. https://doi.org/10.1016/j.jaac.2015.07.001

Sawyer, M. G., Rey, J. M., Arney, F. M., Whitham, J. N., Clark, J. J., & Baghurst, P. A. (2004). Use of health and school-based services in Australia by young people with attention-deficit/hyperactivity disorder. *Journal of the American Academy of Child and Adolescent Psychiatry, 43*(11), 1355–1363. https://doi.org/10.1097/01.chi.0000138354.90981.5b

Sayal, K., Mills, J., White, K., Merrell, C., & Tymms, P. (2015). Predictors of and barriers to service use for children at risk of ADHD: Longitudinal study. *European Child and Adolescent Psychiatry, 24*(5), 545–552. https://doi.org/10.1007/s00787-014-0606-z

Schell, J. (2008). *Game design mechanics. The Art of Game Design A book of lenses* (Vol. Masters). Retrieved from http://ocw.mit.edu/courses/comparative-media-studies/cms-608-game-design-spring-2008/index.htm

Shealy, K. M., Davidson, T. M., Jones, A. M., Lopez, C. M., & de Arellano, M. A. (2015). Delivering an evidence-based mental health treatment to underserved populations using telemedicine: The case of a trauma-affected adolescent in a rural setting. *Cognitive and Behavioral Practice, 22*(3), 331–344. https://doi.org/10.1016/j.cbpra.2014.04.007

Thurston, I. B., & Phares, V. (2008). Mental health service utilization among African American and Caucasian mothers and fathers. *Journal of Consulting and Clinical Psychology, 76*(6), 1058–1067. https://doi.org/10.1037/a0014007

US Census. (2010). 2010 Census. Retrieved from https://ask.census.gov/faq.php?id=5000&faqId=5971

Webb, C., Hayes, A. M., & Deblinger, E. (2014). Trauma-focused cognitive behavioral therapy for youth: Effectiveness in a community setting. *Psychological Trauma: Theory, Research, Practice, and Policy, 6*(5), 555–562. https://doi.org/10.1037/a0037364

Winston, F. K., & Jacobsohn, L. (2010). A practical approach for applying best practices in behavioural interventions to injury prevention. *Injury Prevention, 16*(2), 107–112. https://doi.org/10.1136/ip.2009.021972

Smith, P., Yule, W., Perrin, S., Trahah, T., Dalgleish, T., & Clark, D.M. (2007). Cognitive-behavioral therapy for PTSD in children and adolescents: A preliminary randomized controlled trial. *Journal of American Academy of Child and Adolescent Psychiatry, 46*, 1051–1061. https://doi.org/10.1097/CHI.0b013e318067e288

Yuen, E. K., Gros, K., Welsh, K. E., McCauley, J., Resnick, H. S., Danielson, C. K., . . . Ruggiero, K. J. (2015). Development and preliminary testing of a web-based, self-help application for disaster-affected families. *Health Informatics Journal, 22*(3), 659–675. https://doi.org/10.1177/1460458215579292

28 Eye Movement Desensitization and Reprocessing (EMDR)

Kerstin Bergh Johannesson, Margareta Friberg Weschke, and Abdulbaghi Ahmad

Introduction

Eye movement desensitization and reprocessing (EMDR) is a trauma-focused psychotherapeutic method developed by the American psychologist Francine Shapiro for the treatment of traumatic memories. A first controlled study was published in 1989 (Shapiro, 1989) and since that time a large number of randomized controlled trials as well as clinical case studies have been published.

EMDR therapy is appreciated by many clients for being a gentle therapeutic method. It represents an alternative approach to prolonged exposure (PE), which might be considered more demanding and stressful for the patient because it involves the repeated voluntary recollection of the disturbing traumatic memory. EMDR on the other hand does not demand a detailed narrative of the most horrendous part of the trauma, nor extended exposure, nor daily homework. Some comparative treatment studies even indicate that EMDR might be a faster method than comparative cognitive behavioral therapy (CBT) methods (e.g., Chen et al., 2015; Rothbaum, Astin, & Marsteller, 2005; Power et al., 2002). However, many researchers have criticized EMDR for not being theory based. Following its discovery, it was far from clear what the underlying specific mechanism of action of this intervention was. Indeed, EMDR is considered to share mechanisms with many other therapeutic methods. Meanwhile, the evidence for the efficacy of EMDR as a treatment for PTSD has steadily increased, eventually leading to its recognition as an empirically based intervention. For example, Bisson, Cosgrove, Lewis, and Roberts (2015) found that EMDR was just as effective as trauma-focused cognitive behavior therapy (TF-CBT) and non-TF-CBT in the treatment of PTSD, and that each of these interventions was more efficacious than other types of therapy. Meta-analyses have confirmed that EMDR is an equally effective method for treating traumatized individuals as PE, CBT, and pharmacotherapy (e.g., SSRIs; Cusack et al., 2016; Bisson, Roberts, Andrew, & Cooper, 2013; Powers, Halpern, Ferenschak, Gillihan, & Foa, 2010; Watts et al., 2013).

The recommendation by the World Health Organization (WHO, 2013) was that EMDR, just like trauma-focused cognitive behavioral therapy (CBT) and stress management, is indicated as an empirically supported intervention for adults with PTSD. The recommendation for the treatment of children with PTSD was similar, although the strength of evidence was low for EMDR.

So far, the vast majority of the research on the efficacy of EMDR has been conducted in adult populations, with only a few studies having been conducted on the effects of this treatment in traumatized children and adolescents. In this chapter, we first describe the basic EMDR protocol and special adaptations that have been made to apply this intervention in children and adolescents. Next, we review the empirical support for EMDR as a treatment for PTSD, with a special focus on research that has been conducted in youth populations.

The EMDR Protocol and Its Application in Children and Adolescents

The first phase in the standard EMDR protocol (Shapiro, 2001), *history taking* (can take from one to several sessions depending on the complexity of client), consists of getting a detailed picture of the traumatic event(s) and its psychological sequelae, previous difficult life experiences, and a general picture of the clinically relevant features, such as psychological resources, attachment patterns, and specific vulnerabilities. This leads eventually to a treatment plan with identified traumatic memories for processing.

The second phase of the protocol, *preparation*, provides psycho-education on trauma reactions, describes the EMDR method, and strengthens the therapeutic alliance. The method could be described for clients in the following way:

> Disturbing memories can be stored in the brain in isolation. They can get locked into the nervous system with the original images, sounds, thoughts and feelings. The distressing material just keeps repeatedly getting triggered. This prevents learning / healing from taking place. In another part of the brain, most of the needed information for resolving this problem might be stored, but the two parts cannot connect. Once EMDR starts, a linking takes place. New information can come to mind and the problems can come to an adaptive resolution.

The client is informed about the treatment procedure and the possible benefits and side effects of the method. The bilateral stimulation, such as conducting lateral eye movements induced by the therapist, is demonstrated. This means that the client will track the hand of the therapist with the eyes from side to side. A stabilization technique is introduced to enable the client to relax after intense processing and to regulate strong affect in general. The "safe/calm place" exercise – during which clients visualize a positive inner resource and identify consecutive relaxing feelings that are strengthened by a few sets of slow bilateral stimulation – is commonly applied as a part of the preparation phase.

The third phase, *assessment*, is about identifying the components of the traumatic memory that have been chosen for processing. The client is asked to recall the disturbing, traumatic memory and select a representative picture of the event. The client is asked to formulate a negative belief that is related to this picture and then to identify a more desired alternative positive belief. The positive belief is evaluated on the Validity of Cognition (VOC) scale, which assesses how valid the statement appears in connection to the picture, where 1 indicates that the cognition feels "not believable at all" and 7 indicates that the cognition feels "totally believable." Thereafter, the client is asked to focus on the disturbing memory again and report what feelings the picture and the negative belief evoke. To determine the severity of the memory, the client is asked to score the Subjective Units of Distress Scale (SUDS), which ranges between 0 = "no disturbance at all" and 10 = "the highest disturbance you can imagine." Finally, the clients are asked where in the body they can feel the distress.

The fourth phase, *desensitization*, consists of asking the client to bring up the representative picture of the traumatic memory together with the negative cognition and the body sensation while conducting lateral eye movements induced by the therapist. The eye movements are usually horizontal but can also be diagonal. If eye movements are not comfortable for some reason, tactile or auditory stimulation can be applied, such as tapping on the upper side of the hands of the client, or using headphones that give a beeping sound that goes from ear to ear. After every set of finger movements, the patient is asked to take a deep breath, and to report what comes to mind without evaluating whether it seems right or wrong. The same procedure is repeated until the patient comes with neutral, positive, or no further statements. This desensitization procedure is repeated until the SUDS is diminished to 0 when recalling the original memory.

The fifth phase in the procedure, *linking to the positive cognition*, occurs when the client evaluates the validity of the originally chosen positive belief in connection with the reprocessed memory by means of the VOC. The ultimate goal is to link into more adaptive information into the memory network, thereby making the positive cognition feel totally believable. This is effectuated by continued processing of the memory with bilateral stimulation in the same way as previously done during desensitization, but this time the reprocessed traumatic incident is explicitly associated with the positive belief.

During the sixth phase, *body scan*, an evaluation is done to determine whether any remaining distress or disturbance exists on the body level. If so, the distressing bodily sensations are processed by further bilateral stimulation.

The seventh phase, *closure*, is concerned with ending the session following a special procedure, including a short debriefing. The aim is to restore the stability of the client as much as possible before leaving the session. If the session has been particularly demanding, the client may need to conduct a calming exercise before leaving the session.

The eighth phase, *re-evaluation of the processed memory*, takes place when the client returns for the next session, which is considered the final step in the standard protocol. If the processing of the traumatic memory appears to be incomplete, a continuation of the desensitization procedure is needed.

General Consideration Concerning EMDR with Children

One of the most important factors in the preparation for treating a child with EMDR therapy is assessing if the child is secure enough within their family or the care environment. An ongoing traumatizing situation where there is a risk for further abuse needs to be dealt with first. Thus, if there is family violence or physical, verbal, or sexual abuse, this has to be handled in a professional way before the EMDR treatment is started. It is important to remember that a child is dependent on a family or caregivers and usually has a specific role within the family system.

The standard EMDR protocol can usually be applied from age 9 years (Tinker & Wilson, 1999), whereas younger children need a more adapted protocol. Every phase in the procedure may need specific adjustments to meet every child's specific needs and conditions. Various adaptations have been made to the EMDR protocol (Adler-Tapia & Settle, 2016; Ahmad, Larsson, & Sundelin-Wahlsten, 2007; Ahmad & Sundelin-Wahlsten, 2008; Gomez, 2012; Morris-Smith & Silvestre, 2013; Tinker & Wilson, 1999). The need for participation of the caregiver might be indicated, especially when treating younger children. Parents can serve as either informants or participants in the sessions. Since processing can continue spontaneously between sessions, the parents need to be able to handle possible reactions in an appropriate way.

The presence of parents during treatment sessions is a matter of clinical judgment and can differ from one child to another. For example, consideration needs also to be taken if the parent suffers from PTSD symptoms. It may be necessary to treat the caregiver first or during parallel sessions to prevent them, for example, from having a flashback during the child's session. Small children may need safe attachment persons as their "safe place," while older children, if parents are present, may avoid sharing sensitive information to "protect" parents or to avoid feared negative consequences.

Information and instructions have to be formulated in language that is easy for the child to understand. The child should also be given the means to express themselves in a developmentally appropriate way. Of course, this can be done verbally, but also by means of drawings or play material. Measures should be taken not to stress the child with demands that may provoke a negative reaction. Still, the therapist needs to be consistent in their approach, and in case such negativity occurs they may offer the child a short break before returning to the processing. Tuning in with the child during treatment is very important. Therapists should have good knowledge of developmental psychology and experience of working with children.

Specific Adaptations for Children in the Different Phases of the Protocol

Phase 1: history taking. The trauma history and the developmental history are usually obtained from parents or other caregivers. If necessary, other informants such as teachers, day care personnel, the family doctor, or social workers can also be consulted. If possible, depending on the age of the child, information could also be obtained directly from them. One reason is that the trauma of the child is not necessarily identical with what the parents are reporting. Children have less information and perspective on life and cannot always judge if a situation is "life-threatening." It may not be entirely clear to them that "the danger is over," for example, when a parent had to go to the hospital because of acute stomach pains that turned out to be benign. For the adults, the crisis is over because "it was nothing serious" and the pain was gone. However, the child could be stuck with the memory of mother's pain and abrupt departure to the hospital, with a belief that they can be abandoned at any time. During this phase, parents also need to be informed about the EMDR therapy, and their role in the treatment of the child has to be established.

Phase 2: preparation. In this phase, further contact is established with the child. This can take place with or without parents present in the room. The focus is on the concerns of the child. The parent can be called upon as a "back-up" to what the child tries to tell, but the parent should not be allowed to take over. A respectful listening to the child's troubles and a gentle interviewing about symptoms usually lay a foundation for a good working alliance. It is important not to press the child and to be as easygoing as possible.

Information about PTSD or reactions to frightening experiences should be given in an age-appropriate way. The child is also informed about EMDR in a simple way and is encouraged to try a stabilization exercise such as the "safe place." For a child aged 2–4 years, a safe place can be a body sensation of closeness and warmth from the mother's body when sitting on her lap or listening to her singing a well-known lullaby, which can be strengthened by bilateral stimulation. If the child is old enough, they can draw a picture of something that makes them feel very safe and that renders pleasant bodily sensations. Older children can visualize an inner picture of a safe place, which is related to a pleasant experience.

The child is also shown a STOP-signal, which they can use to indicate when there is a need for a short break. Again, with younger children this can be done in a more playful manner.

Phase 3: assessment. A specific memory of a troublesome situation is selected by the child. To get more details about the event, the child can draw it, demonstrate what happened using puppets and toys, or the therapist could ask the parent to tell it as a story.

When applicable, a negative cognition connected to the memory is obtained. The therapist will usually support the child to find a negative belief that is at least somewhat irrational. Comic strip characters with thought balloons can be helpful to learn more about children's thoughts and feelings. Cards with examples of positive and negative thoughts and with positive and negative emotions can be employed with children who can read. The SUDS may have to be adjusted to the child's age: either concrete scoring categories can be introduced or pictures can be used to evaluate the level of distress associated with the traumatic picture.

Phase 4: desensitization. Bilateral stimulation with children younger than ages 8–9 years is often performed by tactical stimulation because younger children usually have difficulty with making eye movements (Morris-Smith & Silvestre,

2014). The child can be actively involved in the stimulation by tapping on the hands of the therapist. Other types of bilateral stimulation can also be used, such as sounds.

In contrast to adults, strong emotional reactions are unlikely to occur in children treated with EMDR. Compared to adults, children have fewer associative connections; need shorter sets of eye movements or other bilateral stimulation; and, consequently, sessions will be shorter in time (5–20 minutes). The content of the session may also differ as children display less emotional facial expressions and have more concrete language and thinking as compared to adults (Tinker & Wilson, 1999).

Phase 5: linking to positive cognition. During phase five, the aim is to pair the original target with more adaptive thoughts expressed as the positive cognition. This is done by conducting sets of bilateral stimulation until the thought feels completely true. If the child has not been able to come up with a positive cognition, which is often the case for children younger than age 8 years, the therapist could assist the child in formulating one. For example, a positive cognition could be an expression to enable feeling good about oneself. Storytelling with a happy ending, reframed from the troublesome experience, could be the way to process for a toddler, where the happy ending activates a pleasant or happy feeling, which is again accompanied by bilateral stimulation.

Phase 6: body scan. From the age of 8, youth usually can perform the body scan; this task is usually too difficult for younger children. For these children, the recommendation is to just go on with the installation of the positive cognition until they feel relaxed.

Phase 7: closure. The closure phase may include some playful activity or relaxing procedure. If necessary, the safe place or some other stabilizing method can be employed. Closure may take place with the parent/caregiver being present. The parent / caregiver is also reminded that processing could continue following the session and that the child might show some reactions afterward. So, they are asked to observe the child between the sessions and to notice any changes in behavior or emotion.

Phase 8: reevaluation. Reevaluation is performed together with the caregivers since children may not be fully aware of changes. It is therefore necessary to get feedback from parents in relation to the target memory, which was desensitized and processed during the previous session.

Evidence Base for EMDR

Most treatment studies on EMDR have been conducted in adult populations. In the first study describing the effects of this intervention, Shapiro (1989) demonstrated that traumatic memories could be successfully desensitized in 22 volunteer participants aged 11 to 53 years (M = 37 years) suffering from PTSD. At that time, the method was called eye movement desensitization (EMD) because the procedure was only focused on the desensitization process as effected by the bilateral movements of the eyes. Later the method was renamed EMDR, after noticing the additional, more cognitive restructuring elements of the reprocessing procedure (Shapiro, 2001). Since this initial work, more outcome research was conducted, including a number of randomized controlled trials comparing the efficacy of EMDR in treating PTSD with other evidence-based interventions. The results of these studies have been nicely summarized in the meta-analyses that were described in the introduction of this chapter.

When it comes to the efficacy of EMDR for children and adolescents with PTSD, it should be noted that the evidence base is considerably smaller. Nevertheless, the results of this research are in keeping with the adult literature and demonstrate that EMDR is a feasible and potentially effective treatment option for traumatized youth.

Apart from a number of case studies describing positive experiences with EMDR in traumatized youngsters, a pilot investigation by Oras and colleagues (2004) incorporated an EMDR intervention in traditional psychodynamic therapy for 13 refugee children in Sweden who had developed PTSD due to a variety of severe traumatic experiences (e.g., torture, imprisonment, witnessing family or other people being assaulted or killed). Pre- to posttreatment assessments revealed significant reductions in PTSD symptoms and depression and a clear improvement in global functioning.

Since then, a number of more controlled studies have also been published. For example, Rubin et al. (2001) evaluated the effectiveness of adding EMDR to the usual treatment regimen in 39 child guidance center clients aged 6 to 15 years who displayed emotional and behavioral symptoms related to an experienced trauma. Twenty-three children were allocated to the center's routine intervention package involving individual play therapy, group therapy, and family therapy, plus EMDR, whereas 16 children received only the routine package. The results revealed that in general children with elevated symptom scores at pretest displayed a decline (with a moderate effect size) in internalizing and externalizing symptoms. Most importantly, however, there were no significant differences between both intervention groups, indicating that EMDR had little effect beyond the standard treatment package. However, a similar investigation by Soberman, Greenwald, and Rule (2002) in 29 traumatized boys with conduct problems in residential or day treatment did reveal positive effects of this treatment procedure. The boys were randomized into standard care or standard care plus three trauma-focused EMDR sessions, and it was demonstrated that the EMDR group showed large and significant reduction of memory-related distress and problem behavior, as well as trends toward reduction of post-traumatic symptoms, whereas the control group showed only slight improvement.

In another study, Chemtob, Nakashima, and Carlson (2002) explored the efficacy of EMDR in 32 children aged 6 to 12 years who met the clinical criteria for PTSD after being exposed to a hurricane disaster. Half of the children was immediately treated with three sessions of EMDR (immediate treatment group), while the other half received the intervention after the first group had finished (delayed treatment group). Both groups of children displayed substantial reductions in PTSD, anxiety, and depression symptoms following the EMDR intervention, and these gains were maintained at a six-month follow-up.

Ahmad et al. (2007) conducted a randomized controlled trial with 33 children and adolescents aged between 6 and 16 years with a DSM-IV diagnosis of PTSD in relation to a type I (single trauma such as road accident) or a type II trauma (multiple, repeated trauma such as maltreatment). Youth were randomly assigned to EMDR (maximum 8 weekly sessions) or a wait-list group getting EMDR treatment two months after the pretreatment test. The results indicated that improvement in PTSD-related symptom scores were somewhat more robust in the EMDR group as compared to the wait-list group, although the only statistically significant difference was found for re-experiencing symptoms.

Jaberghaderi, Greenwald, Rubin, Zand, and Dolatabadi (2004) were the first to contrast the effects of EMDR with those of another potentially powerful intervention for youth with PTSD. In this research, 14 Iranian girls aged 12 to 13 years who had been sexually abused were randomized to either EMDR or CBT, with the maximum length of the treatment being 12 sessions. Both interventions produced large improvements in PTSD symptoms and modest improvements in behavioral symptoms. No significant difference in efficacy between the two interventions was found, although the positive change in the EMDR group was produced in fewer sessions than the positive change in the CBT group.

A further comparison between EMDR and CBT was made by De Roos et al. (2011) in a population of 52 children and adolescents aged 4 to 18 years who had been referred to a mental health setting after being exposed to an explosion in a fireworks factory. In both treatment groups, youth received up to four individual treatment sessions along with up to four sessions of parental guidance pre- to posttreatment; follow-up assessments indicated that EMDR and CBT were equally effective in reducing PTSD symptomatology, anxiety, depression, and behavior problems, although again treatment gains of EMDR were reached in fewer sessions.

In another randomized controlled trial by Diehle et al. (2015), 47 youth aged 8 to 18 years who had been exposed to multiple traumas were assigned to eight sessions of either EMDR or TF-CBT. The primary outcome measure was a clinician-administered PTSD scale; on this scale, equally large reductions of symptoms were found in both treatment conditions. On some secondary outcome measures (i.e., comorbid symptoms of depression and hyperactivity), TF-CBT – but not EMDR – produced significant improvement. In this study, no support was found for previous findings (De Roos et al., 2011; Jaberghaderi et al., 2004), suggesting that treatment duration was shorter for EMDR.

A final relevant and large study was recently carried out by De Roos et al. (2017) among 103 children and adolescents aged 8 to 18 years who had been referred to mental health treatment centers after having experienced various types of single-incident traumatic events (i.e., physical abuse / assault, sexual abuse, accident / injury, loss, disaster). Youngsters were randomly allocated to one of three groups: EMDR, cognitive behavioral writing therapy (CBWT), or a wait-list condition. Both treatments were well tolerated and relative to the wait-list condition produced large effects on the primary outcome measure of PTSD symptoms. At posttreatment, 92.5 percent of the participants in the EMDR condition and 90.2 percent of those receiving CBWT no longer met the diagnostic criteria for PTSD. All gains were maintained at a 12-month follow-up. Relative to the wait-list group, other positive treatment effects were noticed for both treatment conditions with regard to negative trauma-related appraisals, anxiety, depression, and behavior problems, and these gains were also maintained at follow-up. Interestingly, again the outcome indicated that gains were accomplished with significantly less therapist contact time for EMDR than for CBWT.

So far, two meta-analyses have been conducted to quantify the efficacy of EMDR in traumatized youth across various empirical studies (Gilles et al., 2016; Rodenburg et al., 2009). Fourteen studies including 758 participants in total were included in Gilles et al., 2016, with symptoms of PTSD, depression, and anxiety as outcome measures. Only two of the included studies had applied EMDR as the studied treatment method. Hence, logically this meta-analysis does not include the most recent outcome studies (e.g., De Roos et al., 2017). Nevertheless, its conclusions remain consistent with the current status of evidence for EMDR among children and adolescents with PTSD. That is, EMDR is not less effective than other interventions including (TF-)CBT in the treatment of PTSD among children and adolescents, although the evidence on which this conclusion is based is so far of fairly low quality. Most of the included studies were rated to be possibly prone to various types of biases (e.g., selection bias, attrition bias). In addition, the number of studies is low and the sample sizes are generally small, interventions were rarely blinded, and methods were not clearly described.

Mechanisms of Action / and Predictors / Moderators of Treatment Response

No clear mechanism of action has been identified for EMDR. However, several theories have been developed to try to explain how this approach is working in practice. Shapiro herself (2001; Solomon & Shapiro, 2008) describes the working mechanism of EMDR in terms of processing the disturbing memory and bringing it to an adaptive resolution. She proposes that this occurs through the integration of adaptive information stored in existing memory networks into the traumatic memory. However, the specific mechanisms by which this occurs are not known (Maxfield, 2008).

Leeds (2016) has provided an overview of the hypothesized mechanisms that may account for the positive effects produced by EMDR. The *orienting response hypothesis* means that an alerting reaction and an investigatory response are activated by a novel stimulus, in this case: the eye movements. The orienting response is suggested to produce a subcortical appraisal in the limbic system (Siegel, 2012) and with the absence of actual danger the alerting response is followed by a de-arousal response in the autonomic system, ultimately leading to an increase in feelings of safety and well-being. In EMDR therapy, this could mean that eye movements prevent avoidance and facilitate continued attention to the traumatic memory, activate emotional processing, and facilitate incorporation of new trauma-relevant information (Armstrong & Vaughan, 1994, 1996).

The *REM analogue hypothesis* (see Stickgold, 2002, 2008) claims that EMDR therapy activates a form of memory processing that is normally sleep dependent.

REM sleep seems to activate more distant memory associations compared with non-REM sleep or during normal waking states. During EMDR therapy, a REM-like state is brought about that permits the integration of traumatic memories into associative cortical networks without interference from hippocampal mediated episodic recall (Stickgold, 2002).

The *inter- and intra-hemispheric activation hypothesis* was initially proposed by Russel (1992). One of the mediators of the information processing during EMDR therapy has been supposed to carry out synchronizing neural activity of both brain hemispheres (Christman et al., 2003; Nieuwenhuis et al., 2013) by means of the bilateral stimulation.

The *mindfulness/prefrontal attentional flexibility/metacognitive awareness hypothesis*, which assumes that the instruction given to the client at the beginning of the EMDR procedure to just notice what comes to mind without evaluating, reflects a way of promoting a state of mindfulness and free association. Further, neurobiological studies have indicated that bilateral eye movements directly contribute to improvement in attentional flexibility and executive functioning central to mindful noticing, coupling the amygdala-anterior cingulate areas with the prefrontal cortex (Keller et al., 2014, Yaggie et al., 2015).

A final hypothesis is that EMDR challenges the *working memory* by creating a dual task: thinking about and imagining the traumatic events while conducting eye movements or engaging in some other bilateral stimulation task. Because the capacity of the working memory is limited, the net effect is that the client is less able to retrieve a vivid memory of the trauma, which makes it more susceptible to emotional change (Engelhard, 2012). Several studies have demonstrated that elements of the working memory hypothesis are consistent with the observed treatment effects of EMDR (Guntner & Bodner, 2008; van den Hout et al., 2001). However, a limitation of these studies is the frequent use of nonclinical subjects who do not meet criteria for PTSD and conditions that do not fully match those used in the standard EMDR therapy protocol.

At present, none of these accounts may provide a sufficient and satisfactory explanation for the mechanism(s) of action operating during EMDR, and so it is important that future research is conducted to clarify this important issue. However, moderating factors should be considered concerning the influence of outcome of treatment response. Degree of dissociation and number of psychiatric comorbidities have been associated with treatment nonresponse (Bae, Kim, & Park, 2016). Other mediators that have been suggested are signs of rigid defenses, such as denial and idealization that might be common in some personality disorders (Mosquera & Knipe, 2015).

Clinical Case Illustration

Ted is a 5-year-old boy whose mother contacted the female therapist by phone and shortly described Ted's traumatic experience and his problems with nightmares, bed-wetting, and refusal to go outside. During the first session, mother presented Ted's developmental history and trauma history without Ted being present. She was asked about the present situation and if the child was safe where he lived now, which was the case. EMDR was considered an option and mother was informed about EMDR therapy and she confirmed her interest in having her son treated in this way. She was also instructed of her role during the sessions, that is, to provide safety for her child but not to intervene in the process unless the therapist invited her to comfort her son or provide some brief information if needed. She was informed that she was allowed to respond to the child if he was seeking her support. The responsibility for the session would be on the therapist. Mother was also asked to keep a log of her observations between the sessions to provide feedback to the therapist over the phone, or briefly at the beginning of the next session.

Ted lived with his mother and two younger sisters (aged 1 and 3 years) in an apartment house with external access balconies. To get downstairs, they had to pass the doors of some neighbors. For a couple of months, Ted has had several symptoms after an upsetting incident with an elderly male neighbor. Ted has had nightmares, wet his bed, and refused to go out. Also, he had been constantly watching over his siblings, expressing concern that they might get hurt. He had been clinging to his mother saying that he was afraid that she might die. In preschool, he had jumped when his teachers had touched him. Mother initially expected that his fears would decline over time, but nothing had improved.

A few days later, Ted and mother met the therapist together. Ted was asked if he knew why they were here and he nodded and said: *He tried to kill me*. The therapist invited Ted to explain what had happened. Ted seemed to feel at ease and with a little help from the mother, he told his story: Outside their house was a playground where a group of children apparently had been teasing the old man a lot and maybe several times. It was unclear if Ted had been part of this at an earlier occasion. However, on this particular day when passing the old man's door on his way out, the door suddenly slashed open and Ted was harshly drawn into the man's apartment. He was brutally pressed against the wall and was told in a very angry voice that he would never be let out unless he told the names of the other boys. Ted was so terrified that he wet his pants.

Ted was uneasy during recalling the incident and was asked to show with his hands how bad he felt when recalling the story. Therapist showed "Just a little" (hands closed together) or "Worst thing in the world" (arms wide open). Ted opened his arms a lot (estimated SUDS = 10). The therapist said she understood that it felt awful and that he might need some help not to have to think about that all the time, but that they first were going to do some exercises to help find a good feeling.

Safe place exercise

THERAPIST:	*Tell me about a place where you feel safe and secure and your body feels really good.*
TED:	*The sofa looking at TV.*
THERAPIST:	*Alone or with someone else?*
TED:	*Mum, and my sisters, and Harry (the dog).*
THERAPIST:	*That sounds nice. Is it OK if I tap on your hands while you think about the sofa and your siblings and Harry?*

TED:	*Yes.*
	The therapist gives a small number of alternating taps on Ted's left and right hand.
THERAPIST:	*How is your body now?*
TED:	*Good.*
THERAPIST:	*Can you hear any sounds?*
TED:	*Swamp Bob on TV.*
	The Installation of the safe place continues until Ted is content and relaxed. Ted and the therapist give his experience the name "The Safe place" or "The Sofa."
THERAPIST:	*This is like a place in your head that you can go to when things feel just too bad.*
	Since Ted seems curious and cooperates well, the therapist decides to continue processing the bad experience.
THERAPIST:	*Shall we see if we also can make your bad memory a little less scary?*
	Ted nods.
THERAPIST:	*We will do it about the same way as with the sofa but this time I first need you to begin with thinking about what happened. Do you want to draw it on a paper or can you see it in your head?*
	Ted says he sees it in his head.
THERAPIST:	*Is it like a picture? Some kids tell me it is like a film going over and over again. How is it for you?*
TED:	*I see the picture.*
THERAPIST:	*What is the worst part in that picture?*
TED:	*That he is going to kill me.*
THERAPIST:	*Well, you are alive now. Do you want mum to move over to you?* (Mother moves to sit beside him.)
	Therapist asks mother if the man is still a neighbor.
MOTHER:	*No, he moved several weeks ago, and he is actually sorry for what he did.*
THERAPIST:	*So, it is over now?*
MOTHER:	*Yes. He does not dare to come back!!*
THERAPIST:	*You seem to be a strong mum that would protect your child.*
THERAPIST (TO TED):	*If you need to pause you just do like this* (therapist shows a stop sign with her hand).
	Ted, however, never uses the stop sign for having a break but instead for stopping the tapping when he is eager to tell something.
THERAPIST:	*Now, when you look at the picture in your head and believe he is going to kill you* (negative cognition) *what would you rather think than that he is going to kill you? What good thought would you rather like to have?*
TED:	*I should not have gone out that day!*

THERAPIST:	The therapist decides to leave out the positive cognition not to stress Ted and will get back to it later.
THERAPIST:	*So, look at the picture and remember the words "he is going to kill me." Show me how bad it feels to think about it.*
	Ted shows his hands wide apart.
THERAPIST:	*Where do you feel it in your body?*
	Ted clenches his fists.
THERAPIST:	*OK. Look at the picture, think, "he is going to kill me" and feel how hard you clench your hands, and I will tap on your knees.*

Therapist taps around 15 double taps in each set unless Ted makes the stop sign because he needs to tell something. His associations, both facts and wishes, go from being stuck to being able to move, from helplessness to power, in different scenarios. Quite soon he remembers being let out running back into his own apartment, calling for mum and for protection.

Ted likes using the sign of the hands and spontaneously shows SUDS "ratings" during the processing until he claps his hands together (SUDS = 0). When therapist asks for the SUDS in relation to the incident she just refers to *"thinking of the old man, how scary is it now?"* After rechecking the SUDS, the therapist constructs a positive cognition *"I am safe now"* from the previous discussion and installs it by means of taps.

The validity of the positive cognition, VOC, is left out because it is too complicated for Ted to understand.

At the next session, Ted was cheerful and told the therapist that he had had no nightmares during the week. He was still a little uneasy in his body when thinking of the old man. He was happy to continue with the tapping and the uneasiness resolved very quickly.

To ensure adequate processing of the trauma, the therapist asked Ted about other scary situations to help him make additional mental connections. This was performed since young children have not developed associative channels between different memories as much as adults usually have.

THERAPIST:	*Think of another time when you were so scared that you thought you would die!*
	Ted remembered when he was small and was afraid of a water puddle because he thought he could drown in it. This memory was successfully processed.

At follow-up Ted again indicated some mild uneasiness, which he demonstrated by forming a ring with his thumb and his index finger. After a couple of additional sets of tapping, he covered the middle of the ring with modeling clay, which he showed the therapist, indicating that the uneasiness was now totally gone. Ted was, like many children, hungry, thirsty, and tired after a session but very proud of what he had accomplished.

EMDR for Other DSM-5 Disorders

The latest edition of the *Diagnostic and Statistical Manual of Mental Disorders* (DSM-5; American Psychiatric Association, 2013) lists besides PTSD several clinical conditions in the section named "Trauma and Stressor-Related Disorders" (American Psychiatric Association, 2013) that might be possible indications for a treatment with EMDR, as they are also based on aversive, threatening, or stressful life experiences. First of all, *disinhibited social engagement* and *reactive attachment disorder* both have to do with dysregulated attachment patterns being caused by a lack of appropriate caregiving during childhood (American Psychiatric Association, 2013). There is some preliminary evidence from case studies that EMDR may be a promising treatment for these disorders (Wesselmann, 2012), but obviously controlled treatment outcome research is needed to enlarge the evidence base.

Adjustment disorder is another type of psychopathology for which EMDR could certainly be a suitable intervention, especially because EMDR has been shown to achieve treatment effects within a relatively short period of time. A couple of studies have already indicated that EMDR is more effective than behavioral therapy in the treatment of adjustment disorder in adults (Mihelich, 2000; Oppermann-Schmid, 2014), but no research can be found regarding its effective application in children suffering from this condition.

Since its introduction, EMDR has also been advanced as a treatment for anxiety disorders (e.g., De Jongh, Ten Broeke, & Renssen, 1999). Although positive effects have been documented, the main conclusion of the research so far is that EMDR is less effective than exposure-based behavioral therapy in treating most phobias. However, due to the shortage of controlled outcome research and the limitations in existing studies, the relative efficacy of EMDR for the treatment of anxiety disorders remains to be answered (De Jongh & Ten Broeke, 2009). Exceptions might be those phobias that are clearly trauma based, or based on a clear-cut aversive learning experience (e.g., travel phobia; De Jongh et al., 2011; emetophobia (vomiting phobia), medical phobias; De Jongh, 2012).

Challenges and Recommendations for Future Research in These Areas

The guidelines of the World Health Organization (World Health Organization, 2013) for treatment of trauma-related conditions found EMDR therapy and TF-CBT as the two most efficacious PTSD treatments. This means that compared to other treatment approaches such as pharmacotherapy and non-trauma-focused interventions, EMDR and TF-CBT interventions have been identified as more effective in reducing PTSD symptomatology (Bisson 2013; Seidler & Wagner 2006, Department of Veterans Affairs & Department of Defense, 2017). However, it should be noted that this conclusion is largely based on studies of relatively moderate to low quality, suggesting that more rigorous research is needed. In addition, the efficacy of EMDR in participants with more complex symptom presentations requires more investigation (Ehring et al., 2014; Spinazzola, Blaustein, and Van der Kolk, 2005). Further, as this chapter has made clear, more controlled studies on the EMDR treatment of children and adolescents with PTSD should be conducted, preferably with larger samples with a representative age and gender distribution. Also, the role for EMDR needs to be explored further, provided in either an individual or group format, as an intervention for people in emergency situations (Buydens, 2014; Luber, 2015). Some examples can already be found of EMDR being used in the aftermath of crises and catastrophes for helping adults as well as children and adolescents (e.g., Acaturk et al., 2016; Artigas et al., 2009; Brown et al., 2017; Fernandez et al., 2007; Saltini et al., 2017; Tang, Yang, Yen, & Liu, 2015; Zaghrout-Hodali, Alissa, & Dodgson, 2008).

Guidelines for Training in EMDR

A clinical background is necessary for the effective application of EMDR. Attendance at trainings is limited to licensed mental health professionals whose qualifications are recognized in the country in which they reside. Exact entry requirements differ slightly from country to country. Participants are encouraged to start practicing EMDR with clients right after training. However, to ensure ethically sound and robust clinical practice, to enhance treatment fidelity, and to maximize and enhance client / patient protection and quality control, standards for a practitioner accreditation procedure have been set by EMDR membership associations. In addition, the accreditation standards are considered to substantially assist research fidelity.

Key Practice Points and Recommended Resources for Practice

- EMDR therapy seems to be an effective and time-saving therapeutic method for the treatment of PTSD and other conditions caused by adverse life events.
- Especially children suffering from war and terror experiences could benefit from EMDR treatment. EMDR needs to be properly implemented in the mental health system making use of facilitators well trained in providing this treatment method.
- Given its potential use in crisis situations all over the world, it may be needed to develop culturally adapted EMDR treatment protocols.
- More high-quality research is required on the efficacy and effectiveness of EMDR, particularly in children and adolescents exposed to war and catastrophes, attachment trauma, early childhood abuse, and adverse medical conditions.

References

Acarturk, C., Konuk, E., Cetinkaya, M., Senay, I., Sijbrandij, M., Gulen, B., & Cuijpers, P. (2016). The efficacy of eye movement desensitization and reprocessing for post-traumatic stress disorder and depression among Syrian refugees: Results of a randomized controlled trial. *Psychological Medicine, 46*(12), 2583–2593.

Adler-Tapia, R., & Settle, C. (2016). *EMDR and the art of psychotherapy with children: Infants to adolescents treatment manual* (2nd edn.). New York: Springer.

Ahmad, A., Larsson, B., & Sundelin-Wahlsten, V. (2007). EMDR treatment for children with PTSD: Results of a randomised controlled trial. *Nordic Journal of Psychiatry, 61*(5), 349–354.

Ahmad, A., & Sundelin-Wahlsten, V. (2008). Applying EMDR on children with PTSD. *European Journal of Child and Adolescent Psychiatry, 17*(3), 127–132.

American Psychiatric Association. (2013). *Diagnostic and statistical manual of mental disorders* (5th ed). Arlington, VA: Author.

Andrade, J., Kavanagh, D., & Baddeley, A. (1997). Eye-movements and visual imagery: A working memory approach to the treatment of post-traumatic stress disorder. *British Journal of Clinical Psychology, 36*, 209–223.

Armstrong, N., & Vaughan, K. (1994, June). An orienting response model for EMDR. Paper presented at the meeting of the New South Wales Behaviour Therapy Interest Group, Sydney, Australia.

Armstrong, M. S., & Vaughan, K. (1996). An orienting response model of eye movement desensitization. *Journal of Behavior Therapy and Experimental Psychiatry, 27*, 21–32.

Artigas, L., Jarero, I., Alcalá, N., & López Cano, T. (2009). The EMDR integrative group treatment protocol (IGTP). In M. Luber (ed.), *Eye movement desensitization and reprocessing (EMDR) scripted protocols: Basic and special situations* (pp. 279–288). New York: Springer.

Bae, H., Kim, D., & Park, Y. C. (2016). Dissociation predicts treatment response in eye-movement desensitization and reprocessing for posttraumatic stress disorder. *Journal of Trauma and Dissociation, 17*(1), 112–119. doi:10.1080/15299732.2015.1037039

Bisson, J., Cosgrove, S., Lewis, C., & Robert, N. (2015). Post-traumatic stress disorder. *British Medical Journal, 351*, h6161. doi:10.1136/bmj.h6161

Bisson, J., Roberts, N., Andrew, M., & Cooper, R. (2013). Psychological therapies for chronic post-traumatic stress disorder (PTSD) in adults. *Cochrane Database of Systematic Reviews, 12*, CD003388. doi:10.1002/14651858.CD003388.pub4.

Brown, R. C., Witt, A., Fegert, J. M., Keller, F., Rassenhofer, M., & Plener, P. L. (2017). Psychosocial interventions for children and adolescents after man-made and natural disasters: A meta-analysis and systematic review. *Psychological Medicine, 47*(11), 1893–1905. doi:10.1017/S0033291717000496

Buydens, S. L., Wilensky, M., & Hensley, B. J. (2014). Effects of the EMDR protocol for recent traumatic events on acute stress disorder. *Journal of EMDR Practice and Research, 8*(1), 2–12.

Chemtob, C. M., Nakashima, J., & Carlson, J. G. (2002). Brief treatment for elementary school children with disaster-related posttraumatic stress disorder: A field study. *Journal of Clinical Psychology, 58*, 99–112. http://dx.doi.org/10.1002/jclp.1131; PMID: 11748599

Chen, L., Zhang, G., Hu, M., & Liang, X. (2015) Eye movement desensitization and reprocessing versus cognitive-behavioral therapy for adult posttraumatic stress disorder: Systematic review and meta-analysis. *Journal of Nervous Mental Disorders, 203*(6), 443–451. doi:10.1097/NMD.0000000000000306

Christman, S. D., Garvey, K. J., Propper, R. E., & Phaneuf, K. A. (2003). Bilateral eye movements enhance the retrieval of episodic memories. *Neuropsychology, 17*(2), 221–229.

Cusack, K., Jonas, D. E., Forneris, C. A., Wines, C., Sonis, J., Middleton, J. C., ... Gaynes, B. N. (2015). Psychological treatments for adults with posttraumatic stress disorder: A systematic review and meta-analysis. *Clinical Psychology Review, 43*, 128–141. doi:10.1016/j.cpr.2015.10.003

Department of Veterans Affairs & Department of Defense. (2017). *Clinical practice guideline for the management of posttraumatic stress disorder and acute stress disorder.* Washington, DC: Veterans Health Administration.

de Jongh, A. D. (2012). Treatment of a woman with emetophobia: A trauma focused approach. *Mental Illness, 4*(1), 10–14. doi:10.4081/mi.2012.e3

de Jongh, A., Holmshaw, M., Carswell, W., & van Wijk, A. (2011). Usefulness of a trauma-focused treatment approach for travel phobia. *Clinical Psychology and Psychotherapy, 18*(2), 124–137. doi:10.1002/cpp.680

de Jongh, A., & Ten Broeke, E. (2009). EMDR and the anxiety disorders: Exploring the current status. *Journal of EMDR Practice and Research, 3*(3), 133–140. doi:10.1891/1933-3196.3.3.133

de Jongh, A., Ten Broeke, E., & Renssen, M. R. (1999). Treatment of specific phobias with eye movement desensitization and reprocessing (EMDR). *Journal of Anxiety Disorders, 13*(1), 69–85. doi:10.1016/S0887-6185(98)00040-1

de Roos, C., van der Oord, S., Zijlstra, B., Lucassen, S., Perrin, S., Emmelkamp, P., & de Jongh, A. (2017). Comparison of eye movement desensitization and reprocessing therapy, cognitive behavioral writing therapy, and wait-list in pediatric posttraumatic stress disorder following single-incident trauma: A multicenter randomized clinical trial. *Journal of Child Psychology and Psychiatry,* 58(11), 1219–1228. doi: 10.1111/jcpp.12768. [Epub ahead of print].

de Roos, C., Greenwald, R., den Hollander-Gijsman, M., Noorthoorn, E., van Buuren, S., & de Jongh, A. (2011). A randomised comparison of cognitive behavioural therapy (CBT) and eye movement desensitisation and reprocessing (EMDR) in disaster-exposed children. *European Journal of Psychotraumatology,* 2. doi:10.3402/ejpt.v2i0.5694.

Diehle, J., Opmeer, B. C., Boer, F., Mannarino, A. P., & Lindauer, R. J. L. (2015). Trauma-focused cognitive behavioral therapy or eye movement desensitization and reprocessing: What works in children with posttraumatic stress symptoms? A randomized controlled trial. *European Child & Adolescent Psychiatry, 24*(2), 227–236. doi:10.1007/s00787-014-0572-5

Ehring, T., Welboren, R., Morina, N., Wicherts, J.M., Freitag, J., & Emmelkamp, P.M.G. (2014). Meta-analysis of psychological treatments for posttraumatic stress disorder in adult survivors of childhood abuse. *Clinical Psychological Review, 34*(8), 645–657. doi:10.1016/j.cpr.2014.10.004

Engelhard, I. M. (2012). Making science work in mental health care. *European Journal of Psychotraumatology,* 3. doi:10.3402/ejpt.v3i0.18740

Fernandez, I. (2007). EMDR as treatment of post-traumatic reactions: A field study on child victims of an earthquake. *Educational Child Psychology, 24*, 65–94.

Gillies, D., Maiocchi, L., Bhandari, A. P., Taylor, F., Gray, C., & O'Brien, L. (2016). Psychological therapies for children and adolescents exposed to trauma. *Cochrane Library*. doi:10.1002/146541858.CD012371.

Gomez, A. (2012). *EMDR therapy and adjunct approaches with children: Complex trauma, attachment, and dissociation* (1st edn.). New York: Springer Publishing Company.

Gunter, R. W., & Bodner, G. E. (2008). How eye movements affect unpleasant memories: Support for a working-memory account. *Behaviour Research and Therapy, 46*(8), 913–931. doi:10.1016/j.brat.2008.04.006

Jaberghaderi, N., Greenwald, R., Rubin, A., Zand, S. O., & Dolatabadi, S. (2004). A comparison of CBT and EMDR for sexually-abused Iranian girls. *Clinical Psychology & Psychotherapy, 11*(5), 358–368. doi:10.1002/cpp.395

Keller, B., Stevens, L., Lui, C., Murray, J., & Yaggie, M. (2014). The effects of bilateral eye movements on EEG coherence when recalling a pleasant memory. *Journal of EMDR Practice and Research, 8*(3), 113–128. doi:10.1891/1933–3196.8.3.113

Leeds, A. (2016). *A Guide to the Standard EMDR Therapy Protocols for Clinicians, Supervisors and Consultants* (2nd edn., chap. 2, pp. 28–48). New York: Springer Publishing Company.

Luber, M. (2015). *EMDR therapy and emergency response.* New York: Springer Publishing Company.

Maxfield, L., Melnyk, W. T., & Hayman, G. C. A. (2008). A working memory explanation for the effects of eye movements in EMDR. *Journal of EMDR Practice and Research, 2*(4), 247–261. doi:10.1891/1933–3196.2.4.247

Mihelich, M. L. (2000) Eye movement desensitization and reprocessing treatment of adjustment disorder. *Dissertation Abstracts International: Section B: The Sciences and Engineering, 61*(2-B), 1091.

Morris-Smith, J. A., & Silvestre, M. (2014). *EMDR for the next generation: Healing children and families.* Reading, UK: Academic Conferences and Publishing International Limited. ISBN:978–1-909507–92-0

Mosquera, D., & Knipe, J. (2015). Understanding and treating narcissism with EMDR therapy. *Journal of EMDR Practice and Research, 9*(1), 46–63. doi.org/10.1891/1933–3196.9.1.46

Nieuwenhuis, S., Elzinga, B. M., Ras, P. H., Berends, F., Duijs, P., Samara, Z., & Slagter, H. A. (2013) Bilateral saccadic eye movements and tactile stimulation, but not auditory stimulation, enhance memory retrieval. *Brain and Cognition, 81*(1), 52–56.

Oppermann-Schmid, F. (2014). EMDR with adjustment disorder. In EMDR research symposium (France Haour, Chair). Symposium presented at the 15th EMDR Europe Association Conference, Edinburgh, Scotland.

Oras, R., de Ezbeleta, S. C., & Ahmad, A. (2004) Treatment of traumatised refugee children with eye movement desensitization and reprocessing in a psychodynamic context. *Nordic Journal of Psychiatry, 51*(3), 199–203.

Pfefferbaum, B., Sweeton, J. L., Newman, E., Varma, V., Nitiéma, P., Shaw, J. A., ... Noffsinger, M. A. (2014) Child disaster mental health interventions, part I: Techniques, outcomes, and methodological considerations. *Disaster Health 2*(1), 46–57.

Power, K., Keith Brown, T. M., Buchanan, R., Sharp, D., Swanson, V., & Karatzias, A. (2002). A controlled comparison of eye movement desensitization and reprocessing versus exposure plus cognitive restructuring versus waiting list in the treatment of post-traumatic stress disorder. *Clinical Psychology and Psychotherapy*, *9*(5), 299–318.

Powers, M. B., Halpern, J. M., Ferenschak, M. P., Gillihan, S. J., & Foa, E. B. (2010). A meta-analytic review of prolonged exposure for posttraumatic stress disorder. *Clinical Psychological Review*, *30*(6), 635–641. doi:10.1016/j.cpr.2010.04.007

Rodenburg, R., Benjamin, A., de Roos, C., Meijer, A. M., & Stams, G. J. (2009). Efficacy of EMDR in children: A meta-analysis. *Clinical Psychology Review*, *29*(7), 599–606. doi:10.1016/j.cpr.2009.06.008

Rothbaum, B. O., Astin, M. C., & Marsteller, F. (2005). Prolonged exposure versus eye movement desensitization and reprocessing (EMDR) for PTSD rape victims. *Journal of Traumatic Stress*, *18*(6), 607–616. doi:10.1002/jts.20069

Rubin, A., Bischofshausen, S., Conroy-Moore, K., Dennis, B., Hastie, M., Melnick, L., ... Smith, T. (2001). The effectiveness of EMDR in a child guidance center. *Research on Social Work Practice*, *11*(4), 435–457. doi:10.1177/104973150101100402

Russell, M. C. (1992). *Towards a neuropsychological approach to PTSD: An integrative conceptualization of etiology and mechanisms of therapeutic change*. Unpublished doctoral dissertation, Pacific Graduate School of Psychology, Palo Alto, CA.

Saltini, A., Rebecchi, D., Callerame, C., Fernandez, I., Bergonzini, E., & Starace, F. (2017). Early eye movement desensitisation and reprocessing (EMDR) intervention in a disaster mental health care context. *Psychology, Health and Medicine*, 23, 285–294. doi:10.1080/13548506.2017.1344255

Seidler, G. H., & Wagner, F. E. (2006) Comparing the efficacy of EMDR and trauma-focused cognitive-behavioral therapy in the treatment of PTSD: A meta-analytic study. *Psychological Medicine*, *36*(11), 1515–1522. doi:10.1017/S0033291706007963.

Shapiro, F. (1989). Efficacy of the eye movement desensitization procedure in the treatment of traumatic memories. *Journal of Traumatic Stress Studies*, *2*, 199–223.

Shapiro, F. (2001). *Eye movement desensitization and reprocessing, basic principles, protocols and procedures* (2nd edn.). New York: The Guilford Press.

Siegel, D. J. (2012). *The developing mind: How relationships and the brain interact to shape who we are* (2nd edn.). New York: The Guilford Press.

Soberman, G. B., Greenwald, R., & Rule, D. L. (2002). A controlled study of eye movement desensitization and reprocessing (EMDR) for boys with conduct problem. *Journal of Aggression, Maltreatment and Trauma*, *6*(1), 217–236. doi:10.1300/J146v06n01_11

Solomon, R. M., & Shapiro, F. (2008). EMDR and the Adaptive Information Processing Model. *Journal of EMDR Practice and Research*, *2*(4), 315–325.

Spinazzola, J., Blaustein, M., & van der Kolk, B. A. (2005) Posttraumatic stress disorder treatment outcome research: The study of unrepresentative samples? *Journal of Traumatic Stress*, *18*(5), 425–436. doi:10.1002/jts.20050.

Stickgold, R. (2002). EMDR: A putative neurobiological mechanism of action. *Journal of Clinical Psychology*, *58*(1), 61–75. doi:10.1002/jclp.1129.

Stickgold, R. (2008). Sleep-dependent memory processing and EMDR action. *Journal of EMDR Practice and Research*, *2*(4), 289–299. doi:10.1891/1933-3196.2.4.289

Tinker, R., & Wilson, S. (1999). *Through the eyes of a child*. New York: Norton & Co.

Tang, T. C., Yang, P., Yen, C. F., & Liu, T. L. (2015). Eye movement desensitization and reprocessing for treating psychological disturbances in Taiwanese adolescents who experienced Typhoon Morakot. *Kaohsiung Journal of Medical Sciences*, *31*(7), 363–369. doi:10.1016/j.kjms.2015.04.013

van den Hout, M., Muris, P., Salemink, E., & Kindt, M. (2001). Autobiographical memories become less vivid and emotional after eye movements. *British Journal of Clinical Psychology, 40*(Pt. 2), 121–130.

Watts, B. V., Schnurr, P. P., Mayo, L., Young-Xu, Y., Weeks, W. B., & Friedman, M. J. (2013). Meta-analysis of the efficacy of treatments for posttraumatic stress disorder. *Journal of Clinical Psychiatry, 74*(6), 541–550. doi:10.4088/JCP.12r08225

Wesselmann, D., Davidson, M., Armstrong, S., Schweitzer, C., Bruckner, D., & Potter, A. E. (2012). EMDR as a treatment for improving attachment status in adults and children. *European Review of Applied Psychology, 62*(4), 223–230.

World Health Organization. (2013). *Guidelines for the management of conditions specifically related to stress.* Geneva: WHO.

Yaggie, M., Stevens, L., Miller, S., Abbott, A., Woodruff, C., Getchis, M., . . . Daiss, S. (2015). Electroencephalography coherence, memory vividness, and emotional valence effects of bilateral eye movements during unpleasant memory recall and subsequent free association: Implications for eye movement desensitization and reprocessing. *Journal of EMDR Practice and Research, 9*(2), 78–97. doi:10.1891/1933-3196.9.2.78.

Zaghrout-Hodali, M., Alissa, F., & Dodgson, W. (2008). Building resilience and dismantling fear: EMDR group protocol with children in an area of ongoing trauma. *Journal of EMDR Practice and Research, 2*(2), 106–113. doi:10.1891/1933-3196.2.2.106

29 Innovation in Early Trauma Treatment

The Child and Family Traumatic Stress Intervention (CFTSI)

Steven Marans, Carrie Epstein, Hilary Hahn, and Megan Goslin

Introduction

Childhood trauma constitutes a major public health issue that affects the lives of millions of children every year (Finkelhor, Turner, Shattuck, Hamby, & Kracke, 2015; Listenbee et al., 2012). When unrecognized and untreated, children who are traumatically overwhelmed by unanticipated experiences of violence, including interpersonal trauma, child abuse, accidental injury, chronic illness or injury, or natural or human-made disasters are at high risk for failures of recovery that result in PTSD and other trauma-related, long-term disorders (Briggs, Nooner, & Amaya-Jackson, 2014; Carlson & Dalenberg, 2000). The poor outcomes that follow failures of recovery from traumatic dysregulation include chronic PTSD, depressive and anxiety disorders, academic difficulties, alcohol and drug abuse, delinquency, difficulties with intimate relationships, perpetration of and victimization by interpersonal violence, and personality disorders, as well as increasing risk for serious medical conditions including ischemic heart and chronic pulmonary diseases (Anda et al., 2006; Felitti et al., 1998; Foa & Meadows, 1997; Marans, 2013; Southwick & Charney, 2012). Additionally, the children who are most vulnerable to these long-term, post-traumatic sequelae are those who have experienced multiple types of potentially traumatizing events during their young lives (Anda et al., 2006; Schalinski et al., 2016)

Several risk factors can heighten the severity of early post-traumatic reactions and predict long-term outcomes, including preexisting developmental and mental health difficulties, history of traumatic exposure and other adverse events, and physical and emotional proximity to the index event. Identifying when children are traumatized, increasing communication between traumatized children and their caregivers, and decreasing symptomatology are central protective factors in reducing suffering and decreasing the likelihood of developing longer-term post-traumatic disorders (Ozer, Best, Lipsey, & Weiss, 2003; Trickey, Siddaway, Meiser-Stedman, Serpell, & Field, 2012). When children are alone and do not have words to describe their traumatic reactions, symptomatic behavior may be their only means of expression. When the capacity to regulate is traumatically compromised, children become particularly reliant on caregivers to help recognize and articulate their post-traumatic experience.

This is complicated when caregivers are unable to recognize the links between recent distressing events and the new or increased symptoms they may observe in their children. Furthermore, this task may be especially complicated when caregivers themselves are traumatically impacted (Gewirtz, Forgatch, & Wieling, 2008; Scheeringa & Zeanah, 2001). Caregivers may require education, support, and practical skills to optimize their ability to support their traumatized children, as well as the opportunity to receive their own trauma-focused treatment, when indicated.

The urgent need to improve and increase early identification of children impacted by trauma, as well as the initiation of early interventions that can support recovery, is demonstrated in the sheer numbers of traumatized children whose lives and developmental potentials may be derailed when their acute symptomatic experiences are not recognized or addressed by caregivers. While there are well-established trauma-focused treatments for children who have developed chronic PTSD and related disorders (Dorsey, Briggs, & Woods, 2011; Gillies et al., 2016), the Child and Family Traumatic Stress Intervention (CFTSI) is currently the only evidence-based treatment that addresses the clinical phenomena and challenges that children and caregivers face during the peri-traumatic phase (up to 90 days) that follows the experience of unanticipated, overwhelming events (Leenarts, Diehle, Doreleijers, Jansma, & Lindauer, 2013).

Overview of the Issue – The Need for Innovation

The traumatic situation is one in which there is a sudden, unanticipated realization of the worst of our shared human fears / dangers. According to the fifth edition of the *Diagnostic and Statistical Manual of Mental Disorders* (DSM-5), a traumatic experience is a situation in which a person directly experiences, witnesses, or learns about an event that involves actual or threatened death, serious injury, or sexual violence. The unanticipated nature of these confrontations immobilizes the individual's usual methods for decreasing danger and anxiety, leaving the traumatized individual frozen, out of control, and helpless. In these circumstances, there is a significant interruption of the reciprocal interaction between the prefrontal cortex and amygdala leading to compromises in a traumatized individual's capacities to maintain a balance between executive functioning and affective regulation (Maren & Holmes, 2016; Southwick & Charney, 2012). As a result, affected individuals are far less able to control emotional, cognitive, somatic, and behavioral responses to overwhelming levels of stimulation. Symptoms develop in the following four categories: (1) re-experiencing, (2) avoidance, (3) hyperarousal, and 4) cognitive distortions.

Post-traumatic reactions occur in three phases following precipitating events: the acute phase, the peri-traumatic phase, and the longer-term phase. Each phase is defined by specific characteristics of timing and of post-traumatic reactions that serve as a clinical roadmap in determining the optimal intervention strategies. The acute phase of trauma response occurs within moments to the first 24 to 36 hours and is characterized by acute traumatic disruption of affective, cognitive, somatic, and behavioral regulation, which contributes to an experience of loss of control, helplessness, and suffering. Typical acute reactions often seen in children are emotional numbing or lability; disorganized thinking and attention; somatic responses (including increased heart rate, fast respiratory rate, physical discomfort); and sometimes either agitated, hyper-motor activity or passive, withdrawn presentation. These reactions are often exacerbated by the upheaval in routines of daily life that frequently continue well beyond the conclusion of the original threat to safety and well-being. The clinical phenomena of this phase suggest intervention strategies focused on identification of those at risk, stabilization, and assessment and triage of additional services and assistance.

The peri-traumatic phase refers to the days and weeks following a traumatic event. In this period, symptoms persist, but dysregulation is demonstrated through a more organized presentation of symptoms. Peri-traumatic symptoms reflect a child's continued vulnerability to dysregulation, as well as their unconscious attempts to reverse the feelings of helplessness created by the traumatic experience and to regain a sense of control. These peri-traumatic symptoms result in high costs to the child. For example, intrusive thoughts and somatic hyperarousal can significantly interfere with sleeping and eating, academic performance, relationships with family and peers, and extracurricular activities, thus depleting the child's sense of competence and mastery that is so central to progressive development. Similarly, the child's depressive withdrawal and irritability can prevent them from receiving the social support that is so critical to recovery.

There are additional high costs to the child. Traumatic reminders of original overwhelming events can trigger symptoms such as hyperarousal and can lead to avoidance of activities and settings in an effort to assert protective action long after the original danger is no longer present. Similarly, opposition to demands of parents and other adults in positions of authority may serve, as other symptoms do, to reverse the experience of passivity that is a fundamental part of the child's traumatic loss of control. However, the child's original traumatic experience is, in fact, perpetuated in the persistence of post-traumatic symptoms and in the impact they have on areas of functioning that are so central to general feelings of competence, mastery, and well-being. Children's difficulties in recognizing their symptoms and traumatic origins, as well as identifying traumatic reminders, can significantly contribute to this experience (Marans, 2013; Pynoos, Steinberg, & Piacentini, 1999; Southwick & Charney, 2012).

In addition to the suffering and immediate costs of the peri-traumatic phase, this failure of recovery greatly increases the likelihood of long-term post-traumatic disorders (Epstein, Hahn, Berkowitz, & Marans, 2017; Ozer et al., 2003). For these reasons, the peri-traumatic phase is a critical time in which to capitalize on what is known about risk and protective factors in order to intervene and support recovery. The clinical phenomena of the peri-traumatic phase suggest intervention strategies focused on reestablishing structure and predictability in daily living, increasing communication, and mastering control over symptoms before they become entrenched and develop into established traumatic stress disorders. While there are well-established, evidence-based clinical interventions that address the long-term phase of post-traumatic reactions, until more recently, no evidence-based treatment models addressed the challenges and opportunities presented by the peri-traumatic phase. CFTSI was developed in recognition of both the challenges and the opportunities.

The longer-term phase of trauma response refers to the months following a traumatic event and reflects failures of recovery in earlier phases. In this phase, trauma symptoms have become chronic, significantly impacting the individual's development, impairing established modes of functioning, often with profound impact on personality organization that can result in deficits in adaptive capacities. The long-term phase marks the period in which PTSD and related disorders are diagnosed. For the purposes of this chapter, we focus on peri-traumatic phase phenomena as the context for the development of the CFTSI.

CFTSI: Procedure and Implementation

CFTSI is a treatment model with proven effectiveness in reducing traumatic stress symptoms and reducing or interrupting PTSD and related disorders (Berkowitz, Stover, & Marans, 2011), which was developed specifically for implementation with children, adolescents, and their caregivers during the peri-traumatic period and early phase of PTSD of trauma response, soon after a potentially traumatic event or the recent formal disclosure of physical or sexual abuse (such as in a forensic interview). CFTSI focuses on increasing caregiver support of the child by enhancing communication between the child and caregiver about the child's trauma symptoms, and providing strategies to help children and families master trauma reactions. In addition, CFTSI improves screening and initial assessment of children impacted by traumatic stress, offers an opportunity to assess the child's needs, and seamlessly introduces longer-term treatment when indicated. CFTSI is a manualized treatment (Berkowitz, Epstein, & Marans, 2012) that is accompanied by a standardized training protocol. Treatment applications of CFTSI for young children aged 3 to 6 years (Marans, Epstein, & Berkowitz, 2014), as well as for children recently placed in foster care (Epstein, Marans, & Berkowitz, 2013) have also been developed. CFTSI is listed in US Substance Abuse and Mental Health Services Administration's (SAMHSA) National Registry of Evidence-based Programs and Practices (NREPP), as well as in the California Evidence-Based Clearinghouse for Child Welfare.

Use of Standardized Assessment Tools as Part of the Clinical Intervention

CFTSI was developed as a structured and predictable treatment that offers strategies to help the child and caregiver gain mastery and control in the peri-traumatic phase of post-traumatic reactions. The CFTSI model uses standardized clinical assessment instruments as clinical tools to facilitate focused clinical dialogues that help increase the child's and caregiver's recognition of and communication about symptoms. In addition, the model employs well-established, developmentally informed cognitive behavioral strategies to help decrease identified affective, somatic, cognitive, and behavioral symptoms. These cognitive behavioral techniques can be especially effective in reducing distorted and inaccurate thoughts (self-blame, distorted self-image, and continued anticipation of danger) that often follow traumatic events and contribute to a host of other symptoms. Their aim is to increase children's conscious awareness of these distortions so that they can view challenging situations more clearly and respond in more helpful and effective ways.

The use of structured clinical assessments throughout the CFTSI treatment offers opportunities to support the child, caregiver, and CFTSI clinician in their efforts to regularly discuss and systematically monitor the course of symptoms, as well as the effectiveness of the cognitive behavioral strategies. In this way, CFTSI provides order and predictability for the child by replacing chaotic post-traumatic experience with structure, words, and an opportunity to be heard by the caregiver, their primary source of support.

CFTSI Screening Process

To determine if a child could benefit from CFTSI, a clinician administers a brief standardized trauma symptom assessment instrument, the Child Post-traumatic Stress Symptoms Scale (CPSS; Foa, Johnson, Feeny, & Treadwell, 2001) with the child's primary caregiver (or caregivers), as well as separately with the child to screen for trauma symptoms. This is done as part of a clinical interview, and not as a self-report process. During the peri-traumatic phase, the level of trauma symptomatology in children can be widely varied. For that reason, and because CFTSI is an early trauma-focused treatment, if either the child or the caregiver reports one new trauma symptom or an increase in a preexisting trauma symptom following the recent traumatic event, CFTSI may be an appropriate treatment for that child. The non-offending caregiver's full participation in the CFTSI treatment is essential to meet CFTSI clinical goals, and this is elaborated next.

Session 1: Meeting with Caregiver

During the first session of CFTSI, the clinician meets alone with the primary caregiver and begins by providing education about the phenomena of trauma and trauma symptoms, as well as the impact of traumatic experiences on children. As part of this discussion, the clinician has an opportunity to explain and discuss key elements of trauma phenomena as well as the ways in which symptomatology itself perpetuates the child's sense that life is unpredictable and out of control. This discussion develops as an intellectual scaffold that can serve as a shared point of reference throughout the treatment as well as a basis for the caregiver's increased capacity to better observe trauma symptoms in their child, and often in themselves.

Building on this discussion, the clinician explains that CFTSI focuses on helping both the caregiver and child improve communication about the child's trauma symptoms, identifying cognitive behavioral strategies to lower trauma symptoms, and thus regaining a sense of control. The clinician then explains the CFTSI treatment process, including the importance of communication between caregiver and child about symptoms and the importance of strategies that can help reduce these symptoms. Additionally, the clinician provides a session-by-session outline of CFTSI treatment. By explaining the rationale and the process of CFTSI, and by making explicit what is going to happen, the clinician introduces structure and predictability to counter the original traumatic experience of loss of control.

In Session 1, the clinician next administers brief standardized assessment instruments to determine the caregiver's trauma history, as well as the current state of the caregiver's own post-traumatic responses. The clinician explains this assessment in the context of a discussion with the caregiver about the fact that greater awareness of their own experiences and areas of personal, post-traumatic vulnerabilities can help them fulfill the significant role that caregivers play as mediators of children's experiences. This explanation is also an opportunity to reinforce the specific ways that they can support their child's recovery by identifying, understanding, and communicating with the child about peri-traumatic symptoms as, together, they learn about and implement strategies that can help decrease those symptoms and accompanying distress. Additionally, administering these structured assessments of the caregiver's traumatic reactions can help raise the caregiver's capacities to observe their own symptomatology as well helping to determine whether the caregiver could themselves benefit from treatment.

As part of this first session, the clinician also administers a systematic case management survey to assess current external stressors that adversely affect family functioning in ways that may further interfere with or complicate the recovery process. Referrals to appropriate community resources are provided to address these real-world burdens. And, because traumatic and developmental history plays a role in what is aroused during the post-traumatic experience, the clinician then uses a structured approach to gather information about the child's development, including a review of past traumatic events and health, as well as of current levels of functioning. Next, the clinician uses standardized assessment tools as the basis for a discussion with the caregiver about their impression of the child's level of trauma symptoms. Included in this discussion are questions about how the caregiver became aware of these symptoms (e.g., whether the caregiver observed them, or whether the child told the caregiver about experiencing them). This discussion can also be useful in helping inform the clinician's initial assessment of the caregiver's observational capacities and the current level of caregiver-child communication about symptoms.

Session 2: Meeting with Child

In the second session of CFTSI, the clinician meets individually with the child and, in a similar fashion to Session 1, begins by providing education about trauma and reviewing possible reactions that children commonly experience following a traumatic event. Again, by creating a frame of reference anchored in an understanding of the phenomena of trauma, the clinician can initiate a discussion about why the child is coming to therapy, explain the rationale for CFTSI, describe the treatment process and outline of the sessions, and clarify what the goals of treatment will be. In this way, the clinician is able to prompt the child to organize their post-traumatic experience and give the treatment a structure and predictability to begin to reverse the original post-traumatic sense of loss of control.

Using brief standardized assessment instruments as clinical tools – including the Trauma History Questionnaire (Berkowitz & Stover, 2005), the Post-traumatic Checklist – Civilian Version (Weathers, Litz, Herman, Huska, & Keane, 1994), and the Mood and Feelings Questionnaire (Angold & Costello, 1987) – to provide structure to the discussion, the clinician gathers information about the child's trauma history and assesses the child's impression of their level of trauma symptoms. As part of this discussion, the clinician explores with the child whether the child has communicated with anyone, particularly the caregiver, about any of their trauma symptoms. In this way, the clinician learns more about the child's perspectives on current levels of communication with the caregiver about child's trauma symptoms. The clinician ensures that the child understands that in the next CFTSI session, the clinician will be meeting with the child and caregiver together to compare and contrast both of their reports about the child's trauma history and level of trauma symptoms and to discuss them together. The clinician explains to the child that communicating with the caregiver about their symptoms will help the caregiver have a more complete understanding of the child's post-traumatic experience and can help the caregiver learn ways to support the child. In addition, the clinician emphasizes to the child that coping strategies that they will discuss and practice during the next session will lower the child's symptoms and increase their sense of control.

Session 3: Conjoint Meeting with Child and Caregiver

During CFTSI Session 3, the clinician meets with the caregiver and child together to begin a discussion about child's trauma reactions by comparing and contrasting the caregiver's and child's reports about the child's trauma history and trauma symptoms. The goals for this session are to increase caregiver support by initiating a discussion about the child's symptoms and post-traumatic experience, to help the child learn ways to communicate more effectively about their symptoms and feelings related to the traumatic experience, and to increase the caregiver's understanding and appreciation of the child's experience. In this way, the child and caregiver have an opportunity to compare each other's observations and develop a fuller, better understanding about the child's level of trauma symptoms and distress.

During this part of the discussion, the clinician also helps them determine when different symptoms are occurring, in part, to help them identify possible specific trauma reminders that may be triggering some of these symptoms. The goal is to not only improve their ability to identify symptoms but to also anticipate and realize the situations in which trauma symptoms may most likely occur. Building on the recognition of these symptom contexts, the clinician then helps the child and caregiver develop strategies to better anticipate symptoms and to communicate to each other when symptoms are actually happening. This shared recognition and communication serve as important steps in helping the child and caregiver gain mastery, reduce symptoms, and, in turn, regain a sense of control.

Next, the clinician helps identify the most concerning and problematic trauma symptom(s) the child is experiencing that will be the focus of clinical interventions and coping strategies, such as anxiety, oppositional and / or aggressive behavior, depressive withdrawal, intrusive thoughts, or issues with sleeping. As part of this discussion, the clinician introduces coping strategies that target the most concerning trauma symptom(s) that have been identified to help the child start regaining their sense of control. Strategies may include reestablishing daily routines, rituals, and rules; learning relaxation and affect regulation techniques; reviewing behavior management techniques and effective parenting skills; and learning cognitive coping and cognitive behavioral techniques. After reviewing the coping strategies, the clinician works with the child and caregiver to practice them in session, in preparation for their implementing the strategies at home and other settings.

Session 4: Conjoint Meeting with Child and Caregiver

In CFTSI Session 4, the clinician meets again with the child and caregiver together. After reviewing with them their observations and experiences of the past week, the clinician then readministers the standardized clinical instruments to assess the child's level of distress. Throughout, the clinician points out and supports any demonstration of concordance because of better communication between the child and caregiver about the child's trauma symptoms. In this way, the clinician encourages communication attempts about the child's symptoms. The clinician then discusses with the child and caregiver whether, when, and how well the coping strategies learned in the previous session worked in reducing symptoms and distress. Based on that discussion, the clinician may suggest modifications to the original coping strategies and / or may introduce additional coping strategies to address additional trauma symptoms, as clinically indicated.

Session 5: Conjoint Meeting with Child and Caregiver/Case Disposition

The final session of CFTSI follows the same format as Session 4, with the key additions of case disposition and a discussion of next steps. Similar to Session 4, the clinician discusses with the child and caregiver their observations and experiences of the past week and assesses the child's current level of trauma symptoms by readministering the clinical assessment instruments. Again, the clinician points out and encourages demonstrations of concordance in their reports as a result of better communication. Additionally, Session 5 provides another opportunity to practice the coping strategies reviewed in the last session and to introduce additional coping strategies that might help further lower previously or newly identified symptoms. During these discussions, the clinician determines if there is a need for further trauma-focused treatment or any other additional mental health evaluation and / or treatment, as indicated by presenting symptoms. In either situation, the clinician discusses with the child and caregiver any recommendations and plans to address the additional needs that have been identified.

Post-CFTSI Assessments

After the completion of Session 5, the clinician conducts a post-CFTSI assessment. While the case disposition planning that occurred during Session 5 was based on the status of the child's symptoms, the clinician readministers the original screening instrument with the caregiver and child separately, immediately after the final CFTSI session is completed. Comparing the pre- and post-screening assessments has been useful and informative for families in either further confirming the child's mastery of trauma reactions or reinforcing the need for further treatment. In addition, comparing the pre- and post-assessments can be useful to clinicians, supervisors, and their agencies in tracking CFTSI effectiveness, as well as identifying any challenges to implementation that may require further discussion, support, and / or consultation. Finally, the caregiver is asked to complete a survey to indicate how helpful CFTSI has been to the family.

Possible Additional Sessions

While CFTSI is generally conducted in five treatment sessions, each typically lasting between 50 and 60 minutes, sometimes it is clinically indicated to add one to three additional CFTSI sessions. For example, additional sessions can be used to address challenges that include (1) engaging a caregiver who is initially angry and less supportive of the child and / or blames the child for the circumstances surrounding the traumatic experience; (2) helping a symptomatic caregiver learn coping strategies to decrease their own distressing trauma symptoms that may also interfere with their ability to attend to the distress of their child; (3) helping a cognitively impaired caregiver or child to more fully understand and participate in treatment; or (4) exploring and addressing the concerns of a child who is initially hesitant to talk with the caregiver about trauma symptoms or other issues that may be relevant to the focus of the treatment.

Illustrating the CFTSI Model: The Case of Juan

Juan was a 10-year-old Mexican-American boy who was referred after he experienced an armed robbery at the family's store. The police learned that Juan had walked in during the robbery and saw his parents lying face down on the floor with a gun to his mother's head. The robber had threatened to kill him if he did not leave, and his mother cried for him to run away. Initially frozen, Juan ultimately obeyed his mother and reluctantly fled the store, wondering whether his parents would be killed the moment he left. During the CFTSI screening, Juan's mother, Carmen, identified a moderate level of symptoms, though she acknowledged that she was unsure whether additional symptoms were present for her son. Juan himself reported multiple trauma reactions, which were happening several times per day.

Session 1

The first step in the first CFTSI session with the mother, providing psycho-education about trauma, helped deepen Carmen's appreciation of Juan's experience since the robbery. Most notably, she reported that he seemed more withdrawn and he refused to play outside. She also noted that she had not initially linked some of his uncharacteristic irritability and oppositionality to the robbery, and she guiltily acknowledged losing her temper when he had recently refused to shovel snow from the driveway as he typically did to help the family. This acknowledgment provided an opportunity for the clinician to provide education about the multiple ways that traumatic experiences can impact the entire family and to note that trauma reactions are not always readily identified as such, by either parent or child, especially when parents are struggling with their own fears and symptoms. During the assessment of her own trauma reactions, Carmen endorsed a very high level of symptoms. She was very responsive to the psycho-education that the clinician provided about the link between a parent's own symptoms and their child's recovery, and she participated in problem solving to identify formal and informal supports to assist her in her recovery.

Despite her own high levels of distress, in response to the structured developmental survey, Carmen could provide detailed information about Juan's past and current functioning, as well as his trauma history. One significant detail was that she mentioned that as a preschooler Juan had experienced increased separation anxiety for several months following an earlier (less violent) robbery of the family's store. The systematic review of case management issues also proved helpful to Carmen in terms of identifying the multiple stressors that she had been dealing with since the robbery. This review facilitated problem-solving discussions that included helping the family find appropriate legal resources to address concerns regarding the potential deportation of Juan's father, an undocumented immigrant.

Session 2

At the start of CFTSI Session 2, Juan seemed anxious but ready to engage with the clinician. He acknowledged that prior to the screening session, he had been trying hard to avoid thinking about or discussing the robbery or his trauma symptoms. The clinician introduced a discussion about common aspects of trauma reactions including the symptom of avoidance. The clinician communicated her appreciation for the fact that avoidance represented Juan's understandable best attempt to manage reactions that felt overwhelming to him. Having created a shared frame of reference regarding trauma phenomena, the clinician explained to Juan both the format of CFTSI and ways in which the model could help him find ways to reduce the symptoms and distress he had been experiencing since the robbery. Guided by the CFTSI clinician's use of assessment tools, Juan was able to identify multiple trauma symptoms, including anxiety, difficulty concentrating, guilt that he had not stopped the robbery from occurring, and worry that a similar event could happen again. As part of this systematic assessment, Juan reported that he had been particularly reluctant to talk about his symptoms with his mother because he was very concerned about upsetting her.

Session 3

At the beginning of CFTSI Session 3, Juan and Carmen appeared tense and they said little. The clinician opened the session by predicting and describing the goals of the session. She acknowledged that while it is often hard for children and parents to discuss distressing symptoms, increasing communication between them about the symptoms would be a very important part of reducing both Juan's isolation as well as the symptoms that continued to make him feel so frightened and out of control. In this context, the clinician helped Juan and his mother review each of their perspectives on Juan's current symptomatology and past traumatic experiences, pointing out to them where there were similarities and significant discrepancies in their reports.

After initial hesitation, both Juan and Carmen became very engaged in this discussion and each appeared increasingly more visibly relaxed. Together with the clinician, they identified some of the most distressing symptoms for Juan. Difficulty concentrating at school was chief among Juan's sources of distress and shame as his previous academic success had been such a source of mastery and pride. Further discussion revealed that Juan's difficulty concentrating was secondary to intrusive thoughts and images of the robbery. To address these symptoms of intrusive thoughts, the clinician introduced thought interruption and guided imagery strategies, practicing these with Juan and his mother.

Additionally, Juan and his mother identified generalized anxiety and avoidance as key symptom areas. Juan acknowledged that he was not going outside without his parents or playing with friends because he worried about his and his family's safety. This discussion helped identify specific traumatic reminders that were causing some of Juan's symptoms. For example, it emerged that Juan had been avoiding his chore of shoveling snow because the act of shoveling triggered memories of the robber entering the family's store, which happened while Juan was shoveling the sidewalk outside. Developing an understanding that Juan's fear, rather than his defiance, had led him to refuse to do this chore the past week was significant in helping Juan's mother increase her empathy and her curiosity about whether other conflicts that the family had recently experienced had also been related to Juan's anxiety. To address the physiological symptoms of Juan's experiences of anxiety, the clinician introduced the coping strategy of focused breathing and practiced this with Juan and his mother in the session. They agreed to continue to practice this together at home, in the morning and as part of Juan's bedtime routine.

Session 4

In Session 4, Juan and his mother entered the room and immediately appeared more relaxed than in prior sessions. During this session, Juan and his mother reported an overall reduction in multiple symptoms. They had practiced focused breathing together multiple times over the past week. Juan reported that he had successfully used guided imagery when he had had an intrusive thought during math class and had found it helpful. His pride and relief at beginning to return to being the strong student that he had been were palpable. Knowing that shoveling would be hard for him, Juan and his father began doing the job together.

With an increased general sense of control, Juan was also able to describe cognitive distortions organized around his self-blame for not stopping the robbery. In contrasting the differences between this fantasy and the reality that he could not in fact stop the robber, the CFTSI clinician was able to help Juan recognize the role that these distorted thoughts played in his attempts to reverse the original absence of control. With Juan's greater appreciation for the role his distortions were playing in reversing the original traumatic experience of loss of control, Juan was more open to using strategies that would help him interrupt his painful intrusive thoughts of self-blame. Juan also seemed relieved by his mother's assertion of authority as she reminded him of the fact that it is hers and his father's job to protect the family. Carmen also informed him, for the first time, about concrete steps that the parents had taken to ensure the safety of the family and the security of the store.

Session 5 and Post-CFTSI Assessment

By CFTSI Session 5, Juan's trauma symptoms had decreased significantly. After completing this session, during which the clinician reviewed the case disposition and recommendations, the clinician readministered the original symptom screening instrument with Juan and separately with his mother and compared the pre- and post-treatment levels of trauma symptoms with them. Juan and his mother confirmed a significant decrease in Juan's symptoms compared to the beginning of treatment. His symptoms were below clinically significant levels. Juan seemed relieved to have resumed a focus on developmentally appropriate activities, such as schoolwork, friendships, and helping out around the house. He seemed to be letting go of the need to be the family's protector and allowing his parents to resume that role. Carmen conveyed her pride at having been able to consider her son's needs and to deliver support and ultimately relief to Juan. She agreed to a referral for her own mental health treatment at that point, noting that she had initially thought that it would be too hard for her to face what had happened to her but now she knew that she could do it.

Three-Month Follow-Up

The clinician discussed with Carmen and Juan scheduling a three-month follow-up appointment, explaining that given that CFTSI is an early intervention, it would be helpful to meet again after a period of time to ensure that Juan's improvements were enduring. At the time of this follow-up meeting, the clinician first met with Carmen, who reported that Juan's symptoms had not reemerged and that overall the family was doing well. She also noted that at a family picnic several weeks prior to the follow-up appointment, Juan had become very upset after witnessing a violent fight between his aunt and her boyfriend. Immediately afterward, Juan had sought out his mother about his worried feelings, and together they had practiced coping strategies they had learned during CFTSI. Carmen also continued to report significantly lower levels of her own trauma reactions.

The clinician then met with Juan, who presented a similar picture and did not endorse any persisting clinically significant trauma symptoms. When the clinician asked Juan what he felt had helped him address the reactions he had been experiencing both after the robbery and also after the scary incident at the barbeque, Juan was able to articulate that he had sought out his mother's help, conveyed his symptoms to her, and used the coping strategies he had learned as part of CFTSI.

Evidence Base for the Innovation

CFTSI investigators are utilizing diverse methodological approaches to build the evidence base for the innovation, including a randomized clinical trial (RCT) and chart review of completed cases. Additionally, an open trial of cases receiving treatment in varied settings across the United States is currently underway. As part of this latter strategy, we have developed ways of integrating evaluation methodology with clinical training and implementation efforts.

As part of our efforts to evaluate the efficacy of CFTSI, a randomized controlled trial (RCT) was completed in 2009 (Berkowitz et al., 2011). The CFTSI RCT was conducted in New Haven, Connecticut, with patients aged 7–18 years, referred primarily by the police and the pediatric emergency department. Precipitating events included witnessing violence, assault, motor vehicle accidents, dog bites, and other injuries; referrals for treatment were typically made from 3 to 7 days post event. It is important to note that the majority of subjects enrolled in the CFTSI RCT were not receiving treatment for single-event trauma but rather reported significant trauma histories averaging six types of trauma events prior to the one that precipitated referral for CFTSI. The RCT compared children receiving CFTSI ($N = 53$) to children in a protocolized comparison condition ($N = 53$) that included providing psycho-education about trauma and general discussion about symptoms with the child and caregiver. The study focused on whether or not subjects met criteria for the diagnosis of PTSD immediately after the interventions and at 3 months following the end of treatment, as measured by the UCLA PTSD Reaction Index (Pynoos, Rodriguez, Steinberg, Stuber, & Frederick, 1998). Logistic regression was performed to study group differences in PTSD diagnosis at 3 months following the end of treatment ($N = 82$) while controlling for new traumatic events. CFTSI was found to reduce the odds of full PTSD diagnosis by 65 percent and partial diagnosis by 73 percent (Berkowitz et al., 2011). It is particularly interesting to consider the strength of the study findings in light of the similarities in content and dose in intervention and comparison protocols. Although further study is required to understand the mechanisms of action in the CFTSI model, it appears that the structured nature of the intervention and a specific focus on increasing communication between child and caregiver about symptoms and on learning effective strategies to master traumatic reactions are significant factors.

Two additional studies of CFTSI utilized a chart review approach to study CFTSI cases completed in the Child Advocacy Center (CAC) setting. While the limitations of the chart review methodology are acknowledged, these studies offer additional support for the hypothesis that CFTSI meaningfully reduces post-traumatic symptomatology and increases caregiver-child communication in the peri-traumatic phase of traumatic response. Moreover, as the chart review studies were conducted on cases completed in busy, urban treatment settings, these studies also substantiate the supposition that CFTSI is effective even when implemented in the "real world," beyond the confines of closely monitored protocols and controls that are operational during a controlled trial. The sample for both chart review studies was 114 caregiver-child dyads in which children aged 7–16 years had disclosed sexual abuse in a forensic setting and CFTSI treatment had been recommended and accepted; de-identified data was extracted from charts following completion of CFTSI. The first study (Oransky, Hahn, & Stover, 2013) examined caregiver and child agreement regarding child exposure to potentially traumatic events, children's PTSD and mood symptoms, and children's functional impairment while controlling for caregivers' PTSD symptoms. Investigators found that children reported significantly higher rates of PTSD and mood symptoms at baseline as compared to caregivers, and that discrepancies were significantly, positively correlated with children's reported levels of PTSD and depressive symptoms as well as functional impairment. In addition, investigators found that caregiver PTSD symptom severity was significantly and positively associated with caregiver reports of children's PTSD symptoms, depressive symptom severity, and functional impairment (Oransky et al., 2013). The second chart review study evaluated whether reduction in traumatic stress symptoms immediately following intervention as established in the CFTSI RCT would be similarly demonstrated in a CAC population (Hahn, Oransky, Epstein, Smith Stover, & Marans, 2015). Following the RCT, CFTSI investigators discontinued the use of the PTSD-RI as the main outcome measure for CFTSI, instituting in its place the Child Post-traumatic Symptom Scale (Foa et al., 2001). Pre- to post-comparisons revealed significant reductions of child traumatic stress symptoms as measured with the CPSS. In addition, caregiver and child ratings of child's symptom severity on the CPSS were compared at baseline and post-intervention to assess levels of agreement on independent ratings of child's symptom severity. At baseline, children reported higher levels of traumatic stress symptoms compared to caregivers; following CFTSI, there were no significant differences between child and caregiver ratings of child traumatic stress symptom severity. Child's baseline symptom severity and trauma history as measured using the Trauma History Questionnaire (Berkowitz & Stover, 2005) were found to be significantly and positively associated with symptom severity following CFTSI, while caregiver's baseline PTSD symptoms as assessed using the Posttraumatic Checklist – Civilian Version (Weathers et al., 1994) were not associated with child's post-intervention symptom severity. This finding is initial evidence of the way in which CFTSI may be effective in supporting recovery among children whose caregivers demonstrate post-traumatic symptomatology (Hall et al.,

2006; Kassam-Adams, Garcia-Espana, Miller, & Winston, 2006; Nugent, Ostrowski, Christopher, & Delahanty, 2007; Shemesh et al., 2005), which is a key area of interest for CFTSI investigators. As noted earlier, additional research is needed to determine the mechanisms of action within the CFTSI model and to determine the relative contributions of constituent elements of the model hypothesized to be contributing to children's recovery.

Although further randomized trials will undoubtedly be helpful in hypothesis testing to answer key questions, significant challenges to funding such trials as well as replicating RCT results outside the laboratory setting exist. These concerns have prompted CFTSI investigators to look beyond traditional research methodologies to seek complementary strategies for answering questions of interest. The CFTSI Site Sustainability Project (CSSP) is one such strategy. CSSP was launched in 2014 with two linked goals to (1) capitalize on naturally emerging data to continue to build the evidence base for the model in the very settings and under the same circumstances in which treatment is typically provided and (2) support individual clinicians and agencies in their efforts to implement and sustain CFTSI with fidelity. CFTSI investigators adapted an open-source web-based data collection platform to specifically follow the path of the CFTSI clinical intervention and support these two goals. As clinicians implement CFTSI, they enter de-identified client-level data that are derived in the course of providing treatment. It may also be that the process of entering data serves to support and reinforce training received on CFTSI protocols and increase adherence. Importantly, pre-, post-, and follow-up data emerge naturally from the provision of CFTSI treatment. Thus, as dissemination continues, data on large numbers of cases become available to investigators and can be analyzed using innovative applications of meta-analytic approaches.

In addition to the enormous opportunities afforded by CSSP to evaluators and clinicians alike, agencies and programs are also beneficiaries. Information entered is used to generate implementation metrics, including comparative reports on numbers of cases screened, started, and completed, as well as those CFTSI cases that may have dropped out or failed to start treatment following a determination of eligibility at the point of screening. Monthly metrics reports are created for each unique CFTSI team and delivered to clinicians and agency leaders, as well as the CFTSI consultant working with the team. These reports inform and support teams' quality improvement efforts. The intrinsic value that agencies and programs derive from participation in CSSP has resulted in continued participation far beyond agencies' completion of training requirements, likely attributable to the specific benefits CSSP offers users at all levels. These benefits include automated scoring and graphic representations of symptom assessments readily accessible to clinicians, reports about status of model implementation for supervisors, and data about the impact of CFTSI at the agency level – including data about both symptom reduction and caregiver satisfaction with treatment – for program leaders and agency stakeholders. The Caregiver Satisfaction Survey is a series of questions and scaled responses about the extent to which families believed they received information and help regarding, for example, trauma and symptoms, skills that increased coping, and strategies for better child-parent communication. The survey responses serve as an additional important source of data about CFTSI's general efficacy, active treatment ingredients as well as supporting continuous quality improvement from the perspective of families themselves. In addition, when clinicians request that families review their experiences, they also continue to engage families as active participants in the CFTSI process.

Future Directions

As dissemination of CFTSI continues, an increasing number of programs are beginning to implement the model, while with the support of CSSP and the Core Development Team, existing CFTSI programs are successfully sustaining the model within their agencies. The open trial data set continues to grow and promises to offer enormous potential benefits for investigating a range of questions about the model. Inherently flexible and easily modifiable, the CSSP platform may also be utilized to pursue various questions of interest in collaboration with subsets of current or future agency partners who may be interested, and available to engage, in research with CFTSI investigators using a variety of complementary methodological approaches. Additional research to further substantiate the effects attributable to CFTSI with respect to reduction in trauma symptoms for children, reduction in trauma symptoms for caregivers, and increase in child-caregiver communication changes would be valuable. The CFTSI research agenda also calls for studies designed to identify the mechanisms of action by which change occurs, and the moderators that influence changes seen for both children and their caregivers as a result of CFTSI treatment.

Key Practice Points and Recommended Resources for Practice

Specific strategies have been developed to help ensure that programs will be able to successfully adopt and sustain practice of the CFTSI model with fidelity following the initial training and consultation. The CFTSI team guides programs in assessing their organizational readiness to adopt and implement a model serving children in the peri-traumatic phase of trauma. As a result of this process, programs have significantly improved with respect to key indicators of sustainability, including initial start-up of CFTSI implementation, completion of training requirements, and continued implementation of the model after CFTSI-specific training and consultation have concluded.

CFTSI is provided by master's, PhD, or MD-level mental health clinicians. Training in CFTSI assumes that clinicians already have training in the phenomena of trauma and trauma reactions, client engagement skills, and child development. Training in the CFTSI model is grounded in "learning through doing," and a commitment to supporting sustainability of the practice of CFTSI with fidelity over time. With that in mind, training in CFTSI includes the following components: (1) attending a 2-day in-person interactive CFTSI training conducted by CFTSI Master Trainers and/or the co-developers; (2) participating in a minimum of 9 out of 12 one-hour follow-up consultation conference calls held over a period of approximately 6 months following the initial CFTSI training; (3) completing a minimum of 3 CFTSI cases during the time period of the 12 consultation calls; and (4) participating in the CFTSI Site Sustainability System, which involves collecting and submitting metrics data electronically to the Childhood Violent Trauma Center at the Yale University School of Medicine. Significant interest in CFTSI has been demonstrated by mental health professionals and leaders of organizations that serve children in the peri-traumatic and early PTSD phase of trauma response, as evidenced by the continuous and growing demand for training in the model.

References

Anda, R., Felitti, V., Bremner, J., Walker, J., Whitfield, C., Perry, B., ... Giles, W. (2006). The enduring effects of abuse and related adverse experiences in childhood. *European Archives of Psychiatry and Clinical Neuroscience, 256*(3), 174–186.

Angold, A., & Costello, E. J. (1987). *Mood and Feelings Questionnaire (MFQ)*.

Berkowitz, S., Epstein, C., & Marans, S. (2012). *The Child and Family Traumatic Stress Intervention Implementation Guide for Providers*. Yale University.

Berkowitz, S., & Stover, C. S. (2005). *Trauma history questionnaire parent and child version*. New Haven: Yale Child Study Center Trauma Section.

Berkowitz, S., Stover, C. S., & Marans, S. (2011). The Child and Family Traumatic Stress Intervention: Secondary prevention for youth at risk of developing PTSD. *Journal of Child Psychology and Psychiatry and Allied Disciplines, 52*(6), 676–685. doi:10.1111/j.1469–7610.2010.02321.x

Briggs, E. C., Nooner, K., & Amaya-Jackson, L. (2014). Assessment of childhood PTSD. In M. J. Friedman, T. M. Keane, & P. A. Resick (eds.), *Handbook of PTSD* (2nd edn., pp. 391–405). New York: Guilford Press.

Carlson, E. B., & Dalenberg, C. J. (2000). A conceptual framework for the impact of traumatic experiences. *Trauma Violence and Abuse, 1*(1), 4–28.

Dorsey, S., Briggs, E. C., & Woods, B. A. (2011). Cognitive behavioral treatment for posttraumatic stress disorder in children and adolescents. *Child and Adolescent Psychiatric Clinics of North America, 20*(2), 255–269. doi:10.1016/j.chc.2011.01.006

Epstein, C., Hahn, H., Berkowitz, S., & Marans, S. (2017). The Child and Family Traumatic Stress Intervention. In M. A. Landolt, M. Cloitre, & U. Schnyder (eds.), *Evidence-based treatments for trauma related disorders in children and adolescents* (pp. 145–166). Cham, Switzerland: Springer International Publishing.

Epstein, C., Marans, S., & Berkowitz, S. (2013). *The Child and Family Traumatic Stress Intervention treatment application for children in foster care*.

Felitti, V. J., Anda, R. F., Nordenberg, D., Williamson, D. F., Spitz, A. M., Edwards, V., ... Marks, J. S. (1998). Relationship of childhood abuse and household dysfunction to many of the leading causes of death in adults: The Adverse Childhood Experiences (ACE) Study. *American Journal of Preventative Medicine, 14*(4), 245–258.

Finkelhor, D., Turner, H. A., Shattuck, A. M., Hamby, S. L., & Kracke, K. (2015). Children's exposure to violence, crime, and abuse: An update. *Juvenile Justice Bulletin* (Sept.), 1–13.

Foa, E. B., Johnson, K. M., Feeny, N. C., & Treadwell, K. R. (2001). The Child PTSD Symptom Scale: A preliminary examination of its psychometric properties. *Journal of Clinical Child Psychology, 30*(3), 376–384. doi:10.1207/s15374424 jccp3003_9

Foa, E. B., & Meadows, E. A. (1997). Psychosocial treatments for posttraumatic stress disorder: A critical review. *Annual Review of Psychology, 48,* 449–480. doi:10.1146/annurev.psych.48.1.449

Gewirtz, A., Forgatch, M., & Wieling, E. (2008). Parenting practices as potential mechanisms for child adjustment following mass trauma. *Journal of Marital and Family Therapy, 34*(2), 177–192. doi:10.1111/j.1752–0606.2008.00063.x

Gillies, D., Maiocchi, L., Bhandari, A. P., Taylor, F., Gray, C., & O'Brien, L. (2016). Psychological therapies for children and adolescents exposed to trauma. *Cochrane Database of Systematic Reviews, 10,* CD012371. doi:10.1002/14651858.cd012371

Hahn, H., Oransky, M., Epstein, C., Smith Stover, C., & Marans, S. (2015). Findings of an early intervention to address children's traumatic stress implemented in the child advocacy center setting following sexual abuse. *Journal of Child & Adolescent Trauma,* 1–12. doi:10.1007/s40653-015-0059-7

Hall, E., Saxe, G., Stoddard, F., Kaplow, J., Koenen, K., Chawla, N., ... King, D. (2006). Posttraumatic stress symptoms in parents of children with acute burns. *Journal of Pediatric Psychology, 31*(4), 403–412. doi:10.1093/jpepsy/jsj016

Kassam-Adams, N., Garcia-Espana, J. F., Miller, V. A., & Winston, F. (2006). Parent-child agreement regarding children's acute stress: The role of parent acute stress reactions. *Journal of the American Academy of Child and Adolescent Psychiatry, 45* (12), 1485–1493. doi:10.1097/01.chi.0000237703.97518.12

Leenarts, L. E., Diehle, J., Doreleijers, T. A., Jansma, E. P., & Lindauer, R. J. (2013). Evidence-based treatments for children with trauma-related psychopathology as a result of childhood maltreatment: A systematic review. *European Child and Adolescent Psychiatry, 22*(5), 269–283. doi:10.1007/s00787-012-0367-5

Listenbee, R., Torre, J., Boyle, G., Cooper, S., Deer, S., Durfee, D. T., ... Taguba, A. (2012). *Report of the Attorney General's National Task Force on Children Exposed to Violence.* Washington, DC: United States Department of Justice. www.justice.gov/defendingchildhood/cev-rpt-full.pdf

Marans, S. (2013). Phenomena of childhood trauma and expanding approaches to early intervention. *International Journal of Applied Psychoanalytic Studies, 10*(3), 247–266. doi:10.1002/aps.1369

Marans, S., Epstein, C., & Berkowitz, S. (2014). *The Child and Family Traumatic Stress Intervention treatment application for young children.*

Marens, S., & Holmes, A. (2016). Stress and fear extinction. *Neuropsychopharmacology, 41* (1), 58–79. doi:10.1038/npp.2015.180

Nugent, N. R., Ostrowski, S., Christopher, N. C., & Delahanty, D. L. (2007). Parental posttraumatic stress symptoms as a moderator of child's acute biological response and subsequent posttraumatic stress symptoms in pediatric injury patients. *Journal of Pediatric Psychology, 32*(3), 309–318. doi:10.1093/jpepsy/jsl005

Oransky, M., Hahn, H., & Stover, C. S. (2013). Caregiver and youth agreement regarding youths' trauma histories: Implications for youths' functioning after exposure to trauma. *Journal of Youth and Adolescence, 42*(10), 1528–1542. doi:10.1007/s10964-013-9947-z

Ozer, E. J., Best, S. R., Lipsey, T. L., & Weiss, D. S. (2003). Predictors of posttraumatic stress disorder and symptoms in adults: A meta-analysis. *Psychological Bulletin, 129*(1), 52–73.

Pynoos, R., Rodriguez, N., Steinberg, A. M., Stuber, M., & Frederick, C. (1998). *The UCLA PTSD reaction index for DSM IV (Revision 1)*. Los Angeles: University of California, Los Angeles Trauma Psychiatry Program.

Pynoos, R., Steinberg, A., & Piacentini, J. (1999). A developmental psychopathology model of childhood traumatic stress and intersection with anxiety disorders. *Biological Psychiatry, 46*(11), 1542–1554.

Schalinski, I., Teicher, M. H., Nischk, D., Hinderer, E., Müller, O., & Rockstroh, B. (2016). Type and timing of adverse childhood experiences differentially affect severity of PTSD, dissociative and depressive symptoms in adult inpatients. *BMC Psychiatry, 16*, 295. doi:10.1186/s12888-016-1004-5

Scheeringa, M. S., & Zeanah, C. H. (2001). A relational perspective on PTSD in early childhood. *Journal of Traumatic Stress, 14*(4), 799–815.

Shemesh, E., Newcorn, J. H., Rockmore, L., Shneider, B. L., Emre, S., Gelb, B. D., ... Yehuda, R. (2005). Comparison of parent and child reports of emotional trauma symptoms in pediatric outpatient settings. *Pediatrics, 115*(5), 582–589. doi:10.1542/peds.2004-2201

Southwick, S. M., & Charney, D. S. (2012). *Resilience: The science of mastering life's greatest challenges*. Cambridge: Cambridge University Press.

Trickey, D., Siddaway, A. P., Meiser-Stedman, R., Serpell, L., & Field, A. P. (2012). A meta-analysis of risk factors for post-traumatic stress disorder in children and adolescents. *Clinical Psychology Review, 32*(2), 122–138. doi:10.1016/j.cpr.2011.12.001

Weathers, F., Litz, B., Herman, D., Huska, J., & Keane, T. (1994). *The PTSD checklist-civilian version (PCL-C)*. Boston, MA: National Center for PTSD.

30 Pediatric Post-Traumatic Stress Disorder

Pharmacological Augmented Treatments

Antra Bami, Judith Fernando, and Craig L. Donnelly

Introduction

Post-traumatic stress disorder (PTSD) is a complicated condition involving dysregulation of multiple neurobiological systems influencing cognitive, affective, and behavioral domains of functioning. PTSD entered the diagnostic nomenclature with the introduction of the *Diagnostic and Statistical Manual of Mental Disorders*, 3rd edn. (DSM-III; American Psychiatric Association, 1980) in 1980. In the general adult population, the prevalence rate of PTSD is 6.8 percent (Kessler, Berglund et al., 2005), which equates to about 15 million adults in the United States. The disorder was not immediately recognized as a disorder in childhood. However, subsequent applications of the diagnostic criteria in child and adolescent populations in epidemiological studies indicate that PTSD is also common among youth. Trauma exposure affects approximately two-thirds of children and approximately 13.4 percent of those exposed to trauma will develop some post-traumatic stress symptoms (Copeland, Keeler, Angold, & Costello, 2007).

Overview and the Need for Innovation

Diagnostic Criteria and Clinical Presentation

One of the major revisions made in the DSM-5 is concerned with the diagnostic criteria of PTSD. It is no longer classified as an anxiety disorder and instead has been moved to a separate category of trauma- and stress-related disorders. While the way PTSD is conceptualized primarily remains consistent across the iterations of the DSM, the changes in DSM-5 mark a more comprehensive and developmentally sensitive approach.

Criterion A in DSM-5 redefined what constitutes a traumatic event such that the unexpected death of a family member or a close friend due to natural causes is no longer included and exposure to traumatic content through media such as television, movies, or pictures is disqualified. DSM-5 also eliminated Criterion A2 regarding the subjective reaction to the traumatic event due to the finding that it lacks predictive validity for both adults and preschool children (Friedman, Resick, Bryant, & Brewin

2011). Furthermore, DSM-5 has expanded the diagnostic clusters to four as opposed to three in DSM-IV, essentially to separate negative cognition from avoidance into its own category. Finally, the change most significant to the pediatric populations was the inclusion of a new developmental subtype of PTSD called post-traumatic stress disorder in preschool children. Using this developmentally sensitive set of criteria for diagnosis has shown to yield approximately three to eight times more children qualifying for PTSD compared to DSM-IV (Scheeringa, Weems, Cohen, Amaya-Jackson, & Guthrie, 2011; Scheeringa, Myers, Putnam, & Zeanah, 2012).

The clinical presentation of PTSD in childhood is extraordinarily heterogeneous, often with a bewildering array of symptoms. This is especially true for traumatic experiences that occur prior to or around the establishment of language in children, where trauma may be "encoded" in motor or emotional memories and may thus "prime" stress-related brain HPA axis responsivity and other physiologic responses that are elicited in the absence of language-based memory recall. Post-traumatic stress disorder is indeed a great imitator in psychiatry, both because of its variability in expression and because of its complicated comorbidities. For example, in meeting the minimum symptom criteria for the disorder, there are at least 1,750 combinations or ways in which children can present clinically. The type, magnitude, proximity to, and duration of exposure to traumatic events, as well as factors intrinsic to the individual child and parents, are important in the development and expression of PTSD (Mylle & Maes, 2004; Pfefferbaum, 1997, 2005). Terr (2003) has suggested a useful distinction between single-incident trauma (type I trauma) and chronic, recurrent traumatic exposure (type II trauma). Indeed, it is likely that PTSD describes a family of related disorders that are biologically distinguishable and thus differentially treatable.

Pediatric PTSD is a psychiatric disorder that is prone to both under- and over-diagnosis, especially when assessments are superficially or inexpertly conducted. For example, a traumatic exposure history in combination with current externalizing behavioral symptoms does not necessarily imply a diagnosis of PTSD. Conversely, children who present with an externalizing behavioral disorder in conjunction with anxiety symptoms and aggression are often not fully evaluated for PTSD. Diagnosing PTSD requires a high index of suspicion.

Once a diagnosis of PTSD is made and comorbid conditions identified, the treatment plan is then developed. Identification of target symptoms involves grouping target symptom clusters and their associated functional impairments and segregating them according to treatment modality, this is, biological versus psychotherapeutic versus environmental. This may involve setting up a stimulus hierarchy for cognitive behavior therapy (CBT) or identifying symptoms of mood, anxiety, insomnia, or agitation that will be targeted with medication. Unfortunately, rating scales cannot be relied upon to precisely guide treatment selection decisions regarding which symptoms may be more amenable to medication intervention. The decision about whether to begin pharmacotherapy is multi-determined and may involve lack of accessibility to evidence-based psychotherapy, severity of symptoms (e.g., hallucinations, severe flashbacks / dissociation, nightmares), degree of functional impairment, acuity of symptom onset, psychological distress associated with symptoms, and significant comorbid conditions such as depression – all of which would argue for medication intervention. Pharmacotherapy is sometimes warranted, even in the absence of established CBT or psychotherapy, in such cases where severe agitation, disruptive aggression, significant sleep alteration, or depression limits the behavioral functioning of the child or the child's capacity to engage in psychotherapy.

Segregation of target symptoms between those likely to be responsive to pharmacologic and those needing psychotherapeutic interventions is key. It is useful to specify not only the target symptom and impairment but also the target treatment goal. For example, one might identify frequent traumatic nightmares and initial insomnia as the target symptoms and decreased latency to sleep and infrequent nightmares as the treatment goals. Identifying a specific instrument that is sensitive to treatment change is helpful. A brief instrument such as the Child Posttraumatic Stress Disorder Reaction Index or Trauma Symptom Checklist for Children may be a good choice to measure treatment-related changes in symptoms. For convenience and specificity, an individually tailored and operationally defined list of target symptoms / impairments, with a three-point Likert scale for each item (e.g., no / mild symptoms, moderate symptoms, severe symptoms) can be devised and agreed upon by the treating clinician and child / family. It is important to include both children and parents in constructing such a scale to comprehensively identify and track symptom response to treatment.

Description of the Approach to Innovation

Psycho-Education

Certainly, the initial step in the treatment of pediatric PTSD is psycho-education of the child, parents, and adult caregivers about the nature of the disorder. Treatment should never be a mysterious process. Psycho-education provides the opportunity to discuss with the child and adult caregiver the exact nature of the diagnosis and to define specific treatment targets, impairments, and goals, as well as a clear rationale for all interventions.

Pharmacological Agents

Theories of the neurobiology of stress and trauma have been extensively reviewed (Bremner, Davis, Southwick, Krystal, & Charney, 1993; Charney, Deutch, Krystal, Southwick, & Davis, 1993; Langeland & Olff, 2008). A body of literature has emerged to guide treatment decisions in both child and adult PTSD (Asnis, Kohn, Henderson, & Brown, 2004; De Bellis & Putnam, 1994; Foa, Davidson, & Frances, 1999; Friedman & Southwick, 1995; Stein, Ipser, Seedat, Sager, & Amos, 2006; Yehuda, 1998). The physiological systems involved in trauma include the immune system, the neuroendocrine system, and the central nervous system (CNS). These systems work in a dynamic, integrated fashion to regulate cognition, memory, affect, and behavior. Of these, the neurotransmitter systems of the CNS are the most relevant to psychopharmacological interventions.

At least seven neurobiological systems mediate the mammalian stress response and may be involved in PTSD (Friedman & Southwick, 1995). These include the adrenergic, dopaminergic, serotonergic, gamma-amino butyric acid (GABA) / benzodiazepine, opioid, N-methyl d-aspartate (NMDA), and neuroendocrine systems (the latter including the hypothalamic-pituitary adrenal (HPA), growth hormone, thyroid, and gonadal axes). A rational approach to the pharmacologic treatment of pediatric PTSD symptoms can be informed by understanding medication effects on these neurobiological systems. Because of the lack of empirical studies in pediatric PTSD, it is difficult to recommend a clear treatment hierarchy. There is admittedly scant empirical support in the pediatric treatment literature for any pharmacotherapeutic treatment strategy. Severity or acuity of symptoms and partial or nonresponse to psychotherapeutic interventions are the chief reasons for entering the pharmacologic treatment domain.

Pharmacology has two central roles to play in pediatric PTSD treatment. The first is to target disabling symptoms so that the traumatized child may pursue a normal growth and developmental trajectory. The second is to help traumatized children tolerate emotionally distressing material and work through the distress in both psychotherapy and life. Given the complex pathophysiology of PTSD, effective pharmacotherapy may require a multisystem approach in which several agents are used to target separate clusters of symptoms of PTSD and / or the accompanying comorbidities. This is described in more detail under specific pharmacological agents and in Figure 30.1. As noted, pharmacotherapy may be an early treatment consideration in the face of severe agitation, aggressiveness, self-mutilative behaviors, disorganization, or debilitating symptoms of insomnia, depression, or anxiety.

Evidence Base for Innovation

Translation from Basic/Clinical Science to Practice

Surprisingly little empirical evidence is available about the effectiveness of pharmacotherapeutic agents in pediatric PTSD. In the adult literature, PTSD practice guidelines (Ursano, 2004) provide substantial information and multiple levels of evidence to support medication use. However, the evidence in the pediatric population continues to lag behind the adult literature. Over a 37-year period from 1980 to 2017, there were 27 articles on medication treatment of pediatric PTSD published. Only six studies were randomized controlled clinical trials. The small size of the evidence base for medication use in children dilutes conclusions about which medications are most efficacious for this population (Cosima et al., 2017; Langeland & Olff, 2008). The following section reviews classes of medication with regard to their function and effects in relation to target PTSD symptoms.

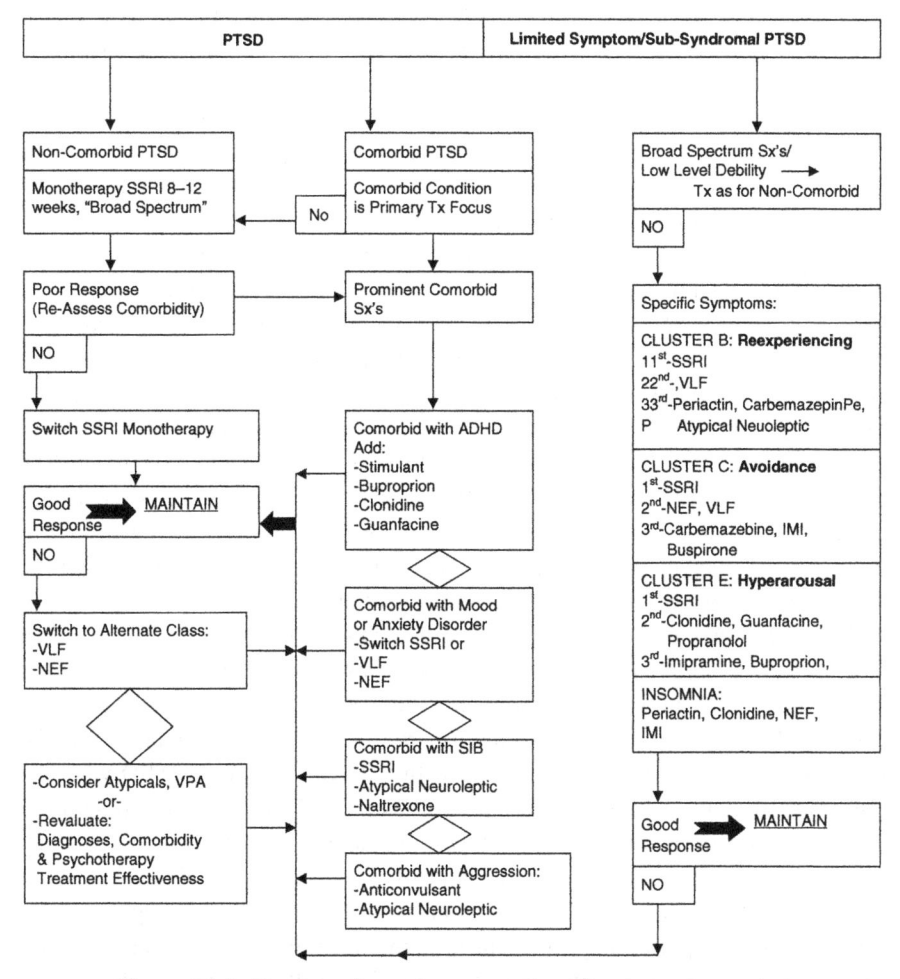

Figure 30.1 *Pharmacologic Treatment Algorithm for Pediatric PTSD*

Adrenergic Agents

The catecholamines norepinephrine, epinephrine, and dopamine are involved in sympathetic arousal, anxiety, frontal lobe activation, mood regulation, reward dependence, working memory, thinking, and perceiving. Adrenergic agents such as the α-2 agonists clonidine and guanfacine, α-1 antagonist prazosin, and the β antagonist propranolol reduce sympathetic arousal as seen in "fight or flight" reactions in mammals. As such, these medications may be effective in the treatment of hyperarousal, impulsivity, and activation seen in PTSD (De Bellis & Putnam, 1994; Langeland & Olff, 2008; Marmar, Foy, Kagan, & Pynoos, 1993). In an open-label trial of 17 children with severe chronic PTSD (13 male, 4 female; mean age 10.4, range 6.0–14.2) relatively low doses of clonidine (0.05–0.10 mg two times daily) were found to provide significant improvement in anxiety, arousal, concentration, mood, and behavioral impulsivity

(Perry 1994). Harmon and Riggs (1996) reported that the use of a clonidine transdermal patch effectively reduced PTSD symptoms in all 7 patients (preschoolers, aged 3–6 years who had severe physical and / or sexual abuse and neglect) in their open-label trial. In a single case study, Horrigan and Barnhill (1996) reported the effectiveness of guanfacine, an alpha-adrenergic agent, in reducing PTSD-associated nightmares in a 7-year-old child who had been exposed to extreme levels of domestic violence and physical abuse at the hand of her father. In an uncontrolled A-B-A design study, Famularo, Kinscherff, and Fenton (1988) found that propranolol significantly reduced PTSD symptoms over the 5 weeks of treatment (2.5 mg/kg/day) in 8 of 11 children with physical, sexual, or both types of abuse. Intrusion and arousal symptoms appeared to be the most responsive to treatment in this study. In a single case study, Brkanac, Pastor, and Storck (2003) noted that prazosin (4 mg nightly) caused a cessation of nightmares and global clinical improvement in a 15-year-old adolescent with PTSD. Akinsanya, Marwaha, and Tampi (2017) in a systematic review of prazosin use in children and adolescents identified 6 case reports of children ranging from 7 to 16 years (Brkanac et al., 2003; Fraleigh, Hendratta, Ford, & Conner, 2009; Oluwabusi, Sedky, & Bennett, 2012; Racin, Bellonci, & Coffey, 2014; Strawn, DelBello, & Geracioti, 2009; Strawn & Keeshin 2011) that showed marked improvement in nightmares as well as hyperarousal and intrusive symptoms of PTSD when prazosin was used at doses between 1 and 4 mg nightly with treatment duration and follow-up ranging from 4 weeks to 11 months. In the two cases (one was a 16-year-old female with a 2-year history of PTSD who had been assaulted with a knife at age 14 and sexually abused by three unfamiliar older males and in the other case a 15-year-old female who had ongoing sexual abuse by a family member since the age of 8) reported by Oluwabusi et al. (2012), the patients were also on sertraline for mood disorder or bupropion for anxiety, but they reported improvement in nightmares only after adding prazosin. In three of the cases, discontinuation of prazosin resulted in increased intensity and frequency of PTSD associated nightmares in children and adolescents who had reported remission of these nightmares while on prazosin.

In adults, both clonidine and propranolol have also demonstrated success in treating PTSD symptoms such as nightmares, insomnia, and hyper-startle as well as intrusive memories and general hyperarousal. Reduction of CNS adrenergic tone through use of these agents to target re-experiencing and hyperarousal symptoms is a rational treatment strategy. Additionally, the α-2-adrenergic agents may be more effective than the psychostimulants for attention deficit / hyperactivity disorder (ADHD) symptoms in maltreated or sexually abused children with PTSD as they exert a "dampening down" affect or nor-adrenergic mediated arousal symptoms (De Bellis & Putnam, 1994). De Bellis's group hypothesizes that alpha-2 presynaptic receptor blockade, such as provided by clonidine or guanfacine, may modulate or dampen down noradrenergic tone in the locus ceruleus – an activation center for arousal – and thus reduce PTSD symptoms of hyperarousal, in addition to treating ADHD symptoms. Stimulants lack this property.

Dopaminergic Agents

There have been several reports in the literature of the utilization of dopamine-blocking agents for symptoms of PTSD in youths. Horrigan and Barnhill (1999) conducted an open-label trial using risperidone in 18 boys (mean age 9.28 years) in residential treatment with PTSD and significant comorbid psychiatric disorders (83 percent of the children were diagnosed with ADHD and 35 percent with bipolar disorder). It was found that 13 of the 18 children experienced a remission of PTSD symptoms with risperidone. Meighen, Hines, and Lagges (2007) reported a case series of three young children (aged 2–3 years) diagnosed with acute stress disorder, who were treated with risperidone. They found a significant reduction in hyperarousal, re-experiencing, and dissociative symptoms as well as an improvement in emotional responsiveness. Keeshin and Strawn (2009) in a case report of a 13-year-old boy with chronic PTSD related to sexual abuse and neglect reported significant improvement of PTSD symptoms (decreased intrusive and hyperarousal symptoms) with adjunctive use of risperidone, although his treatment was complicated by transient hyperprolactinemia.

Stathis, Martin, and McKenna (2005) reported the effectiveness of quetiapine (50–200 mg/day) in a 6-week case series of six adolescents aged 15–17 years in a youth detention center who met criteria for PTSD. They found significant reduction in overall PTSD symptoms and a reduction in dissociation, anxiety, depression, and anger using the Trauma Symptom Checklist for Children. Clozapine (mean daily dose 102 mg/day) was reported to reduce polypharmacy with mood stabilizers and antidepressants in a residential population of adolescents with diagnoses of bipolar affective disorder, intermittent explosive disorder, and PTSD (Kant, Chalansani, Chengapa, & Dieringer, 2004). In a case series of six adolescent treatment-resistant males, with chronic PTSD and psychotic symptoms, clozapine (400–800 mg/day) led to an overall improvement in psychiatric symptoms, self-report and behavioral presentation in four of the six adolescents (Wheatley, Plant, Reader, Brown, & Cahill, 2004).

Given their significant side effect profile and scant evidence as to their utility in PTSD, the atypical, dopaminergic-blocking neuroleptics should be reserved for only the most debilitating cases when other agents have failed or when symptoms of paranoid behavior, para-hallucinatory phenomena, intense flashbacks, self-destructive behavior, explosive or overwhelming anger, psychotic symptoms, severe self-mutilation, or aggressiveness are limiting recovery.

Serotonergic Agents

The neurotransmitter serotonin (5-hydroxytryptamine (5-HT)) is widely distributed in the CNS and subsumes a variety of influences on satiety, mood, aggression, anxiety, as well as compulsive and impulsive behaviors. Serotonin is an important neurotransmitter in psychiatric symptoms commonly associated with PTSD such as aggression, obsessive / intrusive thoughts, alcohol and substance abuse, depression, and suicidal behavior (Friedman, 1990). Suicidal behavior is known to be associated with both childhood maltreatment and low 5-HT functioning (Benkelfat, 1993; Van der Kolk, Perry, & Herman, 1991). Panic attacks, dissociative episodes, and flashbacks appear to be related to serotonin function as well (Southwick, Yehuda, Giller, & Charney, 1994). Thus, there are significant phenomenological overlaps between PTSD symptoms and their comorbid conditions that share mediation by serotonergic systems.

Sertraline and paroxetine have US Food and Drug Administration (FDA) indications for PTSD in adults (Brady, Pearlstein et al., 2000; Marshall, Beebe, Oldham, & Zaninelli, 2001). However, no selective serotonin reuptake inhibitors (SSRIs) have US FDA approval for use in children with PTSD. In children, fluoxetine is approved for depression, while the SSRIs fluoxetine, sertraline, and fluvoxamine are approved for obsessive-compulsive disorder. SSRIs appear to be useful in children with PTSD because many of these children exhibit symptoms associated with serotonergic dysregulation such as anxiety, depression, obsessional thinking, compulsive behaviors, aggression, and alcohol or substance abuse (Friedman, 1990).

Robb et al. (2010) conducted a large multicenter double-blind randomized controlled trial to determine the safety and efficacy of sertraline in children and adolescents (aged 6–17 years) who met DSM-IV criteria for PTSD. The UCLA-PTSD-I scale was used to measure symptoms in this 10-week study that used doses of sertraline of 50–200 mg/day. The study concluded that the treatment efficacy of sertraline was not superior to placebo in the treatment of PTSD in children and adolescents. Significantly, it is noteworthy that the positive results from adult trials may not be generalizable to childhood PTSD. This is consistent with the results found by Cohen, Mannarino, Perel, and Sharon (2007) who looked at sertraline (50–200 mg/day) in a randomized clinical trial with 24 participants with PTSD who were aged 10–17 years. They compared trauma-focused cognitive behavioral therapy (TF-CBT) + sertraline versus TF-CBT + placebo and found comparable results in both groups, with both groups showing a statistically significant reduction in PTSD symptoms. Finally, Stoddard and his colleagues (2011) examined the ability of sertraline to prevent the onset of PTSD symptoms in children who were burn victims. In this 24-weeks double-blind randomized placebo-controlled trial, 26 children (aged 6–20 years) admitted to a pediatric burn center (meeting the DSM-IV A1 criterion for acute trauma experience) received either a 25–150 mg/day dose of sertraline or placebo medication. The study found sertraline to be somewhat more effective than placebo in the prevention of PTSD symptoms according to the parent reports, but the opposite was found in the child reports. While the reason for the aberrant findings of the child report data remains unclear, it is important to keep in mind that a high placebo response rate appears to be more common in child and adolescent trials of central nervous system disorders such as depression and non-PTSD anxiety compared to adult trials (Bridge, Birmaher, Iyengar, Barbe, & Brent, 2009).

Citalopram (20 mg/day) was studied by Seedat, Lockhat, Kaminer, Zungu-Dirwayi, and Stein (2001) in a 12-weeks open-label trial of eight participants who were aged 12–18 years who had developed moderate to severe PTSD from various traumatic experiences. The youngsters reported a 38 percent reduction in PTSD symptoms on the Clinician Administered PTSD Scale (CAPS); however, self-reported depressive symptoms did not improve. Seedat et al. (2002) performed a second study with citalopram (20–40 mg/day) in an 8-weeks open-label trial that included 38 children and adolescents as well as adults. The researchers found no difference in outcomes for the youths versus the adults, and both groups showed a significant mean decrease in CAPS and Clinical Global Impressions-Severity (CGI-S) scores at endpoint indicating improvement. Robert and colleagues (2008) compared fluoxetine (0.29 + 0.16 mg/kg/day) to imipramine (1.00 + 0.29 mg/kg/day) to placebo in a 1-week randomized double-blind placebo-controlled trial with 60 participants aged 4–18 years who met the criteria for ASD. Placebo was found to be just as effective as imipramine or fluoxetine.

Common side effects in the studies with the SSRIs were gastrointestinal, behavioral activation, epistaxis, headache, and akathisia, but in general this type of medication is well tolerated and safe. However, there is a black box warning regarding increased suicidal ideation and behavior rates in children treated with SSRIs based on studies of these agents with depression. SSRIs have no FDA label indication for treating PTSD in youth; thus their use is "off label." Despite this, SSRIs remain one of the most commonly prescribed psychotropic medications for children and adolescents for depression and anxiety disorders as well as PTSD. They can be conceptualized as "broad spectrum" agents with multiple beneficial actions.

Other serotonergic medications are more rarely used, again off label, for treating PTSD in youth. One example is nefazodone, a serotonergic antagonist antidepressant that was studied by Doman and Anderson (2000) in an open-label trial with adolescents with PTSD. This study found nefazodone to be particularly effective in reducing symptoms of hyperarousal, anger, aggression, insomnia, and concentration. They reported an average effective dose of 200 mg twice per day. Nefazodone was well tolerated in doses up to 600 mg/day. However, nefazadone is rarely used in children and adolescents due to an FDA mandated black box warning of problems with hepatic toxicity.

Another example is cyproheptadine, which is an antihistaminic 5-HT antagonist that has shown utility in reducing trauma-related nightmares in a small number of adult patients (Brophy, 1991; Harsch, 1986; Rijnders, Laman, & Van Diujn, 2000). In a single case study of a 9-year-old male with ADHD, ODD, and PTSD, Gupta et al. (1998) noted cessation of nightmares and improvement in sleep with cyproheptadine. Because of its sedative action and generally safe side effect profile, it may be a useful agent in sleep-onset problems and in treatment of nightmares in children with PTSD.

Adrenergic and Serotonergic Agents: Tricyclic Antidepressants and Venlafaxine

Robert, Blakeney, Villarreal, Rosenberg and Meyer. (1999) reported on the use of low-dose imipramine (1 mg/kg) to treat symptoms of ASD in children with burn injuries. In this study, 25 children aged 2–19 years were randomized to receive either chloral hydrate (as a placebo) or imipramine for 7 days. Ten of 12 subjects receiving imipramine experienced a greater than 50 percent remission of ASD symptoms, whereas only 5 of 13 subjects responded to chloral hydrate. In this study, sleep-related flashbacks and insomnia appeared to be particularly responsive to treatment showing significant decreases. Tcheung et al. (2005) showed that either imipramine or fluoxetine could be effective in reducing symptoms of ASD. Using retrospective chart review data of 128 pediatric burn patients, it was noted that 84 of 104 patients responded to initial treatment with imipramine and 18 of 24 patients responded to initial treatment with fluoxetine. Among the 26 patients who were nonresponders to their initial treatment, 12 still responded to the alternate medication. As previously noted, Robert and colleagues (2008) compared fluoxetine to imipramine to placebo in a 1-week randomized double-blinded placebo-controlled trial and found that 1-week "treatment" with placebo was just as effective as imipramine or fluoxetine.

The tricyclic antidepressants (TCAs) appear to reduce symptoms of re-experiencing and depression related to PTSD. In children and adolescents, imipramine may be an effective agent for ASD symptoms. This agent is particularly useful in treatment of traumatic experiences or flashbacks related to sleep onset and sleep maintenance (Robert et al., 1999). The TCAs have been supplanted by the SSRIs as first-line pharmacotherapy in the treatment of depression and anxiety in childhood. SSRIs have a better safety and side effect profile in most patients. Additionally, the TCAs have an apparent lack of effectiveness in childhood depression. As such, TCAs should be reserved for second- or third-line treatment in pediatric PTSD.

Miscellaneous Agents and Those Agents Affecting Multiple Neurotransmitters: Anticonvulsants, Bupropion, and Psychostimulants

Trauma exposure may induce sensitization or kindling phenomena in limbic nuclei in the human CNS. A number of successful open-label trials have been conducted with antikindling / anticonvulsive agents with adult PTSD patients. Lithium, carbamazepine, and divalproex sodium may reduce extreme mood lability and anger dyscontrol.

Loof, Grimley, Kuller, Martin, and Shonfield (1995) reported on the use of carbamazepine (300–1200 mg/day, serum levels 10–11.5 µg/mL) in 28 children and adolescents with sexual abuse histories of whom half had comorbid ADHD, depression, ODD, or poly-substance abuse and were treated with concomitant medications (e.g., methylphenidate, clonidine, sertraline, fluoxetine, or imipramine). By treatment end, 22 of 28 patients were free of PTSD symptoms. The remaining six were significantly improved in all PTSD symptoms except for abuse-related nightmares. Steiner et al. (2007) conducted a randomized controlled trial comparing high-dose divalproex sodium (500–1500 mg/day) to low-dose divalproex sodium (250 mg/day) in 12 juvenile offenders (ages unclear) with conduct disorder and PTSD. The high-dose divalproex sodium group was found to have a significantly greater reduction in intrusion and avoidance symptoms compared to the low-dose group.

Anticonvulsants are more commonly used in children and adolescents with seizure disorders or severe mood instability such as seen in bipolar disorder, though they may be a useful intervention for debilitating avoidance or numbing hyperarousal and sleep dysregulation in children with PTSD, or where overwhelming anger and aggressiveness or explosiveness predominates. Several double-blind, placebo-controlled trials have evaluated the use of topiramate as monotherapy as well as adjunctive treatment for PTSD in adults with some positive data (Tucker et al., 2007; Yeh et al., 2011); however, no clinical trials to date examine the efficacy of topiramate in the pediatric population.

The brain areas that are involved in the stress response also mediate motor behavior, affect regulation, arousal, sleep, startle response, attention, and cardiovascular function. Hence, it is not unusual for traumatized children, particularly those exposed to chronic trauma-like maltreatment, to exhibit a constellation of anxiety plus ADHD and other disruptive behavior symptoms. Some clinicians will consider the use of α agonists in these situations, hoping to avoid stimulant-induced exacerbation of anxiety and PTSD. Anecdotal experience suggests many traumatized children have favorable responses to α agonists as well as to psychostimulants, such as methylphenidate or dextroamphetamine. The symptoms best targeted are hyperactivity, impulse dyscontrol, and attention impairment. Bupropion is often considered a second-line agent for ADHD symptoms and may be a useful agent when affect dysregulation or depressed mood co-occurs with ADHD symptoms in children with PTSD (Daviss, 1999).

It is therefore important to remember that there is not necessarily a one-to-one correspondence between pharmacological effect and neurotransmitter system. For example, SSRIs may effectively reduce PTSD-related symptoms that are not essentially serotonergic in nature, owing to the complex interrelations between neurobiological systems. Table 30.1 presents a summary of levels of evidence for specific medications used to treat PTSD in youth as well as the target symptoms most likely to show a treatment response. Much work remains to be done to identify which medications in which patients for which PTSD symptom constellations are indicated as first-line treatments.

Strawn et al. (2010) report that two of the placebo-controlled trials did not support the use of SSRIs in the treatment of children and adolescents with PTSD. SSRIs are, however, an indicated treatment for anxiety and depressive disorders that are often comorbid in the pediatric population with PTSD.

Antiadrenergic agents have some support for the management of intrusive and hyperarousal symptoms based on the extrapolation from adult studies and open-label trials in children. Currently available data also support the need of a trial of an adjunctive second-generation antipsychotic (e.g., quetiapine, risperidone) or the mood stabilizer carbamazepine for the pediatric population with PTSD

Strawn's (2010) group also noted that several of the antipsychotics (e.g., risperidone and quetiapine) used to treat the child, adolescent, and adult populations are potent antagonists at the alpha 1 receptors. Currently the data for use in this population are limited to case report–level evidence. Therefore, in this pediatric population with PTSD, it is vital to have double-blind placebo-controlled trials with centrally acting alpha 1 and beta receptor antagonists and alpha 2 agonists.

Table 30.1 *Current Psychopharmacological Treatments for PTSD in Children and Adolescents: Levels of Evidence for Medication Use and Their Specific Target Symptoms and Response*

Medication	Level of Evidence[a]	Notes
Antiadrenergics		
Prazosin	IV	↓Intrusive / hyperarousal symptoms
Clonidine	IV	↓Reenactment symptoms
Guanfacine	IV	↓Intrusive symptoms
Propranolol	IV, 1 Negative RCT for secondary prevention	↓Hyperarousal symptoms
Second-generation antipsychotics		
Quetiapine	IV	↓TSCC scores and anxiety, depression and anger
Risperidone	IV	↓Intrusive / hyperarousal
Antiepileptic drugs		
Carbamazepine	IV	
Divalproex	IV	
SSRIs		
Sertraline	2 Negative RCTs	
Citalopram	IV	
Other agents/ class		
Cyproheptadine	IV	↓Intrusive symptoms
Benzodiazepines	No evidence to support use	

[a]Level of evidence: level I, systematic review or multiple randomized controlled trails; level II, randomized controlled trails; level III, individual case control studies; level IV, case-series; level V, expert opinion or based on physiology.
Symbol: ↓ = decrease.
Abbreviations: RCT = randomized controlled trail, SSRI = selective serotonin reuptake inhibitor, TSCC = Trauma Symptom Checklist for Children

Source: Reprinted from Strawn, J. R., Keeshin, B. R., DelBello, M. P., Geracioti, T. D., Jr, and Putnam, F.W. (2010). Psychopharmacologic treatment of posttraumatic stress disorder in children and adolescents: A review. *Journal of Clinical Psychiatry, 71*, 932–941.

Clinical Case Illustration

Eliza, an 8-year-old female, presented to the outpatient child psychiatry clinic with a chief complaint of aggressive and disruptive behavior worsening over the past 6 months. Eliza had a prior history of being diagnosed with oppositional defiant disorder and anxiety disorder, not otherwise specified (with features of separation, generalized, and social anxiety) at age 5 and had a short course of supportive play-based psychotherapy lasting 3 months at that time. She received no prior medication therapy. Eliza lived with her mother, who had a history of PTSD, ADHD, and depression. Father's whereabouts were unknown. Father reportedly had a diagnosis of ADHD and "anger problems" and had been physically and verbally abusive to both mother and Eliza during the first four years of Eliza's life, when the parents were together.

Eliza's behavior apparently worsened 6 months prior to presentation, coincident with mother's boyfriend and his two sons aged 12 and 14 years starting every other weekend visits with Eliza and her mother in their home. Mother described Eliza's behavior as becoming increasingly irritable after these visits began. Eliza would show defiance and argumentativeness and had frequent temper tantrums at home over minor issues. She exhibited some social withdrawal at school and seemed irritable and less interested in usual pleasurable activities according to her teacher. Eliza appeared more distractible than usual and her grades declined over this period.

Psychiatric evaluation revealed that Eliza was experiencing significant sad and irritable mood symptoms for most of the day nearly every day. She reported that her mother's boyfriend's sons had been "mean" to her, that they would often hold her down, touch her private parts, and hold a pillow over her face such that she thought she would suffocate. Eliza was afraid to tell her mother as the boys had threatened to kill her pet cat if she told on them. These episodes reminded her of mistreatment at the hands of her biological father. Eliza acknowledged having flashbacks, intrusive memories, nightmares, and feelings of rage that she could not control regarding these incidents with the boys. ADHD rating scales at home and at school indicated moderate levels of symptomatology; especially prominent were distractibility and impulsivity.

Eliza met diagnostic criteria for PTSD, ADHD combined type, and mood disorder, not otherwise specified. A report was filed with the state's Division of Children, Youth and Families owing to the abusive behavior on the part of the boyfriend's sons. Visits and contact with the boys were stopped. Eliza and her mother were provided psycho-educational materials and explanations for the diagnoses of PTSD and ADHD. They were engaged in a collaborative discussion of a multiple modality treatment plan including options for medication. Eliza was enrolled in individual therapy with a therapist experienced in conducting TF-CBT. The therapist also provided support and coaching for Eliza's mother. Eliza was started on guanfacine 0.5 mg twice a day with up titration to 1 mg bid over two weeks that yielded benefit in terms of reducing her ADHD symptoms by 50 percent on rating scales. The guanfacine was also helpful in reducing Eliza's symptoms of hyperarousal and agitation by her own report. Subsequently, she was started on sertraline 25 mg per day targeting her irritable, dysphoric, sad mood. Sertraline was up titrated over 6 weeks to 100 mg per day with noted improvement in mood and decreased irritability.

Eliza's case is instructive as it reflects a commonly seen presentation of multiple comorbid disorders and externalizing behaviors, some of which are reflective of trauma. Eliza likely had PTSD when she first presented for evaluation at age 5.

Subsequent trauma both reactivated earlier symptoms and led to the development of full-blown PTSD along with co-occurring mood symptoms. Eliza had genetic loading for ADHD and these symptoms worsened subsequent to her re-traumatization. Guanfacine may have been a better choice in Eliza's case than a stimulant medication as it not only helped reduce ADHD symptoms but also may have provided additional "dampening down" of her hyperarousal symptoms. Sertraline, in combination with TF-CBT, appeared beneficial in reducing Eliza's irritability and dysphoric mood. Of course, most important was the identification and removal of the ongoing traumatization.

Commentary of Related DSM-5 Disorders: Advancements and Directions

Just like adults with PTSD, children and adolescents with this disorder often meet criteria for other psychiatric problems (Brady, 1997; Breslau, Davis, Andreski, & Peterson, 1991; De Bellis, 1997; Goenjian et al., 1995; Kessler, Berglund et al., 2005; Perkonigg et al., 2005). Copeland et al. (2007) showed in a study of 1,420 children aged 9 to 13 years that children exposed to trauma had almost double the rates of a comorbid psychiatric disorder than children who were not exposed to trauma. Disruptive behavior disorders, anxiety disorders, and substance use disorders were the most common comorbid conditions in these children.

Multiple studies have noted the comorbidity between PTSD and depressive disorders (Goenjian et al., 1995; Goenjian et al., 2005), as well as between PTSD and externalizing disorders (Cuffe, McCullough & Pumariega, 1994; Ford et al., 2000; Glod & Teicher, 1996; Marsee, 2008; Scheeringa & Zeanah 2008). Younger children with PTSD may present with classical features of ADHD (Cuffe et al., 1994; De Bellis & Putnam, 1994; De Bellis et al., 1999; McLeer, Callaghan, Henry, & Wallen, 1994; Loof et al., 1995; Weinstein, Staffelbach, & Biaggio, 2000). More serious externalizing disorders, such as conduct disorder and oppositional-defiant disorder, are also commonly comorbid with PTSD (Arroyo & Eth, 1985; Scheeringa & Zeenah 2008; Steiner, Garcia, & Matthews, 1997) Similarly, the relationship between PTSD and substance use disorders in children has been noted in several studies (Arroyo & Eth, 1985; Brent et al., 1995; Loof et al., 1995; Williams et al., 2008).

Children with PTSD may be more likely to have comorbid conditions because traumatic insults occur in developmentally sensitive periods. Early-life trauma is particularly toxic in its effects on development. In younger children, these may manifest as attachment disorders, impaired social skills, aggressiveness, severe oppositionality, impulsivity, and sexualized behaviors, depending on the nature of the trauma. Comorbid attachment disorders often result from the more chronic type II childhood traumas.

Owing to a more sophisticated appreciation and sensitivity to child development, DSM-5 has taken PTSD out of the anxiety disorders and included it in a broader section of trauma and stressor-related disorders. Increasing attention is being paid to traumatic events in early childhood as laying the groundwork in older children and adolescents for the development of anxiety disorders, depression, somatization, dysthymia, alcohol abuse, and substance abuse. Understanding development and psychiatric comorbidity has important implications for the optimal matching of pharmacotherapy to symptoms, and for the potential early intervention and prevention of development of subsequent disorders.

Challenges and Recommendations for Future Research

It is clear that prevalence of PTSD, associated morbidity, and long-term emotional and behavioral sequelae in children and adolescents are widely reported; yet, medications are utilized despite limited evidence in youth and are often extrapolated from adult psychopharmacological evidence. Given the differences between children and adults in their response to certain medications discussed earlier, it is imperative to use caution when using findings from adult studies to treat the pediatric population for PTSD. Targeted medication use in children with PTSD has a role to play in the overall treatment strategies for youth with the disorder. While there are "no skills in pills," and medication cannot replace well-conducted psychotherapy (in particular TF-CBT), medication can alleviate significant emotional and behavioral distress and dysfunction, allowing children to both function better in their everyday lives and engage more meaningfully in psychotherapy. Future research will be directed to isolating specific treatment effects in specific symptom presentations that will determine which types of mediation and which types of psychotherapy are most efficacious in well-described clinical populations of children with PTSD.

Key Practice Points and Recommended Resources for Practice

There are many gaps in the current state of knowledge about the psychopharmacology of pediatric PTSD. Empirical evidence is not systematic and is scant in various areas. Clinicians should take a rational approach to the pharmacological treatment of pediatric PTSD. This approach can be based on a convergence of evidence from the adult and child / adolescent literature as well as an understanding of the basic neurobiological mechanisms of the pharmacological agents.

In selecting pharmacologic agents for pediatric PTSD, it is helpful to work stepwise. First, there must be an accurate diagnosis of PTSD or subsyndromal PTSD symptoms that are debilitating enough to warrant pharmacological intervention. Second, comorbid conditions such as depression, ADHD, and attachment disorder must be identified. Third, clinicians must identify the target symptoms for treatment and specify reasonable treatment goals (e.g., reduction in sleep latency, frequency of nightmares, or avoidance behavior). Fourth, selection of therapeutics entails segregation of targets for psychosocial (e.g., TF-CBT) from biological (e.g., pharmacological) intervention. These will often overlap. Both psycho-education and TF-CBT should usually be in place before consideration is given to pharmacotherapy. Ideally, TF-CBT, including narrative exposure and trauma processing, is used in individual or group treatment, often in combination with family-oriented support or psychodynamically based interventions. Medications are unlikely to be effective in settings where trauma exposure or abuse is ongoing in the life of a child or where there is no framework in place for dealing with the aftermath of traumatic experiences. Unfocused, loosely conceived psychotherapy is to be avoided, as it can inadvertently act to re-traumatize. Pharmacological intervention can be used to facilitate psychotherapy by decreasing hyperarousal and avoidance. Medication intervention should be considered early in the treatment process when severe and debilitating symptoms are present, limiting function or interfering with therapy.

In selecting pharmacological interventions in pediatric PTSD, the most debilitating symptoms should be treated first, balanced with a weighing of the symptoms most likely to be responsive to pharmacotherapy. Reduction in even one symptom, for example, insomnia, may provide significant relief and improvement in overall functioning. The use of targeted multi-pharmacotherapy should be used when necessary.

As a general approach, treatment should begin with a broad-spectrum agent such as an SSRI, which covers symptoms of affect dysregulation, panic, comorbid depression, and anxiety. SSRIs are the only agents that appear to be consistently effective for avoidance, numbing, and dissociation symptoms. If ADHD symptoms are also present, the adjunctive use of a stimulant or bupropion should be considered. The agents clonidine and guanfacine, as well as imipramine and cyproheptadine, should be considered if insomnia, hyper-startle, or hyperarousal symptoms are problematic.

In cases of SSRI nonresponse, consideration should be given to using venlafaxine or nefazadone, as these agents appear to be safe and have consensus support for their use. Inevitably, more effective pharmacological interventions will be identified as systematic clinical trials are undertaken in children and adolescents with PTSD.

References

Akinsanya, A., Marwaha, R., & Tampi, R. R. (2017). Prazosin in children and adolescents with posttraumatic stress disorder who have nightmares: A systematic review. *Journal of Clinical Psychopharmacology, 37*(1), 84–88.

American Psychiatric Association. (1980). *Diagnostic and statistical manual of mental disorders* (3rd edn., text rev.). Washington, DC: Author.

Asnis, G. M., Kohn, S. R., Henderson, M., & Brown, N. L. (2004). SSRIs versus non-SSRIs in post-traumatic stress disorder. *Drugs, 64*(4), 383–404.

Arroyo, W., & Eth, S. (1985). Children traumatized by Central American warfare. *Post-traumatic Stress Disorder in Children,* 101–120.

Benkelfat, C. (1993). Serotonergic mechanisms in psychiatric disorders: New research tools, new ideas. *International Clinical Psychopharmacology, 8*(Suppl 2), 53–56.

Brady, K. T. (1997). Posttraumatic stress disorder and comorbidity: Recognizing the many faces of PTSD. *The Journal of Clinical Psychiatry, 58*(Supp.), 12–15.

Brady, K. T., Killeen, T. K., Brewerton, T., & Lucerini, S. (2000). Comorbidity of psychiatric disorders and posttraumatic stress disorder. *The Journal of Clinical Psychiatry, 61* (Suppl), 22–32.

Brady, K., Pearlstein, T., Asnis, G. M., Baker, D., Rothbaum, B., Sikes, C. R., & Farfel, G. M. (2000). Efficacy and safety of sertraline treatment of posttraumatic stress disorder: a randomized controlled trial. *JAMA, 283*(14), 1837–1844.

Bremner, J. D., Davis, M., Southwick, S. M., Krystal, J. H., & Charney, D. S. (1993). Neurobiology of posttraumatic stress disorder. *Review of Psychiatry, 12*, 183–204.

Brent, D. A., Perper, J. A., Moritz, G., Liotus, L., Richardson, D., Canobbio, R., ... Roth, C. (1995). Posttraumatic stress disorder in peers of adolescent suicide victims: Predisposing factors and phenomenology. *Journal of the American Academy of Child & Adolescent Psychiatry, 34*(2), 209–215.

Breslau, N., Davis, G. C., Andreski, P., & Peterson, E. (1991). Traumatic events and posttraumatic stress disorder in an urban population of young adults. *Archives of General Psychiatry, 48*(3), 216–222.

Bridge, J. A., Birmaher, B., Iyengar, S., Barbe, R. P., & Brent, D. A. (2009). Placebo response in randomized controlled trials of antidepressants for pediatric major depressive disorder. *American Journal of Psychiatry, 166*(1), 42–49.

Brkanac, Z., Pastor, J. F., & Storck, M. (2003). Prazosin in PTSD. *Journal of the American Academy of Child & Adolescent Psychiatry, 42*(4), 384–385.

Brophy, M. H. (1991). Cyproheptadine for combat nightmares in post-traumatic stress disorder and dream anxiety disorder. *Military Medicine, 156*, 100–101.

Charney, D. S., Deutch, A. Y., Krystal, J. H., Southwick, S. M., & Davis, M. (1993). Psychobiologic mechanisms of posttraumatic stress disorder. *Archives of General Psychiatry, 50*(4), 294–305.

Cohen, J. A., Mannarino, A. P., Perel, J. M., & Staron, V. (2007). A pilot randomized controlled trial of combined trauma-focused CBT and sertraline for childhood PTSD symptoms. *Journal of the American Academy of Child & Adolescent Psychiatry, 46*(7), 811–819.

Copeland, W. E., Keeler, G., Angold, A., & Costello, E. J. (2007). Traumatic events and posttraumatic stress in childhood. *Archives of General Psychiatry, 64*(5), 577–584.

Cosima, L., Koechlin, H., Zion, S., Werner, C., Pine, D. S., Kirsch, I., ... Kossowsky, J. (2017) Efficacy and safety of selective serotonin reuptake inhibitors, serotonin-norepinephrine reuptake inhibitors, and placebo for common psychiatric disorders among children and adolescents: A systematic review and meta-analysis. *JAMA Psychiatry*, August 30, 2017, E1–E10.

Cuffe, S. P., McCullough, E. L., & Pumariega, A. J. (1994). Comorbidity of attention deficit hyperactivity disorder and post-traumatic stress disorder. *Journal of Child and Family Studies, 3*(3), 327–336.

Davidson, J. R. (1997). Biological therapies for posttraumatic stress disorder: An overview. *The Journal of Clinical Psychiatry, 58*, 29–32.

Daviss, W. B. (1999). Efficacy and tolerability of buproprion in boys with ADHD and major depression or dysthymic disorder. *Journal of Child and Adolescent Psychopharmacology Update, 1*(5), 1–6.

De Bellis, M. D. (1997). Posttraumatic stress disorder and acute stress disorder. In R. T. Ammerman & M. Hersen, eds., *Handbook of prevention and treatment with children and adolescents: Intervention in real world contexts* (pp. 455–494). New York: Wiley.

De Bellis, M. D., Keshavan, M. S., Clark, D. B., Casey, B. J., Giedd, J. N., Boring, A. M., & Ryan, N. D. (1999). Developmental traumatology part II: Brain development. *Biological Psychiatry, 45*(10), 1271–1284.

De Bellis, M.D., & Putnam, F.W. (1994). The psychobiology of childhood maltreatment. *Child and Adolescent Psychiatric Clinics of North America, 3*, 663–678.

Doman, S. E., & Andersen, M. S. (2000). Nefazodone for PTSD. *Journal of the American Academy of Child & Adolescent Psychiatry, 39*(8), 942–943.

Famularo, R., Kinscherff, R., & Fenton, T. (1988). Propranolol treatment for childhood posttraumatic stress disorder, acute type: A pilot study. *American Journal of Diseases of Children, 142*(11), 1244–1247.

Foa, E. B., Davidson, J. R., & Frances, A. (1999). Treatment of posttraumatic stress disorder. *The Journal of Clinical Psychiatry, 66*(Supplement 16), 1–76.

Ford, J. D., Racusin, R., Ellis, C. G., Daviss, W. B., Reiser, J., Fleischer, A., & Thomas, J. (2000). Child maltreatment, other trauma exposure, and posttraumatic symptomatology among children with oppositional defiant and attention deficit hyperactivity disorders. *Child Maltreatment, 5*(3), 205–217.

Fraleigh, L. A., Hendratta, V. D., Ford, J. D., & Connor, D. F. (2009). Prozosin for the treatment of posttraumatic stress disorder–related nightmares in an adolescent male. *Journal of Child and Adolescent Psychopharmacology, 19*(4), 475–476.

Friedman, M. J. (1990). Interrelationships between biological mechanisms and pharmacotherapy of posttraumatic stress disorder. *Posttraumatic Stress Disorder: Etiology, Phenomenology, and Treatment, 1*, 204–225.

Friedman, M. J. (1995). Toward pharmacotherapy for post-traumatic stress disorder. In M. J. Friedman, D. S. Charney, & A. Y. Deutch, *Neurobiological and clinical consequences of stress: From normal adaptation to PTSD* (pp. 465–481). Philadelphia: Lippincott-Raven.

Friedman, M.J., Resick, P.A., Bryant, R.A., & Brewin, C.R. (2011). Considering PTSD for DSM-5. *Depression and Anxiety, 28*(9), 750–769

Glod, C. A., & Teicher, M. H. (1996). Relationship between early abuse, posttraumatic stress disorder, and activity levels in prepubertal children. *Journal of the American Academy of Child & Adolescent Psychiatry, 35*(10), 1384–1393.

Goenjian, A. K., Pynoos, R. S., Steinberg, A. M., Najarian, L. M., Asarnow, J. R., Karayan, I., ... Fairbanks, L. A. (1995). Psychiatric comorbidity in children after the 1988 earthquake in Armenia. *Journal of the American Academy of Child and Adolescent Psychiatry 34*(9), 1174–1184

Goenjian, A. K., Walling, D., Steinberg, A. M., Karayan, I., Najarian, L. M., & Pynoos, R. (2005). A prospective study of posttraumatic stress and depressive reactions among treated and untreated adolescents 5 years after a catastrophic disaster. *American Journal of Psychiatry, 162*(12), 2302–2308.

Gupta, S., Popli, A., Bathurst, E., Hennig, L., Droney, T., & Keller, P. (1998). Efficacy of cyproheptadine for nightmares associated with posttraumatic stress disorder. *Comprehensive Psychiatry, 39*(3), 160–164.

Harmon, R. J., & Riggs, P. D. (1996). Clonidine for posttraumatic stress disorder in preschool children. *Journal of the American Academy of Child & Adolescent Psychiatry, 35*(9), 1247–1249.

Harsch, H. H. (1986). Cyproheptadine for recurrent nightmares. *The American Journal of Psychiatry, 143*, 1491–1492.

Horrigan, J. P., & Barnhill, L. J. (1996). The suppression of nightmares with guanfacine [letter]. *Journal of Clinical Psychiatry, 57*, 371.

Horrigan, J. P., & Barnhill, L. J. (1999). Risperidone and PTSD in boys. *Journal of Neuropsychiatry, 11*, 126–127.

Kant, R., Chalansani, R., Chengappa, K. R., & Dieringer, M. F. (2004). The off-label use of clozapine in adolescents with bipolar disorder, intermittent explosive disorder, or posttraumatic stress disorder. *Journal of Child and Adolescent Psychopharmacology, 14*(1), 57–63.

Keeshin, B. R., & Strawn, J. R. (2009). Risperidone treatment of an adolescent with severe posttraumatic stress disorder. *Annals of Pharmacotherapy, 43*(7–8), 1374–1374.

Kessler, R. C., Berglund, P., Demler, O., Jin, R., Merikangas, K. R., & Walters, E. E. (2005). Lifetime prevalence and age-of-onset distributions of DSM-IV disorders in the National Comorbidity Survey Replication. *Archives of General Psychiatry, 62*(6), 593–602.

Kessler, R. C., Chiu, W. T., Demler, O., & Walters, E. E. (2005). Prevalence, severity, and comorbidity of 12-month DSM-IV disorders in the National Comorbidity Survey Replication. *Archives of General Psychiatry, 62*(6), 617–627.

Langeland, W., & Olff, M. (2008). Psychobiology of posttraumatic stress disorder in pediatric injury patients: A review of the literature. *Neuroscience & Biobehavioral Reviews, 32*(1), 161–174.

Looff, D., Grimley, P., Kuller, F., Martin, A., & Shonfield, L. (1995). Carbamazepine for PTSD. *Journal of the American Academy of Child & Adolescent Psychiatry, 34*(6), 703–704.

Marsee, M. A. (2008). Reactive aggression and posttraumatic stress in adolescents affected by Hurricane Katrina. *Journal of Clinical Child & Adolescent Psychology, 37*(3), 519–529.

Marshall, R. D., Beebe, K. L., Oldham, M., & Zaninelli, R. (2001). Efficacy and safety of paroxetine treatment for chronic PTSD: A fixed-dose, placebo-controlled study. *American Journal of Psychiatry, 158*(12), 1982–1988.

Marmar, C. R., Foy, D., Kagan, B., & Pynoos, R. S. (1993). An integrated approach for treating posttraumatic stress. In R. S. Pynoos (ed.), *Post-traumatic stress disorder: A clinical review*. Lutherville, MD: Sidrar Press.

McLeer, S. V., Callaghan, M., Henry, D., & Wallen, J. (1994). Psychiatric disorders in sexually abused children. *Journal of the American Academy of Child & Adolescent Psychiatry, 33*(3), 313–319.

Meighen, K. G., Hines, L. A., & Lagges, A. M. (2007). Risperidone treatment of preschool children with thermal burns and acute stress disorder. *Journal of Child and Adolescent Psychopharmacology, 17*(2), 223–232.

Mylle, J., & Maes, M. (2004). Partial posttraumatic stress disorder revisited. *Journal of Affective Disorders, 78*(1), 37–48.

Oluwabusi, O. O., Sedky, K., & Bennett, D. S. (2012). Prazosin treatment of nightmares and sleep disturbances associated with posttraumatic stress disorder: Two adolescent cases. *Journal of Child and Adolescent Psychopharmacology, 22*(5), 399–402.

Perkonigg, A., Pfister, H., Stein, M. B., Höfler, M., Lieb, R., Maercker, A., & Wittchen, H. U. (2005). Longitudinal course of posttraumatic stress disorder and posttraumatic stress disorder symptoms in a community sample of adolescents and young adults. *American Journal of Psychiatry, 162*(7), 1320–1327.

Perry, B. D. (1994). Neurobiological sequelae of childhood trauma: Post-traumatic stress disorders in children. *Catecholamine Function in Post Traumatic Stress Disorder: Emerging Concepts*, 233–255.

Pfefferbaum, B. (2005). Aspects of exposure in childhood trauma: The stressor criterion. *Journal of Trauma & Dissociation*, 6(2), 17–26.

Racin, P. R., Bellonci, C., & Coffey, D. B. J. (2014). Expanded usage of prazosin in pre-pubertal children with nightmares resulting from posttraumatic stress disorder. *Journal of Child and Adolescent Psychopharmacology*, 24(8), 458–461.

Rijnders, R. J., Laman, D. M., & Van Diujn, H. (2000). Cyproheptadine for posttraumatic nightmares. *American Journal of Psychiatry*, 157(9), 1524-a.

Robert, R., Blakeney, P. E., Villarreal, C., Rosenberg, L., & Meyer, W. J. (1999). Imipramine treatment in pediatric burn patients with symptoms of acute stress disorder: A pilot study. *Journal of the American Academy of Child & Adolescent Psychiatry*, 38(7), 873–882.

Robert, R., Tcheung, W. J., Rosenberg, L., Rosenberg, M., Mitchell, C., Villarreal, C., ... Meyer, W. J. (2008). Treating thermally injured children suffering symptoms of acute stress with imipramine and fluoxetine: A randomized, double-blind study. *Burns*, 34(7), 919–928.

Scheeringa, M. S., & Zeanah, C. H. (2008). Reconsideration of harm's way: Onsets and comorbidity patterns of disorders in preschool children and their caregivers following Hurricane Katrina. *Journal of Clinical Child & Adolescent Psychology*, 37(3), 508–518.

Scheeringa, M. S., Weems, C. F., Cohen, J. A., Amaya-Jackson, L., & Guthrie, D. (2011). Trauma-focused cognitive-behavioral therapy for posttraumatic stress disorder in three- through six-year-old children: A randomized clinical trial. *Journal of Child Psychology and Psychiatry*, 52(8), 853–860.

Scheeringa, M. S., Myers, L., Putnam, F. W., Zeanah, C. H. (2012) Diagnosing PTSD in early childhood: An empirical assessment of four approaches. *Journal of Traumatic Stress*, 25(4), 359–367.

Seedat, S., Lockhat, R., Kaminer, D., Zungu-Dirwayi, N., & Stein, D. J. (2001). An open trial of citalopram in adolescents with post-traumatic stress disorder. *International Clinical Psychopharmacology*, 16(1), 21–25.

Seedat, S., Stein, D. J., Ziervogel, C., Middleton, T., Kaminer, D., Emsley, R. A., & Rossouw, W. (2002). Comparison of response to a selective serotonin reuptake inhibitor in children, adolescents, and adults with posttraumatic stress disorder. *Journal of Child and Adolescent Psychopharmacology*, 12(1), 37–46.

Southwick, S. M., Yehuda, R., Giller, E. L., Jr., & Charney, D. S. (1994). Use of tricyclics and monoamine oxidase inhibitors in the treatment of PTSD: A quantitative review. *Catecholamine Function in Post-traumatic Stress Disorder: Emerging Concepts*, 293–305.

Stathis, S., Martin, G., & McKenna, J. G. (2005). A preliminary case series on the use of quetiapine for posttraumatic stress disorder in juveniles within a youth detention center. *Journal of Clinical Psychopharmacology*, 25(6), 539–544.

Stein, D. J., Ipser, J. C., Seedat, S., Sager, C., & Amos, T. (2006). Pharmacotherapy for post traumatic stress disorder (PTSD). The Cochrane Library. *Journal of Traumatic Stress*, 20(6).

Steiner, H., Garcia, I. G., & Matthews, Z. (1997). Posttraumatic stress disorder in incarcerated juvenile delinquents. *Journal of the American Academy of Child & Adolescent Psychiatry, 36*(3), 357–365.

Steiner, H., Saxena, K. S., Carrion, V., Khanzode, L. A., Silverman, M., & Chang, K. (2007). Divalproex sodium for the treatment of PTSD and conduct disordered youth: A pilot randomized controlled clinical trial. *Child Psychiatry & Human Development, 38*(3), 183–193.

Strawn, J. R., DelBello, M. P., & Geracioti, T. D., Jr. (2009). Prazosin treatment of an adolescent with posttraumatic stress disorder. *Journal of Child and Adolescent Psychopharmacology, 19*(5), 599–600.

Strawn, J. R., & Keeshin, B. R. (2011). Successful treatment of posttraumatic stress disorder with prazosin in a young child. *Annals of Pharmacotherapy, 45*(12), 1590–1591.

Strawn, J. R., Keeshin, B. R., DelBello, M. P., Geracioti, T. D., Jr., & Putnam, F. W. (2010). Psychopharmacologic treatment of posttraumatic stress disorder in children and adolescents: A review. *Journal of Clinical Psychiatry, 71*, 932–941.

Stoddard, F. J., Jr., Luthra, R., Sorrentino, E. A., Saxe, G. N., Drake, J., Chang, Y., ... Sheridan, R. L. (2011). A randomized controlled trial of sertraline to prevent posttraumatic stress disorder in burned children. *Journal of Child and Adolescent Psychopharmacology, 21*(5), 469–477.

Tcheung, W. J., Robert, R., Rosenberg, L., Rosenberg, M., Villarreal, C., Thomas, C., ... Meyer III, W. J. (2005). Early treatment of acute stress disorder in children with major burn injury. *Pediatric Critical Care Medicine, 6*(6), 676–681.

Terr, L. C. (2003). Childhood traumas: An outline and overview. *Focus, 1*(3), 322–334.

Tucker, P., Trautman, R. P., Wyatt, D. B., Thompson, J., Wu, S. C., Capece, J. A., & Rosenthal, N. R. (2007). Efficacy and safety of topiramate monotherapy in civilian posttraumatic stress disorder: A randomized, double-blind, placebo-controlled study. *Journal of Clinical Psychiatry, 68*(2), 201–206.

Van der Kolk, B. A., Perry, J. C., & Herman, J. L. (1991). Childhood origins of self-destructive behavior. *The American Journal of Psychiatry, 148*(12), 1665.

Weinstein, D., Staffelbach, D., & Biaggio, M. (2000). Attention-deficit hyperactivity disorder and posttraumatic stress disorder: Differential diagnosis in childhood sexual abuse. *Clinical Psychology Review, 20*(3), 359–378.

Wheatley, M., Plant, J., Reader, H., Brown, G., & Cahill, C. (2004). Clozapine treatment of adolescents with posttraumatic stress disorder and psychotic symptoms. *Journal of Clinical Psychopharmacology, 24*(2), 167–173.

Williams, J. K., Smith, D. C., Gotman, N., Sabri, B., An, H., & Hall, J. A. (2008). Traumatized youth and substance abuse treatment outcomes: A longitudinal study. *Journal of Traumatic Stress, 21*(1), 100–108.

Yeh, M. S., Mari, J. J., Costa, M. C. P., Andreoli, S. B., Bressan, R. A., & Mello, M. F. (2011). A double-blind randomized controlled trial to study the efficacy of topiramate in a civilian sample of PTSD. *CNS Neuroscience & Therapeutics, 17*(5), 305–310.

Yehuda, R. (1998). Recent developments in the neuroendocrinology of posttraumatic stress disorder. *CNS Spectrums, 3*(S2), 22–29.

31 Enhanced Family-Based Interventions for Children Who Have Been Traumatized by Physical Abuse and Neglect

Cynthia Cupit Swenson

Introduction

Child abuse and neglect (CAN) is a form of childhood trauma that is increasingly recognized as a significant public health problem throughout the world (United Nations Children's Fund, 2012). In cases where the CAN is less severe and appened fairly recently, short-term child interventions and parent training in managing child behavior may be are sufficient to solve the problem. As serious clinical challenges such as significant parent trauma, substance abuse, intimate partner violence, long-standing child behavior problems, and post-traumatic stress disorder among family members become part of the picture, child protection services (i.e., usually a government agency that investigates abuse and neglect and manages the case and out-of-home placements) is tasked with helping families find services that can reduce their risk of re-abuse and out-of-home placement by addressing these problems. Doing so is quite a challenge because multiple providers may be needed. The time, expense, and coordination required to see multiple providers in a week may make this approach to services impossible for many families. Also, trying to coordinate expansive services for a family and communicate with many different providers is often not feasible for child protection social workers. The unintentional outcome of multiple providers and uncoordinated services can be removal of children from the family due to inability to meet these hefty requirements.

In this chapter, we show that in complex child abuse and neglect cases, child behavioral or emotional difficulties require a much broader treatment than child-focused interventions (i.e., parent, child, family, social network treatment) to reduce the risk of re-abuse and out-of-home placement. Further, complex cases benefit from a coordinated effort rather than multiple providers who are not linked for coordination and communication. The treatment required for cases with multiple serious clinical needs must be comprehensive enough to address the breadth of the risk factors that led to the report of the CAN or that are maintaining the family problems. Multiple research-supported treatments with multiple family members are needed to bring about behavioral changes and sustain those changes. Sustainability of change is needed for families to go forward on their own without future child protection monitoring.

Multisystemic Therapy for Child Abuse and Neglect (MST-CAN; Swenson, Schaeffer, Henggeler, Faldowski, & Mayhew, 2010) is one example of a family and ecologically based treatment for complex cases. As such, we expound on MST-CAN's theoretical framework, describe the clinical model, and present the quality assurance system whose function is to sustain long-term model adherence so that the treatment can be delivered in practice how it was delivered in research trials.

Overview of the Issue – The Need for Innovation

A growing body of scientific literature shows that multiple risk factors correlate with CAN. These risk factors are apparent across multiple systems and include the child, parent, family, and social network.

Child Factors

Although children do not cause adults to abuse or neglect them, several child factors raise the risk of abuse or neglect. For example, children who are generally noncompliant or exhibit externalizing behavioral problems such as aggression are at heightened risk of abuse (Black, Heyman, & Slep, 2001). Further, children with disabilities (e.g., communication disorders, health impairment, behavioral disorders) have been shown to be 1.7 times more likely to experience CAN than children without disabilities (Corr & Santos, 2017; Jonson-Reid, Drake, Kim, Porterfield, & Han, 2004; Sullivan & Knutson, 2000).

Parent Factors

A host of parent factors increase the risk that they will abuse or neglect their own children. In particular, mental health difficulties such as depression, anxiety, PTSD, and certain personality disorders have been shown to increase risk (Brown, Cohen, Johnson, & Salzinger, 1998; Sidebotham & Heron, 2006). A number of studies have examined the intergenerational transmission of abuse or neglect. Findings indicate that not all parents who were abused as children go on to abuse their own offspring. Meta-analytic studies show a moderate effect size in predicting parental acts of physical abuse and a small effect size in predicting acts of neglect (Stith et al., 2009). Aside from direct abuse of their child, parents who have personally experienced abuse may bring risk or harm to their children by engaging in relationships with abusive people (Burton, Purvin, Garrett-Peters, Elder, & Giele, 2009). For example, people who have experienced significant trauma and as a result do not develop the capacity to see risk in relationships may end up in intimate partner violence situations. Further, for some parents, substance abuse will play a role in abuse or neglect of their child (Dubowitz et al., 2011; Jonson-Reid et al., 2010).

Family Factors

Family factors that increase the risk of CAN relate to family structure, parenting skills, and partner relations. Single parents are at increased risk of CAN (Berger, Paxson, & Waldfogel, 2009; Sedlak et al., 2010). This is not a surprising finding given the increased stress that one person might experience with managing children, bills, a household and school alone. With regard to parenting skills, parents who abuse or neglect engage in less interaction with their children (Thomas & Zimmer-Gembeck, 2011), display harsher discipline practices (Koenig, Cicchetti, & Rogosch, 2000), and have less knowledge about child development (Dore & Lee, 1999). Parents who neglect their offspring also have poorer caregiving and stress management skills (Coohey, 1998). Intimate partner violence (IPV) is a family factor that significantly raises the risk of abuse or neglect and serious harm. The co-occurrence of CAN with IPV has been shown to range from 18 percent to 67 percent (Appel & Holden, 1998; Jouriles, McDonald, Slep, Heyman, & Garrido, 2008). In the case of IPV by men toward women, the risk of abuse of the child is not only from the primary aggressor of IPV but also from the mother who is recipient of the IPV (Coohey & Braun, 1997).

Social Network Factors

Social network factors that increase risk of abuse typically involve social isolation. Families that engage in CAN have fewer social connections with their community and their extended family (Coulton, Crampton, Irwin, Spilsbury, & Korbin, 2007). In particular, families that neglect have been characterized as having few social networks and briefer romantic relationships (Coohey, 1996).

Implications of a Multiple Systems Etiology in the Need for Innovation

The implications of scientific studies showing a multi-determined etiology is that when a family is referred for treatment due to CAN, an assessment of risk factors across systems must be conducted. If the risk is identified as due to one factor such as low parenting skills, then the intervention may only involve a parent training. When considering families that have been through child protection services multiple times or across a long period, it is likely that the risk factors will be multiple. For example, one family may experience: (1) a child showing aggressive behavior; (2) a second child experiencing depression; (3) a caregiver struggling with opioid use, depression, and low parenting skills; (4) partner conflict; (5) challenges with paying bills; and (6) lack of social support. To effectively prevent further abuse or neglect, each of these risk factors will need to be considered in the intervention plan. An understanding of risk factors specific to a given family helps guide the needed interventions to reduce or eliminate risk of re-abuse.

In addition to addressing risk factors for re-abuse, a thorough assessment of mental health symptoms is needed. For example, due to their experiences, children may have mental health concerns such as PTSD, anxiety disorders, depression, or disruptive behavior disorders (Cyr, Euser, Bakermans-Kranenburg, & Van Ijzendoorn, 2010; Kim, Cicchetti, Rogosch, & Manly, 2009). These mental health issues may not increase the risk for abuse per se but certainly represent a treatment need that if properly addressed can promote child and family healing. If not addressed, these mental health issues may follow children into adulthood and manifest as long-term mental health problems that may impact their own parenting behaviors (Dube et al., 2001; Sidebotham & Heron, 2006; Springer, Sheridan, Kuo, & Carnes, 2007).

Description of the Approach to Innovation

MST-CAN is a research-supported ecological model for families that have experienced recent physical abuse and/or neglect and are being followed by child protection services. In this approach, the target child (i.e., child who is subject to the abuse) is between the ages of 6 and 17. It should be noted that many MST-CAN target children have siblings younger than age 6, and these siblings also receive services under this model. MST-CAN is currently completing work to extend the age of target children downward. The target child and all family members receive treatment according to the risk factors involved and the needs of each family member. MST-CAN has been the subject of rigorous empirical evaluation, dissemination in multiple countries, and implementation research for the past 20 years. The California Evidence-Based Clearinghouse has rated the model as supported by research for child welfare (-www.cebc4cw.org/).

The goals of MST-CAN are to (1) keep families together (i.e., prevent out-of-home placement), (2) ensure that children are safe, (3) prevent a recurrence of the abuse or neglect, (4) reduce mental health difficulties in both caregivers and children, and (5) increase social support for the families. MST-CAN strives to achieve these goals through a strong theoretical base, guiding principles that support model adherence, a structured service delivery model, and an organized analytic process for assessing risk factors, and using identified risk factors to develop and prioritize interventions that are research supported.

Theoretical Base

MST-CAN is an adaptation of Multisystemic Therapy (MST; Henggeler, Schoenwald, Borduin, Rowland, & Cunningham, 2009) that was originally developed to treat delinquent youth with serious clinical problems (e.g., at risk of incarceration or institutionalization) and their families. MST and all its adaptations are based on Bronfenbrenner's (1979) social-ecological model. Bronfenbrenner's model posits that children are at the center of various systems (e.g., parents and siblings, extended family, school, community). Each system influences the child and the child in turn influences each system. As such, the assessment of referral behaviors must consider risk factors in each of the systems to fully understand with whom interventions should be conducted.

Nine Guiding Principles

According to Henggeler and colleagues (2009), nine principles form a common thread throughout treatment. These principles encompass core characteristics of treatment implementation (Swenson, Henggeler, Taylor & Addison, 2009).

1 *The primary purpose of assessment is to understand the fit between the identified problems and their broader systemic context.* MST assessment is not focused so much on diagnosis but rather on the "fit factors" or risk factors that are hypothesized or observed to correlate strongly with or cause the referral behaviors of concern. The risk factors are assessed across all systems. For example, child neglect in a referred family may be due to parental substance abuse, impact of trauma on a parent, low skills in parenting, low support system, and parental conflict. The identified fit factors guide the team on what interventions need to take place.

2 *Therapeutic contacts emphasize the positive and use systemic strengths as levers for change.* MST is a strengths-based treatment model that focuses on what is going well in a family and builds on those strengths. MST does not engage in or promote in any way negative behaviors or verbalizations toward a family or any system (e.g., child protection) with which the family is involved.

3 *Interventions are designed to promote responsible behavior and decrease irresponsible behavior among family members.* Through MST, skills are taught to replace behaviors that are not helpful and support is given to families to practice new skills daily and evaluate the outcome of using a new skill.

4 *Interventions are present focused and action oriented, targeting specific and well-defined problems.* Interventions are not generally talk-therapy interventions. With MST it is critical for people to see their changes taking place and improvements being made, and this is done by objectively measuring outcomes of interventions being implemented in the here and now.

5 *Interventions target sequences of behavior within and between multiple systems that maintain the identified problems.* When conflict occurs, MST works with the family and all systems involved to understand point by point what occurred and where in the sequence of events the family, parent, child, teacher could have done something different to have a positive outcome.

6 *Interventions are developmentally appropriate and fit the developmental needs of youth.* Through MST, interventions should be understandable to parents and youth. Expectations of therapists must be aligned with actual skills and level of functioning of family members. For example, parents are not asked to set up rules and consequences as a parenting strategy but are taken through the process together with the therapist to increase the likelihood that the new skill will be taken up.

7 *Interventions are designed to require daily or weekly effort by family members.* MST therapists do not expect to have a session with parents or youth, review the concerns, and end it there. MST therapists hold the expectation that parents will carry out the interventions with the therapist and away from the therapist on a daily basis for the new skill to become a part of daily life.

8 *Intervention effectiveness is evaluated continuously from multiple perspectives, with providers assuming accountability for overcoming barriers to successful outcomes.* With each intervention carried out, MST measures outcomes to make sure that progress is occurring. Interventions are measured with all ecology members involved. For example, a youth has not been attending school. An intervention is implemented to increase school attendance. The therapist will ask the parent if the child has attended school but will also ask the teacher or check school attendance records. As such, everyone involved is communicating so that outcomes are assured. If outcomes are not being attained, it is the responsibility of the clinical team to determine why (i.e., what are the fit factors to lack of progress) and implement interventions to overcome the barriers to progress. If the interventions are attaining outcomes, the team's responsibility is to understand why the progress is occurring.

9 *Interventions are designed to promote treatment generalization and long-term maintenance of therapeutic change by empowering caregivers to address family members' needs across multiple systemic contexts.* MST is not a "do for someone" intervention. From the start of treatment, parents are expected to take the skills learned and implement them to help their child. The team is a guide and a support to the family's change. In every intervention, families are empowered to take care of their own problems.

As research has been conducted on efficacy, effectiveness, and implementation of MST in the real world, attention has focused on ensuring model fidelity so that it is implemented in the real world how it was implemented in research trials. Research on MST has shown that adherence to these nine principles relates to achieving clinical outcomes with families (Schoenwald, Sheidow, Letourneau, & Liao, 2003). Monthly interviews with families to assess adherence to the nine principles is a key aspect of the MST-CAN quality assurance system.

A Structured Service Delivery Model

MST-CAN follows a similar service delivery approach to Standard MST. Treatment sessions are generally conducted in the family's home or community. Therapists work on the basis of a flexible schedule so that they can meet families at convenient times. A flexible-hours, home-based treatment removes the barriers that are imposed by lack of transportation and having to meet within outpatient clinic hours. Being able to participate in treatment in the evening can be what makes it possible for some families to schedule and attend treatment sessions. In addition to the typical three sessions per week per family, therapists share an on-call rotation to be able to provide 24 hours a day, 7 days a week assistance for family crises.

MST-CAN is implemented via a team approach. The team consists of a full-time supervisor whose purpose is to train, support, and supervise the team in carrying out the model and has the lead in establishing and maintaining positive relationships with child protection services and the community. The supervisor does not carry a clinical caseload. Three masters-level clinicians carry a caseload of no more than four families each for a total of twelve families seen by a team at any given time. A family case manager is available to all families and focuses primarily on practical needs such as housing, jobs, budgeting. The family case manager also does whatever is needed to support the clinical work such as collecting urine drug screens for caregivers who are participating in substance abuse treatment within MST-CAN. The team has access to a psychiatrist or an advanced practice registered nurse (20 percent time) to assist with psychiatric or medical interventions that might be needed.

As noted, the clinicians carry a caseload of four families each. They are responsible for providing interventions for all family members who have clinical needs. In MST-CAN programs, the average number of family members treated within each family has been five. A special emphasis is on adult treatment since the family was referred to treatment because of adult behavior – abuse or neglect.

The MST Analytic Process

MST-CAN follows the MST analytic process that serves as a road map for treatment planning and intervention. Next, the various steps in this analytic process are described.

An Environment of Alignment and Engagement of Family and Key Participants.
Engagement of families is not a treatment step per se but more a process that continues from beginning to end of treatment. Families that come under the guidance of child protection services often feel a low sense of trust and may fear losing their children. Families may also feel low hope that their situation will change. The team's first responsibility is to listen to the family, get to know them, and work to instill hope. In many cases, the low trust can be expressed by the parent withdrawing and not answering the door or phone. MST-CAN therapists must have an attitude of not giving up so that families do not give up. The relationship the family develops with their therapist and team can at times be a factor in having the strength to engage in treatment when difficult topics are addressed such as conflict, trauma, or loss. It is essential for each of the family members to feel respected and heard. Caregivers bring to the table their best skills in relationships. Many experiences in the lives of caregivers may make engaging in conflict an automatic behavior. Sometimes the conflict is directed toward the therapist. The therapist will need to maintain the strength and professionalism to not engage in conflict and instead model calm behavior.

In working closely with child protection services, the MST-CAN team can help foster positive feelings on the part of child protection services toward the family and on the part of the family toward child protection services. Smoothing the waters in this relationship can boost engagement.

A critical part of engagement is to understand the family's cultural background. Doing so means understanding their cultural practices and traditions and ways of viewing the world, problems, and parenting. Understanding a family's culture also involves knowing who is in their life and community and who will be involved in treatment. It will be important to know whom they view as a social support and whom they are in conflict with. The development of a genogram is useful for providing an overview that the therapist and MST-CAN expert who works with the team can reflect on regularly to keep in mind extended family members, their relationships, and what role they might serve in treatment. Once the social supports or ecology members are known, efforts are made to engage them in treatment, with permission from the caregiver. All members of the ecology, the school, and child protection services give their perception on the reason the family was referred for treatment.

Referral Behavior. The first step in the analytic process is attaining a concrete understanding of the referral behaviors. In MST-CAN cases, the referral is due to physical abuse or neglect. Prior to meeting the family, the supervisor and primary therapist should be clear on what specifically happened in the family that led to a report to child protection services. Baseline information is attained on frequency, intensity, and duration of the referral behaviors.

Once there is a clear understanding of the referral behaviors, the therapist can proceed to complete a full clinical intake. In addition to a full history of the caregivers and the target child, trauma assessments are completed to understand the role that trauma might play in mental health symptoms. Pertinent to the MST process, the therapist assesses the strengths (protective factors) and needs (risk factors) of the caregivers and the target child(ren) across the various systems (e.g., individual, school, work, family, peers). Strengths and needs are reviewed periodically as new information surfaces.

Desired Outcomes of Family and Other Key Participants. Each person in the ecology is provided the opportunity to describe their desired outcomes for treatment. Efforts are made to understand the outcomes at a concrete level. For example, the desired outcome of "behave better" might mean to reduce aggression or to complete homework. These are two very different behaviors and understanding "behave better" objectively allows for appropriate interventions.

Development of Overarching Goals. The desired outcomes attained from all in the ecology are reviewed by the team for consistency to determine the four to five top goals. These *overarching goals* must be concrete and measureable as they define the outcomes required to bring treatment to a close. The overarching goals are reviewed weekly as part of the treatment plan and quality assurance process. All weekly interventions must tie directly to these overarching goals.

Conceptualization of Fit. The primary goal of assessment in MST is to understand the factors that are driving the key problems a family is experiencing. In MST-CAN programs, "fit factors" that relate to physical abuse or neglect are always assessed. These risk or correlating factors are called "fit factors" because they guide the team to see how certain factors (e.g., substance abuse, trauma, low problem-solving skills) fit with the current problem behavior (e.g., child neglect). Based on information from multiple sources, fit factors across multiple systems (e.g., family, individual, school, work, peers) are hypothesized. Evidence is considered whether hypothesized fit factors are driving the problem; when the hypothesis is backed by evidence (e.g., family report, observation), those fit factors are brought forward as the subject of intervention. In complex cases, many fit factors (e.g., substance abuse, trauma symptoms, low parenting skills, caregiver conflict) may be present. Therefore, the fit factors must be prioritized according to those that are considered to be the strongest drivers of the problem behavior. Research-supported interventions are then applied to fit factors.

Intermediary Goals. The fit factors that are targeted for change receive primary attention in weekly interventions. Weekly goals are set and are considered to be intermediate outcomes to achieving the desired changes in the overarching goals. For example, an overarching goal is to reduce parental neglect and the team identifies parental substance abuse as the primary driver of neglect. Weekly intermediary goals are set toward implementing strategies to reduce substance use and are evaluated by urine drug screens.

Intervention Development and Implementation. Interventions that have research support and match with the prioritized fit factors are developed in well-thought-out action steps that can reasonably be conducted in a week's time. Then the intervention is implemented with all participants monitoring actual outcomes throughout the treatment period.

Assessment of Advances and Barriers to Intervention Effectiveness. Through weekly supervision and consultation, the success of the intervention is evaluated. If advances are not made, the team's role is to determine the barriers to success and to do whatever is needed to get the intervention on a successful track.

Research-Supported Interventions Commonly Used in MST-CAN

As noted earlier, interventions implemented within the context of MST-CAN are those that have research support for resolving risk factors that relate to CAN. As MST-CAN has been rigorously researched and disseminated, common risk factors have been seen across families with complex problems. The common risk factors have led to interventions applied to every family regarding safety and clarification of the abuse and neglect and interventions applied to some families when specific mental health issues are present. In general, the interventions implemented involve family therapy and behavioral and cognitive behavioral approaches.

Interventions Applied to All Families

Families that have indicated cases of abuse or neglect by definition have safety issues that need attention. All families participate in intensive safety interventions. In early sessions, a family safety plan is developed with all family members and child protection services together so that families have strategies to rely on to support safety. If a caregiver is abusing substances, the safety plan will include the caregiver leaving the home until a negative urine drug screen is produced. Safety protocols are implemented weekly such as safety checklists completed by walking through the house with the caregiver to attend to any safety needs. For example, the team works with the caregiver to ensure that prescription medications are in safe places. Safety plans are updated weekly and if safety issues are present, the team completes fit circles with the family to understand the barriers to safety and develop a plan to overcome them.

Research on CAN has shown that when parents place responsibility for abuse and neglect on the child, the risk for re-abuse is high (Bradley & Peters, 1991; Bugental, Mantyla, & Lewis, 1989; Feshbach, 1989). Clarification of the abuse (Lipovsky, Swenson, Ralston, & Saunders, 1998) involves the parent taking responsibility for the CAN and writing a letter of responsibility and apology to the child and family. The clarification letter is a teaching tool that looks at and corrects unhelpful thoughts, and so there may be several drafts before the letter is complete. A family clarification meeting is held to give the caregiver a chance to read the letter to the family. This intervention has been very popular among families but also has been shown to relate to reduced parental distress and decreased drug and alcohol abuse among families with children placed out-of-home who were working toward their return (Swenson, Randall, Henggeler, & Ward, 2000).

Interventions Tailored to the Needs of Families

As noted earlier, interventions for emotional and behavioral problems of caregivers and / or children are targeted to the particular risk factors they are experiencing. Low caseloads and the capacity for multiple treatment sessions weekly allow therapists the luxury of implementing more than one evidenced-based intervention simultaneously. For adults experiencing PTSD, prolonged exposure (Foa & Rothbaum, 1998) is used. Reinforcement-based treatment (Tuten, Jones, Schaeffer, Wong, & Stitzer, 2012) is conducted with caregivers experiencing substance abuse (Swenson & Schaeffer, 2012). For caregivers who are having difficulty managing anger due to poorly developed skills, cognitive behavioral treatment for anger management is used (e.g., Feindler, Ecton, Kingsley & Dubey, 1986).

In families experiencing abuse or neglect, children may or may not experience behavioral or emotional problems. Resolving parent mental health issues may resolve child behavioral issues but at times, parent-based interventions and / or child-focused interventions may be needed. For example, if the parent has poor parenting skills, child noncompliance can typically be managed by implementing behavioral parenting strategies (Henggeler et al., 2009). If the behavioral or emotional difficulties are PTSD related, Trauma Focused Cognitive Behavioral Therapy (Cohen, Mannarino, & Deblinger, 2006) is implemented with the child and parent.

Standard MST (Henggeler et al., 2009) is largely based on structural and strategic family therapy (Haley, 1987; Minuchin, 1974). Families that participate in MST-CAN often will have difficulties with problem solving and communication (Swenson et al., 2009). When these issues are present in families and skills are inadequate, families will complete behavioral family therapy training to specifically develop problem-solving abilities and improve family communication (Robin, Bedway, & Gilroy, 1994).

In summary, MST-CAN is a family-based treatment model for families that are being followed by child protection services due to an indicated report of physical abuse and / or neglect. Families referred to MST-CAN will have serious and multiple clinical needs and many may have long-standing problems. The MST-CAN model takes the clinical team through an analytic process to determine treatment goals and the focus of interventions. The interventions implemented are those that address the fit factors (i.e., risk factors) that are strongly related to referral behaviors and that have research support.

The MST-CAN Quality Assurance System

To implement the clinical model in ways consistent with the research (i.e., model adherence), a strong quality assurance (QA) system is a mandatory part of MST-CAN implementation. Components of QA include training, supervision, consultation, audiotape review, and caregiver interview.

Prior to taking a caseload, MST-CAN team members complete a total of 13 days of training including 5 days on the standard MST core model, 2 days on MST-CAN protocols, 2 days on reinforcement-based treatment for caregivers who are abusing substances, 2 days on treatment for adult trauma, and two days on treatment for child trauma. In addition to team members, child protection services' caseworkers and supervisors are invited to attend parts of the training so that they can be clear on the model. Other booster training takes place quarterly on site and is led by the MST-CAN expert assigned to the team.

MST-CAN team supervision and consultation with the MST-CAN expert occur weekly. These 1.5-hour sessions are intensively focused on family safety, the fit of referral behaviors, success of interventions being implemented, and problem-solving barriers to attaining clinical outcomes. Therapists conducting trauma treatment audiotape all sessions and receive session feedback from the MST-CAN supervisor and an MST-CAN expert.

Therapist adherence to MST principles and MST-CAN protocols is measured through caregiver interviews conducted by a trained interviewer independent of the team. The adherence interview questions result in a score that provides an adherence cut off. Therapists receive regular feedback on their adherence scores and set goals to increase adherence. The supervisor and expert have the responsibility of helping the therapists make therapeutic adjustments to ensure adherence to the nine principles.

Evidence Base for Innovation

The evidence for MST-CAN is based on rigorous research with emerging work on dissemination. MST-CAN evidence is based on a randomized efficacy trial

(Brunk, Henggeler, & Whelan, 1987) and a randomized effectiveness trial (Swenson et al., 2010).

Brunk and colleagues (1987) randomized 43 families in which children aged 6 to 9 were the subject of substantiated cases of abuse or neglect to either MST or a group-based behavioral parent training. The families that received MST showed greater pre-post changes on resolving family problems, increasing parenting effectiveness, and restructuring parent-child relationships. Parents who received the group-parent training showed better outcomes with regard to decreasing social problems. The latter result was hypothesized to be related to the social support that a group setting provides. However, group settings are temporary, and it seemed that more effort was needed to help families access natural social supports.

The work of Brunk and colleagues (1987) was the first to apply Standard MST to a population experiencing abuse and neglect. Though this study was university based and did not include some of the current-day adaptations for MST-CAN, the study informed more recent effectiveness work. Brunk's study highlighted the importance of measuring re-abuse, out-of-home placement, and parent and child mental health functioning way forward. In addition, this early work underscored the need to address natural social supports, to treat child and adult mental health problems with evidence-based strategies, and to work collaboratively with child protection services. The work of Brunk and colleagues (1987) gave confidence that MST is an efficacious model for families experiencing abuse and neglect. Adaptations were needed clinically and an evaluation of MST with families experiencing abuse and neglect needed to be conducted in the real world.

After five years of delineating an adapted clinical model and piloting it with families, Swenson and colleagues (2010) conducted a study funded by the National Institute of Mental Health. They randomized 86 families that had substantiated cases of physical abuse to MST-CAN or enhanced outpatient therapy (EOT). The latter treatment involved participation in the group called Systematic Training for Effective Parenting (Dinkmeyer, McKay, McKay, & Dinkmeyer, 1998; Gibson, 1999), therapist special efforts to engage families (e.g., weekly phone calls to remind participants of the group meetings, transportation), and referral and connection to any treatment that was needed by the caregiver, child, or family. Youth who were the subject of the abuse were aged 10 to 17.

The effectiveness study featured a 98 percent recruitment rate and strong treatment retention rates (MST-CAN: 98 percent, EOT: 83 percent). Outcomes were assessed at five points in time across 16-months after the baseline assessment. Intent-to-treat analyses showed that MST-CAN was more effective for reducing youth internalizing problems (PTSD, dissociation, and total symptoms on the Child Behavior Checklist), out-of-home placements, and number of placement changes for youth who had to be placed due to safety issues. Fewer MST-CAN youth had an incident of re-abuse than EOT youth, but base rates were low and the difference was not statistically significant. For caregivers, MST-CAN appeared more effective for reducing parenting behaviors that characterize maltreatment (i.e., minor assault, severe assault, neglectful parenting, and psychological aggression). Also, caregivers were more likely to use nonviolent parenting strategies. With regard to social support, MST-CAN was significantly more effective for increasing perceived social support from members of the natural ecology.

The randomized trials conducted thus far have established MST-CAN as a research-supported evidence-based intervention for families experiencing physical abuse and / or neglect and multiple serious clinical needs. Currently, dissemination research to determine feasibility, acceptability, and clinical outcomes is taking place in the United States and five other countries (England, Switzerland, Holland, Norway, and Australia). In the next section, I illustrate MST-CAN in action through a clinical case example of a typical family referred to this program.

Clinical Case Illustration

The description of this case will follow the steps of the MST analytic process. This clinical case is exemplary for the common experiences of families referred to MST-CAN but due to confidentiality considerations for this vulnerable population, it is not an actual case.

Referral

The Welch family was referred for treatment by child protection services following a substantiated report of child neglect by the mother. Roger (aged 10 years) and Dee (aged 6 years) lived with their mother, Hope, while their father was in prison following a drug distribution conviction. The children were late for school almost every day and often reported being hungry. They also were generally ill dressed and unkempt, and Roger had a toothache that had not been attended to. Roger displayed behavioral problems at school and home for which the mother was not intervening. This was the third report in the prior two years that had been received by child protection services. Also significant to the history is that three years prior to this report, the father had an indicated case for child physical abuse after pushing Roger down too brutally. The father attended an anger management group and lived with the family until he was arrested.

Engagement

The first task of the clinical team was to engage the family. The team supervisor and child protection caseworker went to the family home together to discuss the program with the mother to assure her that she had a choice to start MST-CAN or some other treatment. This joint meeting took away concerns the family might have about being forced into an intensive treatment. The mother decided to sign on with MST-CAN. Even though she strongly desired participation in the treatment, she was concerned about addressing her mental health issues. She believed that if she discussed her problems, child protection services would remove her children. She had experienced significant trauma and was worried that if she were asked to talk about it, she would go crazy. Her fears and low trust for therapists and child protection services led her to not open the door at the first treatment appointment. The team continued to call and text her and dropped by the house to leave notes for another week. They also mailed her a card letting her know they were looking forward to working with her. After she received the card, she phoned the team and set up an appointment, which she kept. The team was well aware that people who have been through significant trauma may show inconsistent engagement. So, engaging the family would be a process that would continue throughout treatment.

Assessment

The goals of the assessment were to (1) understand the family's background and view of the world to see how treatment would work best for them; (2) obtain a clear and concrete definition of the referral behaviors; (3) get a picture of the strengths and needs of the target child, Roger, and other family members; (4) clearly delineate any social supports for the family and who is in the extended family and friendship group; (5) understand safety issues and barriers to safety; (6) examine fit factors for the referral behaviors – that is, drivers of the referral behaviors; and (7) attain desired treatment outcomes by all in the ecology plus the child protection caseworker and MST-CAN therapist. In addition to the MST-CAN intake, the assessment included a formal adult and child trauma assessment to determine traumatic events mother and Roger had experienced.

Strengths, Background, and Needs of Mother. Hope cared deeply for her children and truly wanted to change the family's situation. When the children were in school, she worked part-time at a local restaurant although it was hard for her to leave the house. She enjoyed music. Although she had to drop out of high school to get out of a difficult childhood home situation, she was strong in math skills and wanted to complete a high school education. She had two close friends and was in close contact with her maternal grandmother.

Hope came from a family background where women were viewed as subservient to men. Her father was violent toward her mother most of Hope's life. Her father and a paternal uncle sexually abused her; when she disclosed, the family told her she was making it up. When Child protection services investigated, Hope's parents made her recant the accusation. The lack of support for her abuse disclosure coupled with the forced recantation left her feeling that she could trust no one to keep her safe. In particular, she had low trust in child protection services because they could not "see through her recanting" and had failed to remove her from an unsafe situation. She continued to be sexually abused until she could find a way to leave home at age 16. She lived at times on the streets until the man who was to be Roger's father took her in. She stopped talking about the sexual abuse completely from that time on. Surprisingly because the team asked about sexual abuse and seemed to genuinely care about what she had gone through in her life, mother again disclosed the sexual abuse she experienced as a child.

At the time of referral, Hope was having difficulty disciplining the children. Dee was generally well behaved, but Roger did not follow her directions and when he started name-calling and putting her down, she tended to shut down and experience flash backs of the intimate partner violence she had experienced. Her trauma symptoms were greatly impacting her parenting. She also had been drinking at night after the children went to bed and had difficulty getting up in the morning.

Roger's Strengths and Needs. Roger had many strengths. He had a couple of friends with whom he often spent time. He also got along well with his sister and helped watch over her.

With regard to needs, Roger displayed clear behavioral difficulties at home. He did not obey to the rules set by his mother and was verbally aggressive toward her when she tried to correct him or give him directives. He would call her names, tell her to shut up, and threaten to hit her. Mother reported that Roger had never actually hit her. Roger reported feeling angry and sad all the time. He had very angry memories of the intimate partner violence that had been directed at his mother and felt he should have done something to stop it. He was also angry with his mother for being sad all the time.

Family Strengths and Needs. Despite conflicts that occurred between Roger and his mother, the family had a close relationship and enjoyed activities together. As noted earlier, the maternal grandmother was a source of social support to the family. The main family issues related to low structure and low parenting. The family also struggled financially.

School Strengths and Needs. Roger and Dee liked school and were both performing well academically. They both liked their teachers and enjoyed after-school activities. Roger showed interest and talent in drumming in music class. He was also interested in running but was not connected to this sport. Roger had behavioral difficulties at school. He argued with classmates on a daily basis and in particular was verbally negative to two girls in his class, calling them names.

Overarching Goals

Considering the strengths and needs and desired outcomes of the family and all in the ecology, the family set the following overarching goals: (1) eliminate neglect – mother would get the children to school on time, ensure that they had sufficient food, and that they got to all medical/dental appointments; (2) improve family structure and discipline at home; (3) reduce mother's mental health difficulties; and (4) improve Roger's behavior at home and school.

Fit of the Referral Problem and Interventions for the Fit Factors

Referral Behavior #1: *Neglect.* The fit assessment indicated that Hope was struggling to get the children to school on time because her nighttime drinking led to her sleeping in mornings. A fit assessment of the drinking led to the understanding that mother was experiencing post-traumatic stress symptoms in relation to the sexual abuse as a child and IPV as an adult. She was drinking daily to "drown out the memories." The drinking behavior was addressed by means of the following interventions: (1) support Hope in a period of medical detox and then engage her in a full course of home-based RBT to eliminate alcohol use. Maternal grandmother agreed to stay with the children while mother was in detox for a week and (2) conduct prolonged exposure with Hope to address the traumatic events she experienced and that were causing significant symptoms related to anxiety.

Referral Behavior #2: *Low family structure and parental discipline.* The drivers (fit factors) for low family structure and parental discipline were twofold. Hope had never experienced setting up rules or a discipline plan and so her parenting skills needed development. In addition, her post-traumatic stress disorder impacted her parenting. When Roger called her a name or used a verbally abusive tone similar to his father, Hope said this "stopped me dead in my tracks" as Roger's behaviors were a trauma trigger. She felt overwhelming anxiety, withdrew, and did not carry out the directives. Again, a two-step intervention was taken: (1) a behavioral parent training was implemented to assist Hope in developing a family schedule, setting rules, and delivering consequences. A particular focus was on changing Roger's verbal aggression at home; and (2) prolonged exposure was conducted with Hope to address her trauma symptoms.

Referral Behavior #3: *Hope's mental health difficulties.* Hope's symptoms of anxiety, depressed mood, re-experiencing, avoidance, and hyperarousal were driven by the traumatic events she had experienced in the past. In addition, the alcohol abuse impacted all areas of her functioning and was the main way of coping she had developed to deal with the trauma symptoms. The trauma-related symptoms and alcohol abuse were overlapping drivers, which – as we have seen earlier – were also drivers for the neglect. As such, RBT and prolonged exposure were the primary interventions delivered to improve mental health functioning. In addition, the development of coping skills was conducted by providing Hope with instruction in mindfulness meditation and the use of cognitive behavioral therapy–based cognitive restructuring to replace unhelpful cognitions. Hope also participated in the skills training portion of Trauma Focused–CBT (TF-CBT) with Roger and in these sessions she also learned coping skills.

Referral Behavior #4: *Roger's behavioral problems at school.* The analysis revealed that Roger's ongoing sadness and PTSD symptoms were a result of the IPV, which made it difficult for him to get along with others. To address the PTSD symptoms, the gold standard for child treatment, TF-CBT was used.

Clinical Outcomes

After initial challenges, the family engaged in treatment and satisfactorily completed various interventions, having attained the overarching goals. Weekly safety planning helped Hope maintain a peaceful household. The child protection caseworker worked closely in alignment with the team and family, which helped Hope develop trust. A particular concern was whether child protection services would view an alcohol relapse as a sign to remove the children. The team and child protection services in concert prevented out-of-home placement. Through RBT, Hope became abstinent from alcohol and maintained this abstinence over six months by the end of treatment. Trauma treatment at first was a risky time for relapse and the team and grandmother put social supports in place after the difficult sessions. Hope overcame her PTSD symptoms, which helped solidify her sobriety. Hope and the team worked together on setting up a family structure and learning more effective parenting skills to provide consequences for aggression and rewards for not displaying such behavior. The parenting interventions were helpful in eliminating Roger's aggression at home. The MST-CAN team also worked with the family to connect Roger to a running sports club and to strengthen his connection to music, as he needed more prosocial activities. Through TF-CBT, Roger eliminated PTSD symptoms and the relief he felt was seen at home and school in improved behavior. Finally, Hope completed a clarification letter and read it to Dee and Roger. This acceptance of responsibility was crucial to Roger who had believed he was responsible for the IPV and for making sure his mother was ok. The clarification released him from this pressure. The addition of the grandmother and the mother's friends in treatment helped provide a strong plan for sustainability of treatment gains. At the end of treatment, child protection services closed the case as a success.

Commentary on Related DSM-5 Disorders

As we have implemented MST-CAN, children, adults, and their family members have primarily experienced the social and emotional difficulties we noted earlier. The experience of abuse or neglect is certainly not restricted to these mental health challenges. An entire host of mental health difficulties may be present for adults and children such as anxiety disorders, PTSD, severe depression, and conduct disorder. Regardless of the mental health disorder experienced, with MST-CAN the process of assessment and intervention development is the same. Importantly, in all cases the assessment conducted during MST-CAN focuses on fit factors rather than the diagnosis of a disorder. Research-supported interventions for fit factors are then implemented. For example, if the primary fit factor is caregiver depression, research-supported cognitive therapy for adult depression is used. Behaviors are treated rather than psychiatric disorders.

Challenges and Recommendations for Future Research

Once a treatment model has been rigorously evaluated and found to be effective, a key goal of those who would like to be a part of change in the field and broad change for families is to determine how to disseminate that model to common clinical practice. Dissemination carries many challenges such as funding, engagement of stakeholders, shifting non-evidence-based providers to make a switch to research-supported services, and including a quality assurance model to ensure fidelity. Though these issues are challenging, one of the greatest challenges in implementing complex and comprehensive models that involve learning multiple research-supported interventions such as MST-CAN is training the workforce. When families are experiencing complex, serious clinical needs and ongoing crises, stabilizing the situation to be able to implement interventions takes a great deal of patience, care, solid core clinical skills, and a bit of "thick skin." When the learning curve is steep, therapists can become frustrated and require a great deal of support to maintain feelings of competence. Waxing and waning of engagement for families with serious clinical needs can be disheartening and taxing for therapists who are trying to learn core skills or for any therapist for that matter.

Future research needs are to examine ways to implement research-supported treatments with fidelity and to determine how to train the clinical workforce and support them in ways that prevent turnover. Of course, in the child abuse and neglect field, additional research is needed on effective models for some types of maltreatment that get short shrift (i.e., neglect, psychological abuse). Much of this work is contingent on availability of adequate funding for randomized trials and clinical services.

Key Practice Points

Focusing on ecological- and family-based treatments, the following points are offered for practice:

- Families with difficulties trusting will need significant work helping them trust enough to participate in treatment. Therapists must be patient and persistent with engaging families.
- Understanding a client's culture and family background is essential to not making cultural missteps in treatment that can hamper engagement.
- Knowing the family social supports and engaging them in treatment early will help with engagement and sustainability.
- With families under monitoring of child protection services, safety is a primary treatment goal and should be considered in every session.
- Families with serious and multiple clinical problems can safely address more than one problem at a time (e.g., substance abuse + trauma).
- Implementing a complex treatment model takes buy-in from agency directors and other people who are in decision-making positions.
- Seeking training and support from a mentor to implement treatments that have research support is essential to maintaining treatment fidelity.

Acknowledgments

This article was supported by National Institute of Mental Health Grant R01MH60663 to Cynthia Cupit Swenson. Dr. Swenson is a consultant in the development of MST-CAN programs through MST Services, LLC, which has the exclusive licensing agreement through Medical University of South Carolina for the dissemination of MST technology.

The Medical University of South Carolina owns intellectual property rights to the MST treatment model. As such, the university receives royalties related to the treatment implementation.

References

Appel, A.E., & Holden, G.W. (1998). The co-occurrence of spouse and physical child abuse: A review and appraisal. *Journal of Family Psychology*, *12*, 578–599.

Berger, L.M., Paxson, C., & Waldfogel, J. (2009). Mothers, men, and child protective services involvement. *Child Maltreatment*, *14*, 263–276.

Black, D. A., Heyman, R. E., & Slep, A. M. S. (2001). Risk factors for child physical abuse. *Aggression and Violent Behavior*, *6*, 121–188. doi:10.1016/S1359-1789(00)00021-5

Bradley, E. J., & Peters R. D. (1991). Physically abusive and nonabusive mothers' perceptions of parenting and child behavior. *American Journal of Orthopsychiatry*, *61*, 455–460.

Bronfenbrenner, U. (1979). *The ecology of human development: Experiments by design and nature*. Cambridge, MA: Harvard University Press.

Brown, J., Cohen, P., Johnson, J. G., & Salzinger, S. (1998). A longitudinal analysis of risk factors for child maltreatment: Findings of a 17-year prospective study of officially recorded and self-reported child abuse and neglect. *Child Abuse and Neglect*, *22*, 1065–1078.

Brunk, M., Henggeler, S. W., & Whelan, J. P. (1987). Comparison of multisystemic therapy and parent training in the brief treatment of child abuse and neglect. *Journal of Consulting and Clinical Psychology*, *55*, 171–178. doi:10.1037/0022-006X.55.2.171

Bugental, D. B., Mantyla, S. M., & Lewis, J. (1989). Parental attributions as moderators of affective communication to children at risk for physical abuse. In D. Cicchetti & V. Carlson (eds.), *Child maltreatment: Theory and research on the causes and consequences of child abuse and neglect* (pp. 254–279). New York: Cambridge University Press.

Burton, L. M., Purvin, D., Garrett-Peters, R., Elder, G. H., & Giele, J. Z. (2009). Longitudinal ethnography: Uncovering domestic abuse in low-income women's lives. In G. H. Elder & J. Z. Giele (eds.), *The craft of life course research* (pp. 70–92). New York: Guilford Press.

Cohen, J. A., Mannarino, A. P., & Deblinger, E. (2006). *Treating trauma and traumatic grief in children and adolescents*. New York: Guilford Press.

Coohey, C. (1996). Child maltreatment: Testing the social isolation hypothesis. *Child Abuse and Neglect*, *20*, 241–254.

Coohey, C. (1998). Home alone and other inadequately supervised children. *Child Welfare*, *77*, 291–310.

Coohey, C., & Braun, N. (1997). Toward an integrated framework for understanding child physical abuse. *Child Abuse and Neglect*, *21*, 1081–1094.

Corr, C., & Santos, R.M. (2017). Abuse and young children with disabilities: A review of the literature. *Journal of Early Intervention*, *39*, 3–17. doi:10.1177/1053815116677823

Coulton, C. J., Crampton, D. S., Irwin, M., Spilsbury, J. C., & Korbin, J. E. (2007). How neighborhoods influence child maltreatment: A review of the literature and alternative pathways, *Child Abuse and Neglect, 31*, 1117–1142.

Cyr, C., Euser, E.M., Bakermans-Kranenburg, M.J., & Van Ijzendoorn, M.H. (2010). Attachment security and disorganization in maltreating and high-risk families: A series of meta-analyses. *Development and Psychopathology, 22*, 87–108.

Dinkmeyer, S., McKay, G. D., McKay, J. L., & Dinkmeyer, D. (1998). *Systematic training for effective parenting of teens.* Circle Pines, MN: American Guidance Services.

Dore, M. M., & Lee, J. M. (1999). The role of parent training with abusive and neglectful parents. *Family Relations, 48*, 313–325.

Dube, S. R., Anda, R. F., Felitti, V. J., Chapman, D. F., Williamson, D. F., & Giles, W. H. (2001). Childhood abuse, household dysfunction, and the risk of attempted suicide throughout the lifespan: Findings from the Adverse Childhood Experiences Study. *Journal of the American Medical Association, 286*, 3089–3096.

Dubowitz, H., Kim, J., Black, M. M., Weisbart, C., Semiatin, J., & Magder, L.S. (2011). Identifying children at high risk for a child maltreatment report. *Child Abuse and Neglect, 35*, 96–104.

Feindler, E. L., Ecton, R. B., Kingsley, D., & Dubey, D. R. (1986). Group anger-control training for institutionalized psychiatric male adolescents. *Behavior Therapy, 17*, 109–123. doi:10.1016/S0005-7894(86)80079-X

Feshbach, N. D. (1989). The construct of empathy and the phenomenon of physical maltreatment of children. In D. Cicchetti & V. Carlson (eds.), *Child maltreatment: Theory and research on the causes and consequences of child abuse and neglect* (pp. 349–373). New York: Cambridge University Press.

Foa, E. B., & Rothbaum, B. O. (1998). *Treating the trauma of rape: Cognitive behavioral therapy for PTSD.* New York: Guilford Press.

Gibson, D. G. (1999). *A monograph: Summary of the research related to the use and efficacy of the Systematic Training for Effective Parenting (STEP) program 1976–1999.* Circle Pines, MN: American Guidance Services.

Haley, J. (1987). *Problem-solving therapy* (2nd edn.). San Francisco: Jossey-Bass.

Henggeler, S. W., Schoenwald, S. K., Borduin, C. M., Rowland, M. D., & Cunningham, P. B. (2009). *Multisystemic therapy for antisocial behavior in children and adolescents* (2nd edn.). New York: Guilford Press.

Jonson-Reid, M., Drake, B., Kim, J., Porterfield, S., & Han, L. (2004). A prospective analysis of the relationship between reported child maltreatment and special education eligibility among poor children. *Child Maltreatment, 9*(4), 382–394.

Jouriles, E. N. McDonald, R., Slep, M. S., Heyman, R. E., & Garrido, E. (2008). Child abuse in the context of domestic violence: Prevalence, explanations, and practice implications. *Violence & Victims, 23*, 221–235.

Kim, J., Cicchetti, D., Rogosch, F. A., & Manly, J. T. (2009). Child maltreatment and trajectories of personality and behavioral functioning: Implications for the development of personality disorder. *Development and Psychopathology, 21*, 889–912.

Koenig, A. L., Cicchetti, D., & Rogosch, F. A. (2000). Child compliance/noncompliance and maternal contributors to internalization in maltreating and nonmaltreating dyads. *Child Development, 71*, 1018–1032.

Lipovsky, J. A., Swenson, C. C., Ralston, M. E., & Saunders, B. E. (1998). The abuse clarification process in the treatment of intrafamilial child abuse. *Child Abuse and Neglect, 22*, 729–741. doi:10.1016/S0145-2134(98)00051-9

Minuchin, S. (1974). *Families and family therapy*. Cambridge, MA: Harvard University Press.

Pears, K. C., & Capaldi, D. M. (2001). Intergenerational transmission of abuse: A two-generational prospective study of an at-risk sample. *Child Abuse and Neglect, 25*, 1439–1461.

Robin, A. L., Bedway, M., & Gilroy, M. (1994). Problem solving communication training. In C. W. LeCroy (ed.), *Handbook of child and adolescent treatment manuals* (pp. 92–125). New York: Lexington Books.

Schoenwald, S. K., Sheidow, A. J., Letourneau, E. J., & Liao, J. G. (2003). Transportability and multi-systemic therapy: Evidence for multilevel influences. *Mental Health Services Research, 5*, 223–239.

Sedlak, A. J., Mettenburg, J., Basena, M., Petta, I., McPherson, K., Greene, A., & Li, S. (2010). *Fourth national study of child abuse and neglect (NIS-4): Report to Congress executive summary*. Washington, DC: US Department of Health and Human Services.

Sidebotham, P., & Heron, J. (2006). Child maltreatment in the children of the nineties: A cohort study of risk factors. *Child Abuse and Neglect, 30*, 497–522. doi:10.1016/j.chiabu.2005.1

Springer, K. W., Sheridan, J., Kuo, D., & Carnes, M. (2007). Long-term physical and mental health consequences of childhood physical abuse: Results from a large population-based sample of men and women, *Child Abuse and Neglect, 31*, 517–530. doi:10.1016/j.chiabu.2007.01.003

Stith, S. M., Liu, T., Davies, L. C., Boykin, E. L., Alder, M. ., Harris, J. M., ... Dees, J. E. (2009). Risk factors in child maltreatment: A meta-analytic review of the literature. *Aggression and Violent Behavior, 14*, 13–29.

Sullivan, P. M., & Knutson, J. E. (2000). Maltreatment and disabilities: A population-based epidemiological study. *Child Abuse and Neglect, 24*, 1257–1273.

Swenson, C. C., Henggeler, S. W., Taylor, I. S., & Addison, O. (2009). *Multisystemic therapy and neighborhood partnerships: Reducing adolescent violence and substance abuse* (reprinted paperback edn.). New York: Guilford Press.

Swenson, C. C., Randall, J., Henggeler, S. W., & Ward, D. (2000). Outcomes and costs of an interagency partnership to serve maltreated children in state custody. *Children's Services: Social Policy, Research, and Practice, 3*, 191–209.

Swenson, C. C., Schaeffer, C. M., Henggeler, S. W., Faldowski, R., & Mayhew, A. (2010). Multisystemic therapy for child abuse and neglect: A randomized effectiveness trial. *Journal of Family Psychology, 24*, 497–507.

Thomas, R., & Zimmer-Gembeck, M. J. (2011). Accumulating evidence for parent-child interaction therapy in the prevention of child maltreatment. *Child Development, 82*, 177–192.

Tuten, M., Jones, H. E., Schaeffer, C. M., Wong, C. J., & Stitzer, M. L. (2012). *Reinforcement based treatment (RBT): A practical guide for the behavioral treatment of drug addiction*. Washington, DC: American Psychological Association.

United Nations Children's Fund (2012). *Measuring and monitoring child protection systems: Proposed core indicators for the East Asia and Pacific Region*, Strengthening child protection series No. 1. Bangkok: UNICEF East Asia and Pacific Regional Office (EAPRO)

32 Treatment of PTSD and Comorbid Disorders

Vanessa E. Cobham and Rachel Hiller

Introduction

In the context of trauma exposure and more specifically (for the purpose of this chapter) the diagnosis of post-traumatic stress disorder (PTSD), comorbidity is common. In diagnostic terms, comorbidity refers to the co-occurrence of two or more current or lifetime psychiatric disorders. The issue of comorbidity is a highly significant one clinically – at the very least complicating, and often negatively impacting, the course and prognosis of disorders, as well as treatment outcomes. Comorbidity also brings with it the need for greater thoughtfulness in relation to treatment decisions. For instance, are there conditions that need to be treated separately? Is there an optimal order in which to treat comorbid conditions?

Unfortunately, much of what is known about PTSD and comorbidity (in terms of prevalence, treatment implications, and treatment outcome research) is based on work done with adults. Studies investigating PTSD comorbidity in children and adolescents have been less common, with arguably the most robust research having been conducted with preschoolers, and fewer studies in general examining the issue in older youth (Fan, Zhang, Yang, Mo, & Liu, 2011). For this reason, throughout this chapter, research focusing on adults will be reviewed where research focusing on children and adolescents is either limited or entirely lacking.

Specifically, this chapter will identify the conditions most commonly comorbid with PTSD, present models proposed to explain the development of non-PTSD conditions in the aftermath of trauma exposure, and discuss the impact of comorbidity on the expression of PTSD and treatment outcomes. We will then present two cases designed to illustrate key treatment strategies in the management of two of the most common comorbid presentations: PTSD + depression and PTSD + substance use disorders (SUD). Finally, challenges and recommendations for future research in this field and key practice points and recommended resources for practice will be discussed.

Understanding the Scale of the Issue: Prevalence Rates

By late adolescence, as many as 80 percent of young people have been exposed to at least one potentially traumatic event (PTE), with approximately 15 percent of trauma-exposed young people going on to develop post-traumatic stress disorder (PTSD; Alisic et al., 2014; Copeland, Keeler, Angold, & Costello, 2007; Nooner et al., 2012).

When considering comorbidity with PTSD, several important methodological limitations common to research in this area are important for the reader to keep in mind. To begin with, many studies use self-report questionnaires of the conditions being assessed (including post-traumatic stress symptoms; PTSS), rather than validated diagnostic interviews. Second, the vast majority of studies report on samples that have been exposed to one potentially traumatic event (PTE; e.g., a motor vehicle accident) or a series of traumatic events (e.g., sexual abuse). This opens up the question of generalizability of results across different trauma exposures. Third, many studies investigating comorbidity necessarily only assess for particular conditions (e.g., anxiety or depression), as opposed to screening more widely, impacting on our ability to understand the true extent and range of comorbidities. Finally, the vast majority of studies do not report on dates of onset of post-trauma conditions in relation to one another, with studies failing to accurately document whether comorbid conditions may have predated the index event(s). In summary, the area of PTSD comorbidity in children and youth is one in which much further work is required.

The adult literature tells us that PTSD is particularly likely to be comorbid with depressive disorders, substance use disorders (SUDs), and anxiety disorders, such as social anxiety (Brady, 1997; Brady, Killeen, Brewerton, & Lucerini, 2000). As an example, in a large sample ($N = 1127$) of adults seeking treatment for anxiety and mood disorders, PTSD was the single diagnosis associated with the highest rates of current (92 percent) and lifetime (100 percent) psychiatric comorbidity (Brown, Campbell, Lehman, Grisham, & Mancill, 2001). In this study, PTSD was associated with a significantly elevated rate of lifetime mood disorders (77 percent), anxiety disorders (62 percent), and SUDs (38 percent). In other studies, up to 65 percent of adults diagnosed with PTSD have also been reported to meet criteria for a SUD (Krystal et al., 2011; Pietrzak, Goldstein, Southwick, & Grant, 2011).

Generally speaking, the same patterns of comorbidity are seen in children and adolescents, with some obvious developmental differences. As noted earlier, the few studies that have been conducted with preschool-aged children represent some of the most rigorous work in the area of PTSD comorbidity. Scheeringa, Zeanah, Myers, and Putnam (2003) examined a sample of children aged 20 months to 6 years ($N = 62$) who had been exposed to a range of PTEs (including motor vehicle accidents, accidental injury, witnessing violence, and abuse). Among the children diagnosed with PTSD, respectively 75 percent, 63 percent, and 38 percent also met the criteria for comorbid oppositional defiant disorder (ODD), separation anxiety disorder (SAD), and attention-deficit/hyperactivity disorder (ADHD), respectively. In contrast to the adult literature, the rate for comorbid major depression in preschoolers was only 6 percent. In common with most of the research (whether with adults or youth), this study did not record dates of onset for comorbid conditions – meaning that it is possible that at least some of the comorbid conditions may have predated the PTSD. However, important strengths of this study are its inclusion of participants with a broad range of trauma exposures and its use of a diagnostic interview that allowed assessment of a broad range of possible comorbidities. Building upon their earlier work, Scheeringa and Zeanah (2008) carefully documented the onset of all disorders in a study of young (i.e., aged 3–6 years) children ($N = 70$) who had been exposed to Hurricane Katrina, allowing a clearer picture of PTSD comorbidity – which occurred in 88.6 percent of children with PTSD – to be obtained. Regarding this comorbidity, it was found that approximately half was accounted for by new, post-hurricane conditions. For children with PTSD following the hurricane, the most common *new* comorbid diagnoses were major depressive disorder (MDD; 60 percent), ODD (56 percent), SAD (50 percent), and ADHD (29 percent). Importantly, no cases of new, post-hurricane non-PTSD diagnoses occurring in the absence of PTSD were reported, meaning these comorbidities did not develop until PTSD was also present. This finding has significant treatment implications, suggesting that focusing on PTSD, rather than the comorbidity, may represent the most parsimonious strategy when working with young children in a post-disaster context. These findings have been replicated and extended in a sample of 130 children aged 1–6 years who had experienced unintentional burns (De Young, Kenardy, Cobham, & Kimble, 2012). Of those children who developed PTSD, comorbidity was the norm one month after the event (73 percent), with the most common comorbid diagnoses being MDD, ODD, SAD, and specific phobia. Of those children who retained a diagnosis of PTSD six months after the event, 85 percent continued to meet criteria for at least one comorbid diagnosis, with ADHD, ODD, and SAD being significantly more likely to occur in this group. This clearly suggests that when treatment is not received, PTSD comorbidity persists over time, alongside the primary PTSD diagnosis.

High rates of comorbidities continue to present for older children and adolescents with PTSD. A number of large surveys of children and adolescents have shed light on the high rates of comorbidities in this age range – particularly anxiety, depressive disorders, and SUDs. A phone survey of more than 4,000 12–17-year-olds living in the United States (referred to as the National Survey of Adolescents) found that of boys with PTSD, 47 percent also met criteria for experiencing a major depressive episode, while 30 percent met criteria for substance abuse or dependence. For girls with PTSD, 71 percent met criteria for a comorbid major depressive episode, while 24 percent experienced comorbid substance abuse or dependence (Kilpatrick et al., 2003). A 2012 review of PTSD in adolescents found up to 50 percent of youth with PTSD may meet criteria for comorbid SUDs (Nooner et al., 2012). Following natural disasters, such as the Wenchuan Earthquake in China (Fan et al., 2011) or the 2010 Haitian Earthquake (Cénat & Derivois, 2015), a number of studies involving hundreds of young people have found high and sustained rates of self-reported PTSS and depression, as well as PTSS and a range of anxiety disorders (e.g., separation anxiety, school phobia, social phobia).

Overall, rates of both PTSD and comorbidities are considered to be particularly elevated in samples that would typically be regarded as having been exposed to more complex traumas including youth whose PTSD necessitated a psychiatric inpatient admission, detained and arrested youth, war-exposed refugee youth, and youth who have experienced maltreatment including physical and/or sexual abuse. These more complex samples are particularly important to consider, as it has long been held that exposure to repeated PTEs (such as childhood sexual abuse or multiple-war traumas), as opposed to single PTEs, is likely to result in different and more complex symptom profiles, including a range of comorbidities. In studies of detained and incarcerated youth, the vast majority of participants who met criteria for PTSD on a diagnostic interview also met criteria for at least one comorbid psychiatric disorder (more than 90 percent in one study), with significantly higher rates of comorbidity reported for youth with PTSD compared to youth with no PTSD (Abram et al., 2007; Ruchkin, Schwab-Stone, Koposov, Vermeiren, & Steiner, 2002). The most common comorbid diagnoses were MDD, generalized anxiety disorder (GAD), SAD, past ADHD, conduct disorder, alcohol abuse, and drug abuse. Adolescents with PTSD who require inpatient treatment have been found to demonstrate similar patterns of comorbidity to those who are incarcerated – with high rates of comorbid MDD and conduct disorder reported (Allwood, Dyl, Hunt, & Spirito, 2008; Vivona et al., 1995), as well as more frequent suicidal ideation and attempts (Lipschitz et al., 1999). Refugee children who have been exposed to conflict and then been resettled in another country have been found to experience high rates of comorbid PTSD and depression (Mghir, Freed, Raskin, & Katon, 1995; Thabet, Abed, & Vostanis, 2004; Weine et al., 1995). Other studies of youth living in war zones indicate that when diagnostic criteria for PTSD are met, the risk for comorbid anxiety as well as depression is significantly elevated (Elbedour, Onwuegbuzie, Ghannam, Whitcome, & Abu Hein, 2007; Khamis, 2008). The diagnosis of PTSD also confers additional risk for comorbidity among children exposed to parental maltreatment, physical abuse, and sexual abuse. Specifically, children with PTSD in the context of maltreatment have been found to be at elevated risk for ADHD, anxiety disorders, brief psychotic disorders, and suicidal ideation (Famularo, Fenton, Kinscherff, & Augustyn, 1996). Children and adolescents who have developed PTSD following exposure to sexual abuse, physical abuse, or both are at increased risk for comorbid anxiety and mood disorders – specifically, dysthymia, major depressive disorder, separation anxiety disorder, and overanxious disorder (Ackerman, Newton, McPherson, Jones, & Dykman, 1998; McLeer et al., 1998).

In summary, the majority of children and adolescents who develop PTSD will also have at least one comorbid psychiatric diagnosis. While anxiety, oppositional defiance, conduct disorders, and ADHD are key comorbidities in preschool and early childhood, by adolescence depressive disorders and substance abuse are particularly important to consider. Overall, most studies suggest that older adolescents are at greater risk of developing PTSD and comorbidities, while multiple comorbidities may be particularly elevated and complex where young people have been exposed to multiple PTEs (e.g., child abuse).

Making Sense of Comorbidity in the Face of Trauma

As previously noted, one of the limitations common to PTSD comorbidity research – whether in adults or children and adolescents – is the failure to assess dates of onset of comorbid conditions. This means that in some studies, it is not possible to know whether the comorbid conditions actually existed prior to the onset of the PTSD. Other studies report on the prevalence of new, post-index event conditions, but with insufficient detail to determine the temporal order in which different conditions may have developed.

It is important to understand the relationships between PTSD and comorbid conditions in the aftermath of trauma exposure, as this has potential implications for treatment decisions. In an area in which very little work has been done, McMillen, North, Mosley, and Smith (2002) have made an invaluable contribution – proposing four possible models to explain the psychiatric comorbidity so commonly found with PTSD. In the first model, PTSD was hypothesized to be the primary outcome of trauma exposure, with the presence of PTSD then resulting in the development of secondary, comorbid disorders (e.g., individuals may use alcohol or drugs to self-medicate their PTSD symptoms, potentially resulting in a substance use disorder). In the second model, trauma was hypothesized to lead to multiple possible disorders (with PTSD being viewed as one possible disorder among many), with non-PTSD disorders developing independently of PTSD (Breslau, Davis, Peterson, & Schultz, 1997, 2000). In the third model, diagnostic comorbidity following trauma was hypothesized to be explained by symptom overlap (with major depression and generalized anxiety disorder commonly used as examples). Finally, in the fourth model, a preexisting disorder was hypothesized to make an individual vulnerable to the development of PTSD.

McMillen et al. (2002) investigated these models with adult flood survivors in one of the few studies in which dates of onset of (comorbid) disorders (i.e., PTSD, GAD, MDD, panic disorder, and SUDs) both prior to and following exposure to a PTE were carefully monitored. Another important methodological strength of this study was that individuals with partial PTSD were studied in addition to individuals meeting full diagnostic criteria for PTSD. This is important because research indicates that there is little to no difference in terms of distress and impairment between individuals meeting full DSM-IV criteria (i.e., display sufficient symptoms to meet all three criteria of re-experiencing, avoidance, and increased arousal) compared to those demonstrating partial PTSD (i.e., only display sufficient symptoms of two of the three symptom clusters; e.g., Carrion, Weems, Ray & Reiss, 2002). McMillen et al. (2002) reported that 100 percent of individuals who developed new, non-PTSD disorders following the flood demonstrated significant PTSS (with more than 50 percent meeting criteria for full PTSD). On the basis of their findings, the authors concluded that only the first model described earlier was supported by their data. That is, the best explanation for comorbidities is that PTSD contributes to the development of other disorders in the aftermath of trauma.

A second study that has attempted to untangle PTSD and comorbid conditions in the aftermath of exposure to a PTE was conducted with preschoolers aged 3–6 years (Scheeringa, 2015). Importantly, this study examined children who had been exposed to three types of PTEs – single incident events ($n = 62$; most commonly motor vehicle accidents), Hurricane Katrina ($n = 85$), and repeated events ($n = 137$; most commonly witnessing domestic violence). A number of methodological strengths of this study are worth noting: it is the largest study to examine the issue of comorbidity in young children following exposure to a PTE; it includes children who experienced exposure to a range of different PTEs; the onset of comorbid disorders in relation to earliest PTE experienced was recorded; standardized diagnostic interviews were used; children with partial and full PTSD were included; and the total occurrence of each type of trauma event was documented. Scheeringa (2015) replicated McMillen et al.'s (2002) finding that it was rare for other psychiatric disorders to develop in the absence of PTSD or elevated PTSS. Because this sample was broader in terms of exposure to PTEs (included young children who had been exposed to single incident as well as repeated events), the support for McMillen et al.'s (2002) first model (i.e., that PTSD leads to other psychiatric disorders) can be generalized more widely.

In relation to the development of other internalizing comorbidities, there is also a growing body of literature that shows the same psychological processes that link the experience of trauma to the development and maintenance of PTSD, may also underlie the concurrent or subsequent development of non-PTSD internalizing symptoms. The interested reader is referred to Angelakis and Nixon (2015) for an in-depth review of this overlap in relation to adult PTSD + depression. In the child and adolescent field, how a young person interprets the meaning of the PTE (i.e., maladaptive appraisals or cognitions about the world being very unsafe or young persons being very vulnerable) has been identified as a potential transdiagnostic mechanism that also underlies post-trauma non-PTSD internalizing symptoms (e.g., anxiety and depression symptomatology). The association between trauma-related maladaptive appraisals and non-PTSD internalizing has been replicated in samples who have experienced sexual abuse and maltreatment (Leeson & Nixon, 2011; Mannarino & Cohen, 1996), in a community sample of adolescents (Liu & Chen, 2015), and following single-incident accidental PTE (Hiller et al., 2018). Thus, while there is robust empirical evidence for the role of processes such as maladaptive cognitions for the development of PTSD, there is also developing preliminary support that this process may be related to the concurrent development and maintenance of non-PTSD internalizing problems.

Of course, the temporal development of comorbidities will likely differ for individuals. Nevertheless, evidence that similar psychological processes may underlie the development of non-PTSD symptoms, along with evidence from the child and adult fields of high rates of "new" comorbidities that develop only in the presence of PTSD, again suggests that comorbidities are most likely to develop as a consequence of the PTSD, or at the very least, alongside the PTSD. Such evidence supports clinical guidelines that even in the presence of comorbidities, treating the PTSD should remain the focus of any psychological intervention.

An important possible exception to this conclusion relates to substance use disorders. Although McMillen et al. (2002) examined the comorbidity of alcohol and drug use disorders, this was in the very specific context of a natural disaster. The study by Scheeringa (2015) was with preschoolers, for whom the assessment of substance use disorders was not developmentally relevant. In terms of their temporal relationship to each other, the evidence is less clear around PTSD and SUDs than it seems to be for PTSD and other comorbid conditions. Some research has found that trauma exposure and PTSD predates the development of SUDs in adolescents, with one common theory being that the substance use develops as a consequence of repeated self-medication of PTSD symptoms (Bujarski et al., 2012; Khantzian, 1997). Certainly, exposure to PTEs in childhood has been found to be associated with higher risk for illicit substance use, and a childhood trauma history represents a risk factor when it comes to substance use in adolescence (Carliner et al., 2016). On the other hand, other studies have found that SUDs precede trauma exposure, with one study finding that 50 percent of a community sample of 18-year-olds had developed a SUD before being exposed to a PTE (Giaconia et al., 2000). A common hypothesis proposed to explain this temporal sequence is that the patterns of risky behavior associated with substance use also put youth at increased risk of exposure to PTEs. The interested reader is referred to Simmons and Suarez (2016) for a review of these issues. It is likely that the relationship between PTSD and SUDs (in terms of both onset and function) varies across cases, with clinicians needing to be mindful of a likely "reciprocally reinforcing and bidirectional relationship" (Simmons & Suarez, 2016, p. 725) between post-traumatic symptomatology and substance use. A thorough assessment focusing on dates of onset is critical in working with youth with this particular pattern of comorbidity.

The Impact of Comorbidity on the Expression of PTSD and Treatment Outcomes

While there is widespread endorsement of the idea that the presence of comorbid disorders both makes the clinical presentation of PTSD more complex and has an adverse impact on the treatment of PTSD, there is actually little empirical data that address the issue of the impact of PTSD comorbidity. The existing literature on the impact of comorbidities on treatment outcomes has particularly focused on depressive disorders and SUDs. In relation to PTSD + depression, the research is mixed on how this comorbidity may impact either the expression of PTSD or treatment outcomes. There is some evidence that PTSD with clinical-level depressive disorders is likely to be more severe and more complex to treat, with some, albeit mixed evidence from the adult literature that this group is more likely to drop out or disengage from treatment of PTSD (e.g., McDonough et al., 2005; Schottenbauer et al., 2008; Stein et al., 2012). There are a range of mechanisms that may explain poorer treatment outcomes for PTSD + depressive disorders, including poorer emotion regulation and more entrenched or severe maladaptive cognitions / appraisals. A particular candidate relevant for PTSD + depressive disorders could also be emotional numbing (e.g., the reduced ability to experience emotions). Emotional numbing is central to depressive disorders and PTSD. Research has shown that increased emotional numbing can impede the individual's ability to "optimally engage" in treatment, with subsequent consequences for treatment outcomes (Angelakis & Nixon, 2015). It is also noteworthy that adolescents with a trauma history are more likely to experience treatment-resistant depression compared to adolescents without such a history (Heim, Shugart, Craighead, & Nemeroff, 2010). Thus, assessing for comorbid depressive disorders is likely to be an important component of any assessment of post-trauma mental health. Of note, given the elevated rate of suicidal ideation and attempts in youth with trauma histories and PTSD, it is also critical to assess for suicidality and self-harm, even in cases where depressive symptoms may not be prominent (Gerson & Rappaport, 2013).

In relation to PTSD + SUDs, research suggests that once established, each disorder serves to maintain and exacerbate the other (Back, Brady, Jaanimägi, & Jackson, 2006; Mills, 2009; Simmons & Suárez, 2016) leading to a chronic course of illness and significant treatment complications (Farrugia et al., 2011). For example, exposure to reminders of the traumatic event will often result in increased substance cravings in youth, with PTSD symptom severity associated with more intense substance cravings (Coffey et al., 2002, 2010; Saladin et al., 2003). Adolescents with this comorbidity have significantly more perceived health problems, internalizing symptomatology, and more impaired interpersonal relationships compared to those with a SUD alone (Giaconia et al., 2000). These youth are more likely to be consumers of multiple systems (e.g., special education, child protection, and juvenile justice; Suarez, Belcher, Briggs, & Titus, 2012), and more likely to be at risk of attempting suicide (Brent et al., 2002). In terms of treatment implications, detoxification or withdrawal from substances can potentially exacerbate PTSD symptoms (Brady, 1997). Conversely, focusing on an individual's trauma narrative – an essential ingredient of evidence-based interventions for PTSD – may (as noted earlier) exacerbate symptoms or potentially trigger relapse (via self-medication) in individuals in recovery from a substance use disorder (Brady, 1997). Another important consideration relates to psychopharmacological approaches to treatment of either the PTSD and / or other comorbid conditions (e.g., depression or anxiety), as it will be important to consider the potential for both abuse and drug interactions. Finally, in relation to treatment considerations, we know from the adult literature that treatment providers view an individual with comorbid PTSD + SUDs as significantly more difficult to treat than an individual with either disorder alone, with self-rated confidence in being able to treat this comorbidity being very low (Adams et al., 2016).

Treatment Approaches

Treating Comorbid PTSD and Depressive Disorders

While we know that major depressive disorder or (subclinical) depressive symptoms are common with PTSD, there is less well-developed evidence for the best treatment for this comorbidity. There is also clear overlap between some key symptoms, such as sleep problems, low mood, and poor concentration (Thabet et al., 2004) and growing evidence that transdiagnostic processes may underlie the development of both disorders. Thus, perhaps unsurprisingly, most evidence for the treatment of PTSD in young people shows that standard trauma-focused cognitive and behavioral treatments (as discussed elsewhere in this book) will also lead to a reduction in comorbid internalizing symptoms, including depression (Deblinger, Mannarino,

Cohen, Runyon, & Steer, 2011; Goldbeck, Muche, Sachser, Tutus, & Rosner, 2016; Smith et al., 2007). While there is little evidence to inform which components of the treatment may also be successfully targeting depressive symptoms, there is likely to be clear overlap in negative cognitions (e.g., feelings of blame, guilt, general low mood) that would be targeted in the cognitive component of the treatment. Similarly, most cognitive and behavioral treatments for PTSD will involve processing the memory of the trauma, confronting avoidant coping strategies, and in doing so support the individual to re-engage in previously enjoyable activities. In some ways, these components may act as a behavior activation task (central to the treatment of depression, discussed later).

However, there is a caveat to the finding of depression symptoms reducing from targeting PTSD-only. That is, this research rarely differentiates clinical-level comorbidity from elevated but not clinical-level depressive symptoms. For more complex or severe presentations, an innovative therapeutic approach may be necessary, capturing both the treatment of the PTSD and comorbid major depression. Unfortunately, the empirical literature provides little consensus on this, with research exploring adjuncts to trauma-focused cognitive and behavioral therapies scarce in both the adult and child and adolescent fields. One study by Angelakis (2014) piloted a novel treatment targeting both PTSD and major depression, compared to treatment of PTSD-only, in a group of adults who had experienced a range of traumas, from childhood sexual or physical abuse to an assault in adulthood or traumatic loss. They used cognitive processing therapy, a cognitive and behavioral treatment for PTSD, both as a stand-alone treatment and alongside additional behavioral activation treatment sessions, targeting depressive symptoms. The researchers found that all treatments were successful in reducing both PTSD and major depressive disorder, although incorporating the additional behavioral activation component, after the treatment of PTSD, led to even greater improvements in both PTSD and depression symptoms. These findings, while preliminary, suggest that additional sessions, particularly focused on behavioral techniques used in the treatment of depression, may add further benefit for those with comorbid major depression. Next we present a case study of a 13-year-old boy who presented with comorbid PTSD and depression and suggest some treatment approaches for targeting this comorbidity.

Case Study: PTSD and Depression

Jacob is a 13-year-old boy who was involved in a serious motor vehicle accident. The accident resulted in his sister being seriously injured and a fatality in the other car. Jacob broke his leg although his parents were uninjured. His sister remained in the hospital for one month after the accident. Jacob was in the hospital for less than a week, but he remained out of school for almost a month, while his parents focused on their children's physical recovery. Almost immediately following the accident, Jacob showed signs of a post-traumatic stress reaction. He was having highly distressing nightmares about car accidents. While he told his parents he was sleeping well, they could see from the computer history that he was spending hours awake in the middle of the night, surfing the internet. Jacob would get back in the car but would not sit in the same seat where he was during the accident, and his parents noticed he would often have his eyes closed. His parents would not drive on the same road as the accident occurred so they did not all have to face the reminder of what happened. Over a month later, these symptoms were still present but Jacob's mood was also low. Jacob's parents noticed that he was staying in his room more, was very "snappy" or easily irritable, and seemed to have either lost his appetite or had no interest in joining the family for meals. All of these behaviors were very unlike him before the accident. He seemed to have particularly lost interest in seeing his friends, often ignoring their phone calls and making excuses for them not to visit. Previously he had enjoyed BMX riding, an activity he had not been able to do while his leg was in a cast. However, even after the cast was removed and Jacob was given clearance by the doctor, he seemed uninterested in going back to riding, preferring to stay in his room. Jacob continued to have days out of school, often complaining of a stomachache or headache and asking to stay home. When at school, his teachers noticed that he was "less energetic" at break times and seemed much quieter than his usual self.

Psycho-Education. Given Jacob's presentation, which developed following his involvement in the car accident and persisted for many months after, Jacob was referred to a psychologist for possible assessment of PTSD. His initial assessment also captured that he met criteria for a comorbid major depressive disorder. Thus, as part of the psycho-education component of treatment, he was provided with information on depression, as well as PTSD. This included psycho-education on each disorder separately, as well as their overlap. For Jacob, there were some clear overlaps in the conceptualization of both his PTSD and depression. His broken leg had meant he was physically unable to get back to pre-accident routines and, in particular, his BMX riding and school. By trying to escape his flashbacks and cues that might remind him of the accident, Jacob had also become much more restricted in his movements, preferring to stay inside for long periods of time. His sister's injury severity also meant that his parents had a reduced capacity to support Jacob in processing his experiences, while Jacob also felt immense guilt that he was less injured than his sister and that he was unable to help the person who died.

Treatment of PTSD. Current clinical and empirical evidence shows that treating the PTSD should be the priority in most cases, particularly in Jacob's case, where the depression developed concurrently with the PTSD, and perhaps because of consequences of his PTSD. Therefore, Jacob was treated using trauma-focused CBT, the first-line recommended treatment for child PTSD (National Institute for Health and Clinical Excellence [NICE], 2005; an example of a useful clinical reference is Smith et al., 2009).

As Jacob's PTSD symptoms began to improve, his clinician also introduced two strategies to target his depression, namely behavioral activation (pleasant activities scheduling) and mindfulness. These additional treatment components are taken from the standard cognitive and behavioral treatment for depression in children and adolescents (useful clinical references include Curry et al., 2000; Sburlati et al., 2014; Verduyn et al., 2009). While here his depressive symptoms were addressed concurrently, during the second half of his PTSD treatment, it may also be appropriate to address the depression in additional sessions after the PTSD treatment is completed, given that the depression symptoms may reduce alongside the standard PTSD treatment. Unfortunately, we currently lack robust empirical evidence to guide this decision.

Mindfulness. Mindfulness has received significant attention in the mental health literature over the past decades. It can be found in many cognitive and behavioral treatments, including mindfulness-based cognitive therapy, acceptance and commitment therapy, and dialectical behavior therapy. The practice has particularly been studied in relation to depression relapse (Kuyken et al. 2016; Van der Velden et al., 2015), suggesting it has potential as an innovative technique to target comorbid depression and PTSD. Relaxation techniques, such as those practiced via Mindfulness, have received some support in the trauma literature, as part of a cognitive and behavioral approach (see Cohen et al., 2000), while mindfulness-based CBT, specifically, has also received empirical support with adult trauma-exposed populations, particularly military veterans (e.g., King et al., 2013; Owens et al., 2012), as well as adult survivors of child abuse (e.g., Earley et al., 2014). Jacob's clinician introduced some mindfulness practice in an early session to help him manage his mood and promote better sleep (for a useful clinical resource, see Witkiewitz et al., 2016). In this case, a simple body scanning and mindful breathing activities were used. Jacob was encouraged to practice his body scanning activity at nighttime, including if he woke during the night, while his mindful breathing was encouraged to help him regulate his emotions whenever he was feeling distressed.

Behavioral Activation/Pleasant Activity Scheduling. Pleasant activity scheduling forms a key component of cognitive and behavioral therapy for depression. The goal of activity monitoring and pleasant activity scheduling is to demonstrate to the young person the link between depression / mood and inactivity, as well as how activity can be used to improve mood. The idea being that low rates of positive reinforcement via social interaction or day-to-day pleasant activities are often a contributing factor to the development and maintenance of depression. Jacob's social withdrawal (first caused by injury-related school nonattendance and reduced availability of his parents, then exacerbated as he withdrew further from friends and family and ceased his BMX riding) was resulting in low rates of social interactions, relative to his pre-accident experience. Of course, when a young person is depressed, they are less likely to seek out pleasant activities and, at least initially, may get less enjoyment out of the activity. In Jacob's case, this cycle was relatively clear – his low mood and feelings of guilt led to his withdrawing from seeking out his friends, which further exacerbated his depressed mood, which still further reduced his enjoyment of activities and seeking out of interactions, and so on.

As a first step, Jacob's clinician introduced him to the idea of pleasant activity scheduling, socializing him to the reciprocal relationship between mood and activity. Together they generated a list of possible pleasant activities, based on past activities that Jacob used to enjoy and other activities he might have wanted to achieve. At the end of this chapter, the interested reader will find some references to key clinical resources for establishing pleasant activity scheduling. Activities cover two categories – social activities and success-oriented activities. Social activities should involve spending time with other people, like meeting up with a friend or calling a friend on the phone, while success activities allow us to feel a sense of achievement or competence, like learning a new activity or going back to an activity that was previously enjoyed. Jacob's main activities were his BMX riding, inviting a friend over, taking his dog for a walk, and learning to play a new song on his guitar. Jacob and his clinician discussed that because of his low mood, he might find some of these activities less enjoyable than he used to but with practice and perseverance his mood would hopefully improve as his activity levels increased. After this was introduced, his homework was to create a baseline of his activities and mood. Using a checklist of the activities, each day he rated (1) which activities (if any) he engaged in, (2) his enjoyment of the activity, and (3) his mood before and after the activity. This provided his clinician with a baseline of his activity level and also helped demonstrate the link between his activity and mood.

In the following session, Jacob and his clinician developed a pleasant activity schedule, where they scheduled in activities from his list throughout the week. Again, Jacob rated his enjoyment of the activity and his mood before and after the activity. In Jacob's case, examples of his activities were his best friend coming over to play a new video game and a BMX ride in the local area with his uncle. Alongside his treatment specifically targeting his PTSD, Jacob continued to work with his clinician to monitor and extend his pleasant activity schedule, increasing his engagement in pleasant activities, almost like a graded exposure task. Here, the ultimate goal is to not only see an increase in engagement in pleasant activities but also an increase in the enjoyment of these activities.

Treating Comorbid PTSD and SUD

Based on concern regarding the capacity of individuals with comorbid PTSD and SUD to manage the distressing emotions likely to be elicited by PTSD treatment, treatment guidelines have traditionally recommended that PTSD treatment should commence only after a significant period of abstinence has been achieved. In the vast majority of cases, this is an unrealistic scenario. To begin with, it is well documented among young adults with this comorbidity that PTSD symptoms intensify when an individual abstains from substance use, increasing their risk of relapse (Back, Brady, Jaanimägi, et al., 2006; Bradizza, Stasiewicz, & Paas, 2006). In addition, studies with adults focusing on the temporal sequencing of changes in PTSD and SUD symptoms have clearly demonstrated that the PTSD must be treated to achieve lasting improvements in substance use outcomes (Back, Brady, Jaanimägi et al., 2006; Back, Brady, Sonne, & Verduin, 2006; Bradizza et al., 2006). On the basis of these findings, an integrated approach (that is, treatment of both disorders simultaneously by the same clinician) to the treatment of comorbid PTSD and SUD is now advocated (Cohen, Mannarino, Zhitova, & Capone, 2003; Mills et al., 2012; Simmons & Suárez, 2016). Such an approach allows for PTSD to be treated in a manner that can be tolerated by the individual, while concurrently addressing the substance use. Unfortunately, at this point in time, no empirically validated integrated treatment approaches exist for adolescents with this comorbidity.

However, gold-standard interventions do exist for each of the disorders individually. For PTSD (as discussed elsewhere in this book), the intervention with the most robust evidence base is trauma-focused CBT (TF-CBT). In relation to the treatment of SUD, the combination of family therapy, motivational enhancement (or motivational interviewing; MI), and CBT has been found to be effective in reducing adolescents' substance use (Bukstein et al., 2005; Simmons & Suárez, 2016). Cohen and colleagues (2003) recommend that in treating comorbid PTSD + SUD in adolescents, clinicians draw upon elements that are either common to empirically validated interventions for abuse-related PTSD and SUD in adolescents or have been drawn from empirically supported integrated treatment protocols used with adult participants. The specific treatment components identified by Cohen et al. (2003) include a consistent and trusting therapeutic relationship with the youth and the family; psycho-education about PTSD and SUD; stress management skills; affect regulation skills; cognitive restructuring; social skills; problem-solving, drug refusal, and safety skills; imaginal and in vivo exposure; parental involvement and parenting skills; random urine drug screening; adjunctive psychopharmacologic treatments; and possible referral to adjunctive adolescent-only AA programs. To the best of our knowledge, only one adolescent-specific integrated treatment – the trauma systems therapy for adolescent substance abuse (TST-AS) has been described (Suárez, Ellis, & Saxe, 2014) – although empirical data on the intervention do not appear to be available at this point. The TST-SA consists of five modules based on an approach that incorporates CBT, motivational interviewing (Miller & Rollnick, 2002), and family-focused behavioral and system-oriented interventions (Henggeler, Clingempeel, Brondino, & Pickrel, 2002) and was primarily developed for adolescents with histories of complex trauma (typically interpersonal in nature) and substance use problems. The intervention is described as flexible (with a dual assessment of emotional dysregulation and environmental stability determining the phase at which treatment begins for each adolescent and their family), with treatment length ranging from 3 to 9 months depending on the severity and complexity of the presentation. In the absence of an empirically supported integrated program for adolescents, it is necessary to refer back to the adult literature. Even here, there is relatively little research published on integrated treatment approaches.

Thus, to date, in the adult literature, only two integrated treatment approaches have been reported to demonstrate efficacy relative to treatment as usual for adults demonstrating PTSD + SUD: *Seeking Safety* (Najavits, Schmitz, Gotthardt, & Weiss, 2005) and Concurrent Treatment of PTSD and Substance Use Disorders Using Prolonged Exposure (*COPE*; Back et al., 2012; Mills et al., 2012; Najavits et al., 2005). The *Seeking Safety* program has been piloted with 33 female adolescents; however, the utility of the program with a younger age group was unclear. Thus, while the intervention produced positive outcomes in relation to substance use, there was no change in PTSD symptoms (Najavits, Gallop, & Weiss, 2006). The most likely explanation for these discrepant outcomes is that *Seeking Safety* does not incorporate the gold-standard treatment for adolescent PTSD – trauma-focused CBT involving imaginal and in vivo exposure within a safe environment (Cohen et al., 2003; Foa, McLean, Capaldi, & Rosenfield, 2013; Perrin, 2013). In comparison to the *Seeking Safety* program, *COPE* was specifically designed for adults who have experienced any form of trauma and any kind of substance use. In relation to the PTSD, the cognitive behavioral approach used in *COPE* can be described as trauma focused, in that it relies heavily on imaginal and in vivo exposure to the trauma narrative and trauma reminders, respectively. In RCTs with adults characterized by extensive histories of trauma exposure and poly-drug use, *COPE* has been found to produce superior outcomes in terms of PTSD symptom severity compared to treatment as usual, with reductions in PTSD symptoms associated with reductions in severity of substance dependence (Mills et al., 2012; Ruglass et al., 2017). *COPE* thus appears to offer promise for clinicians working with adolescents with PTSD + SUD. The program consists of 13 individual sessions lasting 90 minutes covering psycho-education, motivational enhancement, and CBT that targets both the PTSD and the SUD. In *COPE*, the first four sessions are spent on providing psycho-education to the client about each disorder and the ways in which they might interact, working on motivational enhancement, and providing CBT to address the substance use (although all of these components are referred back to and built upon continuously throughout the intervention). In vivo and imaginal exposure are introduced in sessions 5 and 6, respectively, and remain part of each subsequent session. Cognitive therapy to address the PTSD commences in session 8 and is implemented in tandem with the exposure work. The final session of the intervention focuses on reviewing strategies learned and gains made, relapse prevention, and termination. Based on the content in the empirically supported (but adult-focused) *COPE*, the recommendations put forward by Cohen et al. (2003) and the description of TST-SA provided by Suárez et al. (2014), we present a case study of a 16-year-old girl presenting with comorbid PTSD + SUD, with suggestions regarding key treatment strategies (e.g., motivational enhancement) for targeting this comorbidity. Other important elements of an integrated approach to the treatment of PTSD + SUD in adolescents – such as family therapy – are beyond the scope of this chapter.

Case Study: PTSD and SUD

Alissa is a 16-year-old girl in her last year of school. She currently lives at home with her biological mother, her stepfather, and her two younger half-siblings. A year ago, Alissa disclosed to her mother that a close male family friend had sexually abused her over a period of 6 months beginning at age 14. The abuse ranged from inappropriate touching of Alissa by the perpetrator to nonconsensual vaginal intercourse. Since the abuse began at age 14, Alissa has been experiencing many symptoms of PTSD. Initially, the most significant of these was nightmares about the abuse. Alissa found the nightmares terrifying, and she would try to stay awake as long as possible each night in an effort to avoid them. Shortly after the abuse began, Alissa also started using substances in a gradually escalating way. In an attempt to get some sleep that she hoped would be nightmare-free, Alissa took half a dozen sleeping tablets from her parents' medicine cabinet. The relief of being fully unconscious was hard to describe – no thoughts, no memories, no nightmares. After experimenting with the sleeping tablets, Alissa gradually sought out new friends, with whom she drank alcohol (mainly beer) in an effort to get the same effect. Her parents were aware at the time that their daughter was staying out later than her curfew and experimenting with alcohol. Although they spoke to her about their concerns a number of times, at this point, her parents had no knowledge of the abuse or Alissa's PTSD symptoms and saw her alcohol use as being within the parameters of "normal" adolescent experimentation. Currently, in terms of her PTSD symptoms, Alissa avoids being alone with any male, including her stepfather and is constantly on the watch for male behavior that she interprets as potentially threatening (e.g., if a male peer looks at her for too long). Alissa experiences flashbacks to incidents of the abuse and becomes very distressed if she has to go anywhere on her own. Alissa avoids places within the house where the abuse occurred (e.g., the downstairs bathroom). Following her lead, nobody in the family talks about what happened to Alissa. In terms of her current substance use, Alissa smokes two or three joints across the course of the day most days, takes a crushed 10 mg diazepam tablet every night, and drinks a couple of cans of beer most days. Alissa steals money from home to buy the diazepam and marijuana from a dealer at her high school. Her parents have noticed that she is increasingly aggressive, difficult to wake in the mornings, and sometimes looks intoxicated. There is a high level of conflict in the house and her parents have insisted that she see a mental health clinician if she wants to remain living at home.

Psycho-Education and Motivational Enhancement. Following a thorough assessment, the clinician makes two preliminary recommendations: (1) Alissa and her family engage in family therapy with another treatment provider within the practice and (2) parent-supported individual therapy focusing simultaneously on Alissa's PTSD and substance use is commenced. In developing a shared formulation with Alissa and her parents, the clinician relies heavily on psycho-education, providing information about each of the disorders individually and their likely interactions. It is important for Alissa and her parents to understand the order in which Alissa's symptoms have developed and the likely self-medication function that Alissa's substance use is serving. Equally important for them to understand is the likelihood that her substance use places Alissa at increased risk of being exposed to future PTEs. Understanding the relationship between Alissa's PTSD and her SUD is a critical part of the formulation of her difficulties. As part of the assessment, the clinician also gauged Alissa's readiness for change. Like most adolescents, Alissa is not in therapy voluntarily. This means that alongside the psycho-educational content, it will be critical to work on motivational enhancement.

Motivational interviewing (MI) or enhancement is based on the assumption that people are only motivated to change the things that provoke a sense of discomfort and / or inconsistency, and that the explicit exploration and resolution of ambivalence about change is a necessary goal unto itself. The principles of MI include developing discrepancies (between client behaviors and client goals and / or values), support and empathy, "rolling with resistance," and supporting self-efficacy (Miller

& Rollnick, 2002). Motivational enhancement with Alissa would involve taking a nonjudgmental stance to encourage her to identify the problems she is already experiencing and the potential future consequences and risks associated with her substance use. She would also be encouraged to try and imagine a different future, to identify the advantages associated with changing her substance use behaviors, and to develop confidence in her ability to change. It will be important for Alissa's parents to understand the concept of readiness for change – and the difficulty involved in behavioral change – and to be prepared to support Alissa in moving toward positive change. However, intrinsically, the process of exploring and resolving ambivalence about change is a deeply personal one, and movement in terms of readiness for change can be facilitated and supported, but not forced. Alissa's parents will need to be aware of this.

Cognitive Behavioral Therapy (CBT). CBT for SUD focuses on helping clients identify the thoughts and cues that are associated with and / or trigger their problematic substance use. It is important to emphasize that although different weight will be given to the different problems at different points in an integrated treatment approach, in reality, the PTSD and SUD are highly related and this relationship will frequently be discussed within any given session. For example, through completion of a thoughts and feelings diary, Alissa may realize that her substance use tends to be preceded by the expectation that she will feel better (in terms of her PTSD symptoms) after using. Other associated thoughts that may come to light include "I won't be able to sleep if I'm not using because the nightmares will come back" and "I need the [substances] to be able to cope with what happened to me [the abuse] ... without that, I couldn't cope ... I would fall apart." Socratic questioning would be used to help Alissa examine her distorted thinking patterns. It would be important for Alissa's parents to be aware of the strategies she is learning in these sessions so that they can encourage and support her to use these strategies outside of the therapy setting. A means of providing this information to her parents would need to be negotiated with Alissa (e.g., she may provide them with a verbal summary of new strategies as they are taught – in this way, she remains in control of how much of her personal content is shared while the parents are aware of the strategies to support). Within CBT sessions, Alissa would also learn about cravings for drugs and strategies for coping with urges to use. As part of this work, she would be asked to identify and anticipate triggers for cravings (people, places, things, situations, feelings or anything else that she associates with using) and high-risk situations. For Alissa, a clear high-risk situation is the time leading up to going to sleep. She is also able to identify that seeing her peers use drugs is a trigger for her, as is conflict with her parents. Alissa would be asked to monitor the situations in which she feels the urge to use, as well as the thoughts and feelings associated with these situations. Avoiding exposure to triggers or high-risk situations is the easiest way to manage cravings. However, this is not always possible – going to sleep at night being a good example of this. Given that Alissa's thoughts and fear in this high-risk situation relate to the recurrence of abuse-related nightmares, useful strategies might include challenging her thoughts around the probability of nightmares occurring every night and providing psycho-education about the likely positive impact of trauma-focused CBT on the occurrence of the nightmares (that is, once Alissa begins exposing herself to the trauma narrative she has been avoiding, her nightmares are likely to reduce in frequency). Positive self-talk, distraction, imagery, controlled breathing, and reviewing the advantages and disadvantages of using (generated during the MI sessions) are other strategies that can become part of Alissa's plan for coping with cravings. In this part of therapy, Alissa would set goals relating to reducing her substance use or abstaining altogether. She would learn and practice a variety of skills including problem solving, emotion regulation, and substance refusal. Other skills that may be relevant for Alissa include communicating effectively and (where necessary) assertively with peers and family members, social skills, and anxiety management. Contingency management (the use of stimulus control and positive reinforcement to influence the likelihood of behavior occurring in the future) is a key element of a behavioral approach to substance use disorders. Thus Alissa may be able to earn inexpensive rewards for engaging well in therapy sessions and meeting her treatment goals. Once Alissa is making progress with her substance use, in vivo and imaginal exposure and trauma-focused CBT would commence.

Useful resources (including worksheets for use with clients with SUD) are listed at the end of the chapter.

Challenges and Moving Forward

When reviewing the empirical evidence base for comorbidities with PTSD, two things are clear: (1) we know that comorbidities are the norm, rather than an exception, with PTSD and (2) we know very little about how standard cognitive and behavioral treatments for PTSD might be modified to improve outcomes where there are complex comorbidities. This is the case across the trauma and PTSD field in general, but it is particularly pronounced when it comes to child and adolescent PTSD. Certainly, in clinical practice, it would be rare to see a young person who "only" meets criteria for PTSD. Thus, many clinicians would be well experienced in managing a range of comorbidities and providing a more integrated treatment approach (an important likely exception relates to the management of PTSD + SUD, where research indicates that clinicians working with adults with this comorbidity have low levels of confidence in treating these clients). Research must now "catch-up" to allow the development of more robust clinical guidelines on the most effective and time-efficient way to target these comorbidities.

Going forward, a particular challenge to comorbidity research is determining the course of the comorbid disorder. Many mental health problems have a shared vulnerability, whether that may be a genetic vulnerability, environmental vulnerability (e.g., poor social support), or a combination of factors. Regardless, understanding why comorbidities are so common remains an important area of consideration. Here we are presented with a classic "chicken – egg" dilemma. Does a preexisting history of mental health problems place a person at increased risk of developing PTSD after trauma exposure, or does the development of PTSD place a young person at risk of developing other mental health problems? McMillen and colleagues (2002) have gone some way in answering this, in the earlier presented models of comorbidity – suggesting comorbidities often develop as a consequence of PTSD. However, far more research is needed to inform our clinical practice. Such information has important ramifications for our knowledge and theories of the development and maintenance of PTSD in young people. If particular preexisting mental health problems place a young person at increased risk of developing PTSD, it may allow for more effective monitoring and timely intervention for this group. If the development of PTSD places some young people at risk of developing other comorbidities – whether that be behavior problems, depression, anxiety, or substance abuse – such evidence would not only help mental health professionals more strongly advocate for the need for access to trauma-focused cognitive and behavioral treatments but also may allow us to better understanding and target those young people with PTSD who are at most risk of complex comorbidities. Given comorbidities are generally associated with a more severe presentation, which can be more resistant to even our best psychological treatment, the latter point would be particularly important if it could allow the targeting of PTSD before the onset of other disorders.

While understanding the course of comorbidities has important theoretical and clinical implications, what we really need to know is what represents best practice in targeting comorbidities. Here the empirical evidence is particularly scarce. The effectiveness of cognitive and behavioral treatments for child and adolescent PTSD is reasonably well established, across countries, age groups, and trauma types – including with young people who have experienced a single accidental trauma (e.g., car accident), a single nonaccidental trauma (e.g., sexual assault), child maltreatment (e.g., ongoing interpersonal abuse), and war-related trauma (e. g., former child soldiers, refugees). Going forward, it would be useful for research to now focus on developing treatment guidelines for young people with PTSD and comorbidities that can provide clinical guidance on how and when to intervene with these groups and allow us to improve on our ability to target post-trauma mental health for those young people who present with a more severe or complex presentation.

Clinical Recommendations

- Assessment needs to take the likelihood of comorbidity into account where the presentation seems to be PTSD (and assessment for comorbidity should be broad rather than narrow). A clear picture regarding the temporal sequence of onset of different disorders needs to be obtained during the assessment.
- For most comorbidities, the evidence base and clinical guidelines suggest treating the PTSD should remain the treatment priority. The presence of comorbidities should not inadvertently lead to avoidance of beginning trauma-focused treatment (i.e., that involves exposure or re-living of the event(s) – as discussed in detail in a previous chapter).

- In some cases, cognitive behavioral therapies for PTSD, as the stand-alone treatment, will lead to a reduction in comorbidities (e.g., depression, anxiety, behavioral problems). An exception to this may be in the case of comorbid substance use disorders.
- Where the comorbidity is significant, such as where depressive symptoms are having a substantial effect on daily functioning, a treatment approach that includes components that target the comorbidity can be useful. In some cases, this may be an adjunct or additional session at the end of the course of trauma-focused CBT. In some cases, it may be beneficial to integrate this focus with the trauma-focused CBT, so sessions targeting comorbidities are embedded throughout the treatment program, and ultimately allow the client to better access the trauma-focused treatment. Common comorbidities such as depressive disorders, substance use disorders, and anxiety disorders all have gold-standard cognitive and behavioral treatment approaches that could be incorporated into PTSD treatment.
- For comorbid substance abuse, it seems more useful to use an integrated approach, in which the PTSD and SUD are addressed during the same course of therapy, by the same clinician. Critical ingredients to be considered in the treatment of this comorbidity include family therapy, psychoeducation, motivational enhancement, and cognitive behavioral therapy for SUD. This work appears to be best placed before as well as alongside standard treatment of PTSD, particularly given that substance use is likely being used as a (maladaptive) coping strategy (e.g., to numb intrusive memories of the trauma).

Clinical References

Examples of Clinician Guides for Depression Modules

Sburlati, Lyneham, Schniering, & Rapee. (2014). *Evidence-based CBT for anxiety and depression in children and adolescents: A competencies based approach.* Wiley-Blackwell.

Curry, J. F. et al. (2000). Treatment for Adolescents with Depression Study (TADS): Cognitive behavior therapy manual. Available online http://tads.dcri.org/wp-content/uploads/2015/11/TADS_CBT.pdf

Verduyn, C., Rogers, J., & Wood, A. (2009). *Depression: Cognitive behaviour therapy with children and young people.* Routledge.

A Brief Guide to Evidence-Based Mindfulness

Witkiewitz et al. (2016). *Mindfulness. Advances in psychotherapy – evidence-based practice,* Vol. 37. Hogrefe Publishing. ISBN: 978-0-88937-414-0.

Example of a Clinical Guide for Treatment of PTSD

Smith, P., Perrin, S., Yule, W., Clark, D. M. (2009). *Post traumatic stress disorder: Cognitive therapy with children and young people.* Routledge.

Working with Substance Use Disorders in Adolescents
www.orygen.org.au/Skills-Knowledge/Resources-Training/Resources/Free/Reference-Library/Substance-Use-Disorder
www.orygen.org.au/Skills-Knowledge/Resources-Training/Resources/Free/Evidence-Summaries/Motivational-Interviewing/The-Effectiveness-of-Motivational-Interviewing-for?ext=.
http://www.parentingstrategies.net/alcohol/guidelines
http://www.therapistaid.com/therapy-worksheets/substance-use/adolescents

References

Abram, K. M., Washburn, J. J., Teplin, L. A., Emanuel, K. M., Romero, E. G., & McClelland, G. M. (2007). Posttraumatic stress disorder and psychiatric comorbidity among detained youths. *Psychiatric Services*, *58*(10), 1311–1316. doi:10.1176/ps.2007.58.10.1311

Ackerman, P. T., Newton, J. E., McPherson, W. B., Jones, J. G., & Dykman, R. A. (1998). Prevalence of post traumatic stress disorder and other psychiatric diagnoses in three groups of abused children (sexual, physical, and both). *Child Abuse and Neglect*, *22*(8), 759–774.

Adams, Z. W., McCauley, J. L., Back, S. E., Flanagan, J. C., Hanson, R. F., Killeen, T. K., & Danielson, C. K. (2016). Clinician perspectives on treating adolescents with co-occurring post-traumatic stress disorder, substance use, and other problems. *Journal of Child and Adolescent Substance Abuse*, *25*(6), 575–583. doi:10.1080/1067828X.2016.1153555

Alisic, E., Zalta, A. K., van Wesel, F., Larsen, S. E., Hafstad, G. S., Hassanpour, K., & Smid, G. E. (2014). Rates of post-traumatic stress disorder in trauma-exposed children and adolescents: meta-analysis. *British Journal of Psychiatry*, *204*, 335–340. doi:10.1192/bjp.bp.113.131227

Allwood, M. A., Dyl, J., Hunt, J. I., & Spirito, A. (2008). Comorbidity and service utilization among psychiatrically hospitalized adolescents with posttraumatic stress disorder. *Journal of Psychological Trauma*, *7*, 104–121.

Angelakis, S. (2014). *Comorbid posttraumatic stress disorder and major depressive disorder: The usefulness of a combined treatment approach.* (PhD), Flinders University, Australia.

Angelakis, S., & Nixon, R. D. V. (2015). The comorbidity of PTSD and MDD: Implications for clinical practice and future research. *Behaviour Change*, *32*(1), 1–25. doi:10.1017/bec.2014.26

Back, S. E., Brady, K. T., Jaanimägi, U., & Jackson, J. L. (2006). Cocaine dependence and PTSD: A pilot study of symptom interplay and treatment preferences. *Addictive Behaviors*, *31*(2), 351–354. doi:10.1016/j.addbeh.2005.05.008

Back, S. E., Brady, K. T., Sonne, S. C., & Verduin, M. L. (2006). Symptom improvement in co-occurring PTSD and alcohol dependence. *Journal of Nervous Mental Disease*, *194*(9), 690–696. doi:10.1097/01.nmd.0000235794.12794.8a

Back, S. E., Killeen, T., Foa, E. B., Santa Ana, E. J., Gros, D. F., & Brady, K. T. (2012). Use of an integrated therapy with prolonged exposure to treat PTSD and comorbid alcohol dependence in an Iraq veteran. *American Journal of Psychiatry, 169*(7), 688–691. doi:10.1176/appi.ajp.2011.11091433

Bradizza, C. M., Stasiewicz, P. R., & Paas, N. D. (2006). Relapse to alcohol and drug use among individuals diagnosed with co-occurring mental health and substance use disorders: A review. *Clinical Psychology Review, 26*(2), 162–178. doi:10.1016/j.cpr.2005.11.005

Brady, K. T. (1997). Posttraumatic stress disorder and comorbidity: Recognizing the many faces of PTSD. *Journal of Clinical Psychiatry, 58 Suppl 9*, 12–15.

Brady, K. T., Killeen, T. K., Brewerton, T., & Lucerini, S. (2000). Comorbidity of psychiatric disorders and posttraumatic stress disorder. *Journal of Clinical Psychiatry, 61 Suppl 7*, 22–32.

Brent, D. A., Oquendo, M., Birmaher, B., Greenhill, L., Kolko, D., Stanley, B., ... Mann, J. J. (2002). Familial pathways to early-onset suicide attempt: risk for suicidal behavior in offspring of mood-disordered suicide attempters. *Archives of General Psychiatry, 59*(9), 801–807.

Breslau, N., Davis, G. C., Peterson, E. L., & Schultz, L. (1997). Psychiatric sequelae of posttraumatic stress disorder in women. *Archives of General Psychiatry, 54*(1), 81–87.

Breslau, N., Davis, G. C., Peterson, E. L., & Schultz, L. R. (2000). A second look at comorbidity in victims of trauma: The posttraumatic stress disorder–major depression connection. *Biological Psychiatry, 48*(9), 902–909.

Brown, T. A., Campbell, L. A., Lehman, C. L., Grisham, J. R., & Mancill, R. B. (2001). Current and lifetime comorbidity of the DSM-IV anxiety and mood disorders in a large clinical sample. *Journal of Abnormal Psychology, 110*(4), 585–599.

Bujarski, S. J., Feldner, M. T., Lewis, S. F., Babson, K. A., Trainor, C. D., Leen-Feldner, E., ... & Bonn-Miller, M. O. (2012). Marijuana use among traumatic event–exposed adolescents: Posttraumatic stress symptom frequency predicts coping motivations for use. *Addictive Behaviors, 37*(1), 53–59. doi:10.1016/j.addbeh.2011.08.009

Bukstein, O. G., Bernet, W., Arnold, V., Beitchman, J., Shaw, J., Benson, R. S., ... Issues, W. G. (2005). Practice parameter for the assessment and treatment of children and adolescents with substance use disorders. *Journal of the American Academy of Child and Adolescent Psychiatry, 44*(6), 609–621.

Carliner, H., Keyes, K. M., McLaughlin, K. A., Meyers, J. L., Dunn, E. C., & Martins, S. S. (2016). Childhood trauma and illicit drug use in adolescence: A population-based national comorbidity survey replication-adolescent supplement study. *Journal of the American Academy of Child and Adolescent Psychiatry, 55*(8), 701–708. doi:10.1016/j.jaac.2016.05.010

Carrion, V. G., Weems, C. F., Ray, R., & Reiss, A. L. (2002). Toward an empirical definition of pediatric PTSD: The phenomenology of PTSD symptoms in youth. *Journal of the American Academy for Child and Adolescent Psychiatry, 41*(2), 166–173.

Coffey, S. F., Saladin, M. E., Drobes, D. J., Brady, K. T., Dansky, B. S., & Kilpatrick, D. G. (2002). Trauma and substance cue reactivity in individuals with comorbid posttraumatic stress disorder and cocaine or alcohol dependence. *Drug and Alcohol Dependence, 65*(2), 115–127.

Coffey, S. F., Schumacher, J. A., Stasiewicz, P. R., Henslee, A. M., Baillie, L. E., & Landy, N. (2010). Craving and physiological reactivity to trauma and alcohol cues in posttraumatic stress disorder and alcohol dependence. *Experimental Clinical Psychopharmacology, 18*(4), 340–349. doi:10.1037/a0019790

Cohen, J. A., Mannarino, A. P., Berliner, L., & Deblinger, E. (2000). Trauma-focused cognitive behavioral therapy for children and adolescents: An empirical update. *Journal of Interpersonal Violence, 15*(11), 1202–1223.

Cohen, J. A., Mannarino, A. P., Zhitova, A. C., & Capone, M. E. (2003). Treating child abuse-related posttraumatic stress and comorbid substance abuse in adolescents. *Child Abuse and Neglect, 27*(12), 1345–1365.

Cohen, Y., Spirito, A., Sterling, C., Donaldson, D., Seifer, R., Plummer, B., ... Ferrer, K. (2000). Physical and sexual abuse and their relation to psychiatric disorder and suicidal behavior among adolescents who are psychiatrically hospitalized. *Journal of Child Psychology and Psychiatry, 37*(8), 989–993.

Copeland, W. E., Keeler, G., Angold, A., & Costello, E. J. (2007). Traumatic events and posttraumatic stress in childhood. *Archives of General Psychiatry, 64*(5), 577–584. doi:10.1001/archpsyc.64.5.577

Cénat, J. M., & Derivois, D. (2015). Long-term outcomes among child and adolescent survivors of the 2010 Haitian earthquake. *Depression and Anxiety, 32*(1), 57–63. doi:10.1002/da.22275

De Young, A. C., Kenardy, J. A., Cobham, V. E., & Kimble, R. (2012). Prevalence, comorbidity and course of trauma reactions in young burn-injured children. *Journal of Child Psychology and Psychiatry, 53*(1), 56–63. doi:10.1111/j.1469-7610.2011.02431.x

Deblinger, E., Mannarino, A. P., Cohen, J. A., Runyon, M. K., & Steer, R. A. (2011). Trauma-focused cognitive behavioral therapy for children: Impact of the trauma narrative and treatment length. *Depression and Anxiety, 28*(1), 67–75. doi:10.1002/da.20744

Earley, M. D., Chesney, M. A., Frye, J., Greene, P. A., Berman, B., & Kimbrough, E. (2014). Mindfulness intervention for child abuse survivors: A 2.5-year follow-up. *Journal of Clinical Psychology, 70*(10), 933–941.

Elbedour, S., Onwuegbuzie, A. J., Ghannam, J., Whitcome, J. A., & Abu Hein, F. (2007). Post-traumatic stress disorder, depression, and anxiety among Gaza Strip adolescents in the wake of the second Uprising (Intifada). *Child Abuse and Neglect, 31*(7), 719–729. doi:10.1016/j.chiabu.2005.09.006

Famularo, R., Fenton, T., Kinscherff, R., & Augustyn, M. (1996). Psychiatric comorbidity in childhood post traumatic stress disorder. *Child Abuse and Neglect, 20*(10), 953–961.

Fan, F., Zhang, Y., Yang, Y., Mo, L., & Liu, X. (2011). Symptoms of posttraumatic stress disorder, depression, and anxiety among adolescents following the 2008 Wenchuan earthquake in China. *Journal of Traumatic Stress, 24*(1), 44–53. doi:10.1002/jts.20599

Farrugia, P. L., Mills, K. L., Barrett, E., Back, S. E., Teesson, M., Baker, A., ... Brady, K. T. (2011). Childhood trauma among individuals with co-morbid substance use and post traumatic stress disorder. *Mental Health and Substance Use, 4*(4), 314–326. doi:10.1080/17523281.2011.598462

Foa, E. B., McLean, C. P., Capaldi, S., & Rosenfield, D. (2013). Prolonged exposure vs supportive counseling for sexual abuse-related PTSD in adolescent girls: A randomized clinical trial. *Journal of the American Medical Association, 310*(24), 2650–2657. doi:10.1001/jama.2013.282829

Gerson, R., & Rappaport, N. (2013). Traumatic stress and posttraumatic stress disorder in youth: Recent research findings on clinical impact, assessment, and treatment. *Journal of Adolescent Health, 52*(2), 137–143. doi:10.1016/j.jadohealth.2012.06.018

Giaconia, R. M., Reinherz, H. Z., Hauf, A. C., Paradis, A. D., Wasserman, M. S., & Langhammer, D. M. (2000). Comorbidity of substance use and post-traumatic stress disorders in a community sample of adolescents. *American Journal of Orthopsychiatry*, *70*(2), 253–262.

Goldbeck, L., Muche, R., Sachser, C., Tutus, D., & Rosner, R. (2016). Effectiveness of trauma-focused cognitive behavioral therapy for children and adolescents: A randomized controlled trial in eight German mental health clinics. *Psychotherapy and Psychosomatics*, *85*(3), 159–170. doi:10.1159/000442824

Heim, C., Shugart, M., Craighead, W. E., & Nemeroff, C. B. (2010). Neurobiological and psychiatric consequences of child abuse and neglect. *Developmental Psychobiology*, *52*(7), 671–690. doi:10.1002/dev.20494

Henggeler, S. W., Clingempeel, W. G., Brondino, M. J., & Pickrel, S. G. (2002). Four-year follow-up of multisystemic therapy with substance-abusing and substance-dependent juvenile offenders. *Journal of the American Academy of Child and Adolescent Psychiatry*, *41*(7), 868–874. doi:10.1097/00004583-200207000-00021

Hiller, R.M., Creswell, C., Meiser-Stedman, R., Lobo, S., Cowdrey, F., Lyttle, M. D., ... Halligan, S. L. (2018). A longitudinal examination of the relationship between trauma-related cognitive factors and internalising and externalising psychopathology in physically injured children. *Journal of Abnormal Child Psychology*. Online First.

Khamis, V. (2008). Post-traumatic stress and psychiatric disorders in Palestinian adolescents following intifada-related injuries. *Social Science & Medicine*, *67*(8), 1199–1207. doi:10.1016/j.socscimed.2008.06.013

Khantzian, E. J. (1997). The self-medication hypothesis of substance use disorders: A reconsideration and recent applications. *Harvard Review of Psychiatry*, *4*(5), 231–244. doi:10.3109/10673229709030550

Kilpatrick, D. G., Ruggiero, K. J., Acierno, R., Saunders, B. E., Resnick, H. S., & Best, C. L. (2003). Violence and risk of PTSD, major depression, substance abuse/dependence, and comorbidity: Results from the National Survey of Adolescents. *Journal of Consulting and Clinical Psychology*, *71*(4), 692–700.

Kimbrough, E., Magyari, T., Langenberg, P., Chesney, M., & Berman, B. (2010). Mindfulness intervention for child abuse survivors. *Journal of clinical psychology*, *66*(1), 17–33.

King, A. P., Erickson, T. M., Giardino, N. D., Favorite, T., Rauch, S. A., Robinson, E., ... Liberzon, I. (2013). A pilot study of group mindfulness-based cognitive therapy (MBCT) for combat veterans with posttraumatic stress disorder (PTSD). *Depression and anxiety*, *30*(7), 638–645.

Krystal, J. H., Rosenheck, R. A., Cramer, J. A., Vessicchio, J. C., Jones, K. M., Vertrees, J. E., ... Group, V. A. C. S. N. (2011). Adjunctive risperidone treatment for antidepressant-resistant symptoms of chronic military service-related PTSD: A randomized trial. *Journal of the American Medical Association*, *306*(5), 493–502. doi:10.1001/jama.2011.1080

Kuyken, W., Warren, F. C., Taylor, R. S., Whalley, B., Crane, C., Bondolfi, G., ... Segal, Z. (2016). Efficacy of mindfulness-based cognitive therapy in prevention of depressive relapse: An individual patient data meta-analysis from randomized trials. *JAMA Psychiatry*, *73*(6), 565–574.

Leeson, F. J., & Nixon, R. D. (2011). The role of children's appraisals on adjustment following psychological maltreatment: A pilot study. *Journal of Abnormal Child Psychology*, *39*(5), 759–771. doi:10.1007/s10802-011-9507-5

Lipschitz, D. S., Winegar, R. K., Nicolaou, A. L., Hartnick, E., Wolfson, M., & Southwick, S. M. (1999). Perceived abuse and neglect as risk factors for suicidal behavior in adolescent inpatients. *Journal of Nervous Mental Disease, 187*(1), 32–39.

Liu, S. T., & Chen, S. H. (2015). A community study on the relationship of posttraumatic cognitions to internalizing and externalizing psychopathology in Taiwanese children and adolescents. *Journal of Abnormal Child Psychology, 43*(8), 1475–1484. doi:10.1007/s10802-015-0030-y

Mannarino, A. P., & Cohen, J. A. (1996). Abuse-related attributions and perceptions, general attributions, and locus of control in sexually abused girls. *Journal of Interpersonal Violence, 11*(2), 162–180. doi:10.1177/088626096011002002

McLeer, S. V., Dixon, J. F., Henry, D., Ruggiero, K., Escovitz, K., Niedda, T., & Scholle, R. (1998). Psychopathology in non-clinically referred sexually abused children. *Journal of the American Academy of Child and Adolescent Psychiatry, 37*(12), 1326–1333. doi:10.1097/00004583-199812000-00017

McMillen, C., North, C., Mosley, M., & Smith, E. (2002). Untangling the psychiatric comorbidity of posttraumatic stress disorder in a sample of flood survivors. *Comprehensive Psychiatry, 43*(6), 478–485. doi:10.1053/comp.2002.34632

Mghir, R., Freed, W., Raskin, A., & Katon, W. (1995). Depression and posttraumatic stress disorder among a community sample of adolescent and young adult Afghan refugees. *Journal of Nervous Mental Disease, 183*(1), 24–30.

Miller, W., & Rollnick, S. (2002). *Motivational interviewing: Preparing people for change* (2nd edn.). New York: Guilford Press.

Mills, K. L. (2009). "Between pain and nothing, I choose nothing": Trauma, post-traumatic stress disorder and substance use. *Addiction, 104*(10), 1607–1609. doi:10.1111/j.1360-0443.2009.02675.x

Mills, K. L., Teesson, M., Back, S. E., Brady, K. T., Baker, A. L., Hopwood, S., ... Ewer, P. L. (2012). Integrated exposure-based therapy for co-occurring posttraumatic stress disorder and substance dependence: A randomized controlled trial. *Journal of the American Medical Association, 308*(7), 690–699. doi:10.1001/jama.2012.9071

Najavits, L. M., Gallop, R. J., & Weiss, R. D. (2006). Seeking safety therapy for adolescent girls with PTSD and substance use disorder: A randomized controlled trial. *Journal of Behavioral Health Services and Research, 33*(4), 453–463. doi:10.1007/s11414-006-9034-2

Najavits, L. M., Schmitz, M., Gotthardt, S., & Weiss, R. D. (2005). Seeking Safety plus Exposure Therapy: An outcome study on dual diagnosis men. *Journal of Psychoactive Drugs, 37*(4), 425–435. doi:10.1080/02791072.2005.10399816

National Institute of Clinical Excellence. (2005). Posttraumatic stress disorder: Management. (Clinical guidelines 26). Retrieved from -www.nice.org.uk/guidance/cg26

NICE (2005). Post-traumatic stress disorder (PTSD): The management of PTSD in adults and children in primary and secondary care. Clinical Guideline 26. London: National Institute for Health and Clinical Excellence. Available at www.nice.org.uk.

Nooner, K. B., Linares, L. O., Batinjane, J., Kramer, R. A., Silva, R., & Cloitre, M. (2012). Factors related to posttraumatic stress disorder in adolescence. *Trauma Violence Abuse, 13*(3), 153–166. doi:10.1177/1524838012447698

Owens, G. P., Walter, K. H., Chard, K. M., & Davis, P. A (2012). Changes in mindfulness skills and treatment response among veterans in residential PTSD treatment. *Psychological Trauma: Theory, Research, Practice, and Policy, 4*(2), 221.

Perrin, S. (2013). Prolonged exposure therapy for PTSD in sexually abused adolescents. *Journal of the American Medical Association, 310*(24), 2619–2620. doi:10.1001/jama.2013.283944

Pietrzak, R. H., Goldstein, R. B., Southwick, S. M., & Grant, B. F. (2011). Prevalence and Axis I comorbidity of full and partial posttraumatic stress disorder in the United States: Results from Wave 2 of the National Epidemiologic Survey on Alcohol and Related Conditions. *Journal of Anxiety Disorders, 25*(3), 456–465. doi:10.1016/j.janxdis.2010.11.010

Ruchkin, V. V., Schwab-Stone, M., Koposov, R., Vermeiren, R., & Steiner, H. (2002). Violence exposure, posttraumatic stress, and personality in juvenile delinquents. *Journal of the American Academy of Child and Adolescent Psychiatry, 41*(3), 322–329. doi:10.1097/00004583-200203000-00012

Ruglass, L. M., Lopez-Castro, T., Papini, S., Killeen, T., Back, S. E., & Hien, D. A. (2017). Concurrent treatment with prolonged exposure for co-occurring full or subthreshold posttraumatic stress disorder and substance use disorders: A randomized clinical trial. *Psychotherapy and Psychosomatics, 86*(3), 150–161. doi:10.1159/000462977

Saladin, M. E., Drobes, D. J., Coffey, S. F., Dansky, B. S., Brady, K. T., & Kilpatrick, D. G. (2003). PTSD symptom severity as a predictor of cue-elicited drug craving in victims of violent crime. *Addictive Behaviors, 28*(9), 1611–1629.

Scheeringa, M. S. (2015). Untangling psychiatric comorbidity in young children who experienced single, repeated, or Hurricane Katrina traumatic events. *Child Youth Care Forum, 44*(4), 475–492. doi:10.1007/s10566-014-9293-7

Scheeringa, M. S., & Zeanah, C. H. (2008). Reconsideration of harm's way: Onsets and comorbidity patterns of disorders in preschool children and their caregivers following Hurricane Katrina. *Journal of Clinical Child and Adolescent Psychology, 37*(3), 508–518. doi:10.1080/15374410802148178

Scheeringa, M. S., Zeanah, C. H., Myers, L., & Putnam, F. W. (2003). New findings on alternative criteria for PTSD in preschool children. *Journal of the American Academy of Child & Adolescent Psychiatry, 42*(5), 561–570. doi:10.1097/01.CHI.0000046822.95464.14

Simmons, S., & Suárez, L. (2016). Substance abuse and trauma. *Child and Adolescent Psychiatric Clinics of North America, 25*(4), 723–734. doi:10.1016/j.chc.2016.05.006

Smith, P., Yule, W., Perrin, S., Tranah, T., Dalgleish, T., & Clark, D. M. (2007). Cognitive-behavioral therapy for PTSD in children and adolescents: A preliminary randomized controlled trial. *Journal of the American Academy of Child and Adolescent Psychiatry, 46*(8), 1051–1061. doi:10.1097/CHI.0b013e318067e288

Stein, N. R., Dickstein, B. D., Schuster, J., Litz, B. T., & Resick, P. A. (2012). Trajectories of response to treatment for posttraumatic stress disorder. *Behavior Therapy, 43*(4), 790–800.

Suarez, L. M., Belcher, H. M., Briggs, E. C., & Titus, J. C. (2012). Supporting the need for an integrated system of care for youth with co-occurring traumatic stress and substance abuse problems. *American Journal of Community Psychology, 49*(3–4), 430–440. doi:10.1007/s10464-011-9464-8

Suárez, L., Ellis, B., & Saxe, G. (2014). Integrated treatment of traumatic stress and substance abuse problems among adolescents. In J. Ehrenreich-May & B. Chu (eds.),

Transdiagnostic treatments for children and adolescents: Principles and practice. New York: Guilford Press.

Thabet, A. A., Abed, Y., & Vostanis, P. (2004). Comorbidity of PTSD and depression among refugee children during war conflict. *Journal of Child Psychology and Psychiatry, 45*(3), 533–542.

Van der Velden, A. M., Kuyken, W., Wattar, U., Crane, C., Pallesen, K. J., Dahlgaard, J., ... Piet, J. (2015). A systematic review of mechanisms of change in mindfulness-based cognitive therapy in the treatment of recurrent major depressive disorder. *Clinical Psychology Review, 37*, 26–39.

Vivona, J. M., Ecker, B., Halgin, R. P., Cates, D., Garrison, W. T., & Friedman, M. (1995). Self- and other-directed aggression in child and adolescent psychiatric inpatients. *Journal of the American Academy of Child and Adolescent Psychiatry, 34*(4), 434–444.

Weine, S. M., Becker, D. F., McGlashan, T. H., Laub, D., Lazrove, S., Vojvoda, D., & Hyman, L. (1995). Psychiatric consequences of "ethnic cleansing": Clinical assessments and trauma testimonies of newly resettled Bosnian refugees. *American Journal of Psychiatry, 152*(4), 536–542. doi:10.1176/ajp.152.4.536

33 Transdiagnostic Treatment for Youth with Traumatic Stress

Hilit Kletter, Victor G. Carrion, and Carl F. Weems

Introduction

In a chapter devoted to trans *diagnostic* treatment, it is important to begin with the fact that traumatic stress is an experience, and not a disorder or diagnosis. Traumatic stress can lead to a variety of psychological outcomes. For example, exposure to traumatic experiences can trigger a number of negative outcomes in youth, including depression, anxiety, traumatic grief, aggressive behavior, and other externalizing and internalizing behavior problems (Carrión, Weems, Ray, & Reiss, 2002; Scheeringa, Zeanah, Myers, & Putnam, 2003). The central disorder in this literature, of course, is post-traumatic stress disorder (PTSD). Some treatment outcome research aims to address the trauma experience as a whole (e.g., abuse or neglect), whereas other research focuses on specific effects of the experience, most often PTSD. It is in this respect that any intervention that focuses on the trauma or the cues associated with negative reactions to the trauma is, by this fact, transdiagnostic. The very diversity of outcomes associated with a traumatic event, however, comes with several unique challenges for intervention and prevention. This chapter aims to provide a brief overview of interventions for youth exposed to trauma and present some avenues toward a better understanding of transdiagnostic treatment for this population.

Overview of the Issue

Estimates suggest that more than 25 percent of youth in the United States are exposed to a traumatic event by age 16 (Costello, Erkanli, Fairbank, & Angold, 2002). Community surveys of Flemish youth aged 11–19 have reported exposure to major stressful events to be even greater at between 47 and 72 percent (Bal, Crombez, Van Oost, & De Boudeaudhuji, 2003). Some of the most commonly investigated events include natural disasters, sexual abuse, physical abuse / maltreatment, violence exposure, war, bombing, kidnapping, traffic accidents, and loss (e.g., death of a loved one). Youth may also be in situations where they are secondary victims or witnesses to trauma, such as seeing domestic violence or someone killed through community and school violence.

The events described here are often referred to as traumatic although the term "trauma" is also used to describe psychological reactions to the event. This can lead to some confusion given the point noted earlier that traumatic events are experiences, not disorders or syndromes (see also Finkelhor & Berliner, 1995). A range of psychological reactions are common in youth and not all young people develop serious psychological problems following trauma (e.g., Bonnano, Brewin, Kaniasty, & La Greca, 2010; Kendall-Tackett, Williams, & Finkelhor, 1993; Weems & Graham, 2014). Some demonstrate relatively positive adjustment and proficient functioning despite their experiences, including the experience of post-traumatic growth (e.g., increased self-understanding, belongingness, personal strength, spirituality, quality of relationships, and appreciation of life; Calhoun & Tedeschi, 2006; Prati & Pietrantoni, 2009; Weems & Graham, 2014), although this may not persist for the long term and may be limited to certain areas of functioning (Haskett, Nears, Sabourin Ward, & McPherson, 2006).

Research has tended to define PTSD using the diagnostic criteria from the *Diagnostic and Statistical Manual of Mental Disorders* (currently in its 5th edition; DSM-5; American Psychiatric Association, 2013), which specifies symptoms of re-experiencing, avoidance, negative cognitions / mood, and arousal following a traumatic event. The recent revision in the DSM-5 relocates PTSD in a new chapter on trauma- and stressor-related disorders, and trauma is now defined as exposure to actual or threatened death, serious injury, or sexual violence in one (or more) of the following ways: (1) directly experiencing the traumatic event(s); (2) witnessing, in person, the event(s) as it(they) occurred to others; (3) learning that the traumatic event(s) occurred to a close family member or close friend, and in the case of actual or threatened death of a family member or friend, the event(s) must have been violent or accidental; (4) experiencing repeated or extreme exposure to aversive details of the traumatic event(s) (e.g., first responders collecting human remains; police officers repeatedly exposed to details of child abuse; APA, 2013). These changes reflect a desire to move away from subjective intensity toward objective criteria in defining trauma; however, research is needed to further develop and create an empirical taxonomy of traumatic stressors (Taylor & Weems, 2009).

The treatment studies on traumatic stressors have tended to select participants on the basis of exposure to one or more of the previously mentioned events who also have elevated symptoms of post-traumatic stress and / or meet full diagnostic criteria for PTSD. While this approach has advanced our understanding of treatment responses for particular types of trauma, it has also meant that the research has often not been able to capture the nuances and complexities identified earlier. For example, there is a tendency to examine outcomes for sexual abuse separately from other types of abuse and maltreatment, which ignores the fact that different types of maltreatment tend to co-occur (although some treatments have good outcomes across a variety of different trauma types; Chaffin, 2006; Cohen, Mannarino, Murray, & Igelman, 2006). Furthermore, participants in such studies are often selected to ensure the sample reflects a "pure" trauma experience, yet we know that multiple or recurrent events are common (Finkelhor, Ormrod, & Turner, 2007; Goodyear-Brown, Fath, & Myers, 2012) and that there is a high level of comorbidity in the effects of trauma (Cohen, Mannarino, Berliner, & Deblinger, 2000; Goodyear-Brown et al., 2012; Stallard, 2006).

Treatments for childhood PTSD include trauma-focused cognitive behavioral therapy (TF-CBT), eye movement desensitization and reprocessing (EMDR), pharmacological interventions, and several specific psychosocial interventions (e.g., Carrión, Kletter, Weems, Berry, & Rettger, 2013; Scheeringa & Weems, 2014; Scheeringa, Weems, Cohen, Amaya-Jackson, & Guthrie, 2011; Taylor & Weems, 2011; Weems et al., 2009). TF-CBT is the most widely investigated and used treatment for childhood PTSD (Kowalik, Weller, Venter, & Drachman, 2011; Silverman et al., 2008). TF-CBT was originally developed for sexually abused children but has since been adapted for children exposed to different types of trauma (Cohen et al., 2006). Several TF-CBT studies have shown it to be efficacious in treating traumatized youth (Cohen, Deblinger, Mannarino, & Steer, 2004; Cohen et al., 2000; Deblinger, Lippman, & Steer, 1996; Jaberghaderi, Greenwald, Rubin, Zand, & Dolatabadi, 2004; King et al., 2000).

While there is a growing body of research on transdiagnostic treatment approaches for emotional disorders in youth, studies as yet tend not to include traumatized individuals, and there is limited research on transdiagnostic interventions specifically for childhood trauma (Ehrenreich-May & Chu, 2013). A few examples of transdiagnostic treatments for childhood trauma are described here. For example, Suarez, Ellis, and Saxe (2013) adapted trauma systems therapy for adolescent substance abuse (TST-SA). The intervention views both trauma and substance abuse as "dysregulated emotional and behavioral states that occur in context of a potentially unstable, and at times threatening environment." The core components of TST that aim to change the social environment that perpetuates trauma symptoms and improve self-regulation are supplemented with motivational enhancement, psycho-education about the interaction between substance abuse and trauma symptoms, behavior management strategies for caregivers, and empirically supported substance use components. Greenwald (2013) has developed The Fairy Tale Model as a transdiagnostic, trauma-informed treatment taught to therapists in the form of a fairy tale in which each part of the story corresponds to a phase of treatment. Components of the intervention include recognition of the effects of trauma / loss on presenting problems, enhancing motivation, improving stability and self-management, resolving trauma / loss memories, and anticipating future challenges. The model is appropriate for all ages and has been found effective in reducing a number of symptoms including anxiety, depression, PTSD, and behavioral problems (i.e., aggression, oppositional behavior, substance use, crime, and academic / work failure).

Dialectical behavior therapy (DBT), originally developed for suicidal adults, has been adapted for use with adolescents with PTSD. DBT emphasizes a balance between change and acceptance and focuses on emotional dysregulation as a common theme in psychological distress rather than specific symptoms. DBT has been shown to reduce both PTSD symptoms and self-injurious behaviors in traumatized adolescents (Berk, Shelby, Avina, & Tangeman, 2013). Emerging evidence exists for the use of mindfulness-based interventions in conjunction with trauma-focused treatments to address co-occurring symptoms such as anxiety, depression, and emotional dysregulation. For example, a pilot study of acceptance and commitment therapy (ACT) found the intervention to be effective in the reduction of PTSD symptoms in adolescents (Woidneck, Morrison, & Twohig, 2013). ACT uses mindfulness exercises to target avoidance of traumatic memories by increasing willingness to tolerate traumatic emotions and thoughts. Another mindfulness intervention, mindfulness-based stress reduction (MBSR), which fosters a nonjudgmental approach to emotions, cognitions, and physiological reactions, has also been found effective for traumatized adolescents (Sibinga, Webb, Ghazanian, & Ellen, 2016).

As previously mentioned, many different responses to trauma exist but the majority of interventions have centered on PTSD. Cue-centered therapy (CCT) was developed to focus on trauma cues and reactions to these cues rather than solely on the traumatic event or PTSD symptoms (Carrión et al., 2013). CCT recognizes that especially for youth exposed to chronic adversity, it may not make sense to process traumatic events in isolation. CCT incorporates findings from the neuroscience of trauma exposure as well as insight and component CBT techniques rendering it a distinguishable intervention for trauma-exposed youth. Further description of this treatment will be provided in the sections that follow.

Related DSM-5 Disorders: Advancements and Directions

As mentioned earlier, DSM-5 moved PTSD from the anxiety disorders into a section for trauma- and stressor-related disorders (APA, 2013). Changes to the PTSD diagnosis take into account developmental variations in symptom manifestation and a separate subtype for children younger than age 6 is now included. Other significant changes to the diagnosis include the elimination of criterion A2 (intense fear, helplessness, or horror), division of avoidance and numbing into two separate criteria, and elimination of the acute versus chronic designation. In addition, symptoms of self or other blaming, persistent negative emotional states, and reckless or self-destructive behaviors have been added.

CCT as a Transdiagnostic Treatment for Traumatized Youth

CCT is a manualized protocol designed for youth aged between 8 and 18 years who have experienced repeated exposure to traumatic events (Carrión et al., 2013). CCT consists of 15 weekly, individual sessions (with some joint sessions with the caregiver) with an approximate duration of 45 minutes. Acknowledging that 80 percent of youth with PTSD have comorbidity (e.g., anxiety, depression, ADHD), this intervention seeks to address any emotional disorder vulnerability for which the accumulation of stressors throughout life (which is labeled as the "allostatic load") was a precursor. The allostatic load is the "wear and tear" our bodies experience from the accumulation of trauma and other stressors (McEwen, 2000). When the load exceeds our coping capacity (both psychological and physical), there is risk for development of trauma symptoms. As trauma is known to invade almost every domain of functioning, CCT is transdiagnostic in that it focuses on domains such as social support, strengthening the caregiver / child relationship (attachment), and improving emotional and behavioral regulation. The main goal of CCT is to build strength and resilience by empowering the child by providing knowledge regarding the relationship between history of trauma exposure and current affective, cognitive, behavioral, or physiological responses. Children and caregivers learn about the significance of traumatic stress, how adaptive responses become maladaptive, how to cope with rather than avoid ongoing stress, and the importance of verbalizing their life experiences. The treatment process involves overall competence building, reduction of physical symptoms of anxiety, modification of cognitive distortions, and facilitation of emotional expression. In CCT, youth and caregivers learn to recognize and effectively manage maladaptive responses that occur in response to traumatic reminders (i.e., "cues").

CCT incorporates several unique components. First, through the use of a life time line, CCT aims to address the impact of the allostatic load, examining the direct influence of circumscribed traumatic events as well as other daily or life stressors. Second, several CCT sessions focus on teaching both youth and caregivers about the conditioning process that occurs through the repeated exposure to trauma, resulting in increased sensitivity of fear and anxiety networks (see later section on translational evidence). Third, having identified key functions altered by trauma, CCT seeks to enhance these functions through specific elements and the complete experience of the treatment. Examples of specific elements include insight-oriented assignments that help youth link their trauma histories to emotions, thoughts, physiological reactions, and behaviors, thereby helping them to better regulate trauma reactions (executive functions), a life time line exercise (memory), and completion of feeling sheets (emotional expression). As will be evident from the section on mediators and moderators of treatment change, parents have emerged as a critical pathway for increased intervention success. In CCT, caretakers help identify cues, receive psycho-education on stress and trauma, receive a mid-therapy update from the child about skills learned and treatment progress and are encouraged to facilitate exposure. Finally, in addition to utilizing behavioral, cognitive, and emotional approaches to develop new responses, CCT adds a physiological approach recognizing that many traumatized youth are sensitive to their interoceptive cues (e.g., increased heart rate, sweating). Physiology is distinguished from emotion as youth may physically feel one way but interpret that in a different way emotionally. For example, an angry child who is dissociating may report feeling OK, despite having an accelerated heart rate (Koopman et al., 2004).

A randomized controlled trial in 13 high-risk, low-income schools in San Francisco and East Palo Alto examined the efficacy of CCT as a short-term intervention for youth exposed to repeated, ongoing traumatic experiences (Carrión et al., 2013). Sixty-five participants aged 8–17 years were randomly assigned to CCT or a wait-list control group. Assessments were conducted pre-, mid-, and posttreatment as well as at a three-month follow-up. Child PTSD symptoms were assessed by both child and caregiver self-report using the UCLA-PTSD Reaction Index for DSM-IV (Pynoos, Rodriguez, Steinberg, Stuber, & Frederick, 1998). Child anxiety and depression were assessed through self-report using the Revised Children's Manifest Anxiety Scale (Reynolds & Richmond, 1985) and Children's Depression Inventory (Kovacs, 1992). Caregiver anxiety and depression were assessed through self-report using the Beck Anxiety Inventory (Beck, Epstein, Brown, & Steer, 1988) and Beck Depression Inventory (Beck, Steer, & Brown, 1996). Results showed reduced post-traumatic stress (as measured by means of child and caregiver report), anxiety, depression, and an overall improvement in functioning as rated by the therapists. In addition, caregivers in the treatment group had a significant decrease in anxiety. These gains were maintained at three-month follow-up.

Translation from Basic / Clinical Science to Practice

The following section discusses the brain regions implicated in childhood trauma and how specific components of transdiagnostic treatments for traumatized youth address the deficits seen in these regions. Throughout childhood, brain development occurs during specific stages, known as critical periods, in which specific brain structures are receptive to input from environmental stimuli (Pennington, 2009). The formation and organization of neural connections are shaped by experience and failure to form connections that result in selective elimination or "pruning" of unused neurons (Sowell, Trauner, Gamst, & Jernigan, 2002). Neuroimaging studies suggest structural and functional abnormalities in three key regions of the brain in traumatized youth. The therapeutic targets and techniques in CCT and similar trauma interventions are linked to these three areas. That is, threat and fear processing are related to the amygdala, encoding and retrieving memories are associated with the hippocampus, and executive function has a connection to the frontal lobes.

The amygdala is a brain region of the anterior portion of the temporal lobes. It is thought to be involved in the evaluation of the emotional significance of incoming stimuli (Tottenham, 2012; Tottenham & Sheridan, 2010). In a study examining response to facial expressions (angry, fearful, sad, happy, and neutral), the amygdala was more quickly activated in response to angry faces in trauma-exposed youth as compared to healthy controls (Garret et al., 2012). This suggests that prior trauma may prime the amygdala to respond faster to trauma-related stimuli. In addition, compared to healthy controls, the trauma-exposed youth had greater activation of the amygdala in response to neutral faces. This may reflect ambiguity or a negative interpretation of neutral stimuli for trauma-exposed individuals. Studies suggest that there are no amygdala volume differences between youth with PTSD and healthy controls (Carrión et al., 2001; De Bellis et al., 1999, 2001, 2002). There is fairly clear evidence that the amygdala develops (and structurally grows in size) until late childhood (Uematsu et al., 2012). However, development of the amygdala may be altered by exposure to early life stress (Tottenham, 2012; Tottenham & Sheridan, 2010). Specifically, maturational differences in amygdala volumes among different patient populations with high or traumatic stress exposure (Mehta et al., 2009; Tottenham, 2012; Tottenham & Sheridan, 2010) suggests that exposure to traumatic stress may moderate the association between age and amygdala volumes (Weems, Klabunde, Russell, Reiss, & Carrión, 2015; Weems, Scott, Russell, Reiss, Carrión, 2013). In a series of studies, older youth with trauma and PTSD symptoms had significantly larger right amygdala volumes (controlling for total brain volumes and gender), whereas, younger youth (lower quartile) with PTSD showed smaller volumes than controls (Weems et al., 2013, 2015) such that traumatic stress may delay, accelerate, or prolong typical growth patterns. By facilitating a connection between history, emotion, and behavior through some of the treatment exercises, CCT aims to improve amygdala connections and regulate its emotional function properties such that youth become less sensitized to trauma-related cues.

The second brain region implicated in childhood trauma is the hippocampus. This area is critical for emotional memory formation. Studies examining hippocampal volumes in traumatized youth have obtained mixed results. For example, one meta-analysis found that hippocampal volumes do not differ in maltreated youth compared to controls based on both cross-sectional studies and one longitudinal study (Woon & Hedges, 2008). Other longitudinal studies, however, have noted that PTSD severity and cortisol levels, independently, predicted reductions in hippocampal volume over a 12- to 18-month interval (Carrión, Weems, & Reiss, 2007). During a memory retrieval task, traumatized youth had reduced activation of the right hippocampus compared to healthy controls (Carrión, Haas, Garrett, Song, & Reiss, 2010). Severity of avoidance and emotional numbing symptoms correlated with reduced left hippocampal activation during retrieval in the traumatized group. Avoidance of thoughts and cues associated with the trauma may manifest in the lack of memory processing of those thoughts and cues. CCT engages the child in approach methods that activate the retrieval of memories that may have been partially encoded or not encoded at all.

The third brain region associated with childhood trauma is the prefrontal cortex (PFC). Abnormalities have also been found within the PFC of traumatized youth as compared to healthy controls including larger left frontal lobe volume and decreased left ventral and left inferior prefrontal gray volumes suggesting reduced emotional regulation in these youth (Carrión, Weems, Richert, Hoffman, & Reiss et al., 2010; Carrión et al., 2001). One study, however, found no PFC differences between traumatized youth and healthy controls (De Bellis et al., 1999). One possible explanation for the difference in findings between these studies may be type and duration of trauma. In a later study, De Bellis and colleagues (2000) measured the relative concentration of N-acetylaspartate and creatine, markers of neural integrity, within the medial prefrontal cortex (mPFC). In traumatized youth compared to healthy controls, abnormal neuronal metabolism was suggested by the reduced concentration of N-acetylaspartate compared to creatine. This result indicates that the neuronal loss observed in traumatized youth may lead to lack of extinction of the conditioned fear response, thus contributing to the pathogenesis of PTSD. In an fMRI task assessing sustained attention and response inhibition (pressing a button for letters shown, except for the letter "X"), maltreated youth with PTSD showed decreased activation of the middle frontal cortex (involved in cognitive processing) but increased activation in the medial PFC (involved in emotional processing) suggesting that traumatized youth engage more emotional processing for a task that requires executive functions (Carrión, Garrett, Menon, Weems, & Reiss, 2008). Insight into the conditioning process that associates cues to behavior may help facilitate inhibition of an automatic response. Through the process of psychoeducation early in treatment, and its reinforcement throughout, CCT and other trauma interventions such as TF-CBT aim to enhance function of areas associated with executive function. Other components of these interventions such as identifying cues and developing adaptive new responses may also enable this process.

As discussed earlier, impairments in various brain regions have been associated with childhood trauma. However, the brain is capable of repairing connections through generation of new neurons in response to novel experiences, such as therapeutic experiences (Cicchetti & Cannon, 1999). Evidence-based interventions for trauma symptoms have been suggested to improve brain function by promoting cortical neurogenesis (De Bellis & Thomas, 2003). By providing coping tools and developing empowerment and self-efficacy, children exposed to trauma interventions such as CCT and TF-CBT may become more capable of not letting future stressors lengthen or inappropriately shift critical periods of brain development. Of course, longitudinal developmental studies are necessary to demonstrate the efficacy of such interventions in improving brain function. To this end, we are currently conducting a trial examining the brain function correlates of experiencing CCT, TF-CBT, and treatment as usual via functional near-infrared spectroscopy (FNIRS).

Mediators and Moderators of Change

The childhood trauma literature suggests several moderators and mediators of treatment outcome for transdiagnostic interventions of traumatized youth. As reviewed by Taylor, Graham, and Weems (2015), most of the research investigating possible moderators of treatment for trauma-exposed youth has been done in the context of meta-analyses (Harvey & Taylor, 2010a, 2010b; Silverman et al., 2008). For example, Silverman et al.'s (2008) meta-analysis revealed several moderating influences on the effect sizes obtained for the outcome variable of post-traumatic stress symptoms, in terms of type of treatment and type of trauma. That is, CBT produced a much higher effect size ($d = .50$) than non-CBT interventions ($d = .19$). Further, the average effect size was larger for sexual abuse treatments ($d = .46$) than for treatments of other types of trauma ($d = .38$). Parent involvement in treatment compared with control conditions (wait-list and active controls combined) had little moderating influence on post-traumatic stress outcomes (but did moderate other outcomes such as anxiety and depression). Harvey and Taylor's (2010a, 2010b) meta-analysis focused exclusively on treatments for sexually abused children and adolescents. Again, CBT approaches produced a larger PTSD / trauma treatment effect ($g = 1.37$) as compared to eclectic ($g = .40$) and other approaches ($g = .74$; Hedges's g is a variation of Cohen's d that corrects for bias due to small sample sizes; Hedges, 1991; Hedges & Olkin,

1985). Family ($g = 2.11$) and individual ($g = 1.31$) treatments had better effects than group-based therapies ($g = .89$), and treatments that incorporated some family involvement produced better outcomes ($g = 1.44$) than those in which family was not involved ($g = .67$). This would suggest that some family or non-offending parental involvement in therapy is beneficial, at least in the context of sexual abuse trauma.

A few individual studies have investigated either moderators or mediators of treatment outcomes for youth with PTSD. Research thus far has suggested gender (Tol et al., 2010; Quota, Palosaari, Diab, & Punamaki, 2012), social support (Tol et al., 2010), peri-traumatic dissociation (Quota et al., 2012), maternal depressive symptoms (Nixon, Sterk, & Pearce, 2012; Weems & Scheeringa, 2013), unhelpful traumatic beliefs (Nixon et al., 2012), and maternal PTSD symptoms (Weems & Scheeringa, 2013; Nixon et al., 2012) as potential moderators of treatment success.

Suggested mediators of treatment outcomes for traumatized youth include maladaptive cognitions and parental depression. These studies will be described in more detail later. Smith and colleagues (Smith et al., 2007) tested changes in maladaptive cognitions as a mediator between individual TF-CBT and PTSD symptoms in 24 youth aged 8–18 years who were exposed to single-incident traumatic events (e.g., motor vehicle accidents, interpersonal violence, witnessing violence). After 10 weekly individual sessions, 92 percent of participants no longer met criteria for PTSD compared to 42 percent of the wait-list participants, and treatment effects were maintained at six-month follow-up. Furthermore, the effects of CBT were partially mediated by changes in maladaptive appraisals about the trauma and its aftermath. However, misappraisals and changes in post-traumatic stress symptoms were measured simultaneously, limiting the ability to make temporal conclusions, which is so critical for establishing mediation. It is also unknown if changes in maladaptive cognitions would mediate symptoms in youth exposed to multiple traumatic experiences. Recently, Neil, Weems, and Scheeringa (2016) conducted formal tests of mediation to determine whether there were indirect effects of change in child PTSD symptoms on change in parent depression symptoms, and vice versa, across treatment sessions. The data came from a randomized treatment trial offering a 12-session manual-based CBT treatment to youth with PTSD (Scheeringa & Weems, 2014). Maternal depression significantly decreased over the course of treatment and had an indirect effect on child PTSD symptom change. Evidence for the reciprocal relationship, child symptom change having an indirect effect on parent symptom change, was also found. Findings highlight the potential benefits of child therapy on parents and the reciprocal benefits of improved parent symptoms on the child.

CCT Case Example

Referral Question

Dan is a 9-year-old Caucasian boy who was referred for treatment due to extreme anxiety that developed in response to multiple traumatic experiences. Dan's biological parents were afflicted by drug addiction and he was born addicted to methamphetamine. He suffered severe physical abuse and neglect before being removed from their care. After that, he was in several foster families and had arrived to his adoptive family 17 months prior to assessment. Dan was diagnosed with leukemia one month before the adoption process began; he had four weeks of chemotherapy left at the start of psychological treatment. He was referred to treatment at this point in time due to continued worries he had about medical procedures and death as well as intrusive memories about the prior abuse he experienced with his biological family.

Assessment

Dan and his adoptive mother (AM) were seen together to assess both trauma-specific and comorbid symptoms. AM reported that Dan was easily frustrated, feared sleeping in the dark and losing control, had low self-esteem, and panicked at any little problem. He banged his fists on his legs and rubbed his hands when anxious. Additional symptoms included avoidance of talking about the past, shame, detachment, and lying (which, according to AM, he learned from his biological mother). Dan's functioning was assessed in several domains (e.g., regressive behaviors, social, cognitive). When he arrived at his adoptive family at age 7.5, Dan walked on all fours, did not know how to feed himself, had poor hygiene, and grunted instead of speaking. His speech was delayed until age 4. While AM described Dan as "very loving" and wanting to have friends, she noted that most of his peers were friends with him just because she was teaching at his school and they liked her. He preferred to interact with peers much younger than himself, letting them take the lead. Further, Dan was significantly behind with his vocabulary and struggled with logic and processing. Dan's social support systems were also assessed. Dan reported feeling very supported by his church community. He also felt supported by his friends, teachers, and medical team. Finally, the therapist assessed the impact of Dan's traumatic experiences on his and his family's functioning. The adoptive family was constantly dealing with Dan's misattributions of blame and fear of getting in trouble. Additionally, Dan's diagnosis of leukemia put a major strain on the family as they could not afford treatment and therefore halted the adoption process a month before finalization so that the state would continue to pay for his care. Dan was unaware of this.

Phase 1 (Sessions 1–3): Psycho-Education and Coping Toolbox

In the first session, Dan and AM were educated about trauma reactions, the development of traumatic cues through classical conditioning, research showing the effectiveness of trauma interventions, and treatment components and expectations. In the following two sessions, Dan was seen alone. These sessions were conducted in the hospital as Dan had developed an infection secondary to his leukemia. Dan was introduced to the concept of a coping toolbox and taught strategies including deep breathing, progressive muscle relaxation, guided imagery, mindfulness, and cognitive restructuring. Dan was also introduced to the use of a feeling thermometer to rate level of distress in order for him to be able to identify when to use a coping strategy. He was also encouraged to develop his own coping tools that included sports, drawing, video games, and talking with friends. Dan was assigned to practice these tools and in the following session they were reviewed, and Dan decided what to include in his toolbox. Dan found deep breathing, cognitive restructuring, and video games effective in helping him cope. While in the hospital, he also visualized his room at home with all his stuffed animals, which made the stay more bearable.

Phase 2 (Sessions 4–7): Chronic Traumatic Stress History and Cognitive Restructuring

This phase involved the therapist guiding Dan in narrating his traumatic experiences while focusing on identification of emotions, thoughts, and traumatic cues. Dan spoke about the abuse and neglect he experienced with his biological parents and continued abuse by his first foster family. He also spoke about his diagnosis and treatment of leukemia. He expressed feelings of anger, sadness, shock, and fear. He shared beliefs that something was wrong with him, that he should have rescued his brother, that he had caused the leukemia, and that bad things always happened to him. Cues identified throughout the narrative included needles, being teased, cheating, and arguing. Dan was also given feelings worksheets in between sessions to further help him link his traumatic emotions to current behaviors and cues. In addition, Dan and the therapist mapped out the events in his life and Dan rated each as positive, neutral, or negative to help him place his traumas in context of his greater life experiences. Once his trauma history narrative and life time line were complete, the therapist assisted Dan in restructuring his cognitive distortions using the strategies he had learned previously. Dan was able to reframe his thoughts to "It's not my fault," "Mostly good things have happened to me," and "God's teaching me to be strong." The therapist also worked with Dan on shifting his view from victim to survivor. Dan noted that despite his difficult experiences, he now had a family that wanted him. He stated, "Fear is an option but not a solution and the past was bad but now I have tools to help me."

Phase 3 (Sessions 8–12): Exposure to Traumatic Cues

This phase began with the therapist meeting with Dan and AM to discuss Dan's progress, share skills learned, and prepare AM for her role in supporting Dan to use his coping strategies during the exposure phase. Dan demonstrated his coping tools to AM and shared his narrative and life time line with her. AM updated that Dan was not crying as frequently and saying he was not good enough at doing things. He was less scared of chemotherapy and teachers reported that he no longer had a negative attitude. In the next session, the therapist met with Dan alone to finalize his cue list and prepare for exposure by completing a cue-response worksheet to identify how each of his cues had an impact on his emotions, thoughts, physiological reactions, and behaviors. The therapist also worked with Dan on identifying alternative responses from his toolbox to try during the exposures and these included deep breathing, guided imagery, cognitive reframing, and progressive muscle relaxation. Dan reported that some of his prior cues no longer bothered him and that now he could work on maladaptive behaviors, such as lying, getting in trouble, and not understanding something.

The next three sessions involved gradual exposure to cues including yelling, lying, getting in trouble, and not knowing something. Prior to the beginning of each exposure, a baseline rating of Dan's level of distress was obtained using the feeling thermometer. He was first asked to imagine each cue and a distress level for each exercise was obtained. Coping strategies were applied as needed to lower his distress. The following week, exposure was conducted in the same manner except this time the therapist role-played with Dan to simulate his cues. Dan's initial distress ratings were 9–10 (scale of 1–10 with 10 indicating the higher level of distress) and through these exercises he was able to lower his distress by using his coping strategies to lower ratings (1–3). He stated in this session, "I like the exposure. You're helping a lot with my stress." Dan was then assigned to practice the exposures in vivo at home with the aid of AM. In the next session, the therapist met with Dan to discuss the success of the in vivo exposure. Dan reported that while he had the opportunity to use his coping strategies when being teased, he forgot to do so. The therapist helped him identify ways he could remember his coping strategies such as carrying an index card with a list of all his tools, having a special name for each tool, and routine daily practice. The therapist also assisted Dan with identifying solutions to other potential obstacles to use of his tools. Dan stated that he felt embarrassed doing progressive muscle relaxation in front of others as they might think he was "weird"; hence, the therapist worked with him to adapt certain steps to make them less conspicuous. New tools that Dan identified from his exposures included walking away, ignoring, repeating a mantra, and twirling his fingers, and these were added to his coping toolbox.

Phase 4 (Sessions 13–15): Processing the Chronic Traumatic Stress History and Termination

In the final phase of treatment, Dan was asked to retell his trauma history in the same manner as before though this time he was to incorporate the skills he had learned in treatment. The therapist noted changes in traumatic reactions, which included not being as sad as before and realizing it was not his fault. Dan stated that while he still did not like to talk about his trauma, he found it easier to do so. The final two sessions were dedicated to termination. In the first, the therapist met jointly with Dan and AM to summarize treatment progress, discuss Dan's strengths, and provide final recommendations. At end of treatment, Dan had completed chemotherapy and was receiving maintenance treatment for his leukemia. His adoptive family was moving ahead to finalize the adoption process and he was looking forward to his adoption ceremony. AM reported that Dan was more aware of his feelings and they were continuing to do exposures at home. He was also able to be more present in the moment. Dan had a difficult time parting from the therapist and cried in the final session. The therapist acknowledged his feelings, reviewed his success in treatment, and relabeled termination as a graduation process. The therapist also helped him identify how he might use his coping strategies for future situations.

Challenges and Recommendations for Future Research

While transdiagnostic treatment approaches such as CCT appear promising for addressing the many outcomes of childhood trauma, further research is needed to compare these approaches with PTSD-specific interventions. The conclusions about the efficacy of transdiagnostic approaches to trauma treatment in youth are based on a small number of studies often with limited sample sizes. It is especially unclear if such approaches are appropriate for PTSD. Most of the studies on transdiagnostic trauma interventions for youth have been done with schoolage children and adolescents; thus, additional research is needed to determine applicability to other age groups, for example, very young children. Finally, it remains unclear whether certain child characteristics are contra-indications for transdiagnostic treatment or what should be included in such treatment. As noted earlier, to begin to answer these questions, the authors have a randomized-controlled trial underway that examines CCT, TF-CBT, and treatment as usual to determine which phases of treatment are most effective; how child characteristics influence treatment outcome; and to identify neuro-markers for treatment outcome.

References

American Psychiatric Association. (2013). *Diagnostic and statistical manual of mental disorders* (5th edn.). Arlington, VA: American Psychiatric Publishing.

Bal, S., Crombez, G., Van Oost, P., & De Boudeaudhuji, I. (2003). The role of social support in well-being and coping with self-reported stressful events in adolescents. *Child Abuse and Neglect*, 27, 1377–1395.

Beck, A. T., Epstein, N., Brown, G., & Steer, R. A. (1988). An inventory for measuring clinical anxiety: Psychometric properties. *Journal of Consulting and Clinical Psychology*, 56, 893–897.

Beck, A. T., Steer, R. A., & Brown, G. K. (1996). *Manual for the Beck Depression Inventory* (2nd edn.). San Antonio, TX: The Psychological Corporation.

Berk, M.S., Shelby, J., Avina, C., & Tangeman, K.R. (2013). Dialectical behavior therapy for suicidal and self-harming adolescents with trauma symptoms. In S. Timmer & A. Urquina (eds.), *Evidence-based approaches for the treatment of maltreated children* (pp. 215–236). Dordrecht, Netherlands: Springer Science.

Bonnano, G. A., Brewin, C. R., Kaniasty, K., & La Greca, A. M. (2010). Weighing the costs of disaster: Consequences, risks, and resilience in individuals, families, and communities. *Psychological Science in the Public Interest*, 11, 1–49.

Calhoun, L. G., & Tedeschi, R. G. (2006). The foundations of posttraumatic growth: An expanded framework. In L. G. Calhoun & R. G. Tedeschi (eds.), *Handbook of posttraumatic growth: Research and practice* (pp. 3–23). Mahwah, NJ: Lawrence Erlbaum Associates Publishers.

Carrión V. G., Weems, C. F., Eliez, S., Patwardhan, A., Brown, W., Ray, R. D., & Reiss, A. L. (2001). Attenuation of frontal asymmetry in pediatric posttraumatic stress disorder. *Biological Psychiatry, 50*, 943–951.

Carrión V. G., Garrett, A., Menon, V., Weems, C. F., & Reiss, A. L. (2008). Posttraumatic stress symptoms and brain function during a response-inhibition task: An fMRI study in youth. *Depression & Anxiety, 25*, 514–526.

Carrión V. G., Weems, C. F., Richert, K., Hoffman, C. C., & Reiss, A. L. (2010a). Decreased prefrontal cortical volume associated with increased bedtime cortisol in traumatized youth. *Biological Psychiatry, 68*, 491–493.

Carrión V. G., Haas, B. W., Garrett, A., Song, S., & Reiss, A. L. (2010b). Reduced hippocampal activity in youth with posttraumatic stress symptoms: An fMRI study. *Journal of Pediatric Psychology, 35*, 559–569.

Carrión, V. G., Kletter, H., Weems, C. F., Berry. R. R., & Rettger, J. P. (2013). Cue-centered treatment for youth exposed to interpersonal violence: A randomized controlled trial. *Journal of Traumatic Stress, 26*, 654–662.

Carrión, V. G., Weems, C. F., Ray, R. D., & Reiss, A. L. (2002). Toward an empirical definition of pediatric PTSD: The phenomenology of PTSD symptoms in youth. *Journal of American Academy of Child and Adolescent Psychiatry, 41*, 166–173.

Carrion, V. G., Weems, C. F., & Reiss, A. L. (2007). Stress predicts brain changes in the children: A pilot longitudinal study on youth stress, posttraumatic stress disorder, and the hippocampus. *Pediatrics, 119*, 509–516.

Chaffin, M. (2006). The changing focus of child maltreatment research and practice within psychology. *Journal of Social Issues, 62*, 663–684.

Cicchetti D., & Cannon T. D. (1999). Neurodevelopmental processes in the ontogenesis and epigenesis of psychopathology. *Developmental Psychopathology, 11*, 375–393.

Cohen, J. A., Deblinger, E., Mannarino, A. P., & Steer, R. A. (2004). A multisite, randomized controlled trial for children with sexual abuse-related PTSD symptoms. *Journal of the American Academy of Child and Adolescent Psychiatry, 43*, 393–402.

Cohen, J. A., Mannarino, A. P., Berliner, L., & Deblinger, E. (2000). Trauma-focused cognitive behavioral therapy for children and adolescents: An empirical update. *Journal of Interpersonal Violence, 15*, 1202–1223.

Cohen, J. A., Mannarino, A. P., Murray, L. K., & Igelman, R. (2006). Psychosocial interventions for maltreated and violence-exposed children. *Journal of Social Issues, 62*, 737–766.

Costello, J. E., Erkanli, A., Fairbank, J. A., & Angold, A. (2002). The prevalence of potentially traumatic events in childhood and adolescence. *Journal of Traumatic Stress, 15*, 99–112.

De Bellis M.D., Keshavan, M. S., Clark, D. B., Casey, B. J., Giedd, J. N., Boring, A. M., … Ryan, N. D. (1999). Developmental traumatology: II. Brain development. *Biological Psychiatry, 45*, 1271–1284.

De Bellis M.D., Keshavan, M. S., Spencer, S., & Hall, J. (2000). *N*-Acetylaspartate concentration in the anterior cingulate of maltreated children and adolescents with PTSD. *American Journal of Psychiatry, 157*, 1175–1177.

De Bellis M.D., Hall, J., Boring, A. M., Frustaci, K., & Moritz, G. (2001). A pilot longitudinal study of hippocampal volumes in pediatric maltreatment-related posttraumatic stress disorder. *Biological Psychiatry, 50*, 305–309.

De Bellis M.D., Keshavan, M. S., Shifflett, H., Iyengar, S., Beers, S. R., Hall, J., & Moritz, G. (2002). Brain structures in pediatric maltreatment-related posttraumatic stress disorder: A sociodemographically matched study. *Biological Psychiatry, 52*, 1066–1078.

De Bellis, M. D. & Thomas, L. A. (2003). Biologic findings of post-traumatic stress disorder and child maltreatment. *Current Psychiatry Reports, 5*, 108–117.

Deblinger, E., Lippmann, J., & Steer, R. (1996). Sexually abused children suffering posttraumatic stress symptoms: Initial treatment outcome findings. *Journal of the American Professional Society on the Abuse of Children, 1*, 310–321.

Ehrenreich-May J. & Chu, B. (eds.) (2013). *Transdiagnostic treatments for children and adolescents: Principles and practice* (pp. 339–362). New York: Guilford Press.

Finkelhor, D., & Berliner, L. (1995). Research on the treatment of sexually abused children: Review and recommendations. *Journal of the American Academy of Child and Adolescent Psychiatry, 34*, 1408–1423.

Finkelhor, D., Ormrod, R. K., & Turner, H. A. (2007). Poly-victimization: A neglected component in child victimization. *Child Abuse and Neglect, 31*, 7–26.

Garrett A., Carrión, V., Kletter, H., Karchemskiy, A., Weems, C. F., & Reiss, A. L. (2012). Brain activation to facial expressions in youth with PTSD symptoms. *Depression & Anxiety, 29*, 449–459.

Goodyear-Brown, P., Fath, A., & Myers, L. (2012). Child sexual abuse: The scope of the problem. In P. Goodyear-Brown (ed.), *Handbook of child sexual abuse: Identification, assessment, and treatment* (pp. 3–28). Hoboken, NJ: John Wiley & Sons, Inc.

Greenwald, R. (2013). *Progressive counting within a phase model of trauma-informed treatment*. New York: Routledge.

Harvey, S. T., & Taylor, J. E. (2010a). A meta-analysis of the effects of psychotherapy with sexually abused children and adolescents. *Clinical Psychology Review, 30*, 517–535.

Harvey, S. T., & Taylor, J. E. (2010b). Erratum to "A meta-analysis of the effects of psychotherapy with sexually abused children and adolescents." *Clinical Psychology Review, 30*, 517–535. *Clinical Psychology Review, 30*, 1049–1050.

Haskett, M. E., Nears, K., Sabourin Ward, C., & McPherson, A. V. (2006). Diversity in adjustment of maltreated children: Factors associated with resilient functioning. *Clinical Psychology Review, 26*, 796–812.

Hedges, L. V. (1991). Statistical considerations. In H. Cooper & L. V. Hedges (eds.), *The handbook of research synthesis* (pp. 29–40). New York: Russell Sage Foundation.

Hedges, L. V., & Olkin, I. (1985). *Statistical methods for meta-analysis*. San Diego: Academic Press Inc.

Jaberghaderi, N., Greenwald, R., Rubin, A., Zand, S. O., & Dolatabadi, S. (2004). A comparison of CBT and EMDR for sexually-abused Iranian girls. *Clinical Psychology and Psychotherapy, 11*, 358–368.

Kendall-Tackett, K. A., Williams, L. M., & Finkelhor, D. (1993). Impact of sexual abuse on children: A review and synthesis of recent empirical studies. *Psychological Bulletin, 113*, 164–180.

King, N. J., Tonge, B. J., Mullen, P., Myerson, N., Heyne, D., Rollings, S., & Ollendick, T. H. (2000). Treating sexually abused children with posttraumatic stress symptoms: A randomized clinical trial. *Journal of the American Academy of Child & Adolescent Psychiatry, 39*, 1347–1355.

Koopman, C., Carrión, V., Butler, L. D., Sudhakar, S., Palmer, L., & Steiner, H. (2004). Relationships of dissociation and child abuse and neglect with heart rate in delinquent adolescents. *Journal of Traumatic Stress, 17,* 47–54.

Kovacs, M. (1992). *Manual of the Children's Depression Inventory.* Toronto, Ontario, Canada: Multi-Heath Systems.

Kowalik, J., Weller, J., Venter, J., & Drachman, D. (2011). Cognitive behavioral therapy for the treatment of pediatric posttraumatic stress disorder: A review and meta-analysis. *Journal of Behavior Therapy and Experimental Psychiatry, 42,* 405–413.

McEwen, B. S. (2000). Allostatis and allostatic load: Implications for neuropsychopharmacology. *Neuropsychopharmacology, 22,* 108–124.

Mehta, M.A., Golembo, N. I., Nosarti, C., Colvert, E., Mota, A., Williams, S. C., Rutter, M., & Sonuga-Barke, E. J. (2009). Amygdala, hippocampal, and corpus callosum size following severe early institutional deprivation: The English and Romanian adoptees study pilot. *Journal of Child Psychology and Psychiatry, 50,* 943–951.

Neil, E. L., Weems C. F., & Scheeringa, M. S. (2016). CBT for child PTSD is associated with reductions in maternal depression: Evidence for bidirectional effects. *Journal of Clinical Child and Adolescent Psychology, 47,* 410–420.

Nixon, R. D. V., Sterk, J., & Pearce, A. (2012). A randomized trial of cognitive behavior therapy and cognitive therapy for children with posttraumatic stress disorder following single-incident trauma. *Journal of Abnormal Child Psychology, 40,* 327–337.

Pennington, B. F. (2009). How neuropsychology informs our understanding of developmental disorders. *Journal of Child Psychology and Psychiatry, 50,* 72–78.

Prati, G., & Pietrantoni, L. (2009). Optimism, social support, and coping strategies as factors contributing to posttraumatic growth: A meta-analysis. *Journal of Loss and Trauma, 14,* 364–388.

Pynoos, R., Rodriguez, N., Steinberg, A., Stuber, M., & Frederick, C. (1998). *UCLA PTSD Index for DSM-IV.* Los Angeles: UCLA Trauma Psychiatric Program.

Quota, S. R., Palosaari, E., Diab, M., & Punamaki, R. (2012). Intervention effectiveness among war-affected children: A cluster randomized controlled trial on improving mental health. *Journal of Traumatic Stress, 25,* 288–298.

Reynolds, C. R., & Richmond, B. O. (1985). Factor structure and construct validity of "What I Think and Feel: The Revised Children's Manifest Anxiety Scale." *Journal of Personality Assessment, 43,* 281–283.

Scheeringa, M. S., & Weems C. F. (2014). Randomized placebo-controlled D-Cycloserine with cognitive behavior therapy for pediatric posttraumatic stress. *Journal of Child and Adolescent Psychopharmacology, 24,* 69–77.

Scheeringa, M. S., Weems, C. F., Cohen, J., Amaya-Jackson, L., & Guthrie, D. (2011). Trauma-focused cognitive-behavioral therapy for posttraumatic stress disorder in three through six year-old children: A randomized clinical trial. *Journal of Child Psychology and Psychiatry, 52,* 853–860.

Scheeringa, M. S., Zeanah, C. H., Myers, L., & Putnam, F. W. (2003). New findings on alternative criteria for PTSD in preschool children. *Journal of the American Academy of Child and Adolescent Psychiatry, 42,* 561–570.

Sibinga, E. M., Webb, L., Ghazanian, S. R., & Ellen, J. M. (2016). School-based mindfulness instruction: An RCT. *Pediatrics, 137,* 2015–2532.

Silverman, W. K., Ortiz, C. D., Viswesvaran, C., Burns, B. J., Kolko, D. J., Putnam, F. W., & Amaya-Jackson, L. (2008). Evidence-based psychosocial treatments for children and adolescents exposed to traumatic experiences. *Journal of Clinical Child and Adolescent Psychology, 37*, 156–183.

Smith, P., Yule, W., Perrin, S., Tranah, T., Dalgleish, T., & Clark, D. M. (2007). Cognitive-behavioral therapy for PTSD in children and adolescents: A preliminary randomized controlled trial. *Journal of the American Academy of Child and Adolescent Psychiatry, 46*, 1051–1061.

Sowell E. R., Trauner, D. A., Gamst, A., & Jernigan, T. L. (2002). Development of cortical and subcortical brain structures in childhood and adolescence: A structural MRI study. *Developmental Medicine and Child Neurology, 44*, 4–16.

Stallard, P. (2006). Psychological interventions for post-traumatic reactions in children and young people: A review of randomized controlled trials. *Clinical Psychology Review, 26*, 895–911.

Suarez, L., Ellis, H., & Saxe, G. (2013). Integrated treatment of traumatic stress and substance abuse problems among adolescents. In J. Ehrenreich-May & B. Chu (eds), *Transdiagnostic treatments for children and adolescents: principles and practice* (pp. 339–362). New York: Guilford Press.

Taylor, J. E., Graham, R. A., & Weems C. F. (2015). Moderators and mediators of treatments for youth with traumatic stress. In M. Maric, P. J. M. Prins, & T. H. Ollendick (eds.), *Mediators and moderators of youth treatment outcomes* (pp. 41–64). New York: Oxford University Press.

Taylor, L. K., & Weems, C. F. (2009). What do youth report as a traumatic event? Toward a developmentally informed classification of traumatic stressors. Psychological Trauma, *1*, 91–106.

Taylor, L. K. & Weems, C. F. (2011). Cognitive-behavior therapy for disaster exposed youth with posttraumatic stress: Results from a multiple-baseline examination. *Behavior Therapy, 42*, 349–363.

Tol, W. A., Komproe, I. H., Jordans, M. J., Gross, A. L., Susanty, D., Macy, R. D., & de Jong, J. T. (2010). Mediators and moderators of a psychosocial intervention for children affected by political violence. *Journal of Consulting and Clinical Psychology, 78*, 818–828.

Tottenham, N. (2012). Human amygdala development in the absence of species-expected caregiving. *Developmental Psychobiology, 54*, 598–611.

Tottenham, N., & Sheridan, M. A. (2010). A review of adversity, the amygdala and the hippocampus: A consideration of developmental timing. *Frontiers in Human Neuroscience, 3*, 1–18.

Uematsu, A., Matsui, M., Tanaka, C., Takahashi, T., Noguchi, K., Suzuki, M., & Nishijo, H. (2012). Developmental trajectories of amygdala and hippocampus from infancy to early adulthood in healthy individuals. *PloS One, 7*, e46970.

Weems, C. F., Taylor, L. K., Costa, N. M., Marks, A. B., Romano, D. M., Verrett, S. L., & Brown, D. M. (2009). Effect of a school-based test anxiety intervention in ethnic minority youth exposed to Hurricane Katrina. *Journal of Applied Developmental Psychology, 30*, 218–226.

Weems, C. F. & Graham, R. A. (2014). Resilience and trajectories of posttraumatic stress among youth exposed to disaster. *Journal of Child and Adolescent Psychopharmacology, 24*, 2–8.

Weems, C. F., Klabunde, M., Russell, J. D., Reiss, A. L., & Carrion, V. G. (2015). Post-traumatic stress and age variation in amygdala volumes among youth exposed to trauma. *Social Cognitive and Affective Neuroscience, 10*, 1661–1667.

Weems, C. F., & Scheeringa, M. S. (2013). Maternal depression and treatment gains following a cognitive behavioral intervention for posttraumatic stress in preschool children. *Journal of Anxiety Disorders, 27*, 140–146.

Weems, C. F., Scott, B. G., Russell, J. D., Reiss, A. L., & Carrión, V. G. (2013). Developmental variation in amygdala volumes among children with posttraumatic stress. *Developmental Neuropsychology, 38*, 481–495.

Woidneck, M. R., Morrison, K. L., & Twohig, M. P. (2013). Acceptance and commitment therapy for the treatment of posttraumatic stress among adolescents. *Behavior Modification, 38*, 451–476.

Woon, F. L., & Hedges, D. W. (2008). Hippocampal and amygdala volumes in children and adults with childhood maltreatment-related posttraumatic stress disorder: A meta-analysis. *Hippocampus, 18*, 729–736.

34 Dissemination and Implementation of Evidence-Based Treatments for Childhood PTSD

Alison Salloum

Introduction

Dissemination and implementation of effective, efficient, and accessible treatments for childhood trauma are imperative given the prevalence and devastating effects of childhood trauma. Approximately 16 percent of youth exposed to trauma will develop post-traumatic stress disorder with rates varying from 8.4 percent to 32.9 percent. Girls with interpersonal trauma have the highest rates (Alisic et al., 2014). Childhood trauma can lead to serious negative neurobiological, psychological, cognitive, emotional, and health outcomes (De Bellis & Zisk, 2014). Impairment caused by childhood trauma may continue into adulthood with links to poor physical and mental health (Anda et al., 2006). In addition to a lifetime of human suffering caused by childhood trauma, the economic burden of child maltreatment including costs associated with child welfare, child and adult health care, criminal justice, education, and productivity is more than $120 billion with estimates ranging to more than $500 billion (Fang, Brown, Florence, & Mercy, 2012). Therefore, as effective treatments are developed to minimize or prevent the deleterious effects of childhood trauma, the focus must be on rapidly disseminating and implementing these treatments to reduce the enormous costs of childhood trauma.

Many children with mental health disorders do not receive services, especially minority youth from low-income families (Kataoka, Zhang, & Wells, 2002). Kovess-Masfety et al. (2017) found that across Europe, approximately one-fourth of youth with mental disorders in the past 12 months had received mental health services with differences in service utilization by high- (31.5 percent) and low- (18.9 percent) resourced countries. While high-income countries often have established systems of care for childhood mental health, there are still major service gaps. Low-income countries that often have the greatest need for mental health services for youth often have the fewest services (World Health Organization, 2005). Many children who have experienced childhood trauma may receive traditional therapy approaches rather than evidence-based practices (EBPs) designed specifically for childhood trauma due to numerous barriers associated with their uptake. Barriers to EBPs being provided include, but are not limited to, insufficient funding, payment plans, lack of advocacy and incentives for EBPs, gaps between research and practice, market-based treatments that lack the empirical evidence needed for EBPs, and therapists' attitudes toward EBPs (Chaffin & Friedrich, 2004). Therefore, dissemination and implementation of EBPs for childhood trauma need to improve and address barriers to providing and receiving treatment so that all children have access to empirically supported interventions.

School-Based Settings for EBPs for Childhood Trauma

Schools provide an ideal setting for implementing EBPs for youth to address mental health needs. In fact, Farmer, Burns, Phillips, Angold, and Costello (2003) found that from a national sample of youth in the United States, the education system was the most common pathway into mental health services. Services in school may provide access to treatment to youth who may not otherwise receive mental health services. However, barriers are associated with school treatment options such as obtaining parental consent and child assent to participate in mental health services (Stein et al., 2007). Gathering active consents (i.e., parents sign and return the consent form indicating agreement for their child to participate) can be time consuming as well as costly and yield a lower response rate than passive consents (i.e., parents sign and return the consent form only if they do not want their child to participate). However, ethical issues with passive consent must be considered. In addition to consent, parental participation in treatment at school is often limited. Parental participation in treatment for childhood PTSD is beneficial and is often a main component of treatment. However, having parents participate in school-based EBPs is often a challenge. For example, when the Cognitive Behavioral Intervention for Trauma in Schools (CBITS; for online training see https://cbitsprogram.org/) was implemented within the schools, only 37 percent of parents attended one or more parent group session (Kataoka et al., 2003). Nonetheless, school-based trauma-focused treatment without parental involvement can still be beneficial to the child (Fitzgerald & Cohen, 2012) and an effective approach to providing access to trauma-focused EBPs. While school-based intervention for trauma may address access, EBP implementation challenges remain.

Barriers to Providing EBPs for Childhood Trauma in Clinical Settings

Many of the common barriers to implementing EBPs for other childhood disorders and problems (e.g., lack of resources and transportation, stigma, limited trained providers including those who do not speak the native language of the client, and public awareness of the problem; World Health Organization, 2005) are also common to providing EBPs for childhood trauma. Two common barriers to disseminating and implementing EBPs for childhood trauma are briefly discussed: costs and trained workforce.

First, costs can present a barrier to treatment for the provider of the EBPs and to the client receiving the treatment. Gaining access to treatment, especially for low-income families, is often limited due to the cost of treatment. Logistical barriers that are associated with costs to families can also pose a problem such as the cost of transportation, not being able to take off work for appointments, and needing childcare. Stable financial support for mental health services for children and adolescents is a concern worldwide. In low-income countries, the out-of-pocket expense for parents can be quite high. For example, the World Health Organization (2005) estimated that the out-of-pocket expenditures for child mental health services in African countries was 71.4 percent compared to 12.5 percent in Europe. For providers, the extra time and training necessary to correctly implement EBPs may be a financial burden. As agencies and policy makers make decisions about implementation of EBPs, it is important that estimates of the incremental (additional) costs and staff time needed are considered. A breakthrough series collaborative approach (which also may be called a learning collaborative) is an intensive quality improvement model for dissemination and implementation consisting of teams from multiple agencies that engage in several in-person trainings, consultation and support, and utilize data as feedback for improvement, Using a breakthrough series collaborative approach for disseminating and implementing trauma-focused cognitive behavioral therapy (TF-CBT, an EBP for childhood trauma; Cohen, Mannarino, & Deblinger, 2017) in community-based mental health clinics in the United States, the average clinic team (7.8 staff) spent 2,127 hours during a year of implementation with non-labor direct costs averaging $4,513 (range = $2,580–$8,311). The average incremental costs to clinics was $85,575 (range = $34,697–$130,063 (Lang & Connell, 2017)). However, Greer, Grasso, Cohen, and Webb (2014) found that the average one-year cost for high-end services (e.g., crisis bed, crisis intervention, day hospital, day treatment, inpatient hospital, residential treatment, wrap-around and intensive outpatient services) in the United States was five times higher for trauma-exposed youth who received treatment as usual than trauma-exposed youth who received TF-CBT. These results suggest that while delivering an EBP may seem costly, the costs of not providing an EBP for childhood trauma may be even higher.

Second, having a trained workforce to implement the EBPs for childhood trauma is another potential barrier to treatment. Training providers in EBPs often takes a lot of time especially since evidence suggests that supervision after initial training is critical for effective implementation (Sholomskas et al., 2005). Training alone is not sufficient for effective implementation. For example, Jensen-doss, Cusack, and de Arellano (2008) found that among 66 therapists who attended a TF-CBT training conducted via a 5-week (2-hour) closed-circuit television broadcast, there was no significant evidence via chart review that use of TF-CBT techniques increased after the training. However, therapists did indicate that CBT approaches were more effective for traumatized youth than other modalities. Interestingly, even though the training was mandatory and therapists could watch the videos at a later time if they missed the live web training, only 46.9 percent viewed all five training sessions. The findings suggest that while beliefs about using CBT to treat childhood trauma were positive, changing practice and utilization requires more intensive training and supervision. Contributing to the problem of not having enough trained providers in EBP for childhood trauma is the turnover rate in many provider organizations. For example, in a case study implementing TF-CBT in Philadelphia, six groups (182 therapists and 34 supervisors) have been trained in TF-CBT since 2011. However, only 46 percent of the trained therapists and 44 percent of the trained supervisors remained in their positions over a four-year period (Beidas et al., 2016). In low-resourced countries, the number of trained providers in EBP for childhood trauma may be very limited, and language barriers may also inhibit accessing effective treatment (World Health Organization, 2005). Given the barriers of costs to providers and clients and a limited trained workforce, effective models for implementing EBPs are needed as are newer service delivery approaches that address barriers to providing and receiving treatment.

Methods for Dissemination and Implementation

Prior to the implementation of any form of EBP, there needs to be an understanding of what the EBP is, why there is a need for it, a culture and climate that is flexible and open to change, and a commitment to adopting the new practice (Self-Brown, Whitaker, Berliner, & Kolko, 2012). Resource guides that provide information about why EBPs are needed and the information organizations need to adopt an EBP can be helpful. In an attempt to increase interest and implementation and dissemination of EBPs in child advocacy centers (CACs) for abused children in the United States, the National Child Traumatic Stress Network (NCTSN) in partnership with the National Children's Alliance published a guide for directors of CACs to help plan and implement trauma-informed, empirically supported treatments (Child Welfare Committee National Child Traumatic Stress Network & National Children's Alliance, 2008). The Child Sexual Abuse Task Force and Research and Practice Core of the NCTSN has developed an implementation guide for TF-CBT that addresses why agencies and therapists should implement TF-CBT, a description of TF-CBT, implementation steps, what stakeholders (e.g., program administrators, supervisors, therapists, families and children, community referral sources, and payers) need to know, organizational readiness, delivery issues, and how to maintain fidelity (Child Sexual Abuse Task Force and Research & Practice Core, 2004). Addressing organizational readiness is important for the implementation of EBPs for childhood trauma as it may save money and time by addressing barriers before training. However, depending on the time and extent of preparing an organization to implement an EBP, it may also increase time and money to the implementation costs (Cohen & Mannarino, 2008).

TF-CBT is a widely disseminated EBP for children with post-traumatic stress symptoms and related trauma problems, and it has been implemented with children and adolescents (aged 3 to 18 years) from diverse backgrounds. Although TF-CBT was developed and first implemented in the United States (e.g., Sigel et al., 2013), it has now been disseminated to and implemented in other countries such as Norway (Jensen et al., 2014), Germany (Goldbeck, Muche, Sachser, Tutus, & Rosner, 2016), Zambia (Murray et al., 2015), and Tanzania (O'Donnell et al., 2014) with studies demonstrating effective outcomes in these various countries. The number of empirically published articles on the effectiveness of TF-CBT helps build a case for why an EBP, and specifically TF-CBT, should be implemented for children who are experiencing post-traumatic stress symptoms. Given the wide dissemination and implementation of TF-CBT, this chapter includes several methods that have been utilized to help disseminate and implement it. Such techniques include an online training program (TF-CBT*Web;* see https://tfcbt2.musc.edu/); live trainings with EBP-approved trainers; train the trainer programs to increase access to trainers; ongoing live, web, and / or phone consultations; learning collaboratives; and mixed models, such as web-based training, live training, and ongoing consultations (Cohen & Mannarino, 2008). TF-CBT has established certification criteria that include many of the lessons learned about dissemination and implementation of TF-CBT. For example, practitioners must have at least a master's degree in a mental health field and hold a professional license to practice in their area, complete the TF-CBT web-based course, participate in a live two-day TF-CBT course with an approved trainer, participate in follow-up consultation calls or a learning collaborative, complete three TF-CBT cases with children or adolescents, utilize standardized measures to assess progress with each case, and pass a knowledge-based test on TF-CBT (see https://tfcbt.org/tf-cbt-certification-criteria/).

Studies on TF-CBT provide lessons learned about methods for dissemination and implementation. For example, in the United States, information from 17 statewide TF-CBT dissemination projects suggests that funding per year, years of funding, total costs, total consultation calls, and use of outcome measures did not significantly differ between a learning collaborative that consisted of system-wide training at all levels (e.g., therapists, supervisors, and managers) and live training plus consultation calls with therapists. There were also no significant differences by type of training and the number of therapists trained. Importantly, these statewide efforts demonstrated that large numbers of therapists (200–300) could be trained over several years to implement TF-CBT regardless of the method of training.

Training costs can be mitigated if methods such as partnering with state agencies or other organizations that can leverage funding, changing policies to promote implementation of EBP, providing incentives to providers, and helping prepare administrators for what will be needed for successful implementation (Sigel et al., 2013) are used. In another statewide dissemination study, Fritz et al. (2013) found that clinicians who participated in consultation calls after the web-based TF-CBT training and live training were more knowledgeable about TF-CBT and more competent in delivering it than those who did not participate in consultation calls but completed the web-based and live training. To go beyond knowledge gained from trainings, consultation is important for implementation competency so that therapists can ask questions about specific cases, role-play or rehearse strategies before using specific methods with clients, and discuss implementation issues in relation to real cases in diverse settings.

Assessing the knowledge and skills level of practitioners when implementing treatment for childhood trauma must also include identifying any specific components that may need additional specialized training. Research shows that clinicians who report using TF-CBT do not always utilize all of its components. For example,

Allen and Johnson (2012) surveyed clinicians and found that the most widely used components of TF-CBT were relaxation and psycho-education; the least likely to be used were teaching behavioral management, developing a trauma narrative, and cognitive restructuring (of note, in vivo desensitization, conjoint parent-child sessions, and enhancing personal safety were not assessed in the study). Similarly, Woody, Anderson, D'Souza, Baxter, and Schubauer (2015) found that helping the child develop a trauma narrative, having a conjoint session where the child shares the trauma narrative, and modifying cognitions were the least implemented components. In a study with trainers of TF-CBT (Hanson et al., 2014), the trainers identified the trauma narrative and the cognitive coping components as two challenging components to help clinicians implement with fidelity and competence. Specialized training and booster trainings may be needed to help therapists achieve the competency needed to implement the more challenging components such as the trauma narrative and cognitive coping and processing.

Other methods for dissemination and implementation may include training counselors in low-resourced communities to deliver the treatment and providing implementation toolkits. For example, in a randomized clinical trial comparing TF-CBT to treatment as usual (TAU) among orphan and vulnerable children in Zambia, Murray et al. (2015) used an apprenticeship approach to train lay counselors in TF-CBT. This approach included training 20 adult counselors (all of whom had at least a high school education) via a 10-day on-site training of counselors and supervisors followed by weekly meetings with supervisors and counselors and weekly consultation with TF-CBT experts for supervisors. Fidelity was documented during the meetings and local supervisors helped counselors implement various components. Results indicated that TF-CBT was superior in decreasing PTSD symptoms and impairment as compared to TAU and that training of lay counselors with fidelity to treatment is feasible. In a qualitative study with 19 trainers of TF-CBT, Hanson et al. (2014) gathered preliminary feedback about the utility of an e-toolkit via iPad or tablet to assist with the implementation of TF-CBT. Trainers were positive about this approach, noting that it could improve child-therapist alliance, fidelity, competence, and engagement and be utilized when implementing TF-CBT at home visits. Possible disadvantages noted were using technology to reinforce avoidance and technology challenges in utilizing its functions. Training on the use of the technology was recommended so that it enhances rather than impedes implementation.

Preliminary Evidence for Stepped Care TF-CBT

Alternative delivery systems of EBPs for childhood trauma that have already been widely disseminated with promising implementation strategies may be one approach for addressing barriers to accessing EBPs for childhood trauma and increasing the uptake of these interventions. Given that costs to providers and clients and limited trained workforce are common barriers to children receiving EBPs for childhood trauma, alternative delivery systems that address these barriers may improve access to effective treatment. Currently, Stepped Care TF-CBT (Salloum et al., 2015; Salloum et al., 2016) is being developed and tested as an alternative service delivery of TF-CBT for some children and is designed to be less costly than the standard approach of delivering TF-CBT (i.e., weekly therapist-led session). Stepped Care TF-CBT includes Step One, also known as *Stepping Together* (Salloum, Scheeringa, Cohen, & Amaya-Jackson, 2009, 2010), which is a parent-led therapist-assisted treatment where the parent and child meet with the therapist every other week for six weeks (i.e., three therapy sessions), and conduct 11 at-home parent-child meetings where the parent and child work in an activity book that was based on the Preschool PTSD Treatment manual (Scheeringa, Weems, Cohen, Amaya-Jackson, & Guthrie, 2011). As the parent and child complete the parent-child meetings at home, the therapist provides weekly phone support to help guide the parent in completing the meetings with the child. Parents can also sign in to a website to learn more about the effects of trauma on children (psycho-education) and demonstrations of how to complete the parent-child meetings. Step One addresses all of the components of standard TF-CBT including psycho-education, parenting skills, relaxation, affective expression and modulation, cognitive coping, trauma narrative, in vivo exposure, conjoint meetings, and safety but in a different manner than having the therapist direct these components.

As part of the *Stepping Together* parent-child workbook, the parent and child engage in in vivo exposures that are referred to in the book as "Next Step activities." The in vivo exposures are called "Next Steps" to minimize the use of professional jargon and let the parent know that these next steps are needed to address the trauma reminders. The Next Steps are based on the assessment summary, including avoidance of trauma reminders, and what is called a "scary ladder." The scary ladder is developed by having the parent and child review the brief trauma narrative that was created in the *Stepping Together* (Salloum et al., 2009, 2010) activity book, and then lists events from the least scary to the most scary. The therapist then works with the parent in sessions 2 and 3 to set up Next Step activities (i.e., in vivo exposures) that are completed in parent-child meetings 5–10. Before the Next Steps are completed, the child also draws scenes of the trauma that are listed on the scary ladder and then engages in brief imaginal exposure of the identified scene.

After Step One (e.g., three therapy sessions, completion of the *Stepping Together* workbook that occurred over 11 parent-child meetings, weekly phone support, and a web-based psycho-education component), an assessment is conducted to determine if the child responded to treatment (Salloum, Scheeringa, Cohen, & Storch, 2015), or if the child needs to step up to the second step (e.g., Step Two), which consists of therapist-directed standard TF-CBT. Children who responded to treatment enter into the maintenance phase where the child and parent have one parent-child meeting a week for six weeks to practice the tools they learned in Step One (i.e., behavior plans with rewards; relaxation techniques; identifying, labeling, and communicating feelings with the caregiver).

Stepped care interventions need to include first steps that are based on empirical support and result in a high proportion of children responding to the treatment so that children's suffering is not prolonged. It is also important to have mechanisms in place to guide clinicians with data-driven algorithms for when a child needs to step up to the next level of care (e.g., Salloum, Scheeringa et al., 2015). In a current study on stepped care TF-CBT, we are studying baseline tailoring variables that can be used to guide children to the best level of care before treatment starts (i.e., standard TF-CBT or stepped care TF-CBT), and time varying tailoring variables that can be used to indicate when a child in *Stepping Together* needs to step up to standard TF-CBT. Baseline tailoring variables will help us identify certain child / family / trauma or environmental characteristics that are associated with response versus nonresponse to Step One and may serve as indicators of how to best match the child to Step One or standard TF-CBT. Being able to tailor the child's treatment will result in an adaptive intervention where we match children to the best level of care.

Pilot studies on stepped care TF-CBT with children aged 3 to 7 years ($n = 35$) and 8 to 12 years ($n = 22$) found that approximately 63 percent (intent-to-treat analysis) responded to Step One and went to the maintenance phase, thus not needing therapist-directed TF-CBT treatment. Results suggest comparable improvements between stepped care and standard care TF-CBT in outcomes (e.g., post-traumatic stress symptoms, severity, internalizing and externalizing symptoms), except significant improvements were not met for externalizing symptoms for younger children. As a result, the revised model includes an additional session with the therapist for children who have externalizing symptoms in the clinical range. There was also no difference in acceptability of treatment among parents who participated in stepped care TF-CBT and standard TF-CBT. Importantly, in terms of therapist and patient time and costs, costs were 51.3 percent to 62.4 percent lower for children who participated in stepped care TF-CBT versus standard TF-CBT (Salloum, Small et al., 2015; Salloum et al., 2016). Having an alternative delivery system that (1) uses data to tailor the child to the best level of care prior to treatment; (2) addresses some barriers to treatment such as time, costs, and limited trained therapist; (3) includes components and treatments that are empirically based; and (4) is based on components that are already being widely disseminated and implemented may increase the uptake in community practice. *Stepping Together* is still in the early stages of development and testing, and more research with larger samples and with long-term follow-up data is needed. However, stepped care approaches that build on EBPs that are already being disseminated and implemented may increase accessibility of treatment and require less training if the providers have training in the basics of the standard EBPs.

Case Example of Stepping Together as Step One of Stepped Care TF-CBT

Thomas (fictitious name), a 12-year-old boy, was physically abused by his father and witnessed domestic violence between his mother and father. On one occasion when Thomas and his father were playing soccer with several other fathers and sons, his father became upset with Thomas after the game and threw him up against a building near the soccer field and attempted to strangle him while telling him that he was going to kill him. The father eventually let go of Thomas and left him standing there while he drove away in his car. When the mother found out what happened to Thomas, she took him to the hospital to be evaluated and Thomas and his mother did not return to the home. The father was arrested with a no-contact order in place. After this incident, the mother broke up with the father and moved to a different state. Upon seeking therapy, Thomas and his mother were living at the mother's sister's home, as she did not have her own housing or a job.

Thomas met criteria for post-traumatic stress disorder. He presented with seven symptoms that included (1) recurrent/intrusive memories: the mother stated that Thomas thought about the incident with his father and talked about it at least 2–3 times per week; (2) nightmares: the mother reported that Thomas had nightmares almost every night within the past month; (3) physiological reactivity upon exposure: the mother reported that Thomas had expressed having more stomach aches and headaches; (4) feeling detached: the mother reported that Thomas did not want to be around many new people and had problems with trusting others; (5) negative emotions: both Thomas and his mother expressed that Thomas felt some sadness and guilt about the traumatic incident with his father; (6) inability to recall aspects of trauma: Thomas reported that he sometimes could not remember everything that had happened during the incident with his father; and (7) anhedonia / diminished interest: Thomas reported that he no longer liked to play soccer like he did in the past, which was an activity he gladly shared with his father prior to this event. The mother reported that if Thomas went on the soccer field, he did not run after the ball or play hard. The mother also reported that Thomas seemed worried when she occasionally left him alone, and he was always asking where she was going and when she would return. These symptoms affected his relationship with mother, as he started becoming defiant toward her. Table 34.1 provides the baseline, mid, and post-assessment data, and the measures that were used on these occasions.

In-Office Session 1. The therapist met with Thomas and his mother to address psycho-education, parenting, and relaxation. Parenting consisted of helping the parent praise Thomas when he demonstrated positive behavior and establishing a behavior plan to minimize his defiant behaviors such as when he would "talk back" and refuse to comply with tasks the mother would ask him to do such as wash his hands and face when he woke up. The parent was given part one of the *Stepping Together* (Salloum et al., 2009, 2010) parent-child activity book.

Parent-Child Meetings 1–4. Thomas and his mother had four parent-child meetings that addressed relaxation exercises, feeling identification, rating, and expression such as identifying feelings of sad, mad, scared, and happy and rating how much of these feelings he was experiencing based on a scale of none to a whole lot and then letting his mother know his feelings and rating, and constructing a brief narrative of the traumatic event by completing an activity sheet that inquired about specifics of the event. Parent and child then completed the "scary ladder" where the parent and child rated the events during the trauma narrative that were least scary to most scary (see Table 34.2). The book *Stepping Together* provides specific instructions for the parent as to how to create a scary ladder. The parent-child meetings took place in

Table 34.1 *Case Example (Thomas): Assessment Data as Obtained During the Stepping Together Treatment*

Measure	Baseline	Mid-assessment	Post-assessment
K-SADS, PTSD module	7 PTSD symptoms	0 PTSD symptoms	0 PTSD symptoms
	1 area of impairment	0 areas of impairment	0 areas of impairment
	Met diagnosis for PTSD	No PTSD	No PTSD
CBCL Externalizing	4 (normal range)	Not assessed	4 (normal range)
CBCL Internalizing	18 (clinical range)	Not assessed	7 (normal range)
TSCYC-PTS	56 (clinical range)	28 (non-clinical)	28 (non-clinical)
UCLA PTSD Reaction Index	20[a]	0	0
CGI-S	3 (moderate)	0 (no illness)	0 (no illness)
CGI-I	Not applicable	1 (free of symptoms)	1 (free of symptoms)

Note. KSADS = Kiddie Schedule for Affective Disorders and Schizophrenia (K-SADS-PL, 2013); CBCL = Child Behavior Checklist (Achenbach & Rescorla, 2001); TSCYC = Trauma Symptom Checklist for Young Children, Posttraumatic Stress Total (Briere et al., 2001); UCLA PTSD Reaction Index For Children and Adolescents- DSM-5 (Steinberg et al., 2013). CGI-S = Clinical Global Impression-Severity (National Institute of Mental Health, 1985); CGI-I = Clinical Global Impression-Improvement (Guy, 1976). The mid-assessment occurred after Step One and the post-assessment occurred after the maintenance phase.
[a] The range for the total PTSD symptoms is 0 to 80, with higher scores indicating higher frequency of PTSD symptoms. Clinical cutoff scores for the updated measure (i.e., UCLA PTSD Index – DSM-5) have not been established yet.

their room at the aunt's home where they were living. The parent was provided a password to sign into the *Stepping Together* website where there is a video demonstration of three relaxation exercises (e.g., deep breathing, muscle relaxation, and positive imagery). The *Stepping Together* website has a link to the National Child Traumatic Stress Network for Parents and Caregivers (see www.nctsn.org/) so that the mother could learn more about the effects of trauma on children. The therapist provided two phone calls to check in with the mother about how the parent-child meetings were going.

In-Office Session 2. The therapist met with Thomas and his mother and reviewed their activity book. The therapist focused on in vivo exposure and helped the parent establish four Next Steps (i.e., in vivo exposure exercises) based on the first four items listed on the scary ladder. The therapist gave the parent part two of the *Stepping Together* activity book that includes information about how to complete parent-child meetings five through eight and explained to the parent and child the importance of completing the activities including the Next Steps.

Parent-Child Meetings 5–8. Thomas and his mother completed the next four parent-child meetings. These four meetings continued to utilize relaxation and feeling identification and expression. Thomas let his mother know that he did not want to meet anymore because he wanted to forget everything and refused to do the Next Steps. The mother explained the importance of facing his trauma triggers and

Table 34.2 *Scary Ladder and Next Step Activities for Case Example*

Scary Ladder	Parent-Child Meeting	NEXT STEPS
Most Scary When he was in my face choking me and I could not breathe at all	10	Thomas went to play soccer at a different location than in meeting 9. He repeated the Next Step for meeting 9 but increased the time and intensity of running. Afterward, he and his mother discussed how this felt and if any of the men at the field looked like his father.
Most Scary When he was in my face choking me and I could not breathe at all	9	Thomas practiced his deep breathing exercises and also discussed feelings with mom. Thomas then went to play soccer and was instructed to run very fast after the ball to the point where his breathing increased. When playing Thomas was also instructed to say to himself, "I am going to realize my dad is not here and I am safe and notice mom is safe too." After the game, the mother asked Thomas if there was anyone who looked like his dad. The goal was to have Thomas realize that when he took deep breaths or became winded when running, he was not choking. Also, similar to meeting 7, he was to realize that just because other men looked similar to his dad, his dad was not there and these men did not hurt him.
Almost Most scary When he told me to come here (trigger: being left alone)	8	The mother left Thomas for 30 minutes in the care of his aunt but did not tell him exactly when she would return. The goal was for Thomas to use his coping skills and to realize that just because he does not know exactly when his mother will return, she is okay and that this did not mean that something bad had happened to her.
Medium Scary When he started walking up to me and I saw his angry face (avoidance: avoiding people during soccer game that look similar to dad)	7	The mother showed Thomas a photograph of dad for 5 minutes, and then they went to the park where there would be men who looked similar to his father. The goal was for the child to realize that the just because certain men may look like his father, this does not mean that these men are dangerous.
Medium Scary My dad yelling at me in the middle of game (trigger: loud noises)	6	Thomas and his mother went to the soccer field and both mom and child yelled loudly about playing soccer such as "kick the ball to me" and so on. Afterward the parent and child discussed that loud noises and yelling do not necessarily mean danger. The Next Step was to help the child test out his belief that hearing yelling means danger. The parent discussed with Thomas differences between loud dangerous yelling and non-dangerous yelling.
Not too Scary: Playing soccer	5	Thomas and his mother went to the soccer field and Thomas played for about 5 minutes on the field.

Note. The Next Steps were developed with the parent and were based on the child's Scary Ladder and baseline assessment report.

completing the activity book together. They agreed to have the parent-child meetings at McDonald's, away from the aunt's home, and complete the Next Step before going back to the home. Thomas liked the treat of going to McDonald's and being out of his aunt's home and agreed to complete the rest of the parent-child meetings, including the Next Steps. During these meetings they also discussed what it means to feel safe and developed a safety plan together, such as being aware of surroundings, talking with his mother if he does not feel safe, calling 911 (e.g., police) if his father shows up, and not participating on social media accounts including not visiting his father's Facebook page. Their safety plan was reviewed at each parent-child meeting. This also provided time for them to talk about the domestic violence that had occurred in the past.

In-Office Session 3. The therapist reviewed with the parent and child the *Stepping Together* workbook, provided supportive counseling with the mother, and helped establish the next two Next Steps.

Parent-Child Meetings 9–11. Thomas and his mother completed the last three parent-child meetings and activities in *Stepping Together*. Meeting 9 included finalizing the safety plan and drawing, imagining, and completing a Next Step. Meeting 10 consisted of the last Next Step and discussing how Thomas would cope in the near and far future if there were trauma reminders (e.g., relapse prevention). Meeting 11 consisted of reviewing the entire *Stepping Together* activity book and celebrating the completion.

Assessments. The parent and child completed the mid-assessment and due to their positive response to treatment, they entered the maintenance phase where they continued to have one parent-child meeting a week to strengthen their relationship and communication, and to practice relaxation exercises and the affect identification and modulation skills that they learned while completing *Stepping Together*. The parent and child completed a post-assessment after the six-week maintenance phase.

Time. The three in-office sessions lasted about an hour to an hour and a half. A total of four phone calls occurred over an 8-week period totaling 55 minutes. The program was to be completed in 6 weeks, but due to the parent's schedule, the time period was extended by 2 weeks. The total time the therapist assisted the parent and child was 4 hours and 30 minutes. Compared to standard TF-CBT (approximately 18 hours), the timesavings for the therapist was 75 percent.

The total time the parent assisted the child was 9 hours and 6 minutes (55 minutes spent on phone calls with the therapist, 3 hours and 27 minutes in the in-office sessions, 4 hours and 39 minutes spent in parent-child meetings, and 5 minutes spent waiting in-office for treatment). The travel time to and from each in-office session was 56 minutes round trip (168 minutes), thus the total time the parent spent with Step One was 11 hours and 54 minutes. Compared to standard TF-CBT, and including drive time, the timesavings for the parent was 59.2 percent.

Training. The therapist providing the Step One treatment was a master's level clinician in a community-based agency. She was trained in standard TF-CBT and was working toward her certification in TF-CBT. Therefore, the therapist was already trained in the components of TF-CBT (e.g., psycho-education, parenting skills, relaxation, affect identification, and modulation skills, cognitive coping, trauma narrative, and cognitive process, in vivo exposure, conjoint sessions, and enhancing safety) and did not require further training on these components. The training on Step One consisted of reading *Stepping Together* (Salloum et al., 2009, 2010), the parent-child activity book, reading the therapist manual that lists steps to be completed in each of the three sessions and general questions to ask during the brief phone calls, tips for motivating parents to complete the parent-child meetings based on lessons learned, and a one-day specialized training in in vivo exposures. Similar to other strategies for implementation, consultation was provided to help the therapist learn how to set up in vivo exposures.

Conclusion

There are many evidence-based interventions for children experiencing PTSD. As dissemination and implementation efforts are underway to train clinicians in these interventions, efforts are also needed to deliver these treatments in ways that make EBP for childhood trauma accessible, efficient and affordable. School-based settings provide one approach to implementing EBP for childhood trauma as school-based mental health can reach more children who may not otherwise receive treatment. Disseminating research on effective methods for implementation or lessons learned can help other providers as they plan to implement an EBP for childhood trauma in different settings. Methods to increase implementation of EBPs for childhood trauma include live trainings by EBP experts, web-based trainings, learning collaboratives or other methods to provide on-going consultation (e.g., live, via conference calls or online platforms) as providers are implementing a specific EBP, train-the-trainer programs, and e-toolkits or other uses of technology to help providers learn EBPs. Service delivery methods that build upon providers' knowledge of effective treatments are needed to address barriers to treatment, as are alternative methods of providing EBPs for childhood trauma. Given the prevalence of childhood trauma around the world, we must find multiple solutions that address the needs of all children to receive accessible, affordable, efficient, and effective treatment for childhood trauma.

References

Achenbach, T. M., & Rescorla, L. A. (2001). *Manual for the ASEBA School-Age Forms & Profiles*. Burlington, VT: University of Vermont, Research Center for Children, Youth, & Families.

Alisic, E., Zalta, A. K., van Wesel, F., Larsen, S. E., Hafstad, G. S., Hassanpour, K., & Smid, G. E. (2014). Rates of post-traumatic stress disorder in trauma-exposed children and adolescents: Meta-analysis. *The British Journal of Psychiatry, 204*, 335–340. doi:10.1192/bjp.bp.113.131227

Allen, B., & Johnson, J. C. (2012). Utilization and implementation of trauma-focused cognitive-behavioral therapy for the treatment of maltreated children. *Child Maltreatment, 17*(1), 80–85. doi:http://dx.doi.org/10.1177/1077559511418220

Anda, R. F., Felitti, V. J., Bremner, J. D., Walker, J. D., Whitfield, C., Perry, B. D., ... Giles, W. H. (2006). The enduring effects of abuse and related adverse experiences in childhood. A convergence of evidence from neurobiology and epidemiology. *European Archives of Psychiatry and Clinical Neuroscience, 256*(3), 174–186. doi:10.1007/s00406-005-0624-4

Beidas, R. S., Adams, D. R., Kratz, H. E., Jackson, K., Berkowitz, S., Zinny, A., ... Evans, A., Jr. (2016). Lessons learned while building a trauma-informed public behavioral health system in the City of Philadelphia. *Evaluation and Program Planning, 59*, 21.

Briere, J., Johnson, K., Bissada, A., Damon, L., Crouch, J., Gil, E., ... Ernst, V. (2001). The Trauma Symptom Checklist for Young Children (TSCYC): Reliability and association with abuse exposure in a multi-site study. *Child Abuse & Neglect, 25*(8), 1001–1014.

Chaffin, M., & Friedrich, B. (2004). Evidence-based treatments in child abuse and neglect. *Children and Youth Services Review*, (11), 1097.

Child Sexual Abuse Task Force and Research & Practice Core, National Child Traumatic Stress Network. (2004). *How to implement trauma-focused cognitive behavioral therapy*. Durham, NC and Los Angeles, CA: National Center for Child Traumatic Stress.

Child Welfare Committee National Child Traumatic Stress Network & National Children's Alliance. (2008). *CAC directors' guide to mental health services for abused children*. Los Angeles, CA & Durham, NC: National Center for Child Traumatic Stress.

Cohen, J., & Mannarino, A. P. (2008). Disseminating and implementing trauma-focused CBT in community settings. *Trauma, Violence, & Abuse, 9*(4), 214–226. doi:10.1177/1524838008324336

Cohen, J. A., Mannarino, A. P., & Deblinger, E. (2017). *Treating trauma and traumatic grief in children and adolescents* (2nd edn.). New York: Guilford Press.

De Bellis, M. D., & Zisk, A. (2014). The biological effects of childhood trauma. *Child and Adolescent Psychiatric Clinics of North America, 23*(2), 185–222, vii. doi:10.1016/j.chc.2014.01.002

Fang, X., Brown, D. S., Florence, C. S., & Mercy, J. A. (2012). The economic burden of child maltreatment in the United States and implications for prevention. *Child Abuse and Neglect*, (2), 156.

Farmer, E. M., Burns, B. J., Phillips, S. D., Angold, A., & Costello, E. J. (2003). Pathways into and through mental health services for children and adolescents. *Psychiatric Services, 54*(1), 60–66. doi:10.1176/appi.ps.54.1.60

Fitzgerald, M. M., & Cohen, J. A. (2012). Trauma-focused cognitive behavioral therapy for school psychologist. *Journal of Applied School Psychology, 28*, 294–315.

Fritz, R. M., Tempel, A. B., Sigel, B. A., Conners-Burrow, N. A., Worley, K. B., & Kramer, T. L. (2013). Improving the dissemination of evidence-based treatments: Facilitators and barriers to participating in case consultation. *Professional Psychology-Research and Practice, 44*(4), 225–230. doi:10.1037/a0033102

Goldbeck, L., Muche, R., Sachser, C., Tutus, D., & Rosner, R. (2016). Effectiveness of trauma-focused cognitive behavioral therapy for children and adolescents: A randomized controlled trial in eight German mental health clinics. *Psychotherapy and Psychosomatics*, *85*(3), 159–170. doi:10.1159/000442824

Greer, D., Grasso, D. J., Cohen, A., & Webb, C. (2014). Trauma-focused treatment in a state system of care: Is it worth the cost? *Administration and Policy in Mental Health and Mental Health Services Research*, (3), 317. doi:10.1007/s10488-013-0468-6

Guy, W. (1976). *ECDEU assessment manual for psychopharmacology*. Washington, DC: US Department of Health, Education, and Welfare.

Hanson, R. F., Gros, K. G., Davidson, T. M., Barr, S., Cohen, J. A., Deblinger, E., ... Ruggiero, K. J. (2014). National trainers' perspectives on challenges to implementation of an empirically-supported mental health treatment. *Administration and Policy in Mental Health and Mental Health Services Research*, *41*(4), 522–534. doi:http://dx.doi.org/10.1007/s10488-013-0492-6

Jensen, T. K., Holt, T., Ormhaug, S. M., Egeland, K., Granly, L., Hoaas, L. C., ... Wentzel-Larsen, T. (2014). A randomized effectiveness study comparing trauma-focused cognitive behavioral therapy with therapy as usual for youth. *Journal of Clinical Child and Adolescent Psychology*, *43*(3), 356–369. doi:10.1080/15374416.2013.822307

Jensen-doss, A., Cusack, K. J., & de Arellano, M. A. (2008). Workshop-based training in trauma-focused CBT: An in-depth analysis of impact on provider practices. *Community Mental Health Journal*, *44*(4), 227–244. doi:http://dx.doi.org/10.1007/s10597-007-9121-8

K-SADS-PL. (2013). *Advanced Center for Intervention and Services Research (ACISR) for early onset mood and anxiety disorders*. Western Psychiatric Institute and Clinic. Child and Adolescent Research and Education (CARE) Program. New Haven: Yale University.

Kataoka, S. H., Stein, B. D., Jaycox, L. H., Wong, M., Escudero, P., Tu, W., ... Fink, A. (2003). A school-based mental health program for traumatized Latino immigrant children. *Journal of the American Academy of Child and Adolescent Psychiatry*, (3), 311.

Kataoka, S. H., Zhang, L., & Wells, K. B. (2002). Unmet need for mental health care among U.S. children: Variation by ethnicity and insurance status. *American Journal of Psychiatry*, *159*(9), 1548–1555. doi:10.1176/appi.ajp.159.9.1548

Kovess-Masfety, V., Van Engelen, J., Stone, L., Otten, R., Carta, M. G., Bitfoi, A., ... Husky, M. (2017). Unmet need for specialty mental health services among children across Europe. *Psychiatric Services*, *68*(8), 789–795. doi:10.1176/appi.ps.201600409

Lang, J. M. & Connell, C. M. (2017). Measuring costs to community-based agencies for implementation of an evidence-based practice. *The Journal of Behavioral Health Services & Research*, *44*(1), 122–134. doi:http://dx.doi.org/10.1007/s11414-016-9541-8

Murray, L. K., Skavenski, S., Kane, J. C., Mayeya, J., Dorsey, S., Cohen, J. A., ... Bolton, P. A. (2015). Effectiveness of trauma-focused cognitive behavioral therapy among trauma-affected children in Lusaka, Zambia: A randomized clinical trial. *Journal of the American Medical Association Pediatrics*, *169*(8), 761–769. doi:10.1001/jamapediatrics.2015.0580

National Institute of Mental Health. (1985). Clinical global impressions. *Psychopharmacology Bulletin, 21*, 839–843.

O'Donnell, K., Dorsey, S., Gong, W., Ostermann, J., Whetten, R., Cohen, J. A., ... Whetten, K. (2014). Treating maladaptive grief and posttraumatic stress symptoms in orphaned children in Tanzania: Group-based trauma-focused cognitive-behavioral therapy. *Journal of Traumatic Stress, 27*(6), 664–671. doi:10.1002/jts.21970

Salloum, A., Scheeringa, M. S., Cohen, J. A., & Amaya-Jackson, L. (2009; 2010). *Stepping Together: Parent-Child Workbook for Children (for young children ages 3 to 7 and children ages 8 to 12) after Trauma*. Unpublished books: asalloum@usf.edu.

Salloum, A., Scheeringa, M. S., Cohen, J. A., & Storch, E. A. (2015). Responder status criterion for stepped care trauma-focused cognitive behavioral therapy for young children. *Child Youth Care Forum, 44*(1), 59–78. doi:10.1007/s10566-014-9270-1

Salloum, A., Small, B. J., Robst, J., Scheeringa, M. S., Cohen, J. A., & Storch, E. A. (2015). Stepped and standard care for childhood trauma: A pilot randomized clinical trial. *Research on Social Work Practice*. doi:10.1177/1049731515601898

Salloum, A., Wang, W., Robst, J., Murphy, T. K., Scheeringa, M. S., Cohen, J. A., & Storch, E. A. (2016). Stepped care versus standard trauma-focused cognitive behavioral therapy for young children. *Journal of Child Psychology and Psychiatry, 57*(5), 614–622. doi:10.1111/jcpp.12471

Scheeringa, M. S., Weems, C. F., Cohen, J. A., Amaya-Jackson, L., & Guthrie, D. (2011). Trauma-focused cognitive-behavioral therapy for posttraumatic stress disorder in three-through six year-old children: A randomized clinical trial. *Journal of Child Psychology and Psychiatry, 52*(8), 853–860. doi:10.1111/j.1469-7610.2010.02354.x

Self-Brown, S., Whitaker, D., Berliner, L., & Kolko, D. (2012). Disseminating child maltreatment interventions: Research on implementing evidence-based programs. *Child Maltreatment, 17*(1), 5–10. doi:10.1177/1077559511436211

Sholomskas, D. E., Syracuse-Siewert, G., Rounsaville, B. J., Ball, S. A., Nuro, K. F., & Carroll, K. M. (2005). We don't train in vain: A dissemination trial of three strategies of training clinicians in cognitive–behavioral therapy. *Journal of Consulting and Clinical Psychology*, (1), 106.

Sigel, B. A., Kramer, T. L., Conners-Burrow, N. A., Church, J. K., Worley, K. B., & Mitrani, N. A. (2013). Statewide dissemination of trauma-focused cognitive-behavioral therapy (TF-CBT). *Children and Youth Services Review, 35*(6), 1023–1029. doi:10.1016/j.childyouth.2013.03.012

Stein, B. D., Jaycox, L. H., Langley, A., Kataoka, S. H., Wilkins, W. W., & Wong, M. (2007). Active parental consent for a school-based community violence screening: Comparing distribution methods. *The Journal of School Health, 77*(3), 116–120.

Steinberg, A. M., Brymer, M. J., Kim, S., Briggs, E. C., Ippen, C. G., Ostrowski, S. A., ... Pynoos, R. S. (2013). Psychometric properties of the UCLA PTSD reaction index: Part I. *Journal of Traumatic Stress, 26*(1), 1–9. doi:10.1002/jts.21780

Woody, J. D., Anderson, D. K., D'Souza, H. J., Baxter, B., & Schubauer, J. (2015). Dissemination of trauma-focused cognitive-behavioral therapy: A follow-up study of practitioners' knowledge and implementation. *Journal of Evidence-Informed Social Work, 12*(3), 289–301. doi:10.1080/15433714.2013.849217

World Health Organization. (2005). *Atlas child and adolescent mental health resources: Global concerns: Implications for the future* (ISBN 92 4 156304 4). Geneva: Switzerland WHO Press.

35 New Wave Therapies for Post-Traumatic Stress Disorder in Youth

Michelle R. Woidneck, Ellen J. Bluett, and Sarah A. Potts

Introduction

The goals of this chapter are to synthesize the accumulating evidence for newer-generation therapeutic approaches being used in the treatment of childhood post-traumatic stress disorder (PTSD), to describe the general tenets of these approaches, and to provide practical steps to support implementation of these therapies in practice. We provide a general overview of the history of the literature, including a brief description of the traditional treatments for childhood PTSD and limitations of existing treatments. We next provide a rationale and overview of new wave mindfulness-based interventions (MBIs) as a therapeutic approach, outline core features of these treatments, present preliminary evidence for these interventions, and discuss mediators and moderators of change. We present a clinical case illustration to demonstrate the clinical utility and example implementation of these practices in a youngster who had developed PTSD after being involved in a traffic accident. Finally, we conclude with a description of challenges and recommendations for future research and highlight key practice points.

Overview and the Need for Innovation

To date, a cognitive conceptualization of the development and maintenance of PTSD largely dominates the literature (Ehlers & Clark, 2000) and thus has informed the main approaches for interventions such as trauma-focused cognitive behavioral therapy (TF-CBT), eye movement desensitization and reprocessing (EMDR), prolonged exposure (PE), and cognitive processing therapy (CPT). The effectiveness of existing interventions has been well documented for adults (Cusak et al., 2016) and youth (Silverman et al., 2008). However, these treatments are not without limitations. For instance, attrition and nonresponse rates have been particularly problematic, with dropout rates averaging around 20 percent (Imel, Laska, Jakupcak, & Simpson, 2013) and nonresponse rates in the adult literature reaching 50 percent (Schottenbaurer, Glass, Arnkoff, Tendick, & Gray, 2008). Clinical trials among youth have also shown that a subgroup of individuals with PTSD may not adequately benefit from CBT or PE approaches, as several studies have revealed from 16 percent to 40 percent of youth diagnosed with PTSD at pretreatment continued to meet the diagnostic criteria at posttreatment (e.g., Cohen, Deblinger, Mannarino, & Steer, 2004; King et al., 2000). Given the rate of attrition and frequency of partial and / or nonresponders to existing PTSD interventions, as well as individual differences that likely influence one's receptiveness and responsiveness to treatment, ongoing expansion and enhancement of available treatment options are needed.

As treatments for PTSD have continued to evolve, newer interventions largely based on mindfulness principles and practices continue to gain attention in the field at large, as well as within the research with PTSD specifically. While the specific techniques across different MBIs may vary, several distinctive features are typically present among these approaches. The features of MBIs have expanded upon existing behavioral, cognitive, and cognitive behavioral traditions and emphasize mindfulness- and acceptance-based processes, tend to rely on methods that are more experiential than didactic in nature, and consider contextual factors rather than a mechanistic framework (see Dimidjian et al., 2016). A central feature of MBIs also includes targeting internal experiences indirectly using strategies such as mindfulness or acceptance of their presence rather than targeting the content of these experiences directly. MBIs, also sometimes referred to in the literature as new wave treatments, third wave treatments, or acceptance- and mindfulness-based treatments, include but are not limited to acceptance and commitment therapy (ACT), mindfulness-based stress reduction (MBSR), mindfulness-based cognitive therapy (MBCT), as well as mind-body interventions, such as yoga, tai chi, qigong, and meditation in various forms. While there are certainly important distinctions among therapies within the mindfulness- and acceptance-based traditions, several universal concepts and processes are worthy of highlighting.

Description of the Approach to Innovation

Function versus Form. Traditional cognitive behavioral approaches largely influenced by the work of Aaron Beck have historically viewed psychopathology as the result of distorted thought patterns. Therefore, these treatments have utilized cognitive change processes, such as cognitive challenging and / or restructuring, with the primary aim of symptom reduction or remission (Beck, 2005). MBIs differ in that they aim to change the way in which an individual relates to internal experiences (i.e., thoughts, feelings, memories, sensations, urges) with the goal of altering how the internal experiences function for the individual. In the case of PTSD, memories about a prior trauma are often experienced as distressing and function as an event that must be avoided or altered. Rather than attempting to change the meaning, frequency, and / or distress of the memory, a new wave approach aims to cultivate an individual's ability to observe the memory and associated internal experiences with openness and nonjudgment. From this stance, an individual can recognize an internal experience *as* an internal experience that will arise and pass in its own time. From this vantage point, a traumatic memory no longer functions as an event that must be avoided, but rather as an inner event that can be willingly experienced and observed. This shift decreases the power the memory possesses over an individual and thereby increases the flexibility of behavioral responding in the presence of the memory. While the content, frequency, and / or severity of distressing psychological experiences may change when using a new wave intervention, these changes are not the primary treatment target and are considered second-order treatment effects.

Mindfulness. As noted earlier, mindfulness is a fundamental process within new wave approaches. John Kabat-Zinn, a pioneer in the field of mindfulness, defines mindfulness by highlighting the psychological process central to new wave therapies. He describes mindfulness as "the awareness that emerges through paying attention, on purpose, in the present moment, and non-judgmentally to the unfolding of experiences moment by moment" (2003, p. 145). Consistent with the previous example, MBIs aim to alter the relationship individuals have with their thoughts by increasing the ability to observe thoughts and emotions in a nonjudgmental, nonreactive, accepting manner.

Mindfulness may be targeted in a variety of ways. Meditation is often utilized to cultivate mindfulness and can refer to a broad range of practices. However, central to all meditation practices is attentional training or, simply stated, being intentional with attention. Practices may include voluntarily focusing on a chosen object or experience (e.g., breath) and / or nonreactive observation of the content of internal experiences as they unfold moment to moment. Movement meditations, such as yoga, tai chi, and qigong, emphasize attention to physical and emotional stimuli through use of breathing and physical poses.

Acceptance. Acceptance involves openly allowing the presence of inner experiences as they occur in the moment. The process of acceptance is volitional and should not be confused with tolerating, wanting, or agreeing. Rather, acceptance involves an acknowledgment of any given present-moment internal event and choosing to willingly experience the inner event without defense, thereby decreasing the power and behavioral control of inner experiences. Accepting the presence of any given thought, memory, or feeling is distinctly different from approving of or agreeing with the experience. Further, it should be emphasized that acceptance refers only to internal experiences. For example, learning to willingly experience *the memory* of a past traumatic event, such as abuse, is distinctly different from accepting the past abuse as admissible and is also different from resigning to remain in a currently abusive situation. It is possible to learn to willingly experience the memory of abuse when it arises and to also view the abuse itself as an unacceptable action. Similarly, it is possible to learn to willingly experience the memory of abuse and to also take necessary actions toward ending an abusive relationship.

Values. As noted earlier, symptom reduction is considered a second-order treatment outcome among MBIs rather than the primary treatment focus. The primary focus among these approaches tends to be increased functioning and improved overall quality of life. Thus, an overarching goal is to develop ways to have any given internal experience without it interfering with one's living. To do so, treatment emphasizes both the identification and clarification of personal values. Values constitute one's life worth living by providing guidance and direction in life. Ultimately, promoting a values-driven life becomes the central focus of treatment, rather than a reduction in symptoms per se. As an example, imagine a teenager experiencing PTSD symptoms in response to a motor vehicle accident, including avoidance of driving or attaining a driver's license. If through the course of therapy, the teen identifies freedom and independence as personal values and acknowledges that the ability to drive is in accordance with these values and is an important aspect of creating a life worth living, then a logical treatment goal may include the attainment of a driver's license. The actions toward this goal will likely evoke distressing internal experiences for the teen; however, a new wave approach is less concerned with the distress that arises and more so with helping develop necessary skills for simultaneously experiencing distress while engaging in values-consistent action.

Evidence-Base for MBIs

MBIs with Youth. Research on the efficacy of MBIs has primarily focused on adult populations. MBIs have been shown to be efficacious in treating a variety of psychological difficulties among adults, such as depression (e.g., Grossman, Niemann, Schmidt, & Walach, 2004), anxiety (e.g., Dalrymple & Herbert, 2007), and chronic pain (e.g., Dahl, Wilson, & Nilsson, 2004). Only recently research has begun to explore MBI outcomes among younger populations. In this section, we provide a brief summary of the existing empirical support for MBIs with child and adolescent samples. Given the limited data in this domain, we will also give a brief overview of the relevant research in the adult literature to help guide our understanding and recommendations regarding the potential appropriateness of MBIs as a treatment of PTSD for youth.

To our knowledge, three meta-analyses exploring the effects of MBIs with youth have been conducted to date (Borquist-Conlon, Maynard, Brendel, & Farina, 2017; Kallapiran, Koo, Kirubakaran, & Hancock, 2015; Zoogman, Goldberg, Hoyt, & Miller, 2014). Zoogman et al. (2014) conducted the first meta-analysis, which included 20 published studies (13 randomized controlled trials (RCTs), 6 treatment-only design, and 1 open-controlled trial) testing MBIs with clinical and nonclinical child and adolescent populations. The meta-analysis included studies that utilized MBSR, MBCT, as well as more general mindfulness meditation practices (e.g., breathing awareness, mindful movement). Results of the combined clinical and nonclinical samples indicated an overall small, positive effect of MBIs. However, when considering clinical samples alone, results revealed an effect in the moderate range. Specifically, MBIs demonstrated small, significant effects for youth diagnosed with mood disorders (Biegel, Brown, Shapiro, & Schubert, 2009) and externalizing disorders (Bogels, Hoogstad, van Dun, de Schutter, & Restifo, 2008), and moderate, significant effects for youth diagnosed with comorbid anxiety and learning disabilities (Beauchemin, Hutchins, & Patterson, 2008). Interestingly, the overall effectiveness of MBIs among youth with anxiety disorders alone produced much smaller, yet significant effects (Semple, Reid, & Miller, 2005). In addition, results from one study suggested that MBIs may be helpful for improving executive functioning in youth (Flook et al., 2010). Outcomes among different MBI types were nonsignificant, limiting conclusions regarding effectiveness of specific MBIs. Overall, the results of this meta-analysis suggest that MBIs are a practical treatment option for youth.

A second meta-analysis explored the effectiveness of specific MBIs on mental health symptoms and quality of life in both clinical and nonclinical child and adolescent populations (Kallapiran et al., 2015). This meta-analysis included five RCTs using MBSR or MBCT with nonclinical samples, three RCTs using ACT with clinical populations, and three RCTs using another MBI (e.g., yoga, mindfulness, meditation) with nonclinical populations. Results indicated that MBSR and MBCT interventions were more effective than non-active control treatments (e.g., wait-list control, psycho-education) in improving stress, anxiety, and depression among nonclinical populations. ACT interventions showed an overall small, yet significant effect that was equally as effective as the active treatment comparisons (including CBT) for anxiety management, depression, and quality of life in clinical populations. Other MBIs (yoga, mindfulness, meditation) were also effective in improving anxiety and stress, but not depression, in nonclinical populations compared to non-active control groups (e.g., psycho-education). Notably, ACT and MBSR appeared to fulfill the necessary requirements to be considered an empirically supported therapy as outlined by Chambless and Hollon (1998).

A more recent systematic review and meta-analysis provided support for MBIs as an effective treatment alternative for youth struggling with more severe anxiety disorders, including PTSD (Borquist-Conlon et al., 2017). This meta-analysis included five recent studies (two RCTs and three quasi-experimental designs), two of which targeted PTSD in youth, while three included youth with generalized anxiety disorder, social anxiety disorder, and unspecified anxiety disorder. The combined effect size for all five studies fell in the moderate range. The two PTSD-specific studies demonstrated significant, positive effect sizes ranging from small (Catani et al., 2009) to large (Gordon, Staples, Blyta, Bytyqi, & Wilson, 2008). Given the focus of this chapter, the two RCTs that included youth with PTSD, along with the one published study examining ACT for youth with PTSD, are discussed in greater detail below.

Catani et al. (2009) randomized 31 children who presented with a preliminary PTSD diagnosis to a meditation-relax group or narrative-exposure therapy group. The meditation-relax condition (MBI group) used present-moment awareness techniques, meditation, breathing, relaxation techniques, and a daily hour-long home practice. The narrative-exposure therapy condition encouraged the child, with the help of a therapist, to construct a detailed account of the traumatic experience. Interventions included six 60–75-minute sessions delivered three times a week for two weeks. Both groups showed a significant decrease in mean PTSD scores post-treatment, and no significant differences were found between conditions. Additionally, 71 percent of children in the MBI group and 81 percent in the exposure condition maintained treatment gains at six-month follow-up. Overall, results of this study showed MBI and an exposure intervention to be equally effective in reducing PTSD symptoms in children, a notable finding given that exposure-based therapies are the current gold-standard treatment for PTSD.

Gordon et al. (2008) explored the effectiveness of a mind-body skills program to treat PTSD in adolescents. Eighty-two participants were randomized to a 12-session mind-body behavioral program, wait-list control, or a delayed-start treatment group. The mind-body behavioral program included present-moment awareness training, meditation, breathing techniques, guided imagery, body scan technique, and relaxation skills. At posttreatment, those in the intervention group showed significantly lower PTSD scores compared to the wait-list control group, and these improvements were maintained at three-month follow-up. The delayed-start group also evidenced significant decreases in PTSD scores, but only after receiving the intervention. These findings suggest that the reduction in PTSD scores was attributable to the intervention itself rather than a result of natural reductions in symptomology across time alone. Results from this study provide preliminary evidence for the effectiveness of MBI in reducing PTSD symptoms in adolescents.

To date, only one study has examined ACT for adolescents with post-traumatic stress. Using a multiple-baseline design, this studied administered 10 sessions of ACT with seven adolescents with post-traumatic stress. Results showed significant reductions in post-traumatic stress, with a 60 percent mean reduction in PTSD symptoms on a clinician-administered PTSD measure and a 73.3 percent mean reduction on a self-report measure of PTSD (Woidneck, Morrison, & Twohig, 2014).

The progression of research exploring the effectiveness of MBIs among youth is promising. Taken together, the existing literature provides preliminary support for use of MBIs with children and adolescents. Given the limited data available, however, additional research examining the efficacy of MBIs for youth with PTSD is clearly needed.

MBIs and PTSD. As evidenced previously, the existing literature examining the efficacy of MBIs for youth with PTSD is extremely limited. Fortunately, research on MBIs for adults with PTSD has gained considerable attention in the past decade. In this section, we provide a brief summary of the research on MBIs for PTSD. While an exhaustive empirical review is beyond the scope of this chapter, an overview of the existing literature is both necessary and informative in understanding how these interventions may be applied to children.

Lang et al. (2012) reviewed the evidence of three meditative practices (mindfulness, mantra, and compassion meditation) for the treatment of PTSD in adults. The authors categorized interventions based upon the purported mechanisms of change for each meditative practice. According to this review, *mindfulness* aims to improve both attentional control and present-moment awareness, *mantra repetition* aims to increase relaxation and reduce physiological arousal, and *compassion meditation* aims to increase positive emotion and social connectedness. Based on a review of the studies available at the time, the authors found mindfulness practices to have the most promising evidence as an effective intervention for PTSD. Mantra repetition practices had limited data available; however, one RCT compared mantra repetition plus care-as-usual to care-as-usual alone. Results showed greater reductions in PTSD symptoms in the mantra-repetition group (small to medium effect sizes) compared to the care-as-usual group (Bormann, Thorp, Wetherall, Golshan, & Lang, 2013). Lastly, no studies investigating compassion meditation as a treatment for PTSD had been conducted at the time of the review. Lang et al. (2012) concluded that while empirical support for MBIs was limited, the interventions were generally well tolerated by participants and produced minimal side effects. In addition, MBIs were found to be beneficial for providers because of their ease of application, cost-effectiveness, and accessibility as an adjunctive therapy.

A comprehensive review by Banks, Newman, and Saleem (2015) examined the efficacy of MBIs for adult populations with PTSD. Of the twelve studies included, eight implemented MBSR, one implemented MBCT, and two implemented other MBIs (mindful meditation training, mindfulness-based stretching, and deep breathing). In addition, the study utilized a standard measure of quality to compare studies with varying methodological design. Overall, study quality ranged from poor to good, with a greater number rated as poor. Due to the variation in study quality, results were reported by research design type (pilot studies, non-controlled trials, controlled trials, RCTs). Of the four pilot studies included, results showed improvements in PTSD symptoms; however, statistically significant change was undetermined due to the small sample size. Three non-controlled treatment trials examined the efficacy of MBSR provided in a group format. Across the three studies, results showed positive improvements in PTSD symptoms with effect sizes ranging from medium to large; however, all participants were concurrently receiving another treatment, thus making it difficult to draw conclusions about effectiveness and generalizability. One controlled trial compared MBCT in group format to treatment-as-usual (psycho-education) and found significant changes in PTSD symptoms and negative cognitions in the MBCT group but no changes in the treatment-as-usual group. Finally, three of four RCTs reviewed found improvements in PTSD symptoms. The RCT that did not find significant improvements in PTSD symptoms included a sample with chronic PTSD.

Taken together, results suggest there is preliminary evidence for MBIs for the treatment of PTSD in adults; however, there is a need for more robust research and refined treatment designs. Overall, most participants across studies showed improvements on PTSD symptoms at posttreatment, and these improvements were maintained at follow-ups ranging from 2 to 30 months. Notably, MBIs appeared to have the largest effect on symptoms associated with avoidance. Further, minimal adverse events were reported. While results from the Banks et al. (2015) review are encouraging, there are several important limitations. Many of the included studies had notable methodological limitations, including small sample sizes, lack of randomization, unevenly matched control groups, and ongoing therapy for more than half of the sample. Finally, a meta-analysis was not possible due to the heterogeneity of the studies included.

One review to date has examined the utility of mind-body interventions for the treatment of PTSD (Kim, Schneider, Kravitz, Mermier, & Burge, 2013). For their review, the authors defined mind-body practices as "interventions with components of interaction among the mind, body, and behavior, with the intent to integrate these three components in the pursuit of improved physical functioning and mental and physical health" (p. 827). Studies that implemented MBSR, meditation, breathing, or physical practices, including yoga, tai chi, qigong, were included in the study. Of the 16 studies reviewed, 12 reported significant positive effects of mind-body intervention on reduction of PTSD symptoms. However, studies included in this review were heterogeneous in nature and varied greatly in rigor, design, and duration, making it difficult to draw conclusions about mind-body interventions generally. While results are encouraging, additional research of mind-body interventions for PTSD is needed.

The only meta-analysis to date examined a total of 10 RCTs of MBIs for adults with PTSD (Hilton et al., 2017). The primary aim of the study was to offer quantitative estimates of the efficacy of MBIs (MBSR, MBCT, mindfulness meditation, yoga, tai chi, qigong, mantra meditation, self-compassion) for the treatment of PTSD. Of the studies included, five RCTs utilized MBSR, three utilized yoga, and two utilized mantra repetition. Pooled analysis of eight studies showed statistically significant reductions in PTSD symptoms for those receiving an adjunctive MBI compared to control groups (treatment-as-usual, education, present-centered therapy). Adjunctive MBIs also showed statistically significant reductions in depression. Furthermore, results were positive but not statistically significant for reductions in anxiety and improvements in quality of life. Importantly, the effect estimates were low for PTSD symptoms and moderate for depression, which was likely due to the limited availability and varying quality of the study data included in the analyses. As with the previous reviews, this study was not without limitations. For example, most studies included a clinician-administered measure of PTSD, while others only included self-report measures (e.g., depression, anxiety, quality of life). Also of note, five of the ten studies had quality ratings of "poor," therefore limiting the degree to which results could be extrapolated.

Taken together, current research suggests that MBIs hold promise as a treatment for PTSD. However, nearly every systematic review highlighted the variability in quality, design, and sample size of the studies conducted in this area. Therefore, to draw conclusions about the efficacy of MBIs, more research is needed with an emphasis on RCTs.

Mediators and Moderators of Change

Identified mediators and moderators of change contribute to overall clinical judgment by suggesting the most appropriate interventions for a specific presentation or client type and highlighting the most valuable treatment components, or processes / mechanisms of change. The majority of existing published RCTs lack process-of-change analyses, which contributes to the current challenge of identifying mechanisms of change within MBIs. Additionally, conceptualizing and measuring potential mechanisms can be challenging given the differences in theoretical models and intervention components (Chiesa & Malinowski, 2011; Gu, Strauss, Bond, & Cavanaugh, 2015). Furthermore, the variance in definition, application, and intended utility of mindfulness among MBIs may present a challenge for identifying overarching mediators and moderators of change. However, this concern is currently in question given that some data suggest the processes of mindfulness are relatively uniform regardless of intervention approach (Swain, Hancock, Hainsworh, & Bowman, 2015). A brief discussion of available data regarding potential MBI mechanisms of change with youth populations will be followed by a summary of known mechanisms of change within adult populations.

Few studies to date have explored mediators or moderators of change in adolescent populations (e.g., Swain et al., 2015; Zoogman et al., 2014). Preliminary findings suggest specific client factors moderate treatment outcome, including age and clinical versus nonclinical emphasis. Zoogman et al. (2014) found age moderated MBI treatment and outcome, such that older adolescents (e.g., aged 12–21 rather than 6–8 years) showed stronger treatment effects. This relationship may be best explained by the natural strengthening of cognitive and abstract abilities that accompany growth (e.g., Schnieder & Lockl, 2002). Presence of a clinical diagnosis, rather than nonclinical emphasis, has also been suggested to moderate MBI treatment and outcome. While individuals with severe psychological presentations often have opportunities for significant improvement from baseline functioning, Zoogman et al. (2014) also suggest the stronger outcomes found in clinical samples might be explained by the fact that MBIs tend to teach less "pathological uses of attention" (p. 302) and instead emphasize perspective, self-discovery, and values-based behavior. Interestingly, no published data suggest moderation effects of session length or frequency, and significant variance certainly exists in dosage among treatments.

In addition to significant moderators of treatment outcome, two preliminary mediators have also been purported. In a review article of five MBI studies in adolescent populations, acceptance was found to account for the relationship between MBI intervention and outcome for adolescents with anxiety. This suggests acceptance is a key mechanism through which MBIs operate (Swain et al., 2015) and provides a rationale for measuring acceptance to monitor treatment impact. In the same review, the ACT "hexaflex model" (i.e., a treatment model including six core processes of change) mediated the relationship between treatment and the following outcomes: clinical severity rating, anxiety symptoms, and depression symptoms (Swain et al., 2015).

Although MBI change mechanism data do not currently exist within adolescent PTSD populations, the available longitudinal data from youth with post-traumatic symptoms can be applied. A recent study found the relationship between childhood sexual abuse and post-traumatic symptoms was partially mediated by mindfulness (Daigneault, Dion, Hebert, & Bourgeois, 2016), suggesting mindfulness held an important role in coping with the post-traumatic experience. Data suggested a person with greater mindfulness ability who encounters a trauma (e.g., sexual abuse) may experience more symptoms initially (e.g., anxiety, anger), while a person with lower mindfulness ability may find the abuse as more tolerable in the moment. However, at a later time (e.g., while engaging in MBCT), a person with greater mindfulness ability is more likely to evidence *decreased* PTSD symptoms. This suggests that for individuals with PTSD, level of mindfulness ability may be an important consideration when beginning treatment and may help with treatment expectations (e.g., a person low in mindfulness may find it particularly challenging at first to contact memories and emotions). This relationship is also aligned with previous research in adult populations (e.g., Rosenthal, Hall, Palm, Batten, & Follette, 2005).

Not surprisingly, the evidence base for purported mediators and moderators for MBIs are predominantly within adult populations. Mindfulness ability (Gu et al., 2015; Nila, Holt, Ditzen, & Aguilar-Raab, 2016) and repetitive negative thinking (e.g., rumination and worry; Ehring, Razik, & Emmelkamp, 2011) are two known MBI mediators. In a systematic review of mindfulness mediation RCTs with clinical and nonclinical samples, mindfulness was found to fully mediate the relationship between MBSR/MBCT treatments and the following outcomes: depression, anxiety, and stress (Gu et al., 2015). Results also suggested decreased rumination / worry as a significant mediator for MBSR / MBCT and the following outcomes: depression, stress, anxiety, and global symptoms of psychopathology. Nila et al. (2016) found that overall mindfulness ability fully mediated the relationship between MBSR and distress tolerance (e.g., set of skills for effectively managing challenging emotions).

Given the limited focus on intervention change mechanisms to date, future studies might consider including an alternate treatment comparison (e.g., measuring factors that boost treatment effects). Greater exploration on change mechanisms in MBI and PTSD research might establish stronger clinical decision making (Bean, Ong, Lee, & Twohig, 2017), such as more targeted interventions (e.g., for whom) and inclusion of key intervention components (e.g., how and what).

Clinical Case Illustration

Background and Symptoms. Eva, a 14-year-old White female, was referred for therapy following a motor vehicle accident (MVA). Prior to the MVA, Eva attended school regularly, earned average to above average grades, and participated on a year-round elite swim team. Eva and her mother, the driver, were involved in a rollover accident after hitting black ice while driving to an out-of-town swim meet. Eva sustained a minor cut to the side of her head and experienced body soreness for multiple days post-MVA. Her mother lost consciousness for several minutes at the time of the accident, sustained a mild traumatic brain injury; broken collarbone; and experienced whiplash, body soreness, and chronic headaches for several months.

Eva presented for treatment shortly after the start of a new school year (six months post-MVA) with concerns related to separation anxiety, school avoidance, and post-traumatic stress symptomology. Eva experienced post-traumatic stress symptoms immediately following the MVA, including intrusive images about the accident, physiological (e.g., headache, ears ringing) and psychological (e.g., fear, anxiety) reactions in response to trauma reminders, and occasional nightmares and difficulty sleeping. She described a sense of responsibility, as from her perspective, the accident only occurred because of travel for her swim meet. Eva expressed guilt that her mother sustained more severe injuries. She endorsed hypervigilance while riding in cars and avoided car rides during inclement or ominous weather. Eva experienced separation anxiety from her mother immediately following the accident, which significantly escalated upon the start of a new school year. She additionally began to exhibit school avoidance at this time (five months post-MVA), and her grades were subsequently declining. Eva's engagement in social activities became increasingly limited in the months following the MVA. When she did engage in such activities, she was unable to enjoy herself, felt distracted, and often engaged in safety behaviors, such as repeatedly checking in with her mother via text messages or phone calls. Eva continued to participate in swimming but refused to compete in out-of-town competitions post-MVA. Eva was hypersensitive to her mother's well-being and experienced increased anxiety and post-traumatic stress symptomology in response to her mother's ailments and / or somatic complaints. Additional trauma reminders included seeing or hearing about MVAs (e.g., on TV / movies or actual accidents), hearing or seeing sirens, body position or movements similar to those experienced at the time of the accident, the sound of breaking glass, hearing music that had been playing at the time of the accident, loved ones driving long distances, and stormy weather.

Treatment Focus. The start of treatment began with rapport building and thorough assessment of symptoms and functional impairment, including identification of contextual factors related to increased impairment and dysfunction as well as decreased impairment and more adaptive functioning. Psycho-education on the stress response and post-traumatic stress reaction was provided to Eva and her parents. A rationale for mindfulness was provided, and this was a primary focus early and throughout the treatment process.

Mindfulness was introduced as strategies to encourage Eva to reconnect with the here-and-now through nonjudgmental, intentional awareness of present-moment stimuli using the five senses. Mindfulness techniques were taught and practiced during and outside of sessions to strengthen Eva's ability to connect with present-moment stimuli, to facilitate experiential awareness of the difference between events in the present versus events in the past, and to cultivate an observer perspective of internal experiences. Multiple mindfulness strategies were incorporated throughout the course of treatment, including mindfulness of breath, identifying and labeling sensory experiencing (e.g., identification of what can be seen / heard / touched in the present), as well as labeling internal experiences that arose during mindfulness practice. For example, when Eva became distracted by memories of her accident or sensations of anxiety during mindful breathing exercises, she audibly or internally said "remembering" or "anxiety" and then redirected her attention to her breath. More advanced mindfulness exercises included cultivating the ability to observe internal experiences as they arise and pass. Exercises targeting this included imagining thoughts as clouds floating through the sky or leaves floating down a stream. Additional exercises to target memories or images included envisioning these images as a YouTube or Instagram video that one can pause, rewind, fast forward, watch in slow motion, or view with any given filter, and so on. The goal of mindfulness was emphasized as becoming aware of and strengthening observation of present-moment experiences versus attainment of any given feeling state (e.g., relaxation) or efforts to escape or distract from any given thought or feeling. It was explained that although this may (or may not) occur during mindfulness practice, any given pleasurable feeling state can be considered a "nice side effect" rather than the goal itself.

A large focus of treatment also included identification of personal values, interests, and aspirations. Eva was clear that friendships and family relationships were important to her. She identified physical health and fitness as areas of importance. Knowledge and personal growth also emerged as important values. She identified goals of graduating high school and attending college and identified an aspiration of swimming for a specific out-of-state college team as well.

These values and goals provided a necessary framework for the remainder of treatment. Exercises aimed at cultivating acceptance were anchored in a clear value, thereby altering the purpose and function of distress. For example, Eva acknowledged that regular school attendance was necessary to work toward her goals of graduation and attending college. Therefore, at the outset of imaginal and in vivo exercises targeting school attendance, bigger picture goals (i.e., graduating, attending college) and values (knowledge, personal growth) were highlighted as the larger purpose of the exercise. Clarification of this purpose serves to cultivate acceptance, or the willingness to experience any given distressing thought or feeling that may arise during imaginal or in vivo exercises. Questions such as "would you be willing to allow this anxiety (or identified distressing internal experience) if doing so is in the service of moving toward your identified value and / or goal?" were commonplace throughout the course of treatment.

While exposure exercises, including imaginal exposure, in vivo exposure, and / or completion of a trauma narrative, may be a component of MBI (and was a component in this sample case), the emphasis is not on reducing the intensity or frequency of distress. Alternatively, exposure aims to cultivate the ability to mindfully and willingly be with any given internal experience to increase the capacity to take effective values-based action and create a life worth living. To achieve this goal, it is essential to decrease the power (versus intensity) of interfering emotions, and to thereby cultivate flexibility. Thus, a new wave approach may conceptualize exposure exercises as "acceptance" or "willingness" exercises. In Eva's case, values-congruent interventions targeted increasing both school attendance and engagement in pleasurable and meaningful activities (e.g., attending social activities and out-of-town swim meets). This meant developing Eva's ability and willingness to contact fearful stimuli in more functional manners. For example, spending increasingly longer periods of time at school without engaging in safety-checking behaviors such as repeated check-ins with her mother. Exercises incorporating imaginal or in vivo exposure to trauma reminders were always implemented with the goal of cultivating flexibility and enhancing overall quality of life. Acceptance and mindfulness strategies were utilized as a means of achieving this overarching goal.

Challenges and Recommendations for Future Research

The current state of the evidence of MBIs for the treatment of PTSD among youth is sparse and possesses multiple limitations. At this time, it is impossible to confidently draw conclusions about the efficacy of MBIs for PTSD in youth. Additional research is clearly needed. Future studies should employ rigorous research designs, including RCTs with adequate control groups. While there is an abundance of qualitative studies examining MBIs for adults and youth with PTSD, there is a notable gap in meta-analytic studies. Thus, more quantitative research is needed. Many existing studies incorporate MBIs as an adjunctive intervention, which precludes our understanding of the effectiveness or utility of MBIs as stand-alone treatments. Thus, future research should investigate MBIs as the sole or primary intervention. Following the determination of effective stand- alone MBIs, research efforts should focus on comparison or head-to-head trials, as well as replication.

Many questions remain unanswered regarding MBIs applied to PTSD. Research is needed to determine the effectiveness of MBIs for various subpopulations of trauma survivors (e.g., physical abuse, MVA, natural disaster, sexual abuse). Further, the most appropriate time to implement MBIs following trauma exposure or the potential for MBIs in prevention of later development of PTSD symptomology following trauma exposure is currently unknown. Future research should explore these variables as they relate to symptom development and course. Yet another challenge in interpreting the existing data is the heterogeneity among MBIs (e.g., duration of treatment, setting). Hilton et al. (2017) suggest establishing adherence measures to help understand and compare complementary or alternative treatments with existing evidence-based treatments for PTSD. Finally, additional research is needed to determine the amount of intervention needed for maximum results.

Key Practice Points

There are several factors to consider when implementing MBIs with youth with PTSD. We provide a set of important considerations here:

- *Client fit.* Clinicians must first ensure that safety has been established and that the client is not experiencing ongoing trauma exposure. Additionally, assessment of the client's ability to focus and engage in exercises is needed to determine appropriateness of fit.
- *Safe environment.* Ensure the client perceives a safe therapeutic environment to minimize hypervigilance. This can be achieved through careful attention to rapport, mindfully attending to client verbal and nonverbal feedback, and ongoing assessment.
- *Choice.* Maximize client choice and control over the therapeutic environment. Invite the client to determine who is present for sessions and arrangement of seating.
- *Consent.* Procedures and expectations can be given at the start of sessions and exercises, and clients might be reminded of choice to refuse any exercise at any time without consequence.

- *Format and structure.* Careful consideration should be given to the format and structure of certain mindfulness practices, such as providing the option to complete exercises with eyes open or closed. Consideration should also be given for movement-based practices, which may require modification for poses or postures that may be triggering.
- *Exercise time / length.* Mindfulness might be introduced via short durations (1–5 minutes) at the outset of treatment to assess a client's readiness for MBIs. While mindfulness in adult populations might build to include longer practices, exercises greater than 20 minutes may not be developmentally appropriate for youth, or for those who struggle with emotion regulation, low distress tolerance, or frequent re-experiencing (Vujanovic, Niles, Pietrefesa, Schmertz, & Potter, 2011).
- *Timing of exercises.* Clinicians may be advised to delay introduction of certain mindfulness exercises until clinical symptoms have stabilized and emotion regulation / toleration skills have been developed.
- *Clinician expertise.* An appropriate level of training and experience is needed to competently administer MBIs. Clinicians may additionally consider developing a personal mindfulness practice and / or encourage parents / guardians to engage in mindfulness practices.
- *General rule of thumb.* When working with youth with PTSD, a clinician is wise to start slowly, increase gradually, assess regularly, and modify appropriately.

References

Banks, K., Newman, E., & Saleem, J. (2015). An overview of the research on mindfulness-based interventions for treating symptoms of posttraumatic stress disorder: A systematic review. *Journal of Clinical Psychology, 71*, 935–963.

Bean, R. C., Ong, C. W., Lee, J., & Twohig, M. P. (2017). Acceptance and commitment therapy or PTSD and trauma: An empirical review. *The Behavior Therapist, 40*, 145–150.

Beauchemin, J., Hutchins, T. L., & Patterson, F. (2008). Mindfulness meditation may lessen anxiety, promote social skills, and improve academic performance among adolescents with learning disabilities. *Complementary Health Practice Review, 13*, 34–45.

Beck, A. T. (2005). The current state of cognitive therapy: A 40-year retrospective. *Archives of General Psychiatry, 62*, 953–959.

Biegel, G. M., Brown, K. W., Shapiro, S. L., & Schubert, C. M. (2009). Mindfulness-based stress reduction for the treatment of adolescent psychiatric outpatients: A randomized clinical trial. *Journal of Consulting and Clinical Psychology, 77*, 855.

Bögels, S., Hoogstad, B., van Dun, L., de Schutter, S., & Restifo, K. (2008). Mindfulness training for adolescents with externalizing disorders and their parents. *Behavioural and Cognitive Psychotherapy, 36*, 193–209.

Bormann, J. E., Thorp, S. R., Wetherell, J. L., Golshan, S., & Lang, A. J. (2013). Meditation-based mantram intervention for veterans with posttraumatic stress disorder: A randomized trial. *Psychological Trauma: Theory, Research, Practice, and Policy, 5*, 259–267.

Borquist-Conlon, D. S., Maynard, B. R., Brendel, K. E., & Farina, A. S. (2017). Mindfulness-based interventions for youth with anxiety: A systematic review and meta-analysis. *Research on Social Work Practice, 24*, 1–11.

Catani, C., Kohiladevy, M., Ruf, M., Schauer, E., Elbert, T., & Neuner, F. (2009). Treating children traumatized by war and tsunami: A comparison between exposure therapy and meditation-relaxation in North-East Sri Lanka. *BMC Psychiatry, 9*, 22.

Chambless, D. L., & Hollon, S. D. (1998). Defining empirically supported therapies. *Journal of Consulting and Clinical Psychology, 66*, 7–18.

Chiesa, A., & Malinowski, P. (2011). Mindfulness-based approaches: Are they all the same? *Journal of Clinical Psychology, 67*, 404–424.

Cohen, J. A., Deblinger, E. Mannarino, A. P., & Steer, R. A. (2004). A multisite randomized controlled trial for children with sexual abuse related PTSD symptoms. *Journal of the American Academy of Child and Adolescent Psychiatry, 43*, 393–402.

Cusack, K., Jonas, D. E., Forneris, C. A., Wines, C., Sonis, J., Middleton, J. C., ... Gaynes, B. N. (2016). Psychological treatments for adults with posttraumatic stress disorder: A systematic review and meta-analysis. *Clinical Psychology Review, 43*, 128–141.

Dahl, J., Wilson, K. G., & Nilsson, A. (2004). Acceptance and commitment therapy and the treatment of persons at risk for long-term disability resulting from stress and pain symptoms: A preliminary randomized trial. *Behavior Therapy, 35*, 785–801.

Daigneault, I., Dion, J., Hebert, M. & Bourgeois, C. (2016). Mindfulness as mediator and moderator of post-traumatic symptomatology in adolescence following childhood sexual abuse or assault. *Mindfulness, 7*, 1306–1315.

Dalrymple, K. L., & Herbert, J. D. (2007). Acceptance and commitment therapy for generalized social anxiety disorder: A pilot study. *Behavior Modification, 31*, 543–568.

Dimidjian, S., Arch, J. J., Schneider, R. L., Desormeau, P., Felder, J. N., & Segal, Z. V. (2016). Considering meta-analysis, meaning, and metaphor: A systematic review and critical examination of "third wave" cognitive and behavioral therapies. *Behavior Therapy, 47*, 886–905.

Ehlers, A., & Clark, D. M. (2000). A cognitive model of posttraumatic stress disorder. *Behavior Research and Therapy, 38*, 319–345.

Ehring, T., Razik, S., & Emmelkamp, P. M. (2011). Prevalence and predictors of posttraumatic stress disorder, anxiety, depression, and burnout in Pakistani earthquake recovery workers. *Psychiatry Research, 185*, 161–166.

Flook, L., Smalley, S. L., Kitil, M. J., Galla, B. M., Kaiser-Greenland, S., Locke, J., & Kasari, C. (2010). Effects of mindful awareness practices on executive functions in elementary school children. *Journal of Applied School Psychology, 26*, 70–95.

Gordon, J. S., Staples, J. K., Blyta, A., Bytyqi, M., & Wilson, A. T. (2008). Treatment of posttraumatic stress disorder in postwar Kosovar adolescents using mind-body skills groups: A randomized controlled trial. *The Journal of Clinical Psychiatry, 69*, 1469–1476.

Grossman, P., Niemann, L., Schmidt, S., & Walach, H. (2004). Mindfulness-based stress reduction and health benefits: A meta-analysis. *Journal of Psychosomatic Research, 57*, 35–43.

Gu, J., Strauss, C., Bond, R., & Cavanagh, K. (2015). How do mindfulness-based cognitive therapy and mindfulness-based stress reduction improve mental health and well-being? A systematic review and meta-analysis of mediation studies. *Clinical Psychology Review, 37*, 1–12.

Hilton, L., Maher, A. R., Colaiaco, B., Apaydin, E., Sorbero, M. E., Booth, M., ... & Hempel, S. (2017). Meditation for posttraumatic stress: Systematic review and meta-analysis. *Psychological Trauma: Theory, Research, Practice, and Policy, 9,* 453–460.

Imel, Z. E., Laska, K., Jakupcak, M., & Simpson, T. L. (2013). Meta-analysis of dropout in treatments for posttraumatic stress disorder. *Journal of Consulting and Clinical Psychology, 81,* 394–404.

Kabat-Zinn, J. (2003). Mindfulness-based interventions in context: Past, present, and future. *Clinical Psychology: Science and Practice, 10,* 144–156.

Kallapiran, K., Koo, S., Kirubakaran, R., & Hancock, K. (2015). Effectiveness of mindfulness in improving mental health symptoms of children and adolescents: A meta-analysis. *Child and Adolescent Mental Health, 20,* 182–194.

Kim, S. H., Schneider, S. M., Kravitz, L., Mermier, C., & Burge, M. R. (2013). Mind-body practices for posttraumatic stress disorder. *Journal of Investigative Medicine, 61,* 827–834.

King, N. J., Tonge, B. J., Mullen, P., Myerson, N., Heyne, D., Rollings, S., ... Ollendick, T. H. (2000). Treating sexually abused children with posttraumatic stress symptoms: A randomized clinical trial. *Journal of the American Academy of Child and Adolescent Psychiatry, 39,* 1347–1355.

Lang, A. J., Strauss, J. L., Bomyea, J., Bormann, J. E., Hickman, S. D., Good, R. C., & Essex, M. (2012). The theoretical and empirical basis for meditation as an intervention for PTSD. *Behavior Modification, 36,* 759–786.

Nila, K., Holt, D. V., Ditzen, B., & Aguilar-Raab, C. (2016). Mindfulness-based stress reduction (MBSR) enhances distress tolerance and resilience through changes in mindfulness. *Mental Health & Prevention, 4,* 36–41.

Rosenthal, M. Z., Hall, M. L. R., Palm, K. M., Batten, S. V., & Follette, V. M. (2005). Chronic avoidance helps explain the relationship between severity of childhood sexual abuse and psychological distress in adulthood. *Journal of Child Sexual Abuse, 14,* 25–41.

Schneider, W., & Lockl, K. (2002). The development of metacognitive knowledge in children and adolescents. In T. J. Perfect & B. L. Schwartz (eds.), *Applied metacognition* (pp. 224–257). Cambridge: Cambridge University Press.

Schottenbauer, M. A., Glass, C. R., Arnkoff, D. B., Tendick, V., & Gray, S. H. (2008). Nonresponse and dropout rates in outcome studies on PTSD: Review and methodological considerations. *Psychiatry, 71,* 134–168.

Semple, R. J., Reid, E. F., & Miller, L. (2005). Treating anxiety with mindfulness: An open trial of mindfulness training for anxious children. *Journal of Cognitive Psychotherapy, 19,* 379–392.

Silverman, W. K., Ortiz, C. D., Viswesvaran, C., Burns, B. J., Kolko, D. J., Putnam, F. W., & Amaya-Jackson, L. (2008). Evidence-based psychosocial treatments for children and adolescents exposed to traumatic events. *Journal of Clinical Child & Adolescent Psychology, 37,* 156–183.

Swain, J., Hancock, K., Hainsworth, C., & Bowman, J. (2015). Mechanisms of change: Exploratory outcomes from a randomized controlled trial of acceptance and commitment therapy for anxious adolescents. *Journal of Contextual Behavioral Science, 4,* 56–67.

Vujanovic, A. A., Niles, B., Pietrefesa, A., Schmertz, S. K., & Potter, C. M. (2011). Mindfulness in the treatment of posttraumatic stress disorder among military veterans. *Professional Psychology: Research and Practice, 42,* 24–31.

Woidneck, M. R., Morrison, K. L., & Twohig, M. P. (2014). Acceptance and commitment therapy for the treatment of posttraumatic stress among adolescents. *Behavior Modification, 38,* 451–476.

Zoogman, S., Goldberg, S. B., Hoyt, W. T., & Miller, L. (2014). Mindfulness interventions with youth: A meta-analysis. *Mindfulness, 6,* 290–302.

Index

AACAP clinical guidelines, 410
academic impact, of research on childhood anxiety, 256
acceptance
  MBIs and, 733
  as moderator of change in PTSD, 739
Acceptance and Commitment Therapy (ACT)
  for OCD, 305, 508
  for PTSD, 700, 732
acceptance exercises, in MBIs, 742
access to internet, 74
access to treatment, xii, 74
accommodation, TF-CBT outcome and, 534
Achenbach System of Empirically Based Assessment (ASEBA), 446
actigraphy, 209
activation syndrome, with SSRIs, 408
adjustment disorder, EMDR for, 603
adrenergic agents, for PTSD, 633
affect regulation, in TF-CBT, 528
agoraphobia, 8
  brief intensive treatments for, 137
  epidemiology of, 8
alpha agonists
  for anxiety disorders, 162
  for PTSD, 639
ambiguous scenarios task, for interpretation bias modification, 110
amygdala, in traumatized youth, 702
anorexia nervosa, with OCD, 318
anticonvulsants, for PTSD, 638
antihistamines, for anxiety disorders, 162, 171
antipsychotics
  for OCD, 303, 415
  for tics in OCD, 455
anxiety
  age of onset of, 5, 6
  comorbidity and, 4, 18
  disease burden of, 3
  epidemiology of, 3
  lack of treatment of, 3
  limitations to research on, xi
  normal versus abnormal, 4
  with OCD, 468
anxiety disorders
  CBT for, 9
  comorbidity between, 4
  differentiation of, 4
  efficacy of standard care for, 15
  EMDR for, 603
  etiology of, 256, 267
  familial transmission of, 183
  impact of, 130, 182
  with OCD, 457
  overlooking of, 3
  in parents, childhood anxiety disorders and, 183
  phenomenology of, research on, 256
  prevalence of, 3, 130, 182
  role of parenting in development of, 183
  standard evidence-based treatment of, 8
  types in children and young people, 5
Anxiety Disorders Interview Schedule for DSM-5: Child and Parent Versions (ADIS-5-C/P), 32
Anxiety Disorders Interview Schedule for DSM-IV (ADIS), 325, 445
  Child and Parent Versions (ADIS-C/P), 314, 316
anxiety disorders with comorbid sleep problems, 206
  case example of targeted behavioral therapy and, 213
  clinical research and practice, recommendations for, 217
  enhancement of CBT by sleep and, 216
  reciprocal nature of sleep problems and anxiety and, 207
  reconceptualization of sleep problems and, 214
  reconciliation of subjective-objective sleep discrepancies and, 209
  sleep-based outcomes following CBT for anxiety disorders and, 211
  sleep measures and, 209
  targeting sleep directly in anxiety-based treatment and, 212
  type of anxiety disorder and, 208
  type of sleep problem and, 208
anxiety severity
  as mediator of mindfulness training exercises, 276
  treatment outcome and, 18
approach-avoidance CBM training, 377

aripiprazole
  for ASD, 450
  for tics in OCD, 455
assessment
  in CFSTI, 613
  of comorbid conditions of OCD, 445
  in EMDR, 591, 594
  functional, family-based approaches for OCD and, 431
  in mindfulness-based treatment for anxiety disorders, 268, 271
  post-CFSTI, 618, 621
assessment of OCD, 294, 409
assessment of PTSD, 550
  avoidance and acceptability of questionnaires and, 559
  for diagnosis, 556
  diagnostic classification systems and, 550
  electronic formats for, 563
  for facilitation of discussion and enhancement of support, 561
  to guide focus of interventions, 562
  key practice points for, 564
  measures used in, 551
  nature of memories and, 557
  to provide feedback to therapist, 562
  respondent choice for, 563
  for screening large numbers of youth, 560
  for symptom monitoring, 557
  trauma history and, 561
attention
  as mediator of mindfulness training exercises, 276
  role in anxiety disorders, 267
  training, 108
attentional bias
  in anxiety disorders, 368
  in OCD, 368, 369
attentional bias modification (ABM), 106, 108, 373
  evidence base for, 111
  mediators and modifiers of change and, 114
attention deficit hyperactivity disorder (ADHD)
  with OCD, 320, 446, 468
  with PTSD, 642
autism spectrum disorder (ASD)
  internet/computer-based therapy for anxiety in, 89
  with OCD, 318, 448, 469
avoidance behaviors, in OCD, 289

BarnInternetprojektet (BiP), effectiveness of, 81
barriers to care
  for anxiety disorders, 107, 131
  for EBPs, 715, 716
  for OCD, 332, 348
  overcoming, 107
  for PTSD, 570

behavioral activation, in treatment of depression with PTSD, 681
Behavioral Assessment Tests (BATs), 40
behavioral observations, for assessment, 40
Behavior Assessment System for Children (BASC), 316, 325
benzodiazepines
  for anxiety disorders, 162, 172
  for OCD, 304
beta-blockers, for anxiety disorders, 162
bibliotherapy for anxiety disorders, 53
  disorder-specific programs for, 57
  evidence base for, 55
  therapist support in, 55
bibliotherapy for OCD, 334, 336
biomarkers, of SSRI response, 414
BiP OCD, 350, 351, 353
body dysmorphic disorder (BDD), OCD with, 316
Body Dysmorphic Disorder Questionnaire (BDDQ), 316
body scan, in EMDR, 592, 595
books
  self-help, for youth with OCD, 334
Bounce Back Now, 574
  evidence base for, 578, 580
brain
  functional improvement through promotion of cortical neurogenesis, 704
  regions implicated in childhood trauma, 702
brain maturation
  sleep and, 208
  stages of, 702
BRAVE-ONLINE program, 87
  design features of, 95
  development of, 95
  effectiveness of, 78
  program content of, 95
  with subgroups of young people or subgroups of anxiety, 88
Brave Program, effectiveness of, 77
Breaking Free from OCD (Derisley et al.), 334
breathing techniques, training, 13
brief intensive treatments for anxiety disorders, 130
  agoraphobia, 137
  barriers overcome by, 133
  clinical case illustration of, 143
  continued exposure practice following, 153
  evidence base for, 134
  failure to respond to, 148
  future research directions for, 148
  GAD, 139
  key practice points for, 151
  long-term impact of, 149
  mediators and moderators of change and, 140
  optimizing parents' roles in, 150
  panic disorder, 137
  planning time for, 152

brief intensive treatments (cont.)
  rapport building and, 151
  SAD, 136
  special developmental considerations for children and, 152
brief intensive treatments for OCD, 392
  brief, high intensity CBT for, 395
  challenges and recommendations for future research and, 402
  clinical case illustration of, 396
  increased session frequency for, 394
  key practice points for, 403
  need for innovation and, 392
brief low intensity interventions, 133
BT Steps (Behavior Therapy Steps), 337
buspirone, for anxiety disorders, 174

Camp Cope-A-Lot, effectiveness of, 83
carbamazepine, for PTSD, 638
cardiovascular physiology measures, for assessment, 41
caregivers
  CFSTI and, 614, 616
  distress in, OCD and, 429
  support from, TF-CBT and, 533
CFSTI Site Sustainability Project (CSSP), 624
child abuse and neglect (CAN)
  child factors and, 651
  family factors and, 652
  parent factors and, 651
  social network factors and, 652
Child/Adolescent Anxiety Multimodal Study (CAMS), for anxiety disorders, 160, 175
Child and Family Traumatic Stress Intervention (CFSTI), 610
  additional sessions for, 618
  caregiver meeting and, 614
  child meeting and, 615
  clinical case illustration of, 618
  conjoint meetings with child and caregiver and, 616
  evidence base for, 622
  future directions for, 625
  key practice points for, 625
  need for innovation and, 611
  post-CFSTI assessments and, 618, 621
  procedure and implementation of, 613
  screening process for, 614
  standardized assessment tools for, 613
Child Anxiety Multi-Day Program (CAMP), for separation anxiety disorder, 135
Child Behavior Checklist (CBCL), 314, 316, 325
child factors, in child abuse and neglect, 651
child management, 14
  as parental role in anxiety disorder therapy, 187
Child Obsessive-Compulsive Impact Scale-Revised (COIS-R), 326
  in OCD, 324

Child Post-Traumatic Cognitions Inventory (CPTCI), 553, 562
Child PTSD Symptom Scale (CPSS), 554, 614
  Interview Version for DSM-5 (CPSS-5-1), 551
  Self-Report Version for DSM-5 (CPSS-5-SR), 552
Children and Young People's Improving Access to Psychological Therapies (CYP IAPT), 252
Children's Depressive Inventory (CDI), 316
Children's Florida Obsessive-Compulsive Inventory (CFOCI), 315, 326
Children's Obsessive-Compulsive Inventory – Revised (ChOCI-R), 326
Children's PTSD Inventory (CPTSDI), 552
Children's Revised Impact of Event Scale (CRIES-8 and CRIES-13), 552, 558
Children's Saving Inventory, 316, 326
Children's Yale Brown Obsessive-Compulsive Scale (CYBOCS), 294, 315, 326
  in OCD, 321, 323, 409
Child Trauma Screening Scale (CTSS), 553
chloral hydrate, for PTSD, 637
citalopram
  for anxiety disorders, 162, 165, 173
  for PTSD, 636
cleaning compulsion, in OCD, 290
clinical decisions, assessment and, 31
Clinical Global Impression – Improvement (CGI-I), 325
  in OCD, 323
Clinical Global Impression – Severity (CGI-S), in OCD, 322, 323, 325
clinical interviews, unstructured, in OCD, 314
clinical training
  in CFSTI, 625
  in EMDR, guidelines for, 604
  in TF-CBT, 541, 719
  treatment fidelity and, 254
Clinician Administered PTSD Scale for Children and Adolescents (CAPS-CA-5), 551
clomipramine
  for anxiety disorders, 171, 174
  for OCD, 299, 303, 415
clonidine, for PTSD, 633, 634
closure, in EMDR, 592, 595
clozapine, for pharmacologic-augmented treatments for PTSD, 635
co-client, as parental role in anxiety disorder therapy, 188
co-clinician, as parental role in anxiety disorder therapy, 188
cognitions, parental, reframing, 188
Cognitive Behavioral Family-Based Treatment (CBFT), 473
cognitive behavioral therapy (CBT)
  approaches for improving outcomes to, xii
  challenges to field, xi

cognitive behavioral therapy (CBT) for anxiety
    disorders
  enhancement by sleep, 216
  sleep-based outcomes following, 211
  in standard evidence-based care, 9
cognitive behavioral therapy (CBT) for OCD, 298, 305
  barriers to, 348
  delivery over web cam, 495
  effectiveness research on, 494
  family-based, 298
  group, 299
  intensive, 299
  interaction with pharmacotherapy, 416
  internet-delivered, 299
  moderators and predictors for, 497
  in outpatient, community-based clinic, 497
  self-help materials as adjunct to, 335
  stepped care studies of, 500
  supervision of supervisors approach for, 496
cognitive behavioral therapy (CBT) for PTSD, 704
  with SUDs, 686
cognitive bias modification (CBM) for anxiety
    disorders, 106
  in adults, 374, 379
  clinical case illustration of, 116
  context in which biases are most malleable and, 121
  current state of research on, 118
  key practice points for, 121
  reliability of bias measurement and, 119
  in youth, 375, 380
cognitive bias modification (CBM) for OCD, 365
  in adults, 376
  assessment and, 371
  challenges and recommendations for future research in, 382
  clinical case illustration of, 380
  evidence base for, 374
  key practice points for, 385
  mediators and moderators of change and, 379
  need for innovation and, 366
  in youth, 377
cognitive enhancement, D-cycloserine for, in OCD, 417
cognitive interpretation bias, 369, 371
cognitive remediation therapy (CRT)
  evidence-base for, 473
  for OCD, 470, 473
cognitive restructuring, in standard evidence-based care, 10
communication
  family, OCD and, 430
  improving, in family-based approaches for OCD, 433
  improving parental skills for, 189
comorbid conditions of OCD, 296, 444
  ADHD as, 446
  affective disorders as, 455
  anxiety disorders as, 457
  ASD as, 448
  assessment of, 445
  case example of, 457
  disruptive behavioral disorders as, 451
  key practice points for, 459
  tic disorders as, 452
  transdiagnostic approaches for OCD and, 468
comorbid conditions of PTSD, 557, 642, 671
  challenges and future directions for, 687
  clinical recommendations for, 688
  determining course of comorbid disorder and, 687
  impact on expression of PTSD and treatment outcomes, 677
  prevalence of, 671
  relationship between PTSD and comorbid conditions and, 674
  SUDs as, 676, 678, 682, 699
  treatment approaches for, 678
Compassion Focused Therapy (CFT), 273
compassion meditation, in PTSD treatment, 736
competence levels, CBT implementation and, 251
component-based transdiagnostic CBT, 228
  evidence base for, 236
compulsions
  definition of, 289
  differentiation between tics and, 453
Concurrent treatment of PTSD and Substance Use Disorders Using Prolonged Exposure (COPE), 683
conduct disorder, with PTSD, 642
conjoint trauma processing sessions, in TF-CBT, 529
Connors Parent/Teacher Rating Scales, 316
consent
  informed, for pharmacologic treatment of anxiety disorders, 172
  parental, as parental involvement in therapy, 187
consenter, as parental role in anxiety disorder therapy, 187
Consolidated Framework for Implementation Research (CFIR), 249
Cool Kids program, 10, 229, 233
  for separation anxiety disorder, 135
Cool-Teens, effectiveness of, 84
coordinator, as parental role in anxiety disorder therapy, 187
Coping Cat, 229, 233
  for anxiety and sleep problems, 212
  for separation anxiety disorder, 135
Coping Coach, 572
  evidence base for, 579, 578
cortico-striato-thalamo-cortico (CSTC) circuitry, in OCD, 292

Cue-Centered Treatment (CCT)
  case example of, 705
  for PTSD, 700, 705
cyproheptadine, for PTSD, 637

D-cycloserine (DCS), for OCD, 304, 417
deep brain stimulation (DBS)
  for OCD, 305
  for tics in OCD, 455
depression
  with OCD, 320, 455
  parental, treatment outcomes in PTSD and, 705
  with PTSD, 642, 678
desensitization, in EMDR, 592, 594
desipramine, for anxiety disorders, 174
developmental periods, sleep and, 218
dextroamphetamine, for ADHD, 447
diagnosis of anxiety disorders, 194
Diagnostic Infant and Preschool Assessment (DIPA), 551
dialectical behavior therapy (DBT)
  for OCD, 510
  for PTSD, 699
diaphragmatic breathing, training, 13
disinhibited social engagement, EMDR for, 603
disruptive behavior disorders
  ERP for, 472
  with OCD, 321, 451
dissemination and implementation (DI) of CBT for OCD, 489
  proposed studies of, 499
  review of CBT outcome literature and, 490
dissemination and implementation (DI) of evidence-based programs for anxiety, 248
  dissemination and, 254
  impact of, 255
  implementation framework for, 248
  research on implementation and, 251
  stages of implementation and, 250
dissemination and implementation (DI) of evidence-based programs for PTSD, 715
  barriers to providing EBPs in clinical settings and, 715, 716
  methods for, 718
  in school-based settings, 716
  stepped care TF-CBT and, 720
dissemination of CBT for anxiety disorders, 242
distress tolerance, modeling, in family-based approaches for OCD, 432
divalproex sodium, for PTSD, 638
dopaminergic agents, for PTSD, 635
duloxetine, for anxiety disorders, 161, 162, 169, 173

economic impact, of research on childhood anxiety, 257
effectiveness research, 491
  on CBT for OCD, 493

efficacy research, 491
  on CBT for OCD, 492
emetophobia, with OCD, 321
emotional memory, activation during sleep, 215
Emotion Detectives Treatment Protocol, 231, 234
  evidence base for, 239
emotion dysregulation, TF-CBT outcome and, 535
emotion, expressed, OCD and, 430
emotion regulation, modeling, in family-based approaches for OCD, 432
environmental sensitivity, 17
error-related negativity (ERN), 42
escitalopram, for anxiety disorders, 162, 165, 173
evidence-based assessment of anxiety disorders, 28
  availability and clinical use of, 31
  behavioral observations for, 40
  cardiovascular physiology measures for, 41
  clinical decisions and, 31
  conceptual foundation of, 28
  modalities for, 30, 32
  neural physiology measures for, 42
  rating scales for, 34
  selecting assessments for, 30
  traditional clinical tools for, 32
evidence-based assessment of OCD, 313
  ancillary area assessment and, 324
  comorbidity and, 315
  differential diagnosis and, 313
  key practice points for, 327
  severity assessment and, 321
evidence-based treatment, xii
  to help children overcome trauma, importance of, 526
evidence-based treatment of anxiety disorders, 3, 248
  child management in, 14
  cognitive restructuring in, 10, 11
  disorder-specific techniques in, 18
  dissemination of, 254
  efficacy of, 15
  gradual exposure in, 11
  group versus individual, 16
  impact of, 255
  implementation framework for, 248
  key practice points for, 19
  outcome predictors for, 17
  parental involvement in, 16
  problem solving in, 14
  psychoeducation in, 9
  relaxation in, 13
  research on implementation of, 251
  stages of implementation of, 250
  types of anxiety disorders in children and young people and, 5
Exploration, Preparation, Implementation, Sustainment (EPIS) framework, 250

exposure
    dissemination of CBT for anxiety and, 254
    in family-based anxiety disorder therapy, 195
    gradual, in standard evidence-based care, 11
exposure and response prevention (ERP)
    clinical case illustration of, 400
    family-based modifications of, 472, 475
    mindfulness augmentation of, for OCD, 514
    modification of, 474, 478
    for OCD, 298, 357, 365, 392, 393
    for tic disorders, 454
    transdiagnostic, for OCD, 471
exposure exercises, in MBIs, 742
expressed emotion (EE), OCD and, 430
extinction learning, enhancement by sleep, 216
eye movement desensitization and reprocessing (EMDR), 590
    challenges and recommendations for future research on, 603
    clinical case illustration of, 599
    considerations with children, 593
    for disorders other than PTSD, 603
    evidence base for, 595
    key practice points for, 604
    mechanisms of action of, 598
    moderating factors for, 599
    for OCD, 305
    protocol for, 591
    resources for, 604
    specific adaptations for different phases of protocol, 593
    training guidelines for, 604

Fairy Tale Model, for PTSD, 699
families
    of children with separation anxiety disorder, 184
    outcomes with TF-CBT, 532
family accommodation, OCD and, 429, 431
Family Accommodation Scale – Parent report (FAS-PR), 326
    in OCD, 324
family-based approaches for OCD, 428
    challenges and recommendations for future research and, 437
    clinical case illustration of, 435
    common elements of, 430
    evidence-based innovations and, 433
    family-related components as targets of, 429
    key practice points for, 438
    predictors and moderators of response and, 435
family-based therapy for anxiety disorders
    evidence base for, 190
family communication dynamics, OCD and, 430
family dysfunction, OCD and, 297
family factors, in child abuse and neglect, 652
family involvement, in OCD treatment, 339
fear extinction, enhancement by sleep, 216

fear hierarchy, gradual exposure and, 11
Fear Survey Schedule for Children-Revised/Short Form of the Fear Survey Schedule for Children-Revised (FSSC-R/FSSC-R-SF), 38
fluoxetine, 173
    for anxiety disorders, 162, 164, 165
    for PTSD, 636, 637, 638
fluvoxamine
    for anxiety disorders, 162, 165, 173
    for PTSD, 636
follow-up, in family-based anxiety disorder therapy, 197
forbidden thoughts, in OCD, 290

gender
    as mediator of self-compassion, 277
    specific phobia and, 7
generalized anxiety disorder (GAD), 6
    age of onset of, 7
    brief intensive treatments for, 139
    OCD with, 316
    sleep problems in, 208
Global Assessment Scale for Children (CGAS), 322
Global Axis of Functioning (GAF), in OCD, 322
glutamatergic agents, for OCD, 304, 415
gradual exposure, in standard evidence-based care, 11
group-based behavioral activation and exposure therapy for youth anxiety and depression, 235
    evidence base for, 239
group behavioral activation and exposure therapy, 231
group treatment, individual treatment versus, 16
Growing Up Mindful, clinical case illustration of, 278
guanfacine, for PTSD, 634

"Helping Your Anxious Child" (Rapee, Spence, Cobham, & Wignall), 55
hippocampus, in traumatized youth, 703
history taking, in EMDR, 591, 593
hoarding
    CRT for, 474
    with OCD, 290, 320
homographs, interpretation bias modification and, 110
hostile criticism, OCD and, 430
hypochondriasis, with OCD, 319

imipramine
    for anxiety disorders, 171, 174
    for PTSD, 637
implementation science, 491, 500
individual impact, of research on childhood anxiety, 257
individual treatment, group treatment versus, 16
inflammation, OCD and, 305

informed consent, for pharmacologic treatment of anxiety disorders, 172
inhibitory learning, 12
  as mediator of intensive CBT, 142
insight, in OCD, 289, 290
integrated behavioral therapy
  for anxiety and depression, 232, 234, 235
  evidence base for, 239
integrated brief behavioral therapy for anxiety and depression, 235
inter- and intra-hemispheric activation hypothesis, of EMDR, 599
intermittent explosive disorder (IED), with OCD, 451
internet/computer-based CBT (I/CCBT), 54, 57
  for adolescents, 58
  for children, 59
  disorder-specific, 60
  therapist contact and, 58, 68
internet/computer-based CBT (I/CCBT) for anxiety disorders, 73
  barriers to adoption of, 93
  brief intensive treatments using, 149
  client satisfaction with, 86
  clinical issues with, 93
  effectiveness of, 75, 87, 88
  future research directions for, 92
  impact on anxiety diagnoses and symptoms, 76
  key practice points for, 98
  mediators and moderators of change and, 90, 357
  mobile applications and, 90
  outcomes with, 98
  rationale for developing, 73
  with subgroups of young people or subgroups of anxiety, 88
  therapist contact and, 86
  therapy dropout and compliance with, 87, 94
  uses of, 74
  virtual reality and, 92
internet/computer-based CBT (I/CCBT) for OCD, 335, 337, 349, 350
  challenges and recommendations for future research and, 358
  clinical case illustration of, 357
  key practice points for, 360
interpretation bias
  in anxiety disorders, 368, 369
  cognitive, 369, 371
  in OCD, 368, 369
interpretation bias modification (IBM), 106, 109
  evidence base for, 112
  mediators and modifiers of change and, 115
interviews
  semi-structured, for assessment, 32
  unstructured, in OCD, 314
in vivo mastery, in TF-CBT, 529

Kids and Accidents, 573
  evidence base for, 578, 579

lamotrigine, for OCD, 304
Level 2 Repetitive Thoughts and Behavior Scale, 315
Life Improvement for Teens (LIFT), 574
linking to positive cognition, in EMDR, 592, 595
lithium, for pharmacologic-augmented treatments for PTSD, 638

maladaptive cognitions, treatment outcomes in PTSD and, 705
mantra repetition, in PTSD treatment, 736
Mastery of Obsessive-Compulsive Disorder: A Cognitive Behavioral Approach (Foa & Kozak), 337
Me and My School self-report questionnaire, 563
memantine, for OCD, 304
memory, activation during sleep, 215
methylphenidate, for ADHD, 447
mind-body interventions, for PTSD, 732
Mindful Attention Awareness Scale for Adolescents, 268
mindfulness
  definition of, 267, 733
  in PTSD treatment, 736
  targeting of, 733
  in treatment of depression with PTSD, 681
Mindfulness-Based Cognitive Therapy, 270
  for PTSD, 732
Mindfulness-Based Cognitive Therapy for Anxious Children (MBCT-C), 270
mindfulness-based interventions (MBIs) for anxiety disorders, 265
  assessment phase of, 268
  caregiver, teacher, and clinician involvement in, 269
  challenges and recommendation for future research on, 281
  clinical case illustration of, 278
  evidence base for, 274
  existing programs, 270
  key practice points for, 282
  as mediator of self-compassion, 277
  mediators and moderators of, 276
  need for innovation and, 266
mindfulness-based interventions (MBIs) for OCD, 511
  augmentation of ERP using, 512, 514
  clinical illustration of, 514
  evidence base for, 512
  mechanisms underlying, 513
  rationale for use of, 512
mindfulness-based interventions (MBIs) for PTSD, 731
  in adults, 737
  approach to innovation and, 732

challenges and recommendations for future research on, 742
clinical case illustration of, 740
common features of, 732
evidence base for, 734
key practice points for, 743
mediators and moderators of change and, 738
need for innovation and, 731
mindfulness-based interventions (MBIs), with youth, 734
Mindfulness-Based Stress Reduction (MBSR), 270
for PTSD, 700, 732
mindfulness exercises, 271, 272
mindfulness/prefrontal attentional flexibility/metacognitive awareness hypothesis, of EMDR, 599
mindfulness techniques, in MBIs, 741
Mindful Self-Compassion (MSC), 273
MindRight, 574
Mini International Neuropsychiatric Interview for Children and Adolescents (MINI-KID/MINI-KID-P), 33
mobile applications
for anxiety disorders, 90
for OCD, 350, 356
for PTSD, 572, 577
Modular Approach to Therapy for Children with Anxiety, Depression, Trauma and Conduct Problems (MATCH-ADTC), 230, 233, 238
modular treatments, 227, 233
evidence base for, 238
Mood and Feelings Questionnaire, 616
motivational enhancement, in treatment of PTSD with SUD, 685
Multidimensional Anxiety Scale for Children (MASC), 34, 316
Multisystemic Therapy for Child Abuse and Neglect (MST-CAN), 650
analytic process of, 656
challenges and recommendations for future research and, 666
clinical case illustration of, 662
evidence base for, 660
goals of, 653
guiding principles of, 654
interventions applied to all families and, 658
interventions tailored to needs of families and, 659
key practice points for, 667
need for innovation and, 651
quality assurance system of, 660
related DSM-5 disorders and, 666
service delivery model for, 655
theoretical base for, 653
muscular desensitization, 13
mutism, selective, 5
myMCT (MY Metacognitive Treatment for OCD), 337

N-acetylcysteine (NAC), for OCD, 304
National Implementation Research Network, 250
nefazodone, for PTSD, 637
neural physiology measures, for assessment, 42
neuropsychological impairment, in OCD, 293
neurosurgery, for OCD, 304
nortriptyline, for anxiety disorders, 174

obsessions, definition of, 289
obsessive-compulsive disorder (OCD)
assessment of, 294, 409
behavioral treatment of, 298
clinical course of, 295
definition of, 289
as developmental disorder, 444
diagnostic criteria for, 289
differential diagnosis of, 294
epidemiology of, 291
etiology of, 291
future research directions for, 305
heritability of, 292
importance of assessment in, 360
neuropsychological profile of, 293
pharmacological treatment of, 299
phenomenology of, 289
psychosocial difficulties in, 297
specifiers in, 289
symptom presentations in, 290
tic-related, 296
treatment outcomes in, 323
Obsessive-Compulsive Inventory – Child Version (OCI-CV), 315, 326
OCD? Not Me!, 335, 350
OC Fighter, 338
one-session treatment (OST), for anxiety disorders, 134, 141, 149
oppositional defiant disorder (ODD)
with OCD, 451, 468
with PTSD, 642
orienting response hypothesis, of EMDR, 598
over-control, parental, childhood and disorders and, 184
overgeneralization, TF-CBT outcome and, 534
overinvolvement of family, OCD and, 430

PANDAS (Pediatric Autoimmune Neuropsychiatric Disorder Associated with Streptococcal Infection), OCD and, 292, 324
Panic Control Treatment for Adolescents (PCT-A), 137
panic disorder (PD), 7
brief intensive treatments for, 137
epidemiology of, 8
PANS (Pediatric Acute-onset Neuropsychiatric Syndrome), OCD and, 293, 324
parental consent, 187

parental involvement
  in PTSD therapy, 704
  in TF-CBT, 533
parental involvement in anxiety disorder therapy, 182
  in brief intensive treatments, 138, 142, 150
  challenges and future research recommendations for, 197
  clinical case illustration of, 193
  contingency management and, 185, 191
  efficacy of CBT and, 16
  evidence base for, 190
  key practice points for, 199
  levels of, 186
  mediators and moderators of change and, 193
  transfer of control and, 185, 191
  types of parental involvement and, 185
parental psychopathology
  depression as, treatment outcomes in PTSD and, 705
  as moderator of change, 193
  treatment outcome and, 18
parent factors, in child abuse and neglect, 651
parenting
  role in development of childhood anxiety disorders, 183
  in TF-CBT, 528
parents
  bibliotherapy and, 55
  dysfunctional behavior of, changing, 189
  improving communication skills of, 189
  involvement in mindfulness-based treatment for anxiety disorders, 269
  as mediators of mindfulness training exercises, 276
  preferences for OCD treatment, 412
  psychopathology of, treating, 189
  reframing cognitions of, 188
  training for, 14
paroxetine
  for anxiety disorders, 162, 173
  for PTSD, 636
Pediatric Anxiety Rating Scale (PARS), 39
Pediatric OCD Treatment Study (POTS), 301
Penn State Worry Questionnaire for Children (PSWQ-C), 38
perfectionism, ERP for, 471, 474
personalized medicine, for OCD treatment, 305
pharmacologic-augmented CBT for OCD, 407
  alternative pharmacologic agents for, 415
  augmentation strategies for, 409
  biomarkers of SSRI response and, 414
  challenges and recommendations for future research and, 420
  clinical management of SSRIs and, 408
  D-cycloserine for, 417
  effectiveness research on, 493
  identifying side effects and, 413
  interaction between CBT and pharmacotherapy and, 416
  key practice points for, 421
  novel strategies for, 417
  pharmacologic monotherapy recommendations and, 407
  predictors and moderators of treatment outcome and, 411
  rapid identification of response to SSRIs and, 413
  traditional strategies for, 411
  treatment preferences and expectancies and, 412
pharmacologic-augmented treatments for anxiety disorders, 160
  challenges and future research recommendations for, 176
  clinical case illustration of, 172
  drugs commonly used in, 173
  evidence base for, 162
  informed consent for, 172
  key practice points for, 178
pharmacologic-augmented treatments for PTSD, 629
  challenges and recommendations for future research on, 643
  clinical case illustration of, 640
  with comorbid disorders, 642
  diagnostic criteria and clinical presentation and, 629
  evidence base for, 632
  key practice points for, 643
  pharmacological agents for, 631
  psychoeducation and, 631
pharmacotherapy
  for OCD, 299, 407
  for tics in OCD, 455
pleasant activity scheduling, in treatment of depression with PTSD, 681
political impact, of research on childhood anxiety, 257
Post-traumatic Checklist – Civilian Version, 616
post-traumatic stress disorder (PTSD)
  barriers to treatment of, 570
  complex, 555
  consequences of failing to treat, 526
  continuum of symptoms in, 526
  diagnostic criteria and clinical presentation of, 629, 698
  differential diagnosis of, 556
  epidemiology of, 697
  evidence base for web and mobile interventions for, 577
  mobile tools to integrate into in-person treatment of, 576
  phases of, 611
  prevalence of, 671
  prevention/early intervention tools for, 572

symptom clusters in, 526, 611
treatments for, 699
web-based programs for, 572, 577
in young children, 554
PRACTICE components of TF-CBT, 527, 542
prazosin, for PTSD, 634
prefrontal cortex (PFC), in traumatized youth, 703
preparation phase, in EMDR, 591, 594
probe detection task, 108
problem solving, 14
propranolol, for PTSD, 634
psychoeducation
   in family-based anxiety disorder therapy, 194
   for pharmacologic-augmented treatments for PTSD, 631
   in standard evidence-based care, 9
   in TF-CBT, 528
   in treatment of depression with PTSD, 680
   in treatment of PTSD with SUD, 685
PTSD Module of Anxiety Disorders Interview Schedule for DSM-IV – Child Version (ADIS for DSM-IV:C), 551

quality assurance system, of MST-CAN, 660
questionnaires, avoidance and acceptability of, in PTSD, 559
quetiapine, for PTSD, 635

rage attacks, with OCD, 451
rating scales, for assessment, 34
REACH for success APP, 91
reactive attachment disorder, EMDR for, 603
reevaluation, in EMDR, 592, 595
relaxation, 13
   in TF-CBT, 528
REM analogue hypothesis, of EMDR, 598
Revised Child Anxiety and Depression Scales Youth and Parent Versions (RCADS/RCADS-P), 36
Revised Children's Manifest Anxiety Scale (RCMAS), 36
riluzole, for OCD, 304
risperidone
   for ASD, 450
   for PTSD, 635
   for tics in OCD, 455

safety enhancement, in TF-CBT, 529
Schedule for Affective Disorders and Schizophrenia for School-Age Children (K-SADS), 33
   Present and Lifetime Versions (KSADS-PL), 314, 316, 325
schizophrenia spectrum disorders, with OCD, 319
school refusal, 6
schools
   CBT implementation in, 251
   EBPs for PTSD provision in, 716

Screen for Child Anxiety Related Disorders (SCARD), 314
Screen for Child Anxiety Related Emotional Disorders/Screen for Child Anxiety Related Emotional Disorders-Revised (SCARED/SCARED-R), 37
screening, for CFSTI, 614
Seeking Safety, 683
selective mutism, 5
selective serotonin reuptake inhibitors (SSRIs)
   activation syndrome and, 408
   for ASD, 450
   for PTSD, 637
selective serotonin reuptake inhibitors (SSRIs) for anxiety disorders, 160, 161, 173
   discontinuation of, 167
   dosing of, 165
   duration of treatment and, 168
   efficacy studies of, 162, 163
   monitoring of, 166
   partial response or treatment failure with, 165
   pharmacokinetics and, 164
   use in children and adolescents, 162
selective serotonin reuptake inhibitors (SSRIs) for OCD, 299, 300, 408
   as adjunct to CBT, 393
   for nonresponders to CBT, 366
self-blame, TF-CBT outcome and, 535
self-compassion approaches for anxiety disorders, 271
   elements of, 273
   evidence base for, 275
   existing programs, 273
   mediators and moderators of, 277
self-compassion exercises, elements of, 273
Self-Compassion Scale, 268
self-efficacy, as mediator of intensive CBT, 141
self-help books, for youth with OCD, 334
self-help treatment for anxiety disorders, 52
   approaches to innovation in, 53
   benefits of, 52
   building goal-directed action and, 65
   challenges and future development for, 67
   clinical case illustration of, 62
   comorbidity and, 66
   engagement and motivation and, 64
   evidence base for, 54
   key practice points for, 69
   managing negative emotion and cognition and, 65
   need for innovation in, 52
   positive coping and, 66
   posttreatment outcomes with, 66
   predictors of change and, 61
   for preschool-aged children, 60
   reducing avoidance and, 65
   relationship building and, 66
   stepped care and, 68

self-help treatment for anxiety disorders (cont.)
   therapist involvement in, 67, 68
self-help treatment for OCD, 332
   in adult populations, 336
   challenges and recommendations for future
      research and, 340
   clinical case illustration of, 339
   evidence base for, 336
   internet-delivered CBT and, 335
   key practice recommendations for, 342
   longevity of, 341
   mediators and moderators of change and, 338
   need for innovation and, 332
   self-help books and, 334
   self-help material as adjunct to
      therapist-delivered CBT and, 335
semi-structured interviews, for assessment, 32
separation anxiety disorder, 6
   brief intensive treatments for, 135
   families of children with, 184
Separation Anxiety Program for Families (TAFF),
   192, 194
serotonergic agents, for PTSD, 635
serotonin-norepinephrine reuptake inhibitors
      (SNRIs) for anxiety disorders, 160, 162, 168,
      169
   discontinuation of, 170
   dosing of, 169
   duration of treatment and, 170
   monitoring of, 169
   use in children and adults, 168
serotonin receptor partial agonists, for anxiety
      disorders, 174
sertraline
   for anxiety disorders, 160, 162, 164, 165, 173
   for PTSD, 636
Session Rating Scale, 562
sexual abuse
   posttraumatic symptoms related to, 739
   TF-CBT for, 530
shared mechanisms, interventions targeting, 234
   evidence base for, 238
sleep
   architecture of, in GAD, 214
   brain maturation and, 208
   context of, need for research on, 218
   memory activation during, 215
sleep-affective relationships, in anxious youth,
   214
sleep problems
   reciprocal nature of sleep problems and anxiety
      and, 207
sleep spindles, social anxiety and, 215
social anxiety disorder (SAD), 5
   brief intensive treatments for, 136
   internet/computer-based therapy for, 89
   lack of response to CBT in, 266
   memory activation during sleep and, 215

sleep problems in, 208
sleep spindles and, 215
Social Effectiveness Therapy for Children
   (SET-C), 164
social network factors, in child abuse and neglect,
   652
*Social Phobia and Anxiety Inventory for Children
   (SPAI-C/SPAI-C-P)*, 38
specific phobias, 7
   age of onset of, 7
   brief intensive treatments for, 134
*Spence Children's Anxiety Scale for Children and
   Parents (SCAS/SCAS-P)*, 37
stepladder, gradual exposure and, 11
Step One, 721
Stepped-Care TF-CBT
   case example of, 722
   preliminary evidence for, 720
Stepping Together, 721
   case example of, 722
*Stop Obsessing! How to Overcome Your
   Obsessions and Compulsions* (Foa &
   Wilson), 337
substance use disorders (SUDs), with PTSD, 642,
   678, 682, 699
support
   from caregiver, TF-CBT and, 533
   improving, in family-based approaches for
      OCD, 433
Swanson, Nolan and Pelham (SNAP)
   Questionnaire, 316
Sydenham's chorea, OCD and, 293
symmetry, in OCD, 290

Talking Back to OCD (March & Benton), 334
Targeted Behavioral Therapy (TBT)
   for anxiety and sleep problems, 212
   case example using, 213
teachers, involvement in mindfulness-based treatment for anxiety disorders, 269
teaching
   in TF-CBT, 529
technological CBT for PTSD, 570
   challenges and recommendations for future
      research on, 582
   clinical case example of, 581
   evidence base for, 577
   facilitation of treatment by, 572
   to integrate into in-person treatment, 576
   key practice points for, 584
   mediators and moderators of, 581
   for prevention/early intervention, 572
   recommended resources for, 584
technology
   assessment of PTSD using, 563
   integration into TF-CBT, 542
teleconferencing interventions, for OCD, 350, 354
temper outbursts, with OCD, 451

therapeutic alliance
　in internet/computer-based therapy, 86
　quality of, outcome and, 17
　TF-CBT and, 534
therapeutic process, in PTSD, feedback to
　　therapist on, 562
therapists
　characteristics of, CBT implementation and,
　　252
　involvement in mindfulness-based treatment for
　　anxiety disorders, 269
therapist support, in bibliotherapy, 55
third wave psychotherapy for OCD, 506
　challenges and recommendations for future
　　research on, 515
　common features of, 507
　key practice points for, 516
　need for innovation and, 506
　types of, 507
tic disorders, 317
　behavioral intervention for, 453
　ERP for, 454, 472, 476
　with OCD, 290, 292, 296, 452, 498
tics, differentiation between compulsions and, 453
topiramate, for OCD, 304
transcranial magnetic stimulation (TMS), for
　　OCD, 305
transdiagnostic approaches for anxiety disorders,
　　9, 226
　clinical case illustration of, 241
　dissemination of, 242
　efficacy of, compared with disorder-specific
　　CBT protocols, 236
　evidence base for component-based protocols
　　and, 236
　evidence base for interventions targeting shared
　　mechanisms, 238
　evidence base for modular protocols and, 238
　goals of, 228
　improving outcomes and, 242
　key practice points for, 243
　mediators of change and, 240
　modular treatments and, 233
　need for innovation and, 227
　predictors of change and, 240, 242
　treatment protocols for, 228
　treatments targeting shared mechanisms and,
　　228, 234, 238
　universally applied therapeutic principles and,
　　227, 228
transdiagnostic approaches for OCD, 467
　challenges and recommendations for future
　　research and, 479
　clinical case illustration of, 477
　comorbidity and, 468
　CRT as, 470
　ERP as, 471
　evidence base for, 473

　key practice points for, 481
　mediators and moderators of change and, 476
　traditional approaches versus, 469
transdiagnostic approaches for PTSD, 697
　ACT as, 700
　brain regions implicated in trauma and, 702
　case example of, 705
　CCT as, 700, 705
　challenges and recommendations for future
　　research and, 709
　DBT as, 699
　Fairy Tale Model as, 699
　MBSR as, 700
　mediators and moderators of change and, 704
　TST-SA as, 699
transdiagnostic CBT (T-CBT), 228
　efficacy compared to disorder-specific CBT,
　　236
trauma-focused CBT (TF-CBT), 525
　barriers to treatment and, 717
　case illustration of, 536
　components of, 527, 542
　dissemination and implementation of, 718
　efficacy of, 532
　emerging innovations, challenges and
　　recommendations for future research and,
　　541
　evidence base supporting, 530
　implementation guides for, 718
　importance of evidence-based therapies and,
　　526
　predictors, moderators, and mediators for, 533
　stepped care, preliminary evidence for, 720
　treatment phases of, 528
Trauma History Questionnaire, 616
Trauma Memory Quality Questionnaire (TMQQ),
　　553
trauma narration and processing, in TF-CBT, 529
Trauma Systems Therapy for Adolescent
　　Substance Abuse (TST-SA), 683, 699
　for SUDs and PTSD, 699
treatment failure, 266
　with pharmacologic treatment, 165
Trennungsangst fuer Familien (TAFF), 192, 194
Triangle of Life, 576, 581
tricyclic antidepressants (TCAs)
　for anxiety disorders, 160, 170
　for OCD, 299
　for PTSD, 638

UCLA PTSD Reaction Index, 554
UCLA PTSD Reaction Index for DSM-5
　Children/Adolescent (UCLA PTSD RI), 552
　Young Children (UCLA PTSD RI YC), 553
Unified Protocol for Adolescents (UP-A), 230, 234
　evidence base for, 238
universally applied therapeutic principles,
　　interventions based on, 227, 228

values, MBIs and, 733
venlafaxine, for anxiety disorders, 168
videoconferencing interventions, for OCD, 350, 354, 355
virtual reality (VR)
    for anxiety disorder treatment, 92
    for OCD treatment, 350, 356
Virtual Reality Exposure Therapy (VRET), 92

web-based programs, for PTSD, 572, 577
word-sentence association paradigm, interpretation bias modification and, 110
working memory hypothesis, of EMDR, 599

Yale-Brown Obsessive Compulsive Scale (Y-BOCS), 294
Yale Global Tic Severity Scale (YGTSS), 316
Youth Anxiety Measure for DSM-5 (YAM-5), 39